SECOND EDITION

PEDIATRIC PHARMACOLOGY

Therapeutic Principles in Practice

SUMNER J. YAFFE, M.D.

Director
Center for Research for Mothers and Children
National Institute of Child Health and Human Development
Bethesda, Maryland

JACOB V. ARANDA, M.D., Ph.D., F.R.C.P.(C)

Professor of Pediatrics and of Pharmacology and Therapeutics
McGill University, School of Medicine;
Director
Developmental Pharmacology and Perinatal Research Unit
Montreal Children's Hospital, Department of Pediatrics
Montreal, Quebec

W.B. SAUNDERS COMPANY

Harcourt Brace Jovanovich, Inc.

Philadelphia, London, Toronto, Montreal, Sydney, Tokyo

W. B. SAUNDERS COMPANY
Harcourt Brace Jovanovich, Inc.

The Curtis Center
Independence Square West
Philadelphia, Pennsylvania 19106

Library of Congress Cataloging-in-Publication Data

Pediatric pharmacology : therapeutic principles in practice / [edited by] Sumner J. Yaffe,
    Jacob V. Aranda. — 2nd ed.
      p.   cm.
    Includes bibliographical references and index.
    ISBN 0-7216-2971-7
    1. Pediatric pharmacology. I. Yaffe, Sumner J., II. Aranda, Jacob V.
    [DNLM: 1. Drug Therapy—in infancy & childhood. WS 366 P369]
  RJ560.P4   1992
  615.5'8-083—dc20
  DNLM/DLC
  for Library of Congress   91-37728
                                                       CIP

Editor: Judith Fletcher

PEDIATRIC PHARMACOLOGY
Therapeutic Principles in Practice   ISBN 0-7216-2971-7

Printed in Mexico.

Last digit is the print number: 9 8 7 6 5 4 3 2 1

Dedicated to
Anita and Ian
and
Betty, Kenneth, and Christopher
for their unswerving love and support

CONTRIBUTORS

GAD ALPAN, M.D.
Assistant Professor, Department of Pediatrics, College of Physicians and Surgeons, Columbia University, New York, New York
Drug Treatment of Neonatal Apnea

MONIQUE ANDRE, M.D.
Pediatric Neurologist, Department of Neonatology, Maternity Hospital, Nancy, France
Anticonvulsants in the Newborn Infant

JACOB V. ARANDA, M.D., Ph.D., F.R.C.P.(C.)
Professor of Pediatrics and of Pharmacology and Therapeutics, McGill University Faculty of Medicine and Attending Neonatologist and Director, Developmental Pharmacology and Perinatal Research, Montreal Children's Hospital, Montreal, Canada
Introduction and Historical Perspectives; Drug Treatment of Neonatal Apnea

B. M. ASSAEL, M.D.
Associate Professor of Pediatrics, Clinica Pediatrica, Universita di Milano, Milan, Italy
Aminoglycoside Antibiotics

ANNABELLE AZANCOT-BENISTY, M.D., Ph.D.
Fetal Cardiology Department, Faculté Lariboisuie, St. Louis, Hôpital Robert Débré. Head, Physiology Department, Cardiovascular Physiology, Fetal Cardiology Unit, Hôpital Robert Debré, Paris, France
Fetal Pharmacology and Therapy: Supraventricular Arrhythmias as an Example

CHESTON M. BERLIN, Jr., M.D.
University Professor of Pediatrics, Professor of Pharmacology and Chief, Division of General Pediatrics, Milton S. Hershey Medical Center, The Pennsylvania State University, Hershey, Pennsylvania
The Excretion of Drugs and Chemicals in Human Milk

C. WARREN BIERMAN, M.D.
Clinical Professor of Pediatrics, University of Washington. Director, Division of Allergy, Children's Hospital and Medical Center, Seattle, Washington
Antihistamines

PIERRE BLANCHARD, M.D.
Associate Professor of Pediatrics, Université de Sherbrooke. Head, Division of Neonatology and Assistant Director of Pediatrics, Centre Hospitalier, Université de Sherbrooke, Sherbrooke, Quebec, Canada
Drug Treatment of Neonatal Apnea

JEFFREY L. BLUMER, Ph.D., M.D.
Carrie R. Kohn Professor of Pediatric Critical Care Medicine, Department of Pediatrics, School of Medicine, Case Western University. Chief, Division of Pediatric Pharmacology and Critical Care, Rainbow Babies' and Children's Hospital, Cleveland, Ohio
Drugs Used to Modulate Gastrointestinal Function; Principles of Neonatal Pharmacology

LARS O. BOREUS, M.D.
Professor and Chairman, Department of Clinical Pharmacology, Karolinska Hospital, Stockholm, Sweden
Therapeutic Drug Monitoring

J. CHRISTOPHER CAREY, M.D.
Associate Professor, University of Oklahoma. Chief, Benign Gynecology, Oklahoma Teaching Hospital, Oklahoma City, Oklahoma
Drugs Used in Labor and Delivery

CHARLOTTE S. CATZ, M.D.
Chief, Pregnancy and Perinatology Branch, Center for Research for Mothers and Children, National Institute of Child Health and Human Development, Bethesda, Maryland
Drugs Used in Labor and Delivery

GEORGE P. CHROUSOS, M.D.
Chief, Pediatric Endocrinology Section, Developmental Endocrinology Branch, National Institute of Child Health and Human Development, Bethesda, Maryland
Glucocorticoids

CAROL CISTOLA, M.D.
Department of Obstetrics and Gynecology, University of Arkansas for Medical Science, Little Rock, Arkansas
Physiological Adaptations to Pregnancy: Impact on Pharmacokinetics

SANFORD N. COHEN, A.B., M.D.
Professor of Pediatrics, Department of Pediatrics, Wayne State University School of Medicine. Distinguished Attending Physician, Children's Hospital of Michigan, Detroit, Michigan
Ethics of Drug Research in Children

ELEANOR COLLE, M.D.
Professor of Pediatrics, McGill University. Physician, Montreal Children's Hospital, Montreal, Quebec, Canada
Insulin and Diabetes Mellitus

MICHELE DANISH, Pharm.D.
Assistant Professor, Department of Pharmaceutics, University of Rhode Island College of Pharmacy, Kingston, Rhode Island
Clinical Pharmacokinetics

WILLIAM E. EVANS, Pharm.D.
First Tennessee Professor of Clinical Pharmacy, College of Pharmacy, and Professor of Pediatrics,

College of Medicine, University of Tennessee. Chairman, Pharmaceutical Division and Member, Saint Jude Children's Research Hospital, Memphis, Tennessee
Antineoplastic Agents

FABIAN EYAL, M.D.
Director, Division of Neonatology, Francis Scott Key Medical Center and Johns Hopkins University School of Medicine, Baltimore, Maryland
Drug Treatment of Neonatal Apnea

DELBERT A. FISHER, M.D.
Emeritus Professor of Pediatrics and Medicine, University of California School of Medicine, Los Angeles. Senior Scientist, Research and Education Institute, Harbor-UCLA, Los Angeles. Medical Center, Torrance, California
Thyroid Hormones

F. C. FRASER, M.D., Ph.D., F.R.S.
Professor Emeritus, Centre for Human Genetics, McGill University. Medical Genetics, The Montreal Children's Hospital, Montreal, Quebec, Canada
Teratology

PETER GAL, Pharm.D., F.C.C.P.
Clinical Professor, School of Pharmacy, University of North Carolina at Chapel Hill. Clinical Associate Professor, Department of Family Medicine, University of North Carolina School of Medicine. Director, Pharmacy Education and Research, Greensboro Area Health Education Center. Codirector, Clinical Pharmacology Research and Development Laboratory, Moses H. Cone Memorial Hospital, Greensboro, North Carolina
Therapeutic Drug Monitoring: Theoretical and Practical Issues

R. GHADIALLY, M.B., Ch.B., F.R.C.P.(C.)
Division of Dermatology, Sunnybrook Medical Centre, Toronto, Ontario, Canada
Topical Therapy and Percutaneous Absorption

JAMIE GILMAN, Pharm.D.
Clinical Associate Professor, School of Pharmacy, University of Florida, Gainesville. College of Pharmacy, Southeastern University of Health Sciences. Director, Section of Neuropharmacology, Comprehensive Epilepsy Center and Pharmacokinetics Laboratory, Miami Children's Hospital, Miami, Florida
Therapeutic Drug Monitoring: Theoretical and Practical Issues

RAFAEL GORODISCHER, M.D.
Professor and Chair, Department of Pediatrics, Clinical Pharmacology Unit, Soroka Medical Center, Ben-Gurion University of the Negev, Beer-Sheba, Israel
Cardiac Drugs; Digoxin

ERIC J. GREENGLASS, B.Sc., M.Sc., M.D., F.R.C.P.(C.), F.A.A.P.
Assistant Professor of Pediatrics and Attending Neonatologist, Neonatal-Perinatal Medicine, Loyola University, Chicago, Illinois
Neonatal Pharmacology: Practical Applications; Adverse Effects of Environmental Chemicals and Drugs of Abuse on the Developing Human; The Adverse Effects of Cocaine on the Developing Human

BARBARA F. HALES, Ph.D.
Associate Professor, Department of Pharmacology and Therapeutics, McGill University, Montreal, Quebec, Canada
Teratology: Biochemical Mechanisms

KAREN HEIN, M.D.
Professor of Pediatrics, Albert Einstein College of Medicine. Director, Adolescent AIDS Program, Montefiore Medical Center, Bronx, New York
Drug Therapeutics in the Adolescent

MALCOLM HILL, Pharm.D.
Assistant Professor of Pediatrics and Pharmacy, University of Colorado Health Sciences Center. Clinical Research Pharmacist, Clinical Pharmacology Division, National Jewish Center for Immunology and Respiratory Medicine, Denver, Colorado
Advances in the Pharmacologic Management of Asthma

SUSAN L. HOGUE, Ph.D.
Fellow, Pediatric Pharmacotherapy, Department of Clinical Pharmacology, Center for Pediatric Pharmacokinetics and Therapeutics, The University of Tennessee, Memphis, Tennessee
Pharmacokinetically Based Drug Interactions

SHEILA JACOBSON, M.D.
Fellow in Clinical Pharmacology, University of Toronto. Fellow in Clinical Pharmacology, Hospital for Sick Children, Toronto, Ontario, Canada
Drug Administration in the Newborn Infant

EVELYNE JACQZ-AIGRAIN, M.D., Ph.D.
Pharmacology Clinic, Hôpital Robert Debré, Paris, France
Fetal Pharmacology and Therapy: Supraventricular Arrhythmias as an Example

KEITH JOHNSON, M.D.
Director, Drug Information Center, The U.S. Pharmacopeial Convention, Inc., Rockville, Maryland
Appendix I: Formulary

BERNARD S. KAPLAN, M.B., B.Ch.
Professor of Pediatrics and Medicine, University of Pennsylvania. Director, Division of Nephrology, The Children's Hospital of Philadelphia, Philadelphia, Pennsylvania
Therapeutic Agents and the Kidney: Pharmacokinetics and Complications; Diuretics

SELNA L. KAPLAN, M.D., Ph.D.
Professor of Pediatrics, University of California. Attending Pediatrician, Moffit-Long Hospital, San Francisco, California
Growth Hormone

RALPH E. KAUFFMAN, M.D.
Professor of Pediatrics and Pharmacology, Wayne State University School of Medicine. Director, Division of Clinical Pharmacology, Vice Chairman for Clinical Affairs, Children's Hospital of Michigan, Detroit, Michigan
Drug Therapeutics in the Infant and Child

GIDEON KOREN, M.D., A.B.M.T., F.R.C.P.(C.)
Associate Professor, Pediatrics and Pharmacology. Director, The Motherisk Program, Division of Clinical Pharmacology and Toxicology, The Hospital for Sick Children, Toronto, Ontario, Canada
Drug Administration in the Newborn Infant; Cardiac Drugs; Digoxin

MARKUS J. P. KRUESI, M.D.
Child Psychology Branch, National Institute of Mental Health, Bethesda, Maryland
Psychoactive Agents

MARC H. LEBEL, M.D., F.R.C.P.(C.)
Assistant Professor, Department of Pediatrics, University of Montreal. Attending Physician, Hôpital Sainte-Justine, Montreal, Quebec, Canada
Antifungal Agents for Systemic Mycotic Infections

PIERRE LEBEL, M.D., F.R.C.P.(C.)
Assistant Professor, Department of Microbiology, University of Montreal. Director of Bacteriology, Department of Microbiology, Hôpital Sainte-Justine, Montreal, Quebec, Canada
Antifungal Agents for Systemic Mycotic Infections

CHARIS LIAPI, Ph.D.
Assistant Professor, Department of Pharmacology, Athens University Medical School, Athens, Greece
Glucocorticoids

JAMES G. LINAKIS, Ph.D., M.D.
Assistant Professor of Pediatrics, Brown University. Attending Physician, Departments of Emergency Medicine and Pediatrics, Rhode Island Hospital. Associate Medical Director, Rhode Island Poison Center, Providence, Rhode Island
Antipyretics

IRIS F. LITT, M.D.
Professor of Pediatrics, Division of Adolescent Medicine, Department of Pediatrics, Stanford University School of Medicine, Stanford, California
Compliance with Pediatric Medication Regimens

JOSE MARIA LOPES, M.D., Ph.D.
Head of Neonatology, Fernandes Figueira Institute, Rio de Janeiro, Brazil
Drug Treatment of Neonatal Apnea

FREDERICK H. LOVEJOY, Jr., M.D.
Chief of Patient Services, Department of Medicine, Children's Hospital. Professor of Pediatrics, Harvard School of Medicine Department of Medicine. Associate Physician-in-Chief, Children's Hospital, Boston, Massachusetts
Antipyretics

ANTOINE MALEK, Ph.D.
Women's Hospital, University of Berne, Berne, Switzerland
Physiological Adaptations to Pregnancy: Impact on Pharmacokinetics

INGRID MATHESON, M.Sci.Pharm., Ph.D.
Associate Professor, Department of Pharmacotherapeutics, Faculty of Medicine, University of Oslo, Oslo, Norway
Drug Utilization in Non-Hospitalized Newborns, Infants, and Children

DONALD R. MATTISON, B.A., M.S., M.D.
Dean, Graduate School of Public Health, Professor of Environmental and Occupational Health and Obstetrics and Gynecology, University of Pittsburgh, Pittsburgh, Pennsylvania
Physiological Adaptations to Pregnancy: Impact on Pharmacokinetics

ELAINE L. MILLS, M.D., F.A.A.P.
Associate Professor, Departments of Pediatrics and Microbiology-Immunology, McGill University. Director of Infectious Diseases, Montreal Children's Hospital, Montreal, Quebec, Canada
Antifungal Agents for Systemic Mycotic Infections

LAWRENCE S. MILNER, M.B., B.Ch.
Assistant Professor, University of Nebraska Medical Center. Nephrologist, Division of Nephrology, University of Nebraska Medical Center, Omaha, Nebraska
Therapeutic Agents and the Kidney: Pharmacokinetics and Complications

TAKASHI MIMAKI, M.D.
Assistant Professor, Department of Pediatrics, Osaka Medical College, Takatsuki City, Osaka, Japan
Anticonvulsants

ALLEN A. MITCHELL, M.D.
Research Professor of Public Health (Epidemiology), School of Public Health, Boston University School of Medicine. Lecturer on Pediatrics, Harvard Medical School. Associate Director and Associate in Medicine (Clinical Pharmacology), Children's Hospital, Boston, Massachusetts
Adverse Drug Effects and Drug Epidemiology

MOHAMMED AL-MUGEIREN, M.D., F.R.C.P.(C.)
King Khalid University. Consultant Pediatric Nephrologist, King Khalid University Hospital, Riyadh, Saudi Arabia
Therapeutic Agents and the Kidney: Pharmacokinetics and Complications

JANAK A. PATEL, M.D.
Assistant Professor, Division of Pediatric Infectious Diseases, Department of Pediatrics, University of Texas Medical Branch, Galveston, Texas
Antiviral Chemotherapy; The Penicillins

L. OGRA PEARAY, M.D.
Professor and Chairman, Department of Pediatrics, University of Texas Medical Branch, Galveston, Texas
Antiviral Chemotherapy

ROBERT G. PETERSON, M.D., Ph.D.
Professor of Pediatrics and Pharmacology and Chairman, Department of Pediatrics, University of Ottawa. Chief, Department of Pediatrics, Children's Hospital of Eastern Ontario, Ottawa, Ontario, Canada
Management of Poisoning; Appendix II: SI Units

WILLIAM P. PETROS, Pharm.D.
Clinical Associate, Department of Medicine, Duke University. Coordinator, Gale Gould Center Drug Pharmacology Lab, Bone Marrow Transplant Program, Duke University Medical Center, Durham, North Carolina
Antineoplastic Agents

STEPHANIE J. PHELPS, Ph.D.
Associate Professor, Department of Clinical Pharmacology, Center for Pediatric Pharmacokinetics and Therapeutics, The University of Tennessee, Memphis, Tennessee
Pharmacokinetically Based Drug Interactions

RONALD L. POLAND, M.D.
Professor and Chairman, Department of Pediatrics, The Milton S. Hershey Medical Center, The Pennsylvania State University, Hershey, Pennsylvania
Ethics of Drug Research in Children

ANDERS RANE, M.D., Ph.D.
Professor and Chairman, Section of Clinical Pharmacology, Academic Hospital. Director, Department of Drugs, National Board of Health and Welfare, Uppsala, Sweden
Drug Disposition and Action in Infants and Children

JUDITH L. RAPOPORT, M.D.
Chief, Child Psychiatry Branch, National Institute of Mental Health, Bethesda, Maryland
Psychoactive Agents

MICHAEL D. REED, Pharm.D., F.C.C.P., F.C.P.
Associate Professor of Pediatrics, Department of Pediatrics, School of Medicine, Case Western Reserve University. Director, Pediatric Clinical Pharmacology and Toxicology, Rainbow Babies' and Children's Hospital, Cleveland, Ohio
Drugs Used to Modulate Gastrointestinal Function; Principles of Neonatal Pharmacology

FRANZ W. ROSA, M.D., M.P.H.
Epidemiologist, Office of Epidemiology and Biostatistics, Food and Drug Administration, Rockville, Maryland
Epidemiology of Drugs in Pregnancy

F. RUSCONI, M.D.
Clinica Pediatrica, Universita di Milano, Milan, Italy
Aminoglycoside Antibiotics

BERNARD P. SCHACHTEL, M.D.
Adjunct Professor of Epidemiology and Biostatistics, Department of Epidemiology and Biostatistics, McGill University, Montreal, Quebec, Canada
Analgesic Agents

ALICIA SCHIFFRIN, M.D.
Associate Professor of Pediatrics, McGill University. Academic Staff, Montreal Children's Hospital, Montreal, Quebec, Canada
Insulin and Diabetes Mellitus

BERNARD H. SHAPIRO, Ph.D.
Head and Professor of Biochemistry, University of Pennsylvania School of Veterinary Medicine, Philadelphia, Pennsylvania
Delayed Teratogenic Expression

NEIL H. SHEAR, M.D., F.R.C.P.(C.)
Head, Clinical Pharmacology Staff, Division of Dermatology, Sunnybrook Medical Centre, Toronto, Ontario, Canada
Topical Therapy and Percutaneous Absorption

JAYANT P. SHENAI, M.D.
Associate Professor of Pediatrics, Vanderbilt University School of Medicine. Attending Neonatologist and Director, Newborn Regionalization Program, Vanderbilt University Medical Center, Nashville, Tennessee
Vitamin A Supplementation in the Very Low Birth Weight Infant

JOSEPH R. SHERBOTIE, M.D.
Assistant Professor of Pediatrics, University of Pennsylvania School of Medicine. Attending Nephrologist, Division of Nephrology, The Children's Hospital of Philadelphia, Philadelphia, Pennsylvania
Diuretics

ALAN R. SINAIKO, M.D.
Professor, Departments of Pediatrics and Pharmacology, Division of Nephrology, University of Minnesota Medical School. University of Minnesota Hospital and Clinics, Minneapolis, Minnesota
Antihypertensive Agents

ARNOLD L. SMITH, M.D.
Professor of Pediatrics, Adjunct Professor of Microbiology, University of Washington. Head, Division of Infectious Disease, Children's Hospital and Medical Center, Seattle, Washington
Chloramphenicol

WAYNE R. SNODGRASS, M.D., Ph.D.
Professor of Pediatrics and Pharmacology-Toxicology, University of Texas Medical Branch. Head, Clinical Pharmacology-Toxicology Unit, University of Texas Medical Branch, Galveston, Texas
The Penicillins

HARRIS R. STUTMAN, M.D.
Assistant Professor, Department of Pediatrics, University of California, Irvine. Director, Pediatric Infectious Diseases, Memorial Miller Children's Hospital, Long Beach, California
Cephalosporins

JAMES L. SUTPHEN, M.D., Ph.D.
Associate Professor of Pediatrics, Department of Pediatrics, School of Medicine, University of Virginia. Chief, Division of Pediatric Gastroenterology, University of Virginia Health Sciences Center, Charlottesville, Virginia
Drugs Used to Modulate Gastrointestinal Function

YASUHIRO SUZUKI, M.D.
Faculty Staff, Department of Pediatrics, Osaka University Medical School, Osaka City, Osaka, Japan
Anticonvulsants

STANLEY J. SZEFLER, M.D.
Professor of Pharmacology and Pediatrics, University of Colorado Health Science Center. Director of Clinical Pharmacology, National Jewish Center for Immunology and Respiratory Medicine, Denver, Colorado
Advances in the Pharmacologic Management of Asthma

PAUL VERT, M.D.
Professor of Pediatrics, Université de Nancy, Faculté de Medecine. Head, Department of Neonatology, Maternity Hospital, Nancy, France
Anticonvulsants in the Newborn Infant

ELLIOT S. VESELL, M.D.
Chairman, Department of Pharmacology, Pennsylvania State University College of Medicine, Hershey, Pennsylvania
Pharmacogenetics

PHILIP D. WALSON, M.D.
Professor of Pediatrics, Pharmacology, Pharmacy and Allied Health Services, The Ohio State University. Division Head, Clinical Pharmacology/Toxicology, Columbus Children's Hospital, Columbus, Ohio
Anticonvulsants

SUMNER J. YAFFE, M.D.
Director, Center for Research for Mothers and Children, National Institute of Child Health and Human Development, Bethesda, Maryland
Introduction and Historical Perspectives

FOREWORD
to the Second Edition

In ancient times children were regarded as small adults and received little consideration. When the modern era of medical treatment began with the introduction of penicillin in the late 1940s, no thought was given to the correct dosage for infants and children other than to guess and give less. It took a series of therapeutic disasters (1950–1970) to convince people of the uniqueness of infants and children. For years finding the correct dose of a medication for an infant or child was a confusing process. No authoritative source existed until 1979.

This textbook of pediatric pharmacology was "born" in 1979. The second edition has grown and matured dramatically, reflecting the rapid advances in this subject during the past eleven years.

Seventy of the top international authorities in the field have been chosen to write on sixty subjects of major practical interest to all practicing pediatricians. This is clearly the most authoritative text in the field.

This textbook will often be consulted. It contains all of the information you need to know about a drug and how to use it intelligently. It is well organized, clear, comprehensive, and succinct. The editors have done an excellent job in covering this important field and establishing this book as the classic in its field.

JEROLD F. LUCEY, M.D.

Professor of Pediatrics
Editor of Pediatrics
UVM College of Medicine
Chief, Newborn Services
Medical Center Hospital of Vermont

FOREWORD
from the First Edition

During the past decade, pediatric pharmacology has progressed from a subcomponent of adult therapeutics to a well-defined and recognized medical specialty. Clinical misfortunes, such as the chloramphenicol–gray syndrome and the thalidomide–phocomelia tragedies, dramatically increased appreciation of the concept of drug treatment appropriate for age. The concept has also influenced practice with the increasing realization that the child is not a small adult, but rather a growing organism that undergoes continuous changes, at times rapidly, to achieve biological maturity. There was mounting evidence that, to ensure drug safety and efficacy at all periods of human development, from conception to adolescence, increased research was needed to clarify interactions among medications administered, physiologic events, and disease states.

The proliferation of workshops and conferences dealing with some aspect of children and drugs and the allocation of special sections to the subject within the general, pediatric, and pharmacologic publications attest to the concern of pediatricians and pharmacologists within the field of pediatric pharmacology. Interest seems to have reached a peak during the International Year of the Child, 1979, designated by the United Nations to encourage all countries and individuals to rekindle their commitments to children. Two specialized journals were planned during that year, and work started on *Pediatric Pharmacology,* the first textbook devoted exclusively to this issue. This multi-authored book presents chapters covering a broad panorama, from fundamental pharmacologic principles as they apply to developing organisms, to specific clinical advances. The writers, all recognized authorities in their fields, share a common interest in the well-being of children. The editor has achieved a comprehensive overview of the field by including chapters on ethical issues of drug study involving children, the behavioral aspects of compliance, and drug surveillance in this population.

This text will serve as a useful guide to all professionals responsible for the care of children as well as to those treating diseases in pregnant women. The compilation, in a single volume, of existing knowledge in the field of pediatric pharmacology serves one further purpose: because the book permits an evaluation of progress to date and indicates gaps in knowledge, pediatricians, pharmacologists, and obstetricians may be stimulated through this book to study some new element in pediatric or developmental pharmacology for the benefit of a most important patient—the child.

HENRY L. BARNETT, M.D.

Professor of Pediatrics
Albert Einstein College of Medicine
New York, New York

PREFACE

Pediatric pharmacology and drug therapy may be viewed as manipulative physiology and biochemistry for the fetus, newborn infant, and growing child. This concept is based on the fact that drugs are used to restore and correct physiological and biochemical abnormalities which occur during pre- and postnatal development.

As advances in the knowledge of diseases and their diagnoses are made, the complexities of treatment, particularly by drugs, increase in tandem. Although therapeutic drug exposure in children has remained relatively constant, the number of drugs available to physicians and health care givers continues to increase. There is an increasing variety of antimicrobials, cardiovascular drugs, diuretics, immunosuppressants, antivirals, and other drugs for the management of sick pediatric patients. Safe and effective use of these agents in infants and children requires adequate knowledge of their pharmacologic properties, including drug action, metabolism, and disposition.

The second edition of *Pediatric Pharmacology: Therapeutic Principles in Practice* has been revised significantly to meet the needs of practitioners in the 1990s. The book has expanded from 24 chapters in the first edition to 52 chapters in this edition, plus an appendix on SI Units and a Drug Formulary appendix. The book is designed to provide relevant information on drugs and their uses in newborn infants, older infants, children, and adolescents. It was proposed as a quick reference for busy clinicians, house staff, students, nurses, pharmacists, and health care providers. It was also written as a general and basic reference for teaching pediatric pharmacology. It is hoped that researchers also will find it useful to understand the unique characteristics and dynamic changes in drug requirements and action during a period of intense growth and development.

The mechanisms of drug actions, the evidence of drug efficacy in certain disease states, dose, therapeutic guidelines, and drug toxicities are emphasized. The book was organized to parallel the distinct periods of early human development. Special sections useful in drug therapy such as therapeutic drug monitoring, adverse drug reactions, and epidemiologic considerations are also included. Certain aspects of pediatric drug therapy, particularly those relating to immunoactive drugs and vitamins, are not included owing to lack of information in these areas. We hope to correct these omissions in the next edition as the knowledge base for these agents in pediatrics increases.

Drugs are double-edged swords; although they can cure illnesses and restore health, they can also produce unwanted and, at times, unanticipated toxicities. The rational, intelligent, and safe use of drugs springs mainly from understanding their actions, uses, problems, and limitations. This understanding in turn will permit selection of the appropriate drug and prescription of the optimal dosage. It is our utmost desire that this textbook can help those providers of care to children to maximize the benefits of pharmacologic agents while averting their adverse effects. Thus, this book will help in the promotion of health and well-being in children.

SUMNER J. YAFFE
JACOB V. ARANDA

CONTENTS

SECTION I

GENERAL PRINCIPLES

1

INTRODUCTION AND HISTORICAL PERSPECTIVES

SUMNER J. YAFFE *and* JACOB V. ARANDA

The past several decades have witnessed a revolution in the practice of therapeutics. It has long been recognized that the nature, duration, and intensity of drug action depend not only on the intrinsic properties of the drug, but also on its interaction with the host to whom the drug has been administered for the treatment of disease. Advances in drug development have led to the introduction of highly specific and extremely potent therapeutic agents into the marketplace.

Prompted perhaps by the synthesis of these highly specific and potent chemical entities, there has developed an ever-increasing understanding of the mechanisms of drug disposition—especially those concerned with the biotransformation of xenobiotics. This has led to a burgeoning new discipline: *clinical pharmacology.* Awareness of host factors as major determinants of drug concentration (and hence drug effect) within the organism also has led to an enlightened efficiency in the selection of drug entities and their dosage.

While these advances have been proceeding at a rapid pace in adult medicine, it is evident that pediatric pharmacology has not kept pace and, until very recently, has lagged far behind the research and attention paid to the proper use of therapeutic and diagnostic drugs in adults. Thus a large percentage of the drugs used in sick infants and children are prescribed on empirical grounds. This information gap in pediatric practice was recognized as a crisis by Dr. Charles C. Edwards, former commissioner of the Food and Drug Administration (FDA), when he addressed the 1972 Annual Meeting of the American Academy of Pediatrics.

The National Academy of Sciences in 1973 also emphasized the different nature of the response of an immature organism to pharmacologic agents and suggested that innovative investigative programs were needed to supply information on the use of pharmacologic agents in the pediatric population. As a consequence of this information gap, the concept of the "therapeutic orphan" has arisen in which many drugs with the potential for use in children have been approved for marketing with a disclaimer on the label concerning usage in infants and children, as well as in pregnant women. Awareness of age, sex, genetic makeup, and nutritional status of the pediatric patient as major determinants of drug action and disposition has occurred largely through therapeutic accidents in which adverse effects in infants and children prompted detailed pharmacologic studies. These adverse effects obviously would have been prevented, or at least minimized, if the appropriate pharmacologic studies had been carried out before the drugs were prescribed to the sick infant and child.

Basic research has clearly demonstrated that the stage of development can markedly affect drug metabolism and excretion, as well as absorption and distribution. It is now recognized that the effects of many drugs on infants and children may vary considerably from the effects seen in adults, even when careful calculation is made to arrive at a dosage proportional to either body weight or estimated body surface area. Pharmacologically, children cannot be regarded as "miniature" adults. Intensified or even toxic effects of drugs administered to children may reflect differences either (1) in processes of drug disposition that differ from those which are operative in the adult patient or (2) in receptor sensitivity due to alterations in receptor binding sites or in bond strength. In view of these circumstances, there is a need for special caution in prescribing medication in the treatment of childhood illnesses, particularly when the medication is used for an extended period of time and therefore is capable of affecting the orderly process of development in the growing child or when a newly marketed drug is used.

The administration of a drug to a growing and developing infant or child therefore presents a unique problem to the physician. Not only must there be constant awareness of the changes in drug dosages that are determined by alterations in processes of disposition at different ages, but also there must be cognizance of the fact that the drug may affect the developmental process itself and that this type of drug action may be delayed and not apparent for many years after the drug has been administered.

3

These concepts and generalizations are partly illustrated in Figure 1–1. The dynamic changes in drug elimination and excretion can be appreciated in the case of theophylline, a methylxanthine used as a respiratory stimulant in the newborn and as a bronchodilator in older children and adults. Based on the well-known pharmacokinetic behavior of this drug with advancing postnatal age, the estimated daily dose of theophylline to maintain equivalent plasma concentrations at various ages could range from 4 to 24 mg/liter. Application of the dose recommended for the toddler to the newborn infant would result in toxic plasma concentrations.

Clearly, at all stages of development, one solution to the safe and effective use of drugs is to base the prescription on scientific data obtained for the particular age group under consideration. This applies not only to the newborn infant, where most attention has been focused, but also to the older infant, child, and adolescent, in whom significant physiologic changes are also taking place. The maturation of an organism into an adult is successfully achieved only after the completion of a series of intricate and interlocking events that proceed through a continuum. The sequence begins at conception, and the processes of growth and development advance in a predictable fashion. The sequence is, however, associated with a wide variation in physiologic functions, not only in the same individual, but also between individuals. Thus the response to a pharmacologic agent may vary from patient to patient.

These inter- and intraindividual differences render the task of studying drugs in the pediatric population even more difficult than in the adult population. These difficulties are heightened when consideration of drug administration to pregnant women is included. Truly, this area of drug administration is an appropriate concern for pediatric pharmacology. Indeed, considerations about the safety of foreign compounds administered to pregnant women have been increasingly questioned since the therapeutic catastrophe of thalidomide.

It was the direct response to this misadventure that led to the promulgation of new drug regulations in 1962 in the United States. According to these regulations, a drug must be demonstrated to be safe and effective for the conditions of use prescribed in its labeling. The regulations concerning this requirement state that a drug should be investigated for the conditions of use specified in the labeling, including dosage levels and patient populations for whom the drug is intended. In addition, appropriate information must be provided when the drug is prescribed. The intent of the regulations is not only to ensure adequate labeling information for the safe and effective administration of the drug by the physician, but also to ensure that marketed drugs have an acceptable risk/benefit ratio for their intended uses. As mentioned previously, most labeling for prescription drugs fails to provide information on pediatric dosage and indications or contains a disclaimer stating that use in children is not recommended because of inadequate studies in this age group. The percentage of drugs with labeling disclaimers is even greater for usage during pregnancy than during infancy and childhood.

The recent advances in the diagnosis of fetal maturity and disease and immediate postneonatal morbidity led to treatment during intrauterine life by the administration of drugs directly to the mother, such as steroids for the prevention of respiratory distress syndrome. This approach requires data characterizing the pharmacokinetics and drug disposition of different compounds in the maternal–placental–fetal unit.

Pediatric drug usage has played a key role in therapeutics by influencing the federal regulations concerning how new drugs are approved and marketed. Adverse effects resulting from well-intentioned but uninformed use in sick infants and children have played a significant role in the historical implementation of federal control over the

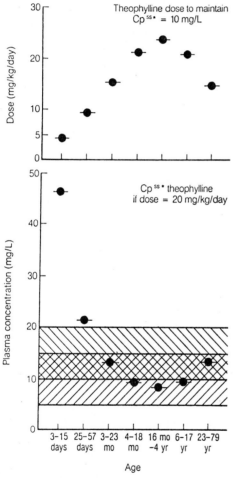

FIGURE 1–1. Theophylline dose requirements and plasma concentrations. *Top panel:* Estimated dose requirements of theophylline (mg/kg/day) to maintain a plasma concentration of 10 mg/L. *Lower panel:* Estimated plasma concentrations of theophylline at steady state if dose is kept at 20 mg/kg/day. Shaded areas indicate tentative therapeutic level for bronchodilatation and anti-apneic activity.

*Cp^{ss} = Plasma concentration at steady state.

(From "Maturational Changes in Theophylline and Caffeine Metabolism and Disposition: Clinical Implications" by J. V. Aranda, in *Proceedings of the Second World Conference on Clinical Pharmacology and Therapeutics,* July 31–August 5, 1983, p. 870, edited by L. Lemberger and M. M. Reidenberg. Copyright by the American Society for Pharmacology and Experimental Therapeutics, Bethesda, 1984. Used with permission.)

drug supply. These statutes, in turn, have directly affected the pharmaceutical industry and have determined to a large extent which therapeutic entities are available to the practitioner. It is therefore of some interest to review milestones in the history of U.S. food and drug law. Although there are differences among nations in mechanisms governing the regulation of drugs, most countries in the Western world employ concepts that are quite similar to those embodied in the U.S. Food and Drugs Act.

For many centuries, societies have been concerned about the purity of the food and drink offered to the public. In the Western world, King John of England proclaimed the first English food law in 1202. This regulation, entitled "The Assize of Bread," prohibited adulteration of bread with such ingredients as ground peas or beans. Regulation of food in the United States was one of the earliest concerns of the newly founded republic, with statutes passed in 1784.

Federal controls over the drug supply started in 1848 with the passage of the Import Drugs Act. This law, enacted to ensure the quality of drugs, was passed when quinine used by the American Army in Mexico for the treatment of malaria was found to be adulterated. The original Food and Drugs Act was passed by Congress in 1906 and signed into law on June 30 of that year by President Theodore Roosevelt. The act prohibited interstate commerce in misbranded and adulterated foods, drinks, and drugs. This was a comprehensive attempt to deal with the widespread problem of food and drug adulteration. During the 26 years preceding the passage of this act, more than 100 bills had been introduced into Congress, but none had passed. Over the next several decades, many changes occurred that determined the functions of the Food and Drug Administration. The most significant event was the passage of the Federal Food, Drug, and Cosmetic Act of 1938. The most important provision of this act required predistribution clearance of the *safety* of new drugs. It is of interest and at the same time tragic to note that the event that motivated this act was the unnecessary death of 107 children following ingestion of an elixir of sulfanilamide. This tragic event clearly demonstrated the need to establish drug safety prior to marketing. The law was a great step forward in the safe and effective usage of drugs. It should be emphasized, however, that the 1938 act continued to use as its legal base the right of the federal government to regulate interstate commerce in adulteration or misbranding of foods, drugs, and cosmetics. Many amendments to the 1938 act have evolved to meet the challenges of public safety resulting from technological development. These include, among others, insulin and antibiotic certification amendments, prescription drug amendments, food additives amendments, and pesticide chemicals amendments.

Significant changes occurred in 1962 with the drug amendments of that year. These followed the tragedies in Europe and Canada that resulted from the use of thalidomide in pregnant women. Note, again, that the motivating agent was a tragedy affecting the young patient, in this case the fetus. These sweeping new amendments added new controls to ensure the quality of all drugs, to simplify drug nomenclature, to improve inspections, to regulate investigational drug use and procedure, to regulate prescription drug advertising, and most important, to require that drugs be shown to be *effective* as well as safe before they are marketed.

A key year in the history of the Food and Drug Administration was 1962. Legislation enacted in that year serves as the basis for the current operations of the FDA. The demonstration of efficacy and safety has been interpreted to require that a manufacturer demonstrate these parameters under circumstances for which the drug is intended for use. This means, for example, that claims of efficacy and safety in an adult male cannot be transferred to a pregnant female or to a developing infant and child unless studies have actually been undertaken during pregnancy and during postnatal life.

The FDA has statutory responsibility for ensuring the safety and effectiveness of marketed drugs for their intended uses and for ensuring that they are accurately and adequately labeled. This includes accurate dosage information and directions for safe usage. The FDA requires that drugs be tested for safety and efficacy before being approved for therapeutic use. This testing has to take into consideration characteristics of the prospective population in which the drug will be employed. Under most circumstances, the claims for efficacy and the demonstration of safety are provided to the FDA by data submitted by the pharmaceutical industry. According to FDA regulations, less than 25 percent of drugs marketed in the United States at the present time can be advertised as safe and effective for use in infants and children. This does not imply that the drugs are contraindicated, unsafe, or disapproved for use in infants and children; rather, it signifies that sufficient data have not been provided to grant approval status for specific clinical indications and uses in the pediatric population. Since neither the safety nor the efficacy of many of these marketed drugs has been demonstrated by clinical trials for use in infants and children, the physician caring for the sick infant and child is faced with this dilemma: (1) Avoid the use of the drug; that is, deprive children of the potential benefits of the therapeutic agents available to adults—known as the "therapeutic orphan" situation—or (2) prescribe the drug despite the lack of certification or approval by the FDA of its safety and efficacy for use in children. Thus the physician is in a quandary. Without the use of the drug, the young patient may be deprived of a significant therapeutic entity. If, on the other hand, the patient uses the drug and an adverse effect occurs, the physician may be subject to medical-legal action. The physician makes the decision for prescribing a therapeutic agent on the basis of either the information contained in the labeling supplied by the manufacturer or data available in the medical literature. New uses (doses and indications) will not be approved by the FDA until "substantial" evidence of safety and efficacy for that indication and for that specific pediatric age group is submitted. This regulatory process may take years or may never occur because there is less incentive to gather and submit data for new uses after a drug has been approved for marketing and the profit motive is no longer operative. Labeling is intended neither to preclude physicians from using their best clinical judgment on behalf of their patients nor to impose medical-legal liability for failure to adhere to the indications that are contained in the label or package insert.

Thus it is evident that there is a complex interplay between clinical, ethical, and legal precepts that brings to perinatal and pediatric pharmacology a series of difficult problems requiring resolution. The North American regulatory agencies, pediatric and clinical pharmacology societies, and other bodies, such as the Institute of Medicine of the National Academy of Sciences, continue to address these issues. Future endeavors of these bodies working together may facilitate the availability of required drugs for the safe and effective treatment of pediatric and neonatal disease. The increasing dialogue between regulatory agencies, academia, practitioners, and the pharmaceutical industry will certainly improve the existing climate for drug development and use in this population.

As previously noted, the most recent significant changes in the Food and Drug Regulations were prompted by therapeutic tragedies affecting children. More recently, the amendments of 1962 declared that new drugs not only must be safe, as required in 1938, but also must be shown to be effective prior to marketing. They also declared that the study of investigational drugs (prior to marketing) must be monitored carefully by the FDA. These 1962 amendments are those under which we operate today and were the direct result of the thalidomide tragedy in which so many infants were malformed following intrauterine exposure to this very effective hypnotic sedative.

In 1963, Dr. Harry Shirkey observed that infants and children are becoming therapeutic or pharmaceutical orphans. The term *therapeutic orphans* refers to the deprivation—actual or potential—of sick children because drugs that might be useful to them are not given as a consequence of statements in the package inserts that such drugs haven't been adequately tested in children. This situation is particularly undesirable both for the sick child and for the prescriber. Unfortunately, it pertains to the majority of prescription drugs marketed today.

Many factors have been implicated in the causes of the therapeutic orphan situation. These include the lack of trained pediatric clinical pharmacologists, inaction due to profit motivation on the part of the drug manufacturers, and societal concerns for the risk of drug studies in general and for the ethicality of drug studies in children in particular. However, many of these factors are no longer applicable, and pediatric clinical pharmacology today is a sophisticated discipline that is very capable of carrying out studies necessary to ensure the evaluation and subsequent use of drugs for infants and children. The drug manufacturers, when spurred by the economic incentives of potential widespread use of a new drug in the pediatric population, have encountered little difficulty in persuading well-trained investigators to study these drugs with well-controlled clinical trials to convince the FDA of substantial evidence of safety and efficacy.

How serious a problem is the therapeutic orphan situation? Firm data regarding this issue are difficult to come by. In 1975, Dr. John Wilson, in a pragmatic assessment, found that 78 percent of prescription drugs carried a label-

ing statement against use in infants and children or were silent with regard to such use because the drugs had not been adequately studied in infants and children in order to assess and get approval on accurate dosages and appropriate indications for use. A decade later, analyses of drugs that had been approved by the FDA showed that 50 percent had pediatric studies undertaken under the sponsorship of the manufacturers. This represented a significant improvement over the 22 percent that had not been subjected to the orphaning clause in the previous decade.

Dr. Franz Rosa, an FDA epidemiologist, surveyed prescription drugs available in 1988. He found that with respect to use in infants, 50 percent have been evaluated in this population. Of this 50 percent, half have been considered safe and efficacious and the remaining half have a caution or risk statement in the label. Fifty percent of the total have not been evaluated, and of these, 60 percent have a label disclaimer and 40 percent have no statement on the label regarding use in infants. This change in the therapeutic orphan situation represents a significant advance from the past, but there certainly is room for improvement.

The current position of the FDA concerning pediatric drug studies is that they should be completed before marketing for (1) drugs that represent a major therapeutic advance and thus are likely to be used in children and (2) drugs that do not represent any major advances but are likely to be used *widely* in children because of their applicability in the treatment of diseases that occur mainly in children. This has particular relevance to the newborn infant in view of the marked advances that have occurred recently in the management of low-birth-weight infants in the intensive care nursery. Application of these guidelines should be flexible in order not to delay the approval and subsequent availability of significant new therapeutic entities for use in adult patients. For example, it is sufficient to indicate that studies are underway in children and not to wait until these studies are completed before giving approval for marketing of major therapeutic advances. In this case, the pediatric studies could be completed after marketing of the adult preparation. However, it is allowable to undertake postmarketing studies in lieu of premarketing studies for those drugs which represent only some advantage over available drugs and are likely to be used in children but not as widely as in (2) above.

Finally, because of limited resources, pediatric studies should not be required for drugs that appear to offer no advantage over those already available; these drugs instead should be marketed with the usual label disclaimers. In this case, manufacturers could voluntarily perform the studies in children if they want to use these drugs in the pediatric population while they are marketing the drug for adults.

In the United States, the FDA has long been aware of the shortage of drugs adequately labeled for use in children (indicating the lack of data upon which to base the substantial evidence of safety and efficacy). As a consequence, government, industry, and the academic community have attempted to develop solutions to this problem. The number of workshops and conferences over the past 15 years indicates the concern with the problem and highlights advances that are being made. The FDA also entered into a contract with the Committee on Drugs of the American Academy of Pediatrics to develop a solution. As a consequence, the committee issued general guidelines for the evaluation of drugs to be approved for use during pregnancy and for the treatment of infants and children.[1] These general guidelines were adopted by the FDA and incorporated into its series of clinical guidelines for drug evaluation as Publication No. 77-3041.[2] These guidelines were updated and revised in 1979 by the Committee on Drugs.[3]

The guidelines identify the research needs in terms of the special techniques that are required to study drugs adequately in young subjects. Emphasis is placed on the need to be aware of unexpected toxicities that may result from immature physiologic and metabolic mechanisms. These toxicities occur because the developmental status of the infant and child is distinct from that of an adult. The toxicities that are predictable in an adult from the drug's known pharmacologic properties are determined from studies. Flexibility in research design is essential to permit modifications necessary to fit the nature of the drug, its intended use, and the age and developmental status of the pediatric patient.

Guidelines for the clinical evaluation of specific classes of drugs also have been developed by the FDA. They emphasize that factors affecting both safety and efficacy may be different in the pediatric population because of both quantitative and qualitative differences that arise from developmental physiologic changes. The development of adequate methods for determination of the drug and its major metabolites in biologic fluids was emphasized, with particular attention to the need for methods that might employ stable isotopes. Certainly, many technological advances have been made in this general area. The variations in pharmacokinetics between the pediatric population and adults have been adequately publicized and have motivated extensive investigation both in Europe and in the United States. These include variations in bioavailability, which would have applicability particularly to oral formulations in view of the continually changing physiology of the gastrointestinal tract in young infants. Emphasis also was placed on different types of drug interactions that might occur in the developing infant and child. Attempts should be made to correlate the pharmacokinetics with the pharmacodynamic responses to a particular drug in order to establish a concentration–response relationship. This is often difficult to accomplish because of the problem of *quantifying* drug effects, particularly in infants and children. Where this information is available, it can be used to monitor and optimize drug therapy.

The importance of experimental design both on practical and ethical considerations has been stressed repeatedly. In common with all research in human subjects, clinical research in children involves the use of a precious resource. It is imperative that investigators make maximum use of the information that can be obtained with as little inconvenience to the patient as possible. It is a general consensus that, whenever possible, investigators beginning new studies in children should thoroughly test their design and analytical techniques on animals and in adult subjects before initiating the pediatric studies. Of course, there are times and indications for pathologic conditions that require treatment that are confined only to the pediatric population. While experimental design in the pediatric population may have to vary from the rigid protocol utilized in adults, it must account for the adequate control of variables with appropriate statistical analysis. In addition, methods and appropriate validation must address not only the assessment of benefit, but also the possibility of unusual adverse effects and a placebo response that may be different from that seen in adults.

Monitoring of clinical studies in infants and children should be intense, and surveillance should be continuous. This, of course, does not differ from that required in the adult population, but in infants and children there is an added element of unanticipated effect present.

The guidelines adopted by the FDA also looked at specific age-dependent factors that might influence the demonstration and evaluation of safety and efficacy. As a result of this, the pediatric population was divided into five (perhaps arbitrarily selected) age groups that were intended to warrant specific consideration. Underlying this approach was the concept that there were complex changes in the anatomy, physiology, biochemistry, and behavior from one stage of development to another over the time frame of growth from conception to adulthood. Each grouping attempted to divide the pediatric patient subset into stages that shared enough characteristics to allow easy distinction of one stage from another. The introduction of this concept was not an attempt to suggest that each drug be tested in each age group; rather, this was an attempt to ensure consideration of the important biologic characteristics of each age group in which the drug would eventually be used under therapeutic circumstances.

These age groups are the intrauterine period (conception to birth), the neonate (birth to 1 month), the infant–toddler (1 month to 2 years), the child (2 years to the onset of puberty), and the adolescent (onset of adolescence to adult life). Within each age group, certain characteristics of the biochemistry and physiology as well as behavior have been identified to alert the investigator to the specific ways in which investigation should be conducted, remembering at all times the uniqueness of each subject at the various stages of development.

In general, the usual testing sequence of a new drug would first involve teenagers, who can consent to participation, and then successively younger children. Exceptions occur when diseases are specific to one age group or another. The neonate must be approached with great care, since even studies in young children may not yield a reliable estimate of adverse effects that may be seen in the neonate. This caution must be given greater emphasis when considering low-birth-weight and very-low-birth-weight infants.

The inadvertent treatment of the fetus by administration of a drug to the mother for a serious medical problem is frequently the first source of information about drug effects in the fetus (neonate). There are many examples of this phenomenon, in which detailed pharmacokinetic investigations of drugs administered in utero have yielded considerable insight into the ability of newborns to handle the drug. Adverse effects in the fetus, of course, depend on its stage of development when the drug was given to the mother. It is simply not enough to look for anatomic birth defects, but attention also should be paid to behavioral effects as well as effects that may arise in the long term.

In 1974, the U.S. Congress established the National Commission for the Protection of Human Subjects of Biomedical and Behavioral Research. A part of their mission was to develop guidelines for the protection of certain categories of research subjects in various segments of the population with impaired ability to give truly informed consent. The report and recommendations of the commission with respect to research involving children were issued in September of 1977.[2] The commission advised that "research involving children is important for the health and well-being of all children and can be conducted in an ethical manner" if certain conditions are met. These included review and determination by an institutional ethical review board that (1) the research is scientifically sound and significant; (2) when appropriate, studies must be conducted first on animals and adult humans and then on older children prior to involving infants; and (3) risks must be minimized by using the safest methods, consistent and sound research design, and by using procedures performed for diagnostic or treatment purposes whenever feasible.

It is apparent from these considerations that much progress has been made in addressing the problems of drug investigation in infants and children. Clinical as well as ethical guidelines have been established. Investigators have been trained, methodologies have been developed, and resources have been made available. Nonetheless, considerable problems remain and others continually arise.

One problem concerns the need to continually educate pediatricians about proper drug use in pediatric patients. All data gained from investigations must be transferred into practical clinical use. A publication by Kennedy and Forbes[4] in the United States examined the national patterns of prescribing drugs for children by office-based physicians. This study divided the population into an infant group and a school-age group. It took advantage of a national disease and therapeutic index system that randomly surveys more than 200,000 office-based physicians. Data were made available concerning the overall use of drugs in ambulatory children. It is surprising that 15 categories of drugs accounted for 80 percent of all drugs prescribed in both population groups studied.

The 15 categories for the two age groups, although similar, showed a few differences. For example, pediatric multivitamins, antidiarrheal drugs, and fungicides appeared in the top 15 categories of drugs used in the infant group and were not present in the school-age group, where topical anti-infective agents, cephalosporins, and desensitizing allergens were present. The major class of drug used in both groups was antibiotics. Surprisingly, despite extensive publicity and label warnings, tetracycline continued to be used in patients under 8 years of age.

There is no way of knowing from this type of survey whether or not antibiotics are overused or misused. However, their extensive prescription (greater than 35 percent of all drugs used) suggests that there might be a problem in association with their use. Of interest is the fact that ampicillin use exceeded that of amoxicillin despite the well-demonstrated superiority of the latter drug at that time.

Concern has arisen in recent years about the effects of "medical progress." This involves the marked improvements in the care of low-birth-weight infants. The development of sophisticated technology, the availability of adequately trained specialists, and the provision of new facilities have been responsible for significant reductions in neonatal mortality and morbidity. Nonetheless, it is important to examine what has taken place. Because of the desperate conditions that exist in the low-birth-weight infant, many treatment methods have been incorporated rapidly into the intensive care nursery without adequate evaluation.

An interesting study concerning this phenomenon in the United States[5] evaluated all of the therapeutic studies published in 1979 in four respected U.S. obstetrical and pediatric journals. The object of the investigation was to determine the quality of the studies, since the treatment methods recommended were widely and rapidly incorporated into clinical practice after publication in respected journals. Evaluation of the quality of the published studies was conducted by a clinical investigator, a biostatistician, a neonatologist, and an obstetrician. Many of the studies failed to meet the criteria for quality perinatal therapeutic research.

Flaws in the design of clinical studies increase the likelihood that treatment methods heralded as improved and published as such will appear ineffective upon subsequent scrutiny. The problem arises that these results may be accepted as valid and incorporated into practice because many physicians are not adequately prepared to evaluate the scientific quality of medical research. Past experience with the misuse of diethylstilbestrol, chloramphenicol, sulfonamide, oxygen, and other agents used in perinatal medicine demonstrates that the fetus and newborn infant are especially vulnerable to the complications of inadequately tested treatment methods. The need for rigorous evaluation of current neonatal treatment methods must be constantly kept in mind; otherwise, ineffective and potentially hazardous treatment methods may be recommended and widely used.

Thus drugs are double-edged swords. While they can save lives, so can they endanger life. Effective and safe drug therapy in neonates, infants, and children requires an understanding of the differences in drug action, metabolism, and disposition that are apparent during growth and development. Virtually all pharmacokinetic parameters change with age. Therefore, pediatric drug dosage regimens must be adjusted for age (major determinant), disease state, sex, and individual needs. Failure to make such adjustments may lead to ineffective treatment or even to toxicity. This book attempts to provide principles and guidelines as well as specific recommendations for the use of the various pharmacologic agents in the perinatal and pediatric population.

REFERENCES

1. American Academy of Pediatrics, Committee on Drugs: General Guidelines for the Evaluation of Drugs to be Approved for Use During Pregnancy and for Treatment of Infants and Children. Evanston, Illinois, American Academy of Pediatrics, 1974
2. U.S. Department of HEW, PHS, FDA: General Considerations for the Clinical Evaluation of Drugs in Infants and Children. (HEW Publication No. (FDA) 77-3041) Washington, U.S. Government Printing Office, 1977
3. American Academy of Pediatrics, Committee on Drugs: Guidelines for the ethical conduct of studies to evaluate drugs in pediatric populations, Pediatrics 60:91–101, 1977
4. Kennedy DL, Forbes MB: Drug therapy for ambulatory pediatrics patients, Pediatrics 70:26–29, 1982
5. Tyson JE, Furzan JA, Reisch JA, Mize SG: An evaluation of the quality of therapeutic studies in perinatal medicine, Pediatrics 102:10–13, 1983

2

DRUG DISPOSITION AND ACTION IN INFANTS AND CHILDREN

ANDERS RANE

Ethical and legal constraints on drug testing in the pediatric population have limited knowledge about drug disposition and action in infants and children. Present drug usage in pediatrics is based on a cautious and conservative empiricism in which therapeutic misadventures have acted as warning signals.

The therapeutic goal of obtaining a specific pharmacologic response with as little risk of adverse effects as possible is best achieved by selecting the appropriate drug and the correct dose and dosage regimen for the disease and individual in question. This is hampered by the large interindividual variability with respect to drug response (pharmacodynamics) and disposition (pharmacokinetics), as well as the disease state and a variety of other patient features. For most drugs, interindividual age-dependent variability and genetic variability in drug response are less pronounced than the variability in drug kinetics. It is also evident that the age-dependent variation in drug kinetics is larger than the genetic variation for most drugs, if one excludes pharmacogenetic polymorphism. The therapeutic disasters with sulfonamides[1] and chloramphenicol[2] involving toxic effects in the newborn after administration of the same (body-weight-related) doses as to adult patients are historical examples of the clinical consequences of altered drug disposition in the young. These events have contributed to the dogma that the developing infant has an augmented response to drugs. This is not always the case, however.

The major cause of age-related changes in drug disposition is the maturational increase in liver and kidney function. Age-dependent variations in plasma protein binding, tissue distribution, gastrointestinal absorption, and other physiologic parameters also contribute to the rapid changes.

It is not within the scope of this chapter to discuss the development of pharmacodynamic expressions in humans. The reader is referred to recent reviews on this topic.[3] Suffice it to say that these aspects of developmental pharmacology are extremely important areas for future research. Although the development of analytical techniques now permits detailed pharmacokinetic studies, there is a dearth of understanding of the concentration–effect relationships in infants and children. It is not possible to extrapolate these relationships from adult patients to children without investigational support.

This chapter discusses how the development of the human organism may affect drug kinetics in infants and children. The text is accompanied by examples from some clinically important pharmacotherapeutic areas.

DRUG METABOLISM AS REFLECTED BY CLINICAL PHARMACOKINETIC DATA

Concepts

Elimination of drugs and other xenobiotics is one means by which an organism terminates their effects. Elimination involves various excretory pathways with or without a preceding chemical alteration, enzymatically or nonenzymatically, of the drug molecule. The elimination processes may be seen as part of the body's defense mechanism. Without these processes, drug accumulation and toxicity would ensue.

The combined efficacy of all elimination processes is quantified by the total-body clearance ($Cl_{I.V.}$) of the drug. This, by definition, is the volume of blood or plasma that is irreversibly cleared of drug per unit of time. If an I.V. dose of the drug (D) is administered to the patient, and the area under the plasma concentration versus time curve ($AUC_{I.V.}$) is assessed, the $Cl_{I.V.}$ may be calculated:

$$Cl_{I.V.} = \frac{D}{AUC_{I.V.}} \qquad (1)$$

The $Cl_{I.V.}$ reflects the sum of the different elimination routes. Thus $Cl_{I.V.}$ may be the sum of hepatic (Cl_H) and renal (Cl_R) clearance as well as possibly other clearance mechanisms.

If the drug is administered orally, the apparent oral clearance (Cl_O) must be corrected for by the fraction (F) of the oral dose that reaches the systemic circulation:

$$Cl_O = \frac{F \times D}{AUC_O} \qquad (2)$$

It follows that $(1 - F)$ is the fraction of the oral dose that is metabolized in the liver and/or gut wall during passage from the gut to the systemic circulation. This phenomenon is called *first-pass elimination* (FPE). If all the drug in the gut is absorbed into the portal vein, then

$$1 - F = E \qquad (3)$$

where E is the hepatic extraction ratio. This is that proportion of the dose entering the liver which is eliminated during one passage through the organ. If only part of the oral dose is absorbed, the deficient absorption must be corrected for in the calculations of E and F.

The relationship between Cl_H, the liver blood flow (Q), and the total intrinsic hepatic clearance (Cl_i) is defined by the perfusion-limited clearance model[4,5] for drug clearance in the liver. This relation is defined as

$$Cl_H = Q \times E = Q\left(\frac{Cl_i}{Q + Cl_i}\right) \qquad (4)$$

The *intrinsic clearance* is defined as the maximum capacity of the liver (or any other organ) to remove drug from the blood in the absence of flow limitations. From Equation 4 it is obvious that changes in *liver blood flow* will preferentially affect the clearance of drugs with high values of Cl_i, which may be observed as changes in plasma half-life ($t_{1/2}$). In contrast, *changes in enzyme activity* will affect the $t_{1/2}$ only of drugs with low values of Cl_i. In addition, such changes will affect the AUC both after oral and after I.V. administration such that the AUC is decreased when the enzyme activity is enhanced.

The drug clearance from an organ is also dependent on drug binding in the blood by modification of Equation 4:

$$Cl_H = Q\left(\frac{f_B \times Cl_i'}{Q + f_B \times Cl_i'}\right) \qquad (5)$$

where f_B denotes the unbound fraction in blood and Cl_i' is the intrinsic hepatic clearance of unbound drug. Drug binding in blood has little importance for the Cl_H if Cl_i' is high. In contrast, drug binding has a limiting (restrictive) influence on Cl_H if the value of Cl_i' is low.[5] As a corollary, hepatic drug extraction from the blood is denoted as nonrestrictive or restrictive, respectively.

Clinical Data

Even if an *in vitro* estimate of Cl_i in terms of enzyme kinetics and expressed as the ratio between V_{max} and K_m in liver microsomes[6] is possible, this information, when available, is of limited value for the *in vivo* situation if the hepatic blood flow is unknown. Therefore, *in vivo* meth-

ods to estimate Cl_i must be employed. By definition, the Cl_O is equivalent to the intrinsic hepatic clearance (Cl_i) of the drug, provided the drug is eliminated only by liver metabolism and is completely absorbed in the gastrointestinal tract. However, very few drugs fulfill these criteria, and in children, no data on the apparent oral clearance of such drugs seem to exist.

The plasma half-life ($t_{1/2}$) may serve as an estimate of the hepatic drug-metabolizing activity only under defined circumstances. The $t_{1/2}$ gives no information about the efficiency of drug-elimination processes even though this parameter has some value for the clinical estimation of duration of effect. If the drug is solely eliminated by means of hepatic metabolism, that is, systemic clearance (Cl_S) = Cl_H, then

$$t_{1/2} = \frac{0.693 \times V_d}{Cl_H} \qquad (6)$$

This relationship demonstrates that $t_{1/2}$ depends on Cl_H as well as on the apparent volume of distribution of the drug (V_d). Assuming that V_d is constant, then the $t_{1/2}$ is virtually proportional to the hepatic enzyme activity (for low-extraction drugs), the hepatic blood flow (for high-extraction drugs), or both (for drugs with intermediate values of Cl_i).

Drug distribution is affected by a variety of physiologic factors, including vascular tissue perfusion, body composition, plasma protein binding, and tissue binding. Since the V_d may be subject to developmental changes, caution must be exercised in interpreting data on $t_{1/2}$ in infants and children.

It may be concluded that hepatic drug clearance is determined by the following factors: (1) enzyme activity, (2) blood flow, and (3) drug binding in blood. If the drug is predominantly eliminated through metabolism, it is important to evaluate the physiologic and environmental factors that influence the development of metabolizing enzymes. It is logical, therefore, to differentiate between *low-extraction* and *high-extraction* drugs. Only then is it possible to make appropriate interpretations of age-dependent changes in pharmacokinetics. A number of drugs have been classified according to this system on the basis of adult human pharmacokinetic data (Table 2–1).

The steady-state concentration (C_{ss}) of a drug administered orally and only metabolized by the liver is given by the following equation:

$$C_{ss} = \frac{F \times D}{Cl_H \times \Delta} \qquad (7)$$

where Δ denotes the dosing interval and F is the drug bioavailability. Rearranging this equation gives

$$C_{ss} = \frac{D}{f_B \times Cl_i' \times \Delta} \qquad (8)$$

This relationship shows that the only biologic determinants of the C_{ss} of a drug that is given orally and solely metabolized by the liver are the Cl_i' and the binding, irrespective of the extraction ratio.[4,30] In this context, any discussion about blood flow is superfluous. Age-dependent plasma binding of drugs is discussed below.

Low-Clearance Drugs

Among the drugs that belong to this group are antiepileptics and certain benzodiazepines. They are frequently used in infants, and their $t_{1/2}$ values are predominantly dependent on the drug-metabolizing enzyme activity. The C_{ss} of these agents is determined by the hepatic enzyme activity and by drug binding in blood according to Equation (8). In as much as the values of f_B and V_d are not age-dependent, the $t_{1/2}$ and C_{ss} may serve as rough estimates of the capacity to metabolize a particular drug. Some of the drugs of this group that have been studied in newborns and adults are listed in Table 2–1.

Both carbamazepine and phenytoin have a similar $t_{1/2}$ in adults and newborn infants of epileptic mothers treated with these agents during pregnancy.[11,21] This is probably due to intrauterine induction of the drug metabolism. For phenytoin, the V_d does not change from the neonatal to the adult stage.[31] Hence the $t_{1/2}$ values indicate that the capacity to metabolize phenytoin in the newborn is well developed at birth.

The V_{max} for oxidation of phenytoin is higher in children than in adults,[32] and the capacity to oxidize phenytoin decreases with age.[33] The clinical use of higher weight-related doses of these antiepileptics in children compared with adults is therefore logical (see below).

Table 2–1 also presents interesting data on the neonatal kinetics of xanthines compared with the fetal *in vitro* activity of hepatic cytochrome P-448.[7,9,10] This form of the drug-oxidizing cytochrome is inducible by methylcholanthrene and other polycyclic hydrocarbons and is believed to catalyze the oxidation of theophylline and caffeine.[34,35] Theophylline and caffeine have comparatively long plasma half-lives in the neonatal period, whereas in adults the corresponding values are only 3.8–8 hours[36,37] and 4 hours,[9] respectively. There is ample evidence that the enzyme activity of cytochrome P-448 *in vitro* is extremely low or undeveloped in the fetal liver,[38] which may explain the observed clinical findings.

High-Clearance Drugs

The $t_{1/2}$ of drugs belonging to this group is dependent very much on hepatic blood flow, whereas enzyme activity plays only a minor role in the elimination of an I.V. dose. However, enzyme activity does determine the AUC and C_{ss} values after single and multiple oral administration, respectively.

Few drugs belonging to this group are used regularly in children. Nevertheless, some kinetic data for these agents have been published and are listed in Table 2–1.

Table 2–2 lists the half-lives of some drugs unclassified with respect to their clearance values. The general impression is that the half-life of most drugs in the neonate is longer than in the adult patient. This strongly suggests that in neonates and infants most investigated drugs have a lower metabolic clearance (as estimated from the $t_{1/2}$) than in the adult. The rate of maturation of metabolic elimination varies from drug to drug. As a corollary, attempts to predict the drug-metabolizing activity in children from adult data are bound to be useless.

DRUG BINDING TO PLASMA PROTEINS

Since a drug's pharmacologic effects and side effects are related to the unbound fraction of drug in blood (f_B), it is relevant to know how f_B varies in different age groups.

TABLE 2–1. COMPARISON OF HALF-LIVES (HOURS) IN NEWBORNS AND ADULTS OF DRUGS WITH LOW OR HIGH HEPATIC EXTRACTION

DRUG	$t_{1/2}$ IN NEWBORNS	$t_{1/2}$ IN ADULTS	REFERENCE
Drugs with Low Hepatic Clearance			
Aminophylline	24–36	3–9	Aranda et al.[7]
Amylobarbitone	17–60	12–27	Krauer et al.[8]
Caffeine	103	6	Aranda et al.[9] Parsons and Neims[10]
Carbamazepine	8–28	21–36	Rane et al.[11]
Diazepam	25–100	15–25	Morselli et al.[12]
Mepivacaine	8.7	3.2	Moore et al.[13]
Phenobarbitone	21–100	52–120	Garrettson and Dayton,[14] Heinze and Kampffmeyer,[15] Jalling,[16] Wilson and Wilkinson,[17] Minigawa et al.,[18] Butler et al.,[19] Lous[20]
Phenytoin	21	11–29	Rane et al.[21]
Tolbutamide	10–40	4.4–9	Nitowsky et al.[22]
Drugs with Intermediate or High Hepatic Clearance			
Bromosulfophthalein	0.16		Wichman et al.[23]
Meperidine	22	3–4	Caldwell et al.,[24] Tomson et al.[25]
Nortriptyline	56	18–22	Sjöqvist et al.[26]
Morphine	2.7	0.9–4.3	Dahlström et al.[27]
Lidocaine	2.9–3.3	1.0–2.2	Mihaly et al.[28]
Propoxyphene	1.7–7.7	1.9–4.3	Wilson et al.[29]

TABLE 2–2. COMPARISON OF PLASMA HALF-LIVES IN NEWBORNS AND ADULTS OF SOME DRUGS THAT ARE UNCLASSIFIED WITH RESPECT TO HEPATIC CLEARANCE

DRUG	$t_{1/2}$ IN NEWBORNS	$t_{1/2}$ IN ADULTS	REFERENCE
Amikacin	2.8	2.9	Lanao et al.[39]
Aminopyrine	30–40	2–4	Reinicke et al.[40]
Bupivacaine	25	1.3	Caldwell et al.[41]
Chloramphenicol	5.1	ND*	Kauffman et al.[42]
Diazepam	25–100	15–25	Morselli et al.[43]
Furosemide	7.7–19.9	0.5	Aranda et al.,[44] Peterson et al.,[45] Cutler et al.[46]
Gentamicin	1.25	ND*	Bravo et al.[47]
Indomethacin	14–20	2–11	Traeger et al.[48]
Oxazepam	21.9	6.5	Tomson et al.[49]
Primidone	7–28.6	3.3–12.5	Kaneko et al.,[50] Morselli[51]
Phenylbutazone	21–34	12–30	Gladtke[52]
Valproic acid	23–35	10–16	Ishizaki et al.,[53] Gugler and von Unruh[54]

*ND = no data.

Most investigated drugs have a lower plasma protein binding in cord/infant plasma than in adult plasma (Table 2–3). Higher binding has been observed for only a few drugs. The clinical implications of the difference in drug binding have yet to be shown. Routine analyses of drugs in plasma generally account only for the total concentration. As long as the drug binding does not change between individuals in the same age group, specific analysis of the unbound fraction is generally not warranted. However, such analysis may have a clinical value in special patients, e.g., if the plasma protein levels are perturbed by compromised kidney function or in liver disease.

As pointed out earlier, the clearance term (Equation 5) is affected by drug binding in blood and plasma. For low-clearance drugs, the hepatic elimination is usually restrictive and the systemic clearance of total drug will depend on binding. The $t_{1/2}$ is prolonged when binding increases. The concentration of unbound drug is essentially unchanged.

On the other hand, for drugs with a high clearance, a decreased binding leads to a higher unbound concentration and more intensive pharmacologic effects.[5] The differential effect of altered drug binding on the total plasma concentration of high-clearance and low-clearance drugs needs consideration in studies of drug concentration–effect relationships.

The steady-state concentration (C_{ss}) of phenytoin that is attained for a given dose per kilogram of body weight is considerably lower in infants than in adults, even though the infant dose is twice as high on a body-weight basis.[74,75] This may be due, in part, to binding alterations, since a lower binding yields a lower total plasma concentration. The low C_{ss} in these infants also may be caused by a higher metabolic rate. The issue of the appropriate *therapeutic concentration* of the drug in these infants is one of great

interest. It is conceivable that the higher f_B compensates partially for the lower total C_{ss} values that are attained.[74]

The lower plasma protein binding observed in neonates or cord blood for many drugs may have several explanations. The plasma protein may be qualitatively or quantitatively different at this age. The albumin concentration in neonates appears to be equivalent to the adult concentration,[76] but α_1-acid glycoprotein concentrations are lower.[69] In addition, hypoproteinemia is frequently observed in premature infants.[76] The possible influence on drug binding of competing ligands has been discussed for bilirubin[74] and free fatty acids.[77] Such factors may be the reason for the lower serum protein binding of many drugs, such as clonazepam.[78] This study demonstrated a lower binding capacity but a higher affinity for clonazepam of serum proteins in adults than in children.

Drug Absorption

Age-related changes in drug absorption are not well understood. In some cases, however, abnormal drug kinetics have been ascribed to such changes. Only a few facts of importance for drug absorption will be discussed here.

The *gastric pH* is alkaline at birth but falls to pH 1–3 within a day or two.[79] Adult levels of gastric acid secretion

TABLE 2–3. PROTEIN BINDING OF SOME DRUGS IN CORD PLASMA IN RELATION TO ADULT PLASMA

LOWER BINDING	HIGHER BINDING
Acid drugs	
Ampicillin[55]	Valproic acid*[53,72]
Benzylpenicillin[55]	(indirect evidence)
Nafcillin[56]	Salicylic acid*[73]
Naproxen[57]	Sulfisoxazole*[60]
Salicylates[58]	Cloxacillin*[63]
Phenytoin[59,60]	Flucloxacillin*[63]
(same or lower binding)	
Phenylbutazone[52]	
Phenobarbitone[61]	
Pentobarbitone[62]	
Cloxacillin[63]	
Flucloxacillin[63]	
Sulfamethoxypyrazine[64]	
Sulfaphenazole[65]	
Sulfadimethoxine[66]	
Sulfamethoxydiazine[66]	
Neutral Drugs	
Digoxin[67]	
Dexamethasone[60]	
Basic Drugs	
Diazepam[68,69]	Diazepam*[60,69]
Imipramine[70]	
Desmethylimipramine[59]	
Bupivacaine[71]	
Lidocaine[69,71]	
Propranolol[69]	
Metocurine*[69]	
D-Tubocurarine*[69]	

*As compared with maternal plasma.

are reached at ages 5–12 years (for a review, see Stewart and Hampton[80]). Even though the nonionic diffusion principle would favor absorption of acidic drugs in the stomach, the quantitatively important absorption takes place in the duodenum. The absorption of penicillin G and semisynthetic penicillins is higher in newborn infants than in adults.[79] This may be explained, in part, by the higher pH in newborn infants.

The *motility of the gut* and the gastric emptying time have been reported to be delayed in newborn infants.[81] Although this may affect the absorption time profile rather than the degree of absorption, it has been proposed as an explanation for the erratic absorption of certain sustained-release theophylline formulations in children.[82] Heimann's data[83] support this assumption. He studied the bioavailability of sulfonamides, digoxin, and some other drugs in infants and children. While the rate of absorption was significantly lower in neonates, the amount of drug absorbed was not correlated with age.

The fetal gastrointestinal tract is rapidly colonized by bacteria after birth. The level of gastrointestinal *microorganism flora* is related to bile acid deconjugation activity and β-glucuronidase activity, both of which are significantly higher in neonates than in adults.[84] Other intestinal enzyme activities that may affect to drug absorption and which are subject to age-dependent alterations include those of lipase and α-amylase,[85] both of which are low in the neonatal period.

DEVELOPMENTAL CHANGES IN METABOLISM PATTERN

As is evident from the preceding discussion, the metabolic disposition of most drugs is reduced in the neonatal period, as judged from the plasma half-lives. However, some drugs do not conform to this trend. Sometimes this may be the result of *in utero* exposure to drugs that induce the fetal metabolizing enzymes. Alternatively, other metabolic pathways that are minor in adults may play a quantitatively more significant role in early life and compensate for the deficient "normal adult" metabolic pathway.

The latter phenomenon is illustrated in Figure 2–1 for two drugs, salicylic acid and acetaminophen (paracetamol). In adulthood, the major metabolic pathway for the latter drug includes glucuronidation. In the early newborn period, glucuronidation is deficient, whereas sulfate conjugation is pronounced.[86–88] This leads to an apparently "normal" half-life in newborns. Another developmental change in metabolism has been demonstrated for salicylic acid.[89] Interestingly, the observations with acetaminophen are consistent with *in vitro* findings in human fetal liver preparations.[90] By using liver microsomal preparations or isolated hepatocytes, it was found that acetaminophen was conjugated with sulfate but not with glucuronic acid.

It is of clinical importance to note that acetaminophen seems to be less poisonous in children than in adults. This may be explained, in part, by the compensatory routes of metabolism, although other mechanisms also may be operating. Age-dependent differences in the quantitative contribution of various conjugation pathways to the overall elimination also have been reported for p-aminobenzoic acid[91] and bromosulfophthalein.[23]

Developmental changes in metabolism also were shown for diazepam and theophylline. As shown in Figure 2–2, the hydroxylation reactions of diazepam are relatively deficient in both premature and full-term neonates.[92] Theophylline is also subject to extensive age-dependent changes in its metabolism (see Figure 2–2). In premature infants, theophylline is eliminated virtually only by direct excretion, which is nonexistent in the adult.[93,94] A small part is methylated to caffeine, consistent with findings in fetal liver preparations.[95] The formation of 1,3-dimethyluric acid gains an increasing importance with age.

It has recently been shown that the different oxidative pathways of caffeine mature at various rates.[96] The N3-demethylation is more important in young infants than in adults, whereas the N1-demethylation is low and develops later than 19 months of age (Figure 2–3).

These observations are not only of academic interest. Since many drugs are bioactivated to toxic metabolites, the differential maturation of various pathways may put the infant at risk only during a limited developmental stage. Further studies to identify such therapeutic situations are required.

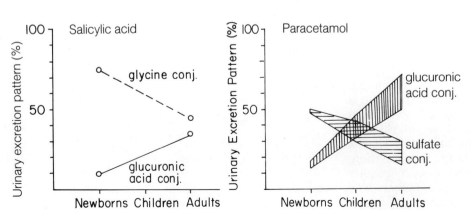

FIGURE 2–1. Age-dependent alterations in metabolism pattern of salicylic acid and paracetamol. (Data from Garrettson et al.,[89] Levy et al.,[86] Miller et al.,[87] and Howie et al.[88])

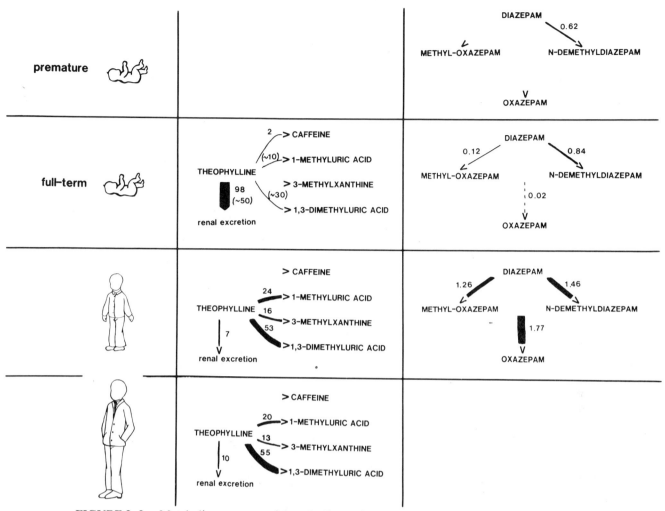

FIGURE 2–2. Metabolism patterns of theophylline (left column) and diazepam (right column) at different developmental stages; from top to bottom, a premature neonate, a full-term neonate, a prepubertal child, and an adult. The numbers indicate the percentage of metabolites retrieved in the urine. (Data from Sereni et al.,[92] Bonati et al.,[93] and Grygiel and Birkett.[94])

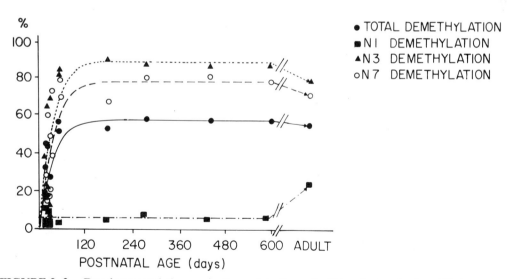

FIGURE 2–3. Developmental changes in the metabolism of caffeine during the first 600 days of life. Demethylation at different positions is given as the ratio of the number of methyl groups absent in the metabolites recovered in the urine related to the number of methyl groups contained in the moles of caffeine from which they originated. (Adapted from Carrier et al.,[96] with permission from the authors and publishers.)

ASPECTS OF DRUG ELIMINATION BY THE KIDNEYS

Some drugs are predominantly eliminated by the kidneys. Dosing of these drugs in children and, in particular, infants is of great concern because of the immaturity of renal function in early life. To some extent, the problem is similar to the decreased renal elimination that occurs in the elderly. Both these "risk groups" of patients at the extremes of age require that the dose and/or dose frequency be decreased to avoid drug accumulation and toxicity. Several nomograms and drug regimens have been developed to facilitate the dosing of these types of drugs in infants.

The glomerular filtration rate (as measured with inulin as a probe agent) is low at birth and reaches adult levels at 5 months of age.[97] The glomerular filtration rate is also a function of the postconceptional age, so there may be a twofold to fourfold difference in values between premature and full-term newborns.[98,99] This difference between inulin clearance in the premature and full-term newborns persists at least throughout the neonatal period.

The tubular secretion rate reaches adult levels somewhat later than the glomerular filtration rate.[97] With para-aminohippuric acid as a test agent, adult rates were obtained by 7 months. With other drugs, the maturity may be achieved at other ages.

This physiologic situation requires special clinical consideration in the use of drugs that are solely dependent on the kidneys for their elimination. This is the case for penicillins[100] and several aminoglycosides,[101] the half-lives of which are extensively prolonged in neonates. The elimination of some cephalosporins, such as ceftriaxone, also has been shown to be significantly prolonged in newborns.[102,103]

Digoxin constitutes an interesting exception to this rule. Its clearance changes in both directions during the first 5 years of life. It is only 1.8 ml/min/kg of body weight during the first week. It then increases to 10.7 ml/min/kg of body weight during the first year and decreases again to 3.8 at the ages of 2–5 years.[104] The half-lives vary consistently with the renal clearance. Variations in apparent volume of distribution (V_d) are less than the clearance changes, and therefore, a renal cause for the observed clearance changes has been proposed. However, the mechanism for this is not well understood.[105]

Dosing of drugs exerting their desired clinical effect *in* the kidney has been extensively discussed. A drug's effect may be insufficient because of deficient kidney function. Furosemide is actively secreted in the tubules and exerts its diuretic effect in the intraluminal space.[106] The recent suggestion by Mirochnik et al.[107] that elevated plasma levels may be required to ensure adequate intraluminal delivery of furosemide therefore seems logical. This also has been suggested for thiazides and organic mercuric compounds.[108,109]

The excretion *patterns* of various drugs may differ in infants and adults. Teleologically, this may serve as a compensatory mechanism for slow renal excretion. This is exemplified by theophylline, which is not excreted as such in adult patients. However, as pointed out earlier, its excretion in infants is significant and would compensate for the impaired elimination observed in infants.[93]

DOSING PRINCIPLES IN CHILDREN

Optimal tailoring of a drug's dose to the newborn infant and child has been subject to discussion over a long period. The several suggestions and dosing rules that have been proposed reveal the complexity of the problem and may reflect the "state of the art" at the time rather than an understanding of the various issues.

No universal dosage rule can be recommended. If age is used as the basis for dosing, errors may be introduced because of the variability in weight among children in the same age group. Administration of a drug based on an infant's weight (Equation 9) is seldom appropriate. With this rule, infants will generally be underdosed.

$$\text{Dose}_{\text{pediatr.}} = \text{dose}_{\text{adult}} \left(\frac{\text{weight}_{\text{pediatr.}}}{\text{weight}_{\text{adult}}} \right) \qquad (9)$$

The "surface rule" gives a better estimate of the appropriate dose for an infant or child. This rule bases the dose on the surface area of the individual. Since surface area is greater relative to volume and weight in small individuals, the dose will be greater than expected from the body weight. As the child grows, the weight increases and so does the surface area, albeit at a slower rate. Although the surface area may be estimated from nomograms using body weight and height, this is usually not convenient. Therefore, an approximation of the dose according to the "surface rule" is obtained if the dose is calculated to follow the weight to the 0.7 power.[110,111]

$$\text{Dose}_{\text{pediatr.}} = \text{dose}_{\text{adult}} \left(\frac{\text{weight}_{\text{pediatr.}}}{\text{weight}_{\text{adult}}} \right)^{0.7} \qquad (10)$$

A table has been published[112] for the convenient calculation of pediatric drug doses according to the surface rule.

The rationale for using the surface rule is not well understood. However, many physiologic parameters, such as cardiac output, respiratory metabolism, blood volume, extracellular water volume, glomerular filtration rate, and renal blood flow, correlate closely with the body surface area. Many of these functions are of direct importance for drug elimination.

Clinical experience with most drugs has shown that dosing according to the surface rule is more appropriate than according to the weight rule. This is evident from the manufacturers' dose recommendations of many of the drugs that are sold today. The clinical "impressions" and experience that infants and small children often need higher doses than adults have now been verified in several pharmacokinetic investigations that indicate incomplete absorption, increased rate of metabolism, or increased renal elimination in such patients as compared with adult patients. A list of drugs that are usually administered at higher doses (on a weight basis) to children than to adults is given in Table 2–4. The reader is referred to the reference literature for the pharmacokinetic explanations.

TABLE 2–4. EXAMPLES OF DRUGS GIVEN IN HIGHER WEIGHT-RELATED DOSES TO CHILDREN THAN TO ADULTS

DRUG	REFERENCE
Phenytoin	Svensmark and Buchthal[113]
Phenobarbitone	Svensmark and Buchthal[113]
Carbamazepine	Morselli[114]
Ethosuximide	Sherwin and Robb[115]
Clonazepam	Rane[120a]
Diazepam	Morselli[114]
Theophylline	Ahrens et al.[116]
Enprofylline	Watson et al.[117]
Digoxin	Morselli et al.[104]
Some anticancer drugs	Evans et al.[118]
Imipramine	Morselli et al.[119]
Clomipramine	Morselli et al.[119]
Haloperidol	Morselli et al.[119]
Chlorpromazine	Rivera-Calimlim et al.[120]

PHARMACOGENETIC ASPECTS OF DRUG METABOLISM

Research in recent years has revealed a number of pharmacogenetic polymorphisms of drug-metabolizing enzymes. Such polymorphisms are of great interest not only from a biochemical point of view, but also clinically, since differences in the incidence of adverse drug reactions and efficacy have been demonstrated in subjects belonging to the different phenotypes. However, virtually nothing is known about the time when the phenotypes express themselves during ontogenesis. This has therapeutic implications in pediatrics, since some of the drugs are used in infants, children, and pregnant women. Deficiency of hepatic N-acetyltransferase was the first polymorphism discovered (for a review, see Weber and Hein[121]). This enzyme metabolizes several drugs, of which isoniazide was the first to be described.[122] Drug-oxidation polymorphisms include two major groups: the debrisoquine/sparteine type, and the mephenytoin type. These are based on genetic differences in the liver microsomal mono-oxygenase enzymes (cytochrome P-450s) that catalyze oxidation of numerous drugs.

The Acetylation Type

The division of adult subjects into two groups of slow acetylators and rapid acetylators has been studied and found to vary largely in different ethnic groups. In fetal liver preparations, *in vitro* studies of clonazepam acetylation could not demonstrate a clear polymorphism. This was partly explained by the large differences in the gestational ages of the fetuses investigated.[123] Similarly, Meisel et al.[124] were unable to demonstrate any polymorphism of fetal liver N-acetyltransferase using procainamide as a substrate.

At least two drugs have been employed in attempts to phenotype infants and children with regard to their acetylator status. The AFMU/1X ratio (5-acetylamino-3-methyluracil/1-methylxanthine), which is used to deter-

mine the acetylator status, was measured in infants who had received caffeine.[96] The antimode is 0.4. It appeared that all but 1 (the oldest) of the 14 infants investigated had ratios below 0.4 and thus appeared to be slow acetylator phenotypes. One infant appeared to be a slow metabolizer at 54 days and a fast metabolizer at 7 months of age. It was concluded that the N-acetylase was not developed and that the caffeine acetylation phenotype cannot be determined in infants less than 1 year of age.

Sulfadimidine also has been used as a probe drug in tests of acetylator phenotype in newborn infants.[125] With this agent, 83 percent of the infants investigated were found to belong to the slow acetylator phenotype, as compared with 50 percent in the adult group of subjects. The different distribution in the young group was partly explained by a deficient dietary intake of pantothenic acid, which is required for the coenzyme A in the reaction. However, other reasons for the age-dependent phenotypic distribution cannot be ruled out.

The late appearance of the adult phenotypic distribution pattern and the predominance of slow acetylators among young infants may result in higher sensitivity to the pharmacologic and toxic effects of the drugs and may be regarded as a potential risk factor. Several drugs that are acetylated are used in the pediatric population, and clinical reseach to identify other polymorphisms is warranted.

The Debrisoquine/Sparteine Type

This polymorphism is inherited through an autosomal recessive gene. Homozygous individuals (poor metabolizers) are characterized by negligible or no metabolism of a variety of drugs. This polymorphism involves the oxidation of members of some very important groups of drugs. Thus several β-adrenoceptor-blocking agents,[126–129] antidepressants,[130] antiarrhythmic agents,[131] and various other drugs are metabolized by this enzyme. In as much as these drugs are given to pregnant women or infants and children, the polymorphism may be of importance for the therapeutic outcome and the risk of adverse drug reactions. So far, nothing is known about when the phenotype develops in children. However, *in vitro* studies in human fetal liver in our laboratory have revealed that the ability to N-demethylate codeine and dextromethorphan seems to precede that of the corresponding O-demethylation reaction.[132] The latter reactions are believed to be catalyzed by the cytochrome P-450 debrisoquine/sparteine. The expression of the responsible cytochrome IID6 would be of interest to study in newborn infants, but no such reports have been published. It seems, however, that the enzyme may be expressed in a minority of investigated fetal liver specimens in the late gestational period.[133]

The Mephenytoin Type

The deficient metabolism of mephenytoin is observed in 2–5 percent of Caucasian and more than 20 percent of Japanese individuals.[134] It is inherited as an autosomal recessive trait. Liver enzymes of poor metabolizers catalyze the stereoselective 4-hydroxylation of S-mephenytoin at a slow rate. It is not known when this polymorphism presents during ontogenesis.

CONCLUSIONS AND PERSPECTIVE

The variations in drug disposition in infants and children are caused predominantly by constitutional and environmental factors, just as in the adult. The physiologic maturation of the organs and the expression of metabolic phenotypes further increase the variability. The complexity of the drug-disposition pattern precludes any attempts to make generalizations from individual cases. Therefore, we have to accept that safe and rational therapeutics must be founded on improved knowledge in different pharmacotherapeutic areas.

The need for new drugs in pediatrics is as great as in adult medicine. Therefore, the performance of controlled clinical studies in children is warranted rather than the "blind" use of new agents in individual patients because such use does not increase our knowledge about the clinical pharmacology of drugs used in the pediatric population.

REFERENCES

1. Silverman WA, Anderson DH, Blanc WA, Crozier DN: A difference in mortality rate and incidence of kernicterus among premature infants allotted to two prophylactic antibacterial regimens. Pediatrics 18:614–621, 1956
2. Weiss CG, Glazko AJ, Weston JK: Chloramphenicol in the newborn infant, a physiologic explanation of its toxicity when given in excessive dose. N Engl J Med 262:787–794, 1960
3. Boréus LO: Principles of Pediatric Pharmacology (Monographs in Clinical Pharmacology). New York, Churchill-Livingstone, 1982, p 118
4. Rowland M, Benet LZ, Graham G: Clearance concepts in pharmacokinetics. J Pharmacokinet Biopharm 1:123–136, 1973
5. Wilkinson GR, Shand DG: A physiological approach to hepatic drug clearance. Clin Pharmacol Ther 18:377–390, 1975
6. Rane A, Shand DG, Wilkinson GR: Disposition of carbamazepine and its 10,11-epoxide metabolite in the isolated perfused rat liver. Drug Metab Dispos 5:179–184, 1977
7. Aranda VJ, Sitar DS, Parsons DV, Loughnan PM; Neims AH: Pharmacokinetic aspects of theophylline in premature newborns. N Engl J Med 295:413–416, 1976
8. Krauer B, Draffan GH, Williams FM, Clare RA, Dollery CT, Hawkins DF: Elimination of amobarbital in mothers and their newborn infants. Clin Pharmacol Ther 14:442–447, 1973
9. Aranda JV, Cook CE, Gorman W, Collinge JM, Loughnan PM, Outerbridge EV: Pharmacokinetics profile of caffeine in the premature newborn infant with apnea. J Pediatr 94:993–995, 1979
10. Parsons WD, Neims AH: Effect of cigarette smoking in caffeine elimination. Clin Res 25:676A, 1978
11. Rane A, Bertilsson L, Palmér L: Disposition of placentally transferred carbamazepine (Tegretol) in the newborn. Eur J Clin Pharmacol 8:283–284, 1975
12. Morselli PL, Principi N, Tognoni G, Reali E, Belvedere G, Standen SM, Sereni F: Diazepam elimination in premature and full-term infants and children. J Perinatal Med 1:133–141, 1973
13. Moore RG, Thomas J, Triggs EJ, Thomas DB, Burnard ED, Shanks CA: The pharmacokinetics and metabolism of the anilide local anaesthetics in neonates. III. Mepivacaine. Eur J Clin Pharmacol 14:203–212, 1978
14. Garrettson LK, Dayton PG: Disappearance of phenobarbital and diphenylhydantoin from serum of children. Clin Pharmacol Ther 11:674–679, 1970
15. Heinze E, Kampffmeyer HG: Biological half-life of phenobarbital in human babies. Klin Wochenschr 49:1146–1147, 1971
16. Jalling B: Plasma and cerebrospinal fluid concentrations of phenobarbital in infants given single doses. Dev Med Child Neurol 16:781–793, 1976
17. Wilson JT, Wilkinson GR: Chronic and severe phenobarbital intoxication in a child treated with primidone and diphenylhydantoin. J Pediatr 83:484–489, 1973
18. Minigawa K, Miura H, Chiba K, Ishizaki T: Pharmacokinetics and relative bioavailability of intramuskular phenobarbital sodium or acid in infants. Pediatr Pharmacol 1:279–289, 1981
19. Butler TC, Mahafee C, Wadell WJ: Phenobarbital: Studies on elimination, accumulation tolerance and dosage schedules. J Pharmacol Exp Ther 111:425–435, 1954
20. Lous P: Blood serum and cerebrospinal fluid levels and renal clearance of phenemal in treated epileptics. Acta Pharmacol 10:261–280, 1954
21. Rane A, Garle M, Borgå O, Sjöqvist F: Plasma disappearance of transplacentally transferred phenytoin in the newborn studied with mass fragmentography. Clin Pharmacol Ther 15:39–45, 1974
22. Nitowsky HM, Marz L, Berzofsky JA: Studies on oxidative drug metabolism in the full-term newborn infant. Pediatr Pharmacol Ther 69:1139–1149, 1966
23. Wichmann HM, Rind H, Gladtke E: Die Elimination von Bromsulphalein beim Kind. Zschr Kinderheilk 103:262–276, 1968
24. Caldwell J, Wakile LA, Notarianni LJ, et al: Transplacental passage and neonatal elimination of pethidine given to mothers in childbirth. Br J Pharmacol Abstract Proceed. of B.P.S., Sept. 1977, 716P, 1978
25. Tomson G, Garle M, Thalme B, Nisell H, Nylund L, Rane A: Maternal kinetics and placental passage of pethidine during labour. Br J Clin Pharmacol 13:653–659, 1981
26. Sjöqvist G, Bergfors PG, Borgå O, et al: Plasma disappearance of nortriptyline in a newborn following placental transfer from an intoxicated mother—evidence for drug metabolism. J Pediatr 80:496–500, 1972
27. Dahlström B, Bolme P, Feychting H, Noack G and Paalzow L: Morphine kinetics in children. Clin Pharmacol Ther 26:354–365, 1979
28. Mihaly GW, Moore RG, Thomas J, et al: The pharmacokinetics of anilide local anaesthetics in neonates, I, Lidocaine. Eur J Clin Pharmacol 13:143–152, 1978
29. Wilson JT, Atwood GF, Shand DG: Disposition of propranolol and propoxyphene in children. Clin Pharmacol Ther 19:264–270, 1976
30. Wilkinson GR, Schenker S: Effects of liver disease on drug disposition in man. Biochem Pharmacol 25:2675–2681, 1976
31. Loughnan PM, Watters G, Aranda J, Neims A: Age-related changes in the pharmacokinetics of diphenylhydantoin (DPH) in the newborn and young infant: Implication regarding treatment of neonatal convulsions. Aust Paediatr J 12:204–205, 1976
32. Eadie MJ, Tyrer JH, Bochner F, Hooper WD: The elimination of phenytoin in man. Clin Exp Pharmacol Physiol 3:217–224, 1976
33. Chiba K, Ishizaki T, Miura H, Minagawa K: Apparent Michaelis-Menten kinetic parameters of phenytoin in pediatric patterns. Pediatr Pharmacol 1:171–180, 1980
34. Lohmann SM, Miech RP: Theophylline metabolism by the rat liver microsomal system. J Pharmacol Exp Ther 196:213–225, 1976
35. Aldridge A, Parson W, Neims AH: Stimulation of caffeine metabolism in the rat by 3-methylcholanthrene. Life Sci 21:967–974, 1977
36. Ellis EF, Yaffe SJ, Levy G: 30th Annual Meeting of American Academy of Allergy. Abstract p. 14 (1974).

37. Ellis EF, Koysooko R, Levy G: Pharmacokinetics of theophylline in children with asthma. Pediatrics 58:542–547, 1976
38. Pelkonen O, Kärki NT: 3,4-Benzpyrene and aniline are hydroxylated by human fetal liver but not by placenta at 6–7 weeks of fetal age. Biochem Pharmacol 22:1538–1540, 1973
39. Lanao JM, Dominguez-Gil A, Dominguez-Gil AA, Málaga S, Crespo M and Nuñu F. Modification in the pharmacokinetics of amikacin during development. Eur J Clin Pharmacol, 23:155–160, 1982
40. Reinicke C, Rogner G, Frenzel, J et al: Die Wirkung von Phenylbutazon und Phenobarbital auf die Amidopyrin-Elimination, die Bilirubin-Gesamt-konzentration im Serum und einige Blutgerinnungsfaktoren bei neugeborenen Kindern. Pharmacol Clin 2:167–172, 1970.
41. Caldwell J, Mofatt JR, and Smith RL: Pharmacokinetics of bupivacaine administered epidurally during childbirth. Br J Clin Pharmacol 3:956–957, 1976
42. Kauffman RE, Miceli JN, Strebel L, Buckley JA, Done AK and Dajani AS: Pharmacokinetics of chloramphenicol and chloramphenicol succinate in infants and children. J Pediatr 98(2):315–20, 1981
43. Morselli PL, Principi N, Tognoni G, Reali E, Belvedere G, Stranden SM and Sereni F: Diazepam elimination in premature and full term infants and children. J Perinatal Med 1:133–141, 1973
44. Aranda JV, Perez J, Sitar DS, Collinge J, Portuguez-Malavasi A, Duffy B and Dupont C: Pharmacokinetic disposition and protein binding of furosemide in the newborn infant. J Pediatr 93:507–511, 1978
45. Peterson RG, Simmons MA, Rumack BH, Levine RL, and Brooks JG: Pharmacology of furosemide in the premature newborn infant. Pediatr 97:139–143, 1980
46. Cutler RE, Forrey AW, Christopher TG and Kimpel BM: Pharmacokinetics of furosemide in normal subjects and functionally anephric patients. Clin Pharmacol Ther 15:588–96, 1974
47. Bravo ME, Arancibia A, Jarpa S, Carpentier PM and Jahn AN: Pharmacokinetics of gentamicin in malnourished infants. Eur J Clin Pharmacol 21:499–504, 1982
48. Traeger A, Nöschel H, Zaumsell J: Zur Pharmokinetic von Indomethazin bei Schwangeren, Kreissenden und deren Neugeborenen Zbi Gynaek 95:635–641, 1973
49. Tomson G, Sundwall A, Lunell NO and Ranc A: Transplacental passage and kinetics in the mother and newborn of oxazepam given during labour. Clin Pharmacol Ther 25:74–81, 1979
50. Kaneko S, Suzuki K, Sato T, Ogawa Y, Nomura Y (1982). The problems of antiepileptics medication in the neonatal period: Is breast-feeding advisable? In Janz D et al (eds.) Epilepsy, Pregnancy, and the Child. New York, Raven Press.
51. Morselli PL (ed): Drug Disposition during Development. New York: Spectrum, 1977
52. Gladtke E: Pharmacokinetic studies on phenylbutazone in children. Farmaco Ed Sci. 23:897–906, 1968
53. Ishizaki T, Yokochi K, Chiba K, Tabuchi T, and Wagatsuma T: Placental transfer of anticonvulsants (phenobarbital, phenytoin, valproic acid) and the elimination from neonates. Pediatr Pharmacol 1, 291–303, 1981
54. Gugler R, and von Unruh, GE: Clinical pharmacokinetics of valproic acid. Clin Pharmacokin. 5:67–83, 1980
55. Ehrnebo M, Agurell S, Jalling B: Age differences in drug binding by plasma proteins: studies on human foetuses, neonates and adults. Eur J Clin Pharmacol 3:189–193, 1971
56. Krasner J, Yaffe SJ: Drug-protein binding in the neonate, in Morselli P. Garattini S, Sereni F (eds): Basic and Therapeutic Aspects of Perinatal Pharmacology. New York, Raven Press, 1975, pp 357–366
57. Borgå O, Tomson G, Alván G and Rane A: Protein binding of naproxen children and adults, Manuscript, 1991
58. Krasner, J, Giaccoia GP, Yaffe SJ: Drug-protein binding in the newborn infant. Ann NY Acad Sci 226:101–114, 1973
59. Ranc A, Lunde PKM, Jalling B, et al: Plasma protein binding of diphenylhydantoin in normal and hyperbilirubinemic infants. J Pediatr 78:877–882, 1971
60. Hamar C and Levy G: Serum protein binding of drugs and bilirubin newborn infants and their mothers. Clin Pharmacol Ther 28 (1):58–63, 1980
61. Boréus LO, Jalling B, Kållberg N: Clinical pharmacology of phenobarbital in the neonatal period, in Morselli P, Garattini S, Sereni F (eds): Basic and Therapeutic Aspects of the Perinatal Pharmacology. New York, Raven Press, 1975, pp 331–340
62. Short CR, Sexton RI, McFarland I: Binding of ^{14}C-salicylic acid and ^{14}O-pentobarbital to plasma proteins of several species during the perinatal period. Biol Neonate 26:58–66, 1975
63. Herngren L, Ehrnebo M, and Boréus LO: Drug distribution in whole blood of mothers and their newborn infants. Studies of cloxacillin and flucloxacillin. Eur J Clin Pharmacol 22:351–358, 1982
64. Sereni F, Perletti L, Marubini E, et al: Pharmacokinetic studies with a long-acting sulfonamide in subjects of different ages. Pediatr Res 2:29–37, 1968
65. Chignell CF, Vesell ES, Starkweather DK, et al: The binding of sulfaphenazole to fetal-neonatal and adult human plasma albumin. Clin pharmacol Ther 12:897–901, 1971
66. Ganshorn A, Kurz H: Unterschiede zwischen der Proteinbindung Neugeborener und Erwachsener und ihre Bedcutund für die pharmakologische Wirkung. Arch Pharm Exp Pathol 260:117, 1968
67. Kim PW, Yanagi R, Krasula RW, Soyka LF, Levitsky S and Hastriter A: Post-mortem digoxin concentration in infants. In Proceedings 47th Ses, 1974
68. Kanto J, Erklola R and Scllman R: Perinatal metabolism of diazepam. Med J 1:641–642, 1974
69. Wood M and Wood AJJ: Changes in plasma drug binding and α_1-glycoprotein in mother and newborn infant. Clin Pharmacol Ther 29(4):522–566, 1981
70. Pruitt AW, Dayton PG: A comparison of the binding of drugs to adult and cord plasma. Eur J Clin Pharmacol 4:59–62, 1971
71. Tucker GT, Boyes RN, Bridenbaugh PO: Binding of anitide-type local anesthetics in human plasma. II. Implications in vivo, with special reference to transplacental distribution. Anesthesiology 33:304–314, 1970
72. Nau H, Helge H, and Luck W: Valproic acid in the perinatal per decreased maternal serum protein binding results in feral accumulation and neo-n displacement of the drug and some metabolites. J Ped. 104:627–634, 1984
73. Hamar G, and Levy G: Factors affecting the serum protein binding of salic acid in newborn infants and their mothers. Pediatr Pharmacol 1:31–43, 1980b
74. Rane A, Lunde PKM, Jalling B, et al: Plasma protein binding of diphenylhydantoin in normal and hyperbilirubinemic infants. J Pediatr 78:877–882, 1971
75. Jalling B, Boréus LO, Rane A, Sjöqvist F: Plasma concentrations of diphenylhydantoin in young infants. Pharmacol Clin 2:200–202, 1970
76. Hyvärinen M, Zeltzer P, Oh W, et al: Influence of gestational age on serum levels of alpha-1 fetoprotein IgG globulin and albumin in newborn infants. J Pediatr 82:430–437, 1973
77. Fredholm BB, Rane A, Persson B. Diphenylhydantoin binding to proteins in plasma and its dependence on free fatty acid and bilirubin concentration in dogs and newborn infants. Pediatr Res 9:26–30, 1975
78. Pacifici GM, Taddeucci-Brunelli G, Rane A: Clonazepam serum protein binding during development. Clin Pharmacol Ther 35:354–359, 1984
79. Weber WW, Cohen SN: Aging effects and drugs in man, in Gillette JR, Mitchell JR (eds): Concepts in Biochemical Pharmacology. New York, Springer-Verlag, 1975, pp 213–233
80. Stewart CF, Hampton EM: Effect of maturation on drug disposition in pediatric patients. Clin Pharm 6:548–564, 1987
81. Gupta M, Brans Y: Gastric retention in neonates. Pediatrics 62:26–29, 1978
82. Hendeles L, Iafrate RP, Weinberger M: A clinical and pharmacokinetic basis for the selection and use of slow-release theophylline products. Clin Pharmacokinet 9:95–135, 1984
83. Heimann G: Enteral absorption and bioavailability in children in relation to age. Eur J Clin Pharmacol 18:43–50, 1980
84. Yaffe SJ, Juchau MR: Perinatal pharmacology. Annu Rev Pharmacol 14:219–238, 1974

85. Lebenthal L, Lee PC, Heitlinger LA: Impact of development of the gastrointestinal tract on infant feeding. J Pediatr 102:1–9, 1983

86. Levy G, Khanna NN, Soda DM, et al: Pharmacokinetics of acetaminophen in the human neonate: Formation of acetaminophen glucuronide and sulfate in relation to plasma bilirubin concentration and D-glucaric acid excretion. Pediatrics 55:818–825, 1975

87. Miller RP, Roberts RJ, Fischer LJ: Acetaminophen elimination kinetics in neonates, children, and adults. Clin Pharmacol Ther 19:284–294, 1976

88. Howie D, Adriaenssens PI, Prescott LF: Paracetamol metabolism following overdosage: Application of high performance liquid chromatography. J Pharm Pharmacol 29:235–237, 1977

89. Garrettson LK, Procknal JA, Levy G: Fetal acquisition and neonatal elimination of a large amount of salicylate. Clin Pharmacol Ther 17:98–103, 1975

90. Rollins D, von Bahr C, Glaumann H, Moldéus P, Rane A: Acetaminophen: Reactive intermediate formation by human fetal and adult liver microsomes and isolated human fetal liver cells. Science 205:1414–1416, 1979

91. Vest MF, Rossier R: Detoxification in the newborn: The ability of the newborn infant to form conjugates with glucuronic acid, glycine, acetate, and glutathione. Ann NY Acad Sci 111:183–197, 1963

92. Sereni F, Morselli PL, Pardi G: Postnatal development of drug metabolism in human infants, in Bossart H, Cruz JM, Huber A, Prodhom LS, Sistek J (eds): Perinatal Medicine. Bern, Hans Huber Publishers, 1972, pp 63–67

93. Bonati M, Latini R, Marra G, Assael BM, Parini R: Theophylline metabolism during the first month of life and development. Pediatr Res 15:304–308, 1981

94. Grygiel JJ, Birkett DJ: Effect of age on patterns of theophylline metabolism. Clin Pharmacol Ther 28:456–462, 1980

95. Aranda JV, Louridas AT, Vitulo BB, Thom P, Aldridge A, Haber R: Metabolism of theophylline to caffeine in human fetal liver. Science 206:1319–1321, 1979

96. Carrier O, Pons G, Rey E, Richard M-O, Moran C, Badoual J, Olive G: Maturation of caffeine metabolic pathways in infancy. Clin Pharmacol Ther 44:145–151, 1988

97. West JR, Smith HW, Chasis H: Glomerular filtration rate, effective renal blood flow and maximal tubular excretory capacity in infancy. J Pediatr 32:10–18, 1948

98. Morselli PL, Franco-Morselli R, Bossi L: Clinical pharmacokinetics in newborns and infants: Age-related differences and therapeutic implications. Clin Pharmacokinet 5:485–527, 1980

99. Guignard J-P: Drugs and the neonatal kidney. Dev Pharmacol Ther 4(suppl I):19–27, 1982

100. Barnett HL, McNamara H, Schultz S, Thompsett R: Renal clearance of sodium penicillin G, procaine penicillin G. Pediatrics 3:418–22, 1949

101. Axline SG, Yaffe SJ, Simon HJ: Clinical pharmacology of antimicrobials in premature infants. Pediatrics 39:97–107, 1967

102. Nakazawa S, Satoh H, Narita A, et al: Evaluation of ceftriaxone administered intravenously in neonates. Jpn J Antibiot 41:225–235, 1988

103. Iwai N, Nakamura H, Miyazu M, et al: Pharmacokinetic and clinical evaluations of ceftriaxone. Jpn J Antibiot 41:262–275, 1988

104. Morselli PL, Assael BM, Gomeni R, Mandelli M, Marini A, Reali E, Visconti U, Sereni F: Digoxin pharmacokinetics during human development in Morselli P, Garattini S, Sereni F (eds): Basic and Therapeutic Aspects of Perinatal Pharmacology. New York, Raven Press, 1975, pp 377–392

105. Nyberg L, Wettrell G: Digoxin dosage schedules for neonates and infants based on pharmacokinetic considerations. Clin Pharmacokinet 3:453–461, 1978

106. Burg M, Stoner L, Cardinal J, Green N: Furosemide effects on isolated tubules. Am J Physiol 225:119–124, 1973

107. Mirochnick MH, Miceli JJ, Kramer PA, et al: Furosemide pharmacokinetics in very low birth weight infants. J Pediatr 112:653–657, 1988

108. Braunlich H, Kersten L: Der Einfluss von Diuretika auf die ren-

109. Frenzel J, Braunlich H, Schramm D, Kersten L: Renale Wirkungen von Cyclopenthiazid in der Neugeborenen Periode. Acta Paediatr Acad Sci Hung 15:157, 1974

110. Dawson WT: Relation between age and weight and dosage of drugs. Ann Intern Med 13:1594–1615, 1940

111. Gyllenswärd Å, Vahlqvist B: Läkemedelsdosering till barn. Nord Med 40:2248–2261, 1948

112. Rane A: Clinical pharmacokinetics of antiepileptic drugs in children. Pharmacol Ther [C] 2:251–267, 1978

113. Svensmark O, Buchthal F : Diphenylhydantoin and phenobarbital: Serum levels in children. Am J Dis Child 108:82–87, 1964

114. Morselli PL (ed): Drug Disposition During Development. New York, Spectrum, 1977

115. Sherwin AL, Robb JP: Ethosuximide: Relation of plasma levels to clinical control, in Woodbury DM, Penry JK, Schmidt RP (eds): Antiepileptic Drugs. New York, Raven Press, 1972, pp 443–448

116. Ahrens RC, Hendeles L, Weinburger M: The clinical pharmacology of drugs used in the treatment of asthma, in Yaffe SJ (ed): Pediatric Pharmacology. New York, Grune & Stratton, 1980, pp 233–280

117. Watson WTA, Simons KJ, Simons FER: Pharmacokinetics of enprofylline administered intravenously and as a sustained-release tablet at steady-state in children with asthma. J Pediatr 112:658–662, 1988

118. Evans WE, Crom WR, Sinkule JA, Yee GC, Stewart CF, Hutson PR: Pharmacokinetics of anticancer drugs in children. Drug Metab Rev 14:847–886, 1983

119. Morselli PL, Bianchetti G, Dugas M: Therapeutic drug monitoring of psychotropic drugs in children. Pediatr Pharmacol 3:149–156, 1983

120. Rivera-Calimlim L, Griesbach PH, Perlmutter R: Plasma chlorpromazine concentrations in children with behavioral disorders and mental illness. Clin Pharmacol Ther 26:114–121, 1979

120a. Rane A: The role of drug metabolism in therapeutic drug monitoring in (TDM), Pediatric aspects, Advances in Therapeutic Drug Monitoring. Tanaka K, Pippinger DE, Mimaki T, Walson PD and Ohgitani S (eds): Enterprise, Tokyo, 1990, p 359

121. Weber WW, Hein DW: N-acetylation pharmacogenetics. Pharmacol Rev 37:25, 1985

122. Price-Evans DA: Human acetylation polymorphism. J Lab Clin Med 63:394, 1964

123. Peng D, Birgersson C, von Bahr C, Rane A: Polymorphic acetylation of 7-aminoclonazepam in human liver cytosol. Pediatr Pharmacol 4:155–159, 1984

124. Meisel M, Schneider T, Siegmund W, Nikschick S, Klebingat K-J, Scherber A: Development of human polymorphic N-acetyltransferase. Biol Res Pregnancy 7:74–76, 1986

125. Szorady I, Santa A, Veress I: Drug acetylator phenotypes in newborn infants. Biol Res Pregnancy 8:23–25, 1987

126. Alvan G, Von Bahr C, Seideman P, Sjöqvist F: High plasma concentrations of beta-receptor blocking drugs and deficient debrisoquine hydroxylation. Lancet 1:333, 1982

127. Dayer P, Kubli A, Kupfer A, Courvoisier F, Balant L, Fabre J: Defective hydroxylation of bufuralol associated with side-effects of the drug in poor metabolisers. Br J Clin Pharmacol 13:750, 1982

128. Lennard MS, Jackson PR, Freestone S, Tucker GT, Ramsay LE, Woods HF: The relationship between debrisoquine oxidation phenotype and the pharmacokinetics and pharmacodynamics of propranolol. Br J Clin Pharmacol 17:679, 1984

129. Raghuram TC, Koshakji RP, Wilkinson GR, Wood AJJ: Polymorphic ability to metabolize propranolol alters 4-hydroxy-propranolol levels but not beta blockade. Clin Pharmacol Ther 36:51, 1984

130. Bertilsson L, Eichelbaum M, Mellström B, Säwe J, Schulz H-V, Sjöqvist F: Nortriptyline and antipyrine clearance in relation to debrisoquine hydroxylation in man. Life Sci 27:1673, 1980

131. Woosley RL, Roden DM, Dai G, Wang T, Altenbern D, Oates J, Wilkinson GR: Coinheritance of the polymorphic metab-

olism of encainide and debrisoquine. Clin Pharmacol Ther 39:282, 1985

132. Ladona MG, Lindström B, Thyr Ch, Peng D and Rane A: Differential fetal development of the O- and N-demethylation of codeine and dextromethorphan in man. Br J Clin Pharmacol, in press, 1991

133. Treluyer JM, Jacqz-Aigrain E, and Cresteil T: Expression of cytochrome P-450 in developing human liver. Abstract. 2nd Congress of European Society of Developmental Pharmacology, Tremezzo, 1990

134. Küpfer A, Preisig R: Pharmacogenetics of mephenytoin: A new drug hydroxylation polymorphism in man. Eur J Clin Pharmacol 26:753, 1984

3

CLINICAL PHARMACOKINETICS

MICHELE DANISH

Pharmacokinetics is the mathematical description of the biologic rate processes by which drug concentrations are altered in the body. This includes the study of the plasma concentration versus time course of a drug following administration and the development of mathematical models to predict these concentrations.

For many systemically acting drugs, the plasma concentration is related to the tissue concentration at the receptor site and the pharmacodynamics of the drug. Knowledge of a drug's physicochemical and pharmacokinetic properties allows the clinician to predict plasma concentrations at any given time after dosage administration and thereby make fairly reliable estimates of the magnitude and duration of drug response in the body. Thus the application of pharmacokinetic principles to dosage selection provides an invaluable tool in reaching the goal of optimal drug therapy for an individual patient. Because of the dramatic physiologic changes occurring from birth through adolescence that may affect drug absorption and disposition, the clinical application of pharmacokinetic principles is a particularly useful tool for the pediatrician.

The purpose of this chapter is to familiarize the clinician with basic pharmacokinetic principles and the application of these principles in a clinical situation. The limitations of pharmacokinetic formulas and dose-adjustment methods also will be discussed.

There are four pharmacokinetic parameters that are critical to the characterization of plasma concentrations after drug administration and therefore are necessary for the determination of appropriate drug dosing regimens: systemic availability, volume of distribution, clearance, and half-life. The methods used to calculate these parameters and the physiologic factors that potentially affect them will be addressed in this chapter.

DRUG TRANSFER: FIRST-ORDER KINETICS

Following drug administration, a drug must cross several membranes to reach its site of action. This transfer is usually accomplished by passive diffusion. The driving force for drug transfer by passive diffusion is the concentration gradient on either side of the membrane. In general, drugs in which the rate of transfer is proportional to the amount of drug remaining to be transferred are described by a *first-order process.*

Drug transfers (between body "compartments") and drug elimination involve rate constants (k) specific for each transfer. Drug transfers can be shown to proceed by first-order kinetics when a semilogarithmic plot of drug concentration versus time results in a straight line. The decline of drug concentration in the plasma is usually accompanied by a parallel decline of drug concentration in the major drug storage tissues. The equation describing the plasma decay curve is

$$\ln C_t = \ln C_0 e^{-kt} \tag{1}$$

where C_t = drug concentration at time t
C_0 = drug concentration at time zero

The slope of the linear portion of the plot represents the elimination rate constant k. It is also possible to calculate k from the half-life ($t_{1/2}$) using Equation 2:

$$k = \frac{0.693}{t_{1/2}} \tag{2}$$

For a drug following first-order kinetics, the half-life is independent of dose, plasma concentration, or route of administration and is often directly related to the duration of pharmacologic effect.

For most drugs, absorption, distribution, metabolism, and renal excretion all proceed as first-order reaction rates.

SYSTEMIC AVAILABILITY

Calculation of Drug Bioavailability

In order to accurately predict drug plasma concentrations and clinical response after administration of a drug to a patient, it is necessary to know the exact amount of drug in the body, i.e., the systemic availability. Administration of a drug by I.V. bolus is assumed to provide 100 percent systemic availability, whereas the systemic availability of all other routes of administration is commonly obtained from the comparison of plasma concentration versus time data following administration of a single dose by the intravascular and extravascular routes. The absolute bioavailability (F) of a drug dosage form is the fraction of the area under the serum concentration curves (AUC) obtained from the comparison

$$F = \frac{AUC_{test\ dose}}{AUC_{I.V.}} \quad (3)$$

F may vary from 0 (no systemic availability of the test dose) to 1 (complete bioavailability).

In calculating AUC, it is assumed that the area between each two data points on the serum concentration versus time plot represent a trapezoid. The sum of the areas of the serial trapezoids of data points collected from time 0 until no more drug can be detected in the plasma (∞) after drug administration is referred to as AUC_0^∞ (Figure 3–1), that is,

$$AUC_0^\infty = \tfrac{1}{2}r(C_0 + C_1)(t_1 - t_0) + \tfrac{1}{2}(C_1 + C_2)(t_2 - t_1) + \cdots + \tfrac{1}{2}r(C_4 + C_N)(t_N - t_4) + C_N/k \quad (4)$$

While the AUC provides a measure of the extent of absorption, the rate of absorption is a critical factor in the determination of bioavailability for drugs given as a single dose or sustained-release preparations. The rate of absorption determines the peak plasma concentration; a drug dosage form that is subject to slow or erratic absorption may never produce the desired therapeutic concentration even though F is approaching or equal to 1. The rate of absorption of a drug may be described by k_a, the absorption rate constant,[1] or by $\bar{t}_a$, the mean transit time for absorption.[2]

Factors Affecting Availability

As mentioned earlier, the route and method of drug administration can significantly affect systemic availability. Intravenous bolus injections of drugs provide 100 percent bioavailability, whereas intravenous infusions are less reliable. Slow infusion rates and distal injection sites may result in large variations in the amount and rate of drug delivered.[3] Significant differences in peak plasma concentrations and the time to peak have been observed following tobramycin infusion in 19 newborns.[4]

Although it is necessary to closely monitor infusion methods to ensure drug delivery, most major discrepancies in systemic availability occur when a drug is administered by an extravascular route. The oral route is the most commonly used method for drug administration in pediatric patients. It is recognized that absorption by this route is influenced by physiologic factors[5] (rate of gastric emptying, gastric pH, food intake, etc.) that may be rapidly changing in the infant.[6] In addition, physicochemical properties of the drug (pK$_a$, molecular weight, lipid solubility) and manufacturing techniques (compression force in tablet production, the presence of stabilizers and fillers, etc.) also may affect absorption.[7]

Oral drugs are also subject to a "first pass" through the liver by means of the hepatic portal vein before entering the general circulation.[8] Some drugs are rapidly metabolized by various enzyme systems upon presentation. Drugs with high extraction ratios (propranolol, nitroglycerin, isoproterenol, etc.) have poor systemic availability after oral administration. Although 90 percent of propranolol is absorbed from a typical oral tablet, only 25 percent is systemically available.[9] The oral dose of a drug subject to a large first-pass effect must necessarily be much larger than the intravenous dose in order to produce similar effects. Theoretically, administration of the drug in its most rapidly absorbable form (i.e., a solution) provides the best systemic availability for these drugs, since the enzymatic systems involved are saturable.

Limited clinical data are available regarding systemic availability of drugs in the pediatric population. The number of plasma samples required to accurately describe the area under the curve has presented ethical constraints for study of very young patients. After the neonatal and early infancy period, there has been no clinical evidence that would suggest alterations in the adult absorption pattern in children; the lack of bioavailability studies in children is therefore not considered significant for patient care.

VOLUME OF DISTRIBUTION

Once absorption is complete, the drug does not remain exclusively in the blood but distributes into various tissues and other fluids. The rate at which a particular tissue–plasma concentration equilibrium is achieved depends on the blood perfusion rate to the organ. The extent to which a drug distributes extravascularly depends on its lipophilicity and its affinity for plasma and tissue

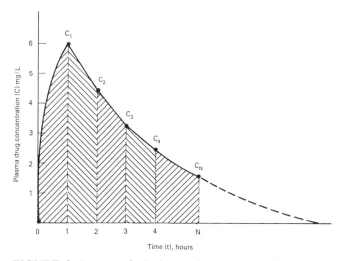

FIGURE 3–1. A typical plasma drug concentration versus time curve for calculation of AUC_0^∞ after a single oral dose.

proteins. The term *volume of distribution* (V_d) is used to identify the proportionality factor relating the amount of drug in the body (A) with the blood or plasma concentration (C):

$$A = V_d C \qquad (5)$$

For the distribution of most drugs, the body can be divided into "compartments" based on tissue vascularity. The drug concentration reaches equilibrium in each compartment at different rates. These compartments can often be classified as the central compartment (V_C), consisting of the plasma and extracellular fluid and highly vascular tissue (red blood cells, lungs, liver, kidney), and a compartment of poorly perfused tissue (V_T) (fat, muscle, and skin). For drugs exhibiting multicompartment kinetics, the relationship can be expressed as

$$V_d = V_C + V_T \qquad (6)$$

For many drugs, the distribution into the peripheral tissue compartment occurs fairly rapidly, and for clinical purposes, pharmacokinetic calculations based on a one-compartment model are adequate.

Calculation of Volume of Distribution

There are many different methods employed to calculate V_d. The values for volume of distribution most frequently found in the literature are based on calculation of $V_{d,area}$:

$$V_{d,area} = \frac{F \times dose}{k \times AUC} \qquad (7)$$

This equation is independent of the number of compartments used to describe the drug's disposition and can be used regardless of the route of drug administration as long as F, the absolute bioavailability, is known. The potential flaw in this calculation method is the appearance of change in V_d when a change in the elimination rate constant k occurs. Another compartment-independent volume term, the volume of distribution at steady state ($V_{d,ss}$), may more accurately reflect drug distribution. When steady state is reached during a multiple dosing situation, the distribution of a drug among various tissues and the plasma is in equilibrium. $V_{d,ss}$ cannot be directly measured, but it can be estimated from the equation of Benet and Galeazzi.[10]

$$V_{d,ss} = \frac{F \times dose \times AUMC}{AUC^2} \qquad (8)$$

The area under the moment curve (AUMC) is obtained from a plot of the product of time and concentration plotted versus time, from time 0 to time infinity. The fraction AUMC/AUC is equal to the mean time a drug resides in the body, called the *mean residence time* (MRT).[11] The calculated values of $V_{d,area}$ and $V_{d,ss}$ are not necessarily equivalent, since $V_{d,ss}$ is independent of changes in the rate of elimination.

Volume of distribution is a convenient tool for calculating an intravenous loading dose. Since the amount of drug in the body at time 0 can be assumed to equal an I.V.

dose, the appropriate I.V. dose can be determined from the equation

$$I.V. \ dose = C_{desired} \times V_d \qquad (9)$$

For a drug that has a prolonged tissue distribution phase, use of this equation may result in early serum levels that are above the minimal toxic concentration. For these drugs, a bolus dose may need to be given as a short infusion. Alternatively, the volume of the central compartment (V_C) may be substituted for V_d in Equation 9. The selection of the appropriate method for administration of a loading dose of a multicompartment-model drug depends on the location of the site of drug action, the central or peripheral compartment.

Factors Affecting Distribution

V_d does not represent a true physiologic volume, but it does have some real physiologic limitations.[12] The minimum V_d value for any drug is equal to the volume of distribution of albumin (7 liters in a 70-kg man). A V_d of approximately 7 liters would occur for a drug highly bound to plasma proteins with no significant tissue binding. If a drug has negligible affinity for plasma proteins, the minimum V_d value would equal extracellular fluid space. There is no upper limit for V_d, and calculation of volume of distribution frequently exceeds total body water. This would indicate significant storage of the drug in peripheral tissue sites.

In newborns, extracellular fluid and total body water represent a much greater percentage of total body weight than that found in adults. Water-soluble drugs will exhibit an increased volume of distribution in newborns when compared with adult liter per kilogram values.[13] Concurrently, the volume of distribution of lipid-soluble drugs may be reduced because of lack of adipose tissue in the neonate.[6] Tissue-binding characteristics also may differ in the pediatric patient. Digoxin has been shown to be much more extensively bound to tissue (and thus have a greater volume of distribution) in infants and children than in adults.[14] This may partially explain the increased tolerance of infants to relatively large doses of digoxin as compared with the adult per-kilogram dose.

CLEARANCE

Calculation of Body Clearance

Just as volume of distribution relates the amount of drug in the body to the plasma concentration, the term *body clearance* (Cl_B) refers to the proportionality factor between the rate of elimination of the drug from the body and the plasma or blood concentration. Clearance is constant for any given plasma concentration as long as the rate of elimination is first order.

Body clearance is a more precise measurement of the body's ability to eliminate drugs than half-life because it has a physiologic basis; i.e., it directly reflects physiologic processes of elimination. Clearance does not measure the quantity of drug eliminated by the body; instead, it quantifies the volume of blood or plasma that could be completely cleared of drug per unit time.

Total-body clearance (Cl_B) is calculated by dividing the total amount of drug systemically available by the area under the plasma concentration versus time for that dose.

$$Cl_B = \frac{F \times \text{dose}}{\text{AUC}} \qquad (10)$$

This equation is compartment-model-independent and can be used after a single dose or during a multiple-dose regimen at steady state. Clearance is the most important pharmacokinetic parameter for appropriate calculation of maintenance doses.

Factors Affecting Clearance

Body clearance can be further defined as the summation of clearances of all organs involved in elimination.

$$Cl_B = Cl_{hepatic} + Cl_{renal} + Cl_{other} \qquad (11)$$

The kidney and/or liver are the major routes of elimination for most drugs. Organ clearance provides a physiologic approach to the concept of drug clearance. The renal clearance of a drug is analogous to the measurement of creatinine clearance. Drug renal clearance depends on renal blood flow, plasma drug–protein binding, and the intrinsic ability of the functioning nephrons to clear a particular compound (i.e., the glomerular filtration, tubular secretion, and reabsorption processes). Thus renal clearance of drugs may be affected by urine pH and urine flow rates.[15] Urine pH should be measured when calculating the renal clearance of weak acids and bases.

Similarly, drug hepatic clearance depends on the hepatic blood flow rate, plasma drug–protein binding, and the intrinsic enzymatic capability to metabolize a drug.

In general, drug metabolism and excretion are impaired in the neonate and infant.[16,17] Unpredictable changes in biotransformation and renal excretion of drugs occur with maturation; to some extent, these changes depend on the clinical condition of the patient, gestational and postnatal age, and the *in utero* or postnatal exposure to drug enzyme inducers or inhibitors. Children 1–5 years of age appear to metabolize many drugs much more rapidly than adults.[18] In older children, a decrease in the rate of drug metabolism to adult levels occurs at or near the time of puberty.

HALF-LIFE

The *plasma half-life* ($t_{1/2}$) of a drug is defined as the amount of time necessary to decrease plasma drug concentrations by 50 percent. For first-order drugs, $t_{1/2}$ is independent of dose. For multicompartment drugs, each disposition phase, as observed on a log plasma concentration versus time curve, has a "half-life." Usually, the terminal portion of the curve (slope = β) is considered to represent the plasma half-life of the drug.

In order to be eliminated from the body, a drug must be present in the plasma as the unbound drug so that it is in direct contact with the organs of elimination. Thus plasma half-life depends on the physiologically based parameters V_d and Cl_B.

$$t_{1/2} = \frac{\ln 2 \, V_d}{Cl_B} \qquad (12)$$

Subsequently, a drug with a very large volume of distribution will probably have a long half-life because of the small fraction of total drug in the vascular system of the body. Conversely, a small volume of distribution does not necessarily signify a rapid half-life because of the role of protein binding and intrinsic metabolic/excretory capacity in determining body clearance.

Plasma half-life is easily conceptualized. Although it is not an independent pharmacokinetic parameter, it is useful in estimation of the time required to eliminate the drug entirely from the body (or any fractional elimination thereof), as well as of the time needed to reach steady state during a multiple-dosing regimen.

APPLICATION OF PHARMACOKINETIC PRINCIPLES TO MULTIPLE DOSE REGIMENS

In most clinical situations, drugs are administered as a series of doses at fixed time intervals or as an infusion. Assuming that a drug's therapeutic "window" is known, an appropriate multiple-dose regimen should maintain plasma concentrations within the range known to produce clinical effectiveness while avoiding subtherapeutic or toxic concentrations.

When drug disposition proceeds as a first-order rate process, V_d, Cl_B, and $t_{1/2}$ are independent of dose or drug plasma level. Thus plasma concentrations during a multiple-dosing regimen can be predicted based on knowledge of the plasma concentration versus time curve after a single dose. This is referred to as the *principle of superposition;* the plasma concentration versus time curve of the second, third, or subsequent doses can be superimposed on the plasma concentration versus time curve of the first dose (Figure 3–2).

When doses of first-order drugs are administered at a fixed dosing interval τ that is shorter than the time required to eliminate all drug from the body (approximately 4–7 half-lives), drug accumulates in the body until a plateau is reached. At the plateau, referred to as *steady state,* the amount of drug entering the body equals the amount of drug eliminated during one dosing interval. The rate at which drug accumulates depends on the half-life; it takes about four half-lives to reach 94 percent of the steady-state plasma concentration and seven half-lives to reach 99 percent of steady state concentrations. At steady

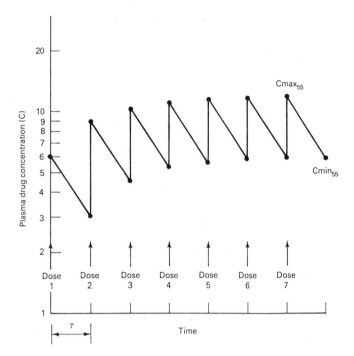

FIGURE 3–2. Log plasma drug concentration versus time data for a drug administered in equal doses by I.V. bolus at a fixed dosing interval τ. In this simulation, τ equals the plasma half-life.

state, the plasma concentrations fluctuate between $C_{\text{max,ss}}$ and $C_{\text{min,ss}}$, the maximum and minimum plasma levels during a dosing interval.

At steady state, the area under the curve for one dosing interval, (AUC^{τ}) is equal to the area under the curve from time 0 to time infinity $(\text{AUC}_{0}^{\infty})$ after a single dose of the drug. The average plasma concentration during steady state $(C_{\text{avg,ss}})$ can be estimated by dividing either AUC_{0}^{∞} after a single dose or AUC^{τ} by the dosing interval τ.

$$C_{\text{avg,ss}} = \frac{\text{AUC}^{\tau}}{\tau} \qquad (13)$$

An easier method to determine $C_{\text{avg,ss}}$ utilizes clearance. At steady state, the rate of elimination equals the dosing rate (rate in = rate out); since clearance is defined as the proportionality factor between the elimination rate and the plasma concentration, at steady state,

$$S \times \text{dosing rate} = C_{\text{avg,ss}} \times \text{Cl}_{\text{B}} \qquad (14)$$

where S is the fraction of a salt containing active drug.

For drugs given by infusion, the dosing rate equals the infusion rate. If aminophylline (85 percent theophylline) is infused at a rate of 0.9 mg/kg/h and the mean literature clearance value of theophylline for a 10-year-old patient (30 kg) is 3 liters/h, the predicted theophylline concentration at steady state will be

$$C_{\text{avg,ss}} = \frac{0.85(27 \text{ mg/h})}{3 \text{ liters/h}}$$
$$= 7.6 \text{ mg/liter}$$

For drugs given at fixed dosing intervals, the dosing rate equals the dose divided by the dosing interval τ. When

given orally, the absolute bioavailability (F) of a drug also must be considered; the equation therefore becomes

$$C_{\text{avg,ss}} = \frac{S \times F \times \text{dose}}{\text{Cl}_{\text{B}} \times \tau} \qquad (15)$$

When adjusting a dose or dosing interval, a period of time equal to four to seven half-lives is needed to reach a new steady state. Administration of a loading dose (Equation 9) followed by the appropriate maintenance dose provides for immediate achievement of the desired steady-state level.

$C_{\text{avg,ss}}$ is compartment-model-independent. The same $C_{\text{avg,ss}}$ can be obtained using many different dosing regimens if the total daily dose remains the same. Dosing schedules of 900 mg q12h, 600 mg q8h, and 300 mg q4h will all produce the same average steady-state plasma concentration. There will be substantial differences in $C_{\text{max,ss}}$ and $C_{\text{min,ss}}$ with the various dosing regimens; the largest fluctuation will be observed with the 12-hour dosing schedule, the longest dosing interval. For drugs with a narrow therapeutic range, computation of $C_{\text{max,ss}}$ and $C_{\text{min,ss}}$ may be needed to ensure achievement of safe and effective plasma concentrations. For intravenous drugs that fit a one-compartment model, $C_{\text{max,ss}}$ and $C_{\text{min,ss}}$ can be readily calculated from the following formulas:

$$C_{\text{max,ss}} = \frac{S \times F \times \text{dose}}{V_{\text{d}}(1 - e^{-k\tau})} \qquad (16)$$

$$C_{\text{min,ss}} = C_{\text{max,ss}} e^{-k\tau} \qquad (17)$$

Equations 16 and 17 could be used to predict plasma concentrations in the following clinical situation. An antibiotic ($S = 0.7$) is administered to a 4-year-old patient (20 kg), 25 mg/kg every 6 hours, by I.V. bolus. The mean literature $t_{1/2}$ and V_{d} for pediatric patients 2–10 years of age are 4 hours and 0.6 liter/kg, respectively. What will the maximum and minimum plasma concentrations of the active drug be at steady state?

$$C_{\text{max,ss}} = \frac{0.7(500 \text{ mg})}{(12 \text{ liters})(1 - e^{-0.17(6)})}$$
$$= 45 \text{ mg/liter}$$
$$C_{\text{min,ss}} = (45 \text{ mg/liter})e^{-0.17(6)}$$
$$= 16 \text{ mg/liter}$$

Equations 16 and 17 also will provide a fairly accurate estimate of $C_{\text{max,ss}}$ and $C_{\text{min,ss}}$ for drugs administered orally if the absorption rate constant is much greater than the elimination rate constant. For sustained-release products, the rate of absorption is not necessarily more rapid than the elimination rate. Equation 15 will still provide an acceptable estimate of $C_{\text{avg,ss}}$; however, $C_{\text{max,ss}}$ would be overestimated and $C_{\text{min,ss}}$ would be underestimated if Equations 16 and 17 are applied to a dosing situation involving a sustained-release product.

NONLINEAR KINETICS

The disposition of some drugs does not exhibit the characteristics of a first-order pharmacokinetic model as outlined in preceding sections. The principle of superposition does not apply to these drugs. Alteration of the dose produces disproportionate changes in the clearance and the average steady-state plasma concentrations.

Certain drugs in this category (e.g., phenytoin, etc.) exhibit Michaelis-Menten kinetics: There is one major metabolic pathway that is saturable. When the maximum metabolic rate (V_{max}) is reached, which may occur at therapeutic doses, the elimination reaction rate proceeds as a zero-order reaction. The amount of drug eliminated does not increase in proportion to the plasma concentration. When the dosing rate exceeds V_{max}, plasma levels continue to rise, never reaching a steady-state level. Values for V_{max} and K_m, the substrate concentration at which V_{max} is half, show wide variations among patients. In the pediatric population, the V_{max} of phenytoin has been found to be inversely related to age.[20] For drugs exhibiting Michaelis-Menten kinetics, nomograms and orbit graphs have been devised to aid in the determination of an individual's V_{max} and K_m.[20-22]

Other drugs eliminated by multiple parallel pathways, such as aspirin and theophylline, frequently exhibit disposition characteristics that strongly suggest the concurrent occurrence of first-order and zero-order elimination reaction processes. Dose adjustment for these drugs should be approached with caution.[23] Although many children receiving theophylline appear to be eliminating the drug in a linear manner, as many as 15 percent of asthmatic children tested have exhibited dose-dependent elimination of theophylline.[24] Monitoring of plasma levels is advisable for any patient not responding as anticipated.

POPULATION PHARMACOKINETICS

Knowledge of a patient's pharmacokinetic response to a drug allows the clinician to individualize the drug dosing regimen and thereby achieve optimal plasma/tissue concentrations. Frequently, in the clinical setting, it is impractical to attempt direct measurement of a patient's clearance and volume of distribution, and as a result, mean literature values are substituted into dosing equations. In most published sources, clearance and V_d values are listed with little, if any, information on the magnitude or causes of potential variability.

In an attempt to overcome these shortcomings, a comprehensive approach to the collection and organization of clinical pharmacokinetic data has been developed.[25,26] In these population pharmacokinetic studies, identifiable patient characteristics are incorporated into pharmacokinetic models. The studies are designed to identify which fixed patient parameters affect a drug's pharmacokinetics and to statistically weigh the importance of these factors. In order to define the relationship between pharmacokinetic parameters and patient characteristics, accurate collection of kinetic and demographic data is required from a defined patient population. The kinetic data utilized usually consist of steady-state concentrations or timed concentration values collected from a large pool of patients. Steady-state concentrations can provide fairly

accurate information on clearance but little information on volume of distribution. Random plasma drug concentrations collected at known times allow the inclusion of routine clinical samples and thereby greatly expand the potential database.[27] Grasela et al.[28] used this method to analyze the phenytoin steady-state concentrations of 322 pediatric and adult patients. A nonlinear function of patient weight (weight$^{0.6}$) was determined to be the best predictor of V_{max}.

There are drawbacks to the application of this type of data analysis. There may be insufficient information from the study population to identify all the influential factors. The magnitude of the variability observed in a population kinetic study also may suggest caution in relying solely on the identified factors for adjusting doses. After adjustment for age, gender, height, weight, and race, the coefficient of variation for V_{max} in the phenytoin data approached 20 percent.[28]

Population pharmacokinetic techniques do provide a valuable tool for drug dosage selection in individual patients. Population-based parameter values adjusted for patient factors are especially useful in patients from whom it is difficult to collect the multiple plasma samples needed for individual characterization of pharmacokinetic parameters (e.g., neonates, infants, and the elderly). Estimation of individual kinetic parameters using a Bayesian feedback system may be necessary for selected patients.[29]

CONCLUSION

The interrelationship of pharmacokinetics and pharmacodynamics, the accessibility of body fluids for the measurement of drug concentrations, and the development of clinically applicable mathematical models provide the rationale for inclusion of pharmacokinetics in therapeutic decisions. The basic principles and equations of applied pharmacokinetics have been reviewed in this chapter. Systemic availability, clearance, volume of distribution, and half-life are the pharmacokinetic concepts that are most useful for the characterization and/or prediction of plasma drug concentrations during multiple dosing. The application of these concepts by means of dosing equations will assist the clinician in the optimal individualization of drug dosage regimens.

ACKNOWLEDGMENTS: I wish to express my appreciation to Dr. Joan Lausier for reviewing this manuscript.

REFERENCES

1. Shargell L, Yu A: Pharmacokinetics of drug absorption, in Applied Biopharmaceutics and Pharmacokinetics, 2d ed. Norwalk, Conn, Appleton-Century-Crofts, 1985
2. Jusko W: Guidelines for collection and analysis of pharmacokinetic data, in Evans W, Schentag J, Jusko W (eds): Applied Pharmacokinetics, 2d ed. Spokane, Wash, Applied Therapeutics, 1986
3. Gould T, Roberts R: Therapeutic problems arising from the use of

the intravenous route for drug administration. J Pediatr 95:465–471, 1979

4. Nahata M, Powell D, Durrell D, et al: Effect of infusion methods on tobramycin serum concentrations in newborn infants. J Pediatr 104:136–138, 1982

5. Welling P: Influence of food and diet on gastrointestinal drug absorption: A review. J Pharmacokinet Biopharm 5:291–334, 1977

6. Stewart C, Hampton E: Effect of maturation on drug disposition in pediatric patients. Clin Pharmacy 6:548–564, 1987

7. Koch-Weser J: Bioavailability of drugs. N Engl J Med 291:503–506, 1974

8. Gibaldi M, Boyes R, Feldman S: Influence of first-pass effect on availability of drugs on oral administration. J Pharm Sci 60:1338–1340, 1971

9. Routledge P, Shand DG: Clinical pharmacokinetics of propranolol. Clin Pharmacokinet 4:73–90, 1979

10. Benet L, Galeazzi R: Noncompartmental determination of the steady state volume of distribution. J Pharm Sci 68:1071–1074, 1979

11. Riegelman S, Collier P: The application of statistical moment theory to the evaluation of *in vivo* dissolution time and absorption time. J Pharmacokinet Biopharm 8:509–534, 1980

12. Qie S: Drug distribution and binding. J Clin Pharmacol 26:583–586, 1986

13. Nahata M, Powell D, Gregoire R, et al: Tobramycin kinetics in newborn infants. J Pediatr 103:136–138, 1983

14. Gorodischer R, Jusko W, Yaffe S: Tissue and erythrocyte distribution of digoxin in infants. Clin Pharmacol Ther 19:256–263, 1976

15. Levy G, Lampman T, et al: Decreased serum salicylate concentrations in children with rheumatic fever treated with antacid. N Engl J Med 293:323–325, 1975

16. Warner A: Drug use in the neonate: Interrelationship of pharmacokinetics, toxicity, and biochemical maturity. Clin Chem 32:721–727, 1986

17. Morselli P, Franco-Morselli R, Bossi L: Clinical pharmacokinetics in newborns and infants. Clin Pharmacokinet 5:485–527, 1980

18. Alvares A, Kapelner S, et al: Drug metabolism in normal children, lead-poisoned children, and normal adults. Clin Pharmacol Ther 17:179–183, 1975

19. Ludden T, Allen J, Valutsky W, et al: Individualization of phenytoin dosage regimens. Clin Pharmacol Ther 21:287–293, 1977

20. Chiba K, Ishizaki T, et al: Michaelis-Menten pharmacokinetics of diphenylhydantoin and application in the pediatric age patient. J Pediatr 96:479–484, 1980

21. Lambie D, Nanda R, et al: Therapeutic and pharmacokinetic effects of increasing phenytoin in chronic epileptics on multiple drug therapy. Lancet 2:386–389, 1976

22. Winter M, Tozer T: Phenytoin, in Evans W, Schentag J, Jusko W (eds): *Applied Pharmacokinetics,* 2d ed. Spokane, Wash, Applied Therapeutics, 1986

23. Wagner J: New and simple method to predict dosage of drugs obeying simple Michaelis-Menten elimination kinetics and to distinguish such kinetics from simple first-order and from parallel Michaelis-Menten and first-order kinetics. Ther Drug Monit 7:377–386, 1985

24. Sarrazin E, Hendeles L, Weinberger M, et al: Dose-dependent kinetics for theophylline: Observations among ambulatory asthmatic children. J Pediatr 97:825–828, 1980

25. Sheiner L, Beal S, et al: Forecasting individual pharmacokinetics. Clin Pharmacol Ther 26:294–305, 1979

26. Whiting B, Kelman A, Grevel J: Population pharmacokinetics: Theory and clinical application. Clin Pharmacokinet 11:387–401, 1986

27. Sheiner LB, Rosenberg B, Marathe V: Estimation of population characteristics of pharmacokinetic parameters from routine clinical data. J Pharmacokinet Biopharm 5:445–479, 1977

28. Grasela T, Sheiner L, Rambeck B, et al: Steady-state pharmacokinetics of phenytoin from routinely collected patient data. Clin Pharmacokinet 8:355–364, 1983

29. Burton ME: Comparison of drug dosing methods. Clin Pharmacokinet 10:1–37, 1985

4

PHARMACOGENETICS

ELLIOT S. VESELL

Even when age, sex, diet, and exposure to environmental agents that induce or inhibit the hepatic drug-metabolizing enzyme system remain constant among subjects, large interindividual variations in drug disposition and response still occur. The magnitude of these interindividual variations in rates of elimination of a drug can range from 4-fold to as much as 40-fold and more depending on both the particular drug and the population studied. In practice, these large differences among normal subjects in rates of drug elimination mean that the same dose of a drug given by the same route can produce toxicity in one subject, a therapeutic effect in another, and failure to obtain any pharmacologic response whatever in a third. Because of these clinically significant differences in both drug disposition and response, the pediatrician must often individualize drug therapy, which means that the appropriate drug and the appropriate dose need to be selected for each child.

The many therapeutic ramifications of large interindividual variations in disposition of numerous drugs make it necessary to attempt the next step of determining the mechanisms responsible for these differences among children. Such investigations are beset with many difficulties that are rooted in the extreme genetic and environmental heterogeneity of children with respect to factors affecting drug disposition. In normal adult humans, however, these factors can often be carefully controlled, and each variable can be manipulated independently of the others. By this technique, the quantitative contribution of each factor to interindividual variations in drug disposition can be studied, and dose–response curves can be constructed for each factor. Over the past decade, such studies have disclosed many factors that can affect drug disposition. Figure 4–1 presents a partial enumeration of such factors, which are connected to indicate the potential for interactions among the 25 environmental and developmental factors in the outer circle as well as among each of these and numerous unspecified genetic factors in the center circle. The extent and magnitude of such interactions change not only with the subject, but even in the same subject with time and condition. Thus these interactions

must be regarded as dynamic in nature and continuously fluctuating in character. Table 4–1 lists the most intensively investigated, and hence best characterized, monogenically transmitted pharmacogenetic conditions. *Pharmacogenetics* is usually defined as the study of genetically controlled variations in drug response. To qualify as pharmacogenetic, the enzymes, proteins, and receptors affected by mutation must directly involve drug metabolism (pharmacokinetics) or drug action (pharmacodynamics), in contrast with many other inborn errors of metabolism, such as gout, diabetes mellitus, or porphyria, where only secondarily to a different type of metabolic defect do drug responses become aberrant.

Epidemiologic studies reveal that about one patient in five enters a hospital in the United States for treatment of an adverse drug reaction. Further, 15 to 30 percent of all hospitalized patients have at least one such reaction.[1] Although wide disparity in patients' responses to drugs is only one of many causes of adverse reactions, it nevertheless constitutes a significant contribution to this major medical problem because it demands individualization of dosages. Multiple factors have been systematically investigated and identified as contributing to wide interindividual variations in drug disposition and response. As indicated in Figure 1, they include age, sex, diet, time of day or season of drug administration, disease, hormonal and nutritional status, stress, and exposure to inducers or inhibitors of the hepatic microsomal drug-metabolizing enzymes, including chronic administration of any one of several hundred drugs.[2-4] Also in the last 20 years, multiple genetic factors altering drug disposition and response in humans have been discovered.[5,6]

MONOGENICALLY INHERITED CONDITIONS DIRECTLY AFFECTING DRUG RESPONSE

Pharmacogenetics deals with clinically significant hereditary variations in response to drugs. These entities

29

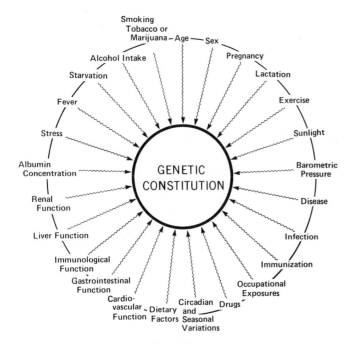

FIGURE 4–1. This circular design suggests the multiplicity of either well-established or suspected host factors that may influence drug response in humans. A line joins all such factors in the outer circle to indicate their close interrelationship. Arrows from each factor in the outer circle are wavy to indicate that effects of each host factor on drug response may occur at multiple sites and through different processes that include drug absorption, distribution, metabolism, excretion, receptor action, and combinations thereof. (Reprinted with permission from Vesell.[4a])

include traditionally recognized hereditary conditions that produce a clinically significant abnormal response to drugs (see Table 4–1). Pharmacogenetic conditions may be divided into those arising from defects in the metabolism of drugs by the body and those arising from abnormal effects on the body due to altered receptor sites on

which the drug acts.[5] "Monogenic" means that the condition is controlled entirely by genes at a single locus on a chromosome, whereas "polygenic" means that more than one locus on a chromosome is involved. Many pharmacogenetic conditions can be regarded as a special or limited form of inborn error of metabolism. Like many other inborn errors of metabolism, several pharmacogenetic conditions were first discovered in children, and for this reason, it seems appropriate to begin with acatalasia.

Abnormal Breakdown of Drugs by the Body

Acatalasia

In 1946, the Japanese otorhinolaryngologist Takahara discovered acatalasia in an 11-year-old Japanese girl. In a series of classic studies, he demonstrated that the defect was transmitted as an autosomal recessive trait.[7–9] His original patient lacked catalase activity in her oral mucosa and erythrocytes, as did three of her five siblings. The patient's parents were second cousins: Consanguinity is a hallmark of autosomal recessive inheritance.

Mild, moderate, and severe expressions of acatalasia have been described.[10] The mild form is characterized by ulcers of the dental alveoli; in the moderate type, alveolar gangrene and atrophy occur; and in the severe form, recession of alveolar bone occurs with exposure of the necks and eventual loss of teeth. The enzyme is deficient in tissues such as mucous membrane, skin, liver, muscle, and bone marrow. Trace levels of catalase activity occur in some patients, and the term *severe hypocatalasia* seems more appropriate than does *acatalasia*.[11] Heterozygotes, who usually have values of catalase activity between those of affected and normal persons, would be classified as having *intermediate hypocatalasia*. In certain Japanese kindreds, some heterozygotes do not exhibit intermediate

TABLE 4–1. MONOGENIC METABOLIC PHARMACOGENETIC CONDITIONS WITH PUTATIVE ABERRANT ENZYME AND MODE OF INHERITANCE (MOST CONDITIONS LEAD TO TOXICITY FROM ACCUMULATION OF PARENT DRUG)

CONDITION	ABERRANT ENZYME AND LOCATION	MODE OF INHERITANCE
1. Acatalasia	Catalase in erythrocytes	Autosomal recessive
2. Slow inactivation of isoniazid	N-Acetyl transferase in liver	Autosomal recessive
3. Suxamethonium sensibility or atypical pseudocholinesterase	Pseudocholinesterase in plasma	Autosomal recessive
4. Phenytoin toxicity due to deficient parahydroxylation	Mixed-function oxidase in liver that parahydroxylates phenytoin	Autosomal dominant
5. Bishydroxycoumarin sensitivity	? Mixed-function oxidase in liver that hydroxylates bishydroxycoumarin	Unknown
6. Acetophenetidin-induced methemoglobinemia	? Mixed-function oxidase in liver that deethylates acetophenetidin	Autosomal recessive
7. Polymorphic serum aryl esterase activity	Serum aryl esterase (paraoxonase)	Autosomal recessive
8. Deficient N-glucosidation of amobarbital	? Mixed-function oxidase in liver that N-hydroxylates amobarbital	Autosomal recessive
9. Polymorphic hydroxylation of debrisoquine in humans	Mixed-function oxidase in liver that 4-hydroxylates debrisoquine	Autosomal recessive
10. Polymorphic hydroxylation of mephenytoin	Mixed-function oxidase in liver that hydroxylates S-mephenytoin	Autosomal recessive
11. Polymorphic methylation	Erythrocyte catechol-O-methyltransferase, thiopurine methyltransferase, and thiolmethyltransferase	Autosomal recessive

levels of catalase activity, but rather have values that overlap the normal range, suggesting heterogeneity.[12]

In 1959, a Korean patient was reported with acatalasia, the first non-Japanese subject to be described.[13] Two years later, Aebi and associates[14] found three affected individuals by screening 73,661 blood samples from Swiss army recruits.[14] All three were healthy and showed none of the dental defects typical of the Japanese cases. The Swiss "acatalasics," unlike the Japanese ones, exhibited residual catalase activity, possibly protecting them against the hydrogen peroxide formed by certain microorganisms thought to be responsible for the oral lesions. The catalase from Swiss subjects also differed from that of normal persons in electrophoretic mobility, pH and heat stabilities, and sensitivity to certain inhibitors. These facts suggest that in Swiss families actalasia is a structural gene mutation.[15] Other variants are likely to have a similar derivation, although more complex regulatory mutations cannot be excluded.

Slow Inactivation of Isoniazid

Although isoniazid (INH) was synthesized in 1921, its bacteriostatic effect was not discovered until 1952. Soon, great differences among subjects were reported in the metabolism of INH, but each patient maintained an unchanged pattern of excretion during long-term therapy.[16,17] Slow inactivators show reduced activity of acetyl transferase, the soluble hepatic enzyme responsible for the metabolism of INH and sulfamethazine,[18] as well as other monosubstituted hydrazines, such as phenelzine and hydralazine.[19] Toxic effects of these drugs occur chiefly in "slow acetylators." Acetylation of procainamide is polymorphic, and thus the effect of this popular antiarrhythmic agent varies appreciably according to the genotype of the patient to whom it is administered.[20] Toxicity as a result of chronic INH administration takes the form of polyneuritis due to vitamin B_6 deficiency; this potential deficiency of pyridoxine to which slow acetylators are particularly susceptible can be overcome easily by giving this compound with INH whenever INH is administered for long periods. Another form of toxicity to which slow acetylators appear to be more disposed than "rapid acetylators" is both the drug-induced and spontaneous forms of disseminated lupus erythematosus. Thus susceptibility to certain diseases may be linked to genetic differences among subjects in the capacity to biotransform drugs and other compounds that do not apparently bear any direct pathogenetic relationship to the diseases. Finally, among 23 chemical dye workers who were chronically exposed to benzidine in a plant located in Yorkshire, England, and who all eventually developed bladder cancer, 22 were slow acetylators.[21] This represents a 40 percent excess of acetylators over matched control subjects in this region, implicating the slow-acetylator phenotype as being at increased risk of contracting bladder cancer.[22]

The sedative nitrazepam also shows a similar variation in response. Acetylation of other drugs, such as para-aminosalicylic acid and sulfanilamide, is accomplished by a different acetylase, and no genetic differences among subjects occur in the metabolism of these drugs. Interestingly, neither the slow nor the rapid acetylase genotype is more liable to resistance to tubercle bacilli or reversion. The half-life of INH ranges from 45 to 80 minutes in the plasma of rapid inactivators, whereas the half-life extends from 140 to 200 minutes in slow inactivators.[23] Although slow acetylators excrete in urine approximately 70 percent of a dose as metabolites, rapid acetylators excrete 97 percent of a dose as metabolites,[24] thereby being exposed to higher concentrations of potentially toxic reactive metabolites. Such toxic intermediates have been implicated as the cause of the severe hepatic necrosis and hepatitis that occur in approximately 1 percent of patients receiving INH chronically for prophylactic purposes.[25,26] The transient elevation of serum transaminases, however, as a result of liver damage in approximately 10–20 percent of patients receiving INH or INH plus rifampin chronically seems to occur predominantly in slow acetylators.[27,28]

Slow inactivation of INH is inherited as an autosomal recessive trait.[29] The best evidence suggests that the different phenotypes result from a structural gene mutation. Diverse geographic and racial distributions of the gene are documented. Most uncommon in Eskimos (5 percent), slow inactivation is only slightly more frequent in Far Eastern populations, where it occurs in approximately 10 percent of Japanese subjects.[30] Slow inactivation is common in blacks and in European populations, in nearly 80 percent of whom the aberrant gene is present either in the homozygous or heterozygous state.[30–33] Approximately half the U.S. population consists of rapid acetylators.

Succinylcholine Sensitivity

Shortly after the muscle relaxant succinylcholine was introduced in 1952 and its use became widespread, patients occasionally were found to be extraordinarily sensitive to it; indeed, several deaths associated with its use were reported.[34] Normally, action of the drug is short (2–3 minutes), and this brevity in normal subjects is due to the exceedingly rapid hydrolysis of succinylcholine by plasma pseudocholinesterase, which catalyzes the sequential removal of choline radicals. Serum pseudocholinesterase activity was reduced in the initially published reports of prolonged apnea. The difficulty can be reversed by transfusion of either normal plasma or a highly purified preparation of human enzyme. The abnormality is the result of a structurally altered enzyme with kinetic properties decidedly different from those of the usual enzyme.[35] The abnormal enzyme exerts no measurable effect on succinylcholine at concentrations of the drug usually present during anesthesia, whereas the normal enzyme shows marked hydrolytic activity.[36]

The atypical enzyme is more resistant than the normal one to many pseudocholinesterase inhibitors; i.e., both fluoride and organophosphorus compounds inhibited the normal and atypical enzyme differentially.[37,38] Dibucaine, also a differential inhibitor of normal and atypical pseudocholinesterases, can distinguish three phenotypes:

homozygous normal individuals, heterozygotes, and affected individuals who could not be separated satisfactorily simply by measuring the pseudocholinesterase activity of their plasma.[35] The percentage inhibition of pseudocholinesterase activity produced by 10^{-5} M dibucaine was designated the *dibucaine number* (DN). Whereas atypical pseudocholinesterase is inhibited only 20 percent, the normal enzyme is inhibited about 80 percent, and heterozygotes exhibit 50–70 percent inhibition. Tetracaine, unlike other previously studied compounds, is hydrolyzed faster by atypical than by normal pseudocholinesterase, and an even larger separation of phenotypes apparently can be achieved with the procaine/tetracaine ratio than with the DN. The discovery of additional genetic variants resulted from using sodium fluoride as an inhibitor.[39]

In some families, the DNs do not follow the typical pattern of inheritance. These persons are thought to be heterozygous for a rare, so-called silent gene. Heterozygotes for this gene exhibit two-thirds of the normal serum cholinesterase activity; they widely overlap normal values. A few rare individuals are presumably homozygous for the silent allele, reflecting complete absence of serum and liver pseudocholinesterase activity.[40] Apparently normal otherwise, these persons lack all four of the usual isozymes of serum pseudocholinesterase; the absence of antigenically cross-reacting material was revealed by immunodiffusion and immunoelectrophoretic studies.

This silent mutation may affect the controlling element of the gene, thereby completely disrupting protein production. Alternatively, a single structural mutation may affect both the active site and the antigenic determinants. Another silent allele has been described in which there is some (about 2 percent) residual enzymatic activity, indicating further heterogeneity.[41]

Family studies suggest that inheritance of various types of atypical pseudocholinesterase occurs through allelic codominant or recessive genes at a single locus.[42,43] Symptoms may occur after treatment with succinylcholine in persons homozygous for any of the variant alleles and in some mixed heterozygotes.[11] At least four alleles have been identified definitely with the 10 resultant genotypes:

$$E_1^u E_1^u, \quad E_1^u E_1^a, \quad E_1^a E_1^a, \quad E_1^s E_1^u, \quad E_1^s E_1^s$$
$$E_1^s E_1^a, \quad E_1^f E_1^u, \quad E_1^f E_1^f, \quad E_1^f E_1^a, \quad E_1^f E_1^s$$

where E_1 signifies the pseudocholinesterase genetic locus and u, a, s, and f indicate the "usual," "atypical," "silent," and "fluoride-sensitive" alleles, respectively. A new allele (E_1^j) has been described that apparently causes reduction of E_1^u molecules by about 60 percent.[44]

The incidence of atypical pseudocholinesterase remains comparatively constant in different geographic areas. Persons who are homozygous recessive for the atypical allele number about 1 in 1500.[45] An exceptionally high incidence of the silent mutation was discovered in a population of southern Eskimos.[46] Prior to this survey in Alaska, only 10 individuals homozygous for the silent gene had been described. The gene frequency of 0.12 in this locality, extending from Hooper Bay to Unalakleet and centered on the lower Yukon River, suggested that 1.5 percent of this Alaskan population was sensitive to succinylcholine. The isolation and consequent inbreeding of these natives may have resulted in the high frequency of the rare silent gene in this region of Alaska, although only 2 of the 11 Eskimo families are known to be related.

Similarity of gene frequencies of atypical pseudocholinesterase in most populations suggests that either little selective advantage is conferred by the various genotypes or the contributing environmental factors are common to widely differing countries. In several abnormalities—such as thyrotoxicosis, schizophrenia, hypertension, acute emotional disorders, and after concussion—plasma pseudocholinesterase activity may be elevated. Increases are also observed as a genetically transmitted condition without apparent clinical consequences but associated with an electrophoretically slower migrating C_4 isozyme (the Cynthiana variant).[47] The person with this variant had plasma pseudocholinesterase activity more than three times higher than normal. Further investigation of his family revealed a sister and a daughter who also had high values. The exceptionally high pseudocholinesterase activity was associated with resistance to the pharmacologic effects of succinylcholine.[48]

The Cynthiana variant may result from either a defect of a regulator gene that controls pseudocholinesterase activity or a duplication of a structural gene. Slightly higher than normal pseudocholinesterase activity associated with a retarded electrophoretic mobility of the main isozyme was found in roughly 10 percent of a random sample of the British population.[49] This slower-moving band was designated C_5. The greatly elevated total plasma pseudocholinesterase activity of the U.S. variants distinguished them from the variants described in England.

Deficient Parahydroxylation of Diphenylhydantoin

Since its introduction, diphenylhydantoin (DPH), now designated phenytoin, has become one of the most popular anticonvulsants. It can cause multiple toxic reactions, however, including nystagmus, ataxia, dysarthria, and drowsiness, reactions that are clearly dose-related. The drug is metabolized in humans mainly by parahydroxylation of one of the phenyl groups to yield 5-phenyl-5'-parahydroxyphenylhydantoin (PPHP), which is conjugated with glucuronic acid and then eliminated in the urine.[50] Many lipid-soluble drugs, such as DPH, are rendered more water-soluble, and hence more excretable, through metabolism by oxidative enzyme systems in liver microsomes. The earliest published example of a genetic defect of mixed-function oxidases in human beings is deficient hydroxylation of DPH, although only one affected family has been described.[51]

A study of two generations of this family revealed two affected and three unaffected members, suggesting that low activity of DPH hydroxylase may exhibit dominant transmission. Toxic symptoms developed in the propositus on a commonly used dosage of 4.0 mg/kg, but not on a dose of 1.4 mg/kg. Abnormally low urine levels of the metabolite PPHP occurred in combination with prolonged high blood levels of unchanged DPH. Apparently, phenylalanine and drugs such as phenobarbital are parahydroxylated by enzymes different from those hydroxylating DPH, since the proband's capacity to parahydroxylate these compounds was normal.

Recently, slow inactivation of INH has been identified as a more important cause of DPH intoxication than heritable deficiency of parahydroxylase activity.[52] In 29 individuals receiving DPH and INH, all five patients who developed symptoms of DPH toxicity were slow INH inactivators. Both INH and para-aminosalicylic acid interfered with DPH parahydroxylation in rat liver microsomes. This example shows how genetic constitution can influence the clinical severity of a drug interaction.

Bishydroxycoumarin Sensitivity

Bishydroxycoumarin sensitivity occurred in a patient receiving the drug for an acute myocardial infarction.[53] On a dose of 150 mg, the patient's plasma bishydroxycoumarin half-life was 82 hours, compared with normal values of 27 ± 5 hours. The patient's mother suffered a spinal cord hematoma, causing permanent paraplegia, while she was receiving a small weekly dose of 2.5–5 mg warfarin. Although familial studies were not performed because of lack of cooperation, this unfortunate event in the treatment of the patient's mother suggests the possibility of hereditary transmission of bishydroxycoumarin sensitivity.

Warfarin and bishydroxycoumarin are extensively hydroxylated in the rat.[54] Genetic factors influence responsiveness to anticoagulants in rabbits, as they do in rats, in which resistance to warfarin as a rodenticide is transmitted as an autosomal dominant trait.[55] The metabolites in humans are not fully characterized, but the patient with bishydroxycoumarin sensitivity just described and his mother may have a metabolic defect involving deficiency of a hepatic microsomal hydroxylase.

Increased sensitivity to coumarin anticoagulants also can result from acquired conditions, including vitamin K deficiency, increased turnover of plasma proteins, and numerous forms of liver disease that impair the subject's capacity to produce vitamin K–dependent clotting factors. Various drugs can increase the prothrombinopenic response to coumarin anticoagulants. Cinchophen may damage liver cells; phenothiazine may produce cholestasis, thereby diminishing absorption of vitamin K; phenylbutazone increases sensitivity by displacing warfarin from plasma albumin; and phenyramidol inhibits the hepatic microsomal enzymes responsible for metabolism of coumarin drugs. Resistance to warfarin derivatives also has been reported.

Acetophenetidin-Induced Methemoglobinemia

Severe methemoglobinemia and hemolysis occurred in a 17-year-old girl after she had taken phenacetin (aceto-phenetidin).[56] Multiple studies excluded heritable erythrocytic disorders, including hemoglobinopathies, and extracorpuscular compounds seemed to be causing hemolysis. As much as one-half the patient's hemoglobin was occasionally in the form of methemoglobin. After administration of phenacetin, large amounts of 2-hydroxyphenetidin and 2-hydroxyphenacetin derivatives were discovered in the girl's urine. In normal persons, more than 70 percent of a dose of 2 gm phenacetin appears in the urine as N-acetyl-para-aminophenol, with only minute amounts of the hydroxylated products that were so prevalent in this patient's urine. One sister, a brother, and both parents of the patient had a normal response to phenacetin, but another sister likewise responded abnormally.

These observations suggest an autosomal recessive inheritance of a defect in which the patient's hepatic microsomal mixed-function oxidases were deficient in deethylating capacity. Instead of being deethylated as in normal persons, phenacetin, in the patient and her 38-year-old sister, was hydroxylated.

The toxicity observed after phenacetin administration was probably produced by these hydroxylated products, since induction of the hepatic microsomal phenacetin-hydroxylating enzymes prior to administration of phenacetin by phenobarbital exacerbated the condition; i.e., severe neurologic symptoms, including bilateral positive Babinski responses, and profound methemoglobinemia developed. After the same pretreatment, a normal volunteer developed neither methemoglobinemia nor neurologic changes.

Deficient N-Glucosidation of Amobarbital

Pursuing their initial observation based on a twin study that showed large interindividual variations in elimination rates of amobarbital to be predominantly under genetic control,[57] Kalow and associates[58] investigated the family of one set of twins with a deficiency in N-hydroxylation, but not C-hydroxylation, of amobarbital. The family study of these twins disclosed that this deficiency was most likely produced through autosomal recessive transmission,[58] although only urinary ratios of these metabolites were measured. Later, this group[59] reported that the urinary metabolite was mistakenly identified as an N-hydroxylamobarbital and that the actual metabolite was instead N-β-D-glucopyranosyl amobarbital. This metabolite showed great variability in the urine of 129 volunteers studied after a single oral dose of amobarbital; one volunteer completely lacked the metabolite, whereas 14 subjects had it as the primary form.[60] Four of these 14 subjects were of Chinese origin, suggesting possible racial differences in the pattern and pathway of metabolite formation.[60] These studies on amobarbital illustrate the utility of searching whenever possible for a monogenic origin of pharmacogenetic conditions, the necessity of performing genetic analyses in families, and the need, whenever more than a single metabolite is produced from the parent drug, to measure rates of metabolite formation rather than only disappearance of the parent drug.

Polymorphic Hydroxylation of Debrisoquine

The antihypertensive drug debrisoquine has been widely used in England but not yet employed in the United States. It was observed that patients receiving debrisoquine vary widely in the hypotensive response to the adrenergic-blocking action of the drug and that a close correlation exists between debrisoquine plasma concentrations and the resultant decline in blood pressure.[61] In 94 unrelated volunteers, the urinary ratio of the parent drug to the primary metabolite, 4-hydroxy-debrisoquine, was measured after a single oral dose of 10 mg debrisoquine.[62] In 3 of these 94 subjects, the ratio was very high, suggesting a possible hepatic microsomal deficiency of N-hydroxylation of debrisoquine. Furthermore, family studies of these three volunteers with abnormally high ratios of debrisoquine to 4-hydroxy-debrisoquine in the 8-hour urinary collection suggested transmission of the metabolic deficiency as an autosomal recessive trait.[62] Most side effects, as well as most pronounced antihypertensive activity, of debrisoquine occurred in the slow metabolizers (those individuals with the highest urinary ratio of parent drug to metabolite). This result, which could have been predicted from the fact that the main metabolite is devoid of antihypertensive action, illustrates both the direct clinical and toxicologic consequences of pharmacogenetic conditions and the need for physicians observing an unusual drug response in a patient to consider genetic factors as a potential cause.

Approximately 7–9 percent of the population in the United Kingdom, Canada, and the United States are deficient metabolizers of debrisoquine. Approximately 6 percent of the population of Ghana and 3 percent of the population of Sweden are also slow metabolizers. In Ghana, heterozygotes were encountered in a higher frequency (36 percent) and homozygotes in lower frequency (58 percent) than elsewhere.[63,64]

Deficient (poor) debrisoquine metabolism is a phenotype controlled by a double dose of an autosomal gene, an affected subject receiving one gene from each parent. The same genotype evidently controls a wide variety of different phenotypes characterized by deficient metabolism of numerous drugs. These drugs, almost all of which are basic, include sparteine,[65–67] nortriptyline,[68,69] phenacetin,[70] phenformin,[71] guanoxan, dextromethorphan, certain β-adrenoreceptor-blocking drugs (such as metoprolol, alprenolol, timolol,[72] and propranolol[73]), perhexiline,[74] and encainide.[75]

Studies on liver biopsies from patients with the deficient phenotype showed absence of a single cytochrome P-450 isozyme that in extensive metabolizers could be clearly visualized on starch gel electrophoresis. This isozyme constituted only a very small proportion of the total liver content of cytochrome P-450.[76,77] Most drugs biotransformed by the debrisoquine cytochrome P-450 are also metabolized by several other pathways, each pathway being catalyzed by a different combination or family of cytochrome P-450 isozymes. Therefore, in the deficient phenotype, genetically controlled reduction of a specific cytochrome P-450 isozyme could have slightly different consequences for different drugs. For a specific drug, the outcome depends not only on the contribution of the deficient pathway to the overall pattern of hepatic drug elimination, but also on whether this particular aberrant pathway involves additional cytochrome P-450 isozymes present in the patient in normal kind and amount. Even within each of the two clearly separable phenotypes of deficient[78] and fast[79] debrisoquine 4-hydroxylation, a broad range of values occurs. Evidence indicates that the phenotype of deficient debrisoquine metabolism arises from the contribution of several different genetic loci.[78]

Since genetically deficient metabolizers of debrisoquine are also at increased risk of toxicity from decreased biotransformation of other drugs, development of a predictive test based on drug-oxidizing capacity would be useful. A subject with deficient debrisoquine metabolism has some degree of retardation in the capacity to biotransform more than 21 other basic drugs degraded in large part by the same hepatic drug-oxidizing pathway through which debrisoquine passes. This knowledge should help to prevent the dose-dependent adverse reactions seen among patients with the deficient phenotype on usual doses of these drugs. In such subjects, doses need to be reduced or alternative drugs selected that are metabolized by other pathways. The debrisoquine polymorphism exemplifies dramatically how genetic constitution determines susceptibility to drug toxicity and how it can serve to prevent toxicity by identifying sensitive subjects prior to drug administration.

Polymorphic Hydroxylation of Mephenytoin

Introduced in 1945 to treat epilepsy, mephenytoin has an antiseizure spectrum similar to that of phenytoin but is associated with significantly more toxicity, which limits its use. Mephenytoin exhibits stereoselective hepatic metabolism. (R)-Mephenytoin is slowly demethylated, whereas the (S)-enantiomer is rapidly demethylated. The demethylated product is pharmacologically active, but the (S)-enantiomer is rapidly 4-hydroxylated by hepatic mixed-function oxidases to an inactive product. However, in approximately 2–3 percent of Caucasian subjects, an autosomal recessive condition exists that causes slow or deficient 4-hydroxylation of the (S)-enantiomer of mephenytoin.[80] In deficient hydroxylators, mephenytoin accumulates, even when given in low doses, to cause sedation.[81] This polymorphism of mephenytoin metabolism differs genetically from that affecting debrisoquine, since subjects who are deficient metabolizers of one drug biotransform the other at normal rates.[81,82] Therefore, defective 4-hydroxylation of mephenytoin arises from an abnormality of a different cytochrome P-450 isozyme from that responsible for debrisoquine 4-hydroxylation. This cytochrome P-450 isozyme has been isolated and investigated, but in deficient metabolizers of mephenytoin, no drug other than mephenytoin has been shown to exhibit retarded elimination.[83] Like the debrisoquine polymorphism, the mephenytoin polymorphism is characterized by marked geographic differences in gene frequencies. However, for the mephenytoin polymorphism,

Chinese subjects exhibit a higher frequency than Caucasians for the gene that confers deficient metabolism.[83] This appears to be the reverse of the situation for the debrisoquine polymorphism.[83]

Polymorphic Methylation

Weinshilboum and Sladek[84] reported that erythrocyte thiopurine methyltransferase (TPMT) exhibited a trimodal distribution of activity in 298 randomly selected subjects. Furthermore, this distribution conformed to a Hardy-Weinberg equilibrium in which variation in TPMT activity is controlled by two alleles at a single locus with gene frequencies of 0.06 and 0.94. Family studies suggested transmission of the genetic control of TPMT activity as an autosomal codominant trait. Future studies are required to determine whether these *in vitro* results on TPMT activity exert effects *in vivo* on the metabolism of thiopurines administered as drugs, such as 6-mercaptopurine. In addition to TPMT, thiolmethyltransferase and catechol-O-methyltransferase in human erythrocytes show genetically controlled variations that are probably also attributable to two alleles at a single locus. Thus methylation phenotype may be one factor responsible for variations in the metabolism of drugs and environmental chemicals in humans.

Polymorphic Distribution of Residual Serum Paraoxonase Activity

The insecticide parathion, while inactive, has as its principal metabolite the potent insecticide paraoxon. Toxicity from paraoxon arises deliberately in insects and accidently in humans as a result of irreversible inhibition of acetylcholinesterase. This inhibition causes high concentrations of acetylcholine at receptors near the neuromuscular junction with resultant paralysis. Like the previously discussed polymorphism of S-methylation, genetic differences among subjects with respect to residual paraoxonase activity have been demonstrated only *in vitro*. Genetic differences in this arylesterase, termed *paraoxonase* or *cholinesterase,* that have been established *in vitro* probably also possess toxicologic significance *in vivo*. Studies performed *in vitro* on residual paraoxonase activity raise the possibility that certain subjects may be more or less susceptible to toxicity on exposure to paraoxon.

Geldmacher-v. Mallinchkrodt and associates[85] incubated sera of 799 unrelated German subjects with paraoxon (3.2×10^{-8} M) at 37°C for 60 minutes. The degree to which paraoxon inhibited serum cholinesterase activity under these conditions varied from 0–67 percent depending on the particular subject. Residual serum cholinesterase activity exhibited a trimodal distribution that conformed to a Hardy-Weinberg equilibrium in which two alleles at a single genetic locus controlled the observed variation. The frequencies of the two alleles p and q at this locus were 0.24 and 0.76, respectively. Approximately 57.9 percent (q^2) of 799 unrelated German subjects had low residual serum cholinesterase activity, 36.1 percent (2 pq) had medium activity, and 6 percent (p^2) had high activity. Low serum paraoxonase activity appeared to be transmitted as an autosomal recessive trait. Although it is unknown whether paraoxonase activity can be induced *in vivo* through chronic exposure to paraoxon and related chemicals, there appears to be no relationship between initial serum paraoxonase activity, age or sex, and residual serum paraoxonase activity determined under the conditions described above.

CONDITIONS IN WHICH DRUGS ACT ABNORMALLY ON THE BODY AS A RESULT OF GENETICALLY ALTERED RECEPTOR SITES

Warfarin Resistance

Genetically controlled resistance to warfarin was found in a patient, age 71 years, receiving anticoagulants for a myocardial infarction.[86] Physical and laboratory examination showed no abnormalities other than a reproducible reduction in his one-state prothrombin concentration to about 60 percent of normal. Anticoagulants were initially withheld because of the patient's low prothrombin time. They were administered after 1 month, at which time the patient proved to be resistant, rather than sensitive, to dicoumarol. A daily dose of 145 mg was required to reduce the prothrombin concentration to therapeutic levels, i.e., nearly 50 standard deviations above the mean.

Detailed studies showed that the drug was absorbed normally from the gastrointestinal tract; kinetic and binding studies also were normal. Even after administration of very high doses, warfarin was not excreted unchanged in the urine or stools, and amounts of a metabolite of warfarin similar to those recovered from the urine of normal subjects who were given equivalent amounts of the drug were recovered from the patient's urine. The patient also showed resistance to bishydroxycoumarin and the indanedione anticoagulant phenindione, but not to heparin.

An enzyme or receptor site with altered affinity for vitamin K or for anticoagulant drugs was postulated by O'Reilly et al.[87] as the mechanism responsible for resistance to warfarin in this patient. Five other members of both sexes of the patient's family over three generations also were resistant to warfarin, suggesting autosomal dominant transmission of the trait. A second large kindred of 18 patients with warfarin resistance in two generations has been reported.[88]

Various environmental conditions lead to resistance to coumarin anticoagulants as phenocopies of the genetic defect. Most commonly, the resistance is related to the simultaneous administration of inducing agents that reduce the blood concentration of anticoagulant drugs by stimulating their metabolism, e.g., barbiturates, glutethimide, chloral hydrate, and griseofulvin.

Glucose-6-Phosphate Dehydrogenase (G-6-PD) Deficiency

Formerly called *primiquine sensitivity* or *favism,* G-6-PD deficiency is the most common hereditary enzymatic abnormality in humans, and it is transmitted as an X-linked recessive disorder. More than 80 physiochemically discrete molecular variants are described, each being associated with slightly different clinical features.[89] Ordinarily, only the male hemizygote shows significant drug-related hemolysis. Female subjects may be affected mildly, as would be predicted from the Lyon hypothesis, or more severely, as in populations wherein the gene frequency is high enough that homozygosity is appreciable. A mild self-limited anemia is associated with the common variant of G-6-PD deficiency found in blacks, in whom drugs can be given repeatedly without danger, since only the susceptible, older red blood cells are removed from the circulation by hemolysis; they are rapidly replaced by resistant, younger cells.

In various Mediterranean G-6-PD deficiency variants, hemolysis affects a larger proportion of the total erythrocyte population and occurs more rapidly after administration of smaller doses of drug. Severity of hemolysis depends not only on the total activity of the mutant G-6-PD, but also on its other properties, including stability. Several properties in addition to symptomatic severity can characterize the variants, including the total erythrocytic G-6-PD activity, enzymatic electrophoretic mobility, and various kinetic measurements. The specific amino acid substitution in G-6-PD A$^+$ and in G-6-PD Hektoen has been elucideated by microfingerprinting techniques.[90,91]

The exact biochemical mechanisms by which a given drug or its metabolites cause hemolysis remain unknown. The metabolism of the erythrocyte is unusual, since it must function without benefit of a nucleus. It still needs sources of energy to maintain concentration gradients of sodium and potassium and for continual reduction of methemoglobin. This energy source is supplied by the glycolytic and oxidative pathways of glucose metabolism. Certain enzymes, including G-6-PD, lose activity as the normal cell ages, and G-6-PD activity declines with cell age faster than normal in G-6-PD-deficient cells. Therefore, older cells of persons with mutations of their G-6-PD are more susceptible to hemolysis than are younger cells.

Reactions catalyzed by G-6-PD lead to the production of nicotinamide adenine dinucleotide phosphate, reduced-form NADPH, a substance necessary for maintenance of sulfhydryl substances, such as glutathione, in the reduced (GSH) state. Sufficient quantities of reduced glutathione appear to be essential for erythrocytic membrane integrity. The sequence of events suggested in drug-induced hemolysis related to G-6-PD deficiency includes, first, the metabolism of the drug to a product more amenable to further oxidation.[92,93] The erythrocyte converts this metabolite to an intermediate oxidant. The latter then damages the erythrocyte membrane (particularly in old cells), perhaps by oxidation of reduced sulfhydryl groups. The younger cells with their higher G-6-PD activities resist the osmotic and oxidant effects of various drugs and their metabolites, whereas the older, more sensitive cells with their greater relative deficiency are eliminated.

Determining *in vitro* the hemolytic potential of new drugs continues to be of prime importance, especially in geographic areas where the incidence of the disorder is high. Numerous tests have been devised, but none is suitable, in availability and cost, for routine screening of large populations.

Hemolysis apparently may occur spontaneously or during infection in certain G-6-PD deficiency variants. Obviously, enough stress can be placed on the metabolism of G-6-PD-deficient erythrocytes to cause hemolysis by several environmental alterations in addition to those produced by drug administration.

Drug-Sensitive Hemoglobins

A life-threatening hemolytic anemia developed in a 2-year-old girl and her father after they received sulfa drugs.[94] Both subjects registered an abnormal hemoglobin content, electrophoretic mobility being between that of hemoglobins A and S.[95] Further studies showed an abnormality in the beta chain, with arginine taking the place of the usual histidine residue at the 63rd position, where the heme group is attached.[96] Fifteen of the 65 relatives examined showed the abnormal hemoglobin feature, designated *hemoglobin Zurich,* a defect transmitted as an autosomal dominant trait. In another family with the same substitution, discovered in Maryland, the severity of the hemolytic episodes was less than in the Swiss cases.[97]

Another drug-sensitive hemoglobin, hemoglobin H, is a special form of α-thalassemia. Composed of four beta chains, hemoglobin H is sensitive to the oxidant drugs described under G-6-PD deficiency. In certain regions, such as Thailand, the frequency of homozygous hemoglobin H is high, i.e., 1 in 300 individuals.

Phenylthiocarbamide-Tasting Ability

The ability to taste phenylthiocarbamide (PTC) is transmitted as an autosomal dominant trait, and tasters may be either heterozygous or homozygous.[98] This polymorphism was discovered in 1932 when Fox,[99] who synthesized the compound, noted that he could not detect a bitter taste from dust of the compound arising as it was poured into a container, whereas a colleague in the same room complained of the bitter taste.

Although this polymorphism seems to be benign, some workers have related the ability to taste PTC to thyroid disease. Administration of PTC can produce goiter in the rat. Compounds related to PTC by possessing the $N-C=S$ group, such as the antithyroid drugs methyl- and propylthiouracil, also have the same biomodality in taste perception exhibited by subjects to PTC. Forty-one percent of 134 patients with nodular goiter were nontasters,[100] an observation confirmed in 447 patients who underwent thyroidectomy for various reasons.[101] In male patients with multiple thyroid adenomas, a marked increase in nontasting frequency also was noted. Nontasters seem to be more susceptible to athyreotic cretinism as well as to adenomatous goiter. These data suggest to some investigators that nontasters may be more susceptible than tasters to environmental goitrogens. The physicochemical basis for the difference in taste perception in affected individuals is unknown.

The frequency of tasting capacity shows geographic variation in that 31.5 percent of Europeans, 10.6 percent of Chinese, and 2.7 percent of Africans are nontasters.[102,103] As with the physicochemical findings, the reasons for these variations in the gene for PTC tasting are equally obscure.

Intraocular Pressure, Steroids, and Glaucoma

A polymorphism may exist in the response of ocular pressure of normal subjects to steroids applied topically. Elevations in intraocular pressure in 80 normal persons after local administration of hr 0.1 percent ophthalmic solution of dexamethasone-21-phosphate for 4 weeks exhibited a trimodal distribution. Familial studies suggested the existence of three genotypes, namely, $P_L P_L$ for low elevations of 5 mmHg or less, $P_L P_H$ for intermediate increases from 6–15 mmHg, and $P_H P_H$ for high increments in pressure of 16 mmHg or more.

In 1968, an association was described between certain types of responses and glaucoma.[104] In a sample of patients with both open-angle hypertensive and low-tension glaucoma, the distribution of responses differed from that in the random sample of normal subjects. A marked reduction in $P_L P_L$ genotypes and a corresponding increase in $P_L P_H$ and $P_H P_H$ genotypes occurred in both conditions and surprisingly in the uninvolved eye of patients with unilateral posttraumatic glaucoma. Familial studies suggested that the response of high elevations of intraocular pressure after administration of dexamethasone was inherited as an autosomal recessive trait. Although glaucoma can occur with genotypes other than $P_H P_H$ and $P_H P_L$, it was concluded that the P_H gene is closely associated with these types of glaucoma.[104] In 1972, a twin study failed to identify a role for genetic factors in intraocular pressure response to glucocorticoids; the results showed that monozygotic twins responded to the same extent as dizygotic twins with respect to intraocular pressure to glucocorticoids.[105]

Malignant Hyperthermia and Muscular Rigidity

In 1962, hyperthermia was reported to be the cause of death in 10 of 38 family members who had received anesthesia for various surgical procedures.[106] This was the first indication that the rare, hitherto seemingly sporadic malignant hyperthermia afflicting persons exposed to various anesthetic agents might be genetically transmitted. More than 200 cases of malignant hyperthermia have been identified and have been shown to have a hereditary basis.[107] The condition is associated with muscular rigidity

and appears to be transmitted as an autosomal dominant trait. It develops during anesthesia with nitrous oxide, methoxyflurane, halothane, ether, cyclopropane, or combinations thereof and is more common in association with the use of succinylcholine as a preanesthetic agent. During anesthesia, body temperature rises rapidly, occasionally reaching 46°C.

The incidence of malignant hyperthermia is in the range of 1 in 20,000 cases of general anesthesia and exhibits no sex preference, but it does occur more in younger than in older anesthetized patients. Approximately two-thirds of the patients die, usually from cardiac arrest. The degree of rigidity is variable, differing from patient to patient, sometimes being absent. This variability may indicate that the term *malignant hyperthermia* refers to several discrete diseases.

Occasionally, rigidity is so marked that the body literally becomes as stiff as a board, progressing without interruption into rigor mortis. Intravenous administration of procaine or procainamide is reported to alleviate the rigidity and fever in certain cases. Curare is ineffective. Interestingly, a limb under tourniquet does not become rigid, suggesting a peripheral rather than a central lesion. Animal models have been produced in dogs treated with halothane and dinitrophenol and in Landrace pigs.

ASSOCIATIONS WITHOUT WELL-ESTABLISHED MENDELIAN MECHANISMS BETWEEN GENETIC FACTORS AND RESPONSE TO DRUGS

Tests *in Vitro* Predict Risk for Drug Toxicity *in Vivo*

Spielberg and colleagues[108,109] developed an intriguing approach consisting of an *in vitro* test to phenotype family members as well as unrelated subjects for the potential to exhibit idiosyncratic drug reactions *in vivo*. They selected acetaminophen and phenytoin for initial investigation because tissue damage from these drugs, although rare, is generally considered to result from reactive intermediates generated during the course of their hepatic metabolism. In the initial studies, human lymphocytes isolated on a Ficoll gradient served as target cells for reactive intermediates produced on incubating for 2 hours varying concentrations of acetaminophen with murine hepatic microsomes and an NADPH-generating system.[109] When enough acetaminophen was added to deplete glutathione (GSH) 80 percent or more, lymphocytes began to die. If either hepatic microsomes or the NADPH-generating system were not included, GSH depletion and cell lysis ceased, indicating that the lymphocytes did not themselves form toxic metabolites of acetaminophen, but rather reacted with such metabolites generated by the murine microsomes.

Lymphocytes from patients who had previously experienced idiosyncratic reactions to drugs *in vivo* were later removed and reexposed to drug under the *in vitro* test conditions described above. These lymphocytes lysed much more frequently than did normal lymphocytes in such a test system. Very rarely, subjects who ingest phenytoin develop an idiosyncratic reaction consisting of fever, rash, hepatotoxicity, and lymphoadenopathy.[110,111] Since this syndrome resembles infectious mononucleosis, rubella, collagen-vascular disease, and even lymphoma, an in vitro test was needed to increase the specificity of diagnosis. Accordingly, Spielberg and associates[112] examined in vitro the lymphocyte toxicity of four anticonvulsants, phenobarbital, phenytoin, mephenytoin, and phenacemide, using the assay described above.

In patients receiving these antiseizure agents chronically, phenobarbital and phenytoin produce idiosyncratic reactions only very rarely, whereas mephenytoin and phenacemide carry a higher risk, causing approximately 1 among 20 cases of all drug-induced liver and bone marrow toxicities.[113] As above, murine hepatic microsomes and NADPH were required in the in vitro mixture together with drug for toxicity to occur in the form of cell lysis.

To explain the development of phenytoin hepatotoxicity among subjects who chronically received phenytoin, Spielberg et al.[114] postulated a defect in the mechanism of normal arene oxide detoxification. In affected subjects, a mutant form of epoxide hydrolase (EH) was hypothesized as the molecular basis for the abnormal drug reaction. This aberrant EH could detoxify arene oxide only very slowly and inefficiently. Phenytoin arene oxides would thus be much longer-lived than usual and therefore tend to form more covalent bonds, thereby damaging various cellular macromolecules. Lymphocytes from three patients with well-established phenytoin toxicity in vivo were investigated in vitro under the conditions of the preceding assay, and the results obtained supported the hypothesis.[114]

Potential causation of human birth defects by arene oxide metabolites of phenytoin was investigated with the same in vitro system described above.[115] Lymphocytes taken from 24 children exposed to phenytoin throughout gestation, as well as from members of their families, were challenged in a blind protocol with phenytoin metabolites derived from a murine hepatic microsomal drug-metabolizing system. Fourteen of the 24 children exhibited a positive test result: a significant increase in lymphocyte death in vitro associated with phenytoin metabolites.[115] Moreover, each child with a positive result had a parent with a positive result, thereby suggesting the possibility of a dominant Mendelian pattern of transmission of this form of phenytoin toxicity. It was concluded that a positive in vitro challenge of phenytoin administration to certain subjects' lymphocytes correlated highly with major birth defects, including congenital heart disease, cleft lip and palate, microcephaly, and so on.

These investigators extended their studies on the potential toxicity of reactive metabolites of acetaminophen and phenytoin to other drugs, including nitrofurantoin.[116] Similar conclusions drawn for different drugs under the conditions of this in vitro test have thus become generalizable, and it now seems that toxicity can arise from numerous drugs that require activation to arene oxides if a particular subject bears a genetically transmitted defect

or block in the conversion of a highly reactive arene oxide to an inactive dihydrodiol. Ultimately, subjects with such genetically transmitted susceptibility to drug toxicities might be identified by the test in vitro before they are exposed in vivo to any offending agents.

Blood Groups

Possible correlations between adverse reactions to drugs and genetic factors were determined by a survey of hospitalized patients.[117,118] In young women developing venous thromboembolism while taking oral contraceptives, a significant deficit was discovered of blood group O individuals relative to those possessing groups A and AB combined.

A correlation was found between ABO blood groups and the development of arrhythmias after administration of digoxin, with decreased risk in blood group O patients relative to non-O patients.

Diphenhydramine in Orientals and Caucasians

Spector et al.[119] showed that the kinetics and psychomotor effects of diphenhydramine differed in Orientals and Caucasians. After either oral or intravenous administration of diphenhydramine, Caucasians had not only plasma drug concentrations twice as high as Orientals at each time point tested, but also more sedation and deterioration in psychomotor performance than did Orientals. Plasma clearance and apparent volume of distribution, but not plasma half-life, of dephenhydramine were higher in Orientals than in Caucasians. Whether these kinetic and dynamic differences in response to diphenhydramine had a genetic cause or were related to such environmental differences as diet, smoking, and so on or a combination of factors could not be resolved in this study.

Depression and Antidepressants

It has been suggested that symptoms of depression are produced by at least two genetically distinct entities and that "endogenous" depressions more frequently benefit from treatment with imipramine, whereas "reactive" depressions improve after administration of monoamine oxidase (MAO) inhibitors.[120] Data supporting this hypothesis are based on similarities in drug response between probands and relatives who also suffered from depression and who also received imipramine, MAO inhibitors, or lithium carbonate. The concordance in drug response among depressed relatives and depressed probands was reported to be statistically greater than expected by chance alone. Studies in different patients tended to confirm these initial impressions.[121]

Striking differences may exist in the genetic background of lithium responders compared with nonresponders. Genetic determination of large interindividual variations in lithium ion distribution was observed in a study of monozygotic and dizygotic twins.[122]

Association Between HLA Haplotype and Drug Response

The human leukocyte antigens (HLA) are genetic determinants on a single chromosome which, taken together, constitute a haplotype. Accordingly, every person has two haplotypes, one inherited from each parent. At least four closely linked loci, only a few centimorgans apart on the short arm of human chromosome 6, control the synthesis of antigens on the surface of leukocytes. Because of their close linkage, the specific genes at these four loci only rarely separate during meiosis through crossover between homologous chromosomes. Of interest is the extreme genetic heterogeneity of these four loci, more than 100 alleles having been identified, theoretically enabling more than 1 million different phenotypes. HLA loci and loci closely linked to them function in immune surveillance, protecting the body from several types of environmental assaults. For example, these genes serve to combat viral and other pathogens and are active in the rejection response to foreign tissues.[123,124] Pertinent to this discussion, certain HLA haplotypes markedly increase susceptibility to diseases associated with immunologic impairment, such as chronic active hepatitis, glomerulonephritis, ankylosing spondylitis, Reiter's syndrome, rheumatoid arthritis, and disseminated lupus erythematosus.[123,124] In certain HLA haplotypes, risk of these disorders, characterized by derangement of normal immunologic mechanisms, can be increased by up to 40-fold above that of the population at large.[123,124]

For reasons as yet unclear, some uncommon alleles at the HLA loci may be much more strongly associated with certain drug responses than other alleles. For example, in schizophrenic patients, HLA-A1 has been reported to be highly associated with a favorable response to chlorpromazine.[125,126] In contrast, HLA-A2 appeared to be associated with an unfavorable response. In patients with affective disorders treated with lithium, HLA-A3 was associated with a high rate of relapse.[127]

With respect to adverse reactions to drugs, in patients with rheumatoid arthritis treated with sodium aurothiomalate, adverse reactions, particularly proteinuria, occurred 32 times more frequently in the HLA-DR3 haplotype.[128] Also, in patients with rheumatoid arthritis, agranulocytosis after levamisole was encountered much more frequently in subjects with the rare haplotype HLA-B27.[129] Hydralazine-induced systemic lupus erythematosus occurred twice to three times more frequently in hypertensive patients with HLA-DR4 haplotype who received the drug.[130] Another genetically determined phenotype, slow acetylation of hydralazine, also is associated with increased susceptibility to lupus.[131] Although the acetylation polymorphism itself does not appear to be linked to any HLA haplotype,[130] potential linkages between other HLA haplotypes and different pharmacogenetic polymorphisms remain to be established and merit study.

Genetic Factors Affecting the Disposition of Commonly Used Drugs

Because most of the conditions just described are rare and produce toxicity after only a few drugs, they probably contribute only to a small extent to the current major medical problem of adverse drug reactions. Another development in pharmacogenetics suggests, however, that among subjects genetic differences that directly affect drug disposition play a prominent role in commonly encountered forms of drug toxicity. This idea was suggested by a series of experiments that examined rates at which healthy adult identical and fraternal twins cleared commonly used drugs administered to them in single doses. These twins were in a basal state with respect to most of the factors listed in Figure 1. This means that they were nonmedicated and living in different households and were not exposed at work or at home to such inducing agents as ethanol consumption or chronic cigarette smoking.

Twins are of two types: Identical twins have identical heredities, since they arise from a single fertilized egg, and are accordingly termed *monozygotic;* whereas fraternal twins arise from two fertilized eggs, are called *dizygotic,* and are no more alike genetically than siblings, except that they are born at the same time. After phenylbutazone, bishydroxycoumarin, antipyrine, halothane, ethanol, diphenylhydantoin, nortriptyline, or salicylate were administered alone, large interindividual variations that existed among unrelated people vanished within sets of identical twins but were preserved in most, but not all, sets of fraternal twins (Figure 4–2). The magnitude of interindividual variations in rates of drug elimination among unrelated people was 30-fold for nortriptyline, 10-fold for bishydroxycoumarin, 4-fold for phenylbutazone and antipyrine, 3-fold for halothane, and 2-fold for ethanol. Family studies on three of these drugs substantiated observations made in twins; in families, predominantly polygenic mechanisms appeared to control large interindividual variations in the disposition of the tested drugs. More studies have to be done using twins and families in which rates of production of metabolites are examined both in blood and in urine rather than simply disappearance of parent drug.

Precise determination of the mode of inheritance is usually quite easy with single-gene traits, especially if they are rare. Family studies are invaluable; alleles segregate during gamete formation and rejoin in offspring to form gene combinations that can be detected by their phenotypic expression.

Polygenic inheritance produces a different picture. Instead of alleles at only a single gene location, alleles at several sites on a chromosome or chromosomes contribute to the formation of the phenotype. The effect of each gene is not as profound as it is with single-gene inheritance; instead, the final expression is a combination of genetic plus environmental effects.

The possibility remains that the long-sustained influence of certain environmental factors could be responsible in some measure for the particular rate of drug disposition of an individual who might otherwise appear to be in a basal state. To explore this possibility, a careful

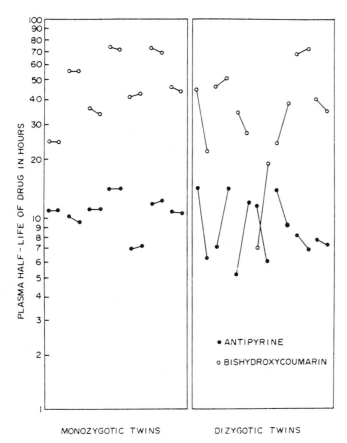

MONOZYGOTIC TWINS   DIZYGOTIC TWINS

FIGURE 4–2. Plasma half-lives of bishydroxycoumarin and antipyrine were measured separately at an interval of more than 6 months in healthy monozygotic (identical) and dizygotic (fraternal) twins. A solid line joins the values for each set of twins for each drug. Note that intratwin differences in the plasma half-life of both bishydroxycoumarin and antipyrine are smaller in monozygotic than in most dizygotic twins. (Reprinted with permission from Vesell.[132])

inquiry into the individual's exposure at home and at work to these factors is necessary. The existence and operation of numerous environmental factors (see Figure 4–1), each with different capabilities of altering the basal, genetically controlled rate of drug disposition, make it exceedingly difficult to attribute quantitatively different portions of the total interindividual variation to specific single environmental factors. The task of partitioning the total interindividual variation in drug elimination of large heterogeneous populations into component parts is further complicated because such seemingly pure "environmental" factors as smoking and diet are closely associated with other environmental factors, as well as with genetic factors. Extrapolation to a large population of the precise contribution of a particular trait, such as vegetarianism, to interindividual variations in rates of drug elimination observed in a selected, small study population can be hazardous. Such extrapolations should be accompanied by a demonstration that the frequency of the particular trait in the study group is similar to its frequency in the larger population. Without such demonstration, the quantitative contribution of the trait cannot be legitimately extrapolated from the small study group to the large population. The simultaneous contributions of multiple

genetic and environmental factors to the particular drug-metabolizing activity of a given individual, as well as the change in relative importance of these different factors with time and condition, such as during aging, fever, disease, dietary change, drug administration, acute or chronic exposure to environmental chemicals, etc., make it exceedingly difficult to quantitate the relative influence of the numerous factors involved at any given time, other than in a transient, relatively basal state. Also, for these reasons, carefully controlled studies are required.

The hereditary control of large variations in drug disposition among healthy, nonmedicated volunteers in a basal state with respect to rates of drug elimination has several potentially useful implications. First, determination of drug half-lives in plasma or saliva might be ascertained before chronic drug administration as a guide to adjusting dosage according to individual requirements, thereby helping to reduce the frequent occurrences of toxicity or undertreatment encountered when the same dose of a drug is given to all subjects. Second, if within a subject correlations existed in capacity to metabolize various drugs, drugs could be grouped into categories. Once the rate of metabolism of one drug in a category has been ascertained, as in debrisoquine polymorphism, the rate of handling all the others in that category could be readily calculated, and judgments as to dosage could again be made. Several investigations suggest that correlations in drug-metabolizing capacity exist for a few, but not the majority of chemically unrelated drugs. One study established correlations between the plasma half-lives of bishydroxycoumarin and phenylbutazone. Another investigation reported correlations between steady-state blood concentrations of desmethylimipramine or nortriptyline and the plasma half-life of oxyphenylbutazone. For certain drugs, therefore, a common rate-limiting step may exist in the several reactions required for drug metabolism within the liver. Some enzyme(s) catalyzing a rate-limiting step common in the oxidation of several drugs could be responsible for these surprising correlations in rates of drug elimination. Attempts to develop further drug categories constitute a major effort in pharmacogenetics.

Third, physicians should be alert for the introduction of environmental factors that might change their patients' genetically determined drug-biotransforming capacity. For example, diseases affecting cardiovascular, thyroid, renal, or hepatic status; environmental exposure on a large scale to such agents as insecticides, nicotine, polycyclic hydrocarbons, or caffeine; and finally, chronic administration of many drugs either alone or in combination can influence the duration and intensity of drug action. Not only in cases of polygenic or multifactorial inheritance are the influences of the environment of consequence. Although it is recognized that intelligence, which probably has some polygenic influence, can be altered by environmental insults such as malnutrition, viruses, and toxic chemicals, it is also important to recognize environmental influences on single-gene conditions. For example, acute intermittent porphyria is an autosomal dominant condition characterized by sudden attacks of burgundy-colored urine. Although bouts may occur without apparent environmental insult, administration of barbiturates is followed by explosive clinical attacks. Similarly, acute exacerbations of diabetes mellitus and gout can be precipitated by environmental changes involving diet, drugs, or both.

Of more theoretical interest is the relationship between genetic differences among subjects in rates of drug metabolism and the production of potentially toxic biotransformation products of a parent drug. In the past, the hepatic drug-metabolizing enzyme system has been regarded as a "detoxification" system because this system converted lipid-soluble parent compounds that could remain indefinitely in the body into more polar metabolites that could be easily excreted in the urine. More recently, however, it has been recognized that this enzyme system can produce potentially toxic, highly reactive metabolites that combine with tissue proteins to produce necrosis, immunologic reactivity, and even cancer. Differences among subjects in pathways by which they degrade drugs, as well as quantitative differences in the enzyme activities of the proteins that catalyze these reactions and pathways, could be involved in the regulation and control of such tissue damage. Thus genetic differences among subjects can render certain individuals more or less sensitive to drug toxicity from these different reactive metabolites.

THERAPY OF GENETIC DISEASES

A fascinating aspect of pharmacogenetics deals with the therapy of genetic lesions. Once an inborn error of metabolism is defined to permit isolation of the primary gene product, theoretically, it should be possible to relieve the metabolic block by administration of the purified protein or DNA obtained from a normal source. Because enzymes are highly efficient catalysts, a very small amount of enzyme might reverse the toxicity arising from such genetic defects. Practical therapeutic problems involve production of a sufficiently stable enzyme or other protein to be administered as a drug and its transport across several membranes into the appropriate cells. Certainly, the most widely known example of protein replacement is the use of insulin in cases of diabetes mellitus; the hormone successfully returns blood sugar levels in these patients to normal. Insulin does not correct the small-blood-vessel disease, however, which continues unabated. This has led some to suggest that the basic defect in diabetes involves more than a simple deficiency of insulin.

Another approach to therapy involves passing a patient's plasma through columns or over sheets of stably bound enzyme to reduce the level of a toxic substrate, thereby favoring the removal of intracellular toxic substrates through reequilibration. Still another approach to enzyme replacement is suggested by the observation that for certain diseases characterized by abnormal accumulation of mucopolysaccharides, mixed cultures of cells from two genetically distinct forms of the disease grow normally. Some molecules pass between contiguous cells, reducing mucopolysaccharide accumulation. It seems reasonable to expect that such molecules, purified and given to patients, might produce therapeutic benefit in certain mucopolysaccharidoses.

The need for replacement would be obviated if organ transplants could supply normal protein to genetically affected subjects. Bone marrow transplantation for various immunologic deficiency states is an example of the replacement technique. Enzyme replacement need not be considered in other cases of inherited defects. As long as the body has some residual enzyme activity present, more of the necessary enzyme product can be obtained by supplying more of the enzyme substrate, as exemplified by administration of vitamin B_{12} to patients with methylmalonic acidemia.

Avoidance of drugs and metabolic intermediates that may be toxic in individuals with various pharmacogenetic conditions is a cardinal therapeutic principle. Particularly liable to toxicity are individuals with G-6-PD deficiency, in whom innumerable drugs initiate an acute anemia due to red blood cell breakage. Limitation of intake of potentially harmful precursors is recommended in phenylketonuria, in which the amino acid phenylalanine is the offending compound. Failure to remove phenylalanine from the diet at the time of birth is followed by the development of severe mental retardation, whereas removal of phenylalanine during the first few years of life results in the development of normal intelligence.

In some disorders, enzyme inhibitors can be given to decrease production of toxic substances. Gout is a genetically transmitted disease characterized by an increased body content of uric acid, by bouts of acute arthritis, and by precipitation of urate in various tissues throughout the body, including the kidney, as a result of limited solubility of uric acid in body fluids. Allopurinol was specifically synthesized to inhibit the enzyme xanthine oxidase, which catalyzes the formation of uric acid. Thus, in treated individuals, uric acid fails to form, and uric acid precursors, which have greater solubility in body fluids, are eliminated from the body.

In other inherited genetic defects, treatment has been directed toward the removal of toxic substances. Two such conditions, Wilson's disease and cystinuria, are treated with penicillamine, which removes copper ions and cystine, respectively. Without treatment, patients with Wilson's disease develop spasticity, tremor, and liver disease as a result of copper accumulation in the brain and liver, and patients with cystinuria develop renal stones composed or pure cystine.

Finally, primary genetic material in the form of DNA or RNA has been provided to human mutant cells in culture to induce production of a normal enzyme absent in the mutant cells. Cultured cells from patients with galactosemia, who lack an enzyme that metabolizes galactose, were infected with a bacterial virus that carried the normal enzyme. The previously deficient cells were then able to synthesize the enzyme. Techniques have been developed for transferring genetic material from one bacterium to another with the eventual incorporation of the transferred piece into the host cell. These experiments offer hope for application in the therapy of genetic disease. At present, severe genetic diseases are usually not amenable to effective therapy. Advances in prenatal diagnosis by means of amniocentesis have resulted generally in therapeutic abortions rather than in early initiation of effective treatment. Genetic therapy may become available in the future through development of some of the approaches outlined here, but much progress must be made before these hopes are realized.

REFERENCES

1. Cluff LE, Thornton GL, Smith J: Epidemiological study of adverse drug reaction. Trans Assoc Am Physicians 78:255, 1965
2. Gillette JR: Factors affecting drug metabolism: Drug metabolism in man. Ann NY Acad Sci 179:43, 1971
3. Conney AH, Welch R, Kuntzman R, et al: Effects of environmental chemicals on the metabolism of drugs, carcinogens and normal body constituents in man. Ann NY Acad Sci 179:155, 1971
4. Vesell ES: Factors altering the response of mice to hexobarbital. Pharmacology 1:81, 1968
4a. Vesell ES: Pharmacogenetics. Biochem Pharmacol 24:445, 1975
5. Vesell ES: Recent progress in pharmacogenetics. Adv Pharmacol Chemother 7:1, 1969
6. Vesell ES (ed): Drug metabolism in man. Ann NY Acad Sci 179:1, 1971
7. Takahara S: Progressive oral gangrene probably due to lack of catalase in the blood (acatalasemia). Lancet 263:1101, 1952
8. Takahara S, Sato H, Doi M, et al: Acatalasemia. III. On the heredity of acatalasemia. Proc Jpn Acad 28:585, 1952
9. Takahara S, Doi K: Statistical study of acatalasemia (a review of thirty-eight cases appearing in the literature). Acta Med Okayama 13:209–219, 1959
10. Takahara S, Hamilton HB, Neel JV, et al: Hypocatalasemia: A new genetic carrier state. J Clin Invest 39:610, 1960
11. Wyngaarden JB, Howell RW: Acatalasia, in Stanbury JB, Wyngaarden JB, Frederickson DS (eds): The Metabolic Basis of Inherited Disease. New York, McGraw-Hill, 1966
12. Hamilton HB, Neel JV: Genetic heterogeneity in human acatalasia. Am J Hum Genet 15:408, 1963
13. Yata H: A case of acatalasemia. Nihou Shika Hyoron 204:7, 1959
14. Aebi H, Heiniger JP, Butler R, et al: Two cases of acatalasia in Switzerland. Experientia 17:466, 1961
15. Aebi H, Suter H: Acatalasemia, in Harris H, Hirschhorn K (eds): Advances in Human Genetics, vol 2. New York, Plenum Press, 1971
16. Hughes HB: On the metabolic fate of isoniazid. J Pharmacol Exp Ther 109:444, 1953
17. Hughes HB, Biehl JP, Jones AP, et al: Metabolism of isoniazid in man as related to the occurrence of peripheral neuritis. Am Rev Tuberc 70:226, 1954
18. Price Evans DAP, White TA: Human acetylation polymorphism. J Lab Clin Med 63:394, 1964
19. Price Evans DAP: Individual variations of drug metabolism as a factor in drug toxicity. Ann NY Acad Sci 123:178, 1965
20. Reidenberg MM, Drayer DE, Levy M, et al: Polymorphic acetylation of procainamide in man. Clin Pharmacol Ther 17:722, 1975
21. Cartwright RA, Glashan RW, Rogers HJ, et al: The role of N-acetyltransferase phenotypes in bladder carcinogenesis: A pharmacogenetic epidemiological approach to bladder cancer. Lancet 2:842, 1982
22. Weber WW, Hein DW: N-Acetylation pharmacogenetics. Pharmacol Rev 37:25, 1985
23. Kalow W: Pharmacogenetics: Heredity and the Reponse to Drugs. Philadelphia, Saunders, 1962
24. Peters J: Relationship between plasma concentration and urinary excretion of isoniazid, in Transactions of the Conference on Chemotherapy of Tuberculosis, 18th Conference, St. Louis Medical Society Auditorium, St. Louis, Missouri, 1959
25. Mitchell JR, Thorgeirsson UP, Black M, et al: Increased incidence of isoniazid hepatitis in rapid acetylators: Possible relation to hydrazine metabolites. Clin Pharmacol Ther 18:70, 1975
26. Mitchell JR, Zimmerman HJ, Ishak KG, et al: Isoniazid liver injury: Clinical spectrum, pathology and probable pathogenesis. Ann Intern Med 84:181, 1976
27. Smith J, Tyrrell WF, Gow A, et al: Hepatotoxicity in rifampin–isoniazid treated patients related to their rate of isoniazid inactivation. Chest 61:587, 1972
28. Lal S, Singhal SN, Burley DM, et al: Effect of rifampicin and isoniazid on liver function. Br Med J 1:148, 1972
29. Price Evans DAP, Manley K, McKusick VA: Genetic control of isoniazid metabolism in man. Br Med J 2:485, 1960
30. Motulsky A: Pharmacogenetics. Prog Med Genet 3:49, 1964
31. Sunahara S: Genetical, geographical and clinical studies of isoniazid metabolism, in Proceedings of the 16th International Tuberculosis Conference, Toronto, 1961
32. Harris HW: Isoniazid metabolism in humans: Genetic control, variation among races, and influence on the chemotherapy of tuberculosis, in Proceedings of the 16th International Tuberculosis Conference, Toronto, 1961
33. Price Evans DAP: Pharmacogenetique. Med Hyg 20:905, 1962
34. Evans FT, Gray PWS, Lehmann H, et al: Sensitivity to succinylcholine in relation to serum cholinesterase. Lancet 262:1229, 1952
35. Kalow W, Genest K: A method for the detection of atypical forms of human serum cholinesterase: Determination of dibucaine numbers. Can J Biochem 35:229, 1957
36. Davies RO, Marton AV, Kalow W: The action of normal and atypical cholinesterase of human serum upon a series of esters of choline. Can J Biochem 38:545, 1960
37. Kalow W, Davies RO: The activity of various esterase inhibitors toward atypical human serum cholinesterase. Biochem Pharmacol 1:183, 1959
38. Harris H, Whittaker M: Differential inhibition of human serum cholinesterase with fluoride: Recognition of two new phenotypes. Nature 191:496, 1961
39. Harris H, Whittaker M: The serum cholinesterase variants: A study of twenty-two families selected via the "intermediate" phenotype. Ann Hum Genet 26:59, 1962
40. Hodgkin WE, Giblett ER, Levin H, et al: Complete pseudocholinesterase deficiency: Genetic and immunologic characterization. J Clin Invest 44:486, 1965
41. Goedde HW, Altland K: Evidence for different "silent genes" in the human serum pseudocholinesterase polymorphism. Ann NY Acad Sci 151:540, 1968
42. Harris H, Whittaker M, Lehmann H, et al: The pseudocholinesterase variants: Esterase levels and dibucaine numbers in families selected through suxamethonium-sensitive individuals. Acta Genet 10:1, 1960
43. Lehmann H, Liddell J: Genetical variants of human serum pseudocholinesterase. Prog Med Genet 3:75, 1964
44. Garry PJ, Oretz AA, Lubraw T, et al: New allele at cholinesterase locus. J Med Genet 13:38, 1976
45. LaDu BN: The isoniazid and pseudocholinesterase polymorphisms. Fed Proc 31:1276, 1972
46. Gutsche BB, Scott EM, Wright RC: Hereditary deficiency of pseudocholinesterase in eskimos. Nature 215:322, 1967
47. Neitlich HW: Increased plasma cholinesterase activity and succinylcholine resistance: A genetic variant. J Clin Invest 45:380, 1966
48. Yoshida A, Motulsky AG: A pseudocholinesterase variant (E Cynthiana) with elevated plasma enzyme activity. Am J Hum Genet 21:486, 1969
49. Harris H, Hopkinson DA, Robson EB, et al: Genetical studies on a new variant of serum cholinesterase detected by electrophoresis. Ann Hum Genet 26:359, 1963
50. Maynert EW: The metabolic fate of diphenylhydantoin in man. J Pharmacol Exp Ther 130:275, 1960
51. Kutt H, Wolk M, Scherman R, et al: Insufficient parahydroxylation as a cause of diphenylhydantoin toxicity. Neurology 14:542, 1964
52. Brennan RW, Dehejia H, Kutt H, et al: Diphenylhydantoin intoxication attendant to slow inactivation of isoniazid. Neurology 18:283, 1968
53. Solomon MH: Variations in metabolism of coumarin anticoagulant drugs. Ann NY Acad Sci 151:932, 1968
54. Ikeda M, Sezesny B, Barnes M: Enhanced metabolism and decreased toxicity of warfarin in rats pretreated with phenobarbital, DDT or chlordane. Fed Proc 25:417, 1966
55. Greaves JH, Ayres P: Heritable resistance to warfarin in rats. Nature 215:877, 1967

56. Shahidi NT: Acetophenetidin sensitivity. Am J Dis Child 113:81, 1967

57. Endrenyi L, Inaba T, Kalow W: Genetic study of amobarbital elimination based on its kinetics in twins. Clin Pharmacol Ther 20:701, 1976

58. Kalow W, Kadar D, Inaba T, et al: A case of deficiency of N-hydroxylation of amobarbital. Clin Pharmacol Ther 21:530, 1977

59. Tang BK, Kalow W: Amobarbital metabolism in man: N-Glucoside formation. Res Commun Chem Pathol Pharmacol 21:45, 1978

60. Kalow W, Tang BK, Kadar D, et al: Distinctive patterns of amobarbital metabolites. Clin Pharmacol Ther 24:576, 1978

61. Silas JH, Lennard MS, Tucker GT, et al: Why hypertensive patients vary in their response to oral debrisoquine. Br Med J 1:422, 1977

62. Mahgoub A, Dring LG, Idle JR, et al: Polymorphic hydroxylation of debrisoquine in man. Lancet 2:584, 1977

63. Woolhouse NM, Andoh B, Mahgoub A, et al: Debrisoquin hydroxylation polymorphism among Ghanaians and Caucasians. Clin Pharmacol Ther 26:584, 1979

64. Woolhouse NM, Eichelbaum M, Oates NS, et al: Dissociation of coregulatory control of debrisoquin/phenformin and sparteine oxidation in Ghanaians. Clin Pharmacol Ther 37:512, 1985

65. Eichelbaum M, Spannbrucker N, Steinecke B, et al: Defective N-oxidation of spartein in man: A new pharmacogenetic defect. Eur J Clin Pharmacol 18:183, 1979

66. Eichelbaum M, Bertilsson L, Sawe J, et al: Polymorphic oxidation of sparteine and debrisoquine: Related pharmacogenetic entities. Clin Pharmacol Ther 31:184, 1982

67. Inaba T, Otton SV, Kalow W: Deficient metabolism of debrisoquine and sparteine. Clin Pharmacol Ther 27:547, 1980

68. Bertilsson L, Eichelbaum M, Mellstrom B, et al: Nortriptyline and antipyrine clearance in relation to debrisoquine hydroxylation in man. Life Sci 27:1673, 1980

69. Mellstrom B, Bertilsson L, Sawe J, et al: (E)- and (Z)-10-hydroxylation of nortriptyline: Relationship to polymorphic debrisoquine hydroxylation. Clin Pharmacol Ther 30:189, 1981

70. Sloan TP, Mahgoub A, Lancaster R, et al: Polymorphism of carbon oxidation of drugs and clinical implications. Br Med J 2:655, 1978

71. Shah RR, Oates NS, Idle JR, et al: Genetic impairment of phenformin metabolism. Lancet 2:1147, 1980

72. Alvan G, von Bahr C, Seideman P, et al: High plasma concentration of β-receptor blocking drugs and deficient debrisoquine hydroxylation. Lancet 1:333, 1982

73. Shah RR, Oates NS, Idle JR, et al: Beta blockers and drug oxidation status. Lancet 1:1019, 1982

74. Shah RR, Oates NS, Idle JR, et al: Impaired oxidation of debrisoquine in patients with perhexiline neuropathy. Br Med J 284:295, 1982a

75. Woosley RL, Roden DM, Duff HJ, et al: Coinheritance of deficient oxidative metabolism of encainide and debrisoquine. Clin Res 29:501A, 1981

76. Davis DS, Kahn GC, Murray S, et al: Evidence for an enzymatic defect in the 4-hydroxylation of debrisoquine by human liver. Br J Clin Pharmacol 11:89, 1981

77. Meier PJ, Mueller HK, Dick B, et al: Hepatic mono-oxygenase activities in subjects with a genetic defect in drug oxidation. Gastroenterology 85:682, 1983

78. Steiner E, Iselius L, Alvan G, et al: A family study of genetic and environmental factors determining polymorphic hydroxylation of debrisoquin. Clin Pharmacol Ther 38:394, 1985

79. Bertilsson L, Aberg-Wistedt A, Gustafsson LL, et al: Extremely rapid hydroxylation of debrisoquine: A case report with implication for treatment with nortriptyline and other tricyclic antidepressants. Ther Drug Monit 7:478, 1985

80. Kupfer A, Preisig R: Pharmacogenetics of mephenytoin: A new drug hydroxylation polymorphism in man. Eur J Clin Pharmacol 26:753, 1984

81. Inaba T, Jurima M, Nakano M, et al: Mephenytoin and sparteine pharmacogenetics in Canadian Caucasians. Clin Pharmacol Ther 36:670, 1984

82. Wedlund PJ, Aslanian WS, McAllister CB, et al: Mephenytoin hydroxylation deficiency in Caucasians: Frequency of a new oxidative drug metabolism polymorphism. Clin Pharmacol Ther 36:773, 1984

83. Omenn GS, Gelboin HV: Banbury Report, Vol. 16. Cold Spring Harbor, New York, Cold Spring Harbor Laboratory, 1984

84. Weinshilboum RM, Sladek SL: Mercaptopurine pharmacogenetics: Monogenic inheritance of erythrocyte thiopurine methyltransferase activity. Am J Hum Genet 32:651, 1980

85. Geldmacher-v Mallinckrodt M, Hommel G, Dumback J, et al: On the genetics of the human serum paraoxonase. Hum Genet 50:313, 1979

86. O'Reilly RA, Aggeler PM, Hoag MS, et al: Hereditary transmission of exceptional resistance to coumarin anticoagulant drugs: The first reported kindred. N Engl J Med 271:809, 1964

87. O'Reilly RA, Pool JG, Aggeler PM: Hereditary resistance to coumarin anticoagulant drugs in man and rat. Ann NY Acad Sci 151:913, 1968

88. O'Reilly RA: The second reported kindred with hereditary resistance to oral anticoagulant drugs. N Engl J Med 282:1448, 1970

89. Motulsky AG, Yoshida A, Stamatoyannopoulos G: Variants of glucose-6-phosphate dehydrogenase. Ann NY Acad Sci 179:636, 1971

90. Yoshida A: Amino acid substitution (histidine to tyrosine) in a glucose-6-phosphate dehydrogenase variant (G6PD Hekteon) associated with overproduction. J Mol Biol 52:483, 1970

91. Yoshida A: A single amino acid substitution (asparagine to aspartic acid) between normal (B+) and the common negro variant (A+) of human glucose-6-phosphate dehydrogenase. Proc Natl Acad Sci USA 57:835, 1967

92. Fraser IM, Tilton BE, Vesell ES: Effects of some metabolites of hemolytic drugs on young and old, normal and G6PD-deficient human erythrocytes. Ann NY Acad Sci 71:644, 1971

93. Fraser IM, Tilton BE, Vesell ES: Alterations in normal and G6PD-deficient human erythrocytes of various ages after exposure to metabolites of hemolytic drugs. Pharmacology 5:173, 1971

94. Hitzig WH, Frick PG, Betke K, et al: Hemoglobin Zürich: A new hemoglobin anomaly with sulfonamide-induced inclusion body anemia. Helv Paediatr Acta 15:499, 1960

95. Frick PG, Hitzig WH, Betke K: Hemoglobin Zürich. I. A new hemoglobin anomaly associated with acute hemolytic episodes with inclusion bodies after sulfonamide therapy. Blood 29:261, 1962

96. Muller CJ, Kingma S: Hemoglobin Zürich: $\alpha_2 A \beta_2$-63 Arg. Biochem Biophys Acta 50:595, 1961

97. Rieder RF, Zinkham WH, Holtzman NA: Hemoglobin Zürich: Clinical chemical and kinetic studies. Am J Med 39:4, 1965

98. Blakeslee AF: Genetics of sensory thresholds: Taste for phenyl thiocarbamide. Proc Natl Acad Sci USA 18:120, 1932

99. Fox, AL: The relationship between chemical constitution and taste. Proc Natl Acad Sci USA 18:115, 1932

100. Harris H, Kalmus H, Trotter WH: Taste sensitivity to PTC in goitre and diabetes. Lancet 257:1038, 1949

101. Kitchin FD, Howel-Evans W, Clarke CA, et al: PTC taste response and thyroid disease. Br Med J 1:1069, 1959

102. Saldanha PH, Becak W: Taste thresholds for phenylthiourea among Ashkenazic Jews. Science 129:150, 1959

103. Barnicot NA: Taste deficiency for phenylthiourea in African Negroes and Chinese. Ann Eugen 15:248, 1950

104. Armaly MF: Genetic factors related to glaucoma. Ann NY Acad Sci 151:861, 1968

105. Schwartz JT, Reuling FH, Feinleib M, et al: Twin heritability study of the effect of corticosteroids on intraocular pressure. J Med Genet 9:137, 1972

106. Denborough MA, Forster JFA, Lovell RH, et al: Anaesthetic deaths in a family. Br J Anaesth 34:395, 1962

107. Kalow W: Topics in pharmacogenetics. Ann NY Acad Sci 179:654, 1971

108. Speilberg SP: In vitro assessment of pharmacogenetic susceptibility to toxic drug metabolites in humans. Fed Proc 43:2308, 1984

109. Speilberg SP: Acetaminophen toxicity in human lymphocytes in vitro. J Pharmacol Exp Ther 213:395, 1980

110. Dhar GJ, Pierach CA, Ahamed PN, et al: Diphenylhydantoin-induced hepatic necrosis. Postgrad Med 56:128, 1974

111. Parker WA, Shearer CA: Phenytoin hepatotoxicity: A case report and review. Neurology 29:175, 1979
112. Spielberg SP, Gordon GB, Blake DA, et al: Anticonvulsant toxicity in vitro: Possible role of arene oxides. J Pharmacol Exp Ther 217:386, 1981
113. Woodbury DM, Penry JK, Schmidt RP: Antiepileptic Drugs. New York, Raven Press, 1972
114. Spielberg SP, Gordon GB, Blake DA, et al: Predisposition to phenytoin hepatotoxicity assessed in vitro. N Engl J Med 305:722, 1981
115. Strickler SM, Miller MA, Andermann E, et al: Genetic predisposition to phenytoin-induced birth defects. Lancet 2:746, 1985
116. Spielberg SP, Gordon GB: Nitrofurantoin cytotoxicity: In vitro assessment of risk based on glutathione metabolism. J Clin Invest 67:37, 1981
117. Jick H, Slone D, Westerholm B, et al: Venous thromboembolic disease and ABO blood type: A cooperative study. Lancet 1:539, 1969
118. Lewis GP, Jirk H, Slone D, et al: The role of genetic factors and serum protein binding in determining drug response as revealed by comprehensive drug surveillance. Ann NY Acad Sci 179:729, 1971
119. Spector R, Choudhury AK, Chiang C-K, et al: Diphenhydramine in Orientals and Caucasians. Clin Pharmacol Ther 28:229, 1980
120. Pare CMB: Differentiation of two genetically specific types of depression by the response to antidepressive agents. Humangenetik 9:199, 1970
121. Pare CMB, Mack JW: Differentiation of two genetically specific types of depression by the response to antidepressant drugs. J Med Genet 8:306, 1971
122. Dorus E, Pandey GN, Frazer A, et al: Genetic determinant of lithium ion distribution. I. An in vitro monozygotic–dizgotic twin study. Arch Gen Psychiatry 31:463, 1974
123. Svejgaard A, Houge M, Jersild C, et al: The HLA system: An introductory survey, in Beckman L, Huage UM (eds): Monographs in Human Genetics, vol 7. Basel, Karger, 1975, p 486
124. Bodmer WF: Inheritance of Susceptibility to Cancer in Man. Oxford, England, Oxford University Press, 1983
125. Smeraldi E, Bellodi L, Sacchetti E, et al: The HLA system and the clinical response to treatment with chlorpromazine. Br J Psychiatry 129:486, 1976
126. Smeraldi E, Scorza-Smeraldi R: Interference between anti-HLA antibodies and chlorpromazine. Nature 260:532, 1976
127. Perris C, Strandman E, Wahlby L: HLA antigens and the response to prophylactic lithium. Neuropsychobiology 5:114, 1979
128. Wooley PH, Griffin J, Panayi GS, et al: HLA-DR antigens and toxic reaction to sodium aurothiomalate and D-penicillamine in patients with rheumatoid arthritis. N Engl J Med 303:300, 1980
129. Schmidt KL, Mueller-Eckhardt C: Agranulocytosis, levamisole, and HLA-B27. Lancet 2:85, 1977
130. Batchelor JR, Welsh KI, Mansilla Tinoco R, et al: Hydralazine-induced systemic lupus erythematosus: Influence of HLA-DR and sex on susceptibility. Lancet 1:1107, 1980
131. Perry HM, Tan EM, Carmody S, et al: Relationship of acetyl transferase activity to antinuclear antibodies and toxic symptoms in hypertensive patients treated with hydralazine. J Lab Clin Med 76:114, 1970
132. Vesell ES: Pharmacogenetic perspectives gained from twin and family studies. Pharmacol Ther 41:532, 1989

5

COMPLIANCE WITH PEDIATRIC MEDICATION REGIMENS

IRIS F. LITT

A patient's behavior following the prescription of medication represents the most vulnerable link in the therapeutic chain and yet receives minimal attention in physician education. If the patient improves, the assumption is that the medication was taken properly, and conversely, lack of improvement is assumed to reflect noncompliance. Rarely is the possibility of compliance difficulty anticipated in advance of the embarrassing reality of therapeutic failure, nor are steps taken to improve the likelihood of patient compliance. The problem of adult patient noncompliance has been explored extensively, whereas most pediatric studies have focused on parental behavior rather than that of the youthful patient.

Lack of compliance creates problems in evaluating quality of care and may be a factor contributing to dissatisfaction with health care. How can the efficacy of a new drug be measured if a patient fails to take the recommended dose or takes it intermittently? Despite all the attention given to it, patient compliance with a medication remains little understood. There is a need to understand compliance behavior better and to develop effective health promotional interventions based on sound theory.

Unfortunately, a myriad of complexities surrounds the issue of measuring compliance with a therapeutic regimen. As Marston[1] notes, it is usually misleading to compare compliance rates from different studies because of the wide variations in operational definitions of compliance among investigators, the lack of truly objective measures of compliance, and the loss of precision that enters into estimates of compliance based on several quite different medical recommendations.

Furthermore, in pediatrics, there exists another dimension of complexity to the compliance problem. Mediating the doctor–patient relationship is the parent, in most cases the mother. In the adult population, estimates suggest that one-third of the patient population fails to comply with the physician's instructions.[2] It is estimated that the overall noncompliance rate in the pediatric clinic population remains about 50 percent and ranges from 20–80 percent. It is often unclear, however, whether it is the parent or the pediatric patient who is responsible.

Although compliance among adult patients has been studied from a variety of vantage points, the literature on pediatric compliance remains limited. Most studies have concentrated on identifying parental characteristics associated with compliance and only recently have begun to explore the role of the child or adolescent patient in determining outcome. Research is further complicated by the fact that full informed consent of experimental subjects has been appropriately mandated by federal statute, rendering it more difficult to study compliance.

This chapter will review the present state of understanding of the determinants of compliance, compliance measures, and intervention strategies geared toward improving compliance. The implications of understanding the phenomenon among child and adolescent patients are broader if one considers the impact of early health-related experiences on establishing patterns of health care behavior in later adulthood.

MEASUREMENT

Since our knowledge of any phenomenon is in large part determined by the validity and reliability of our instrumentation and methods of observation, the findings reported in this chapter must be viewed in light of current compliance measurement technology. The measurement of compliance varies according to type of therapeutic regimen under consideration.

In the clinical setting, noncompliance is frequently assumed when the patient fails to improve or when visable side effects of the prescribed drug disappear. Although suspicion alone usually suffices, further action, ranging from confrontation and/or analysis of blood or urine for levels of the prescribed drug, may be undertaken. In the research area, however, clinical impressions are inadequate and may be misleading.

A common problem in compliance research is the absence of a unique operational definition of compliant behavior. Comparisons of compliance studies are difficult

45

because of variations in the definition of compliance and in the selection of cutoff points for distinguishing compliant and noncompliant behavior. How should compliance be defined? Ideally, there should be a biologic basis for identifying the cutoff point required to distinguish compliance from noncompliance.[3]

To overcome these difficulties, a number of strategies have been used to segment study populations into compliant and noncompliant subgroups: (1) some investigators divide patient populations on a strictly statistical basis; (2) others select a compliance cutoff point arbitrarily, using levels employed by previous studies; and (3) still other investigators avoid classifying patients as compliers or noncompliers but instead consider compliance as a continuous variable. Despite the absence of a rigid definition of compliance and a lack of uniformity that makes it difficult to summarize and compare the findings of various studies, investigators continue to utilize a variety of direct and indirect measures of compliance.

Analysis of Body Fluids

Direct measures include the quantitative or qualitative analysis of body fluids for the drug prescribed, its metabolite, or an inert marker. The most commonly analyzed substance is blood. Serum or plasma levels have been utilized to study anticonvulsants, salicylates, digoxin, phenothiazines, and antiasthmatic preparations. Studies of compliance with penicillin, phenothiazines, isoniazid, salicylates, and other anti-inflammatory drugs have utilized urinary levels as the dependent variable. Recent analytic advances have made it feasible to measure levels of anticonvulsants and lithium in the saliva,[4] although the application of this method to other drugs may be limited because of the effect of residue of ingested drug in the oral cavity.[5] Other studies have documented the excretion of 5,5-diphenylhydantoin and methadone into the semen,[6] adding further to the list of body fluids potentially available for analysis. Similarly, sweat levels of alcohol have been used, and other studies of compliance have involved analysis of drugs in tears. The finding that certain substances such as mefenamic acid, flufenamic acid, and riboflavin fluoresce when excreted in urine examined under ultraviolet light has facilitated compliance research, since the latter may be utilized as a tracer when added to the compound under investigation.[7] Studies utilizing urine testing report compliance as the ratio of tests positive to tests done per patient per period of time times 100 percent.

While these objective measures may at first appear ideal for their stated purpose, their usefulness may be limited by the possibility that specimen collection may itself influence the patient's compliance. This hypothesis was supported by a study of Morrow and Rabin,[8] who found noncompliance greater when specimens were collected during unannounced home visits than at the clinic. Gordis et al.,[9] on the other hand, found good concordance between levels in urine collected at home when compared with those obtained in the clinic setting. Friedman et al.[4] found that home collection by adolescent patients who subsequently mailed in the required specimens did not

appear to change the typical distribution of noncompliance. Individual differences in drug metabolism and bioavailability, in addition to compliance, influence levels in body fluids and potentially confuse study outcomes when used as the basis for compliance studies.

Pill Count

The use of pill counts for the purpose of identifying discrepancies between the amount of medication remaining and that which should have been utilized tends to overestimate compliance. Compliance is thus reported as follows:

$$C = \frac{\text{number of pills taken}}{\text{number of pills prescribed}} \times 100\% \qquad (1)$$

In Bergman and Werner's study[10] of penicillin treatment for streptococcal pharyngitis in pediatric patients, compliance by the 9th day of a 10-day course was good in only 8 percent based on urine testing, whereas utilization of the pill-count method produced a compliance rate of 18 percent. Since patients often forget to return with their medication bottle, it may be difficult to utilize this method for assessing noncompliance. If used, however, it is important to document that the prescription is accurately filled at the outset.[11] Another problem encountered, perhaps more often in adolescents, is the inclination to share medication with a friend. Inquiry into this possibility should be specifically undertaken.

Physician Estimates of Patient Compliance

It would be logical to assume that experienced physicians might become adept at estimating compliance among their own patients. A number of studies have examined this hypothesis, with uniformly disappointing results. The study by Charney et al.[13] of pediatricians in private practice found that these physicians' predictions of compliance were no better than chance alone. Blackwell's review[14] supports the finding of Charney et al. that physicians fail to detect compliance problems on better than a chance basis and that compliance tends to be overestimated. Whether it is because of their need to believe that patients follow their advice or simply because of a low index of suspicion, physicians' estimates of their patients' compliance cannot be relied on as a compliance measure for research purposes.

Outcome

Outcome is often used clinically as a measure of compliance. This approach, however, confuses two distinct phenomena. Response to treatment may be influenced by compliance, but the nature of this relationship remains little understood. When patients in a treatment program appear to get better, there is a tendency to assume a high rate of compliance; conversely, when patients do poorly, the tendency is to assume noncompliance. That patients may improve for reasons other than the prescribed medication, that often less than the full prescribed course may effect clinical improvement, or that very compliant patients may fail to improve[15] suggests some of the limitations of using outcome as the dependent variable for compliance studies. Only independent measures of compliance will help to clarify these relationships.

Self-Reports

The patient interview is commonly used to measure compliance. The validity of the patient interview depends on the skill of the interviewer as well as on the patient's ability to recall certain events, the ability to examine that event, and a willingness to report the event accurately. Several investigators have examined the correlation between patient interviews and various measures of compliance. These studies suggest that poor compliance is underreported by patient interviews. For example, Rickels and Briscol[15] examined verbal reports and pill counts of patients in an outpatient clinic and noted that errors in reporting are greatest with smaller deviations from the prescription and that gross departures are more accurately reported. In their study of patients with uncontrolled hypertension, Sackett et al.[16] report that half the noncompliant patients (those with pill counts of less than 80 percent) could be identified with an interview. Park and Lipman[17] reported that only 50 percent of those patients who deviated from the prescribed dosage of imipramine were willing to disclose this deviation during the interview.

Under the rubric of self-report comes the full range from use of a single question (e.g., "Did you take your pills?") to use of well-designed, standardized instruments geared to a nonjudgmental approach that gives permission for noncompliance (e.g., "We all have trouble remembering to take our medication sometimes. Tell me what you did when this happened to you."). Studies have compared patient self-report with objective measures or with other indirect measures such as pill counts. One such study was that of Francis et al.,[18] in which there was less than a 10 percent discrepancy between interview and pill count, with the latter suggesting noncompliance and the former implying good compliance with oral medication for acute illness. Comparison among measures of self-report by adolescents taking oral contraceptives, urinary fluorescence of an added tablet marker, and serum norethindrone levels showed good concordance in a study by Jay et al.[7] In contrast, Feinstein et al.[19] found marked differences between pill count and interview for those who reported good compliance with penicillin prophylaxis. In another study of penicillin prophylaxis for rheumatic fever, Gordis et al.[9] noted overreporting of compliance when the interview was compared with urine testing for the drug. In summary, interviewing appears to be acceptable to the extent that those who report noncompliance rarely lie, but conversely, this method will tend to overestimate compliance if used alone. We have found, in addition, that adolescent patients' assessments of their past medication compliance is a useful predictor of their future likelihood for compliance.[20]

In conclusion, every measure of compliance suffers one or more methodologic limitations. As a result, in planning a study of compliance, it may be wise to combine two or more measures.

MAGNITUDE OF THE PROBLEM

Estimation of the overall noncompliance rate for a pediatric population is 50 percent, with a range of 20–80 percent. This estimate appears consistent with that for adults. Adolescents' compliance falls into this range as well, with most studies showing approximately 50 percent noncompliance.[21] Although Goldsmith[22] reports that compliance may vary according to regimen, Sackett[23] indicates that the U- or J-shaped curve may be typical of the long-term regimen in asymptomatic conditions, with roughly one-third of the patients taking no medication, one-third taking almost all, and one-third distributed between these extremes. Sackett further notes that one may expect that, on average, only 50 percent of patients on long-term medication will remain compliant. Noncompliance appears unquestionably to be a feature of all self-administered regimens. In fact, Blackwell[14] suggests that every asymptomatic individual on prolonged preventive or maintenance therapy is at risk for noncompliance.

When compliance problems are examined according to types of noncompliance, five patterns emerge. The first, a complete failure to follow the prescribed regimen, comprises between 25 and 50 percent of noncompliant patients and includes two subcategories of patients: (1) those who maintain contact with the physician but take virtually no medication and (2) those who totally drop out of treatment.

A major lack of understanding of the phenomenon of compliance behavior stems from the "dropout" rate reported in most clinical investigations. Cadwell et al.[24] report that in the hypertension division of a hospital clinic, 50 percent of the patients remained in treatment at the end of 11 months and only 17 percent after 5 years. Porter[25] reports a 23 percent attrition rate in a 2-year imipramine trial. In addition to dropout, some patients never even begin the treatment regimen. Boyd et al.,[26] in a hospital outpatient clinic study, found that 18 of 134 patients never filled their prescriptions.

A second pattern of noncompliant behavior involving improper dosage intervals has been reported by several investigators. Boyd et al.[26] found improper dosage intervals in 56 percent of the prescriptions sampled. Hulka et al.[27] reported scheduling errors in 17 percent of medications taken, with the figure dropping to 3 percent when patients with misconceptions about scheduling were eliminated from the sample.

A third noncompliant pattern consists of missed doses, and this is closely related to improper dosage intervals. Boyd et al.[26] found missed doses in 70 percent of the prescriptions sampled, with 50 percent reportedly forgotten and 50 percent knowingly omitted.

Increasing or reducing the dose or daily number of doses comprises the fourth pattern of noncompliance. It appears that the number of doses is more frequently reduced than increased and that dosage amount is no more often increased than it is decreased.[26] Data suggest that inconvenient intrusion of the regimen into the daily routine may lead to intentional noncompliance. This is particularly true of adolescents who are reluctant to be seen by their peers to be taking pills at school, owing to concern that such behavior may be misinterpreted as indicative of drug abuse.

The fifth pattern of noncompliance involves taking medication for the wrong purposes, taking outdated or discontinued drugs, taking more medication than the physician has prescribed, and fabricating test results.

In addition to the preceding patterns of noncompliance, findings indicate that the rate of deterioration of compliance for short-term medication treatment is much higher than that for long-term medication treatment.

Gordis et al.[9] examined the compliance rates of children on long-term penicillin prophylaxis for rheumatic fever prevention. The measurement employed was urinalysis, defined by the presence of the medication in the urine. It was found that 33 percent of the patients complied with the drug regimen, with 32 percent being partially compliant and 35 percent noncompliant. This study provided an interesting analysis of the frequency distribution of the compliance rates for these children. The distribution was roughly U-shaped, with one-third of the sample taking practically no medication, one-third with almost 100 percent compliance, and the other third scattered between these two extremes.

Characteristics of the Condition Being Treated

The type and severity of disease, prior experience with disease, duration of symptoms, susceptibility, and knowledge of illness have all been studied in relationship to patient compliance. In most studies, compliance with prescribed medication is better when the disease is considered severe by the parent or patient. The study by Mattar et al.[11] of compliance with medication for acute otitis media, however, found no correlation between compliance and parents' perception of severity. Other characteristics of the disease associated with good medication compliance include prior experience with the disease, particularly if it resulted in hospitalization, and the perception that one is "susceptible" to it or its recurrence.

Compliance among pediatric patients has been studied in a variety of clinical contexts. In the domain of prevention, data are now available about adolescents' compliance with the use of automotive safety devices and contraceptives. Consistent use of seat belts was found in only 17 percent of teenagers studied before the passage of a mandatory seat belt law.[28] A more recent study by Beck et al.[29] showed a rate of 41 percent. In both studies, however, noncompliance was associated with evidence of depression. Compliance with contraceptive use among sexually active adolescents has been extensively studied over the

past decade.[30] In general, about half of those who receive effective methods of birth control continue to use them for more than 6 months. A variety of demographic, biologic, social, and psychologic factors have been shown to correlate with noncompliance, including lower age, lower socioeconomic status, lower postmenarchal age, infrequent sexual intercourse, multiple partners, low perceived risk of pregnancy, high cost/benefit ratio, lack of peer and parental support, low self-esteem, and lack of autonomy. Interestingly, the presence of drug side effects has not been shown to be a significant factor. DuRant and Jay[30] have developed an integrative model for understanding noncompliance with contraceptives among adolescents.

Compliance among pediatric patients with chronic illnesses who were required to take long-term, often painful, and/or multiple medications appears to vary with the condition being treated, as well as with characteristics of the medication itself.

ASTHMA. The major cause of morbidity in asthma is failure to comply with prescribed chronic therapy. In one study it was found that 75 percent of visits to the emergency room by inner-city children and adolescents with chronic asthma occurred because of poor compliance with theophylline therapy.[31] In an attempt to understand the factors associated with noncompliance among parents of children with asthma, Becker et al.[32] questioned them about their health beliefs. Significant predictors of adherence were the mother's perception of her child as being susceptible to illness, in general, and her not experiencing difficulty with medication administration. Intervention strategies for improving compliance in asthmatics have included teaching self-management skills and a combined program consisting of provision of written drug information and behavioral strategies, including tailoring the regimen and increasing supervision.[33] The first approach did not improve compliance, and although the combined program did result in improved compliance of 78 versus 55 percent approximately 4 months later, it is not possible to know which of its components was responsible or if the apparent gains were sustained over time.

CANCER. Conventional wisdom would suggest that faced with a potentially fatal disease, a patient's compliance with medication designed to cure or palliate would be 100 percent. It is therefore of interest to find that the compliance rate among adults with a complete cancer treatment protocol has ranged from 31–40 percent in various studies.[35] The first study to examine this issue in the pediatric literature was that of Smith et al.,[35] which used 17-ketogenic steroid analysis of the urine and determined a noncompliance rate of 41 percent among adolescents with acute leukemia and lymphoma. A subsequent study by Tebbi et al.[36] of children and adolescents with malignancies found occasional or frequent noncompliance in 19 percent at 2 weeks and 35 percent by 50 weeks of followup, with adolescents having a higher rate of reported missed doses than younger children. In an important study of the care providers' perceptions of their patients' compliance, half the adolescents were judged to be noncompliant, in contrast with the view that all the younger children were either good or very good in their compliance.[37] Factors associated with poor compliance among adolescent patients with cancer include fear of deformity or diminished attractiveness as a result of the medication, radiation, or surgery.[37] Among adolescents who completely refused cancer treatment, Blotcky et al.[38] found that they were "prone to anxiety and cope with present distress by maintaining the belief that their lives are determined by fate or religious convictions." Their mothers scored higher on scales of religiosity and trait anxiety than did mothers of adolescent patients who consented to treatment.[38] In the study by Tebbi et al.,[36] there was poor understanding of the medication schedule among those who were frequent noncompliers. Lansky et al.[39] found sex differences in the psychologic correlates of parents' compliance with their children's cancer regimens. Parents of boys more often described them as vulnerable and were themselves more hostile, anxious, and feeling helpless. These characteristics were associated with better medication compliance. Parents were more likely to give their daughters responsibility for their medication administration, and it was the girls' anxiety that was a predictor of good compliance in this study.

DIABETES. Poor glycemic control is a common problem among adolescents with diabetes mellitus of multiple causes, one of which is poor compliance with insulin administration and glucose monitoring. A study by Wilson and Endres[40] documented poor compliance in adolescents by evidence of fabrication of test results in 40 percent and failure to record test results in 18 percent using blood glucose reflectance meters with memory capabilities. Positing developmental differences in psychologic characteristics as factors in this process, Burns et al.[41] divided their study population into three groups (8–10, 11–13, and 14–16 years of age). They found that among those in the youngest group, feeling in control of one's health and having a low body image were associated with higher levels of glycosylated hemoglobin. Contrary to most other studies, the young adolescents had better glycemic control when their reported self-esteem was lowest. For all age groups studied, self-reports of difficulties in management and adherence with the regimen were correlated with poor control. Jacobson et al.[42] found poorer compliance among adolescents than among preadolescents with diabetes mellitus and a correlation between higher self-esteem and social functioning and better compliance. Adolescents in poor metabolic control were found to have more negative interactions with family members in a study by Schafer et al.[43] The role of the health belief model in explaining nonadherence to diabetic treatment regimens was explored by Brownlee-Duffect et al.[44] Although their so-called younger sample included subjects up to the age of 26 years, their findings are included because they are the only ones addressing this issue. They found that 52 percent of adherence in this group was accounted for by the model. Specifically, significant variance in levels of glycosylated hemoglobin was accounted for by the patients' perceived severity and susceptibility. Among teenagers referred to a tertiary care center because of chronic problems of metabolic control, Orr et al.[45] found excessive school absence, social isolation, and depression to be frequent accompaniments. Among the small group that accepted psychiatric counseling, subjective improvement at followup is reported.

An intervention study designed to improve metabolic control randomized patients to two groups, in one of which the physician, patient, and parent were provided with results of glycosylated hemoglobin determinations. Those who initially had poor control and received feedback improved 12 to 16 months later.

CYSTIC FIBROSIS. Patients with cystic fibrosis reportedly have the highest rate of compliance with medical regimens among children and adolescents with chronic illness. Rates of 20–30 percent of noncompliance are quoted in the literature, most of which has been based on children for whom parents are responsible for medication administration.[46] Czajkowski and Koocher[47] attribute this to the fact that such patients are seldom asymptomatic and the negative consequences of noncompliance are rapidly apparent. In their study, they found a noncompliance rate of 35 percent, higher for females and adolescents. One unique form of noncompliance in adolescents with cystic fibrosis is smoking, which is found in 12 percent.[48] Czajkowski and Koocher's study[47] revealed six coping behaviors that discriminated compliant from noncompliant patients: does not underestimate severity of the illness, seeks information, is involved in school/work, has future goals/orientation, is responsible for medication administration, and is open with peers about illness. Scores on an instrument called the "Medical Compliance Incomplete Stories Test" also correlated with compliance in this sample. Developmental differences were found among the adolescents, with the youngest most involved in coping skills that encouraged peer interactions, those in midadolescence continuing involvement with peers but also becoming concerned about planning for the future, and the oldest most involved with issues related to autonomy and independence.

RISK FACTORS FOR NONCOMPLIANCE

The search for the determinants of noncompliance has been motivated by the hope that identification and understanding of these factors may lead to the development of strategies for prevention and intervention and by the belief that awareness of these risk factors might help physicians identify potentially noncompliant patients. Unfortunately, most factors studied have been analyzed one at a time, and few conceptual models have been proposed for considering combinations of factors and their interrelationships.

Although the phenomenon of compliant behavior remains extremely complex, a number of relationships have been reported consistently in the literature, and most investigators have referred to these factors as determinants of compliant behavior despite their basis in correlational analyses.

These factors cannot, however, be considered as either sufficient or necessary to produce compliance or noncompliance, and thus, while they may serve as useful cues in clinical practice, they are not sufficiently reliable to replace objective measures of compliance. These factors are reviewed and summarized in the following subsections.

Characteristics of the Therapeutic Regimen

The form and schedule of medication, the duration of therapy, its cost, side effects, and pharmacy errors also have been investigated in relation to compliance. One common finding is the decay of compliance rates over time in those with chronic illness. In one study of adults with tuberculosis, all patients were found to be noncompliant 5 years after therapy was begun.[49]

Taylor et al.,[50] after examining 90 percent of an inception cohort 2–3 years after the initiation of drug therapy for hypertension, found only 63 percent of the patients still adhering to the drug regimen.

Complexity of a drug regimen is negatively correlated with patient compliance. It has been shown that the simultaneous prescription of more than one medication reduces the likelihood of compliance, as does the need for prolonged medication. The study by Weintraub et al.[51] supports this finding, for the compliance rates of patients on a digoxin regimen decreased when potassium and a diuretic were added to the therapy. Porter[52] also found compliance rates much lower for patients required to take ferrous sulfate three times a day as compared with those taking it once a day. Fewer drugs, as well as less frequent doses, appear to have a positive effect on a patient's adherence to a drug regimen. Regimens that require behavioral change are typically associated with poorer compliance.

It also has been shown that side effects rarely cause low compliance rates. In a study of hypertensive adults, Podell et al.[53] reported that only 2 of the 53 patients blamed side effects for their noncompliance, as measured by poor blood pressure control. Other studies with adult patients showed no association between noncompliance and side effects.[3]

Finally, it has been shown that neither the cost of nor the form of medication (i.e., pill versus liquid) has a significant effect on compliance. On the other hand, the study by Mattar et al.[11] of pharmaceutic factors affecting pediatric compliance alerts us to the fact that pharmacy errors were responsible for noncompliance in 51 percent of the cases they investigated.

Characteristics of the Patient

A variety of demographic and psychologic characteristics such as age, race, sex, position in the family, previous serious illness, and self-esteem also have been investigated to predict patient compliance. Most studies have shown no relationship between compliance and demographic variables. For example, contrary to the stereotypic view of adolescents as being more noncompliant than others, Litt and Cuskey[54] found no difference between the compliance of adolescents with rheumatoid arthritis and that of prepubertal patients. On the other hand, Becker et al.[55] have shown that while a mother's level of education is not predictive of the administration of medication, it will predicate other variables related to administration, such as knowing the name of the drug, schedule, and date of followup appointment. Radius et al.[56] reported that the number of years of formal education (under 8 years versus over 8 years) were predictive of medication adherence in asthma sufferers. Korsch et al.,[57] in their study of patients with chronic renal disease, found most of the noncompliance among adolescent females. They demonstrated noncompliance to be associated with low self-esteem and socialization, as well as with psychosocial problems prior to onset of illness. These and other psychologic characteristics of noncompliant patients have recently received attention in the literature.[58] It appears that any therapy that results in the teenager looking different from his or her peer group or simply unattractive will not be accepted, regardless of the consequences to health, even among patients with life-threatening illnesses such as cancer. Body image and self-esteem are also important predictors of compliance among adolescents with chronic illness, as well as with preventive regimens. The level of cognitive development may have an impact on a young person's ability to conceptualize hypothetical consequences of compliance. The presence of stressors and differences in coping strategies also will influence compliance. Some have postulated that the degree to which an adolescent patient feels in control of events in his or her life ("internal locus of control") will affect adherence to therapeutic regimens. Research on this issue has resulted in conflictual outcomes.[41]

Patient comprehension and recall should not be assumed, since both are essential for the patient to carry out the prescribed task. Joyce et al.[59] interviewed one group of patients immediately after an office visit and another group 2 weeks later and found no association between the passage of time and loss of information. These authors also found, however, that in both groups, two-thirds of the diagnosis and treatment explanations and one-half of the instructional statements were forgotten and, that information recalled decreased in proportion to the amount given; i.e., "overloading" the patient with information is counterproductive.

Several additional factors may contribute to patient recall and comprehension. Joyce et al.[59] suggest that recall is associated with anxiety; persons with either low or high levels of anxiety forget more, with the moderately anxious patient retaining more. Nonanxious persons may not be motivated to listen to the instructions, may not perceive the seriousness of the illness, or may not see themselves as susceptible to its consequences. Very anxious persons, on the other hand, may not be able to attend to the clinician because excessive anxiety interferes with cognitive processes.

Characteristics of the Family

Family characteristics such as the number of people living at home, socioeconomic status, history of family illness, and communication problems have all been investigated in relation to compliance. While the number of children in the family seems unimportant, one study indicates that the number of adults in a household is positively correlated with compliance.[13]

Socioeconomic status appears unrelated to compliance, with the exception of the study by Korsch et al.,[57] in which the mean income of families of noncompliant patients ($13,000) was lower than that of the compliant ones. Most studies, however, are conducted in clinics with indigent populations, so differences based on socioeconomic criteria may have not been observed because of lack of variability among the sample. It was therefore useful to see results of the study by Emans et al.,[60] which compared adolescent patients in a private practice with those in a clinic setting and found that those in the former with high educational goals had better compliance with oral contraceptives. Prior experience with the illness within the family was positively associated with compliance, as was the owning of a fever thermometer.[61] The existence of "communications problems" within the family was felt to be a predictor of noncompliance in the Korsch et al. study.

On the positive side, the extent to which the patient obtains support from family members has been associated with greater compliance.[62] Oakes et al.[63] reported that the family's expectation that the patient will comply to the prescribed therapeutic regimen tends to be associated with better performance. The influence of the family on compliance may result from the supervisory role it assumes, and supervision has been found to be strongly associated with compliance among adults.

Discussions about family stability and its relationship to health behavior and compliance appear primarily in studies involving a child's adaptation to chronic illness. Families who were able to express their conflicts had hemophiliac children who were well adapted; on the other hand, there is some evidence that family stability is not a factor in compliance. Gordis et al.[64] reported that in the case of rheumatic fever patients, compliance was not related to the number of family problems reported by the mother. They did find, however, that noncompliance was more common in children who came to the clinic alone. Administering medication for an acute ear infection was not found to covary with number of family problems; yet, in the same study, mothers who reported "having trouble getting through the day" were less likely to administer medication.[55]

The mother's pattern of self-medication might be predictive of those she will follow with her child. Using interview and chart-recording techniques, Haggerty et al.[65] analyzed mothers' patterns of self-medication and the patterns of medication of the youngest child in the household. Both over-the-counter and prescribed medications were included in the analysis. On any one day of a 28-day recording cycle, 15.4 percent of the children versus 22.5 percent of their mothers had taken some sort of curative medicine.

Characteristics of the Physician–Patient Relationship

Patient satisfaction with the physician, type of physician, and the patient's perception of physician demeanor, warmth, and friendliness have all been studied to better understand those factors which influence patient compliance. While having a consistent physician was found to result in compliance in two studies, that of Meyer et al.[66] of cystic fibrosis patients found no relationship between physician consistency and compliance. Heinzelmann's study[67] of factors in prophylaxis in treating rheumatic fever, on the other hand, found a negative association between having the same doctor and compliance. Heinzelmann[67] also found compliance to be enhanced when the physician was a specialist rather than a generalist. An interesting comparison between medication compliance with pharyngitis and otitis media by Charney et al.[13] showed better compliance with the latter disease when the private physician had cared for the patient for fewer than 4 years and poorer compliance with penicillin for pharyngitis when care had been rendered for more than 4 years previously.

When the mother had faith in the doctor's ability to make a correct diagnosis, compliance was good, whereas noncompliance was the rule if the mother perceived the doctor as unfriendly or as not understanding her concern about her child's illness.[18] Doctors who described the patient's mother as being "responsible," "organized," and "intelligent" were more likely to describe her as compliant.[13] It is impossible in such a study to distinguish cause from effect, since physicians may have based their personality assessment on the mother's previous compliance behavior. In this context, it is interesting that Becker et al.[61] found the best predictor of compliance to be the mother's agreement with the statement, "I try to do exactly what the doctor tells me to do, without question."

Freeman et al.[68] found that compliance was higher when the physician included more discussion of the child's diagnosed illness rather than of treatment or history taking. They found that parents want the doctor to give information freely; they do not want to feel as if they have to extract information. They also seek doctors with a friendly, social-type approach.

A final factor influencing compliance behavior is satisfaction with care and caretakers. In their study of adolescent patients' compliance with appointment keeping, Litt and Cuskey[69], found that having a consistent physician and scoring high on a standardized adolescent patient satisfaction questionnaire were associated with good compliance. Hurtado et al.[70] report that appointment failures are more common among patients who are hostile to the physician.

Characteristics of the Clinic

Pediatricians in private-practice settings usually obtain better compliance than those in a clinic setting.[60] This finding may be explained by the continuity of care and the establishment of long-term relationships by the private-practice model. However, some features of the clinic setting have been identified as contributors to poor compliance.

Investigators find a consistently negative relationship between waiting time and compliance.[13,19] The four factors most frequently reported include (1) the block scheduling system, (2) physician lateness, (3) patient lateness, and (4) patient no-shows. Effective management procedures within the clinic can control factors 1 and 2, and the fourth factor may be alleviated by use of a mail and/or telephone appointment reminder, although this is a particular problem among adolescent patients.[71]

To this end, a positive, warm atmosphere in the clinic/office can contribute substantially to improving patient satisfaction. Further, Alpert[72] suggests that positive identification with the clinic may be fostered by the entire staff, not just by the primary physician.

METHODS OF IMPROVING COMPLIANCE

The ultimate goal of research into patient compliance behavior is that of improving the likelihood that medication will be utilized in the manner in which prescribed. The need to improve compliance is as important as that of prescribing appropriate therapy.

Educational Strategies

Theoretically, the more a patient understands his or her illness, the better is the rate of compliance. Studies of adolescent patients with chronic illness, however, fail to demonstrate any relationship between the patient's knowledge about the illness or the treatment regimen and medication compliance. Although patients should be made aware of the various aspects and consequences of their illness, evidence indicates that education alone cannot effectively increase patient compliance. Accompanying the strategy of education is the notion of "scare" techniques. The effective use of fear arousal as a technique to improve compliance varies depending on the patient's previous level of fear and coping mechanism used. In general, high levels of fear arousal are counterproductive to the desired goal.[73]

Simplifying the Drug Regimen

Even though no controlled trials have examined the effects of a modified drug regimen on compliance, descriptive studies have supported this strategy as an effective intervention method. Pediatricians have long known that use of injectible penicillin eliminates compliance problems associated with the prescription of oral preparations for the eradication of streptococci. The replacement of a week-long administration of oral medication with a single dose of metronidazole has yielded a higher cure rate of trichomonal vaginitis. Similarly, administration of a single oral dose of ampicillin (3.5 gm) and probenecid (1.0 gm) has been shown to avoid the problem of compliance with longer oral treatment regimens for acute uncomplicated gonococcal infection. The simplification of dosage and drug schedules should enhance compliance, although these strategies have not yet been subjected to rigorous investigation.[74]

Medication Packaging

When the form or dosage schedule cannot be effectively altered, use of some type of patient reminder appears to be helpful. The use of pill containers with preset signal alarm devices was effective in simulated patients. Special packaging of medications in calendar packs or in individual "units of use" (e.g., special package for dinner-time administration) is currently undergoing evaluation. These strategies have not been systematically studied among pediatric patients.

Increased Patient Supervision

Studies involving hypertensive adult patients have shown evidence of improved compliance when various forms of supervision were employed.[75,76] There are few studies that examine this factor among pediatric patients. One study of children and adolescents with juvenile rheumatoid arthritis did, however, demonstrate better medication compliance in patients seen more frequently for clinic visits, regardless of the severity of disease.[54] The use of patient reminders has not been demonstrated as an effective strategy for improving compliance among adolescents.[71]

Peer Support

The importance of peer relationships to adolescents has implications for their medication compliance as well as for other aspects of their lives. Peer counseling has been shown to improve adolescents' compliance with use of oral contraceptives, for example.[77]

Contract Setting

This strategy has been effective in improving compliance with weight-gain programs for patients with anorexia nervosa. Its potential in other therapeutic contexts has not been studied.

DIRECTIONS FOR FUTURE RESEARCH

The most obvious requirement for future research is the development of better criteria of compliant behavior. The problem of noncompliance cannot be dealt with sufficiently if it cannot be defined at a better than chance level. The operationalizations of the definition also should be subject to less variation.

Another aspect worthy of further investigation is the analysis of the critical period for the onset of noncompliance. Examination of the time period in which an individual stops or reduces drug intake could benefit future planning in drug regimens. The issue of generational continuity as well as that of relationships between compliance with medication and such behavior as school performance, drug use, and athletic participation would be useful to understand.

REFERENCES

1. Marston MV: Compliance with medical regimens: A review of the literature. Nurs Res 19:312, 1970
2. Becker MH, Maiman LA: Sociobehavioral determinants of compliance with health and medical recommendations. Med Care 13:10–24, 1975
3. Gordis L: Methodologic issues in the measurement of patient compliance, in Sackett DL, Haynes RB (eds): Compliance with Therapeutic Regimens. Baltimore, The Johns Hopkins University Press, 1976, pp 51–66
4. Friedman IM, Litt IF, King DR, et al: Compliance with anticonvulsive therapy for epileptic youth. J Adolesc Health Care 7:12–17, 1986
5. Danhof M, Breimer DD: Therapeutic drug monitoring in saliva. Clin Pharmacokinet 3:39–57, 1978
6. Leger RM, Swanson BN, Gerber N: The excretion of 5,5-D-phenylhydantoin in the semen of man and the rabbit: Comparison with plasma concentrations of the drug. Proc West Pharmacol Soc 20:69–72, 1977
7. Jay MS, Litt IF, Durant RH: Compliance with therapeutic regimens. J Adolesc Health Care 5:124–136, 1984
8. Morrow R, Rabin DL: Reliability in self-medication with isoniazid I & II. Clin Res 14:362A, 1965
9. Gordis L, Markowitz M, Lilienfeld AM: Studies in the epidemiology and presentability of rheumatic fever. IV. A quantitative determination of compliance in children on oral penicillin prophylaxis. Pediatrics 43:173–182, 1969
10. Bergman AB, Werner RJ: Failure of children to receive penicillin by mouth. N Engl J Med 268:1334–1338, 1963
11. Mattar ME, Markello J, Yaffe SJ: Pharmaceutic factors affecting pediatric compliance. Pediatrics 55:101–108, 1975
12. Davis MS: Variations in patients' compliance with doctors' orders: Analysis of congruence between survey responses and results of empirical investigations. J Med Ed 41:1037–1048, 1966
13. Charney E, Bynum R, Eldredge D, et al: How well do patients take oral penicillin? A collaborative study in private practice. Pediatrics 40:188–195, 1967
14. Blackwell B: Drug therapy: Patient compliance. N Engl J Med 289:249–252, 1973
15. Rickels K, Briscol E: Assessment of dosage deviation in outpatient drug research. Clin Pharmacol Ther 10:153–160, 1970
16. Sackett DL, Haynes RB, Gibson ES, et al: Randomized clinical trial of strategies for improving medication compliance in primary hypertension. Lancet 1:1205–1207, 1975
17. Park LC, Lipman RS: A comparison of patient dosage deviation reports with pill counts. Psychopharmacologia 6:299–302, 1964
18. Francis V, Korsch BM, Morris MJ: Gaps in doctor–patient communication: Patients' response to medical advice. N Engl J Med 280:533–540, 1969
19. Feinstein AR, Wood HF, Epstein JA, et al: A controlled study of three methods of prophylaxis against streptococcal infection in a population of rheumatic children. II. Results of the first three years of the study, including methods for evaluating the maintenance of oral prophylaxis. N Engl J Med 260:697–702, 1959
20. Litt IF: Know thyself: Adolescents' self-assessment of compliance behavior. Pediatrics 75:693–696, 1985
21. Litt IF, Cuskey WR: Compliance with medical regimens during adolescence. Pediatr Clin North Am 27:3–15, 1980
22. Goldsmith CH: The effect of differing compliance distributions on the planning and statistical analysis of therapeutic trials, in Sackett DL, Haynes RB (eds): Compliance with Therapeutic Regimens. Baltimore, The Johns Hopkins University Press, 1966, pp 137–151
23. Sackett DL: The magnitude of compliance and noncompliance, in Sackett DL, Haynes RB (eds): Compliance with Therapeutic Regimens. Baltimore, The Johns Hopkins University Press, 1976, pp 9–25
24. Caldwell JR, Cobb S, Dowling MD, et al: The dropout problem in antihypertensive treatment. J Chronic Dis 22:579–592, 1970
25. Porter AMW: Drug defaulting in a general practice. Br Med J 1:218–222, 1969
26. Boyd JR, Covington TR, Stanaszck WF, et al: Drug defaulting. II. Analysis of noncompliance patterns. Am J Hosp Pharmacol 31:485–491, 1974
27. Hulka BS, Cassel JC, Kupper LL, et al: Communication, compliance, and concordance between physicians and patients with prescribed medication. Am J Public Health 66:847–853, 1976
28. Litt IF, Steinerman PR: Compliance with automotive safety devices among adolescents. J Pediatr 99:484–486, 1981
29. Beck A, Schichor A: Adolescent seatbelt use: A marker of depression and other risk factors. Presented at the Society for Adolescent Medicine Meeting, New York, March 1988
30. Durant RH, Jay MS: A social psychologic model of female adolescents' compliance with contraceptives. Semin Adolesc Med 3:135–144, 1987
31. Chryssanthopoulos C, Laufer P, Torphy DE: Assessment of acute asthma in the emergency room: Evaluation of compliance and combined drug therapy. J Asthma 20:35–38, 1983
32. Becker MH, Rosenstock IM, Radins SM, et al: Compliance with a medical regimen for asthma: A test of the health belief model. Public Health Rep 93:268–277, 1978
33. Baum D, Creer TL: Medication compliance in children with asthma. J Asthma 23:49–59, 1986
34. Lewis C, Linet MS, Abeloff MD: Compliance with cancer therapy by patients and physicians. Am J Med 74:673–678, 1983
35. Smith SD, Cairns, NW, Sturgeon, JR: A reliable method for evaluating drug compliance in children with cancer. Cancer 43:169–173, 1979
36. Tebbi CK, Cummings M, Zevon MA, et al: Compliance of pediatric and adolescent cancer patients. Cancer 58:1179–1184, 1986
37. Dolgin MJ, Katz ER, Doctors SR, et al: Caregivers' perceptions of medical compliance in adolescents with cancer. J Adolesc Health Care 7:22–27, 1986
38. Blotcky AD, Conatser C, Cohen DG, et al: Psychosocial characteristics of adolescents who refuse cancer treatment. J Consult Clin Psychol 53:729–731, 1985
39. Lansky SB, Smith SD, Cairns NU, et al: Psychological correlates of compliance. Am J Pediatr Hematol Oncol 5:87–92, 1983
40. Wilson DP, Endres RK: Compliance with blood glucose monitoring in children with type 1 diabetes mellitus. J Pediatr 108:1022–1024, 1986
41. Burns KL, Green P, Chase HP: Psychosocial correlates of glycemic control as a function of age in youth with insulin dependent diabetes. J Adolesc Health Care 7:311–319, 1986
42. Jacobson AM, Hauser ST, Wolfsdorf JI, et al: Psychologic predictors of compliance in children with recent onset of diabetes mellitus. J Pediatr 110:805–811, 1987
43. Schafer LC, McCaul KD, Glasgow RE: Supportive and nonsupportive family behaviors: Relationships to adherence with metabolic control in persons with type 1 diabetes. Diabetes Care 9:179–185, 1986
44. Brownlee-Duffeck M, Peterson L, Simonds JF, et al: The role of health beliefs in the regimen adherence and metabolic control of adolescents and adults with diabetes mellitus. J Consult Clin Psychol 55:139–144, 1987
45. Orr DP, Golden MP, Myers G, et al: Characteristics of adolescents with poorly controlled diabetes referred to a tertiary care center. Diabetes Care 6:170–175, 1983
46. Zeltzer L, Ellenberger L, Rigler D: Psychological effects of illness in adolescents. II. Illness in adolescents: Crucial issues and coping styles. J Pediatr 97:132–137, 1980
47. Czajkowski DR, Koocher GP: Medical compliance and coping with cystic fibrosis. J Child Psychol Psychiatry 28:311–318, 1987
48. Stern RC, Byard PJ, Tomashefski JF: Recreational use of psychoactive drugs by patients with cystic fibrosis. J Pediatr 3:293–302, 1987
49. Luntz GR, Austin R: New stick test for PAS in urine: Report on use of Phenistix and problems of long-term chemotherapy for tuberculosis. Br Med J 1:1679–1684, 1960
50. Taylor DW, Sackett DL, Haynes RB, et al: Compliance with anti-

hypertensive drug therapy. Ann NY Acad Sci 304:390–403, 1978

51. Weintraub M, Lasagna WYW, Lasagna AU, Lasagna L: Compliance as a determinant of serum digoxin concentration. JAMA 224:481–485, 1973
52. Porter AMW: Drug defaulting in a general practice. Br Med J 1:218–222, 1969
53. Podell RN, Kent DK, Keller KK: Patient psychological defenses and physician response in the long-term treatment of hypertension. J Fam Pract 3:145–149, 1976
54. Litt IF, Cuskey WR: Compliance with salicylate therapy in adolescents with juvenile rheumatoid arthritis. Am J Dis Child 135:434–436, 1981
55. Becker M, Drachman R, Kirscht J: A new approach to explaining sick role behavior in low-income populations. Am J Public Health 64:205–216, 1974
56. Radius S, Becker M, Rosenstock I, et al: Factors influencing mothers' compliance with a medication regimen for asthmatic children. J Asthma Res 15:133–149, 1978
57. Korsch BM, Fine RN, Negrete VF: Noncompliance in children with renal transplants. Pediatrics 61:872–876, 1978
58. Friedman IM, Litt IF: Adolescents' compliance with therapeutic regimens: Psychological and social aspects and intervention. J Adolesc Health Care 8:52–67, 1987
59. Joyce CRB, Capla G, Mason M, et al: Quantitative study of doctor–patient communication. Q J Med 38:183–194, 1969
60. Emans SJ, Grace E, Woods E, et al: Adolescents' compliance with the use of oral contraceptives. JAMA 257:3377–3381, 1987
61. Becker MH, Drachman RH, Kirsch JP: Predicting mothers' compliance with pediatric medical regimens. J Pediatr 81:843–854, 1972
62. Haynes RB: A critical review of the "determinants" of patient compliance with therapeutic regimens, in Sackett DL, Haynes RB (eds): Compliance with Therapeutic Regimens. Baltimore, The Johns Hopkins University Press, 1976, pp 26–50
63. Oakes TW, Ward JR, Gray RM, et al: Family expectations and arthritis patient compliance to a hand resting splint regimen. J Chronic Dis 22:757–764, 1970
64. Gordis L, Markowitz M, Lilienfield A: Why patients don't follow medical advice: A study of children on long-term antistreptococcal prophylaxis. J Pediatr 75:957–968, 1969
65. Haggerty RJ, Roghmann M, Klaus J: Noncompliance and self-medication: Two neglected aspects of pediatric pharmacology. Pediatr Clin North Am 19:101–115, 1965
66. Meyers A, Dolan TF, Mueller D: Compliance and self-medication in cystic fibrosis. Am J Dis Child 129:1011–1013, 1975
67. Heinzelmann F: Factors in prophylaxis behavior in treating rheumatic fever: An exploratory study. J Health Hum Behav 3:73–81, 1962
68. Freeman M, Negrete V, Davis M, et al: Gaps in doctor–patient communication: Doctor–patient interaction analysis. Pediatr Res 5:298–311, 1971
69. Litt IF, Cuskey WR: Satisfaction with health care. J Adolesc Health Care 5:196–200, 1984
70. Hurtado AV, Greenlick MR, Colombo TJ: Determinants of medical care utilization: Failure to keep appointments. Med Care 11:189–198, 1973
71. Cromer B, Chako M: Increasing appointment compliance through telephone reminders: Does it ring true. Dev Behav Pediatr 8:133–135, 1987
72. Alpert JJ: Broken appointments. Pediatrics 34:127–132, 1964
73. Radelfinger S: Some effects of fear-arousing communications on preventive health behavior. Health Educ Monogr 19:2–15, 1965
74. Haynes RB, Sackett DL, Taylor DW, et al: Commentary. Manipulation of the therapeutic regimen to improve compliance: Conceptions and misconceptions. Clin Pharmacol Ther 22:125–130, 1977
75. Wilbur JA, Barrow JG: Reducing elevated blood pressure. Minn Med 52:1303–1306, 1969
76. McKenney JM, Slining JM, Henderson HR, et al: The effect of clinical pharmacy services on patients with essential hypertension. Circulation 48:1104–1111, 1973
77. Jay MS, DuRant RH, Litt IF, et al: The effect of peer counselors on adolescent compliance with oral contraceptives. Pediatrics 73:126–131, 1984

6

ETHICS OF DRUG RESEARCH IN CHILDREN

SANFORD N. COHEN *and* RONALD L. POLAND

The majority of pharmacologic agents and pharmaceutical preparations currently marketed in the United States cannot be advertised as safe and effective for infants and children. Many of the agents and preparations that are commonly prescribed for pediatric patients contain "disclaimers" in their labeling regarding the lack of information concerning appropriate dosage recommendations, side effects, etc. This inequity in the protection afforded children when compared with that available to adults has been termed "unethical."[1,2] Indeed, the U.S. Food and Drug Administration, the regulatory agency charged with the responsibility of certifying that drugs are safe and effective for use as claimed, has established a policy of requiring that new drugs that are likely to be used widely in infants and children must be evaluated properly so that they can be labeled accordingly prior to approval for marketing. The American Academy of Pediatrics published its "guidelines" for the ethical conduct of drug research studies in infants and children in 1977* in an attempt to ease the transition between the current situation and the ideal one, in which labeling of all drugs necessary for the treatment of pediatric patients will contain enough information for their safe and effective use.[1] Nonetheless, there continues to be confusion and debate regarding the moral, ethical, and legal issues that surround drug research and evaluation in infants and children.

All investigators who engage in experiments involving human subjects frequently find themselves in a conflict between their scientific and professional quest for new knowledge and future understanding and their societal (indeed legal) obligation to be mindful and protective of the inviolability of the individual. Thus there is a basic value conflict inherent in investigations in humans. Few areas exemplify this conflict between knowledge and ethics and morality so strikingly as does research in infants and children. Furthermore, research in pediatric populations frequently introduces questions concerning both the

legality of investigators' actions and the responsibility of institutions and society at large to protect the interests of those who lack competence under the law to protect themselves.

Ethics may be defined as the philosophical inquiry into the principles of morality, of right and wrong conduct, of virtue and vice, and of good and evil as they relate to conduct.[3] The moral code that guides all our behavior as a society requires that we "do not harm." Thus, if investigators and/or physicians wish to achieve a positive advantage for society at large, for a segment of society, or even for individual patients, they must do so while taking care that they "do not harm" in the process.

One ethical dilemma of the modern investigator who wishes to study drugs in pediatric populations centers around the definition of "harm" in a research situation. This is further complicated by legal restraints imposed by the centuries-old common-law standard, based on the Magna Carta, that permission to act on a minor or his or her property can only be given when the action can be construed as being to the minor's own benefit. There has been progress in defining "harm" as distinct from "discomfort" or "mere inconvenience." Such a redefinition, if agreed to by a majority of opinion makers and by the members of society, may lead to a modification of the interpretation of this basic legal tenet by the courts and thus to a set of clearer guidelines to the legal as well as the ethical standards of professional behavior.

The philosophy and ethics literature contains spirited exchanges concerning the definition of the more difficult to define concept of "benefit." It has been suggested by some that it is ethically sound for a parent or a guardian to consent to the participation of a minor child for whom he or she is responsible when there is minimal pain and/or hazard involved in such participation and when the overall societal benefits to be derived from the investigation are thought to be major.[2,4,6] One basis of this contention is that the minor, if of age, would consent to such participation, because as a member of society, the minor would realize that he or she "should" or "ought" to par-

---

*Revised document to be published late 1991.

ticipate.[5] According to this formulation, the black-and-white, strict constructionist interpretation of "benefit" is restated to include shades of gray that permit the greater good of society to be considered, as long as appropriate protections exist to ensure that the individual is respected and is not exposed to undue stress and/or risk. Other writers have vigorously disputed this contention.[7,8]

It will be some time before any basic and clear-cut statement of the ethics of drug research on infants and children will emerge from the current debate and before appropriate court opinions can be cited as indicating a basic change in the common-law principles governing the actions of researchers. There are a number of guidelines, however, that can be followed to permit necessary clinical and therapeutic advances to be made in an ethical manner and according to rigorous stands following open discussion by knowledgeable and reasonable people. Indeed, such guidelines are required if our society is to continue to afford maximal protection to the individual (especially to those individuals who are not capable of protecting themselves) and still maintain systems that are equitable (ethical?) to all groups in the society.

Standards for clinical practice have been established over time and have been accepted generally by society. These are based on the scientific as well as the humane objectives and purposes of both society and professional practitioners. Likewise, standards for performance of drug research studies in infants and children are being developed according to the imperative that scientific and humane goals be served by providing treatment modalities for pediatric patients with the same consideration for the protection of the individual afforded others.[9,10] One basic standard, therefore, that must be adhered to in drug research in pediatric populations is that all studies must be carried out according to an appropriate scientific design. Poor scientific design or uncontrolled experimentation can be considered "unethical," according to this construct.

A second basic standard is that the investigator must be both competent and ethical. The competence and ethical nature of the investigator are the most important safeguards for the protection of the interest and well-being of the child subject. The investigator who wishes to conduct studies utilizing human subjects who are in the pediatric age groups must not only be knowledgeable and well trained, but also must understand the feelings and attitudes of the parties involved in the research and be especially sensitive to the special needs and fears of young children.

A third standard requires that the investigator must be fully aware of the need for any research plan to include a consideration of the concept of distributive justice and that this be adhered to in its execution. Thus infants and children should not be exposed to unwarranted risks, no matter how minimal, for the convenience of the investigator, and no subgroup of children (e.g., racial, ethnic, socioeconomic, etc.) should bear a greater share of the research burden than others, except as dictated by the clinical and scientific requirements of the investigation itself or of the disease process under study. A study conducted to evaluate an appropriate dosage schedule for pediatric patients who require a specific form of therapy should therefore include patients from as wide a segment of society as is practical, whereas a study to evaluate dosages of agents used to treat specific diseases should involve individual subjects in reasonable proportion to the risk or incidence of that disease in their subgroup of society.

No investigator can be free from all bias or self-interest when planning a study. However, the individual who proposes to carry out a drug research project in children must strive to present a balanced view of the benefits and of the risks (if any) inherent in the study when seeking informed consent from an individual who is qualified to act on behalf of the minor subject. This standard of conduct requires that there be recognition of the rights of any proposed subject to be informed and to be free to consent or to withhold consent on the basis of the information provided. It also requires that the adult who is legally qualified to act on behalf of the proposed minor subject understand all significant and reasonably expected consequences of participation (both benefits and risks) and have full access to individuals who are qualified to answer questions prior to volunteering a minor as a research subject. In general, once written consent is obtained from the adult who is acting for the proposed minor subject, the subject should be given the opportunity to refuse to participate after he or she is appropriately informed. This standard must be adhered to in all instances when the proposed subject is developmentally and physically capable of understanding the implications of volunteering (i.e., 14 years of age) and whenever a younger or less capable child would require unreasonable coercion or physical restraint to allow the study to be carried out.

The determination of the risks of a proposed study should not only include the known and the predictable effects of the drug as determined from animal studies, prior studies in adults or other children, or observations from clinical practice, but also a broader review of specific concerns for pediatric patients. Some adverse effects may remain latent for years, and the possibility that they may surface later must be weighed in assessing the ethics of a proposed study. Additional types of "risks" that must be considered when a proposal is in preparation or under review include pain, fright, and the separation from parents, friends, or familiar surroundings necessitated by the study protocol. It must be remembered that an invasive procedure per se does not render a study unethical, but that the entire study protocol must be weighed in any effort to determine its ethical quality.

Investigators and reviewers of their work are guided by codes of behavior that are usually stated in such general terms as to be inadequate to cover the complex situations presented by specific research proposals. The basis for specific evaluations and recommendations must therefore be the broader ethical concepts and standards discussed earlier. The practical implementation of these broad ethical concepts in the context of specific research proposals must be delegated to a select institutional review board. Such a board, made up of reasonable, interested, and dedicated individuals, provides important protections for the proposed subjects of biomedical research and for investigators alike.

Any institution under whose auspices clinical research is conducted must ensure that the investigation is reviewed by an appropriately constituted institutional review committee.* When clinical investigations are to be conducted in children by individuals independent of institutions with such a committee, a review committee which will serve the same functions as the institutional review committee should be established to ensure that the proposed investigations are carried out within accepted guidelines and are subjected to appropriate ethical scrutiny.

The institutional review committee affords protection for the subject, for the institution, and for the investigator. The institutional review committee should be composed of medical scientists, other physicians who are not engaged in clinical investigations, representatives of the community, and nonmedical professional groups.

All committees reviewing proposals for investigations in children must include persons who care for children. These persons are likely to be more aware of the special psychologic and social needs of child research subjects and are likely to be better advocates for children's welfare. It may be advisable for institutions to have a separate subcommittee with medical representation composed predominantly, if not exclusively, of pediatricians to review and approve proposed protocols which involve minor subjects.†

Ideally, a specially constituted pediatric institutional review board (PIRB) should be used to evaluate pediatric proposals. The investigator needs to provide the PIRB with all the information that the board might require to appraise the proposed benefits and the potential risks for the individual infant or child who is to be enrolled in the proposed research study. The PIRB must be satisfied that the risks and discomforts that may attend the performance of the research are justified by the potential advantages for each pediatric participant.

The pediatric institutional review board should include persons who are knowledgeable about pediatric medical care, the conduct of clinical research, and the special needs of infants and children. Individuals may be selected from the ranks of clinical researchers, practicing clinicians, lawyers, philosophers (especially ethicists), theologians, and representatives of the community served by the institution. These participants should have an appreciation of the societal value of research as well as of the requirement that infants and children be protected from unreasonable risks and discomforts.

The PIRB must review all proposals for research involving children in the institution it serves. The welfare of the research subjects should always be the primary focus. The board should not approve a proposal for research until it is satisfied that the proposal is scientifically sound, that the proposed procedure for obtaining consent is fair and informative, and that the risks and discomforts attendant on participating in the project are clearly offset by the benefits (or potential benefits) for each research subject. The PIRB's role does not end once a pro-

posal is approved. The board is obligated to monitor the progress of approved research for unexpected outcomes, for changes in protocol, and for compliance with institutional guidelines for the ethical conduct of pediatric research.

If a project involving pediatric subjects is not designed well enough to ensure clear interpretation of potentially useful results, then the risks of the project, no matter how small, cannot be justified. The PIRB must decide whether it is likely that the information obtained will benefit the subject and/or other children in the same category. The board must consider whether the proposal has properly taken into account the theoretical action of the drug being tested and the pathophysiology of the disease being treated. It must decide whether the goals are clearly stated, and if so, whether the approach proposed is one that will likely lead to (an) answers to the investigator's question(s). Consideration must be given to subject selection, group assignment, and the data-gathering process for the board to be assured that the investigator has taken appropriate precautions against bias.

Clear and appropriate definitions for the dependent and independent variables are an important part of the evaluation of scientific merit. The variables should be clinically relevant, definable, and measurable. The list of variables should include any confounders that might bias the results of the study. A discussion of sample size should be included with most, if not all, proposals; i.e., if no "statistically significant" difference is detected between groups at the conclusion of the study, how sure will the investigator be that a clinically significant difference was not overlooked or missed due to the size of the sample? The sample size calculation should be presented in the proposal, and the investigator should include a statement of all assumptions leading to the estimate. A research proposal that is not likely to reach its stated goals, either owing to deficiency of subjects or to an unrealistic research strategy, is not worth starting.

Approval of the consent form is a very important aspect of the work of a PIRB. The form should include a presentation to the parents, guardians, and the subject (where appropriate) of sufficient information concerning the goals and content of the proposal and its risks, discomforts, and benefits for a reasonable person with little or no technical knowledge to be able to make a reasoned decision when asked to volunteer his or her child for participation. The language used in the form should be simple and understandable by persons unfamiliar with medical terms and jargon. It must differentiate the investigational parts of the project from those procedures which are part of standard clinical care for similar pediatric patients. The consent form should provide information that will allow the subject's family (or guardian) to contact the investigator easily during the study period. The form should state clearly that participation is optional and that withdrawal from the study is also an option any time after enrollment. The consent form must make it clear that nonparticipation or withdrawal will not compromise the usual care that will be provided for the potential subject. The institutional policy concerning medical care occasioned by any untoward events that may occur as a consequence of participation in the study should be stated clearly in the form's text.

The PIRB should be sensitive to the possibility that the method of obtaining consent or the incentives that may be used to encourage the enrollment of subjects could appear to be unfairly coercive. Thus, if a physician in charge of the child's care asks for permission to enroll the child in a research project, the parents may feel more obligated to agree than they would if other staff members or researchers make the request. The person asking for permission must allow time for questions and reflection on the part of the parent(s). Reimbursement for expenses is permissible, but if such is proposed, the PIRB must consider whether the reimbursement is reasonable under the circumstances. In one recent instance at our institution, an investigator received support from a pharmaceutical manufacturer to test a new antibiotic proposed for the treatment of otitis media. The manufacturer was very anxious to enhance compliance, especially for follow-up visits. To that end, the plan was to reimburse parents for both transportation and time lost, up to $150 per 3-weeks of compliance with the protocol. Since the subjects were unlikely to spend that much on transportation or to forego that amount of income due entirely to participation in the study, the PIRB felt that parents/guardians would be unduly influenced to volunteer their children's participation by the proposed sum, and the protocol was not approved with that incentive in it.

At times, the bias of the investigator might color the explanation given to the subjects prior to consent. In our own PIRB deliberations, a proposal was submitted in which the subjects were nurses working with children. The consent form explained that the study, which depended primarily on a questionnaire, was designed to "measure the extent to which hopsital administration policies increase the stress of the staff nurse." The review board needs to look for instances of this kind of error and to help the investigator to communicate with potential subjects without contributing bias to the outcome of the study.

Another issue that the PIRB must consider for children enrolling in clinical research projects is the age of assent. If the investigator wishes to enroll children older than 7 years of age, the board must monitor how the investigator will decide whether the assent of the subject is needed. It has been suggested that assent may be appropriate for a normally developed 7-year-old, but that several characteristics of the child and/or the project may be considered in the decision made at that age. A child who can understand what the research entails and who has demonstrated a sense of responsibility for his or her own decisions should be asked to assent. Most authorities agree that the normally developed 14-year-old has the necessary abilities to make a fully informed decision about participation, and such a subject should sign the consent form along with his or her parent/guardian.

The investigator must provide the PIRB with information that at least suggests a favorable benefit/risk ratio for the proposed treatment and control groups. Information about the use of the test agent in adult humans and immature animals or in other pediatric patients will help in assessing the safety. In most cases, the investigation of a drug in the pediatric setting should have been preceded by similar testing in adults. The pros and cons of the use of a placebo or alternative therapy group should be explored. The board should be informed of the treatment the patient will receive if he or she is not enrolled in the proposed project. The investigator should have a reasonable plan for surveillance of subjects for possible untoward effects from the agent under investigation. In many cases there should be a plan for intermediate reviews of results so that there may be early termination of the project when a clear difference between groups has been identified. How these intermediate reviews of the data will be carried out without producing bias during the remainder of the project should be explained to the PIRB.

The investigator needs to justify the use of all nontherapeutic (e.g., diagnostic or data-gathering) interventions in the protocol. If the risks or discomforts of the suggested procedures do not represent only a minor addition to what a subject fitting the selection criteria would ordinarily experience, they may not be justified. The PIRB must be satisfied that the child who is enrolled in the study will not have its well-being, dignity, and/or autonomy compromised by participating.

The PIRB should develop policies and procedures to monitor the possible enrollment of the same infant/child into more than one project at a time. It may be reasonable to enroll an individual in two or more studies under certain circumstances, but the implications of the added protocol(s) on issues of safety and fairness need to be considered in advance. If each project involves blood drawing, for instance, then the total amount to be taken and the number of times the patient's blood is sampled should be no more than can be justified by any single project. In addition, the board should consider the total experience that a child will have while enrolled in multiple projects to decide whether it is reasonable to enroll that child in more than one. It might be helpful to combine protocols whenever possible or to have a "traffic controller" (or moderator) who decides which patients will be asked about participation in which projects. In any event, the board should establish a mechanism to ensure that patients are not abused by being asked to participate in more research protocols than the board feels is reasonable. One mechanism is to have the investigator submit a copy of each consent form to the board so that the board's staff can cross-check to learn whether the same subject has been asked to participate in more projects than is appropriate for the subject. Another method is to have a copy of each consent form attached to the subject's record to alert other investigators to the subject's participation in each research project.

In general, therapeutic research is not carried out in infants and children, but rather the research study is carried out "under therapeutic conditions." This is an important distinction, since it is rare that one would administer drugs for study purposes without there being any therapeutic potential for the child; i.e., children are almost never reasonable subjects of drug research studies before late phase II.[10] When children are recruited as the subjects of drug research, it is usually with the knowledge that there is a real possibility that there will be a therapeutic advantage derived from the drug under study and that the research cannot be called therapeutic in its own right. Rather, the research portion of the study in such a situation is the drawing of blood, or the obtaining of urine, or the conduct of the tests to monitor pharmacokinetics or pharmacodynamics in a situation that basically involves providing therapy for the patient.

The following excerpt from the published guidelines of the American Academy of Pediatrics illustrates the detail that must be observed in categorizing and evaluating pediatric drug research proposals. It includes some discussion of each of the points illustrated and includes a description of the situation in which a placebo-treated group is not only permissible, but may be required.[1]

Drug Research
General Conditions

Therapy is the treatment of a disease. Drug therapy is the use of drugs (as opposed to physical or phychologic means) for the treatment of disease. Thus, if therapy with a marketed drug is used by a physician solely for an individual's benefit, it should not be considered research, even if the drugs cannot be advertised for this indication or purpose. However, if drug therapy is used by a physician for the acquisition of knowledge which may be of benefit to others, as well as for therapy, it is research (albeit research in a therapeutic situation). This type of research is subject to the ethical and medical scrutiny proposed here.

Drug research may be divided into two major, but not mutually exclusive, categories: research under therapeutic conditions (type I research) and nontherapeutic research (type II research). Type I research includes studies of the safety, elimination, metabolism, efficacy, and interactions of drugs given to treat a condition or illness. Type II drug research involves studies on drugs given principally to determine their effect and action unrelated to the therapy of the individual. Because these major categories involve different ethical and medical considerations, different protections may be required for the subjects of each type of research.

Research Under Therapeutic Conditions
(Type I Drug Research)

There are several subcategories in type I drug research:

1. Noninvasive studies that do not include an additional pharmacologic agent to a prescribed treatment regimen.

Example: The patient is given a well-established therapeutic agent for his illness. The investigator studies the metabolism or excretion of the drug in the patient's normal excretory products (e.g., urine, sweat) or observes the patient's behavior, response, or condition after administration of the drug.

2. Invasive studies that do not involve an additional therapeutic agent.

Example: The patient is being given a drug which is the established form of therapy for his illness, but the investigator wishes to procure several blood specimens to establish the kinetics, absorption, and so forth of his drug in the patient's age group.

3. Studies of the efficacy, safety, and dose of an investigational drug in children.

Example: (1) A drug effective for a condition in adults is to be tried for treatment of a child with a similar condi-

tion. The investigator wishes to determine the efficacy of this drug in children with the condition, its safety for the developing organism, and the appropriate drug and dosage regimen for its administration in a child. (2) An agent with potential value in animals or laboratory studies for a condition occurring only in infants and children (e.g., respiratory distress syndrome or infantile spasms) is to be administered to a child subject with this condition to establish pharmacologic parameters, such as safety, efficacy, and metabolism, in the absence of comparable data in adults.

The Committee on Drugs believes that drug studies in infants and children should include detailed evaluations of the pharmacology of the drugs in the various age groups, but there is at least one exception to this requirement. In the foregoing situation, where a disease or condition occurs only in infants and children, it may be reasonable for pilot studies of the efficacy of an investigational drug for the condition to proceed after only minimal pharmacokinetic studies. If pilot studies indicate probable efficacy, the ethics of drug evaluation in children require that an investigator's protocol incorporate detailed research into safety, efficacy, and general pharmacology in succeeding studies.

Whenever possible, research protocols should be designed to permit the results of laboratory studies to be used for the benefit of the research subject. This is especially important in studies of investigational drugs in children; the ethical nature of such studies is clearest when minor subjects can derive benefit from the use of the investigational drug as well as the various tests done as part of the scientific investigation.

4. Studies requiring the use of placebos.

In general, placebos should be used when data cannot be obtained by comparing the efficacy and safety of the drug under study with either a commonly used therapeutic agent for that condition or the natural course of the disease as described from clinical studies. The word "placebo" is not intended to mean "untreated" because any routine treatment must continue in all drug research in children where placebos are used. The conditions under which the use of placebos is ethical in drug research in children include (1) when there is no commonly accepted therapy for the condition and the agent under study is the first one that may modify the course of the disease process; (2) when the commonly used therapy for the condition is of questionable or low efficacy; (3) when the commonly used therapy for the condition carries with it a high frequency of unacceptable side effects; (4) when the incidence and severity of undesirable side effects produced by adding a new treatment to an established regimen are uncertain; (5) when the disease process is characterized by frequently, spontaneous exacerbations and remissions.

5. Long-term prospective studies of the safety of a drug.

When drugs are administered to developing organisms, the effects may be latent for a long time and cannot be predicted from any prior studies or experience.

Example: (1) A drug used in pregnant women must be studied for its effect on the fetus. Follow-up studies of the offspring must also be done to determine if there are late effects. (2) Studies of drugs effective for therapy of acute conditions which are given to pediatric patients over a short period of time require some mechanism for follow-up and evaluation of the research subjects.

Even a brief period of drug administration at a critical period in the development of an individual might lead to long-term effects on behavior, learning, and so forth. Planning pediatric drug research is especially difficult when it involves long-term administration of an agent for chronic management of a disease process (e.g., hyperactivity or asthma). Evaluation of the long term effects on learning, behavior, respiratory function, and other processes must be built into the original design of the study. In long-term prospective studies in children, the drug's action may interfere with cell metabolism; e.g., as with the chemotherapeutic agents used in neoplastic and unremitting viral diseases. Therefore, there must be some mechanism to determine such possibilities as development of new forms of neoplasia at a later age, disturbance of learning processes and other central nervous system functions, or serious compromise of growth and behavior patterns. Thus, even if a new therapeutic agent is lifesaving, the ethics of drug evaluation in children require the investigator to look at the effects of the new drug on the quality of life following treatment and compare them with the effects of other forms of therapy.

Nontherapeutic Research
(Type II Drug Research)

1.   Studies of the pharmacology and toxicology of drugs (1) taken accidentally or in overdoses in infants, children, or pregnant women, and (2) which enter the fetus or newborn infant transplacentally or through breast milk because of necessary therapeutic use by the pregnant woman or nursing mother.

Example: (1) A child ingests a drug prescribed for another person's use. (2) A child is overdosed with a prescription drug or an over-the-counter preparation whose pharmacology and toxicology have not been established in children. (3) A pregnant woman ingests a drug or is given a drug for an illness, and the effect on her fetus is unknown or uncertain. (4) A lactating woman ingests or is given a drug without knowledge of the effect of the drug on the developing infant.

When type II studies are to be conducted after accidental intake of a drug, the conduct of the study may not in any way interfere with the appropriate treatment of the patient's acute condition.

2.   Prospective studies to advance knowledge for the future benefit of the child subject.

Example: A youngster with cystic fibrosis is given a few doses of a new antibiotic so investigators can learn about its pharmacology, despite the fact that he had no infection requiring its use at the time it is administered. This type of study is within the ethical framework stressed in this document *only* when the results of the research can be predicted to lead to more effective and safer therapy of the same individual when this type of treatment is indicated.

3.   Prospective studies to advance knowledge for others. In general, the Committee on Drugs believes that it is not ethical to conduct studies which offer no benefit to the child subject.

However, such studies might be ethically permissible with agents that are available over the counter in the dose and form to be given since such drugs might in any case be in general use. When this type of study is to be carried out, there must be consent from the person acting on behalf of the minor and, except as specified here (at least),

assent from the minor himself/herself. If the studies entail an excess of pain or discomfort for the age group in question over that associated with usual hospital or clinic procedure, they can be carried out only in individuals who have reached the age when consent can be obtained from them as well as from the adult acting on their behalf. When procedures necessitated by the study of over-the-counter drugs will not impose pain or added discomfort, children who are old enough to assent may be considered as subjects. When the procedures will not impose pain or added discomfort and there are data from prior common use concerning the safety of the drug at the dose proposed in the protocol, children below the age of assent may be enrolled in such studies.

Ethical Considerations
Type I Drug Research

1.   Noninvasive type I drug research studies should not pose problems for ethical review. Nevertheless, informed consent must be obtained before this type of study is carried out.

2.   Invasive type I drug research studies need not cause problems for ethical review, if the data to be generated will assist in the treatment of the child under study. However, when this type of study does not assist in the treatment of the child, the institutional review committee must give special attention to the proposal. It must ascertain that any risks are weighed appropriately against the benefits others may derive from the results of the study. In these instances, the consent of the child 13 years or older . . . should be required in addition to consent of the person acting for the child before he/she is enrolled in the study.

3.   Studies of the efficacy, safety, and dose of investigational drugs in children may only be carried out in infants and children with the disease or condition for which the drug is to be tested. When agents are used for conditions occurring only in children (e.g., respiratory distress syndrome), the institutional review committee must review the safeguards provided for the subjects with unusual case. Every attempt must be made to have laboratory evaluations of the progress of the therapy available to the physician responsible for the patient's carte soon enough to be useful clinically. Any systems known to be adversely affected by the agent in adults (from phase I studies) should be monitored carefully.

4.   When placebos are to be used, the subject or someone acting in his/her behalf must be fully informed about the nature of placebos, the design of the experiment, and the reason for the inclusion of a placebo group. Efforts must be made to design the protocol to minimize risks and trauma to the child who may not be receiving the active drug. Furthermore, the protocol should be designed so the active drug will be introduced into the study regimen for each subject at the earliest possible time.

5.   It may not always be possible to complete the long-term follow-up studies suggested here. However, the investigator must provide a plan for follow-up studies prior to the enrollment of subjects. Furthermore, the subjects and the persons acting on their behalf must be informed of this requirement at the time consent is obtained. Investigators are ethically obliged to fulfill this commitment to the subject and society; it is an implied commitment when he/she accepts the privilege of carrying out investigations in children.

Type II Drug Research

1. Studies of drugs taken accidentally, in overdose, or *via* the placenta or breast milk are important in gaining information on the pharmacology and toxicology of drugs in normal infants and children. The accidental ingestion of a drug or the accidental overdosing of a patient provides an unusual opportunity for study of drugs in normal children. It is "unusual" because normal children cannot be used for "phase I" testing and because no individual may ever intentionally be given more than the usual therapeutic doses for study purposes.

The study of this type of patient is an ethical form of opportunism; it may not be of direct benefit to the subject but may be of enormous benefit to others. Protocols to carry out such studies should be designed, approved in advanced, and evaluated carefully by the institutional review committee so they can be kept on file and activated when the opportunity presents itself. The institutional review committee must be especially critical of such protocols to assure that "the need to know" for others does not expose the subject to undue trauma or risk.

2. Detailed conditions under which prospective pediatric drug studies to advance knowledge for others may be carried out have been discussed.

The various codes that have been written since 1945 (e.g., Nuremberg Code, 1947, revised Helsinki Declaration, 1975, etc.) consist of guidelines and rules that are supposed to assist investigators as they design, review, and carry out research in humans. They are inadequate, however, in meeting the needs of investigators and/or reviewers who are faced with numerous complex, interacting questions as they review and carry out their research projects. The codes tend to be static and narrow, and in some instances they are insensitive to the need to provide special protections for children in a research situation. The broader ethical principles referred to earlier and the more generally applicable guidelines cited may be a more appropriate point of departure for investigators and/or reviewers who carry out or supervise drug studies in infants and children.

A special case exists when research involving the human fetus is proposed. Several experimental approaches to the treatment of fetal conditions have been tried during the past few years, and many more are likely to be proposed in the near future. Examples of well-publicized experimental surgical interventions include surgery on fetuses for malformations such as congenital diaphragmatic hernia, hydrocephalus, and urinary tract obstruction. These techniques show some promise, but their benefits are far from proven, and the procedures are in need of further investigation. Biochemical/molecular biological techniques (e.g., enzyme replacment and gene splicing) became feasible and were attempted in the late 1980s. Pharmacologic approaches to fetal conditions, such as the use of drugs for cardiac arrhythmias and of antibiotics for fetal infections, need rigorous testing before they are adopted for fetal care. The principles stated earlier, which protect the infant or child, also apply categorically to the fetus in cases of research in therapeutic situations using subjects before birth. However, the possible effects on the pregnant women of research on her fetus also must be considered by investigators and IRBs and explained adequately to the pregnant woman and her family when consent is sought. The autonomy of a pregnant potential volunteer should always be respected. Consent must be obtained from the pregnant subject for herself as well as for her fetus.

The use of coercion, even in the face of potential fetal demise, is highly controversial and should be avoided. Thus any judicial order that requires a pregnant woman to undergo treatment that might be life-saving for her fetus but requires treatment of her that she may wish to refuse must be seriously questioned. In some cases where expert testimony predicted the demise of a viable fetus if the mother refused treatment (e.g., cesarean section for placenta previa), judges have ordered women to undergo surgery against their wishes for the benefit of their fetuses. In most of these cases, the judgment courts' orders were defied by the women, who refused to consent to the surgery, and the pregnancies ended naturally with the delivery of a living child, despite predictions to the contrary by experts.

The moral value of the life of a viable fetus is very high, but it may come into conflict at times with the values of the pregnant woman. An approach to thinking about this issue might be to liken the pregnant woman's relationship to her fetus to the relationship between an HLA-matched relative and a child with terminal renal disease. Courts have not breached the autonomy of a potential organ donor by ordering that person to donate a kidney to the dying child. The courts may need to reconsider the tendency to try to breach the autonomy of pregnant women in the same light. However, the outcome of this part of the debate notwithstanding, there can be no justification for disregarding the wishes of a pregnant woman when she is being asked to volunteer to participate in a trial of experimental fetal therapy. The experimental nature of the trial precludes any notion of assured benefit to the potential fetal subject, and without fully informed, freely given consent, no woman should become the subject of a research study—whether she is pregnant or not.

The common and statutory laws that govern behavior in our complex society are sensitively protective of the life and welfare of individuals (especially those who are dependent, such as infants and children) but are also very conservative. Thus Justice Holmes said, "Continuity with the past is not a duty, it is a necessity," and Freund added, "The law, for better or worse, is addicted to principle, and thus it constantly fears setting bad precedent."[11]

The relationship between the morality and ethics of society and the law that controls the society is complex. It can probably be simplified here, however, to indicate that, in general, moral principles and ethical precepts that develop in the social milieu cause the (conservative) common law to modify over time in order that the redefined ethics of behavior can be controlled in a predictable and societally beneficial fashion.

Clinical investigators and others in the "caring" professions hew quite comfortably to the moral imperative of "do no harm." The ethical issues involved in clinical experimentation with child subjects can be defined with some precision. What remains is for the law to change in such a way that justice and the inviolability of the individual are protected while the overall good of society and the health care of children in particular are improved. This will occur when responsible investigators and representatives of society at large challenge the established common-law precedents in such a way that "good" new precedents result.

REFERENCES

1. American Academy of Pediatrics, Committee on Drugs: Guidelines for the ethical conduct of studies to evaluate drugs in pediatric populations. Pediatrics 60:91–101, 1977
2. Editorial: Research involving children: Ethics, the law, and the climate of opinion. Arch Dis Child 53:441–442, 1978
3. Ladd J: The task of ethics, in Reich WT (ed.): Encyclopedia of Bioethics. New York, The Free Press, 1979
4. Capron AM: Legal considerations affecting clinical pharmacological studies in children, Clin Res 21:141–150, 1973
5. McCormick RA: Proxy consent in the experimentation situation. Perspect Biol Med 18:2–20, 1974
6. McCormick RA: Experimentation in children: Sharing in sociality. Hastings Center Report 6:41–46, 1976
7. Freedman B: On the rights of the voiceless. J Med Philos 3:196–210, 1978
8. Ramsey P: The enforcement of morals: Nontherapeutic research on children. Hastings Center Report 6:21–30, 1976
9. Lebacqz K: The national commission and research in pharmacology: An overview. Fed Proc 36:2344–2348, 1977
10. Cohen SN: Development of drug therapy for children. Fed Proc 36:2356–2358, 1977
11. Freund PA: Is the law ready for human experimentation? Am Psychol 22:394–399, 1967

BIBLIOGRAPHY

Ackerman TF: Moral duties of investigators toward sick children. IRB 3:1–5, 1981
Klein JO: Medical ethics and controlled clinical trials. Ann Otol Rhinol Laryngol 88(suppl 60):99–106, 1979
Pearn JH: The child and clinical research. Lancet 2:510–512, 1984
Rosner F: The ethics of randomized clinical trials. Am J Med 82:283–290, 1987

7

THERAPEUTIC DRUG MONITORING

LARS O. BOREUS

The logical way of coping with individual variations in drug response would be simply to measure the degree of effect in the patient and then adjust the dose accordingly. Unfortunately, such a straightforward approach is seldom possible, since it is usually difficult to quantify the effect easily and reliably in the routine situation.

One reason why adjustments of the standard dose must be made in some patients is interindividual variation in pharmacokinetics. Especially important are individual differences in the capacity of biotransformation and renal elimination. The pharmacokinetic profile of an individual is genetically determined but also may be highly influenced by age, disease, and various environmental factors, including concomitant drug therapy.

A practical help in attempts to optimize the dose according to the individual need is to measure the blood levels of drug and active drug metabolites in the patient at relevant time points. The rationale of such *therapeutic drug monitoring* (TDM) is that it gives information about the pharmacokinetic features of the individual as related to a large population of patients. This information, combined with careful clinical observation, will give the physician guidance on whether or not a dose adjustment is needed.

TDM has become available as a routine service in clinical work. The analytical techniques needed for selective assay of drugs and drug metabolites have developed rapidly and are no longer restricted to research laboratories.

This chapter will make a critical examination of the present possibilities for a meaningful use of TDM in drug therapy in children. The use of TDM in pediatrics has been the subject of some previous reviews.[1-5]

THE CONCEPT OF THERAPEUTIC DRUG MONITORING

The basis of TDM is the finding that during steady-state conditions and for reversibly acting drugs, the blood (plasma or serum) concentration is better related than the

dose to the pharmacologic effect (for reviews, see Evans et al.,[6] Sjöqvist et al.,[7] and Spector et al.[8]). The concentration/effect relation can be quantitatively determined in clinical trials on relevant patient populations and with sophisticated techniques available only in the research situation. The results of such "population kinetics" studies are expressed as a certain recommended range of concentration. Values well outside this target range suggest a pharmacokinetic deviation from the average, which may be accounted for by an adjustment of the dose or dose schedule.

PHARMACOKINETIC ASPECTS

The wide variation in clinical response between individuals is partly due to pharmacokinetic differences, including drug absorption, drug distribution, and drug elimination (metabolism and excretion). A TDM system is designed to detect such interindividual variations. However, it can only describe the net result of the various part processes involved. For instance, an unexpectedly low plasma value (as compared with a population of similar patients) may involve either poor bioavailability or rapid metabolism and excretion or a combination of these factors. Separate measurement of the part processes usually requires a more extensive kinetic investigation than can be provided by routine TDM.

Target values only apply to the patient population on which they were determined. Since ethical considerations limit the possibilities of controlled clinical trials, especially in children, the recommended therapeutic plasma ranges in the pediatric age groups are usually based more on empiricism than on hard data.

DOSE ADJUSTMENTS BASED ON TDM VALUES

The decision to change drug dosing during continuous therapy in a patient must be based primarily on clinical

63

observation. TDM should be regarded as a support in the process. The experienced physician will combine all types of information and come to a resolution without any type of mathematical calculation. This "trial and error" approach may work well. However, it can take some time to arrive at the optimal dosage with this method. An alternative way would be to calculate the optimal dose using pharmacokinetic equations and data from some initially made measurements in the patient.

This possibility has been widely discussed in the pharmacokinetic literature. Most of the suggested mathematical models have been based on an initial intravenous dose because the kinetic data are then not confounded with the uncertainty of the variable bioavailability that is always associated with oral administration. For example, a patient's total-body clearance and distribution volume may be estimated from an initial constant-rate infusion. This procedure was successfully used for calculation of the subsequent dose of gentamycin with small differences between predicted and measured trough and peak levels.[9] However, using data from the initial oral administration also may work. For instance, the dosage requirements of theophylline in children can be accurately estimated from orally derived pharmacokinetic measurements.[10]

Various kinetic models have been suggested and reported to give accurate results (theophylline,[11] gentamycin,[12] digoxin[13]). A comparison of the different drug dosing methods is found in the review by Burton et al.[14]

A practical difficulty with this kinetic approach is that the initial determination of kinetic data may require special arrangements (I.V. instead of oral administration, relatively extensive blood sampling) that may interfere with or delay effective early treatment. The Bayesian method[15] is somewhat less disturbing for the usual treatment practice because the previous routine TDM values in the patient are utilized for the kinetic information. The calculation is based on the notion that the variation in pharmacokinetic parameters is similar in the individual and in the population. The Bayesian method requires only routine data, is more flexible, and can be computerized. Therefore, it has been recommended for various drugs, such as digoxin,[16] theophylline,[17] phenytoin,[18] and aminoglycosides.[14]

A source of error with most mathematical approaches is the assumption that the patient's kinetic characteristics are stable during the continued therapy. This is often not true in the growing child, especially not during the neonatal period. The capacity for biotransformation and excretion can change so rapidly during the first weeks of life that all mathematical predictions become unreliable.

Thus, even if the mathematical dose calculations look attractive, they have certain disadvantages and will not necessarily speed up the procedure of optimizing the dose. They have not yet been generally accepted as more efficient and cost-effective than the conventional "intuitive" process. To work well, they require the assistance of specially interested consultants in pharmacokinetics. This will increase the cost of the TDM service.

FACTORS THAT COMPLICATE THE INTERPRETATION OF TDM VALUES

The concept of TDM is basically simple, but a number of problems become apparent when individual concentration values are interpreted clinically.

1. *The concentration/effect relationship may vary.* The relation between the drug concentration and effect in experimental laboratory models is usually stable and reproducible; in fact, the sigmoid log concentration/effect curve in isolated organ baths is a classical means in experimental pharmacology for studies of the quantitative action of agonists and antagonists.

However, the situation *in vivo* is complicated by a variety of factors, such as compensatory mechanisms and disease conditions. A well-known example is the response to digoxin, which is increased by hypokalemia, hypercalcemia, and hypothyroidism but decreased by hypocalcemia and hyperthyroidism. Clinical signs of digoxin toxicity may therefore appear even when digoxin levels are within the recommended target range.

During continued treatment, the target receptors themselves may react with up- or down-regulation, which will increase or decrease, respectively, the subsequent response of the effector system. These changes must be accounted for in the correct interpretation of TDM concentration values.

2. *The available information about concentration/effect relationship is incomplete.* Measurements of serum levels in individual patients are of little value if the relation between concentration and degree of effect in the general population is not known. The quality of such data determines the usefulness of TDM.

As will be apparent from the description below, relevant data on the concentration/effect relation are often surprisingly scarce, even for drugs that are usually included in routine TDM programs. The reason for this shortage of good data is that the therapeutic effects of many drugs, e.g., psychoactive compounds, are difficult and costly to assess under realistic clinical conditions. Prospective trials over long time periods and with elaborate protocols are required.

Furthermore, the external validity of even excellent trials is sometimes questionable. Diagnostic criteria and routines for observation of the patient may differ from place to place. The typical difficulty in pediatrics is that results from one age group may not be relevant for another. The recommended target concentrations in newborn infants and small children are often empirical rather than based on prospective clinical trials, which are especially difficult to execute in these age groups.

3. *Compliance and "spontaneous" variation in pharmacokinetics is difficult to control.* How well the patient follows the instructions about the use of the drug (compliance) can never be reliably controlled in outpatients. Irregular intake of the dose will make comparisons of drug concentrations at different times more difficult. The degree of compliance reflects how well the cooperation

between the child, the parents, and the physician works. It is more fruitful to try to promote this interaction than to look upon TDM as a device to measure compliance.

The *interindividual* variation in pharmacokinetics has been studied for many drugs. However, if differences occur over time in the same individual (*intraindividual* variation), this is of equal importance for the practical utilization of TDM data in long-term treatment, such as in epilepsy. Dose adjustments must be considered during a long period of the child's life, and it must be possible to compare concentration values from different consultations. To what extent short-term, "spontaneous" variations in the kinetics of an individual contribute to the intraindividual variation has not been much studied but is a possible source of "noise" in the system.

PSYCHOLOGIC ASPECTS

The purpose of drug monitoring is to provide the physician with pharmacokinetic information. In long-term treatment, especially in epilepsy, TDM also plays an educational role. An open discussion with the parents and patient about the results may promote an understanding of the disease and its treatment. This may improve compliance.

THE INFLUENCE OF AGE

In the pediatric setting, the age factor becomes a dominating difficulty in TDM interpretation. The special pharmacokinetic features of the growing child are discussed in Chapter 2. It is obvious that not only the increasing size of the child, but also the age-related changes in distribution and elimination can influence the dose requirement.

It should be emphasized here that the response to drugs also may show *qualitative* differences in children compared with adults. This is especially obvious with centrally active drugs. Well-known examples are the excitation often seen following phenobarbital administration to infants and the control of hyperkinetic behavior in minimal brain dysfunction by means of amphetamine or methylphenidate. Such pharmacodynamic age differences are not revealed by any TDM system.

DRUG-MONITORING SITUATIONS IN PEDIATRICS

In adult medicine, drug monitoring is utilized in many disease groups. In pediatrics, it is concentrated to (1) treatment of epilepsy and asthma, where long-term therapy is usually required, and (2) drug therapy in the newborn, where pharmacokinetics are special and rapidly changing

and dose adjustments therefore are often required. Antidepressants, neuroleptics, lithium, and antiarrhythmics are common drugs in adult TDM programs that are seldom needed in children.

Since many forms of epilepsy exist in childhood, several different drugs must be utilized, either in monotherapy or in combinations. TDM is very useful in these patients. Short- and long-term changes in plasma levels can be detected, which may explain side effects or treatment failures. Interaction effects also can often be discovered by TDM and dealt with by dose adjustments. The educational effect of regular monitoring on the patient and parents is an additional advantage.

The treatment of *asthma* with theophylline is another obvious area for TDM in children. Theophylline is a potentially toxic drug with a relatively narrow therapeutic interval. Monitoring of the plasma levels may help the physician avoid too high levels (side effects) or too low levels (treatment failure). If a switch to a slow-release product is considered necessary, TDM may be helpful in handling the situation.

The *newborn infant* has a unique pharmacokinetic profile that is described in detail in Chapter 2 in this book. Many drugs are utilized in a newborn intensive care unit,[19] and some of them have known concentration-dependent toxicities. TDM of theophylline or caffeine during prophylaxis of neonatal apnea is well established. Monitoring of the aminoglycoside antibiotics in the treatment of neonatal septicemia is also routine, although the target concentrations are still not well established. For digoxin, it has been even more difficult to define a recommended concentration interval.

It is obvious that the "menu" for pediatric TDM programs must be continuously modified according to the advances in drug therapy in general and to the changes in the drug policies of the local hospital. The laboratory must have the capacity to follow the developments in analytical technology, in pharmacokinetics, and in pediatric drug therapy.

A SUGGESTED TDM PROGRAM IN PEDIATRIC CARE

This section presents a TDM pediatric program. It contains nine drugs, of which seven have reasonably well documented concentration/effect correlations and which should be monitored routinely. Two of them, valproic acid and digoxin, may be useful to assay in special cases.

The generally recommended target plasma concentrations are summarized in Table 7–1, which also contains some remarks of practical importance in the interpretation of TDM values. In the subsequent subsections, the nine drugs are briefly described individually. For more detailed accounts of the pharmacology, the reader is referred to the references indicated in Table 1 and to the regular textbooks of pharmacology. The literature in the area is rapidly expanding. The local TDM laboratory should be consulted for information about recommended

TABLE 7–1. A SUGGESTED PEDIATRIC TDM MENU

DRUG	TARGET CONCENTRATION IN PLASMA (TROUGH VALUES)		COMMENTS	REFERENCE
	Old Units	SI Units		
Phenytoin	10–20 μg/ml	40–80 μmol/liter	Concentration-dependent metabolism: slower elimination at higher plasma levels; interaction can occur with other acidic compounds with high plasma protein binding.	Richens[62]
Carbamazepine	5–10 μg/ml	20–40 μmol/liter	Has an active metabolite; induction of metabolism may occur during combination treatment.	Bertilsson[63]
Phenobarbital	10–30 μg/ml	45–130 μmol/liter	Slow elimination; may induce the metabolism of other drugs.	Booker[64]
Ethosuximide	40–100 μg/ml	300–700 μmol/liter	Slow elimination; optimal concentration varies considerably among patients.	Sherwin[65]
Valproic acid	50–100 μg/ml	350–700 μmol/liter	Concentration/effect relationship poorly established.	Chadwick[32]
Theophylline	10–20 μg/ml	55–110 μmol/liter	Small therapeutic range; rapid elimination, sensitive to induction, methylation to caffeine may occur in the newborn.	Ogilvie[66]
Caffeine	5–15 μg/ml	26–77 μmol/liter	For prevention of apneic spells in the newborn.	Aranda et al.[37]
Digoxin	0.5–2 ng/ml	1–2.5 nmol/liter	Concentration/effect relationship poorly established, especially in the newborn; useful for detection of accumulation in the individual infant.	Wettrell and Andersson[40]
Gentamicin	max 2 μg/ml	max 3.7 μmol/liter	The trough sample may be supplemented with one or several samples, e.g., at 1 hour after administration; the peak value should probably not exceed 12 μg/ml (22 μmol/liter).	Evans et al.[6]

sampling times, types of collecting tubes, and handling of the samples.

PHENYTOIN. It is generally accepted that the anticonvulsant as well as the neurotoxic effects of phenytoin are parallel to the plasma concentrations.[20,21] Higher values than 20 μg/ml (80 μmol/liter) are associated with increasing risk of nystagmus at far-lateral gaze, ataxia, and sedation. The long-term side effects of phenytoin (gingival hypertrophy, coarsening of facial features, hypertrichosis, peripheral neuropathy, and osteomalacia) have been more difficult to relate to plasma concentration. The lower limit of the recommended concentration range (10 μg/ml or 40 μmol/liter) is more uncertain, and some children may be well controlled even at lower values.

There are two pharmacokinetic reasons to monitor the plasma levels of phenytoin. First, the drug is more slowly eliminated at higher levels; the first-order elimination kinetics then tends to approach a zero-order process. This phenomenon *(nonlinear elimination kinetics)* is also found in children[22,23] and is interpreted as enzyme saturation at higher concentrations.[24,25] The practical consequence is that even a small dose change (increase or decrease) may result in an unexpectedly large change in concentration. TDM will detect this. Second, the high protein binding of phenytoin (about 90 percent) makes this drug sensitive to displacement by other acidic drugs or endogenous substances with a high capacity to bind to albumin.

Several phenytoin products are marketed that may have different dissolution rates. A switch from one product to another may therefore change the absorption rate of the drug. Monitoring of phenytoin plasma levels during the dose interval can clarify the situation.

CARBAMAZEPINE. This drug is increasingly used in all types of epilepsy, except absences. It has partly replaced phenytoin because it has a more favorable side-effect profile. However, the recommended plasma level for carbamazepine (20–40 μmol/liter) is somewhat uncertain, since the metabolism of carbamazepine may be induced by the drug itself and by other drugs such as phenobarbital and phenytoin. Thus the addition of these drugs may be associated with a decrease of carbamazepine levels in plasma. In trigeminal neuralgia in adults, where the concentration/effect relation may be more reliably determined, a target range of 24–43 μmol/liter has been suggested.[26]

Another problem in the monitoring of carbamazepine plasma levels is the presence of the active metabolite carbamazepine-10,11-epoxide. The ratio between the concentrations of parent compound and metabolite varies because it is related to the rate of metabolism of both. It is not yet established if TDM should routinely include determinations of both carbamazepine and the epoxide.

Carbamazepine tablets are marketed by several manufacturers, and the extent and rate of bioavailability may differ somewhat between the products. Sustained-release tablets have been introduced in order to avoid too rapid absorption, which may lead to high plasma peaks with increased risk of side effects. Monitoring may, as in the case of phenytoin, provide the information needed to improve the dose schedule.

PHENOBARBITAL. This barbiturate has been used in pediatrics for many years on empirical grounds. It gives relatively predictable plasma levels in children.[27,28] However, the suggested negative effect on cognitive and psychomotor functions during long-term administration in children have made phenobarbital less attractive in the treatment of epilepsy and in the prophylaxis of febrile seizures.[29] In neonatology, it is also used for "brain protection" in asphyxiated newborn infants and is supposed to lessen the risk for intraventricular hemorrhages (presumably by decreasing the blood pressure). In these cases, the suggested doses are high enough to inhibit respiration. The function of TDM in these patients is to avoid too high plasma concentrations.

The most characteristic feature in the pharmacokinetic profile is the slow elimination with a long plasma half-life, which may be 4–5 days in the newborn infant and about 2 days in children. This means that, in steady state, the fluctuations in plasma between trough and peak are small and the time of sampling relative to administration of the last dose is less crucial than for the other drugs in the TDM program.

Phenobarbital is hydroxylated and conjugated with glucuronic acid. Glucoronidation is slow in premature newborn infants,[30] but since all metabolites are inactive, it is enough to monitor the parent compound.

ETHOSUXIMIDE. The place for ethosuximide is in the treatment of petit mal (absence) seizures. Like phenobarbital, it has a long plasma half-life, 25–35 hours in children and about 60 hours in adults. The target range is wide, 300–700 μmol/liter, and the variation in individual need is considerable. Ethosuximide is extensively transformed to hydroxylated and conjugated metabolites, which seem to be inactive. There is no apparent correlation between plasma levels and side effects.

VALPROIC ACID. There is no simple relation between plasma concentration and anticonvulsive or toxic effects of valproic acid.[31] The lower level for effect is in the order of 350 μmol/liter. The upper limit of the mean therapeutic range is even more unclear, but about 700 μmol/liter has been suggested.[32] It is probable that the antiseizure effect is lost when the concentration increases beyond a certain level.

Thus routine TDM is not very helpful for individualization of dose. Measurement of plasma concentrations may, however, be informative in individual patients on combination therapy; valproic acid interacts with phenobarbital, ethosuximide, and phenytoin. Simultaneous measurement of the drugs in combination can often facilitate treatment.

Valproic acid is a simple fatty acid with high plasma protein binding (90 percent), and it has several metabolites that are suspected to have antiepileptic properties.

THEOPHYLLINE/CAFFEINE. The toxic effects of theophylline (nausea, cardiac arrhythmias, and convulsions) are serious and concentration-dependent. This fact alone makes TDM desirable, if not necessary. Furthermore, the clearance rate can vary considerably among patients.[33]

The elimination is rapid and is influenced by various external factors. It is difficult to avoid large fluctuations in plasma concentrations during maintenance therapy in asthma. The clearance in children up to about 16 years of age is, on average, higher than in adults. Therefore, a somewhat higher relative dosage must be used in the young to achieve the recommended plasma concentration of 55–110 μmol/liter. This range is reasonably well established.

Many types of oral sustained-release products have been constructed in order to avoid early peak levels as well as too low values during the early morning hours when theophylline is administered the evening before. TDM can assist in the selection of dose, dose interval, and product in the individual patient.[34]

It has been shown that theophylline, like phenytoin, exhibits *dose-dependent kinetics,*[35] which means that the plasma concentration tends to increase relatively more than expected from the dose increment.

Theophylline is also used in the prevention of recurrent apneic spells in preterm infants. The pharmacokinetics in this age group have been well studied. It has been found that theophylline, which is a dimethylated xanthine, may be N7-methylated by the newborn to the trimethylated xanthine caffeine. It may therefore be logical to monitor both these xanthines when theophylline is used. Caffeine itself can successfully replace theophylline. The dramatic changes in elimination of theophylline and caffeine during the newborn period require plasma monitoring.[36,37] If caffeine is used, TDM is simplified to measurement of only one drug.

DIGOXIN. The pharmacokinetics of digoxin could be reliably studied when radioimmunoassays were introduced in the early 1970s. Newborn infants were found to eliminate digoxin from plasma at a much slower rate than adults (for reviews, see Morselli et al.,[38] Morselli and Bianchetti,[39] and Wettrell and Andersson[40]). The total-body clearance is highly dependent on gestational age and body weight, and the steady-state digoxin concentrations are inversely related to these factors.[41,42] Clearance rapidly increases along with the dramatic development of renal function during the first weeks of life. On the other hand, clearance tends to be *higher* in children between 1 month and 2 years of age. In this age group, therefore, higher doses of digoxin per body weight or body area are probably needed during maintenance therapy as compared both with younger children and with adults.

Studies on adults have shown that during the first 6–8 hours after administration, there is no direct relationship between plasma concentration and intensity of inotropic response. A more stable relationship is established during 12–24 hours after dose. Sampling should therefore not be performed during the first 8 hours after dosing.

A complicating fact is that the relative distribution of digoxin between blood and tissues seems to vary both with age and with muscular activity. The distribution to the heart and red blood cells is higher in young infants.[43] In adults, physical activity increases the skeletal muscle digoxin concentration and decreases the blood concentration.[44] Such distribution phenomena add to the difficulties in interpretation of TDM data on digoxin.

The recommended plasma concentration range, 1–2.5 nmol/liter, is only approximate and is derived mainly from studies on adults. It is not clear if the same levels are optimal in the pediatric age groups. Earlier dose schedules result in the same or even higher concentrations than in the adult. The earlier belief that the myocardium of the infant is more resistant to the action of digitalis is probably incorrect, and reductions of the standard doses have been suggested.[45]

Endogenous digoxin-like immunoreactive substances (EDLS) have been found in plasma from patients not taking digoxin.[46] They are present in newborn infants in concentrations that may cause false-positive measurements.[47] Studies on the origin and chemical nature of EDLS are in progress and will show if these substances influence TDM of digoxin in a clinically significant way. A chemical assay for TDM of digoxin is not available.

Thus routine monitoring of digoxin in children cannot be expected to answer the question of whether the dose is optimal or not. The justification for the assay is to detect accumulation of the drug with threat of toxicity, especially in the newborn infant.

GENTAMICIN AND OTHER AMINOGLYCOSIDE ANTIBIOTICS. TDM for aminoglycosides (gentamicin, tobramycin, amicacin, and netilmicin) is primarily a safety device to avoid too high concentrations of these potentially nefrotoxic and ototoxic drugs. It is routinely used in the treatment of proven or suspected neonatal septicemia, where plasma levels can be expected to vary considerably as a result of the dependence of these antibiotics on renal function for the elimination.

The target concentration may be achieved in the newborn by means of dosage regimens based on postnatal/gestational age and on body weight.[48] Plasma creatinine concentrations is a questionable measure of neonatal renal function[49] and should not be used alone for dose calculation.

It must be recognized, however, that recommended trough and peak values are very difficult to establish because the typical toxicity of aminoglycosides develops slowly and may be hard to distinguish from sequelae of the disease itself. There has been suggestive evidence for a lower toxicity of aminoglycosides in the newborn than in the adult. The target values in Table 1 must therefore be regarded as approximate.

Because of the parenteral administration and rapid elimination of these antibiotics, the optimal sampling time has been much discussed. A minimum is to take a trough sample, but the height of the peak is then unknown. A three-point sampling schedule of aminoglycoside (1, 3, and 5 hours after administration) gives much more information, since extrapolation to both maximum and minimum concentrations may be made.[50] A practical compromise is to take a trough value combined with one sample at 1 hour. However, this gives only an approximate estimate of the real peak level.

The aminoglycosides are not much metabolized and are mainly excreted by glomerular filtration. The plasma half-lives are about 2–3 hours in adults, longer in neonates and shorter in children. A protracted renal elimination of small amounts of drug has been reported that may reflect tissue accumulation. Its relation to the development of toxicity is not known.

OTHER DRUGS. The drugs just reviewed are the most common in present TDM systems in pediatrics. Depending on the specialization and research activities of the hospital, other drugs may need to be included on the menu. Two examples will be mentioned. Monitoring of salicylates in children with juvenile rheumatic arthritis may be useful in order to avoid toxic effects. In status epilepticus, it may be necessary to treat with lidocaine. In such a case, it is advantageous to follow the plasma levels not only of the parent compound, but also of the metabolites, since they possess convulsive action. The withdrawal of lidocaine may therefore involve a delicate balance between the concentrations of the parent drug and its metabolites.

In accidental drug intoxications, e.g., salicylic acid and acetaminophen (paracetamol), the facilities and experience of the TDM laboratory (or a toxicology laboratory) must be utilized to guide the treatment.

DRUG DETERMINATION IN SALIVA

Noninvasive procedures are especially attractive in pediatric care. A TDM system based on saliva rather than on blood sampling should be useful in children who are afraid of the pain associated with needles.

Another advantage would be to facilitate monitoring outside the hospital when the child is at home or at school. In this way, determination could be made around the clock, and the circadian variation could be investigated.

Furthermore, saliva concentration is supposed to reflect the unbound concentration in plasma, which is the fraction of drug that can produce pharmacologic effects. Therefore, a determination of saliva concentration should, theoretically, correlate better to effect than the total plasma concentration.

Despite these various advantages, TDM in saliva has not met with much success. Although there have been some enthusiastic reports, they have concerned monitoring of one or two drugs during carefully controlled, research-like conditions. In routine service, there are several difficulties.

First, a stable ratio between saliva and plasma concentrations may not always apply. It may vary during the dose interval, as for theophylline,[51] or with the pH of the saliva, as with phenobarbital.[52] Since the acidity of saliva can vary individually, the concentration ratio for ionized drugs may differ among patients.

Second, several technical difficulties are involved with saliva sampling. The proportions of secretions from the parotidal, submandibular, and sublingual glands are not controlled in common mixed saliva. The procedure of spitting in a test tube at fixed time points may be difficult in younger children. Stimulation of flow by chewing parafilm or similar material or by application of citric acid may help. This technique has been reported to diminish the variations in the saliva/plasma concentration ratio.[53]

Finally, the drug in saliva may be bound to protein or

cell debris.[54] Furthermore, drug residues remaining in the oral cavity from a previous tablet can entirely destroy a correct assay in saliva.

It must be remembered that the concentration in saliva, for highly protein drugs like phenytoin, is much lower than the total concentration in plasma. Thus the analytical technique must be more sensitive.

Even if a routine program for TDM cannot be based on saliva determinations, it may be helpful in some research situations, e.g., to study the pharmacokinetics of a drug during an entire dose interval. In these cases, the child and the parents must be well instructed and trained. Even so, however, it is hard to imagine drug sampling in saliva alone; from time to time, the saliva/plasma concentration ratio must be determined anyway.

DETERMINATION OF UNBOUND FRACTION OF DRUG

Common practice is to determine the total (unbound plus bound) drug concentration in plasma. However, it is only the unbound (free) fraction that can diffuse to the extracellular fluid and exert pharmacologic action. Measurement of the unbound concentration is of clinical interest for highly bound drugs such as phenytoin ($\sim$90 percent), valproic acid ($\sim$90 percent), and possibly carbamazepine ($\sim$75 percent). Variation in binding may occur for these drugs as a result of displacement by endogenous compounds or by other drugs during combination treatment. For the other drugs in the preceding menu, changes in binding will have insignificant effects on the unbound drug level.

The protein binding of phenytoin has been extensively studied, and there is general agreement that the unbound fraction is very stable in patients on monotherapy. In most clinical situations, the unbound concentration must therefore not be determined,[55] especially since this procedure is more time consuming, involving a previous step of ultrafiltration or dialysis before the assay in the nonprotein water phase. Measurement of the unbound concentration of phenytoin is, however, of clinical value in patients with hypoalbuminemia when displacement phenomena are suspected to operate and in some cases of resistant epilepsy.[56-58]

FUTURE DEVELOPMENTS

TDM is a service function, and its future role is entirely related to the spectrum of drugs that will be used in pediatric patients. Additions of new drugs to the routine program should be made only when the effect (therapeutic and toxic) is clearly concentration-dependent. At the present time, cyclosporine is more systematically introduced, since it has concentration-dependent toxicity. Improved immunologic and chromatographic assays are now available for cyclosporine. Another group of poten-

tial interest is cytostatic drugs. Although the antitumor effect cannot be expected to be simply reflected in the plasma concentration level, the toxic actions on normal tissues may be monitored. Methotrexate in high-dose treatment of childhood leukemia requires plasma-level controls that will show when the antidote, leucovorin, must be administered.

There is a need for further development in analytic technology, particularly with regard to selectivity. The immunologically based assays, such as EMIT (enzyme multiplied immunoassay) and FPIA (fluorescence polarization immunoassay), are rapid and simple to perform but may show cross-reaction with metabolites or endogenous molecules. Digoxin is a typical example (see above). Separation of active isomers from racemic mixtures also may be considered for selected drugs[59,60] when this procedure can be shown to have clinical importance.

Automatization of the assay procedures, including development of dry reagent strip assays, has already come a long way. These procedures are very simple to use but should not be allowed to replace good analytical skill on the part of the technicians. The maintenance of know-how is important for the future quality of the service. In fact, the assay itself is only one factor for the cost-effectiveness of TDM.[61]

Furthermore, the most urgent need in the future development of TDM is not the hardware (the analytical equipment), but the software, in the form of improved techniques for measurement of clinical effects. As mentioned earlier, the quality of the predictions based on TDM values is strongly dependent on good pharmacokinetic studies, where the relevant clinical effects also have been quantitated. Reports on long-term effects and on CNS action are badly needed. Another important task for research is the elucidation of the factors responsible for the intraindividual and interindividual variations in pharmacokinetics. In pediatrics, studies on the role of the age factor should have priority.

CONCLUSIONS

Monitoring of plasma (serum) drug concentrations may help the pediatrician to individualize the dose so that the therapy becomes optimal, i.e., effective with minimal side effects in all age groups. This is of special importance in long-term treatment, in neonatal care, and in the investigation of unclear side effects.

The deficiency of TDM at present is that the correlation between plasma concentration and pharmacologic effect is insufficiently known for many drugs.

A meaningful TDM service in pediatrics requires the following:

1. That the drug concentration is in a simple way correlated with the important clinical effect(s) and that this correlation is known for the relevant age group.
2. That a laboratory takes responsibility for the quality and reproducibility of its assays, for the contin-

ued development of the analysis program, for assisting the pediatrician in the interpretation of the results, and for information about the possibilities and limitations of its service.

REFERENCES

1. Pippenger CE: Rationale and clinical application of therapeutic drug monitoring. Pediatr Clin North Am 27:891–925, 1980
2. Rylance GW, Moreland TA: Drug level monitoring in paediatric practice. Arch Dis Child 55:89–98, 1980
3. Boreus LO: Principles of Pediatric Pharmacology. New York, Churchill-Livingstone, 1982
4. Boreus LO: The role of therapeutic drug monitoring in children. Clin Pharmacokinet 17 (Suppl 1):4–12, 1989
5. Buchanan N: Therapeutic drug monitoring in childhood. Aust Paediatr J 22:19–26, 1986
6. Evans WE, Schentag JJ, Jusko WJ: Applied Pharmacokinetics: Principles of Therapeutic Drug Monitoring, 2d ed. Spokane, Wash, Applied Therapeutics, 1986
7. Sjöqvist F, Borgå O, L'Orme EM: The role of the clinical pharmacological laboratory in improving drug therapy, in Avery GS (ed): Drug Treatment, 3d ed. Auckland, Australia, ADIS Press, 1987
8. Spector R, Park GD, Johnson GF, Vesell ES: Therapeutic drug monitoring. Clin Pharmacol Ther 43:345–353, 1988
9. Sawchuck RJ, Zaske DE, Cipolle RJ, Wargin WA, Strate RG: Kinetic model for gentamicin dosing with the use of individual patient parameters. Clin Pharmacol Ther 21:362–369, 1977
10. Brocks DR, Lee KC, Tam YK, Weppler CP, Bradley JM: A pharmacokinetic dosing method for oral theophylline in pediatric patients. Ther Drug Monit 10:58–63, 1988
11. Pancorbo S, Davies S, Raymond JL: Use of a pharmacokinetic method for establishing doses of aminophylline to treat acute bronchospasm. American J Hosp Pharm 38:851–856, 1981
12. Lesar TS, Rotschafer JC, Strand LM, Solem LD, Zaske DE: Gentamicin dosing errors with four commonly used nomograms. JAMA 248:1190–1193, 1982
13. Jones WN, Perrier D, Trinca CE, Hager WD, Conrad K: Evaluation of various methods of digoxin dosing. J Clin Pharmacol 22:543–550, 1982
14. Burton ME, Vasko MR, Brater DC: Comparison of drug dosing methods. Clin Pharmacokinet 10:1–37, 1985
15. Sheiner LB, Rosenberg B, Melmon KL: Modeling of individual pharmacokinetics for computer-aided drug dosage. Comput Biomed Res 5:441–459, 1972
16. Sheiner LB, Beal SL, Rosenberg B, Marathe VV: Forecasting individual pharmacokinetics. Clin Pharmacol Ther 26:294–305, 1979
17. Sheiner LB, Beal SL: Bayesian individualization of pharmacokinetics: Simple implementation and comparison with non-Bayesian methods. J Pharm Sci 71:1344–1348, 1982
18. Vozeh S, Muir KT, Sheiner LB, Follath F: Predicting individual phenytoin dosage. J Pharmacokinet Biopharm 9:131–146, 1981
19. Aranda J, Collinge JM, Clarkson S: Epidemiologic aspects of drug utilization in a newborn intensive care unit. Semin Perinatol 6:148–154, 1982
20. Kutt H, Winters W, Kokenge R, McDowell F: Diphenylhydantoin metabolism, blood levels, and toxicity. Arch Neurol 11:642–648, 1964
21. Lund L: Anticonvulsant effect of diphenylhydantoin relative to plasma levels. Arch Neurol 31:289–294, 1974
22. Garretson LK, Jusko WJ: Diphenylhydantoin elimination kinetics in overdosed children. Clin Pharmacol Ther 17:481–491, 1975
23. Dodson WE: Phenytoin kinetics in children. Clin Pharmacol Ther 27:704–707, 1980
24. Bochner F, Hooper WD, Tyrer JH: Effects of dosage increments on blood phenytoin concentrations. J Neurol Neurosurg Psychiatry 35:873–876, 1972
25. Atkinson AJ, Shaw JM: Pharmacokinetic study of a patient with diphenylhydantoin toxicity. Clin Pharmacol Ther 14:521–528, 1973
26. Tomson T, Tybring G, Bertilsson L, Ekbom K, Rane A: Carbamazepine therapy in trigeminal neuralgia: Clinical effects in relation to plasma concentration. Arch Neurol 37:699–703, 1980
27. Jalling B: Plasma and cerebrospinal fluid concentrations of phenobarbital in infants given single doses. Dev Med Child Neurol 16:781–793, 1976
28. Lockman LL, Kriel R, Zaske D, Thompson T, Virnig N: Phenobarbital dosage for control of neonatal seizures. Neurology 29:1445–1449, 1979
29. Knudsen FU: Optimum management of febrile seizures in childhood. Drugs 36:111–120, 1988
30. Boreus LO, Jalling B, Kållberg N: Phenobarbital metabolism in adults and in newborn infants. Acta Paediatr Scand 67:193–200, 1978
31. Armour DJ, Veitch GBA: Is valproate monotherapy a practical possibility in chronically uncontrolled epilepsy? J Clin Pharm Ther 13:53–64, 1988
32. Chadwick DW: Concentration-effect relationships of valproic acid. Clin Pharmacokinet 10:155–163, 1985
33. Jenne JW, Wyze R, Rood FS, McDonald FM: Pharmacokinetics of theophylline: Application to adjustment of the clinical dose of aminophylline. Clin Pharmacol Ther 13:349–360, 1972
34. Glynn-Barnhart A, Hill M, Szefler SJ: Sustained-release theophylline preparations: Practical recommendations for prescribing and therapeutic drug monitoring. Drugs 35:711–726, 1988
35. Weinberger M, Ginchansky E: Dose-dependent kinetics of theophylline disposition in asthmatic children. J Pediatr 91:820–824, 1977
36. Aranda JV, Grondin D, Sasyniuk BI: Pharmacologic considerations in the therapy of neonatal apnea. Pediatr Clin North Am 28:113–133, 1981
37. Aranda JV, Beharry K, Rex J, Johannes RJ, Charest-Boule L: Caffeine enzyme immunoassay in neonatal and pediatric drug monitoring. Ther Drug Monit 9:97–103, 1987
38. Morselli PL, Assael BM, Gomeni R, Mandelli M, Marini A, Reali E, Visconti U, Sereni F: Digoxin pharmacokinetics during human development, in Morselli PL, Garattini S, Sereni F (eds): Basic and Therapeutic Aspects of Perinatal Pharmacology. New York, Raven Press, 1975, pp 377–392
39. Morselli PL, Bianchetti G: Cardiovascular agents, in Morselli PL (ed): Drug Disposition During Development. New York, Spectrum, 1977, pp 393–429
40. Wettrell G, Andersson KE: Clinical pharmacokinetics of digoxin in infants. Clin Pharmacokinet 2:17–31, 1977
41. Collins-Nakai RL, Ng PK, Beadry MA, Ocejo-Moreno R, Schiff D, Van Petten GR: Total-body digoxin clearance and steady-state concentrations in low-birth-weight infants. Dev Pharmacol Ther 4:61–70, 1982
42. Hastreiter AR, Simonton RL, van der Horst RL, Benawra R, Mangurten H, Lam G, Chiou WL: Digoxin pharmacokinetics in premature infants. Pediatr Pharmacol 2:23–31, 1982
43. Gorodischer R, Jusko WJ, Yaffe SJ: Tissue and erythrocyte distribution of digoxin in infants. Clin Pharmacol Ther 19:256–263, 1976
44. Joreteg T, Jogestrand T: Physical exercise and digoxin binding to skeletal muscle: Relation to exercise intensity. Eur J Clin Pharmacol 25:585–588, 1983
45. Nyberg L, Wettrell G: Pharmacokinetics and dosage of digoxin in neonates and infants. Eur J Clin Pharmacol 18:69–74, 1980
46. Soldin SJ: Digoxin: Issues and controversies. Clin Chem 32:5–12, 1986
47. Valdes R Jr, Graves SW, Brown BA, Landt M: Endogenous substance in newborn infants causing false-positive digoxin measurements. J Pediatr 102:947–950, 1983
48. Thomson AH, Way S, Bryson SM, McGovern EM, Kelman AW, Whiting B: Population pharmacokinetics of gentamicin in neonates. Dev Pharmacol Ther 11:173–179, 1988
49. Feldman H, Guignard JP: Plasma creatinine in the first month of life. Arch Dis Child 57:123–126, 1982
50. Herngren L, Boreus LO, Jalling B, Lagercrantz R: Pharmacokinetic aspects of streptomycin treatment of neonatal septicemia. Scand J Infect Dis 9:301–308, 1977
51. Danhof M, Breimer DD: Therapeutic drug monitoring in saliva. Clin Pharmacokinet 3:39–57, 1978
52. Cook CE, Amerson E, Poole WK, Lesser P, O'Tuama L: Phenytoin and phenobarbital concentrations in saliva and plasma

measured by radioimmunoassay. Clin Pharmacol Ther 18:742–747, 1976

53. Jusko WJ, Gerbracht L, Golden LH, Koup JR: Digoxin concentrations in serum and saliva. Res Commun Chem Pathol Pharmacol 10:189–192, 1975

54. Reynolds F, Ziroyanis PN, Jones NF, Smith SE: Salivary phenytoin concentrations in epilepsy and in chronic renal failure. Lancet 2:384–386, 1976

55. Rimmer EM, Buss DC, Routledge PA, Richens A: Should we routinely measure free plasma phenytoin concentration? Br J Clin Pharmacol 17:99–102, 1984

56. Theodore WH: Should we measure free antiepileptic drug levels? Clin Neuropharmacol 10:26–37, 1987

57. Baird-Lambert J, Manglick MP, Wall M, Buchanan N: Identifying patients who might benefit from free phenytoin monitoring. Ther Drug Monit 9:134–138, 1987

58. Johno I, Kuzuya T, Suzuki K, Hasegawa M, Nakamura T, Kitazawa S, Aso K, Watanabe K: Is free fraction measurement of phenytoin always necessary in pediatric epileptic patients? Ther Drug Monit 10:39–44, 1988

59. Drayer DE: Pharmacodynamic and pharmacokinetic differences between drug enantiomers in humans: An overview. Clin Pharmacol Ther 40:125–133, 1986

60. Ariens EJ, Wuis EW: Bias in pharmacokinetics and clinical pharmacology. Clin Pharmacol Ther 42:361–363, 1987

61. Voseh S: Cost-effectiveness of therapeutic drug monitoring. Clin Pharmacokinet 13:131–140, 1987

62. Richens A: Clinical pharmacokinetics of phenytoin. Clin Pharmacokinet 4:153–169, 1979

63. Bertilsson L: Clinical pharmacokinetics of carbamazepine. Clin Pharmacokinet 3:128–143, 1978

64. Booker HE: Phenobarbital: Relation of plasma concentration to seizure control, in Woodbury DM, Penry JK, Pippenger CE (eds): Antiepileptic Drugs. New York, Raven Press, 1982, pp 341–350

65. Sherwin AL: Ethosuximide: Relation of plasma concentration to seizure control, in Woodbury DM, Penry JK, Pippenger CE (eds): Antiepileptic Drugs. New York, Raven Press, 1982, pp 637–645

66. Ogilvie RI: Clinical pharmacokinetics of theophylline. Clin Pharmacokinet 3:267–293, 1978

8

TOPICAL THERAPY AND PERCUTANEOUS ABSORPTION

R. GHADIALLY *and* NEIL H. SHEAR

The permeability of the skin to diverse substances is the basis of almost all dermatologic therapy. In disease, alterations in the skin's natural permeability barrier can have unfortunate consequences. Rates of penetration of substances may vary 10,000-fold, with even greater variation in damaged skin.

In normal skin, the intact stratum corneum (SC) serves as a barrier to loss of internal fluids as well as absorption of external agents. The living epidermis and dermis (Figure 8–1) also must be traversed by any topically applied agent before reaching the systemic circulation in the form of dermal capillary beds.

PERCUTANEOUS ABSORPTION

There are three components in the skin "barrier": stratum corneum, viable epidermis, and dermis. The importance of each component has been the subject of extensive debate. Smith et al.[1] in 1919 were the first to locate the barrier as the SC. However, it was not until the 1940s that Burch and Winsor[2,3] showed conclusively that the horny layer was the permeability barrier to water.

Percutaneous absorption involves a series of individual steps. Initially, molecules must be absorbed into the SC from the surface. They must then diffuse (permeate) through the SC and then be absorbed into the viable epidermis and diffuse through epidermis and papillary dermis until they reach capillaries and enter the circulation.

In normal situations, diffusion across the SC is the rate-limiting step. However, if blood flow is severely reduced or stopped, the diffusion is controlled by the transfer of molecules into the capillaries rather than by diffusion through the SC.

Before proceeding further, it is necessary to clarify the various terms used in the study of percutaneous absorption. *Diffusion* is a process by which molecules move from an environment of greater to one of lesser concentration.

The term *permeation,* however, is less specific, meaning only to pass through by an unspecified mechanism. *Adsorption* is the taking up of molecules at phase boundaries that are in contact by physical or chemical forces. *Absorption,* however, means "taking up" by any means and is not limited to surface interaction. A *partition coefficient* is the relative solubility of a drug in the stratum corneum as compared with the vehicle. Absorption of the surface is the initial step in percutaneous absorption. However, it occurs relatively quickly[1] and is of small consequence in the rate of absorption compared with diffusion through the SC.

Diffusion through the SC is a passive process through dead tissue. In the past, it was supported that the bifunctional solubility of the stratum corneum to both polar and nonpolar chemicals resulted from its inherently mosaic filament-matrix (tonofibril-gel) ultrastructure, which allows both aqueous and lipid regions to exist separately within cells.[4] However, it is now known that the corneocytes are surrounded by lipid derived from lamellar bodies.[5] This raises the question of whether cell-to-cell diffusion can occur and by what process. It also explains the differential permeability to lipophilic versus hydrophilic substances. However, after crossing the stratum corneum, transfer into aqueous fluids may be more difficult and may result in the stratum corneum acting as a reservoir for such substances.[6] The rate of diffusion can be determined using Fick's law, which states that the flow across a membrane is directly proportional to the concentrations of the molecule on either side. This can be modified for percutaneous absorption such that

$$J = K_p \times C_s \qquad (1)$$

where J = flux, C = concentration gradient, and K_p = permeability constant of drug through skin.

$$K_p = \frac{K_m \times D_m}{l} \qquad (2)$$

where l = length = thickness of SC, D_m = diffusion constant under given conditions of temperature, hydration,

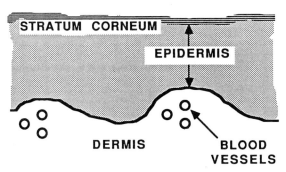

FIGURE 8–1. Structure of skin

etc., and K_m = partition coefficient, or the relative solubility of the drug in the SC compared with the vehicle. Modified,[7] we have

$$J = \frac{K_m \times D_m \times C_s}{l} \qquad (3)$$

The variable of partition coefficient is one that can be altered in drug design to optimize percent absorption. If a drug is not completely in solution, it will only diffuse into the SC slowly. If the drug is in solution with a large excess of solvent, it also will have less tendency to move into the SC.[7] This is an area for therapeutic manipulation.

Once in the SC, the rate of movement depends on the concentration gradient and the diffusion constant. The diffusion constant is a measure of the ease of movement of water through a tissue. The diffusion constant of water in liquid water is 10^{-5} cm²/s. For water in SC, it is 10^{-10}–10^{-9} cm²/s. For viable epidermis, it is 10^{-6} cm²/s, i.e., a thousand times easier than for SC.[8] This is so because the extracellular domains of the SC are hydrophobic as opposed to the hydrophilic extracellular domains of viable epidermis.

Many physicians feel that children absorb topically applied drugs more rapidly than adults and this is why many toxic reactions are reported in children rather than adults. More rapid absorption has not been documented in children. However, surface area/mass ratios are quite likely to be responsible for differences in the systemic dose of drug received.

Weston et al.[14] found that percutaneous absorption of *testosterone* was equivalent in adults and infants. The same authors show that in a total-body topical application, a neonate will receive three times the systemic dose of the medication per milligram of body weight; that is, if

Adult area is 17,000 cm²,

Neonate surface area is 2200 cm²,

Systemic dose (mg/kg) is dose (mg) times percent absorbed divided by body weight (kg),

Adult dose of salicylic acid is 100 mg/70 kg,

Neonate dose is 13 mg/3.4 kg, and

20 percent absorption occurs in adult and neonate, then

$$\text{Systemic dose (adult)} = \frac{100 \text{ mg}}{70 \text{ kg}} \times 0.02$$
$$= 0.28 \text{ mg/kg} \qquad (4)$$

$$\text{Systemic dose (neonate)} = \frac{13 \text{ mg}}{3.4 \text{ kg}} \times 0.02$$
$$= 0.76 \text{ mg/kg} \qquad (5)$$

Increased toxicity in infants has been demonstrated repeatedly in the past.

Kwell (γ-benzene hexachloride) has caused problems in both infants and people with massively excoriated skin. CNS toxicity, including seizures, resulted mainly from ingestion, overexposure, or mishandling of the drug.[15] Infants would be more susceptible to overexposure because of the increased systemic dose per kilogram per topical application.

In the past, deaths from percutaneous absorption of phenol as well as from salicylic acid have occurred, especially when these drugs are applied under occlusive dressings.

FACTORS AFFECTING PERCUTANEOUS ABSORPTION

- Site
- Age
- Hydration of SC
- Damage to SC
- Appendages
- Solute
- Solvent

Site

Differences in percutaneous absorption at different sites result from differences in thickness of the SC and the diffusion constant. Comparisons of different regions are most easily made using water permeation data. For example, plantar skin is 40 times thicker than abdominal skin; however, the diffusion constant is nearly 100 times greater (related to the lower lipid content of plantar skin). The lag time for the initial diffusion through plantar skin is proportional to the square of the thickness. Therefore, the water flux is only 10 times greater in plantar skin than in abdominal skin.[9]

Aging

Aging has little effect on permeability of the skin, except in preterm infants.[10,11] In infants less than 35 weeks old, in whom the SC is not completely formed, permeability is measurably greater.

In animal studies it was found that the stratum corneum, and therefore the permeability barrier, developed during the last quarter of gestation and was completed just before term.[12] At birth, the stratum corneum is indistinguishable from that of the adult and probably has just as complete a barrier function.[13] Preterm infants, however, show increased blanching to topically applied Neo-Synephrine. This is indirectly suggestive of a decreased barrier.

Hexachlorophene (pHisoHex) absorption is 3.1 percent of the topically applied dose.[16] When used on two children suffering from congenital ichthyosis, death resulted from percutaneous absorption of hexachlorophene. In the early 1970s, it was shown that repeated bathing of premature infants with 3 percent hexachlorophene was associated with vacuolar encephalopathy of the brainstem. In the children with ichthyosis, the main factor appeared to be a defective skin barrier to percutaneous absorption. In the premature infant, the low weight, and therefore relatively high systemic dose, was related to the prevalence of vacuolar encephalopathy.

The absorption of 1 percent hydrocortisone has been studied in adults and children. No significant effect was found on urinary steroids, plasma cortisol, blood pressure, or serum glucose.[16–18] However, more potent steroids, such as betamethasone valerate, have been shown to suppress the hypothalamus–pituitary–adrenal (HPA) axis when applied to the neck and waist in young children.[19] These studies suggest that the use of potent steroids may be associated with HPA axis suppression and growth retardation, and therefore, use of more potent corticosteroid should be avoided or used on a short-term basis only.

Hydration of the Stratum Corneum

Hydration of the SC enhances permeability of hydrophilic drugs, and less so lipophilic drugs, by increasing the diffusion constant D_m.

Damage to the Stratum Corneum

Paradoxically, however, extreme drying of the skin increases percutaneous absorption by disruption of the stratum corneum. Preexisting skin disease with fissuring and cracking can work in the same way to cause breaks in the SC and therefore increase percutaneous absorption.

Appendages

It has been shown that percutaneous absorption can occur through hair and sweat ducts. However, the extent of contribution is limited by the fact that appendages only cover 0.1–1 percent of the surface skin.[20] Mackee et al.[21] demonstrated follicular diffusion within 5 minutes of topical application. They found that shunt diffusion predominated only initially.[21] Schuplein[22] also showed that once sufficient time elapses to establish diffusion across the SC, diffusion through the shunts becomes less significant. The extent of appendigeal penetrance, of course, depends on the solute. Highly polar nonelectrolytes that are capable of binding to hydrated keratin, thus hindering diffusion across the SC, are more likely to undergo relatively prominent shunt diffusion.

The Solute

Most topically applied medications are covalent compounds. Many simple polar nonelectrolytes penetrate the SC at the same rate as water, with similar diffusion constants, e.g., ethanol and propanolol.[23] Study of a series of steroids ranging from progesterone to the more polar hydrocortisone showed that the more polar steroids have much lower diffusion constants. This is due to increased binding to keratin.[24] As the steroid becomes more polar, the flux becomes very small and shunt diffusion becomes relatively more important.

For less polar compounds (lipid-soluble nonelectrolytes) with similar diffusion constants, the permeability must be determined by differences in the partition coefficient (Fick's law). However, increasing the lipid solubility of a molecule may increase or decrease permeability depending on the solvent (vehicle used). If the vehicle is less lipophilic than the SC, then permeability will increase, and vice versa. For example, phenol in water has at least four times the permeability of phenol in arachis oil. This increased permeability is due to the relative insolubility of phenol in water versus an increased solubility in tissues. The mixture that most closely approximates the solvent characteristics of the SC is a 50:50 mixture of ethanol and water. For lipophilic substances, the partition coefficient will therefore be approximately unity. By appropriate alterations in the vehicle, lipophilic substances may be made to penetrate thousands of times faster.[25]

Electrolytes from aqueous solutions do not penetrate skin readily. Two factors are thought to decrease ionic permeability through tissue. Hydration around an ion makes it a large unit that will certainly penetrate no faster than water. The charge on the ion is capable of interactions that hinder permeability.

The Solvent

The solvent (vehicle) may have many functions, including retardation of water loss, heat retention, and increased percutaneous absorption. Vehicles that contain oleaginous solids with little or no water are called *ointments;* those with 20–50 percent water are called *creams.*[26] A greater component of water results in a *lotion.* Alternatively, vehicles can be divided into ointments, emulsions (oil in water, water in oil), and gels.

Ointments are usually composed of a fairly lipophilic drug in a base such as petrolatum, mineral oil, waxes, or organic alcohols. An *emulsion* is a two-phase system of two otherwise immiscible substances mixed with the aid of an emulsifier. These are generally more cosmetically acceptable than ointments. They may be water in oil (cold creams) or oil in water (vanishing creams). Emulsifiers coat one of the substances so that one is suspended in the other in the form of tiny droplets. They are also surface-active agents (surfactants), decreasing surface tension. The drug in this environment may exist dispersed as a solution, suspended as particles in a propylene glycol/aqueous phase, or dissolved within tiny micelles of excess surfactant. *Gels* are lotions with no oleaginous phase. They have fatty alcohols or fatty acids loosely aggregated with water, forming a gelatinous matrix at room temperature. With body contact, the gel melts and the water evaporates. This leaves semisolid particles and the active drug on the skin.

Other commonly added components to vehicles include the following:

EMULSIFIERS. These are commonly nonionic surfactants such as span, polysorbate (Tween 20 or 80), or sodium lauryl sulfate. Cationic emulsifying agents are weak emulsifiers, such as quaternary ammonium compounds. Auxiliary emulsifying agents improve the texture of emulsions, e.g., cetyl alcohol, glyceryl monostearate, and polyethylene glycols.

STABILIZERS. Chemicals that help preserve stability over time of both or either the drugs and/or its vehicle are stabilizers. These include preservatives, antioxidants, and chelating agents.

THICKENING AGENTS. These are used to increase the viscosity of a product or to suspend ingredients in a vehicle (emulsion stabilization). Examples are beeswax and carbomers.

HUMECTANTS. These agents are added to vehicles because they are hygroscopic and therefore are purported to draw moisture into the skin. Glycerin, propylene glycol, and sorbitol solution are examples.

TRANSDERMAL DELIVERY OF DRUGS

Transdermal delivery systems deliver drugs to the systemic circulation by means of the skin. The advantages of such a system are that the first-pass effect of the liver on drug metabolism is avoided, although some degree of analogous metabolism may take place in the skin (see Metabolism section). Drugs with a narrow therapeutic range can be maintained at a constant concentration in the plasma, thus reducing side effects and maintaining efficacy. These systems also provide convenient regimens for drugs with short half-lifes. Transdermal delivery is a noninvasive parenteral route for drugs that are unsuitable for oral ingestion or for use in patients who are nauseous or unconscious.

Only certain drugs, however, are suitable for this sort of delivery system. First, the drugs must penetrate the skin at adequate rates so that the rate-limiting step is supply of drug from the system and not the ability of the skin to transport drug. This allows drug input to be constant in all patients despite variations in skin permeability. Usually, agents effective at a parenteral dose of 2 mg/day or less are ideal for this form of therapy. However, 30-cm^2 systems delivering 15 mg/day nitroglycerin have been excellent. The less potent the drug, the higher its permeability through skin must be to achieve a therapeutic rate of delivery through a reasonable area of skin.[27] Second, the drug must not irritate or sensitize the skin.

Four transdermal therapeutic systems are now available. Transdermal scopolamine marketed by Ciba-Geigy was the first transdermal dosage form to become commercially available.[28] This provides 3-day protection against motion sickness with a single application. Similar products for nitroglycerin, clonidine, and 17-β-estradiol are now available. These dosage forms could be of tremendous importance in children who cannot or will not swallow tablets.

XENOBIOTIC METABOLISM BY THE SKIN

Not only may drugs penetrate the skin unchanged, but they also may be metabolized in the skin or interact with receptors present on or in epidermal cells. The skin is therefore not the inert barrier it was traditionally thought to be. The study of drug metabolism in the skin has been difficult because the structural proteins in this tissue are resistant to conventional homogenizing techniques that work well in other tissues. Also, although it has been suggested that the epidermis is the major site of drug metabolism, the scalpel scraping technique leads to dubious purity of the epidermal fraction.

Oxidative reactions demonstrated in the skin include alcohol oxidation, hydroxylation of aliphatic and alicyclic carbon atoms, oxidation of aromatic rings, and deamination and dealkylation. Examples of alcohol oxidation include the oxidation of hydrocortisone to cortisone and of testosterone to androstenedione.[30] The skin is also involved in the metabolic activation of carcinogens such as benzpyrene by oxidation of the aromatic rings.

Reductive reactions also occur in the skin. An example is the carbonyl reduction of 5α-dihydrotestosterone to 5α-androstenediol. Carbon–carbon double-bond reduction occurs in the reduction of hydrocortisone to its metabolite allodihydrocortisol.[31] Also, 5α-reductase is responsible for the reduction of testosterone to 5α-dihydrotestosterone in the skin.

There is little information on conjugation reactions in the skin. However, methylation, sulfate conjugation (of dehydroepiandrosterone), and glucuronide formation have been demonstrated.[30]

The enzyme system responsible for drug metabolism in the skin resembles that of the liver. This system is membrane bound and requires NADPH and oxygen for catalytic activity, as well as exhibiting a pH optimum. The terminal oxidase of the mono-oxygenase system is the heme protein cytochrome P-450. Although the liver is the major site of drug metabolism in the body, it has become evident that significant drug metabolism may occur in extrahepatic tissues.[29] As in the liver, other oxidases exist separately from the mono-oxygenase system. For example, there are the NAD-dependent dehydrogenases. Finally, analogous to the liver, these enzymes are highly inducible.

The epidermal metabolism of polycyclic aromatic hydrocarbons is an important subject in carcinogenesis to which much work has been devoted. When benzpyrene (BP) is applied to skin, it may be metabolized to various metabolites, including phenols, guanines, and dihydrodiols. Some of these reactions detoxify BP, but others activate it to more reactive species, which may interact with cell macromolecules.[33] Carcinogenicity studies of BP and its metabolites have been performed in mouse skin, and BP-7,8-dihydrodiol was found to be more carcinogenic.[34] Covalent DNA binding was greater with BP-7,8-dihydrodiol than with any other BP metabolite, suggesting higher tumorigenic activity.[35]

The distribution of cutaneous drug-metabolizing activity is related both to the anatomic site and to the cutaneous layer. Hydrocortisone 5α-reductase has been detected in human foreskin but not in other sites.[31] There are also differing enzyme activities at different sites. For example, although NAD is uniformly distributed in the epidermis and dermal appendages, the degree of reduction is higher in the epidermis and hair follicles than in the sweat glands and dermis.[36]

DRUG RECEPTORS IN THE SKIN

Drugs also may exert their effect directly in the skin by binding to specific receptors on plasma membranes, in the cytoplasm, or in the nuclear chromatin. Most studies of steroid receptors in the skin have been done with androgens. Like other steroid molecules, the receptors are cytoplasmic, and after modification of the bound hormone, there is attachment to the chromatin of the cell. There is resultant increased beard growth, increased male-pattern baldness, and increased sebum production. Cyproterone acetate and cimetidine will competitively inhibit binding of dihydrotestosterone. The concentration of receptor is greater in genital than nongenital sites, and this variation in concentration is thought to be of greater significance than the circulating testosterone level.[37] Dihydrotestosterone, produced locally by 5α-reductase from testosterone, binds to receptors more avidly than does testosterone. Thus the level of metabolic activity in the skin also may have an overshadowing effect on the circulating testosterone level.

Glucocorticoids also have similar receptors in the skin, and there is a wide variance in receptor concentration, with very high levels, for example, in the foreskin and low levels in the abdomen. Steroids affect all components of the skin, resulting in decreased epidermal-cell replication, proliferation of dermal fibroblasts, and synthesis of matrix components. Before binding to receptors, steroids must enter the cell by simple diffusion, although some cells may have special transport systems for this. They then bind receptors in the cytoplasm, followed by binding of the steroid–receptor complex to nuclear chromatin.[37] Some retinoid actions also may be mediated through intracellular receptor proteins binding to the retinoid as it enters the cytoplasm and translocating it to the nucleus. Both cellular retinoid-binding protein (CRBP) and cellular retinoic acid-binding protein (CRABP) have been isolated.[38,39]

Vitamin D_3 is synthesized photochemically in the skin. Hydroxylation in the liver and then the kidney results in formation of the active hormone. The main receptors are in the intestine, kidney, and bone, but receptors also exist in the skin.[40,41]

Membrane-associated hormone receptors on human epidermal cells include those for adenylate cyclase, epidermal growth factor (EGF), and insulin.

INVERSE PENETRATION

A concept in percutaneous drug movement that is more difficult to study is that of *outward migration,* or *inverse penetration.* Many chemicals vaporize from the skin surface, including elemental gases, water, hydrocarbons, ketones, and alcohols. Little attention has been paid, however, to the outward transcutaneous migration of nonvaporous chemicals such as drugs.[42] This is due to the small quantities of drug in question. However, the use of systemic agents for superficial skin diseases such as acne and dermatophyte infections indicates that such movement takes place.

After oral, I.M., or I.V. administration of a drug, there is assumed an even distribution through the entire skin, whereas with topical application there will be uneven distribution of the drug within the skin, with higher concentrations in the upper layers of the epidermis. If a drug were to be distributed equally within the body, only 10 percent or less of the drug would enter the skin.[43] The quantification of drug in the skin is very difficult, therefore, because of the low amounts involved. Drug migrates from the capillary circulation of the dermis through the dermis to the epidermis. The epidermis and horny layer have a passive role, but factors such as sweating and transepidermal water loss may influence accumulation of the drug. Certain organic compounds are actually excreted in the sweat, including histamine, vitamin K-like substances, amphetamine-like compounds,[44] and griseofulvin.[45]

CONCLUSIONS

The skin is both an inert barrier and a pharmacologically active organ. Consideration of its multifaceted role in drug delivery and drug metabolism is an important step in the development and use of therapeutic agents for skin diseases. Special attention must be paid to children and neonates. Large gaps exist in our knowledge, and it is not sufficient, nor wise, to extrapolate from adult or *in vitro* models.

REFERENCES

1. Smith HW, Clawes HA, Marshall EK: Mustard gas. IV. The mechanism of absorption by the skin. J Pharmacol 13:1–3, 1919
2. Burch EG, Winsor T: Diffusion of water through dead plantar, palmar, and dorsal human skin and through toe nails. Arch Dermatol 53:39–41, 1944
3. Burch EG, Winsor T: Rate of insensible perspiration locally through living and dead human skin. Arch Intern Med 74:437–444, 1946

4. Rasmussen JE: Topical therapy and percutaneous absorption, in Yaffe SJ (ed): Paediatric Pharmacology. New York, Grune & Stratton, 1980, p 305
5. Elias PM: Epidermal lipids, barrier function, and desquamation. J Invest Dermatol 80:40–49, 1983
6. Blank IH: Protective role of the skin, in Fitzpatrick TB, et al (eds): Dermatology in General Medicine, 3d ed. New York, McGraw-Hill, 1987, p 337
7. Vidmar DA: Percutaneous absorption: A review. J Assoc Milit Dermatol 8:57–60, 1982
8. Arndt KA, Mendenhall PV: The pharmacology of topical therapy, in Fitzpatrick TB, et al (eds): Dermatology in General Medicine, 3d ed., New York, McGraw-Hill, 1987, p 2552
9. Elias PM, Cooper ER, Korc A, Brown BE: Percutaneous transport in relation to stratum corneum and lipid composition. J Invest Dermatol 76:297–301, 1981
10. Kligman AM: Perspectives and problems in cutaneous gerontology. J Invest Dermatol 73:39–46, 1979
11. Nachman RL, Esterly NB: Increased skin permeability in preterm infants. J Pediatr 79:628–632, 1971
12. Singer EJ, Wegmann PC, Lehman MD, Christensen S, Vinson LJ: Barrier development, ultrastructure, and sulfhydryl content of the fetal epidermis. J Soc Cosmet Chem 22:119–137, 1971
13. Rasmussen JE: Percutaneous absorption in children, in Dobson RL (ed): 1979 Year Book of Dermatology. Chicago, Year Book Medical Publishers, 1979, pp 15–38
14. Weston RC, Noonan PK, Cole MP, et al: Percutaneous absorption of testosterone in the newborn rehsus monkey: Comparison to the adult. Pediatr Res 11:737–739, 1977
15. Rasmussen JE: The problem of Lindane. J Am Acad Dermatol 5:507–516, 1981
16. Feldman RJ, Maibach HI: Absorption of some organic compounds through the skin in men. J Invest Dermatol 54:399, 1970
17. Goldman L, Cohen W: Total body inunction as topical corticosteroid therapy. Arch Dermatol 85:146–149, 1962
18. Fleischmajer R: The lack of systemic hydrocortisone effects after massive and prolonged external application. J Invest Dermatol 26:11–16, 1962
19. Munro DD: The effects of percutaneously absorbed steroids on hypothalamic–pituitary–adrenal function after intensive use in inpatients. Br J Dermatol 94:67J–76, 1976
20. Idson B: Percutaneous absorption. J Pharm Sci 64:901–924, 1975
21. MacKee GM, Sulzberger MB, Herrmann F, Baer RL: Histologic studies on percutaneous penetration with special reference to the effect of vehicles. J Invest Dermatol 6:43–61, 1945
22. Scheuplein RJ: Mechanism of percutaneous absorption. II. Transient diffusion and the relative importance of various routes of skin penetration. J Invest Dermatol 48:79–88, 1967
23. Blank IH, Scheuplein RJ, MacFarlane DJ: Mechanism of percutaneous absorption. III. The effect of temperature on the transport of nonelectrolytes across the skin. J Invest Dermatol 49:583–589, 1967
24. Scheuplein RJ, Blank IH, Brauner GJ, MacFarlane DJ: Percutaneous absorption of steroids. J Invest Dermatol 52:63–70, 1969
25. Scheuplein RJ, Bronaugh RL: Percutaneous absorption, in Goldsmith LA (ed): Biochemistry and Physiology of the Skin. Oxford, England, Oxford University Press, 1983, p 1255
26. Weston WL: Practical Paediatric Dermatology, 2d ed. Boston, Little, Brown and Company, 1985
27. Chandrasekaran SK, Bayne W, Shaw JE: Pharmacokinetics of drug permeation through human skin. J Pharm Sci 67:1370–1374, 1978
28. Shaw JE, Prevo ME, Amkraut AA, et al: Testing of controlled release transdermal dosage forms. Arch Dermatol 123:1548–1556, 1987
29. Bickers DR, Dutta-Choudhury T, Mukhtar H: Epidermis: A site of drug metabolism in neonatal rat skin. Mol Pharmacol 21:239–247, 1982
30. Pannatier A, Jenner P, Testa B, Etter JC: The skin as a drug-metabolizing organ. Drug Metab Rev 8:319–343, 1978
31. Hsia SL, Hao YL: Metabolic transformations of cortisol-4-[^{14}C] in human skin. Biochemistry 5:1469, 1966
32. Voigt W, Fernandez EP, Hsia SL: Transformation of testosterone in 17-beta-hydroxy-5-alpha-androsten-3-one by microsomal preparations of human skin. J Biol Chem 245:5594, 1970
33. Noonan PK, Wester RC: Cutaneous biotransformation and some pharmacological and toxicological implications, in Marzulli FN, Maibach HI (eds): Dermatotoxicology. Washington, D.C., Hemisphere Publishing Corporation, 1983, 71–89
34. Kapitulunik J, Levin W, Conney AH, Yagi H, Jerina DM: Benzo(a)pyrene 7,8-dihydrodiol is more carcinogenic than benzo(a)-pyrene in newborn mice. Nature 266:378–380, 1977
35. Borgen A, Davey H, Castagnoli N, Crocker T, Rasmussen R, Wang I: Metabolic conversion of benzo(a)pyrene by Syrian hamster liver microsomes and binding of metabolites to deoxyribonucleic acid. J Med Chem 16:502–506, 1973
36. Leider M, Buncke CM: Physical dimensions of the skin: Determination of the specific gravity of skin, hair, and nail. Arch Dermatol 69:563, 1954
37. Ponec J: Hormone receptors in the skin, in Fitzpatrick TB, et al (eds): Dermatology in General Medicine, 3d ed. New York, McGraw Hill, 1987, 367—375
38. Ong D, Chytil F: Cellular retinoic acid-binding protein from rat testes: Purification and characterization. J Biol Chem 253:4551, 1978
39. Ong D, Chytil F: Cellular retinol-binding protein from rat liver: Purification and characterization. J Biol Chem 253:828, 1978
40. Colston K, Hirst M, Feldman D: Organ distribution of the cytoplasmic 1,25-dihydroxycholecalciferol receptor in various mouse tissues. Endocrinology 107:1916–1922, 1980
41. Feldman D, Chen T, Hirst M, Colston K, Karasek M, Cone C: Demonstration of 1,25-dihydroxyvitamin D-3 receptors in human skin biopsies. J Clin Endocrinol Metab 51:1463–1465, 1980
42. Peck C, Conner P, Bolden J, Almirez G, Kingsley E, Mell D, Murphy M, Hill E, Rowland M, Ezra D, Kwiatkowski E, Bradley CR, Abdel-Rahim M: Outward transcutaneous chemical migration: Implications for diagnostics and dosimetry. Skin Pharmacol 1:14–23, 1988
43. Schaefer H, Zesch A, Stuttgen G: Skin Permeability. New York, Springer, 1982
44. Vree TB, Musreus AT, Rossun JM, et al: Excretion of amphetamines in human sweat. Arch Int Pharmacodyn Ther 199:311, 1972
45. Shah, VP, Epstein WL, Riegelman S: Role of sweat in accumulation of orally administered griseofulvin in skin. J Clin Invest 53:1673–1678, 1974

SECTION II

DRUGS AND PREGNANCY

9

PHYSIOLOGIC ADAPTATIONS TO PREGNANCY: Impact on Pharmacokinetics

DONALD R. MATTISON, ANTOINE MALEK, *and* CAROL CISTOLA

In addition to changing size, shape, and center of gravity, there are complex alterations in pulmonary, cardiovascular, renal, gastrointestinal, and hepatic function that occur during pregnancy.[1,2] These physiologic adaptations can alter the uptake, distribution, metabolism, and clearance of drugs that may be used to treat maternal, fetal, or pregnancy-associated diseases (Table 9–1). Physiologic alterations during pregnancy also may alter maternal response to toxicants and toxins. This chapter will review physiologic changes occurring during pregnancy that may alter pharmacokinetics. The effect of these changes on the amounts and concentrations of xenobiotics in maternal and fetal compartments also will be explored using classical pharmacokinetic models.

Models of many types are used in all phases of biologic research.[3] They are simplified systems used to organize our view of biologic structure and function. In an experimental and theoretical sense, models are used to define and predict the responses of complex organisms to external forces or factors. This discussion will explore pharmacokinetic models that can be used to predict human risk for adverse pregnancy outcome following xenobiotic exposure.

Classical pharmacokinetic models begin with compartmental descriptions of the structure of interest. Although they are of value in many situations, these models may be limited in defining the target-tissue dose of a compound. In addition, classical compartmental pharmacokinetic models do not provide a direct approach to account continuously for alterations in physiology, growth, or development. As such, these compartmental models represent static images at a particular time or stage of development. This should not be interpreted as suggesting that pharmacokinetic models are of little value. On the contrary, classical pharmacokinetic models can be and have been used to provide insight into the effects of hormonal alterations, placental function, physiologic changes during pregnancy, growth, and development on xenobiotic absorption, distribution, metabolism, and elimination.

ONE-COMPARTMENT MODEL

A one-compartment model (Figure 9–1), although potentially limited in validity, can be used to describe the effect of physiologic adaptations during pregnancy on the pharmacokinetics of xenobiotics in the maternal organism.[4] Using a one-compartment model, the physiologic alterations that can be studied during pregnancy include the amount of xenobiotic absorbed, the rate of absorption, the volume of distribution, and the rate of elimination.[5]

A one-compartment model may be especially useful in exploring the effect of physiologic changes during pregnancy on treatment for maternal or pregnancy-related disease (Table 9–2). The one-compartment model has been used to explore in detail the impact of pregnancy-related changes on the pharmacokinetics of several commonly used drugs.[4]

Physiologic Variations in Absorption

During pregnancy, there are physiologic changes in several systems that can alter the amount of a xenobiotic absorbed into the maternal organism (Table 9–3). Intestinal motility is decreased, and gastric emptying time is increased,[6] probably a result of the high circulating levels of estrogen. As a result of these changes in gut motility, xenobiotics will spend a longer time in both the stomach and the small intestine. Using the one-compartment model, it is possible to explore the impact of decreased gut motility and increased gastric emptying time on xenobiotic absorption (Figure 9–2).

If the xenobiotic is absorbed through the small intestine, increased residence time in the stomach may delay the time to peak concentration in the maternal compartment. In addition, the xenobiotic may be metabolized in the stomach, so increased residence time will decrease the amount of parent compound available for absorption. If

TABLE 9–1. DISEASES REQUIRING DRUG THERAPY DURING PREGNANCY

MATERNAL DISEASE	PREGNANCY AND FETAL DISEASE
Hematologic:	Abortion:
Anemia	Threatened
Clotting disorders	Recurrent
Cardiovascular:	Labor:
Hypertension	Premature
Arrythmias	Postmature
Respiratory:	Dysfunctional
Asthma	Fetal cardiovascular:
Central nervous system:	Arrythmias
Seizure disorders	Failure
Psychiatric disease	Fetal pulmonary:
Endocrine:	Respiratory distress
Diabetes	Fetal hematologic:
Thyroid	Isoimmunization
Adrenal	Pregnancy-induced hypertension
Pituitary	
Renal:	
Autoimmune	
Collagen-vascular	
Infection	
Pain	
Gastrointestinal	
Cancer	

Source: Modified from Mattison.[4]

the ingested xenobiotic passes through the stomach unaltered, the longer time in the small intestine will increase the fraction absorbed. For example, if only 50 percent of a drug is absorbed during passage through the small intestine in the nonpregnant state and decreased gut motility increases the fraction absorbed to 75 percent, the initial concentration will be increased.

Pulmonary function also changes significantly during pregnancy (Table 9–4). Although the respiratory rate, breaths per minute, is unchanged,[7] the tidal volume, the volume of air exchanged per breath, is increased from 487 to 678 ml, a 39 percent increase. As a result of this increase in minute volume, the amount of inhaled toxins, toxicants, and biologicals is significantly increased during pregnancy.

It is not known if this change in pulmonary dose during pregnancy is responsible for increased maternal or fetal toxicity. However, a study by Gerhardsson and Ahlmark[8] suggests that women are more vulnerable to silicosis than

TABLE 9–2. CONSIDERATIONS FOR DRUG THERAPY DURING PREGNANCY

Treatment for maternal disease:
  Therapeutic effectiveness
  Maternal toxicity
  Effect of therapy on fetus
Treatment for fetal and pregnancy-related disease:
  Effect of therapy on maternal organism
  Therapeutic effects *in utero*

Source: Modified from Mattison.[4]

men. This study explored the age at diagnosis and duration of exposure to the development of silicosis in men and women in Sweden. Over the duration of the study, there was little difference in age at diagnosis for men and women pottery-forming workers. There were, however, significant differences in the relationship between the duration of exposure and diagnosis of silicosis. The mean duration from exposure to diagnosis was significantly ($p < .001$) shorter for women (20.5 ± 8.6 years) than for men (28.1 ± 10.1 years). The authors do not comment on the number of pregnancies or duration of work exposure during pregnancy. However, if these women worked during pregnancy, they would be inhaling substantially greater doses of dust. Interestingly, this phenomenon of shorter latency to onset of pulmonary disease in women also has been observed in the German fire clay industry.[8]

There are also substantial changes in blood flow to different regions of the body during pregnancy. Blood flow to the hand increases approximately sixfold during pregnancy from 3–18 ml/min/100 ml tissue.[9] Blood flow to the foot doubles during gestation, increasing from 2.5–5 ml/min/100 ml tissue. Over this same period of gestation there are only small increases in blood flow to the forearm and leg. The increase in blood flow to the hand may have a significant impact on amount of xenobiotic absorbed; this will be explored using a two-compartment model.

TABLE 9–3. PHYSIOLOGIC ALTERATIONS DURING PREGNANCY THAT MAY ALTER PHARMACOKINETICS

ALTERATION	CHANGE
Absorption:	
Gastric emptying time	Increased
Intestinal motility	Decreased
Pulmonary function	Increased
Cardiac output	Increased
Blood flow to the skin	Increased
Distribution:	
Plasma volume	Increased
Total-body water	Increased
Plasma proteins	Decreased
Body fat	Increased
Metabolism:	
Hepatic metabolism	$\pm$
Extrahepatic metabolism	$\pm$
Plasma proteins	Decreased
Excretion:	
Renal blood flow	Increased
Glomerular filtration rate	Increased
Pulmonary function	Increased
Plasma proteins	Decreased

Source: Modified from Mattison.[4]

PHARMACOKINETICS IN PREGNANCY SINGLE COMPARTMENT MODEL

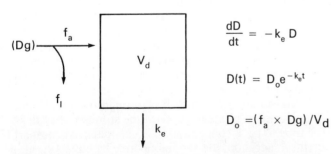

$$\frac{dD}{dt} = -k_e D$$

$$D(t) = D_o e^{-k_e t}$$

$$D_o = (f_a \times Dg)/V_d$$

FIGURE 9–1. One-compartment pharmacokinetic model of pregnancy (D_g, dose given; f_a, fraction absorbed; f_l, fraction lost; V_d, volume of distribution; K_e, elimination rate constant).

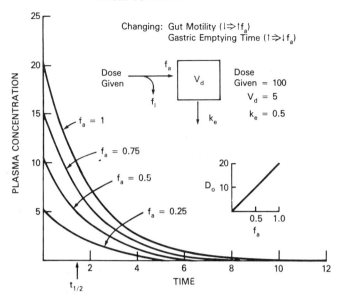

FIGURE 9-2. Effect of increased gastric emptying time and decreased gut motility on initial concentration. Increased residence in the gut may increase metabolism and decrease the fraction absorbed (f_a). Increased time in the intestine, resulting from decreased motility, may increase the fraction absorbed. For example, if $f_a = 0.5$ in the nonpregnant state and increases to 0.75 during pregnancy, the initial concentration will increase from 10 to 15.

Physiologic Variations in Distribution

During pregnancy, there are changes in body weight, total-body water, plasma proteins, body fat, and cardiac output that can alter the distribution of drugs (Tables 9-5 and 9-6) and other xenobiotics.[1,2,4] Maternal cardiac output increases approximately 40–50 percent by the middle of the second trimester and remains elevated throughout gestation. Maternal weight increases from approximately 50 kg at the start of pregnancy to approximately 63 kg at 40 weeks. The total-body water volume increases from 25 liters at the start of pregnancy to 33 liters at term. Maternal extracellular fluid volume increases from 11 liters at the start of pregnancy to 15 liters over the course of pregnancy. Plasma volume increases from 2.5 to 3.8 liters over the 40 weeks of gestation.

Maternal body fat also increases about 25 percent during gestation.[10] At the beginning of pregnancy, the mater-

TABLE 9-4. PULMONARY FUNCTION CHANGES DURING PREGNANCY

FUNCTION	NONPREGNANT	PREGNANT	CHANGE
Respiratory rate	15	16	—
Tidal volume (ml/min)	487	678	+39%
Minute ventilation (ml)	7,270	10,340	+42%
Minute O₂ uptake	201	266	+32%
Vital capacity (ml)	3,260	3,310	—

Source: Data from deSwiet.[7]

nal body contains approximately 16.5 kg of adipose tissue. At 20 weeks, the midpoint of gestation, maternal body fat has increased to 18.5 kg; and by 30 weeks, to 20 kg. There may be a slight decrease in body fat over the last 10 weeks of gestation. This increase in body fat during pregnancy may increase the body burden of lipid-soluble xenobiotics during pregnancy and may have an impact on the delivery of xenobiotics to the infant during lactation.

The increase in plasma volume and total-body water during pregnancy will decrease the concentration of many xenobiotics in the maternal organism (Figure 9-3 and Table 9-7). Consider, for example, caffeine. The volume of distribution in the nonpregnant woman is 25 liters; if the dose is 150 mg, the initial concentration will be 6 mg/liter. During pregnancy, the volume of distribution increases to 25.5, 27.0, 29.0, and 33.0 liters at 10, 20, 30, and 40 weeks. This increase in the volume of distribution will decrease the initial concentration of caffeine to 5.9, 5.6, 5.2, and 4.5 mg/liter. Note that changing volume of distribution is not the only alteration to caffeine metabolism during pregnancy.

If the xenobiotic is a drug given for some therapeutic effect in the maternal organism, increasing the volume of distribution may decrease therapeutic effectiveness (see Table 9-7). Consider, for example, the commonly used antibiotic ampicillin. The volume of distribution for this drug increases from 21 to approximately 35 liters during pregnancy. This will clearly have an impact on the amount of ampicillin needed for therapeutic effectiveness in the treatment of an infection.[4] Note the effect of increasing distribution volume increases even more with ampicillin's higher elimination rate inpregnancy.

Physiologic Variations in Metabolism

The altered hormonal milieu of pregnancy is associated with changes in hepatic and extrahepatic xenobiotic metabolism.[11,12] In addition, during gestation, metabolism by the fetus and placenta may alter maternal levels of the parent xenobiotic or its metabolites (Tables 9-7 and 9-8). Placental and fetal metabolism also may influence fetal or placental toxicity produced by a xenobiotic.

Gillette[13] has evaluated the impact of fetal metabolism on maternal and fetal levels of hypothetical xenobiotics. He suggests that fetal metabolism has only a small effect on the maternal concentration of a lipid-soluble xenobiotic that is rapidly transported into the fetal compartment. The effect of fetal metabolism may lower the fetal concentration by half. If the xenobiotic is slowly transported to the fetus, metabolism in fetal tissues may have an even greater impact on fetal concentration. With a slower rate of transport to the fetus, metabolism reduces fetal concentrations to 20 percent of the concentration if fetal metabolism does not occur. Placental metabolism also may play a similar role in altering maternal and fetal concentration of some xenobiotics.

Physiologic Variations in Elimination

During gestation, alterations in renal blood flow, glomerular filtration rate, hepatic blood flow, bile flow, and

TABLE 9–5. MATERNAL FACTORS THAT INFLUENCE VOLUME OF DISTRIBUTION

GESTATION (weeks)	MATERNAL WEIGHT (kg)	PLASMA VOLUME (liters)	EXTRACELLULAR FLUID VOLUME (liters)	TOTAL-BODY WATER (liters)	BODY FAT (kg)
0	50.0	2.50	11	25.0	16.5
10	50.6 (1.01)	2.75 (1.10)	12 (1.09)	25.5 (1.02)	16.8 (1.02)
20	54.0 (1.08)	3.00 (1.20)	13 (1.18)	27.0 (1.08)	18.6 (1.13)
30	58.5 (1.17)	3.60 (1.44)	14 (1.27)	29.0 (1.16)	20.0 (1.21)
40	62.5 (1.25)	3.75 (1.50)	15 (1.36)	33.0 (1.32)	19.8 (1.20)

The values listed are estimates for the indicated stage of gestation, as well as the nonpregnant value. Numbers in parenthesis are fold change from nonpregnant at that state of gestation.
Source: Modified from Mattison.[4]

pulmonary function may alter maternal elimination of a xenobiotic (see Tables 9–7 and 9–8). During pregnancy, maternal renal plasma flow increases from 500 ml/min/ 1.73 m^2 to approximately 700 ml/min/1.73 m^2. Glomerular filtration rate also increases during pregnancy. At the beginning of gestation, glomerular filtration rate is approximately 100 ml/min/1.73 m^2. By midgestation (20 weeks), the glomerular filtration rate has increased to approximately 150 ml/min/1.73 m^2.[14]

Both the increased renal plasma flow and the increased glomerular filtration rate will increase the elimination rate constant for xenobiotics cleared by the kidney (Figure 9–4). Consider, for example, the antibiotic ampicillin. If the rate constant for elimination is 0.016 h^{-1} at the beginning of gestation and increases to 0.018 h^{-1} at term, ampicillin will be cleared more rapidly during pregnancy. This effect of increased rate of elimination can have a significant impact on drug treatment during pregnancy. For

ampicillin, the combined effect of increased volume of distribution and rate of elimination essentially doubles the amount of drug needed to achieve the same area under the concentration versus time curve (see Table 9–7). Some anticonvulsants are cleared more rapidly during pregnancy than in the nonpregnant state. This means that to maintain plasma anticonvulsant levels within the therapeutic range, it is necessary to increase the dose or the frequency of administration.

Caffeine is a drug whose volume of distribution increases from 25.0–33.0 liters and whose rate of elimination decreases from 0.2–0.066 h^{-1} during pregnancy. As pregnancy advances, the increased volume of distribution decreases the initial concentration of caffeine in maternal plasma. However, the decrease in the elimination rate constant decreases the rate at which the drug is cleared from the body. In fact, to keep the area under the concentration versus time curve constant during pregnancy, it is necessary to decrease the dose of caffeine from 150 mg at the beginning of gestation to 86 mg at midgestation and 68 mg at term.

As a final example in this section, consider a xenobiotic whose volume of distribution increases proportional to maternal weight during pregnancy and whose rate of elimination also increases from 0.10–0.15 h^{-1} during the first trimester proportional to pulmonary or renal elimination (Figure 9–5). As pregnancy advances, the increased volume of distribution decreases the initial concentration of the xenobiotic in maternal plasma (Figure 9–5A). The increase in the elimination rate constant increases the rate at which the xenobiotic is cleared from the body. This suggests that for some xenobiotics, maternal tolerance may actually increase during pregnancy. However, increased renal clearance during pregnancy may, by increasing the dose of xenobiotic delivered, increase toxicity to the maternal bladder epithelium.

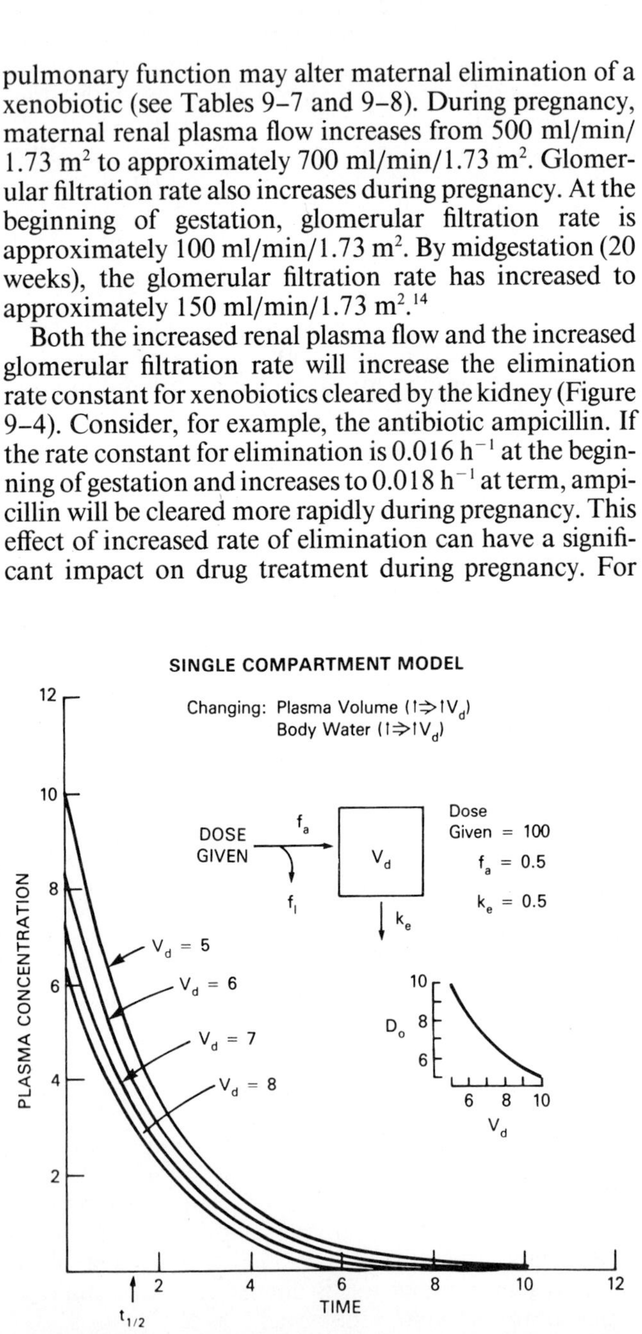

FIGURE 9–3. Effect of increasing plasma volume or total-body water on the initial concentration of a drug (D_0). If volume of distribution (V_d) is 5 liters in a nonpregnant individual and the dose given is 100 mg, then D_0 will be 10 mg/liter. If V_d increases to 8 liters during pregnancy, D_0 will fall to 8 mg/liter. The inset *(lower right)* illustrates the relationship between D_0 and V_d.

TABLE 9–6. EFFECT OF PREGNANCY ON THE VOLUME OF DISTRIBUTION OF SELECTED DRUGS

DRUG	VOLUME OF DISTRIBUTION
Oxacillin	Increased
Ampicillin	Increased
Methaqualone	Unchanged
Phenobarbitol	Increased
Cefalothin	Increased
Meperidine	Decreased

Source: Modified from Mattison.[4]

TABLE 9–7. AMPICILLIN, MEPERIDINE, CAFFEINE, AND FUROSEMIDE PHARMACOKINETICS DURING PREGNANCY

DRUG	GESTATION (weeks)	VOLUME OF DISTRIBUTION (liters)	$t_{1/2}$ (h)	K_e (h⁻¹)	DOSE (mg) FOR EQUAL AUC
Ampicillin	0	20.5	44	0.0158	500
	10	27.8	39	0.0178	764
	20	29.7	39	0.0178	816
	30	32.2	39	0.0178	885
	40	34.4	39	0.0178	945
Meperidine	0	200	3.4	0.2038	50.0
	10	137	3.7	0.1873	31.5
	20	146	3.7	0.1873	33.5
	30	158	3.7	0.1783	36.3
	40	169	3.7	0.1783	38.8
Caffeine	0	25.0	3.5	0.1980	150
	10	25.5	4.7	0.1474	122
	20	27.0	7.2	0.0963	86
	30	29.0	10.0	0.0963	67
	40	33.0	10.5	0.0660	68
Furosemide	0	9.0	1	0.6930	40.0
	10	9.1	1.2	0.5775	33.7
	20	9.8	1.2	0.5775	36.3
	30	10.8	1.2	0.5775	40.0
	40	11.6	1.2	0.5775	42.9

Source: Modified from Mattison.[4]

Placental Alterations During Pregnancy

Following implantation in the primate, the placenta begins to exert control on the maternal organism. An early signal sent by the placenta, human chorionic gonadotropin (hCG), stimulates continued ovarian production of progesterone. In the absence of hCG production or in the face of ovarian inability to respond to hCG, spontaneous abortion may occur. During implantation, therefore, the success of pregnancy depends on interactions between the ovary and placenta. Following establishment of the placenta, it will determine the success of the pregnancy. In other species, however, the ovary plays a more prominent role in the maintenance of pregnancy.[15]

During implantation, the placenta invades the endometrium, which formed under hormonal control of the ovary, and maternal and fetal circulatory systems are created. In primates, the *lobules*—the maternal portion of the placenta—are poorly defined regions separated by incomplete septa. The *cotyledons*—the fetal portion of the primate placenta—are discrete entities. There are generally several cotyledons within each lobule. The gross

TABLE 9–8. EFFECT OF PREGNANCY ON THE RATE OF ELIMINATION

DRUG	RATE OF ELIMINATION
Methicillin	Decreased
Ampicillin	Increased
Cefalothin	Decreased
Gentamicin	Unchanged
Caffeine	Decreased
Cefatrizine	Decreased
Methaqualone	Increased

Source: Modified from Mattison.[4]

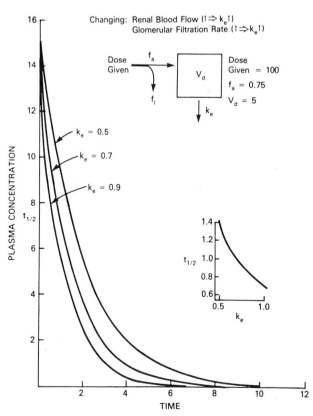

FIGURE 9–4. Effect of increased renal elimination on pharmacokinetics during pregnancy. If the renal elimination rate constant increases from 0.5 to 0.9 h¹ during pregnancy ($t_{1/2}$ decreases from about 1.4 to 0.69 h), the drug or xenobiotic will be cleared from the maternal compartment more rapidly.

ONE COMPARTMENT PHARMACOKINETIC MODEL

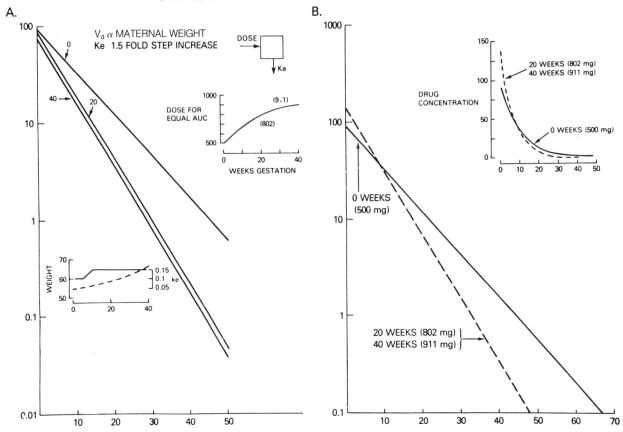

FIGURE 9–5. Impact of increased volume of distribution and elimination rate constant on pharmacokinetics. The vertical axis represents drug concentration; the horizontal axis reresents time. (*A*) The volume of distribution (V_d) is proportional to maternal weight, and the elimination rate constant (K_e) increases from 0.10 to 0.15 h^{-1} at the end of the first trimester. Under these conditions, the dose required to maintain an equal area under the concentration versus time curve (AUC) increases from 500 to 911 mg. (*B*) If the dose of the drug is increased to provide equal AUC, the initial concentration and concentration over the first 10 hours is increased compared with the nonpregnant state. If the drug has a narrow therapeutic window, this increased concentration may increase toxicity or side effects.

and microscopic structure of the placenta is strongly dependent on the species, however, so this description of the primate placenta will not be adequate for many experimental animals.

Exchange of proteins, amino acids, carbohydrates, fats, gases, and xenobiotics between the maternal and fetal circulatory systems occurs across the placenta. Quantitative risk assessment for developmental toxicity must consider species differences in placental type and structure. In addition, quantitative risk estimation must consider differences in placental surface area during pregnancy (Table 9–9), as well as differences in fetal or maternal blood flow rates through their respective circulatory units in the placenta.

Across species, for example, there are substantial differences in placental type. These differences may, in part, account for the high false-positive rate of developmental toxicity seen in the rodent.[16,23] The use of mechanism-based physiologic–pharmacokinetic models, however, may allow these differences to be considered in defining human reproductive hazard and risk assessments.[17]

Comparative surface area across species and during gestation also needs to be considered in formulating a ratio-

nal risk assessment. For example, in the human, the placental surface area increases from about 1.5 m^2 at 100 days of gestation to 15 m^2 at term (see Table 9–9). It is clear that comparative transfer rates, taking into consideration the number of tissue layers, the distance separating circulations, the placental metabolism, and the placental area, must be considered in any quantitative risk assessment exploring embryonic or fetal toxicity. At the present time, research using human fetal tissues from first- or second-trimester pregnancies is quite difficult for

TABLE 9–9. SURFACE AREA OF THE HUMAN PLACENTA DURING GESTATION

GESTATION (days)	SURFACE AREA (m^2)
100	1.5
120	2.5
170	4.7
190	4.9
220	7.3
240	14.0
270 (term)	15.0

ethical, legal, and procedural reasons. Therefore, most research has been restricted to defining placental transfer and metabolism using term human placentas. It is hoped that with the easing of these restrictions and with greater experience in defining placental function using term human placentas, it will be possible to characterize placental function—transport and metabolism—in second- and first-trimester placentas.

By the third trimester, much of the structure of the fetus has been defined; during this period, however, many of the functional characteristics of the fetus are being developed. For example, cellular communication (e.g., neuronal contacts) is being developed, as is the cell number in many organ systems. In addition, the fetus remains vulnerable to cytotoxic or disruptive processes during the third trimester. Finally, during the third trimester, issues of fetal toxicity from environmental exposures remain a substantial concern.

Existing evidence suggests that placental transfer from maternal to fetal circulatory systems occurs for essentially every compound tested.[18] Placental metabolism is less likely, although it has been demonstrated for selected compounds.[19-21] However, when placental metabolism occurs, it may have a significant impact on fetal concentrations[13] and fetal or placental toxicity. In addition to mediating fetal toxicity by transferring the parent compound or metabolites into the fetal circulatory system, placental toxicity by destruction of placental cells or placental functions may have similar disruptive effects on the fetus. For example, in experimental animals, prenatal exposure to cadmium produces fetal death. This effect, however, is not the result of direct fetal toxicity but is the result of placental toxicity.[22] For this reason, xenobiotic uptake and effect on placental function are as important as placental transport of the parent xenobiotic or metabolism and transport of metabolites to the fetus.

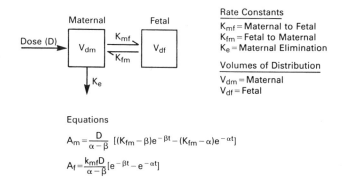

PHARMACOKINETICS IN PREGNANCY
TWO COMPARTMENT MODEL

Rate Constants
K_{mf} = Maternal to Fetal
K_{fm} = Fetal to Maternal
K_e = Maternal Elimination

Volumes of Distribution
V_{dm} = Maternal
V_{df} = Fetal

Equations

$$A_m = \frac{D}{\alpha - \beta} [(K_{fm} - \beta)e^{-\beta t} - (K_{fm} - \alpha)e^{-\alpha t}]$$

$$A_f = \frac{k_{mf}D}{\alpha - \beta} [e^{-\beta t} - e^{-\alpha t}]$$

$$\alpha = \frac{1}{2}[(K_{mf} + K_{fm} + K_e) + \sqrt{(K_{mf} + K_{fm} + K_e)^2 - 4K_{fm}K_e}]$$

$$\beta = \frac{1}{2}[(K_{mf} + K_{fm} + K_e) - \sqrt{(K_{mf} + K_{fm} + K_e)^2 - 4K_{fm}K_e}]$$

FIGURE 9–6. Two-compartment pharmacokinetic model during pregnancy (Modified from Wagner.[5]).

TWO-COMPARTMENT MODEL

Having explored the impact of some of the physiologic changes during pregnancy on pharmacokinetics in the maternal organism, it is instructive to consider the effects of these alterations on the amount of xenobiotic reaching the fetal compartment (Figure 9–6). The two-compartment model used is composed of maternal and fetal tissues.[5] Xenobiotic elimination is only through the maternal compartment. Exchange between maternal and fetal compartments only occurs across the placenta.

The assumptions and parameters used in defining this model are illustrated on Figures 9–7 and 9–8. The volume

PHARMACOKINETICS IN PREGNANCY
TWO COMPARTMENT MODEL

FIGURE 9–7. Parameters of a two-compartment pharmacokinetic model during pregnancy. The maternal (V_{dm}) and fetal (V_{fm}) volumes of distribution are proportional to maternal and fetal weights. The maternal elimination rate constant (K_e) is proportional to renal blood flow and glomerular filtration rate. The rate constants for transfer across the placenta (K_{fm}, K_{mf}) are proportional to the placental weight. Although there may be disagreement about the validity, the maternal and fetal clearances are assumed to be equal in this simulation. Also note that in this simulation a single dose of 1000 mg is given instantaneously into the maternal compartment.

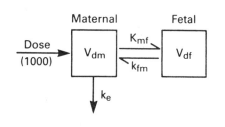

Assumptions
1. $V_{dm} \propto$ Maternal Weight
2. $V_{df} \propto$ Fetal Weight
3. $K_{mf} \propto$ Placental Weight
4. Maternal = Fetal Clearance
   ($K_{mf}V_{dm} = K_{fm}V_{df}$)
5. K_e Increases 3-Fold
   (Linearly with Gestation)

Gestation (weeks)	Maternal Weight (kg)	V_{dm}	Fetal Weight (gm)	V_{df}	Placental Weight	K_{mf}	K_e
0	55	20.0	—	—	—	—	2.0
8	55.5	20.2	1	0.001	20	0.005	2.8
12	56	20.4	14	0.005	30	0.0075	3.2
16	57	20.8	105	0.040	70	0.0175	3.6
20	59	21.5	310	0.113	160	0.040	4.0
24	61	22.2	640	0.234	210	0.0525	4.4
28	63	22.9	1080	0.400	250	0.0625	4.8
32	64.5	23.5	1670	0.600	300	0.075	5.2
36	66	24.0	2400	0.860	330	0.0825	5.6
40	67	24.4	3500	1.20	380	0.0950	6.0

PHARMACOKINETICS IN PREGNANCY
TWO COMPARTMENT MODEL

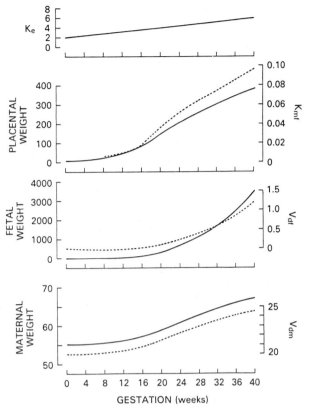

FIGURE 9–8. Physiologic changes during pregnancy. The maternal or fetal parameters (e.g., maternal or fetal weight) are illustrated by the solid lines. The impact of these parameters on pharmacokinetic rate constants is shown by the dotted lines. These volumes of distribution and rate constants are used in the following two-compartment simulation.

of distribution in the maternal (V_{dm}) and fetal (V_{df}) compartments will be proportional to maternal and fetal weights. The rate of elimination from the maternal compartment (K_e) will be proportional to renal plasma flow and glomerular filtration rate. The rate of transfer of xenobiotics between the maternal (K_{mf}) and fetal (K_{fm}) compartments will be proportional to placental weight.

Given the assumptions of this model and its limitations, it is interesting to explore the changing xenobiotic levels in maternal and fetal compartments following a single 1000-mg bolus dose (Figure 9–9). Over the first trimester, through 12 weeks of pregnancy, the maternal and fetal xenobiotic concentrations are essentially identical. This is reflected in a fetal-to-maternal ratio, which is approximately 1. During the second trimester, through 24 weeks of pregnancy, with increasing maternal and fetal volumes of distribution and increasing maternal elimination rate constant, the initial concentrations begin to fall from the nonpregnant value of 50. In addition, beginning at about 16 weeks, the concentration of the xenobiotic falls more rapidly in the maternal compartment than it did during the nonpregnant state. This produces fetal-

to-maternal ratios that become increasingly larger than 1. Note that the increasing fetal volume of distribution is reflected in a decreasing peak fetal concentration of the xenobiotic in the fetal compartment. This two-compartment model can be used to explore exposure scenarios involving dermal or pulmonary exposures during pregnancy (Table 9–10).

Xenobiotic Absorbed Through the Skin

During pregnancy, blood flow to the hand increases approximately sixfold, and blood flow to the foot increases approximately twofold. If the hand is a major site of absorption for the xenobiotic, and if transdermal absorption is influenced by blood flow, there may be as much as a sixfold increase in maternal dose during gestation (see Table 9–10). Using the two-compartment model, the dose absorbed through the hand may increase from 100 mg in the nonpregnant state to 600 mg at 40 weeks of gestation (Table 9–11). Over the same time period during pregnancy, the maternal volume of distribution (V_{dm}) will increase from 5.0–6.3 liters. Fetal volume of distribution (V_{df}) will change from 0.0008 liter at 10 weeks to 0.35 liter at 40 weeks. The rate constant for elimination from the maternal compartment (K_e) will increase from 5.0–7.2 h^{-1} over the 40 weeks of gestation. In this model we will assume that transfer from the maternal to fetal compartment (K_{mf}) occurs 10 times faster than transfer from the fetal to maternal compartment (K_{fm}) and that the rate of transfer is proportional to the placental weight. The parameters for the two-compartment model of pregnancy are summarized on Table 9–11; the results of the calculations are summarized on Table 9–12 and Figures 9–10 and 9–11.

These calculations were done in two different ways: In the first series of calculations (see Figure 9–10), the dose absorbed through the hand is constant throughout pregnancy (100 mg), but volume of distribution, rate of transfer, and rate of elimination are changing (see Table 9–11 and Figure 9–10). In the second set of calculations (see Figure 9–11), the dose absorbed through the hand increases sixfold over the course of gestation along with the previously defined changes in maternal and fetal volume of distribution, maternal elimination rate constant, and placental transfer rates (see Table 9–11 and Figure 9–11). Because of the increase in the dose of xenobiotic absorbed through the hand, there is an increase in concentration in the maternal and fetal compartments (see Table 9–12 and Figure 9–11) compared with the simulation, where maternal dose does not increase (see Table 9–12 and Figure 9–10). In the simulation with fixed dose (see Figure 9–10, *left panels*), the initial amount in the maternal compartment is unchanged during pregnancy (100 mg). The amount in the maternal compartment falls to zero more rapidly as gestation progresses, reflecting the increased rate of elimination (see Table 9–11). The amount in the fetal compartment increases over gestation, a result of increasing placental weight and surface area and therefore increasing maternal-to-fetal transfer. In the simulation with increasing dose (see Figure 9–11,

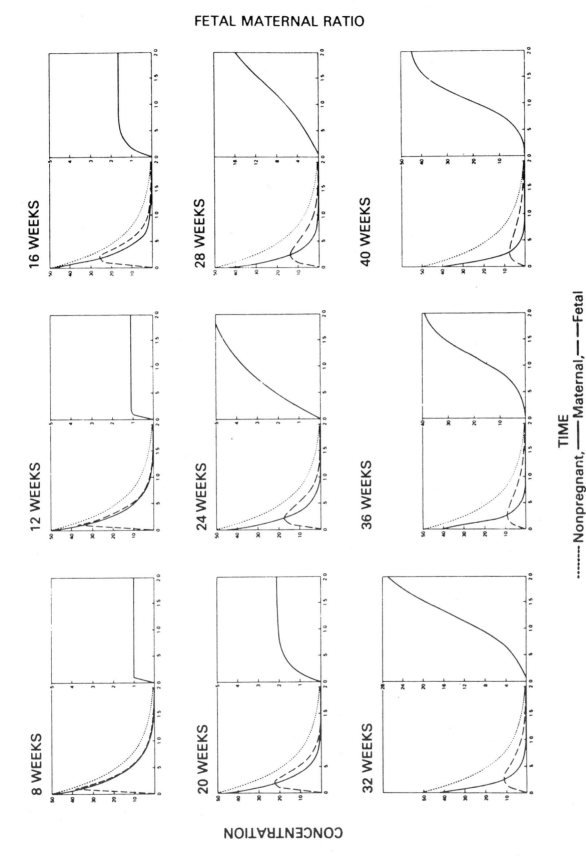

FIGURE 9–9. Pharmacokinetics in pregnancy, two compartment model ($K_{mf} \propto$ placental weight, Ke_1 with gestation). The impact of physiologic changes during pregnancy on concentration of the xenobiotic in the maternal or fetal compartment (*left panel*) or ratios of fetal to maternal concentration (*right panel*). The dotted lines represent the concentrations of the xenobiotic in the maternal compartment in the nonpregnant state. The solid lines represent the concentrations in the maternal compartment at the indicated times during gestation. The dashed lines represent the concentrations of the xenobiotic in the fetal compartment at the indicated times during pregnancy.

TABLE 9–10. PHYSIOLOGIC PARAMETERS USED IN TWO-COMPARTMENT MODEL OF PREGNANCY PHARMACOKINETICS

GESTATION (weeks)	ABSORPTION		DISTRIBUTION			ELIMINATION
	Hand Blood Flow (ml/ min/100 ml tissue)	Pulmonary Function Minute Ventilation (ml/min)	Maternal Weight (kg)	Placenta Weight (gm)	Fetal Weight (gm)	Renal Plasma Flow (ml/min/1.73 m²)
0	3	7,270	50	—	—	500
10	4.5	7,997	51	25	8	760
20	6	8,724	54	160	310	760
30	12	9,451	59	275	1,350	680
40	18	10,340	63	380	3,500	720

TABLE 9–11. XENOBIOTIC ABSORBED THROUGH HAND: PHARMACOKINETIC PARAMETERS

GESTATION (weeks)	DOSE ABSORBED (mg)	V_{dm} (liters)	V_{df} (liters)	K_{mf} (h^{-1})	K_{fm} (h^{-1})	K_e (h^{-1})
0	100	5.0	—	—	—	5.0
10	150	5.1	0.0008	0.25	0.025	7.6
20	200	5.4	0.031	1.6	0.16	7.6
30	400	5.9	0.135	2.8	0.28	6.8
40	600	6.3	0.350	3.8	0.38	7.2

See Figure 9–6 for definition of these pharmacokinetic parameters.

FIGURE 9–10. Effect of changing volumes of distribution, elimination rate constant, and rate constants for transfer between maternal and fetal compartments on amount and concentration of xenobiotic in maternal and fetal compartments. In this simulation, the amount of xenobiotic absorbed through the hand is constant at all stages of gestation. See Figure 9–11 for a similar simulation with increased xenobiotic absorption through the hand during gestation. The pharmacokinetic parameters used in the simulation are defined in Table 9–11. The panels on the left illustrate the amount of xenobiotic in each compartment. The panels on the right illustrate the concentration. (A) Amount, nonpregnant. (B) Concentration, nonpregnant. (C) Amount, 10 weeks pregnant. (D) Concentration, 10 weeks pregnant. (E) Amount, 20 weeks pregnant. (F) Concentration, 20 weeks pregnant. (G) Amount, 30 weeks pregnant. (H) Concentration, 30 weeks pregnant. (I) Amount, 40 weeks pregnant. (J) Concentration, 40 weeks pregnant.

Overleaf

FIGURE 9–11. Effect of increased xenobiotic absorption through the hand during pregnancy. The dose absorbed, volumes of distribution, placental transfer rates, and rates of elimination are defined on Table 9–11. See Figure 9–10 for a similar simulation with constant dose of xenobiotic absorbed. (A) Amount, nonpregnant. (B) Concentration, nonpregnant. (C) Amount, 10 weeks pregnant. (D) Concentration, 10 weeks pregnant. (E) Amount, 20 weeks pregnant. (F) Concentration, 20 weeks pregnant. (G) Amount, 30 weeks pregnant. (H) Concentration, 30 weeks pregnant. (I) Amount, 40 weeks pregnant. (J) Concentration, 40 weeks pregnant.

FIGURE 9–12. Effect of increased pulmonary absorption during pregnancy. This simulation is with a constant pulmonary dose; see Figure 9–13 for simulations with increasing pulmonary dose. Parameters for this two-compartment model are defined in Table 9–13. (A) Amount, nonpregnant. (B) Concentration, nonpregnant. (C) Amount, 10 weeks pregnant. (D) Concentration, 10 weeks pregnant. (E) Amount, 20 weeks pregnant. (F) Concentration, 20 weeks pregnant. (G) Amount, 30 weeks pregnant. (H) Concentration, 30 weeks pregnant. (I) Amount, 40 weeks pregnant. (J) Concentration, 40 weeks pregnant.

FIGURE 9–13. Effect of increased pulmonary absorption during pregnancy. See Figure 9–12 for a simulation with constant pulmonary dose during pregnancy. The parameters for this two-compartment model are defined in Table 9–13. (A) Amount, nonpregnant. (B) Concentration, nonpregnant. (C) Amount, 10 weeks pregnant. (D) Concentration, 10 weeks pregnant. (E) Amount, 20 weeks pregnant. (F) Concentration, 20 weeks pregnant. (G) Amount, 30 weeks pregnant. (H) Concentration, 30 weeks pregnant. (I) Amount, 40 weeks pregnant. (J) Concentration, 40 weeks pregnant.

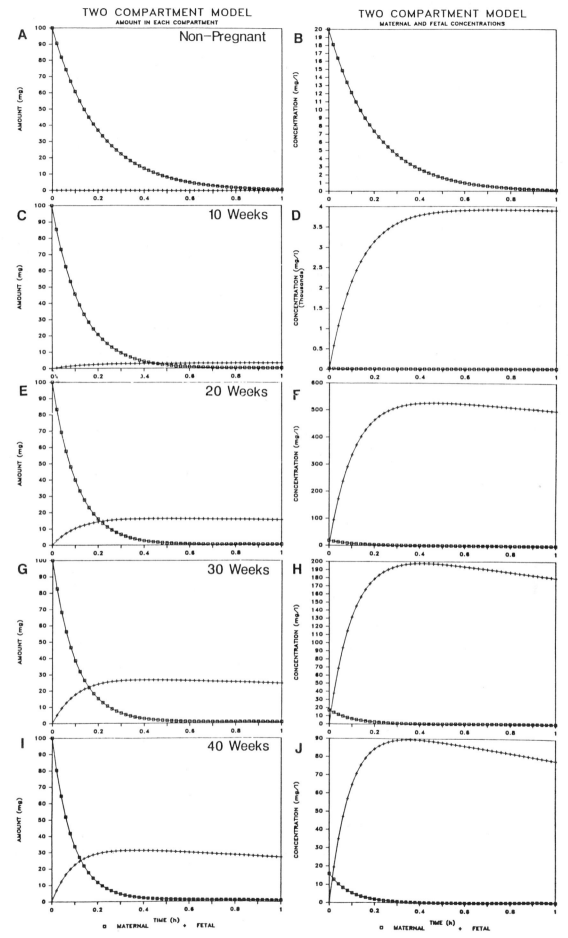

TWO COMPARTMENT MODEL
AMOUNT IN EACH COMPARTMENT

TWO COMPARTMENT MODEL
MATERNAL AND FETAL CONCENTRATIONS

FIGURE 9–10. *See legend on opposite page.*

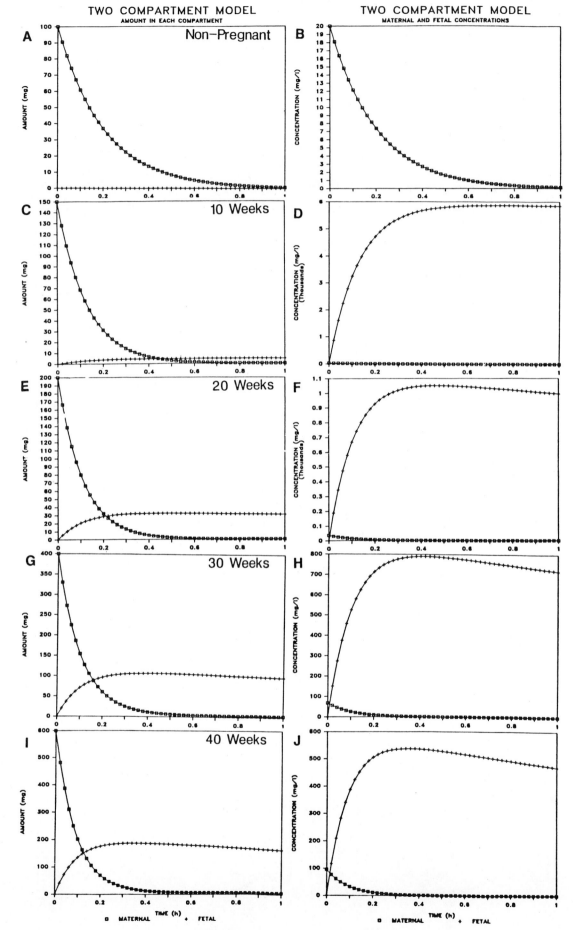

TWO COMPARTMENT MODEL
AMOUNT IN EACH COMPARTMENT

TWO COMPARTMENT MODEL
MATERNAL AND FETAL CONCENTRATIONS

A Non-Pregnant

B

C 10 Weeks

D

E 20 Weeks

F

G 30 Weeks

H

I 40 Weeks

J

□ MATERNAL + FETAL

FIGURE 9–11. *See legend on page 90.*

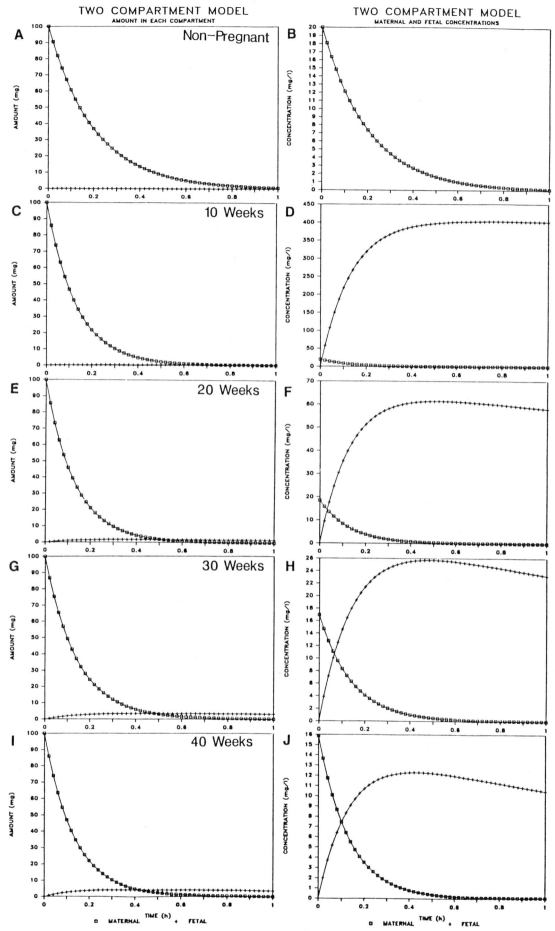

TWO COMPARTMENT MODEL
AMOUNT IN EACH COMPARTMENT

TWO COMPARTMENT MODEL
MATERNAL AND FETAL CONCENTRATIONS

FIGURE 9–12. *See legend on page 90.*

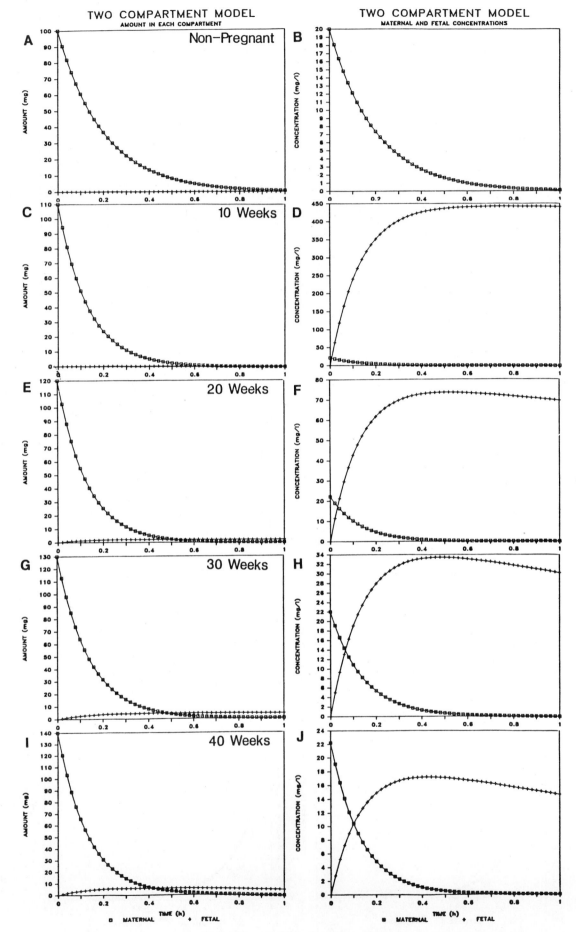

FIGURE 9–13. *See legend on page 90.*

TABLE 9–12. EFFECT OF INCREASED XENOBIOTIC ABSORPTION THROUGH THE HAND

GESTATION (weeks)	AMOUNT OF XENOBIOTIC ABSORBED (mg)		PEAK CONCENTRATION (mg/liter)			
			Maternal		Fetal	
	+	−	+	−	+	−
0	100	100	20.0	20.0	—	—
10	150	100	29.4	19.6	5860	3910
20	200	100	37.0	18.5	1050	526
30	400	100	67.8	16.9	790	198
40	600	100	95.2	15.9	537	89.5

In these simulations, − indicates no change in maternal dose over pregnancy; + indicates increasing maternal dose that is proportional to the increase in blood flow to the hand during gestation.

left panels), the amount absorbed increases proportionately to blood flow in the hand (100 to 600 mg). This produces a sixfold increase in the amount delivered into the fetal compartment.

With both simulations, there is a distinct difference in the time during gestation of peak concentration in maternal and fetal compartments (see Figures 9–10 and 9–11, *right panels,* and Table 9–12). Maximum concentration in the fetal compartment occurs at 10 weeks (see Table 9–12), while peak maternal concentration occurs at 0 weeks in the simulation without increasing dose. In the simulation with increasing maternal dose, however, peak maternal concentration occurs at 40 weeks, while peak fetal concentration still occurs at 10 weeks of gestation. If occupational exposure to a xenobiotic is through skin absorption, increasing absorption may increase the dose delivered to the fetus throughout gestation. Interestingly, however, this two-compartment model predicts that maximum fetal concentration will occur early in gestation. Therefore, in addition to increased vulnerability of the fetus on a biologic basis, the first trimester also may represent a period of pharmacokinetic vulnerability to the fetus. Maternal concentration, however, will continue to increase with increasing absorption so that maximum maternal concentration will occur late in gestation at the time of maximum absorption through the hand.

Xenobiotic Absorbed Through the Lungs

This two-compartment simulation also will explore the effect of increased pulmonary dose during gestation on the amount and concentration of xenobiotic in the maternal and fetal compartments (Table 9–13). In this simulation, the xenobiotic absorbed through the lung is distributed rapidly to both maternal (V_{dm}) and fetal (V_{df}) compartments. The volume of distribution in maternal and fetal compartments is proportional to maternal and fetal weights, respectively (see Table 9–13). The rate of elimination from the maternal compartment (K_e) is proportional to maternal renal blood flow. Transfer between maternal (K_{mf}) and fetal (K_{fm}) compartments is proportional to the placental weight. Since the xenobiotic absorbed is rapidly distributed, the rate constant for transfer between maternal and fetal compartments is assumed to be equal in both directions but increasing with gestation proportional to placental weight and surface area. In these simulations, the amount transferred into the maternal compartment is constant (Figure 9–12, *left panel*) or increases by approximately 40 percent (Figure 9–13, *left panel*) over the course of gestation, proportional to the increase in pulmonary minute volume. Note that because of the characteristics of the rate constants for placental transfer, the amount transferred into the fetal compartment is much smaller in these simulations than in the previous simulations of hand absorption (see Figures 9–10 and 9–11, *left panel*).

In this simulation, like the preceding two-compartment pharmacokinetic simulation, there is a difference in the time during gestation at which maximum maternal and fetal concentrations are reached (Table 9–14 and Figures 9–12 and 9–13, *right panel*). Maximum fetal concentrations occur early in gestation, at 10 weeks in both simulations. Over the rest of gestation, fetal concentrations decrease. As expected, however, the fetal concentrations are higher in the simulation with increased pulmonary absorption. In the maternal compartment, maximum concentration occurs at 0 weeks in the simulation in which increased pulmonary absorption does not occur. If pulmonary absorption increases during gestation, maximum maternal concentrations are achieved at 20 weeks and maintained at 30 and 40 weeks gestation.

TABLE 9–13. XENOBIOTIC ABSORBED THROUGH THE LUNGS

GESTATION (weeks)	DOSE ABSORBED (mg)	V_{dm} (liters)	V_{df} (liters)	K_{mf} (h⁻¹)	K_{fm} (h⁻¹)	K_e (h⁻¹)
0	100	5.0	—	—	—	5.0
10	110	5.1	0.0008	0.025	0.025	7.6
20	120	5.4	0.031	0.016	0.016	7.6
30	130	5.9	0.031	0.16	0.16	6.8
40	140	6.3	0.350	0.38	0.38	7.2

See Figure 9–6 for the definition of these pharmacokinetic parameters.

TABLE 9–14. EFFECT OF INCREASED ABSORPTION THROUGH THE LUNGS

GESTATION (weeks)	XENOBIOTIC ABSORBED (mg)		MAXIMUM CONCENTRATION (mg/liter)			
			Maternal		Fetal	
	+	−	+	−	+	−
0	100	100	20.0	20.0	—	—
10	110	100	21.6	19.6	442	402
20	120	100	22.2	18.5	74	61
30	130	100	22.0	16.9	33	26
40	140	100	22.2	15.9	17	12

In the columns marked +, maternal dose through the lung is increasing during pregnancy. In columns marked −, maternal dose through the lung does not change during pregnancy.

CONCLUSIONS

During pregnancy, there are substantial changes in maternal, placental, and fetal physiology. These physiologic adaptations are necessary for the success of the pregnancy and fetal growth and development and also alter pharmacokinetics. Absorption, distribution, metabolism, transfer between maternal and fetal compartments, and elimination will change for many xenobiotics and drugs during pregnancy. Because many women will want to continue working or will need to continue medication during pregnancy, it is important to define the effect of physiologic adaptations on the amount and concentration of chemicals in the maternal and fetal compartments. Any method for quantitative risk assessment that includes extrapolation across dose, route, or species for maternal, placental, or fetal toxicity must consider these physiologic adaptations and their species specificity.

A number of *in vitro, in vivo,* and theoretical models are being explored that offer promise for understanding drug- or chemical-induced developmental toxicity. These models also offer the opportunity to define common links between species for the formulation of risk assessments with well-characterized uncertainty.

The development of risk assessment in reproductive and developmental toxicology across species, however, will not come without research initiatives in several areas. The areas that are most likely to be productive include (1) development and exploration of pharmacokinetic and physiologic models, (2) validation of the physiologic and pharmacokinetic models with concurrent experimentation using *in vivo* and *in vitro* systems, and (3) development of expert systems for consistent, well-defined prediction of human reproductive risks from animal data.

At the present time, the most compelling need is the development of databases of physiologic, pharmacokinetic, and metabolic parameters within species during gestation and development. Once these data are available, it will be possible to begin development and testing of mechanism-based physiologic and pharmacokinetic models for quantitative risk assessment. The database, alone and together with the physiologic and pharmacokinetic models, also will suggest *in vivo* and *in vitro* experiments to validate the risk estimates and reduce their uncertainty. Finally, the database will be a reusable and continuously growing scientific resource.

ACKNOWLEDGMENTS: We would like to acknowledge the superb typing and organizational skills of Ms. Terri Young.

REFERENCES

1. Hytten FE, Leitch I: The Physiology of Human Pregnancy. Oxford, England, Blackwell, 1971
2. Hytten FE, Chamberlain G: Clinical Physiology in Obstetrics. Oxford, England, Blackwell, 1980
3. Committee on Models for Biomedical Research: Models for Biomedical Research: A New Perspective. Board on Basic Biology, Commission on Life Sciences, National Research Council, National Academy Press, 1985
4. Mattison DR: Physiological variations in pharmacokinetics during pregnancy, in Fabro S, Scialli AR (eds): Drug and Chemical Action in Pregnancy. New York, Marcel Dekker, 1986, pp 37–102
5. Wagner JG: Fundamentals of Clinical Pharmacokinetics. Hamilton, Ill, Drug Intelligence Publications, 1979
6. Hytten FE: The alimentary system, in Hytten FE, Chamberlain G (eds): Clinical Physiology in Obstetrics. Oxford, England, Blackwell, 1980, pp 147–162
7. deSwiet M: The respiratory system, in Hytten FE, Chamberlain G (eds): Clinical Physiology in Obstetrics. Oxford, England, Blackwell, 1980, pp 79–100
8. Gerhardsson L, Ahlmark A: Silicosis in women: Experience from the Swedish Pneumoconiosis Register. J Occup Med 27:347–350, 1985
9. deSwiet M: The cardiovascular system, in Hytten FE, Chamberlain G (eds): Clinical Physiology in Obstetrics. Oxford, England, Blackwell, 1980, pp 3–42
10. Hytten FE: Weight gain in pregnancy, in Hytten FE, Chamberlain G (eds): Clinical Physiology in Obstetrics. Oxford, England, Blackwell, 1980, pp 193–233
11. Lewis PJ: Drug metabolism, in Hytten FE, Chamberlain G (eds): Clinical Physiology in Obstetrics. Oxford, England, Blackwell, 1980, pp 270–286
12. Lewis PJ: Clinical Pharmacology in Obstetrics. Boston, Wright PSG, 1983
13. Gillette JR: Factors that affect drug concentrations in maternal plasma, in Wilson JG, Fraser FC (eds): Handbook of Teratology, vol 3. New York, Plenum Press, 1977, pp 35–77
14. Davison JM: The urinary system, in Hytten FE, Chamberlain G (eds): Clinical Physiology in Obstetrics. Oxford, England, Blackwell, 1980, pp 289–327
15. Ryan KJ: Steroid hormones in mammalian pregnancy, in Greep RO, Astwood EB (eds): Handbook of Physiology: Endocrinology II, part 2. Washington, D.C., American Physiological Society, 1973, pp 285–293
16. Mattison DR, Jelovsek FR: Pharmacokinetics and expert systems as aids for risk assessment in reproductive toxicology. Environ Health Perspect 76:107–119, 1987
17. Fisher JW, Whittaker TA, Taylor DH, Clewell HJ, Andersen ME: Physiologically based pharmacokinetic modeling of the pregnant rat: A multiple exposure model for trichloroethylene and its metabolite, trichloroacetic acid. Toxicol Appl Pharmacol 99:395–414, 1989
18. Schneider H, Dancis J: In vitro perfusion of human placental tissue, in Contributions to Gynecology and Obstetrics. Basel, Karger, 1985
19. Pelkonen O: Developmental drug metabolism, in Jenner P, Testa B (eds): Concepts of Drug Metabolism. New York, Marcel Dekker, 1980, pp 285–309
20. Slikker W Jr, Hill DE, Young JF: Comparison of the transplacental pharmacokinetics of 17β-estradiol and diethylstilbestrol in the subman primate. J Pharmacol Exp Ther 221:173–182, 1982
21. Slikker W Jr, Newport GD, Hill DE, Bailey JR: Placental transfer of synthetic and endogenous estrogen conjugates in the rhesus monkey (Macaca mulatta). Am J Prim. 2:385–399, 1982
22. Levin AA, Plautz JR, di Sant'Agnese PA, Miller RK: Cadmium: placental mechanisms of fetal toxicity. (Suppl 3):308–318, 1981
23. Frankos VH: FDA perspectives on the use of teratology data for human risk assessment. Fund Appl Toxicol 5:615–625, 1985

10
EPIDEMIOLOGY OF DRUGS IN PREGNANCY

FRANZ W. ROSA

Drug epidemiology is concerned with the balance of two general outcomes: (1) benefits and (2) risks. Because there are so many pitfalls in detecting risks, a wise generalization is to assume that no agent has been proven completely safe and should be employed in pregnancy only if it has clear benefits. The diethylstilbesterol (DES) problem exemplifies this. DES was widely assumed to be valuable in improving pregnancy outcome. Only after *in utero*–exposed females turned up 20 years later with adenocarcinoma of the vagina[1] was it pointed out that controlled studies had shown no clear benefits of DES. Despite this example, the same problem persists another 20 years later with progesterone exposures. More and more studies have been done on whether progesterone administration for threatened abortions or other reasons has risks.[2] At the same time, adequately controlled studies have never established whether it has any benefits. An important current question relates to aspirin. Growing knowledge of the relationship of prostacyclin to pregnancy maintenance and of thromboxane to adverse outcome, together with several clinical studies (either with small sample size[3] and/or with inappropriate controls[4]), points toward the possibility of major benefits from low-dose aspirin. The benefits may include improving placental perfusion, preventing preeclampsia, preventing much intrauterine growth retardation, and perhaps preventing much selectively induced premature delivery. This must be balanced against concern that aspirin exposure to term may increase hemorrhagic and possibly other risks in the mother and infant. Despite the fact that the suggestion of important benefits from aspirin is more than 10 years old, as of today, we are still waiting for an adequate study to confirm the benefits.

There are three reasons why drugs do not receive adequate epidemiologic tests for their effects in pregnancy. First is the feeling that testing drugs in pregnant women poses unethical risks for the fetus. Second is the liability hazard. Third, for most drugs, manufacturers feel the market for use in pregnant women is too small to justify the costs of investigation. Therefore, most studies of drug effects in pregnancy depend on poorly controlled postmarketing observations of necessary or accidental pregnancy exposures.

Only a small proportion of drugs have been found to have fetal risks. Time always lapses between the time the drug is marketed and the time that fetal risk is confirmed. Table 10–1 shows the year that human fetal drug injury was strongly suspected or confirmed relative to the year that the drug was marketed for a number of drugs.[5–31]

Fetal risk questions in pregnancy generally fall in two pregnancy periods. First are questions related to organogenesis, usually with periconceptional or first-trimester exposures. These questions sometimes extend beyond the first trimester, since brain organogenesis continues beyond this period, sex hormone receptivity of the fetus persists, susceptibility to thyroid suppression occurs after the 12th week,[6] and ductus arteriosus patency/pulmonary hypertension/tricuspid incompetence relates to last-trimester exposures.

The second period concerns immediate predelivery and delivery exposures for late complications of pregnancy and management of delivery. Late pregnancy exposures affect the neonate, with persisting levels and/or withdrawal effects of the maternally administered agent. Because of the difficulty separating the dose of the agent administered from the fetal/neonatal effect of the maternal condition requiring the treatment, carefully controlled clinical studies are usually required to define the risks versus benefits of these treatments. Clinical aspects of exposures in labor and delivery will be discussed in Chapter 16.

A *confounder* is an exposure associated both with an exposure and with an outcome that can produce a spurious association. Confounders require identification in all types of epidemiologic studies. The most important confounder in drug studies is the indication for which the agent is given. Although in both early and late pregnancy

The views expressed in this presentation are those of the author and do not represent an official statement by the Food and Drug Administration.

TABLE 10–1. DRUGS BY APPROXIMATE YEAR HUMAN FETAL RISK WAS FIRST STRONGLY SUSPECTED

DRUG*	RISK	YEAR MARKETED	YEAR SUSPECTED
Iodides[5]	Goitrous hypothyroidism	1850	1940
Aminoglycosides[6]	Congenital nerve deafness	1945	1950
Aminopterin[7]	Abortion, microcephaly, spina bifida	1953	1950
Testosterone[8]	Virulization of females	1939	1955
Progestins[9]	Virulization of females	1945	1959
Thalidomide[10]	Phocomelia, microtia, etc.	1958	1961
Iodine 131[11]	Thryoid injury	?	1963
Cyclophosphamide[12]	Fetal growth retardation, etc.	1977	1964
Hydantoins[13]	Face, palate, heart, digits	1938	1964
Thiouracils[14]	Goitrous hypothyroidism	1947	1968
Vitamin D[15]	Hypercalcemia, syndrome	1920	1968
Coumarins[16]	Osteochondrodyspasia punctata, etc.	1961	1968
Methadiones[17]	Face, palate, heart	1955	1970
Barbiturates[18]	Face, palate, heart	1903	1970
Tetracyclines[19]	Calcification disturbances	1950	1970
Diethylstilbesterol[1]	Adenocarcinoma vagina, GU defects	1935	1970
Penicillamine[20]	Cutis laxa	1956	1971
Lithium[21]	Ebstein anomaly	1939	1974
Danazol[22]	Virulization female	1977	1979
Valproate[23]	Spina bifida, heart	1977	1982
Etretinate[24]	Skeletal, spina bifida	1980	1982
Isotretinoin[25]	Brain, microtia, cardio aortic	1982	1983
Vitamin A[26]	Microtia, brain, heart	1930	1984
Carbamazepine[27]	Spina bifida	1968	1984
Methimazole[28]	Cutis aplasis scalp	1980	1983
Primidone[29]	Dysmorphia	1965	1983
ACE inhibitors[30]	Neonatal anuria	1980	1983
Prostaglandin inhibitors[31]	Ductus closure	1960	

*References may be reviews rather than the initial identification.

it is important to sort out the effect of the agent from that of the condition being treated, this is particularly difficult with late-pregnancy exposures. Examples of other possible confounders for certain associations are concurrent drug exposures (e.g., antiepileptic combinations) and maternal age. Possible confounders are analyzed by multivariate or stratified analyses.

Following sections describe methods and limitations of drug epidemiology in pregnancy, which for the most part is not based on controlled trials but is dependent on observational research methods. Topics include (1) birth-defect monitoring, (2) exposure cohort studies, (3) evaluation of isolated case reporting, (4) case-control studies, (5) selected exposure and outcome concerns, and (6) needs for the future.

BIRTH-DEFECT MONITORING

Birth-defect monitoring follows temporal and geographic frequencies of birth defects. More than 20 registries are currently coordinated by the International Clearinghouse for Birth Defect Monitoring Systems. About 30 states have birth-defect monitoring systems in various stages of development. The concept of these registries is that a teratogen would lead to an unusual temporal and geographic frequency of particular types of defects. Although some unusual human frequencies have been observed, as yet none were found to be due to a drug teratogen. Two drug teratogenicities were discovered in birth-defect registries, but neither caused a statistically significant effect in the frequency of the defect concerned. Robert and Guiband[23] documented the association between spina bifida and valproic acid by case-control methodology (see following section) rather than by an effect on the prevalence of spina bifida. Examination of an unusual frequency of 11 scalp defects in the Washington State Birth Defect Registry led Milam[28] to find that 3 of these were associated with the antithyroid agent methimazole. Although these 3 unusual cases were sufficient to strongly implicate such an infrequent exposure, it does not appear that they were sufficient to explain the unusual frequency of the defect. It was not documented that the unusual frequency corresponded to changes in the frequency of exposure. Birth-defect frequency monitoring is especially unlikely to identify a drug teratogen, since most drug exposures involve a small proportion of pregnancies during the crucial period of embryogenesis. It is difficult to show that changes in frequencies of defect categories in registries would have identified the thalidomide disaster, although this was accomplished "after the fact" in the Swedish birth-defect registry by tightening the focus from limb-reduction defects to the phocomelia defects that were characteristic of thalidomide teratogenesis.[32]

The scarcity of temporal and geographic variations in birth-defect frequency distributions (with the notable exception of neural tube defects, which show major geographic variations and temporal trends) contrasts with the striking temporal and geographic variations for various types of cancers. For those types of defects which are readily counted, this suggests that environmental factors do not play as important a role as is true for cancers. Although this may provide some indirect reassurance about the limited role of extrinsic exposures, it provides no direct answers about specific drug injuries, because, as mentioned, these exposures occur in too small a proportion of the population to have a detectable influence on defect-monitoring data.

Birth-defect registries can serve as references for obtaining defects for case-control exposure studies (see Case-Control Studies below). However, another major deficiency in monitoring systems is that they are limited to easily identifiable defects present at birth, which constitute only a fraction of fetal exposure risks.

EXPOSURE COHORT STUDIES

Exposure cohort studies examine the frequencies of adverse outcomes among a group of exposures, preferably in comparison with a group of nonexposures (exposure/nonexposure analysis). An advantage to such studies is that they can look at the distribution of many types of outcomes to detect possible associations. Three levels of cohort studies exist. First are cohorts of particular *exposures.* These can compare defects among exposures with defects among nonexposures, but they cannot compare exposures among cases with exposures among noncases (see Case-Control Studies below). These studies may suffer from late registration in pregnancy. Second are cohorts of *pregnancies* in which the frequency of all exposures and adverse outcomes can be examined, but the proportion of drug use associated with pregnancy is not documented. This type of cohort can be used for "nested" case-control studies, as well as for cohort analysis. Pregnancy cohorts again may suffer from late registration in pregnancy after the teratogenic period. Third are cohorts of *populations* in which the frequency of pregnancy exposures in the population can be examined in addition to the frequency of exposures and adverse outcomes in pregnancy. In this type of cohort, case-control analysis also can be nested.

Premarketing prospective *exposure* cohort studies are limited to drugs studied for specific pregnancy indications, such as ovulation inducers (clomiphene and gonadotropins), antiemetics (i.e., Bendectin), and tocolytics (ritodrine). Postmarketing cohorts are gathered from accidental and necessary pregnancy exposures to specific drugs or from an overall cohort of pregnancies, examining effects of any drug exposures. It is necessary to limit cohort studies to prospectively recorded exposures, since exposures reported as a consequence of an outcome are generally biased toward abnormal outcomes. Even large cohorts are limited in size for comparing infrequent outcomes. (Virtually most specific birth-defect outcomes are infrequent.) If many outcomes are being examined, one or more may appear to be associated by chance. Thus a cohort study generally is capable of identifying only a major increase in any specific defect or of raising hypotheses where borderline associations are seen. Meta-analysis of several studies is necessary to see if more defects are occurring with exposures than would be expected.

In an overall cohort of *pregnancies,* the frequency of many exposures during pregnancy as well as the frequency of many possible adverse effects can be examined. Although this type of study of a cohort of pregnancies may appear large, the actual cohorts of exposures for each drug are usually small, and the number of specific outcomes for each exposure is smaller still. Because hundreds of types of exposures are being examined against hundreds of possible outcomes, associations are likely to arise by chance. It is unwise to regard such associations as conclusive unless they are supported by findings in other studies. In the United States, two prospective pregnancy studies developed in the 1960s with National Institutes of Health support incorporated concern growing out of the thalidomide disaster. Both studies had long-term followup. The first study, the Collaborative Perinatal Project, involved 20 institutions in different parts of the United States following more than 50,000 pregnancies with 1500 major birth-defect outcomes.[33] The only drug teratogenic associations were with antiepileptics[34] and one thyroid anomaly associated with iodine 131 exposure. A suggested association of sex hormone exposure with heart defects[35] was discounted by more detailed examination of specific cases in the study.[36] Eight neuroblastic tumors associated with killed polio vaccination also were identified.[37] The second study, the University of California Child Development Study, assembled prospective information on 20,000 pregnancies in the 1960s based on records of a health-maintenance organization (HMO). This study suggested human teratogenicity from sedatives and tranquilizers,[38] but this has not yet been confirmed in other studies.

Population samples in which to examine where and how drugs are used and what adverse effects occur are found in HMOs, socialized medical services, and Medicaid services. Cohort and/or case-control studies can be based in these samples. Although these populations are not fully representative of the general population, they offer the only direct basis for obtaining a population frequency of an exposure and a defect outcome. Since 1980, under an FDA contract, the Computerized On-Line Medicaid Pharmaceutic Surveillance System (COMPASS) has been developed. Advantage is taken of routinely computerized invoices for prescriptions and diagnoses for medical visits in Michigan. A computer tape containing family membership has been used to link maternal records with infant outcome records. In the 4 years 1980–1983, there were 135,000 deliveries, among which 7086 were linked to suspected birth-defect outcomes (about 5 percent). Analysis generally has been limited to 104,000 first deliveries in the maternal case profiles linked with 6500 suspected birth-defect cases. In these, first-trimester histories were available on 55,000 deliveries, of which approximately 3400 were linked to infants with suspected or obvious birth-defect diagnoses. Club foot, metatarsus varus, inguinal and umbilical hernia, and patent ductus arteriosus are not included. Chromosomal defects are handled in a separate file. Maternal outpatient prescriptions by date of dispensing and of contemporaneous diagnoses suggesting prescription indication can be examined relative to the infant outcome. For each generic drug, the total number of linked suspected defects, cardiovascular defects, and spontaneous abortions are tabulated. Estimated relative risks and confidence intervals are developed. The complete frequency distribution of defects has been examined for selected suspected first-trimester exposures (5995 for Bendectin, 472 for diazepam, 327 for cimetidine, 486 for hydroxyzine, 423 for furosemide, 308 for nitrofurantoin, 147 for tretinoin, and all identifiable antiepileptic exposures). The frequency distribution of all first-trimester drug recipients has been examined for selected defects (cardiovascular defects, spina bifida, cleft lip and/or cleft palate, diaphragmatic hernias, and choanal atresia).[39]

Another population sample approach can monitor *population experience* with a known teratogen, such as abortions and deliveries with suspected isotretinoin (Accutane) exposures and suspected fetal circulatory injury with prostaglandin synthesis inhibitors. Among 1064 women prescribed isotretinoin, 55 appeared to have a suspected coinciding pregnancy. Forty of these women had an induced or spontaneous abortion, 2 (possibly 3) had perinatal deaths, and the remainder reached delivery. In two exposures, isotretinoin syndromes have been identified. In the remainder, no defect has been confirmed, although the clinical records obtained were often inadequate, and in no case has it been possible to have a followup examination of the infant suspected to have been exposed. This study suggested the extent pregnancy exposures and adverse outcomes, at least in this population sample, exceeded the rate reported in the general population.[40]

Drug-exposure cohorts have contributed to the identification of only a few fetal risks: aminopterin,[7] thalidomide,[10] antiepileptics,[13] and isotretinoin.[25]

ISOLATED CASE REPORTING

Both cohort studies and case-control studies require time to accumulate sufficient experience for analysis. Human fetal risks are usually initially observed through isolated case reporting by alert clinicians. Although most birth-defect exposure cases occur by chance, a suspicious observation can focus epidemiologic studies. Suspicious observations include *those expected from postnatal therapeutic experience* (e.g., aminoglycoside deafness,[6] androgen virilization,[8,9,22] antithyroid effects,[5,11,14] and prostaglandin synthesisis inhibitor ductus closure[31]), *coincidence of an unusual outcome* (e.g., DES clear-cell adenocarcinoma of the vagina,[1] warfarin osteochonrodysplasia punctata,[16] penicillamine cutis laxa,[20] methimazole scalp cutis aplasia[28]), or a *coincidence with animal findings* (cyclophosphamide,[12] isotretinoin syndrome,[25] and vitamin A[26]). Despite the importance of case reports, these are still not strongly promoted. Both clinicians and medical journal editors may feel that isolated case reports are unscientific. Agencies collecting reports may shield these from publication because of fears of misinterpretation of reports, of unwarranted public reactions, and of legal actions. Thus 25 years after the thalidomide disaster, the most important method of avoiding a similar experience is still underexploited.

Comprehensive case reporting of all birth-defect drug exposures is not feasible. Nonunique defects resulting from long-established use of a drug can be better examined in existing epidemiologic databases than through case reporting. The priorities of case reporting are outcomes with newly marketed agents, unusual outcomes, and especially those unlikely to be recognized at birth.

Case reporting of some established teratogens remains desirable even after the association is known. At present, the only system in place for evaluating the effect of control measures for isotretinoin teratogenicity is continuing case recognition and reporting. Such case reports should describe how and why the exposure occurred.

Since 1969, the FDA has computerized more than 10,000 birth-defect case reports with suspicions of drug causation; 1500 additional reports cover perinatal exposure concerns. Each of these reports is examined upon receipt. Table 10–2 compares the number of human drug-associated birth-defect cases that have appeared in various U.S. epidemiologic systems and those in the FDA Spontaneous Report System. The latter, by drawing suspicious cases from an unlimited (although undefined) denominator, has by far the best potential for quickly noting a suspicious observation, especially from a newly marketed drug that has been used in only a small fraction of the population. An FDA form for case reporting is shown in Figure 10–1. Ordinarily, item 2 should be the mother's age, item 3 the infant's sex, and items 4–6 the birth date. Item 7 for describing reactions should be filled as follows. "Code: anomaly, congenital; Text (describe as fully as possible the nature of the defect). All adverse effects suspected to be due to pregnancy exposures are coded and retrieved as "anomaly, congenital" in the FDA system. The FDA's information system can provide immediate access to the number of "anomaly, congenital" codings for each drug (either trade or generic identification; the generic tabulation is for about 500 agents) and a line listing of the texts for each report for any agent. Within a few hours, microfiches of the original reports also can be obtained. Any personal confidential information about the case or the reporter is removed before the reports are made public. A standard rider is attached to case report releases indicating that the case reports in themselves do not establish causation. This freedom of publication of information collected by national authorities is fully warranted and is an important step toward rapid investigation and identification of new human teratogens.

Case exposure reporting constitutes an unknown proportion of occurrences but is undoubtedly only a small fraction of the total occurrences. The degree of reporting is biased toward limb-reduction defects, litigation cases, previously published questions, newly marketed agents, and events that conceptionally relate in the mind of the reporter to the function of the drug. Underreporting is greater for nonprescription items. The only "controls" are (1) the frequency and defect distribution of reports relative to the marketing of the agency compared with the frequency distribution of reports relative to the marketing

TABLE 10–2. ESTIMATED DRUG BIRTH-DEFECT DETECTION IN U.S. SYSTEMS

	PREGNANCIES	MAJOR DEFECTS	BIRTH DEFECT CASES		
			Suspected[1]	Known[2]	New
Monitoring (CDC, 1970–1982)	1,000,000/yr	15,000/yr	0	0	0
Case-control registries with retrospective exposures:					
CDC Atlanta, 1970–1987	200,000	1,231[3]	10	?	0
Slone Epidemiology Unit, 1978–1988	500,000	8,000[3]	?	?	0
Prospective exposure cohorts:					
NIH Collaborative Perinatal, 1959–1965	52,000	1,457	20	2	13[4]
COMPASS Michigan, 1980–1983	55,000	2,800	20	10	12
Case reporting (FDA, 1969–1991)	80,000,000[5]	10,000	250	500	300[6]

[1]Defects suspected with sex hormones, tetracycline, antiepileptics, benzodiazapines, clomiphene, and antidiabetics.

[2]Defects previously known to be associated with sex hormones, tetracycline, antiepileptics, warfarin, alcohol, radioiodine, and antineoplastics.

[3]Selected defects.

[4]Polio vaccine (8 neuroblastic tumors), antiepileptics (5 defect cases).

[5]Undefined universal denominator of births 1969–1988.

[6]Valproate (89), isotretinoin (83), danazol (12), carbamazapine (22), penicillamine (6), etretinate (4), vitamin A (4), lithium (1), methimazole (4 scalp defects), amiodioquin (2 goiters), ACE inhibitors (5 neonatal anuria), prostaglandin inhibitors (10 suspected ductus closures), primidone (20), clomiphene (2 conjoined twins).

for related agents and (2) the frequency of the exposure for a defect in question compared with the frequency with other defects. Normal outcomes are not available in the spontaneous report system to ascertain their frequency or the frequency of the exposure with normal outcomes. In order to obtain exposure denominators for case defect questions, it may be necessary to have a cohort study. In order to have a comparison of the exposure rate for a defect question, it may be necessary to proceed to a case-control study if exposures are sufficiently frequent and recognizable (see following section). However, some drug teratogenicities still do not have such comparisons and are assumed only on the basis of case reports. These include aminoglycosides deafness,[6] iodine 131 thyroid injury,[11] coumarin osteochondrodysplasia,[16] methadione dysmorphia,[17] penicillamine cutis laxa,[20] lithium Ebstein anomaly,[21] danazol virulization,[22] etretinate teratogenicity,[24] vitamin A teratogenicity,[26] methimazole scalp defects,[28] primidone dysmorphia,[29] and angiotensin-converting enzyme inhibitor anuria.[30]

CASE-CONTROL STUDIES

Case-control studies compare the exposure frequency for a specific defect in question with exposure frequencies in outcomes without the defect. These studies can examine the frequency of a specific exposure question or the frequency distribution of many exposures. With a common, easily recognizable exposure, case-control studies have greater power to evaluate a birth-defect question than exposure cohort studies. Although case-control exposures can be obtained from pregnancy and population cohort studies (see preceding section), they usually depend on retrospective interview data. Recall deficiencies are likely to reduce and possibly bias the quantity and quality of exposure identification.[41] Another problem is that the *timing* of short-term exposures is likely to be poorly recalled. Long-term exposures, such as antiepileptic exposures, contraceptive failures, and ovulation induction, are examples of exposures that can be exceptionally well documented by interview. To optimize interview data, questions are addressed at three levels: (1) asking for exposures by indication, (2) by drug category, and (3) by specific drug. Trade names must be used, because interviewees are seldom aware of the generic name or composition of an agent. Because persons with a birth-defect outcome are biased toward better recall of drug exposures than persons with normal outcomes, it has been necessary to use "other defects" as controls for the defect in question.

Case-control studies have been used mainly to confirm or refute suspected birth-defect associations rather than for initial detection (hypothesis raising). Such a suspicion arises from case reports, from postnatal exposure experience, or rarely, from observations in cohort studies or other case-control studies. Where the frequency distribution of many exposures is compared for a selected birth-defect question with a control, again the possibility of chance associations must be considered. As with cohort studies, meta-analysis of several studies may be desirable. With a high-frequency exposure and a rare but unique outcome, case-control studies can confirm associations with only a handful of cases. Adenocarcinoma of the vagina as a result of DES exposures is an example.[1] However, such a case-control study does not directly show the frequency of the defect with the exposure. In the DES example, although most vaginal adenocarcinoma patients were exposed to DES, a cohort study required more than 500 exposures before such an outcome could be found (other outcomes have been more frequent).[42] For nonunique outcomes (e.g., spina bifida with valproic acid exposures[23]), an estimate of exposure risk can be obtained by applying the estimated relative risk obtained in a case-control study (known as an *odds ratio*) to the expected frequency of the defect without exposure.

DEPARTMENT OF HEALTH AND HUMAN SERVICES
PUBLIC HEALTH SERVICE
FOOD AND DRUG ADMINISTRATION (HFN-730)
ROCKVILLE, MD 20857

ADVERSE REACTION REPORT
(Drugs and Biologics)

Form Approved: OMB No. 0910-0230.

FDA CONTROL NO.

ACCESSION NO.

I.	REACTION INFORMATION

1. PATIENT ID/INITIALS (In Confidence)	2. AGE YRS.	3. SEX	4.-6. REACTION ONSET			8.-12. CHECK ALL APPROPRIATE:
			MO.	DA.	YR.	

7. DESCRIBE REACTION(S)

13. RELEVANT TESTS/LABORATORY DATA

☐ PATIENT DIED

☐ REACTION TREATED WITH Rx DRUG

☐ RESULTED IN, OR PROLONGED, INPATIENT HOSPITALIZATION

☐ RESULTED IN PERMANENT DISABILITY

☐ NONE OF THE ABOVE

II.	SUSPECT DRUG(S) INFORMATION

14. SUSPECT DRUG(S) (Give manufacturer and lot no. for vaccines/biologics)

20. DID REACTION ABATE AFTER STOPPING DRUG?

☐ YES ☐ NO ☐ NA

15. DAILY DOSE

16 ROUTE OF ADMINISTRATION

17. INDICATION(S) FOR USE

21. DID REACTION REAPPEAR AFTER REINTRODUCTION?

18. DATES OF ADMINISTRATION (From/To)

19 DURATION OF ADMINISTRATION

☐ YES ☐ NO ☐ NA

III.	CONCOMITANT DRUGS AND HISTORY

22. CONCOMITANT DRUGS AND DATES OF ADMINISTRATION (Exclude those used to treat reaction)

23. OTHER RELEVANT HISTORY (e.g. diagnoses, allergies, pregnancy with LMP, etc.)

IV. ONLY FOR REPORTS SUBMITTED BY MANUFACTURER	V. INITIAL REPORTER (In confidence)

24. NAME AND ADDRESS OF MANUFACTURER (Include Zip Code)

26.-26a. NAME AND ADDRESS OF REPORTER (Include Zip Code)

24a. IND/NDA. NO. FOR SUSPECT DRUG	24b MFR. CONTROL NO.

26b. TELEPHONE NO. (Include area code)

24c. DATE RECEIVED BY MANUFACTURER	24d. REPORT SOURCE (Check all that apply) ☐ FOREIGN ☐ STUDY ☐ LITERATURE ☐ HEALTH PROFESSIONAL ☐ CONSUMER

26c. HAVE YOU ALSO REPORTED THIS REACTION TO THE MANUFACTURER?

☐ YES ☐ NO

25 15 DAY REPORT? ☐ YES ☐ NO	25a. REPORT TYPE ☐ INITIAL ☐ FOLLOWUP

26d. ARE YOU A HEALTH PROFESSIONAL?

☐ YES ☐ NO

Submission of a report does not necessarily constitute an admission that the drug caused the adverse reaction.

NOTE: Required of manufacturers by 21 CFR 314.80

FORM FDA 1639 (7/86)

PREVIOUS EDITION MAY BE USED

FIGURE 10–1. FDA form for reporting adverse reactions to drugs and biologics. (Food and Drug Administration, Public Health Service, Form FDA 1639 [7/86]. Rockville, Md., Department of Health and Human Services, July 1986.)

NEED FOR STUDIES OF SELECTED EXPOSURES AND OUTCOMES

Throughout this chapter I have preferred to use the term *birth defects* or *fetal risks* rather than *teratogenicity. Teratogenicity,* in both animal and human studies, traditionally refers to irreversible structural defects caused by exposures during organogenesis (as seen in the thalidomide experience). However, a functional transient effect such as neonatal anuria can cause death.[30] Some important pregnancy risk exposures are known to cause intrauterine growth retardation, probably with long-term developmental limitation. Examples of these types of exposure and outcome questions are presented below.

The current importance of clarifying the risks versus benefits of low-dose *aspirin* exposure after the first trimester was mentioned earlier. It is hoped that the large clinical trials of aspirin compared with placebo controls that are about to be completed in the United States and the United Kingdom will soon do this. If the initial studies are confirmed (it is an open question whether they will be confirmed or not), this measure could lead to preventing as many as 80,000 intrauterine growth retardation births and 40,000 selectively induced premature deliveries in the United States annually.

Antiepileptic exposures occur in about 1 in 200 pregnancies, or about 20,000 pregnancies yearly in the United States. Generally, there appears to be a more than 2 percent excess of major birth defects (4 percent of births as opposed to 2 percent in nonexposures) with these exposures. This would be about 400 major birth defects yearly. Antiepileptics can be studied not only in exposure cohort studies, but also advantageously in case-control studies. Exposure is long term and readily identified, and a continuing exposure is more likely to coincide with a critical period of embryogenesis than a short-term drug use in the first trimester of pregnancy. Although associations with cleft lips (with or without cleft palate), heart defects, and other dysmorphias are well documented, and there have been more than 40 cohort and case-control studies of antiepileptics in pregnancy, the relative safety of various antiepileptic regimens is still not clarified. Each cohort of maternal epileptic cases is likely to have too few exposures to each regimen to compare the teratogenicity of different exposures. Concurrent antiepileptic exposures often overlap. These pose questions not only as to which agent is responsible, but also as to the teratogenicity of antiepileptic interactions. National interinstitutional studies have coordinated cohort observations in Japan[43] and France.[44] It is desirable to update these and expand national and international coordination to other countries to resolve questions about the relative safety of different antiepileptic regimens in women at risk.

Behavioral abnormalities, influences on the *autonomic nervous system,* and other *late developmental outcomes,* such as *cancer, sexual maturation,* and *fertility,* are difficult to study, requiring careful long-term followup. However, these can be important, as shown with the DES experience.

Long-term fertility and behavioral effects are suspected with extrinsic *sex hormone* exposures. Furthermore, there may be effects on reproductive performance when the exposed offspring reach maturity. Antiandrogenicity is known in adults with cimetidine, ranitidine, spiranolactone, and ketoconazole. Theoretically, pregnancy exposures could cause lack of normal male development, which has actually been observed in some animal studies. Human case reports have been received only for estrogen and progesterone exposures, and these are no doubt biased by the perception that these female sex hormone exposures would cause "feminization" in males.

Teratogenicity from megadose exposure to *vitamin A* is well known in all species, but the dose required to produce teratogenicity in the human is still not known. Case reporting is poor, and no cohort or case-control studies have been possible. Because of these difficulties, it is proposed that steps to avoid megadose vitamin A exposures should be taken without waiting for teratoepidemiologic studies.[45]

Many women are able to have nearly normal lives because of antimanic maintenance on *lithium.* Nine case reports of a rare cardiovascular defect, Ebstein anomaly, and one small cohort study showing an excess of other cardiovascular defects[46] leave the risks of lithium exposure far from clear. Careful followup of prospectively recorded lithium exposures is highly desirable.

Interaction of exposures may be important. Epidemiologic data suggest that exposure to multiple antiepileptics or to multiple antineoplastic agents may be more important than monoexposure. This is plausible on the basis that certain agents are known to accelerate hepatic microsomal metabolism, increasing teratogenic metabolites such as epoxides.[47] Exposure to alcohol, nicotine, caffeine, marijuana, and industrial chemicals should be considered in interactions. These are difficult to sort out in nonexperimental epidemiologic studies and deserve more attention in experimental animal studies.

Spontaneous abortions are an important component of teratogenic injury, both in animal studies (abortions generally resorbed) and in human observations. Isolated reports of abortions are useless because of the natural frequency of this event. An exposure denominator is essential. Abortions in a prospective exposure denominator were the first indication of isotretinoin human fetal risks.[25] Columbia University has established a large retrospective registry of more than 10,000 spontaneous abortions and a similar number of normal-outcome pregnancy controls.[48] Maternal drug histories are compared with those of normal pregnancy outcomes. Although this registry offers potential, it has not yet identified a drug abortifactants. The study suffers not only from problems of retrospective interview analyses on maternal recall, but also from abortions interrupting the opportunity for first-trimester drug exposure, disturbing comparisons. In the previously mentioned COMPASS system, prospective trends can be compared by month before abortion, by which temporal associations with abortion can be closely explored. Drug exposures prior to 4264 spontaneous abortions were compared with those before induced abortions and with first-trimester exposures of delivered pregnancies. A suspected association of spontaneous abortions with topical imidazole antifungal agents provides an example in this analysis.[49]

Closely associated with abortion outcome is the identification of *chromosomal* injury, since a large proportion of spontaneous abortions show chromosomal abnormalities. A drug-association question has arisen of a possible association between trisomy and ovulation induction.[50] Although this association question remains unresolved, it is an interesting example of the importance of *risk* as opposed to *causation*. The decision to do antenatal testing must be made on the basis of risk estimates, regardless of whether the risk is due to the agent or to conditions under which the agent is given.

Numerous important *drug concerns arise in late pregnancy and during the perinatal period.* These include analgesics and anesthetics, prostaglandins and prostaglandin inhibitors (thromboplastic and antithromboplastic influence effects on fetal maturation and ductus closure), labor-inducing agents, drugs for threatened premature delivery, antihypertensives and other cardiovascular drugs, and drug-abuse problems. Because the effect of most therapeutic agents is so intertwined with the effect of therapeutic indication or other socioenvironmental problems, these questions generally require carefully controlled clinical evaluation.

FREQUENCY OF THERAPEUTIC DRUG USE IN WOMEN IN THE FERTILE AGE RANGE

A national projection of 1990 use of suspected pregnancy risk drugs in women in the fertile age range is shown in Table 10–3.

NEEDS FOR THE FUTURE

The initial epidemiologic studies following the thalidomide episode were only able to identify drug teratogens

TABLE 10–3. ANNUAL NATIONAL APPEARANCES* OF POTENTIAL AND POSSIBLE FETAL RISK RELATED DRUGS FROM NATIONAL DISEASE AND THERAPEUTIC INDEX (1990)

POTENTIAL TERATOGENS	ALL APPEARANCES (× 1000)	FEMALES AGE 20–39 (× 1000)	POTENTIAL TERATOGENS	ALL APPEARANCES (× 1000)	FEMALES AGE 20–39 (× 1000)
Nonsteroidal Anti-inflammatory Agents†	52659	6939	Estrogens DES	162	0
Benzodiazepines	17615	3312	Barbiturates	1820	247
Corticoids, plain (systemic)	25905	3242	Oral Antidiabetics	14692	278
Major Tranquilizers	7778	1462	Clomiphene (Clomid)	519	467
Fungicides Suppositories	1643	1056	Calcium Channel Blockers	26046	522
Progestogens Medroxyprogesterone	107	10	Vitamin A Congeners Isotretinoin	503	170
Anticonvulsants			Cancer Therapy		
Dilantin	3316	370	Methotrexate	773	51
Depakene	116	13	Tamoxifen	936	19
Depakote	789	193	Cytoxan	902	56
Mysoline	252	53	Fluorouracil	1609	60
Tegretol	2343	439	Danazol (Hormones, Sex, Other)	173	98
Antihypertensives			Immunosuppressants		
Aldomet	1749	102	Imuran	490	82
Aldoril	678	11	Cyclosporine	194	9
Catapres	1234	32			
Minipress	1231	32	Penicillamine	98	9
Apresoline	444	3			
Hydralazine	453	9			
Clonidine	837	43			
Minoxidil	131	13	Misoprostol (Cytotec)	1046	60
ACE Inhibitors			Lovastatin	3591	30
Prinivil (lisinopril)	2372	87			
Vasotec (enalapril)	7795	185	Anti-obesity Agents, Other Diethylpropion (Tenuate)	357	149
Zestril (lisinopril)	2431	80			
Capoten (captropril)	6170	66	Anti-thyroid Therapy Propylthiouracil	217	71
Lithium	2502	651			

Source: IMS America, Plymouth Meeting, PA.

*Projected from a national multidisciplinary sample of visits to office based physicians. A drug appearance is the mention of a drug use within a single visit to an office based physician. Based on repeated visits a patient may have several annual drug appearances.

†Does not include aspirin and nonprescription ibuprofen.

that showed very high relative risks for flagrantly apparent defects. These studies had little power to identify low-level risks, which can be important with frequent exposures. Only in the case of DES was attention called to a delayed teratogenic effect. Improvements in case-control methodology and expansion of databases are increasing the potential to identify lower-level teratogenicity. Coordinated enrollment of selected exposures for *expanded cohort studies* has the potential for answering important questions, such as selecting the least teratogenic antiepileptic regimen. Increased *exposure analysis in case registries* also can contribute. Greater exploitation of *routinely computerized experience in population samples,* such as HMOs, Medicaid, and other treatment groups, is a way to obtain the vast data size necessary to analyze selected problems at much less cost than past comprehensive pregnancy cohort studies. *Case reporting* remains the first line for quickly flagging human fetal risks. This needs to be increased, with greater attention to coordinating reports and analyzing suspected coincidences. Defined denominators are slow to accumulate and are always limited in size for identifying risks of rare events and/or low relative risks. Clarification of policy for rapid information exchange (in the face of bureaucratic rigidity and fears of unfounded publicity and litigation) is another requirement for avoiding "further thalidomides." Greater attention to functional, behavioral, and long-term developmental sequelae is necessary to identify problems that are less obvious than the structural abnormalities apparent at birth.

Careful double-blind *clinical trials* to define benefits are also an important need. The potential for low-dose aspirin to avoid placental perfusion problems and low birth weight is currently the outstanding example. Antihypertensives, antibiotics, tocolytics, and antiemetics are other examples. The urgency of such studies must be stressed relative to the continuing fetal risks from irrational management of pregnant women.

REFERENCES

1. Herbst AL, Ulfelder H, Poskanzer DC: Adenocarcinoma of the vagina: Association of maternal stilbestrol therapy with tumor appearance in young women. N Engl J Med 284:878–881, 1971
2. Schardein JL: Congenital abnormalites and hormones during pregnancy. Teratology 22:251–270, 1980
3. Wallenburg HCS, Dekker GA, Makovitz JW, Rotmans P: Low-dose aspirin prevents pregnancy-induced hypertension and pre-eclampsia in angiotensin-sensitive primigravidae. Lancet 1:1–3, 1986
4. Elder MG, de Swiet M, Robertson A, et al: Low-dose aspirin in pregnancy. Lancet 1:410, 1988
5. Parmalee AH, Allen E, Stein IF, Buxbaum H: Three cases of congenital goiter. Am J Obstet Gynecol 40:145–147, 1940
6. Warkany J: Antituberculosis drugs. Teratology 20:133–138, 1979
7. Thiersch JB, Phillips FS: Effect of aminopterin on early pregnancy. Proc Soc Exp Biol Med 74:204–208, 1950
8. Hoffman F, Overzier C, Uhde G: Zur Frage der Hormonalen erzeugug Fotaler Zwittenbildungen beim Menschen. Geburtshilfe Frauenheilkd 15:1061–1070, 1955
9. Grumbach MM, Ducharme JR, Moloshok RE: Fetal masculinizing action of certain oral progestins. J Clin Endocrinol Metab 19:1369–1380, 1959
10. McBride WG: Thalidomide and congenital anomalies. Lancet 2:1358, 1961
11. Fisher WD, Vooress ML, Gardner LI: Congenital hypothyroidism in infant following maternal I(131) therapy. J Pediatr 62:132–146, 1963
12. Greenberg LH, Tanaka KR: Congenital anomalies probably induced by cyclophosphamide. JAMA 188:423–426, 1964
13. Janz D, Fuchs R: Sind Antiepileptische Medikamente wahrend der Schwangerschaft Schadlich. Dtsch Med Wochenschr 89:241–243, 1964
14. Klevit HD: Iatrogenic thyroid disease, in Gardner LI (ed): Endocrine and Genetic Diseases of Childhood. Philadelphia, WB Saunders, 1969, pp 243–252
15. Friedman WF: Vitamin D and the supravalvular aortic stenosis syndrome, in Woollam DHM (ed): Advances in Teratology. New York, Academic Press, 1968, pp 83–96
16. Becker MH, Genieser NB, Finegold M, et al: Chondrodysplasia punctata: Is warfarin therapy a factor? Am J Dis Child 129:365–369, 1975
17. German J, Kowal A, Ehlers KH: Trimethadione and human teratogenesis. Teratology 3:349–362, 1970
18. Meadow SR: Congenital abnormalities and anticonvulsant drugs. Proc R Soc Med 63:121–123, 1970
19. Baden E: Environmental pathology of the teeth, in Gorlin RJ, et al (eds): Oral Pathology, 6th ed. St. Louis, CV Mosby, 1970, pp 189–191
20. Mjolnerod OK, Rassmussen K, Dommerud SA, Gjeruldsen ST: Congenital connective-tissue defect probably due to penicillamine therapy in pregnancy. Lancet 1:673–675, 1971
21. Nora JJ, Nora AH, Toews WH: Lithium, Ebstein's anomaly and other congenital heart defects. Lancet 2:594–595, 1971
22. Rosa FW: Virilization of the female fetus with maternal danazol exposure. Am J Obstet Gynecol 149:99–100, 1984
23. Robert E, Guiband P: Maternal valproate exposure and neural tube defects. Lancet 2:937, 1982
24. Sautier Laboratories: Bilan des effets teratogenes du Tigason et du Roaccutane. Geneva, Letter to physicians, dated July 27, 1983
25. Rosa FW: Teratogenicity of isotretinoin. Lancet 2:513, 1983
26. Rosa FW, Wilk AL, Joshi SR, Kelsey F, Troendle G: Teratology of hypervitaminosis A. ADR Highlight 1984-1, FDA, 1984
27. Rosa FW: Spina bifida in infants of women treated with carbamazepine during pregnancy. N Engl J Med 324:624–665, 1991
28. Milham S: Scalp defects in infants of mothers treated for hyperthyroidism with methimazole or carbimazole during pregnancy. Teratology 32:321, 1985
29. Maybre SA, Williams R: Teratogenic effects associated with maternal primidone therapy. J Pediatr 99:160–162, 1981
30. Rosa FW, Bosco, LA, Graham CF, et al: Neonatal anuria with maternal angiotensin converting enzyme inhibition. Obstet Gynecol 74:371–374, 1989
31. Csaba IF, Sulyok E, Ertl T: Clinical note: Relationship of maternal treatment with indomethacin to persistence of fetal circulation syndrome. J Pediatr 92:484, 1978
32. Kallen B, Rahmani TMZ, Winberg J: Infants with congenital limb reduction registered in the Swedish register of congenital malformations. Teratology 29:73–85, 1983
33. Heinonen OP, Slone D, Shapiro S: Birth Defects and Drugs in Pregnancy. Littleton, Mass., PSG, 1977
34. Monson RR, Rosenberg L, Hartz SC, et al: Diphenhydramine and selected congenital malformations. N Engl J Med 289:1049–1052, 1973
35. Heinonen OP, Slone D, Monson RR, et al: Cardiovascular birth defects and antenatal exposure to female sex hormones. N Engl J Med 298:67–70, 1977
36. Wiseman RA, Dodds-Smith IC: Cardiovascular defects and antenatal exposure to female sex hormones: A reevaluation of some base data. Teratology 30:370–379, 1984
37. Heinonen OP, Shapiro S, Monson RR, et al: Immunization during pregnancy against poliomyelitis and influenza in relation to childhood malignancy. Int J Epidemiol 2:229–235, 1973
38. Milkovitch L, Van den Berg B: Effects of prenatal meprobamate and chlordiazepoxide on human embryonic and fetal development. N Engl J Med 291:1268–1271, 1974
39. Rosa FW: Food and Drug Administration Computerized On-Line Medicaid Pharmaceutical Surveillance Systems (COMPASS) human teratology. Teratology 33:542, 1986

40. Rosa FW: Detecting human retinoid embryopathy. (abstract). Teratology 43:419, 1991

41. Klemitti A, Saxen L: Prospective versus retrospective approach in the search for environmental causes of malformations. Am J Public Health 2071–2075, 1967

42. Lanier AP, Noller KL, Decker DG, et al: Cancer and stilbesterol: A followup of 1719 persons exposed to estrogens in utero and born 1943–1959. Mayo Clin Proc 48:793–799, 1973

43. Nakone T, et al: Multi-institutional study on teratogenicity and fetal toxicity of antiepileptic drugs: A report of a cooperative study group in Japan. Epilepsia 21:663–680, 1980

44. French Chapter of International League Against Epilepsy: Tertogenic risk of antiepileptic drugs with special reference to sodium valproate, in Porter RJ (ed): Advances in Epileptology. New York, Raven Press, 1984, pp 299–307

45. Rosa FW: Megadoses of vitamin A. Teratology 36:272, 1987

46. Kallin B, Tandberg A: Lithium and pregnancy: A cohort study of manicdepressive women. Acta Psychiatr Scand 68:1984–1989, 1983

47. Meinardi H, Lindhout D: Teratogenicity of antiepileptic drugs. Br J Clin Pract Suppl 27:37–41, 1983

48. Kline J, Stein Z, Susser M, Warburton D: Fever during pregnancy and spontaneous abortion. Am J Epidemiol 121:832–842, 1985

49. Rosa FW, Baum C, Shaw M: Pregnancy outcome after first trimester vaginitis drug therapy. Obstet Gynecol 69:751–755, 1987

50. Oakley GP, Flynt GO: Increased prevalence of Down's syndrome (mongolism) among the offspring of women treated with ovulation-inducing agent. Teratology 5:264, 1972

11

TERATOLOGY

F. C. FRASER

This chapter will review the principles of teratology, particularly the genetic aspects of embryonic susceptibility to malformation. A drug is said to be *teratogenic* when it induces a malformation in the embryo. Those who treat women in pregnancy are concerned also with less specific evidence of harm during development, such as abortion, stillbirth, low birth weight, infertility, and psychomotor retardation. Drugs that damage the embryo/fetus in these more general ways are said to be *embryo/fetotoxic.* Although these effects are important, much less is known about them (see Chapters 12 and 13), and the principles to be reviewed here will deal primarily with teratogenicity. For convenience, I shall use the term *embryo* to refer to both the embryo and the fetus.

Estimates of malformation frequency depend on what are considered malformations and how hard they are looked for. The usual definition is a structural anomaly, present at birth, that is severe enough to impair viability or physical well-being, severity being measured by whether the malformation requires treatment. (For statistical purposes, the definition is taken to include deformations and disruptions.) Estimates of malformation frequency at birth cluster around 3 percent.[1] If the children are followed for several years to identify malformations not found at birth (particularly those of the heart), frequency estimates increase by at least twofold. Furthermore, they do not include other manifestations of embryonic damage, such as growth retardation and behavioral deficits (see Chapters 12 and 13). With few exceptions, the frequency of malformations has remained stable over the past few decades,[2] suggesting that increasing drug use and environmental pollution have not had much teratogenic impact. The incidence of ventricular septal defect and of patent ductus arteriosus has been rising for unexplained reasons, whereas that of neural tube defects has been falling, even when the impact of prenatal screening and selective abortion is taken into account.[2]

Causes of malformations can be classified as mutant genes of major effect, chromosomal imbalance, multifactorial (many genes of small effect interacting with environmental factors of small effect), and identifiable environmental teratogens. Since there are genetic predis-

positions to most environmental teratogens, the latter two categories may overlap somewhat.

Monogenic and chromosomal causes may account for about 14 percent of malformations, and about 20 percent are multifactorial.[1] Perhaps 5 percent are related to maternal factors such as rubella, toxoplasmosis, and CMV,[3] diabetes mellitus,[4] and (1 percent) anticonvulsant and other drugs. This leaves a large class of malformations (61 percent) in which the cause is unknown. Thus the teratogenic impact of drug-induced malformations appears to be relatively small, but as mentioned earlier, these figures ignore the fetopathic and behavioral effects (see Chapters 12 and 13) that do not get included in malformation surveys and which may be greatly underestimated.

An agent can cause malformations by altering the genetic code of the DNA (mutation, largely expressed in subsequent generations) or by damaging the somatic tissues of the embryo, e.g., by causing cell death, suppressing enzyme synthesis, altering membrane properties, or inhibiting mitosis (see Chapter 14). Thus most mutagens are teratogens (because they cause not only mutations, but also nonspecific tissue damage), but teratogens are not necessarily mutagenic.

PRINCIPLES OF TERATOLOGY

Whether an agent is likely to cause malformations depends not only on its chemical and physical nature (its innate teratogenicity), but also on the developmental stage at exposure, the dose, the genotype of the embryo and mother, and possible interactions with other environmental factors.[5,6] These principles have been derived largely from animal studies. What little evidence there is suggests that they apply also to human teratogenicity.

Developmental Stage

It is not surprising that the developmental upsets caused by exposure to a teratogen depend on what is going on in the embryo when it is exposed. A drug is not likely to cause cleft palate in an embryo whose palate has already closed. What is not so obvious is that the critical period (the stage at which exposure causes the highest frequency of malformations) may *precede* the period at which the damaged structure is forming. The critical period for cortisone-induced cleft palate in the mouse is 2 days before the palate shelves start to close[7]—equivalent to several weeks in the human embryo.

Data on critical periods are available for only a few human teratogens, particularly thalidomide[8] and rubella.[3] For thalidomide, for example, the susceptible period for malformations is from 20 to 36 days after conception, and the critical period for ventricular septal defect is in the 5th week, about 2 weeks before the septum closes.

Before organogenesis begins (around the end of the 3rd postconceptional week), the embryo has great regulative ability. If exposure to the injurious agent does not kill it, the embryo will reorganize itself to reestablish normal development, so exposure to teratogens in the first 2½ weeks will probably not result in malformations. Nor will exposure after the period of organogenesis, but the embryo will still be susceptible to toxicity. Alcohol, rubella, and warfarin, for example, can damage the embryo long after organogenesis is finished, as discussed in Chapter 12 and 13.

Changes in susceptibility with stage of development also may occur as the mode of maternal/embryonic communication changes. When organogenesis begins, the embryo is lying in a crater in the uterine wall, with little to separate it from the maternal tissues, and nutrition is histiotrophic (from maternally derived macromolecules). Chorioallantoic placentation is established at about 21 days, but nevertheless, histiotrophic nutrition continues until midterm.[9]

Dose

In animal studies, as the dose is gradually increased, a point is reached where malformed embryos appear in numbers above the "background" frequency of the strain being tested. Whether there is a no-effect level is a matter of argument[10]; for malformations, which are threshold characters (see below), one would expect that there should be. At least there are doses where the probability of inducing a malformation is vanishingly small. As the dose is further increased, the frequency of induced malformations continues to increase, and at a given dose, the frequency of fetal lethality will begin to increase. At still larger doses, maternal toxicity will appear, and eventually, maternal lethality occurs. The most effective (and dangerous) teratogens are those which induce malformation at, or close to, the therapeutic level and well below the fetal lethal or maternal toxic range. The most dramatic example is thalidomide, where a single pill may be enough to cause a malformation in the human embryo and it is almost impossible to reach maternally toxic levels.

Of course, the dose of a teratogen that induces malformations depends on the embryo's sensitivity to it, as discussed in the following section. Thus a drug that is harmless to most embryos when used in the therapeutic dose range may cause a malformation in the occasional case where the embryo's (and mother's) genes and particular environment make it unusually sensitive. This is the bugbear of those who would like to be sure that a drug is teratogenically "safe" before it is marketed.

Genotype

The influence of fetal and maternal genotype on teratogenic susceptibility has been well illustrated in the cortisone-induced cleft palate mouse model.[11,12] The same dose of cortisone causes high frequencies of cleft palate in one strain (A/J) and low frequencies in another (C57BL/6J). In crosses between the two strains, the F_1 generation had much higher frequencies of cleft palate when the treated mother was A/J rather than C57BL/6J, showing that maternal as well as fetal genes are important influences on sensitivity.

There are now many examples of genetic differences influencing teratogenic sensitivity, and these involve many teratogens and many types of malformation. They occur both within and between species. A drug that produces malformations in one species may not do so in another. Thus the fact that a drug appears to be nonteratogenic in experimental animals does not mean that it will be safe in people; conversely, a number of drugs that are highly teratogenic in experimental animals do not appear to be so in people, at least at therapeutic doses.

What determines genetic differences in teratogenic susceptibility? There may be differences in how much of the drug reaches the embryonic organs, differences in response of the embryonic tissues to the teratogen, and differences in the embryo's normal developmental pattern.

Differences in how much drug reaches the embryo include pharmacogenetic differences in binding, metabolism, or excretion of the drug (see Chapter 4), placental transport (see Chapter 15), and the way the fetus binds, metabolizes, or excretes the drug (see Chapter 14). Little is known of the underlying genetics. The most extensively studied difference is the aryl hydrocarbon oxidase (Ah) locus, which regulates the inducibility of various cytochrome P-450–mediated mono-oxygenases. Although the locus has been cloned, the genetics are exceedingly complex. Crosses and various backcrosses between inducible and noninducible strains show that in a noninducible mother, benzo[a]pyrene is more toxic/teratogenic to inducible embryos than to their noninducible siblings because the inducible embryos rapidly transform the benzopyrene into toxic metabolites. When the mother is of the inducible strain, the embryonic damage is high irrespective of the embryo's genotype, because there is increased exposure to toxic metabolites, which overrides the embryonic differences in metabolism.[13] With maternal–fetal interaction being so complex, it is not surprising that there are few examples in human beings (see, for example, phenytoin toxicity, as discussed in Chapter 4).

The mouse also provides an example of a genetic difference in teratogenic susceptibility acting through the placenta. The difference between the A/J and C57BL/6J strains in susceptibility to phenytoin-induced cleft lip appears to be mediated by a difference in activity of the placental PHT metabolizing system.[14] The genetics of the system have yet to be worked out.

Strain differences in teratogenic sensitivity also may arise from differences in the degree *to which the embryonic tissues respond,* and there are studies attempting to relate sensitivity to differences in H_2 (the mouse HLA), drug receptors, growth factors, and so forth. This is not an easy task, and the closer one gets to the gene, the more complex the results appear.[15]

Finally, differences in teratogenic susceptibility may result from *differences in the embryo's normal pattern of development.* For example, the A/J strain is more susceptible to cortisone-induced cleft palate than is the C57BL/6J strain because its genes cause the embryonic palate shelves to close at a later stage relative to the embryo as a whole. Since A/J shelves normally close later, it is easier to delay them beyond the point where they are able to close at all.[11,16] Similarly, the A/J embryos later-closing atrial septum makes it more susceptible to amphetamine-induced atrial septal defect,[17] and its face shape (less divergent medial nasal processes) makes it more susceptible to

aspirin-induced cleft lip.[18] For obvious reasons, there are no demonstrated examples in humans, but it is reasonable to suppose that they exist. The message is that even if a drug is not teratogenic to most human embryos, it may malform the occasional one whose genes have made it particularly susceptible.

Interactions of Drugs and Environmental Factors

In experimental teratology, it is well demonstrated that the teratogenicity of a drug may be altered by the concomitant administration of another drug or by a variety of environmental factors, such as diet, type of litter, or noise.[19] Furthermore, two drugs given at nonteratogenic doses may together be teratogenic. Third, a drug may be teratogenic in an embryo heterozygous for a mutant gene that causes a malformation in the homozygote. No comparable human examples are known, but the possibility that they may exist increases the complexity of evaluating

TABLE 11–1. SELECTED TERATOGENS IN HUMANS IMPLICATED WITH VARIOUS DEGREES OF CONFIDENCE

TERATOGENS	CONFIDENCE CLASS*	APPROXIMATE FREQUENCY OF MALDEVELOPMENT
Infections:		
Rubella	1	90% (see text)
Cytomegalovirus	1	1/1000
Herpes simplex (HSV) as teratogen	3	?
Syphilis	1	Very high
Toxoplasmosis	1	~15%
Maternal conditions:		
Diabetes	1	7 (depends on control)
Fever	2	?
Lupus erythematosus	1	Very high
Phenylketonuria, untreated	1	Very high
Drugs, chemicals, and radiation:		
Alcohol (chronic alcoholism)	1	30%
Amphetamines	3	?
Anticoagulants (coumarin)	2	5–10%
Anticonvulsants		
Hydantoin (Phenytoin)	1	10%
Phenobarbital	3	?
Trimethadione	1	? ~20%
Valproic acid	1	~5%
Chemotherapeutic agents	1	High
Cocaine	2	~15%
Hypoglycemics	3	?
Lithium	1	10%
Mercury, organic	1	High
Minor tranquilizers		
Diazepam	2	? (very low)
Meprobamate	3	? (very low)
Penicillamine	2	Moderate
Radiation	1	Dose-dependent
Sex hormones		
Male	1	? Low
Female	2	<1%?
Stilbestrol	1	?
Thalidomide	1	50–80%
Vitamin A congeners		
Isotretinoin (Accutane)	1	20%
Etretinate (Tegison)	2	?
Vitamin A (megadoses)	3	?

*Confidence class 1, no doubt; 2, very likely; 3, possibly.
Source: Modified from Nora and Fraser.[6]

the potential risk of an exposure to a particular drug in a particular pregnancy.

EVALUATION OF TERATOGENICITY

Before being marketed, new drugs must be tested for toxicity in a variety of ways, including tests for teratogenicity in several animal species. It is reassuring if no malformations or other signs of fetal toxicity are induced except at doses far above the therapeutic level, or in the maternally toxic range, but this does not prove safety, as mentioned previously. If teratogenicity is observed, then a decision as to whether to market the drug or not must be made on the basis of how important the benefits may be and how often the drug is likely to be used in pregnancy. Accutane is an interesting example of a drug known to be teratogenic that nevertheless remains on the market, presumably because of its important benefits.

When a new drug is marketed, the manufacturer will naturally wish to keep track of its use during pregnancy for any evidence of an increase in the rate of miscarriages, malformations, or signs of fetotoxicity. However, there is no requirement for systematic, rigorous followup of exposed pregnancies, and it is often impossible to obtain reliable data to show that there is not (or is) an increase in the malformation rate in infants exposed in early gestation to a particular drug.

If a drug is, in fact, teratogenic, this will be most easily detected if the induced malformations are bizarre and occur in a high proportion of exposed embryos, as in the case of thalidomide.[8] It is much more difficult to detect teratogenicity if the malformations are common and the attack rate low. Regrettably, but understandably, there are many drugs on the market for which the data on malformation rates in babies exposed to the drug in early pregnancy are wholly inadequate. Thus drugs may be classified as those which are demonstrably teratogenic, those which have been thoroughly investigated (usually for forensic reasons) and found not to increase the malformation rate detectably (although not found to be safe), and those in which the data are inadequate and one must make more or less informed guesses as to how high a risk of induced malformation has been ruled out. One can usually say, at least for drugs that have been on the market for some time, that the teratogenic risk is probably low or else it would have been detected. It is unwise, however, to say that a drug is teratogenically safe. A number of volumes summarize and evaluate the available data.[20–22] There are also a number of computerized information services that can be consulted with respect to particular exposures.[23,24] Finally, the question of potential teratogenicity of drugs, and of other agents, raises concerns involving decisions to be made by patients about reproduction and by scientists, public health officials, and regulatory agencies about the agents in question.[24] Table 11–1 summarizes information about drugs known to be teratogenic.

For the physician, the message is that it is good practice to refrain from prescribing any drug during pregnancy, even if it is not known to be teratogenic, unless there is a demonstrable need that outweighs the (usually unknown but probably low) risks.

REFERENCES

1. Kalter H, Warkany J: Congenital malformations: Etiologic factors and their role in prevention. N Engl J Med 308:424–431, 491–497, 1983
2. Oakley GP: Incidence and epidemiology of birth defects, in Kaback MM (ed): Genetic Issues in Pediatric and Obstetric Practice. Chicago, Year Book Medical Publishers, 1981
3. Sever J: Perinatal infections and immunity, in Scarpelli DG, Migaki G (eds): Transplacental Effects on Fetal Health. New York, Alan R. Liss, 1988, pp 3–13
4. Mills JL, Knopp RH, Simpson JL, et al: Lack of relation of increased malformation rates in infants of diabetic mothers to glycemic control during organogenesis. N Engl J Med 318:671–676, 1988
5. Wilson JG: Current status of teratology: General principles and mechanisms derived from animal studies, in Wilson JG, Fraser FC (eds): Handbook of Teratology, vol 1. New York, Plenum Press, 1977, pp 47–74
6. Nora JJ, Fraser FC: Medical Genetics: Principles and Practice, 3d ed. Philadelphia, Lea & Febiger, 1989, pp 268–277
7. Biddle FG, Fraser FC: Genetics of cortisone-induced cleft palate in the mouse: Embryonic and maternal effects. Genetics 84:743–754, 1976
8. Lenz W: Drug therapy in pregnancy as an experiment in human teratology, in Fishbein M (ed): Proceedings of the 2nd International Conference on Congenital Malformations, 1963
9. Beck F, Lloyd JB: Comparative fetal transfer, in Wilson JG, Fraser FC (eds): Handbook of Teratology, vol 3: Comparative, Maternal, and Epidemiologic Aspects. New York, Plenum Press, 1977, pp 155–186
10. Gaylor DW, Sheehan DM, Young JF, Mattison DR: The threshold dose question in teratogenesis. Teratology 38:389–391, 1988
11. Fraser FC: The William Allan Memorial Award Address: Evolution of a palatable multifactorial threshold model. Am J Hum Genet 32:796–813, 1980
12. Fraser FC: Research revisited. Cleft Palate J 26:255–257, 1989
13. Shum S, Jensen NM, Nebert DW: The murine Ah locus: In utero toxicity and teratogenesis associated with genetic differences in benzo[a]pyrene metabolism. Teratology 20:365–376, 1979
14. Johnston MC, Sulik KK, Dudley KH: Genetic and metabolic studies of the differential sensitivity of A/J and C57B1/6J mice to phenytoin ("Dilantin") induced cleft lip. Teratology 19:33A, 1979
15. Goldman AS, Herold R, Piddington R: Inhibition of embryonic palatal shelf horizontalization and medial edge-epithelial breakdown by cortisol: Role of H-2 in the mouse. J Craniofac Genet Dev Biol 8:135–145, 1988
16. Vekemans M, Fraser FC: Stage of palate closure as one indication of "liability" to cleft palate. Am J Med Genet 4:95–102, 1979
17. Nora JJ, Somerville RJ, Fraser FC: Homologies for congenital heart diseases: Murine models influenced by dextroamphetamine. Teratology 1:413–416, 1968
18. Trasler D, Machado M: Newborn and adult face shapes related to mouse cleft lip predisposition. Teratology 19:197–206, 1979
19. Fraser FC: Interactions and multiple causes, in Wilson JG, Fraser FC (eds): Handbook of Teratology, vol 1. New York, Plenum Press, 1977, pp 445–463
20. Kelley-Buchanan C: Peace of Mind During Pregnancy, 2nd ed. New York, Facts on File Publications, 1989
21. Schardein JL: Chemically Induced Birth Defects. New York, Marcel Dekker, 1985
22. Shepard TH: A Catalog of Teratogenic Agents, 4th ed. Baltimore, Johns Hopkins University Press, 1989
23. Teratogen Information Service (TERIS), Department of Pediatrics, University of Washington School of Medicine, Seattle, Washington, 98195.
24. Hanson JW, Thomson EJ: Clinical aspects risk assessment and management of transplacental hazards for the fetus: Considerations for public policy, in Scarpelli G, Migaki G (eds): Transplacental Effects on Fetal Health. New York, Alan R. Liss, 1988, pp 327–335

12

DELAYED TERATOGENIC EXPRESSION

BERNARD H. SHAPIRO

Inadvertently, it is the pediatrician who must deal with the often devastating consequences of maternal drug therapy. Scores of drugs, including analgesics, vitamins, sedatives, antibiotics, hormones, antihistamines, appetite suppressants, diuretics, etc., have been reported to cause congenital malformations.[1-3] Add to this list such nontherapeutic drugs as alcohol, nicotine, caffeine, "recreational drugs" (i.e., cocaine, marijuana), environmental pollutants, food additives, etc., and the number of potential teratogens becomes more threatening.

Surely, the easiest way to prevent drug-induced birth defects is to simply avoid drug exposure during pregnancy. Unfortunately, just as ours has become a highly litigious society, it is also a society that does not hesitate to medicate itself. A recent survey[4] of women's attitudes found that "54 percent of those questioned felt that it was better to take drugs than to go through a day tense and nervous, and 48 percent felt it was better to use drugs than to spend a sleepless night." Statistics regarding the use of tranquilizers have shown that in Great Britain in 1980, 1 woman in 5 and 1 man in 10 took mind-altering drugs, with Valium being the most commonly used drug.[5] In the United States in 1977, over 80 million prescriptions were written for chlordiazepoxide (Librium), diazepam (Valium), and flurazepam (Dalmane), meaning that 8000 tons of benzodiazepine were consumed.[6] In 1979, Americans consumed 5 billion pills of tranquilizers,[7] and in 1984, Americans filled 25 million prescriptions for Valium.[8] The enormity of the problem is further dramatized in the United States by the fact that more than 1.2 billion drug prescriptions are written each year; there is unlimited self-administration of over-the-counter drugs, and approximately 500 new products are introduced annually.[2]

Of particular relevance to teratologic studies is the finding that between 750,000 and 1 million American women of childbearing age are regular, high-frequency users of alcohol plus psychoactive drugs; almost 600,000 are current or regular users of barbiturates; almost 200,000 are current or regular users of prescription stimulants and appetite depressants; 125,000 use prescription narcotics; and about 100,000 use prescription antidepressants.[9] These numbers probably pale in comparison with the amounts of nonpsychoactive prescription drugs and over-the-counter medications consumed by young women. This propensity for drug taking appears to be unabated during pregnancy. In 1970, the average number of drugs taken by each pregnant woman in the United States was 8.7.[10] In 1973, a mean of 10.3 different drugs were consumed during pregnancy.[11] And by 1978, the average number of drugs used during pregnancy was 11.[12] In this latter study, 93.4 percent of the pregnant women consumed 5 or more different drugs. Moreover, the average of 11 drugs does not accurately reflect the number of different chemicals to which the fetus is exposed, since many products contain numerous ingredients. It also should be noted that accompanying our dramatic advances in neonatology comes the reality that premature infants born in North America are exposed to around 20 prescribed drugs between conception and discharge from the hospital.[13] One can appreciate the aptness of Goldman's observation[2] "that the unborn child is being incubated in a sea of drugs."

In 1979, the National Foundation–March of Dimes reported that more than 250,000 American babies, about 7 percent of all live births, were born with congenital defects each year.[14] Although it is not possible to determine the number of defects that are drug-induced, if developmental exposure to drugs is a significant cause of birth defects, then it seems reasonable to expect that the increased consumption of drugs during the past few decades would result in an increased number of birth defects. In fact, the National Health Interview Survey[15] reported a 100 percent increase in the number of birth defects in the 25-year period starting in the late 1950s. Of relevance to this chapter is the finding that the majority of birth defects are no longer obvious malformations apparent in the newborn but represent more subtle biochemical and behavioral anomalies, such as learning disabilities, that are not diagnosed until several years after birth.[3,15]

DELAYED TERATOGENIC EFFECTS

Historically, *teratogens* have been considered to be prenatal toxic agents that either kill the embryo or produce congenital malformations during the critical period of organogenesis. Using classical definitions, *congenital malformations* have been defined as anatomic abnormalities present at birth. Since its arrival as a bonafide scientific discipline, and even before that, *teratology,* as derived from the Greek *terat-* , meaning "monster," has emphasized the study of gross anatomic anomalies. Understandably, there has been a major concern for those teratogens which produce obvious and devastating structural malformations.

However, during the past decade, there has grown an increased awareness that many teratogens may act after the period of organogenesis, through birth and into lactation. Since a preponderance of drugs easily pass through the placental "barrier" as well as the mammary epithelium into the milk, the developing mammal remains susceptible to the teratogenic effects of maternally administered drugs from conception through fetal development and parturition and during nursing. With this awareness has come an understanding that teratogens, often at far lower doses than those needed to produce anatomic anomalies, can induce more subtle defects in the biochemistry, physiology, and behavior of the developing animal.[16] Furthermore, many of these subtle defects are not apparent at birth and may lie "dormant" or "latent" in the animal until years later. Like the classic teratogens, those compounds which interfere with normal biochemical, physiologic, or behavioral development are active at only limited critical times during development, and their adverse effects are permanent and irreversible. However, the fetal critical periods for what might be called *subtle teratogens* usually occur sometime after organogenesis, and depending on the species, this may be as late as the postnatal period. Furthermore, the effects of the teratogens are latent. That is, at the time of administration, the teratogen appears to produce a "programming" or "imprinting" defect in a developing tissue or organ. This programming defect need not be expressed until adulthood, since the animal may not require the "program" until that time.

Both clinical and experimental findings have shown the brain to be highly susceptible to the delayed expression of teratogens. Maternal alcohol consumption can result in retarded development, impaired learning capability,[17,18] and a decreased reproductive potential[19] without obvious anatomic anomalies. Prenatal administration of morphine has been reported to alter locomotor activity,[20] tolerance to the analgesic effects of morphine in adulthood,[21] activity in the open-field test, pubertal onset, and the adrenal stress response.[22] Moreover, the prenatal administration of D-amphetamine results in postnatal brain abnormalities in motor behavior and brain biogenic amine levels.[23]

This is not to indicate that the brain is unique in its ability to exhibit latent responses to fetal insults. It has been shown from highly publicized studies in humans[24,25] and animals[26] that exposure *in utero* to diethylstilbestrol (DES) results in subsequent abnormalities in the reproductive structures of both female and male offspring when they become adults. In the case of women, prenatal exposure to maternally administered DES is associated with an enhanced risk of clear-cell adenocarcinoma of the vagina and cervix and a dramatic increase in abnormal vaginal cytology.[24,27] Furthermore, DES daughters have less successful pregnancies,[28] a greater risk of menstrual irregularities,[29] and an increase in psychopathologies, especially depression,[30] during adult life. Two decades had to pass before the congenital defects produced by the DES teratogen were expressed. Just what DES did *in utero* to the appoximately 2 to 4 million exposed American men and women[31] is still a matter of investigation; only the delayed consequences are now sadly clear.

THE CASE FOR ANIMAL MODELS

Realizing how profoundly important and long-lasting are the effects of development on the adult, the concept of delayed teratogenic expression seems almost intuitively irrefutable. How can one deny the tragic consequences of prenatal exposure to DES? In actuality, however, with the exception of the fetal alcohol syndrome and the DES children, there really is not that much compelling scientific evidence establishing delayed teratogenic expression as an important human health problem. Although there are now hundreds of reports showing that countless numbers of drugs can produce latent teratogenic effects in laboratory animals, the skeptic might recall Albert Szent-Györgyi's comment[32] that "a drug is a substance which, if injected into a rabbit, produces a paper."

Numerous drugs identified as teratogens in laboratory species appear to be harmless to the human embryo. However, in defense of animal studies, it should be noted that the converse is not true. That is, all human teratogens have been shown to produce congenital defects in experimental animals.[3] Although somewhat in hindsight, we have now learned that prenatal exposure to DES produces the same reproductive defects in laboratory animals as previously reported in humans.[26] Moreover, it should be noted that drugs considered as nonteratogenic in humans are so classified because they produce no observable structural defects in the newborn. There are very few studies that have examined the long-term effects in humans of *in utero* drug exposure. How do we know that an increasing incidence of infertility in our population is not a delayed result of our increased *in utero* exposure to drugs and environmental toxins? Perhaps certain patterns of aging that are expressed near the end of our lives are a legacy of some developmental insult. The heterogeneous influences and the time frame of our lives make it exceedingly difficult to identify latent teratogenic defects in human populations. In contrast, it seems reasonable to conduct these studies on environmentally and genetically controlled laboratory species whose life spans are sufficiently short to allow for the completion of experimental protocols. If perinatal exposure to a drug at therapeutic-like levels for that species produces long-lasting biochemical or behavioral defects in the adult offspring, it seems judicious to consider the drug as a potential threat to the unborn, requiring additional studies in alternate species and already exposed human populations.

DRUGS AND DOSAGES IN ANIMAL STUDIES

Teratologic studies are often criticized for basing conclusions on the use of suprapharmacologic levels of drugs or environmental agents to which human embryos or fetuses are rarely exposed. A case in point is radiation. Clearly, massive *in utero* exposure to radiation produces the literal meaning of teratology, i.e., monstrosities.[33] Although pregnant women may be exposed to diagnostic levels of radiation,[34] how relevant are these animal studies to the human experience? How much information can we extrapolate from these studies to help us understand the actions of the more common chemical teratogens? Unlike drug teratogens that produce specific anatomic or biochemical lesions at critical times during differentiation,[2,16] the destructive effects of radiation can be broad and nonselective.[33]

Just as teratologic studies should avoid administering drugs at doses large enough to add to the animal's body weight, the opposite also could be a problem. Animal experiments that duplicate human therapeutic serum levels of drugs could be using inappropriately low doses to produce teratogenic defects. Since laboratory animals tend to metabolize drugs more quickly than humans,[35] it

seems prudent to also study drug teratogens at doses that are therapeutic for the particular species under study.

THE TERATOGENICALLY SENSITIVE SEXUAL BRAIN

During the past 15 or more years, we have been interested in the latent effects of teratogens and have concentrated our studies on the sexual development of the brain. It seemed that sexual and reproductive brain functions were excellent parameters for studying the latent effects of imprinting. First, differentiation of the central nervous system extends over a much longer period of time than that of the other major organ systems,[16] so the human brain, which continues to develop for several years after birth,[36] remains vulnerable to teratogenic damage for a prolonged period. Second, most drugs are lipid-soluble, and the developing central nervous system with its high fat content and no functional blood–brain barrier[37] becomes a repository for drugs, resulting in an enhanced sensitivity to low levels of exposure. Lastly, almost by definition, teratogenic effects on reproduction must be latent. The "programs" or "imprints" for reproduction are not required for a long time after embryogenesis, and yet we know that the "programs" for these brain functions (i.e., reproductive cycles, taste preferences, sexual behavior, etc.) are established at the time of brain differentiation.[38,40]

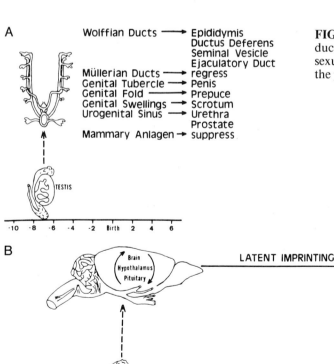

FIGURE 12–1. (*A*) Prenatal masculinization of reproductive anlagen by the fetal rat testes. (*B*) Some of the sexually dimorphic adult brain functions imprinted by the perinatal rat testes.

TABLE 12–1. SEXUAL DIFFERENTIATION OF THE RAT BRAIN

SYSTEM	ORGANIZER	MASCULINE	FEMININE
Gonadotropin secretion	Estrogen	Tonic	Cyclic
Sexual behavior	Estrogen	Ejaculatory	Lordotic
Saccharin preference	Androgen	Diminished	Enhanced
Growth hormone secretion	Androgen	Pulsatile	Tonic

In the classical sense, fetal testosterone,[41,42] or its metabolite dihydrotestosterone,[43] is normally responsible for masculinizing the reproductive structures of the mammalian male as well as the mammalian female when administered during the critical embryologic period of organogenesis (Figure 12–1A). In the same sense, the mammalian brain is also masculinized by testosterone and/or its estrogen metabolites.[44,45] In the case of the rat, endogenous androgens or estrogens in the male or similar exogenous hormones in the female masculinize the developing brain so that the adult exhibits an entire panoply of masculinized brain functions (Figure 12–1B). In particular, the masculinized mammalian brain secretes gonadotropins in a tonic fashion, allows for the display of masculine sexual behavior (e.g., mountings, intromissions, and ejaculations), exhibits a decreased preference for saccharin, and secretes growth hormone in pulsatile bursts (Table 12–1). As with classic teratogens, once these sexual brain functions are imprinted in the developing brain, the results, as seen in the adult, are permanent and irreversible. In contrast, hormonal effects are always transitory when hormones are administered to adults.

In the human, behavioral development, unlike morphogenesis, is shaped by incalculable influences, making it difficult to dissect out the imprinting role of fetal hormones, acting "momentarily," decades earlier, in the mother's womb. Nevertheless, psychosexual studies of adult humans, exposed *in utero* to aberrant levels of sex steroids (e.g., congenital adrenal hyperplasia, testicular feminization, maternal treatment with virilizing progestins or DES), indicate that the human brain is not exempt from the imprinting effects of prenatal sex steroids. Genetic females exposed to elevated androgen levels during the critical period of brain development exhibit masculinized play and grooming behavior as children[46] and are more likely to be bisexual as adults.[47] Boys exposed to subnormal levels of androgens during development appear to have more feminized behaviors.[46,48] Adult women exposed to maternally administered DES were found to exhibit decreased heterosexual activity and motivations and increased bisexuality.[30]

DELAYED TERATOGENIC EXPRESSION OF COMMONLY PRESCRIBED DRUGS

As mentioned earlier, there is a paucity of hard evidence, and equally few conducted studies, demonstrating the delayed teratogenic effects of known human teratogens. Imagine the difficulty of trying to identify an environmental pollutant or drug, ingested for a brief critical period during pregnancy, as the cause of some biochemical or behavioral abnormality expressed in adulthood in an individual seemingly free of any anatomic malformations. Who would suspect that the abnormality expressed in adulthood was actually a congenital defect? This inability even to perceive of a link between cause and effect is responsible for the paucity of studies concerning the latent expression of teratogens.

For the physician, there is a particular moral dilemma in treating pregnant and nursing women whose medical conditions require drug therapy. Moreover, we are all concerned about the teratogenic effects of environmental pollutants. However, what can the individual—physician included—do? Surely this is a societal problem requiring political remedy. The excessive use of over-the-counter medications, alcoholic beverages, smoking, etc. during pregnancy is a serious threat to the unborn, and physicians have unequivocally condemned their excessive use. In contrast, how do you treat women whose medical conditions require drug therapy but who incidentally happen to be pregnant? Who would want to restore the health of a mother at the cost of compromising her child's long-term well-being?

In this regard, there are drugs whose widespread use and teratogenic potential make them likely candidates for long-term teratogenic studies. Cimetidine, a histamine H_2-receptor antagonist, has gained widespread use in the treatment of duodenal ulcers, peptic esophagitis, upper gastrointestinal hemorrhage, and Zollinger-Ellison syndrome.[49,50] Experience with millions of patients has demonstrated that cimetidine is both a highly efficacious and apparently safe drug.[49,51]

Independent of its H_2-receptor antagonistic properties, cimetidine is a mild antiandrogen capable of displacing testosterone and dihydrotestosterone from cytosolic androgen receptors in target tissues, thereby blocking nuclear uptake of the androgen and preventing androgen-directed transcription.[52,53] Indeed, results of toxicologic studies had predicted the antiandrogenic action of cimetidine. Animal studies have shown that daily administration of cimetidine can cause atrophy of the seminiferous tubules as well as the secondary sexual organs and a higher than normal incidence of benign Leydig-cell tumors.[54,55] In agreement with the animal findings, several cases of sexual dysfunction, including impotence,[56,57] gynecomastia,[49,58,59] and galactorrhea,[60] in addition to abnormal secretions of gonadal and pituitary sex hormones,[56,61,62] have been reported in patients treated with cimetidine.

Since cimetidine freely crosses the placenta and is excreted into breast milk,[63,64] its use during pregnancy and lactation raises important concerns regarding the drug's teratogenic potential. Not unexpectedly, pregnant women with peptic acid diseases are often treated with H_2 antagonists, especially cimetidine.[49,65] However, a much larger number of pregnant women frequently experience the gastrointestinal disturbance commonly referred to as "morning sickness" that is palliatively treated with antacids or H_2-receptor antagonists.[65,66] In this regard, since cimetidine is an antiandrogen, its use during pregnancy might result in a teratogenic risk to the male fetus, whose reproductive structures and subsequent sexual function are masculinized by the organizing actions of perinatally secreted testosterone and its metabolites.[42,67] This developmental problem has been studied in animals, but the findings have been contradictory. In one case, it was reported that maternally administered cimetidine produced a profound demasculinization of the dam's male offspring that clearly persisted into adulthood.[68,69] In contradictory studies, it was reported that peripartum exposure to cimetidine caused no deleterious effects on masculine differentiation at either a morphologic, steroidogenic, or behavioral level.[54,70,71] Surprisingly, to my knowledge, not a single followup study or survey has been conducted on the sons of cimetidine-treated mothers.

ANTICONVULSANTS

Other than the anticonvulsants, there are few classes of drugs whose delayed teratogenic potential are so great as to warrant investigation. Approximately 1 out of every 200 women is epileptic,[72] and 95.7 percent of them are on anticonvulsant therapy[73] that is invariably continued throughout pregnancy and lactation.[74,75] In this regard, the evidence indicates that anticonvulsant drugs are responsible for producing a two to three times greater incidence of malformations in the children of epileptic mothers.[76,77] With the exception of the fetal alcohol syndrome, anticonvulsant-induced malformations, specifically the fetal hydantoin syndrome, represent the most commonly recognized teratogen-induced malformations.[78]

Phenytoin (diphenylhydantoin) is probably the most efficacious and widely used anticonvulsant in North America.[79] Considering that phenytoin easily passes through the placenta into the fetal tissues and through the mammary epithelium into the milk,[75,80] there has been a justifiable concern that the drug could be teratogenic. In this regard, animal studies have demonstrated clearly that prepartum administration of phenytoin can produce congenital malformations.[1,3,76,79] Studies in humans[73,74,77,78] have indicated that *in utero* exposure to phenytoin may be responsible for inducing such anatomic malformations as cleft lip and palate, microcephaly or trigonocephaly, and various anomalies of the face and fingers, often referred to as the *fetal hydantoin syndrome*. In addition, there is evidence to suggest that peripartum exposure to phenytoin can produce more subtle long-term biochemical and behavioral defects at doses too low to induce structural malformations.[81,82] It has been reported that in the absence of anatomic malformations, adult rats exposed perinatally to maternally administered phenytoin have several behavioral and neurologic deficits resulting in delayed motor development, persistent locomotor dysfunction, and abnormal maze learning,[81,83] as well as reduced fertility.[13,84] Our findings of normal developmental profiles of serum androstenedione, testosterone, and dihydrotestosterone in phenytoin-exposed male offspring[85] suggest that the delayed reproductive dysfunc-

tions found by others[13,84] are like the behavioral defects,[81,83] a result of phenytoin's teratogenic action on the developing brain.

Unrelated to its anticonvulsant properties, phenytoin is also an inducer of the hepatic mono-oxygenase enzymes that normally metabolize fatty acids, prostaglandins, steroids, and xenobiotics.[86,87] In fact, we have reported that maternal treatment with therapeutic-like doses for the rat of phenytoin induces significant elevations in the Michaelis constants and maximal velocities of hepatic aminopyrine-N-demethylase in the dam's 8-day-old offspring.[88] Similarly, administration of the anticonvulsant to pregnant women has been shown to increase aminopyrine metabolism in their newborn.[89] The long-term effects of early exposure to phenytoin on liver function also have been investigated in animal models. Maternal administration of the anticonvulsant at therapeutic-like doses that do not produce morphologic anomalies was found to cause permanent defects in the drug-metabolizing capacity of the exposed adult offspring.[82] Perhaps of greater significance is the finding that peripartum exposure to subtherapeutic-like doses for the rat of phenytoin produced, in adulthood, so-called "silent" defects in the hepatic mono-oxygenase system. That is, adult rats exposed perinatally to these low doses of phenytoin exhibited very few abnormalities in the basal levels of hepatic drug-metabolizing enzymes. However, when the hepatic mono-oxygenases of these adults were challenged with various threshold doses of phenobarbital, the silent defect became apparent; peripartum exposure to phenytoin resulted in a significant block in the response of the hepatic mono-oxygenases to phenobarbital induction.

In this regard, organisms are constantly exposed to subtle levels of environmental inducing agents (i.e, drugs, carcinogens, food additives, hormones, insecticides, industrial pollutants, etc.) that may be capable of altering the activities of the hepatic drug-metabolizing enzymes. Thus, by disrupting the development of hepatic enzyme induction mechanisms, perinatal exposure to phenytoin may irreversibly alter an important homeostatic mechanism that is normally responsive to daily exposure to low levels of various endogenous and exogenous inducing agents.

Unlike phenytoin, an exclusive anticonvulsant, barbiturates are used in the treatment of at least 77 different disorders and are compounded in about 190 medications.[90] Of particular concern to pediatricians is the fact that tranquilizers and sedatives, such as phenobarbital, represent the major class of drugs prescribed to pregnant women.[91] In a comprehensive review, Reinisch and Sanders[90] state that "based upon epidemiologic data, it is estimated that 25 percent of births in the decades of the 1950s and 1960s were treated with barbiturates. In the 1970s, notwithstanding the widespread use of the benzodiazepines as the minor tranquilizers of choice, we estimate conservatively that a minimum of 10 percent of pregnancies were so treated. Since 105,274,961 live births occurred in the United States between 1950 and 1977, it seems reasonable to project that 22,346,543 offspring were born of barbiturate-treated pregnancies. These numbers only represent an estimate of mothers treated medically with these compounds and do not reflect children of mothers who ingested these drugs for nonmedical reasons.''

Studies using animal models have shown that perinatal exposure to phenobarbital can result in a whole compliment of neural dysfunctions that include subnormal sexual behavior,[92] reduced seizure susceptibility,[93] and locomotor and learning deficits[94,95] associated with CNS damage.[95] In addition, direct administration of phenobarbital to newborns causes a permanent elevation of several drug-metabolizing enzymes,[97,98] resulting in an unresponsiveness to normally therapeutic levels of drugs. Of further clinical significance is the finding that adult offspring of phenobarbital-treated nursing rats have increased aflatox B_1-adduct formation and binding to DNA that could result in an increased risk of cancer.[99]

We have found that prenatal exposure to phenobarbital can produce latently expressed reproductive dysfunctions in male and female rats. In female offspring, the barbiturate caused a delay in the onset of puberty, irregular estrous cycles, and dramatically reduced fertility. Associated with these biologic changes were alterations in serum levels of luteinizing hormone, estradiol, and progesterone, as well as estrogen receptors.[100] In male offspring, *in utero* exposure to phenobarbital caused delayed testicular descent followed by a decreased production and secretion of testosterone and gonadotropins throughout adult life and an associated infertility.[101] The mechanism underlying this delayed teratogenic expression was investigated in the perinates at the time of phenobarbital exposure.[102] We found that the anticonvulsant inhibited testicular secretion of testosterone, resulting in subnormal levels of plasma and brain testosterone at the critical developmental period for brain masculinization (Figure 12–2). It seems reasonable to conclude that the reproductive dysfunctions expressed in the adult were a result of teratogenic interference in the normal sexual differentiation of the perinatal brain.

In the case of humans, phenobarbital has long been considered a teratogen responsible for inducing a number of reproductive and somatic congenital malformations in the offspring of epileptic mothers.[90,103,104] A connection between early exposure to barbiturates and childhood cancer has been suspected. Cancer is the second leading cause of death in the child under 14 years of age, and brain tumors are one of the most frequently occurring cancers in children.[105] Epidemiologic studies have estimated that as many as 8 percent of brain tumors in children may be attributable to the use of barbiturates either by the child or prenatally by the mother.[102] (These findings are quite similar to a more recent report linking the incidence of brain tumors in children to maternal or paternal occupations involving chemical exposure.[107])

Considering that laboratory animals treated perinatally with phenobarbital express behavioral, learning, sexual, hepatic, and reproductive defects in adulthood, and noting the widespread use of the drug during pregnancy and its ability to induce congenital malformations in humans, it seems incredible that not a single long-term followup study has been conducted on an exposed human population.[90]

FOOD ADDITIVES

We have hypothesized that like certain drugs, some food additives, considered to be safe, might similarly be capable of inducing latent defects. (Invariably, *teratogen safe* means "does not produce malformations.") No trivial comparison to the growing use of drugs is our enormous consumption of food additives. We need only go up and down the aisles of our modern supermarkets and examine the exciting carts to appreciate our basic reliance on packaged and processed foods, a reliance that is steadily increasing as more homemakers enter the workplace.

Like preservatives, some form of flavor-enhancing chemical can be found in almost all commercially prepared foods.[108] The ability of neonatally administered aspartate and glutamate, individually or in combination, to induce a developmental syndrome in animals charac-

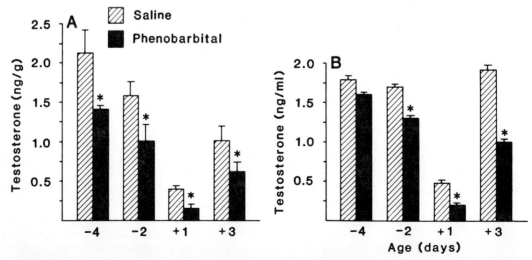

FIGURE 12–2. Testosterone levels in the brains (*A*) and plasma (*B*) of perinates exposed to maternally administered phenobarbital. (From Gupta C, Yaffe SJ, Shapiro BH: Prenatal exposure to phenobarbital permanently decreases testosterone and causes reproductive dysfunction. Science 216:640–642, 1982; copyright 1982 by the AAAS.)

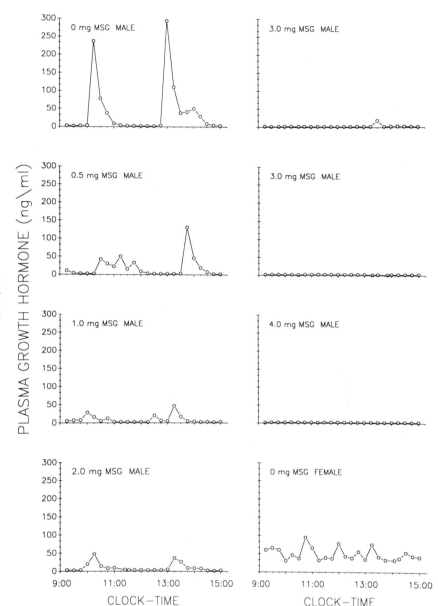

FIGURE 12–3. Plasma levels of circulating growth hormone obtained from individual adult rats neonatally treated with diluent or various doses of MSG.

terized by hypothalamic lesions resulting in growth retardation and obesity has been well recognized for many years.[108,109] Although its teratogenic potential resulted in its voluntary removal from baby food in 1969, it was a belated action for millions of adults who had already consumed MSG (monosodium glutamate) in childhood. Americans continue to consume at least 50 million pounds of it a year[110] which makes it highly likely that human perinates are still being exposed to MSG. The fact that MSG is added to a food is sometimes reported on the label, but the amounts used are never disclosed. Nevertheless, independent analyses have shown that such common store-bought foods as soups contain around 1.1 g MSG/6 oz serving.[111] Indeed, restaurant-served won ton soup may contain 5 g of the additive per cup.[108,109] In the extreme, a recent survey reported that large subgroups in the Korean population consume an average of 4 g MSG per day, with some people eating an incredible 120 g MSG per day. Moreover, Korean restaurants were found to add almost 10 g MSG to a single dish.[112]

Neonatal administration of MSG to rats and mice, as well as rabbits, chickens, guinea pigs, hamsters, cats, and monkeys, produces a well-defined syndrome characterized by neuroendocrine deficiencies causing stunted body growth, obesity, and reduced pituitary size.[108,109] Whereas serum levels of ACTH, prolactin, TSH, FSH, and LH[113,114] are usually normal, or perhaps only slightly depressed, serum concentrations of growth hormone are profoundly reduced in MSG-treated rats.[113,115] Coincidentally, the ultradian rhythms in circulating growth hormone (Figure 12–3) regulate the sexually dimorphic expression of hepatic monooxygenases.[115] In male rats growth hormone, under androgen regulation, is secreted in episodic bursts every 3–4 hours. Between the peaks, growth hormone levels are extremely low or undetectable. In females, peaks are of lower magnitude than in males and occur irregularly, whereas the troughs between the peaks are considerably elevated compared to those in males.[116,117] Exposure to the more tonic feminine secretory pattern of growth hormone produces the lower level of hepatic drug metabolism found in female rats. Conversely, the ultradian rhythm in growth hormone secretion characterized as masculine allows for the occurrence of a 3- to 5-fold higher level of hepatic drug metabolism.[116-118]

Neonatal male rats were treated with MSG at either 0.5, 1.0, 2.0, 3.0, or 4.0 mg/g body weight.[115,117] As adults, rats were catheterized[119] to obtain unstressed, serial blood samples for the determination of ultradian patterns of circulating growth hormone. Although the lower doses had little or no detrimental effects on growth or development, the results demonstrated a dose-dependent, graded biochemical response to all MSG levels. As the administered dose of MSG increased from 0.5 to 4.0 mg, there was a concurrent decline in the amplitudes of the characteristically masculine, episodic bursts of growth hormone, until at the highest 4-mg dose and occasional 3-mg dose, the pulses were no longer detectable (Figure 12–3). Associated with this dose-dependent alteration in the ultradian pattern of growth hormone secretion was a measurable change in the activities of the hepatic drug metabolizing enzymes and their constituent, sex-dependent isoforms of cytochrome P450. As the pulse heights of the hormone declined to 10 to 20 percent of their normal amplitudes (1 mg and 2 mg MSG doses) the levels of drug metabolizing enzymes were maintained, and in many cases, exceeded the levels normally found in males. However, with the loss of all detectable levels of circulating growth hormone (4 mg MSG), hepatic drug metabolizing capacity was reduced to 35 percent of normal.

We have suggested[82] that the sex of the animal may influence the severity of the teratogenic effects. Our findings with MSG clearly support this idea. Similar to what we found with males, neonatal administration of 0.5 to 4.0 mg/g of MSG produced a dose-dependent and graded reduction in the concentration of circulating growth hormone characteristic of the female profile.[116] At the highest dose, circulating growth hormone was undetectable. In contrast to the males, none of the doses of MSG had any effect on the activities of the drug metabolizing enzymes as well as six specific forms of P450.

Our studies with rats and mice have shown dose-dependent teratogenic effects of glutamate as well as aspartate[118] at possible human dietary levels. Either amino acid could produce more subtle developmental defects in growth hormone secretion and drug metabolism than the full-blown obesity and growth retardation normally associated with the syndrome. We are concerned that early exposure to low levels of MSG, as well as certain drugs, from before birth until 5 years of age when hepatic and neuroendocrine differentiation are still incomplete, could permanently alter growth hormone secretion and the expression of hepatic drug metabolizing enzymes. Such defects could unknowingly affect normal maturation and the efficacy of drug therapy or the susceptibility to chemically-induced cancers in adulthood.

CONCLUSIONS

The purpose of this chapter is to introduce the reader to a little known but potentially very serious health hazard to children. I refer to the ability of perinatally consumed drugs and food additives to produce subtle biochemical or microstructural defects, undetectable in the newborn, but expressed years or perhaps decades after exposure. Human studies indicate that a higher than normal incidence of mental retardation and childhood and adult cancers can be attributed to *in utero* exposure to alcohol, narcotics, diethylstilbestrol, phenobarbital, and various industrial chemicals. Similarly, compelling evidence from animal models shows that peripartum exposure to such drugs as diazepam, phenytoin, morphine, cimetidine, phenobarbital, sex steroids, etc. can produce latently expressed abnormalities and diseases in the adult offspring.

The question is not whether *in utero* exposure to drugs can produce latently expressed defects, but how serious is the problem? Unfortunately, pregnant and nursing women take lots of drugs. But how do we establish a cause-and-effect relationship between the onset of an isolated disease and exposure to a teratogen that occurred decades earlier? In truth, this clinical problem is complicated by more than a temporal factor. Latently expressed teratogenic defects are not necessarily associated with congenital malformations or recognized syndromes, making it unlikely for the physician to suspect that the adult disease is in actuality a birth defect. The offending drug may have been considered innocuous when taken and was ingested for only a brief period, albeit a developmentally critical one, so that the consumption is forgotten. Since the actual clinical manifestation expressed in adulthood is merely a consequence of the perinatally induced defect, it becomes more difficult to identify the true developmental lesion(s). Extrapolating from animal models, *in utero* exposure to phenytoin would result in a latently expressed depression in the activities of hepatic drug-metabolizing enzymes. However, the clinical manifestation of this birth defect would be toxicity to generally accepted therapeutic doses of drugs. In contrast, *in utero* exposure to phenobarbital would cause a permanent elevation in the activities of drug-metabolizing enzymes. Not only would the affected individual be refractory to normal drug therapy, but there would be an enhanced conversion of inactive environmental pollutants (e.g., benzopyrene) to carcinogens, resulting in an increased incidence of cancers. Lastly, similar drugs, or for that matter, the same drug, could produce different teratogenic defects if consumed during different periods of gestation. A drug taken early in pregnancy might produce a structural anomaly. After the period of organogenesis, the drug might cause a metabolic defect in the liver. Even later exposure to the same drug might coincide with the critical period for brain differentiation, causing behavioral abnormalities in adulthood. Somewhat tongue-in-cheek, it is possible that some delayed teratogenic defects might never be expressed: the Eskimo with a congenital defect in the homeostatic response to heat stroke or the religious celibate with a teratogen-induced reproductive dysfunction.

Thus the biomedical community, and the pediatrician in particular, must be prepared to face a new kind of health problem. These challenges are not without precedent. With the eradication of infectious diseases, we have had to develop new approaches to combat the increasing threat of nontransmissible diseases. Similarly, we cannot ignore the reality of diseases resulting from the delayed expression of birth defects. We shall find that this type of disease is not unique and is similar in consequence to those subtle genetic defects which predispose the carrier to cancer, heart disease, arthritis, etc. Indeed, these may be the unrecognized health problems of the future.

For the present, a little old-fashioned 1960s consciousness raising would be appropriate. In addition, we should continue to develop animal models as sentinels to warn us of the potential teratogenic dangers of drugs and environmental toxins. Perhaps the threat will become so real that we are moved to shelter our unborn from teratogenic dangers and can eliminate an entire class of disease before we write the textbooks.

REFERENCES

1. Hill RM, Stern L: Drugs in pregnancy: Effects on the fetus and newborn. Drugs 17:182–197, 1979
2. Goldman AS: Drugs and pregnancy, in Yaffe SJ (ed): Pediatric Pharmacology Therapeutic Principles. Orlando, Fla, Grune & Stratton, 1980, pp 101–118
3. Tuchmann-Duplessis H: Drugs and other xenobiotics as teratogens. Pharmacol Ther 26:273–344, 1984
4. Russo NF: Women in the American Psychological Association. Washington, DC, American Psychological Association, 1984
5. Doyle C: Dangers of tranquillity. The Observer (London), Feb 24, 1980, p 45
6. Tallman JF, Paul SM, Skolnick P, Gallager DW: Receptors for the age of anxiety: Pharmacology of the benzodiazepines. Science 207:274–281, 1980
7. Yellow light for tranquilizers. Time, July 21, 1980, p 53
8. Valium by another name. Time, March 11, 1985, p 53
9. Women and Drugs (Research Series 31), National Institute on Drug Abuse. Washington, DC, U.S. Department of Health and Human Services, 1983
10. Bleyer WA, An WY, Sange WA, Raisz LG: Studies on the detection of adverse drug reactions in the newborn. JAMA 213:2046–2048, 1970
11. Hill RM: Drug ingested by the pregnant woman. Clin Pharmacol Ther 14:654–659, 1973
12. Doering PL, Stewart RB: The extent and character of drug consumption during pregnancy. JAMA 239:843–846, 1978
13. Sonawane BR, Yaffe SJ: Delayed effects of drug exposure during pregnancy: Reproductive function. Biol Res Pregnancy 2:48–55, 1983
14. Facts: White Plains, NY, National Foundation–March of Dimes, 1979.
15. Birth defects doubled since '50s, study finds. The Philadelphia Inquirer (Suburban North Edition), July 19, 1983, p 1A
16. Shapiro BH, Goldman AS: New thoughts on sexual differentiation of the brain, in Vallet HL, Porter IH (eds): Genetic Mechanisms of Sexual Development. New York, Academic Press, 1979, pp 221–246
17. Auroux M, Dehaupas M: Influence de la nutrition de la mère sur le développement tardif du systeme nerveux central de la progeniture. I. Amelioration, chez le rat de la capacité d'apprentissage de la progeniture par alcoolisation de la mere. CR Soc Biol 164:1432–1436, 1970
18. Randall L: Teratogenic effects of in utero ethanol exposure, in Blum K (ed): Alcohol and Opiates: Neurochemical and Behavioral Mechanisms. New York, Academic Press, 1977, pp 91–107
19. Stockard CR, Papanicolaou GN: Further studies on the modification of the germ cells in mammals: The effect of alcohol on treated guinea pigs and their descendants. J Exp Zool 26:119–226, 1918
20. Davis WM, Lin CH: Prenatal morphine effects on survival and behavior of rat offspring. Res Commun Chem Pathol Pharmacol 3:205–214, 1972
21. O'Callaghan JP, Holtzman SG: Prenatal administration of morphine to the rat: Tolerance to the analgesic effect of morphine in the offspring. J Pharmacol Exp Ther 197:533–544, 1976
22. Zimmerman E, Sonderegger T, Bromley B: Development and adult pituitary–adrenal function in female rats injected with morphine during different postnatal periods. Life Sci 20:639–646, 1977
23. Hitzemann RA, Hitzemann RJ, Brase DA, Loh HH: Influence of prenatal D-amphetamine administration on development and behavior of rats. Life Sci 18:605–612, 1976
24. Herbst AL, Scully RE, Robboy SJ: Prenatal diethylstilbestrol exposure and human genital tract abnormalities. Natl Cancer Inst Monogr 51:25–35, 1979
25. Henderson BE, Benton B, Cosgrove M, et al: Urogenital tract abnormalities in sons of women treated with diethylstilbestrol. Pediatrics 58:505–507, 1976
26. Bern HA, Jones LA, Mori T, Young PN: Exposure of neonatal mice to steroids: Long-term effects on the mammary gland and other reproductive structures. J Steroid Biochem 6:673–676, 1976
27. O'Brien PC, Noller KL, Robboy SJ, et al: Vaginal epithelial changes in young women enrolled in the National Cooperative Diethylstilbestrol Adenosis (DESAD) Project. Obstet Gynecol 53:300–308, 1979
28. Kaufman RH, Noller K, Adam E, et al: Upper genital tract abnormalities and pregnancy outcome in diethylstilbestrol-exposed progeny. Am J Obstet Gynecol 148:973–984, 1984
29. Peress MR, Tsai CC, Mathur RS, Williamson HO: Hirsutism and menstrual patterns in women exposed to diethylstilbestrol in utero. Am J Obstet Gynecol 144:135–140, 1982
30. Meyer-Bahlburg HFL, Ehrhardt AA: A prenatal hormone hypothesis for depression in adults with a history of fetal DES exposure, in Halbreich U (ed): Hormones and Depression. New York, Raven Press, 1987, pp 325–338
31. DES Task Force Summary Report. Washington, DC, DHEW Publication No. (NIH) 1679–1688, 1978
32. Szent-Györgyi A: Some reminiscences of my life as a scientist. Int J Quantum Chem, 3:7–12, 1976
33. Warkang J: Congenital Malformations: Notes and Comments. Chicago, Year Book Medical Publishers, 1971
34. Tuchmann-Duplessis H: Dangers de l'irradiation Prenatale, in Traité de Radiodiagnostic. Paris, Masson, 1980, pp 439–445
35. Williams RT: Species variations in drug biotransformations, in LaDu BN, Mandel HG, Way EL (eds): Fundamentals of Drug Metabolism and Drug Disposition. Baltimore, Williams & Wilkins, 1972, pp 187–205
36. Moore KL: The Developing Human: Clinically Oriented Embryology. Philadelphia, WB Saunders, 1973
37. Ganong WR: Review of Medical Physiology. Los Altos, Calif, Lange Medical Publications, 1967, p 489
38. Pfeiffer CA: Sexual differences of the hypophyses and their determination by the gonads. Am J Anat 58:195–225, 1936
39. Whallen RE, Edwards DA: Hormonal determinants of the development of masculine and feminine behavior in male and female rats. Anat Rec 157:173–180, 1967
40. Shapiro BH, Goldman AS: Feminine saccharin preference in the genetically androgen-insensitive male rat pseudohermaphrodite. Horm Behav 4:371–375, 1973
41. Goldman AS, Shapiro BH, Root AW: Inhibition of fetal masculine differentiation in the rat by maternal administration of antibodies to bovine LH, cyanoketone, or antibodies to testosterone 3-bovine serum albumin. Proc Soc Exp Biol Med 143:422–426, 1973
42. Goldman AS, Shapiro BH, Neumann F: Role of testosterone and its metabolites in the differentiation of the mammary gland in rats. Endocrinology 99:1490–1495, 1976
43. Wilson JD: Testosterone uptake by the urogenital tract of the rabbit embryo. Endocrinology 92:1192–1199, 1973
44. Shapiro BH, Levine DC, Adler NT: The testicular feminized rat: A naturally occurring model of androgen-independent brain masculinization. Science 209:418–420, 1980
45. MacLusky NJ, Naftolin F: Sexual differentiation of the central nervous system. Science 211:1294–1303, 1981

46. Ehrhardt AA, Meyer-Bahlburg HFL: Effects of prenatal sex hormones on gender-related behavior. Science 211:1312–1318, 1981

47. Money J, Schwartz M, Lewis AG: Adult erotosexual status and fetal hormonal masculinization and demasculinization: 46,XX congenital virilizing adrenal hyperplasia and 46,XY androgen-insensitivity syndrome compared. Psychoneuroendocrinology 9:405–414, 1984

48. Money J, Ehrhardt AA, Masica DN: Fetal feminization induced by androgen insensitivity in the testicular feminizing syndrome: Effect on marriage and maternalism. Johns Hopkins Med J 123:105–114, 1968

49. Sharpe PC, Hawkins BW: Efficacy and safety of cimetidine: Long-term treatment with cimetidine, in Burland WL, Simpkins MA (eds): Cimetidine: Proceedings of The Second International Symposium on Histamine H$_2$-Receptor Antagonists. Amsterdam, Excerpta Medica, 1977, pp 358–366

50. Winship DH: Cimetidine in the treatment of duodenal ulcers. Gastroenterology 74:402–406, 1978

51. Freston JW: Cimetidine I: Development pharmacology and efficacy. Ann Intern Med 97:573–580, 1982

52. Funder JW, Mercer JE: Cimetidine, a histamine H$_2$-receptor antagonist, occupies androgen receptors. J Clin Endocrinol Metab 48:189–191, 1979

53. Sivelle PC, Underwood AH, Jelly JA: The effect of histamine H$_2$-receptor antagonists on androgen action in vivo and dihydrotestosterone binding in the rat prostate androgen receptor in vitro. Biochem Pharmacol 31:677–684, 1982

54. Leslie GB, Walker TF: A toxicological profile of cimetidine, in Burland WL, Simkins MA (eds): Cimetidine: Proceedings of the Second International Symposium on Histamine H$_2$-Receptor Antagonists. Amsterdam, Excerpta Medica, 1977, pp 24–33

55. Leslie GB, Nokes DN, Pollitt FD, et al: A two-year study with cimetidine in the rat: Assessment for chronic toxicity and carcinogenicity. Toxicol Appl Pharmacol 61:119–137, 1981

56. Peden NR, Cargill JM, Browning MCK, et al: Male sexual dysfunction during treatment with cimetidine. Br Med J 1:659, 1979

57. Wolfe MM: Impotence on cimetidine treatment. N Engl J Med 300:94–98, 1979

58. Hall WH: Breast changes in males on cimetidine. N Engl J Med 295:841, 1976

59. Spence RW, Celestin LR: Gynaecomastia associated with cimetidine. Gut 20:154–157, 1979

60. Bateson MC, Browning MCK, Maconnachie A: Galactorrhea with cimetidine. Lancet 2:247–248, 1977

61. Van Thiel DH, Gavaler JS, Smith WI, Paul G: Hypothalamic-pituitary–gonadal dysfunction in men using cimetidine. N Engl J Med 300:1012–1025, 1979

62. Wang C, Lai CL, Lam KC, Yeung KK: Effect of cimetidine on gonadal function in man. Br J Clin Pharmacol 13:791–794, 1982

63. Somogyi A, Gugler R: Cimetidine excretion into breast milk. Br J Clin Pharmacol 7:627–629, 1979

64. Howe JP, McGowan WA, Moore J, et al: The placental transfer of cimetidine. Anaesthesia 36:371–375, 1981

65. Dobbins JW, Spiro HM: Gastrointestinal complications, in Burrow GN, Ferris TF (eds): Medical Complications During Pregnancy. Philadelphia, WB Saunders, 1982, pp 259–263

66. Van Thiel DH, Gavaler JS, Joshi SH, et al: Heartburn of pregnancy. Gastroenterology 72:666–668, 1977

67. Shapiro BH: A paradox in development: Masculinization of the brain without androgen receptors, in Lash JW, Saxen L (eds): Developmental Mechanisms: Normal and Abnormal. New York, Alan R. Liss, 1985, pp 151–173

68. Anand S, Van Thiel DH: Prenatal and neonatal exposure to cimetidine results in gonadal and sexual dysfunction in adult males. Science 218:493–494, 1982

69. Parker S, Udani M, Gavaler JS, Van Thiel DH: Pre- and neonatal exposure to cimetidine but not ranitidine adversely affects adult sexual functioning of male rats. Neurobehav Toxicol Teratol 6:313–318, 1984

70. Walker TF, Bott JH, Bond BC: Cimetidine does not demasculin-ize male rat offspring exposed in utero. Fund Appl Toxicol 8:188–197, 1987

71. Shapiro BH, Hirst SA, Babalola GO, Bitar MS: Prospective study on the sexual development of male and female rats exposed, perinatally, to maternally administered cimetidine. Toxicol Lett 44:315–329, 1988

72. Kalter H, Warkany J: Congenital malformations: Etiologic factors and their role in prevention. N Engl J Med 308:491–497, 1983

73. Kelly TE, Edwards P, Rein M, et al: Teratogenicity of anticonvulsant drugs. II. A prospective study. Am J Med Genet 19:435–443, 1984

74. Janz D: Antiepileptic drugs and pregnancy: Altered utilization patterns and teratogenesis. Epilepsia 23(suppl 1):553–563, 1982

75. Nau H, Kuhnz W, Egger H-J, et al: Anticonvulsants during pregnancy and lactation: Transplacental, maternal, and neonatal pharmacokinetics. Clin Pharmacokinet 7:508–543, 1982

76. Bossi L: Fetal effects of anticonvulsants, in Morselli PL, Pippenger CE, Penry JK (eds): Antiepileptic Drug Therapy in Pediatrics. New York, Raven Press 1983, pp 37–63

77. Kelly T: Teratogenicity of anticonvulsant drugs. I. Review of the literature. Am J Med Genet 19:413–434, 1984

78. Smith DW: Hydantoin effects on the fetus, in Hassel TM (ed): Phenytoin-Induced Teratology and Gingival Pathology. New York, Raven Press, 1980, pp 35–40

79. Wells PG: Physiological and environmental determinants of phenytoin teratogenicity: Relation to glutathione homeostasis, and potentiation by acetaminophen, in MacLeod SM, Okey AB, Speilberg SP (eds): Developmental Pharmacology. New York, Raven Press, 1983, pp 367–371

80. Gabler WL, Falace D: The distribution and metabolism of Dilantin in nonpregnant, pregnant and fetal rats. Arch Int Pharmacodyn Ther 184:45–58, 1970

81. Vorhees CV: Developmental effects of anticonvulsants. Neurotoxicology 7:235–244, 1986

82. Shapiro BH, Lech GM, Bardales RM: Persistent defects in the hepatic mono-oxygenase system of adult rats, exposed perinatally, to maternally administered phenytoin. J Pharmacol Exp Ther 238:68–75, 1986

83. Vorhees CV: Fetal anticonvulsant syndrome in rats: Effects on postnatal behavior and brain amino acid content. Neurobehav Toxicol Teratol 7:471–482, 1985

84. Takagi S, Alleva FR, Seth PK, Balázs T: Delayed development of reproductive functions and alteration of dopamine receptor binding in hypothalamus of rats exposed prenatally to phenytoin and phenobarbital. Toxicol Lett 34:107–113, 1986

85. Shapiro BH, Babalola GO: Developmental profile of serum androgens and estrous cyclicity of male and female rats exposed perinatally to maternally administered phenytoin. Toxicol Lett 36:165–175, 1987

86. Eling, TE, Harbison RD, Becker BA, Fouts JR: Diphenylhydantoin effect on neonatal and adult rat hepatic drug metabolism. J Pharmacol Exp Ther 171:127–134, 1970

87. Heinicke RJ, Stohs SJ, Al-Turk W, Lemon HM: Chronic phenytoin administration and the hepatic mixed function oxidase system in female rats. Gen Pharmacol 15:85–89, 1984

88. Shapiro BH, Bardales RM, Lech GM: Perinatal induction of hepatic aminopyrine-N-demethylase by maternal exposure to phenytoin. Pediatr Pharmacol 5:201–207, 1985

89. Rating D, Jäger-Roman E, Nau H, et al: Enzyme induction in neonates after fetal exposure to antiepileptic drugs. Pediatr Pharmacol 3:209–218, 1983

90. Reinisch JM, Sanders SA: Early barbiturate exposure: The brain, sexually dimorphic behavior and learning. Neurosci Biobehav Rev 6:311–319, 1982

91. Forfar JO, Nelson MM: Epidemiology of drugs taken by pregnant woman: Drugs in the intrauterine patient. Clin Pharmacol Ther 14:632–642, 1973

92. Clemens LG, Popham TV, Ruppert PH: Neonatal treatment of hamsters with barbiturate alters adult sexual behavior. Dev Psychobiol 12:49–59, 1979

93. Sobrian SK, Nandedkar AKN: Prenatal antiepileptic drug expo-

sure alters seizure susceptibility in rats. Pharmacol Biochem Behav 24:1383–1391, 1986

94. Middaugh LD, Santos CA III, Zemp JW: Effects of phenobarbital given to pregnant mice on behavior of mature offspring. Dev Psychobiol 8:305–313, 1975

95. Middaugh LD, Thomas TN, Simpson LW, Zemp JW: Effects of prenatal maternal injections of phenobarbital on brain neurotransmitters and behavior of young C57 mice. Neurobehav Toxicol Teratol 3:271–275, 1981

96. Yanai J, Bergman A: Neuronal deficits after neonatal exposure to phenobarbital. Exp Neurol 73:199–208, 1981

97. Yanai J: Long-term induction of microsomal drug oxidizing system in mice following prenatal exposure to barbiturate. Biochem Pharmacol 28:1429–1430, 1979

98. Bagley DM, Hayes JR: Xenobiotic imprinting of the hepatic mono-oxygenase system: Effects of neonatal phenobarbital administration. Biochem Pharmacol 34:1007–1014, 1985

99. Faris RA, Campbell TC: Exposure of newborn rats to pharmacologically active compounds may permanently alter carcinogen metabolism. Science 211:719–721, 1981

100. Gupta C, Sonawane BR, Yaffe SJ, Shapiro BH: Phenobarbital exposure in utero: Alteration in female reproductive function in rats. Science 208:508–510, 1980

101. Gupta C, Shapiro BH, Yaffe SJ: Reproductive dysfunction in male rats following prenatal exposure to phenobarbital. Pediatr Pharmacol 1:55–62, 1980

102. Gupta C, Yaffe SJ, Shapiro BH: Prenatal exposure to phenobarbital permanently decreases testosterone and causes reproductive dysfunction. Science 216:640–642, 1982

103. Nelson MM, Forfar JO: Associations between drugs administered during pregnancy and congenital abnormalities of the fetus. Br Med J 1:523–527, 1971

104. Speidel BD, Meadow SR: Maternal epilepsy and abnormalities of the fetus and newborn. Lancet 2:839–843, 1972

105. Cutler SJ, Young JL Jr: Third National Cancer Survey: Incidence data. Natl Cancer Inst Mongr 41:102–103, 1975

106. Gold E, Gordis L, Tonascia J, Szklo M: Increased risk of brain tumors in children exposed to barbiturates. J Natl Cancer Inst 61:1031–1034, 1978

107. Peters JM, Preston-Martin S, Yu MC: Brain tumors in children and occupational exposure of parents. Science 213:235–237, 1981

108. Olney JW: Excitatory neurotoxins as food additives: An evaluation of risk. Neurotoxicology 2:163–192, 1981

109. Olney JW: Excitotoxic food additives: Functional teratological aspects. Progr Brain Res 73:283–294, 1988

110. Brody J: Jane Brody's Nutrition Book. New York, W. W. Norton, 1981, pp 476–477

111. Consumer Reports, Dried Soup Mixes (This is Soup?), November 1978, pp 615–619

112. Citizen's Alliance for Consumer Protection in Korea, A study of the use of MSG in Korea, UNICEF, 1986, pp 1–9

113. Terry LC, Epelbaum J, Martin B: Monosodium glutamate: Acute and chronic effects on rhythmic growth hormone and prolactin secretion, and somatostatin in the undisturbed male rats. Brain Res 217:129–142, 1981

114. Dada MO, Blake CA: Monosodium L-glutamate administration: Effects on gonadotrophin secretion, gonadatrophs and mamotrophs in prepubertal female rats. J Endocr 104:185–192, 1985

115. Shapiro BH, MacLeod JN, Pampori NA, Morrissey JJ, Lapenson FP, Waxman DL: Signalling elements in the ultradian rhythm of circulating growth hormone regulating expression of sex-dependent forms of hepatic cytochrome P450. Endocrinology 125:2935–2944, 1989

116. Waxman DJ, Morrissey JJ, MacLeod JN, Shapiro BH: Depletion of serum growth hormone in adult female rats by neonatal monosodium glutamate treatment without loss of female-specific hepatic enzymes P450 2d(IIC12) and steroid 5α-reductase. Endocrinology 126:712–720, 1990

117. Pampori NA, Agrawal AK, Waxman DJ, Shapiro BH: Differential effects of neonatally administered glutamate on the ultradian pattern of circulating growth hormone regulating expression of sex-dependent forms of cytochrome P450. Biochem Pharmacol 41:1299–1309, 1991

118. Agrawal AK, Pampori NA, Shapiro BH: Sex- and dose-dependent effects of neonatally administered aspartate on the ultradian patterns of circulating growth hormone regulating hexobarbital metabolism and action. Toxicol Appl Pharmacol 108:96–106, 1991

119. MacLeod JN, Shapiro BH: Repetitive blood sampling in unrestrained and unstressed mice using a chronic indwelling right atrial catheterization apparatus. Lab Anim Sci 38:603–608, 1988

TERATOLOGY:
Biochemical Mechanisms

BARBARA F. HALES

Since the discovery in the early 1960s that exposure to thalidomide during limb organogenesis could lead to phocomelia,[1] a number of other drugs and environmental chemicals have been identified as teratogens.[2,3] These compounds range from small-molecular-weight compounds such as alcohol, steroid analogues such as androgenic hormones or diethylstilbestrol, a variety of anticancer drugs such as aminopterin, methotrexate, chlorambucil, cyclophosphamide, mechlorethamine, busulfan, and 5-fluorouracil, to vitamin analogues such as 13-cis-retinoic acid (Accutane). Like thalidomide, these chemicals may affect a specific organ system in the developing embryo or fetus at specific stages of organogenesis. Alternatively, they may have more generalized toxic effects on multiple organs. Examples of drugs with such generalized effects include most of the anticancer drugs, where exposure results in a variety of skeletal and soft-tissue defects, or CNS reactive drugs such as the anticonvulsants, which are associated with CNS, facial, and digital anomalies.

For years it was generally believed that only exposure of the fetus actually during organogenesis was likely to result in birth defects. It was thought that early exposure would cause pregnancy loss or have no effect, whereas late exposure was unlikely to harm the fetus in any major way. We now know that early exposure to some chemicals, even very shortly after fertilization, may result in malformations.[4] Later exposure, during the period of major neuronal proliferation, may result in long-term effects on behavior or intelligence.[5]

It was also thought that the conceptus could be harmed only by drugs to which it was exposed by means of the mother or by an indirect effect of the drug on maternal homeostasis. In the past few years, evidence has accumulated to suggest that adverse effects on the progeny also may be a consequence of exposure of the father to drugs, rather than the mother.[6] Exposure of male rodents to anticancer drugs or radiation has been shown to result in the production of malformed progeny.[7-9]

Significantly, the compounds that have been identified as human teratogens represent very diverse chemical structures with a variety of pharmacologic activities. Exposure to thalidomide, a mild analgesic and sedative, may result in limb malformations, but similar limb-reduction malformations also could result from exposure to a vitamin A analogue such as 13-cis-retinoic acid or an anticancer drug with alkylating activity such as cyclophosphamide. It is difficult to imagine how such a variety of chemicals with different structural and pharmacologic properties could cause malformations by the same mechanism. Indeed, despite extensive research, it remains difficult to pinpoint the precise mechanism by which almost any teratogen interferes with development. The main underlying problem is that we have insufficient knowledge about the biochemical mechanisms governing normal embryogenesis.

A number of excellent review articles and books have been written on mechanisms postulated to be involved in drug teratogenesis.[10-13] It is not possible to present each hypothesis or even fairly represent much of the work in this area here. Rather, an attempt will be made to "synthesize" some of the concepts presented by many different investigators into one general hypothesis. *This hypothesis is that teratogenesis (or abnormal development) is due to a drug or chemically induced change in gene expression during development.* Gene expression may be altered as a consequence of a change in the gene itself, i.e., a gene mutation or chromosomal rearrangement or deletion. Alternatively, epigenetic mechanisms may affect gene transcription or translation. The end result will be an altered cell, leading to inappropriate cell death and/or growth; this will result in a malformation if the normal repair mechanisms in the embryo cannot compensate.

GENETIC MECHANISMS

One of the approaches to altering gene expression is to alter the gene itself. There is evidence from a variety of different systems that alteration of the genetic information in an organism will result in abnormal development. Wilson[14] estimated that about 20 percent of all human congenital anomalies are associated with gene mutations and another 5 percent with chromosomal aberrations. One recent study[15] found that genetic causes were responsible for 27.7 percent of the malformations among affected infants. Of these, 3.1 percent of the infants with malformations had phenotypes that could be attributed to single mutant genes.

However, in most instances, it has not been possible to causally link anomalies associated with drug exposure to an identifiable mutation or chromosomal aberration. Based on literature surveys, Schreiner and Holden[16] have concluded that agents which produce chromosomal damage or mutations have a high chance of being teratogens. However, it is also clear that a number of compounds that are negative in cytogenetic and mutagenicity test procedures (e.g., thalidomide and retinoic acid) are teratogenic.[1-3] Clearly, additional steps may intervene between exposure to any teratogen, a gene mutation, and the expression of this mutation as a malformation; nongenetic disruptions also must contribute.

For most drugs that are considered to be potent human teratogens, there is often only a severalfold increase in the relative risk of malformations in an exposed group over that found in the unexposed population. Even when the relative risk of malformations is very high, such as for 13-cis-retinoic acid, this risk has been estimated at 25.[17] Consequently, many of the embryos that are exposed will likely be unaffected.

It becomes important to find out what the factors are that are important in determining the subpopulation at risk to any exposure. One of the drugs for which there is some evidence that the risk of drug-induced malformations is not uniformly distributed, perhaps due to genetic considerations, is the commonly used anticonvulsant diphenylhydantoin. Diphenylhydantoin is thought to require metabolic activation (catalyzed by the cytochrome P-450 mono-oxygenase system or by co-oxygenation with prostaglandin synthetase?) to a reactive metabolite to be teratogenic.[18,19] This putative reactive metabolite also can be metabolically detoxified to an inactive metabolite. The results of studies from the laboratory of Speilberg and coworkers[20] support the hypothesis that pharmacogenetically determined abnormal detoxification of a reactive metabolite of diphenylhydantoin is an important risk factor for major birth defects in fetuses exposed to the drug.

The polycyclic aromatic hydrocarbons are another example of a group of chemicals for which pharmacogenetic differences in metabolic activation appear to play a role in the susceptibility to adverse pregnancy outcomes, including malformations. Nebert and coworkers[21] have demonstrated that the genotype of the mother and the conceptus are both important in determining susceptibility to adverse effects of carcinogens and mutagens such as benzo[α]pyrene; benzo[α]pyrene is metabolically activated to reactive diolepoxides by the Ah locus family of the cytochromes P-450.

Animal Models

Inbred Strains

It has been easier to study genetic influences on developmental defects with animal models rather than in humans. There are now a number of inbred strains of mice with defined and heritable malformations. Strains of mice that develop neural tube malformations as a result of a single-locus mutation with high penetrance include "rib fusions" and "crooked,"[22] "splotch,"[23] and "loop-tail."[24] Other strains do not appear to show single-locus, high-penetrance patterns of inheritance, e.g., "curly tail"[25] and "exencephaly".[26,27] One locus, the T locus on chromosome 17 in the mouse, appears to be of particular interest because of its importance in the development of dorsal midline structures such as the notochord, neural tube, and gut.[28] Heterozygotes (T/+) are short-tailed, the spinal cord is distorted, and vertebrae are often fused or absent. Homozygote embryos (T/T) have severe malformations and die on day 10 of gestation because of a failure to establish placental connections. It seems feasible that many of these model systems in inbred strains of mice are paralleled in humans.

In addition to those strains, where the homozygotes or heterozygotes actually have a characteristic birth defect, it is clear from the classic experiments of Clarke Fraser and his group[29] that genes and teratogens can synergize to "push" some phenomena during development above a threshold leading to a malformation that may not be seen with either alone at the exposure levels used.

Transgenic Animals

With the advent of transgenic animals, technology has advanced to the state where it is possible to look more closely at the interplay between gene mutations and abnormal development. Experiments from several laboratories have demonstrated that the insertion of exogenous DNA (as a result of the integration of a retrovirus) into the genome of a fertilized mouse egg can result in developmental arrest (a recessive lethal mutation). Jaenish and colleagues[30] have shown that in the Mov-13 mouse strain, established from an embryo infected with Moloney murine leukemia virus, the provirus has integrated into and inactivated the $\alpha 1(I)$ collagen gene. The consequence of this disruption of an endogenous gene is embryo death at a specific time during gestation. In another example, microinjection of DNA into the pronuclei of mouse zygotes resulted in a transgenic strain of mice with limb malformations; this mutation has been found to be an allele of a previously described locus, limb deformity (ld).[31] Thus the insertion of foreign DNA may result in gross chromosomal rearrangements or may disrupt or inactivate an essential cellular gene, usually leading to peri-implantation death or malformations. The role of viral DNA insertions in disrupting critical genes leading to malformations among virally infected babies remains to be elucidated.

Among the major new technical developments in developmental genetic experiments is the use of embryonic stem cells, which can be manipulated *in vitro* and then introduced into another embryo.[32] These embryonic stem cells are cells from embryos at the blastocyst stage that are cultured in such a manner that they maintain their undifferentiated status. Specific genes in the embryonic stem cells can be "targeted" for mutation at an increased frequency by homologous recombination. Using both positive and negative selection, the clones with DNA integrated into a specific site can be isolated for further study. β-Galactosidase (LacZ) reporter constructs can be inserted to screen for integration of the sequence and to permit analysis of their expression. The selected embryonic stem cells are reinjected into blastocysts, where they efficiently form chimeras. The marker (LacZ) can be stained, permitting easy analysis of temporal and spatial expression directly in the chimeric mouse embryos. Using these approaches, and with germ-line transmission of the altered gene, new mouse strains in which one can examine the role of specific genes in development are being established.[33,34] When a transgene that does not have a strong promoter and is influenced by the position of integration into the genome is used, it should be possible to probe the mouse genome for active chromosomal domains and thus identify endogenous genes involved in organogenesis and pattern formation.[35] We can imagine how this technology could, at some future date, be used therapeutically to "correct" gene deficiencies.

Genes and Development

With the advent of homologous recombination and polymerase chain reaction technology, it is also possible to start choosing a gene on which to concentrate. Information on the particular genes that might regulate developmental events is beginning to accumulate. One group of genes of great interest is the homeobox gene family. A second group of genes of potential importance in growth and development are the cellular proto-oncogenes.

Homeobox Genes

Homeobox genes contain a 180-base-pair DNA sequence encoding a conserved 60-amino-acid protein-coding sequence. The homeobox sequence has been found in many of the genes that commit cells to follow specific patterns of development in the early embryos of the fruit fly *(Drosophila)* as well as in worms, frogs, and mice.[36,37] Human homeobox genes also have been described.[38] Mutations in homeobox genes may cause specific disruptions of the embryonic segmentation pattern, the dorsoventral axis, neuronal differentiation, development of the visceral musculature, and so on.[39,40] These genes are expressed during development with both spatial and temporal specificity. It is of interest to note that some of the homeobox genes that in fruit flies are associated with segmentation pattern appear to be involved in CNS development in mammals.

The homeodomain proteins appear to be an essential element of many DNA-binding proteins that most likely act as sequence-specific transcription factors.[41] The DNA sequences to which some of these homeodomain proteins bind are very similar, and it seems likely that some of these proteins compete for the same sites, perhaps with differing affinities.[42]

There are many more questions than answers at this stage regarding the role of homeobox genes in regulating normal development, as well as their potential role in mediating birth defects. For example, how do cells come to express different combinations of homeobox gene products during development? We now know that one homeodomain protein can influence the expression of others. Can they also influence the expression of other target genes? How do cellular homeobox proteins determine cellular phenotype? Joyner and Rossant[33] have reported the production of transgenic mice with a mutation in one of the homeobox genes, engrailed (or en-2). Simultaneously, Zimmer and Gruss[34] reported the production of chimeric mice from embryonic stem cells carrying a mutation in a second homeobox gene, Hox 1.1. It is anticipated that more will be learned about the functions of these unique proteins during development of these animals in the future. What remains to be determined is if drugs that are potent teratogens can interact with these genes or their products during development, thus potentially interfering with normal development by disrupting the "regulators" that establish the pattern in the embryo.

Proto-Oncogenes

The second major group of genes to be considered briefly here are the proto-oncogenes or cellular oncogenes. The proto-oncogenes are a wide variety of genes that can influence the cell cycle at different stages and contribute to cell proliferation and differentiation. Several of the proto-oncogene products have now been identified as growth factors, hormone receptors, or tyrosine kinases.[43] Like the homeobox genes, the proto-oncogenes are often expressed in a tissue and developmental stage-specific manner and may play an important role in the growth and development of a variety of tissues.

EPIGENETIC MECHANISMS

It is clear that a large variety of malformations are nonheritable and may involve mechanisms other than a gene mutation or chromosomal rearrangement. In some of these instances, it appears that although the gene itself is not altered, gene expression is affected, either by an effect on gene transcription or on translation. Some of the mechanisms involved may include a specific receptor or a generalized effect on cell homeostasis such as a change in intracellular pH, osmotic balance, or hyperthermia. Alternatively, the effect on the embryo may be mediated by means of an effect on the mother or maternal homeostasis that functionally translates into an effect on the embryo, such as altered nutrition or O_2 tension.

Receptor-Mediated Mechanisms

Effects of a drug or teratogen on gene expression may be mediated by a nuclear receptor for the drug involved. One drug that may fall into this category is retinoic acid, for which nuclear receptors have been identified.[44] Other nuclear receptors for glucocorticoids, estrogens, and androgens also may be involved in the defects associated with these steroids and their analogues.

Isotretinoin, or 13-cis-retinoic acid, is one of the major human teratogens of the 1980s.[17] Retinoids are essential for development, but exposure of animal or human embryos to excess amounts of all-trans or 13-cis-retinoic acid results in a spectrum of defects in the developing organism ranging from neural tube defects to facial and limb defects.[45] Retinoids have long been known to affect cell differentiation and gene expression. Retinoic acid has, in addition, recently been the first chemical to be identified as a morphogen.[46] Retinoic acid is endogenously present in chick limb buds, specifying an anteroposterior axis during limb development. Extraction and application of this retinoic acid to the distal part of the limb bud results in a reproducible and symmetrical pattern of digital malformations.[46] Functional retinoic acid receptors are located in regenerating new limbs,[47] and it has been suggested that positional information may be established through differential receptor activation. Interesting recent experiments with amphibian *(Xenopus)* embryos have resulted in evidence that retinoic acid could also be acting as an endogenous morphogen regulating CNS differentiation, transforming anterior neural tissue to a posterior neural specification.[48] The concentrations of free retinoids appear to be tightly regulated in developing tissues, perhaps both by synthesis and by regulation of a specific binding protein (cellular retinoic acid-binding protein).

One could imagine that by modifying the expression of a particular target gene—maybe a gene whose product is involved in cell–cell communication—one could produce the malformation characteristic of retinoic acid exposure. Retinoids do affect cell–cell communication,[49] and this effect may be involved in their teratogenesis. The mechanism by which retinoic acid affects cell–cell communication is not yet clear.

Cell-surface receptors for neurotransmitters such as acetylcholine, GABA, or serotonin also may be involved in mechanisms of teratogenesis mediated by drugs that interact with them. It is especially interesting that neurotransmitters themselves have the potential to act as regulators of nerve-cell growth and division in the developing nervous system.[50] The expression of the serotonin 1c receptor in fibroblast (NIH 3T3) cells can induce a malignant state of uncontrolled growth.[51]

Non-Receptor-Mediated Mechanisms

Intracellular pH

Nau and Scott[52] have put forward the suggestion that the "common" effect of a large variety of teratogens with divergent chemical structures is an effect on embryonic intracellular pH. The intracellular pH in the embryo during organogenesis is consistently higher than that of the maternal blood; on days 8 and 9 of gestation in the mouse, there is a pH difference of approximately 0.4. Many teratogens are weak acids (thalidomide, valproic acid, retinoic acid, diphenylhydantoin), and this pH difference is sufficient to promote accumulation of these teratogens in the embryo. Thus the embryo is exposed to a higher concentration of the teratogen than would otherwise be predicted. It is not clear if these weak acids act to further decrease embryonic pH and if such a decrease could itself alter cell homeostasis (and gene expression) sufficiently to result in abnormal growth and malformations.

Hyperthermia

There is evidence in humans that a high maternal fever during pregnancy may lead to an increased risk for birth defects.[53] Experimentally, hyperthermia during development has been demonstrated to result in death or abnormal development in the embryos of species ranging from plants to fruit flies to mammals. Usually, an increase in body temperature of approximately 5°C is sufficient to produce neural tube and other malformations. In *Drosophila,* the stage-specific malformations that are produced are called *phenocopies* because of their resemblance to phenotypic mutant defects.[54] In mammalian embryos, neural tube defects are most frequently induced.[55]

Hyperthermia, or "heat shock," is associated with a reduction in the synthesis of normal mRNA and protein and the induction of a group of "conserved" and characteristic heat shock proteins.[56] The synthesis of these proteins also can be induced by exposure to a variety of stress-inducing conditions, including anoxia, certain heavy metals, and other chemicals, as well as teratogens such as diphenylhydantoin.[57] It is interesting to note that exposure to a low, nonteratogenic dose of heat can induce the synthesis of these heat shock or stress proteins and result in tolerance to a subsequent, normally damaging dose of heat. It now appears that cross-tolerance may develop such that a mild heat stress will provide protection against subsequent exposure to a chemical teratogen such as cadmium.[58] Thus the heat shock response appears to have a role in protecting the cells or embryo against chemical insult.

The mechanism by which heat shock induces characteristic malformations is not clear. The immediate effect of heat shock is a stoppage of development. Heat shock blocks cell proliferation and increases cell necrosis, apparently by preventing cells from entering mitosis. It seems likely that heat shock directly affects gene expression. We know that normal protein synthesis is altered and that heat shock proteins are produced. The defects produced, at least in *Drosophila,* may be a consequence of a disruption of the same developmental process that can be altered by a mutation. In *Drosophila,* stage-specific embryonic defects likely resulting from disruption of transcription-controlled processes are produced by short heat shocks of postblastoderm embryos.[59]

Indirect Effects

It is clear that the mother has a role in the mediation of birth defects in the mammalian embryo. In animal experiments, murine strain differences in susceptibility to some specific teratogens can be traced to the mother.[21] One factor may be maternal differences in drug metabolism—drug activation or detoxification. As mentioned earlier, such differences in drug metabolism may be at least partly responsible for differences in susceptibility to aryl hydrocarbon (e.g., benzo[α]pyrene) teratogenicity. In crosses where the mother was from a strain with high aryl hydrocarbon hydroxylase inducibility, the fetus had an increased risk of malformations compared with crosses where the mother had low inducibility.[21]

There is increasing evidence that the placenta and/or yolk sac is a target for some teratogens, such as somatomedin inhibitor[60] and specific antibodies.[61] Experiments reported by Stark and Juchau[62] suggest that the malformations resulting from the effects of one teratogen, nitrosofluorene, on the yolk sac were abnormal axial rotation of the embryo, whereas an abnormal prosencephalon resulted from an effect directly on the embryo.

SUMMARY

The hypothesis that has been presented in this chapter is that teratogenesis (or abnormal development) is due to a drug or chemically induced change in gene expression during development. Although a great deal of information on the biochemical basis for the action of teratogens during development is still lacking, the data that are now available do suggest that there may be more specificity in the targets and effects of drugs during development than previously thought. We now have examples of genes that play critical roles in developmental programming and drugs and other treatments such as heat shock that may interfere with the expression of such genes.

REFERENCES

1. Lenz W, Knapp K: Thalidomide embryopathy. Arch Environ Health 5:100–105, 1962
2. Shepard TH: Catalog of Teratogenic Agents, 6th ed. Baltimore, Johns Hopkins University Press, 1989
3. Schardein JH: Chemically Induced Birth Defects. New York, Marcel Dekker, 1985
4. Generoso WM, Rutledge JC, Cain KT, Hughes LA, Braden PW: Exposure of female mice to ethylene oxide within hours after mating leads to fetal malformations and death. Mutation Res 176:269–274, 1987
5. Otake M, Schull WJ: In utero exposure to A-bomb radiation and mental retardation: A reassessment. Br J Radiol 57:409–414, 1984
6. Robaire B, Trasler JM, Hales BF: Consequences to the progeny of paternal drug exposure, in Lobl TJ, Hafez ESE (eds): Advances in Reproductive Health Care. Lancaster, England, MTP Press, 1985, pp 225–243
7. Trasler JM, Hales BF, Robaire B: Paternal cyclophosphamide treatment of rats causes fetal loss and malformations without affecting male fertility. Nature 316:144–146, 1985
8. Trasler JM, Hales BF, Robaire B: Chronic low-dose cyclophospha-

9. mide treatment of adult male rats: Effect on fertility, pregnancy outcome and progeny. Biol Reprod 34:275–283, 1986
9. Kirk KM, Lyon MF: Induction of congenital malformations in the offspring of male mice treated with x-rays at pre-meiotic and post-meiotic stages. Mutation Res 125:75–85, 1984
10. Juchau MR (ed): The Biochemical Basis of Chemical Teratogenesis. New York, Elsevier/North Holland, 1981
11. Welsch F (ed): Approaches to Elucidate Mechanisms in Teratogenesis. Washington, Hemisphere Publishing, 1987
12. Wilson JG, Fraser FC (eds): Handbook of Teratology, vol 2: Mechanisms and Pathogenesis. New York, Plenum Press, 1977
13. Beckman DA, Brent RL: Mechanisms of teratogenesis. Annu Rev Pharmacol Toxicol 24:483–500, 1984
14. Wilson JG: Teratogenic effects of environmental chemicals. Fed Proc 36:1698–1703, 1977
15. Nelson K, Holmes LB: Malformations due to presumed spontaneous mutations in newborn infants. N Engl J Med 320:19–23, 1989
16. Schreiner CA, Holden HE Jr: Mutagens as teratogens: A correlative approach, in Johnson EM, Kochhar DM (eds): Handbook of Experimental Pharmacology, vol 65: Teratogenesis and Reproductive Toxicology. Berlin, Springer-Verlag, 1983, pp 135–168
17. Lammer EJ, Chen DT, Hoar RM, et al: Retinoic acid embryopathy. N Engl J Med 313:837–841, 1985
18. Martz F, Failinger C III, Blake DA: Phenytoin teratogenesis: Correlation between embryopathic effect and covalent binding of putative arene oxide metabolite in gestational tissue. J Pharmacol Exp Ther 203:231–239, 1977
19. Wells PG, Kupfer A, Lawson JA, Harbison RD: Relation of in vivo drug metabolism to stereoselective fetal hydantoin toxicology in mouse: Evaluation of mephenytoin and its metabolite, nirvanol. J Pharmacol Exp Ther 221:228–234, 1982
20. Strickler SM, Dansky LV, Miller MA, et al: Genetic predisposition to phenytoin-induced birth defects. Lancet 2:746–749, 1985
21. Shum S, Jensen NM, Nebert DW: The murine Ah locus: In utero toxicity and teratogenesis associated with genetic differences in benzo[α]pyrene metabolism. Teratology 20:365–376, 1979
22. Cole WA, Trasler DG: Gene-teratogen interaction in insulin-induced mouse exencephaly. Teratology 22:125–139, 1980
23. Kapron-Bras CM, Trasler DG: Gene–teratogen interaction and its morphological basis in retinoic acid-induced mouse spina bifida. Teratology 30:143–150, 1984
24. Wilson DB, Finta LA: Early development of the brain and spinal cord in dysraphic mice. Anat Embryol (Berl) 160:315–326, 1980
25. Embury S, Seller MJ, Adinolfi M, Polani PE: Neural tube defects in curly-tail mice. I. Incidence, expression and similarity to the human condition. Proc R Soc Lond (Biol) 206:85–94, 1979
26. Wallace ME, Knights PJ, Anderson JR: Inheritance and morphology of exencephaly, a neonatal lethal recessive with partial penetrance, in the house mouse. Genet Res 32:135–149, 1978
27. Macdonald KB, Juriloff DM, Harris MJ: Developmental study of neural tube closure in a mouse stock with a high incidence of exencephaly. Teratology 39:195–213, 1989
28. Bennett D: The T locus of the mouse. Cell 6:441–454, 1975
29. Fraser FC: Interactions and multiple causes, in Wilson JG, Fraser FC (eds): Handbook of Teratology, vol 1. New York, Plenum Press, 1977, pp 445–463
30. Harbers K, Kuehn M, Delius H, Jaenisch R: Insertion of retrovirus into the first intron of alpha(1) collagen gene leads to embryonic lethal mutation in mice. Proc Natl Acad Sci USA 81:1504–1508, 1984
31. Woychik RP, Stewart TA, Davis LG, et al: An inherited limb deformity created by insertional mutagenesis in a transgenic mouse. Nature 318:36–40, 1985
32. Gossler A, Joyner AL, Rossant J, Skarnes WC: Mouse embryonic stem cells and reporter constructs to detect developmentally regulated genes. Science 244:463–465, 1989
33. Joyner A, Skarnes WC, Rossant J: Production of a mutation in mouse En-2 gene by homologous recombination in embryonic stem cells. Nature 338:153–156, 1989
34. Zimmer A, Gruss P: Production of chimeric mice containing embryonic stem (ES) cells carrying a homeobox Hox 1.1 allele mutated by homologous recombination. Nature 338:150–153, 1989

35. Allen ND, Cran DC, Barton SC, et al: Transgenes as probes for active chromosomal domains in mouse development. Nature 333:852–855, 1988

36. Ingham PW: The molecular genetics of embryonic pattern formation in Drosophila. Nature 335:25–34, 1988

37. Gehring WJ: Homeo boxes in the study of development. Science 236:1245–1252, 1987

38. Simeone A, Mavilio F, Acampora D, et al: Two human homeobox genes, c1 and c8: Structure analysis and expression in embryonic development. Proc Natl Acad Sci USA 84:4914–4918, 1987

39. Balling R, Mutter G, Gruss P, Kessel M: Craniofacial abnormalities induced by ectopic expression of the homeobox gene Hox-1.1 in transgenic mice. Cell 58:337–347, 1989

40. Wright CVE, Cho KWY, Hardwicke J, et al: Interference with function of a homeobox gene in Xenopus embryos produces malformations of the anterior spinal cord. Cell 59:81–93, 1989

41. Levine M, Hoey T: Homeobox proteins as sequence-specific transcription factors. Cell 55:537–540, 1988

42. Hoey T, Levine M: Divergent homeo box proteins recognize similar DNA sequences in Drosophila. Nature 332:858–861, 1988

43. Adamson ED: Oncogenes in development. Development 99:449–471, 1987

44. Giguere V, Ong ES, Segui P, Evans RM: Identification of a receptor for the morphogen retinoic acid. Nature 330:624–629, 1987

45. Kamm JJ: Toxicology, carcinogenicity and teratogenicity of some orally administered retinoids. J Am Acad Dermatol 6:652–659, 1982

46. Thaller C, Eichele G: Identification and spatial distribution of retinoids in the developing chick limb bud. Nature 327:625–628, 1987

47. Giguere V, Ong ES, Evans RM, Tabin CJ: Spatial and temporal expression of the retinoic acid receptor in the regenerating amphibian limb. Nature 337:566–569, 1989

48. Durston AJ, Timmermans JPM, Hage WJ, et al: Retinoic acid causes an anteroposterior transformation in the developing nervous system. Nature 340:140–144, 1989

49. Mehta PP, Bertram JS, Loewenstein WR: The actions of retinoids on cellular growth correlate with their actions on gap junctional communication. J Cell Biol 108:1053–1065, 1989

50. Ashkenazi A, Ramachandran J, Capon DJ: Acetylcholine analogue stimulates DNA synthesis in brain-derived cells via specific muscarinic receptor subtypes. Nature 340:146–150, 1988

51. Julius D, Livelli TJ, Jessell TJ, Axel R: Ectopic expression of the serotonin 1c receptor and the triggering of malignant transformation. Science 244:1057–1062, 1989

52. Nau H, Scott WJ Jr: Weak acids may act as teratogens by accumulating in the basic milieu of the early mammalian embryo. Nature 323:276–278, 1986

53. Smith DW, Clarren SK, Harvey MAS: Hyperthermia as a possible human teratogenic agent. J Pediatr 92:878–883, 1978

54. Mitchell HK, Lipps LS: Heat shock and phenocopy induction in Drosophila. Cell 15:907–918, 1978

55. Webster WS, Edwards MJ: Hyperthermia and the induction of neural tube defects in mice. Teratology 29:417–425, 1984

56. Pardue ML, Feramisco JR, Lindquist S (eds): Stress-Induced Proteins. New York, Alan R Liss, 1989

57. Bournias-Vardiabasis N, Buzin CH: Altered differentiation and induction of heat shock proteins in Drosophila embryonic cells associated with teratogen treatment, in Banbury Report 26: Developmental Toxicology: Mechanisms and Risk. Cold Spring Harbor, NY, Cold Spring Harbor Laboratory, 1987, pp 3–16

58. Kapron-Bras CM, Hales BF: Heat shock induced tolerance to the embryotoxic effects of hyperthermia and cadmium in mouse embryos in vitro. Teratology 43:83–94, 1991

59. Eberlain S: Stage-specific embryonic defects following heat shock in Drosophila. Dev Genet 6:179–197, 1986

60. Sadler TW, Phillips LS, Balkan W, Goldstein S: Somatomedin inhibitors from diabetic rat serum alter growth and development of mouse embryos in culture. Diabetes 35:861–865, 1986

61. Jensen M, Lloyd JB, Koszalka TR, et al: Preparation and developmental toxicity of monoclonal antibodies against rat visceral yolk sac antigens. Teratology 40:505–511, 1989

62. Stark KL, Juchau MR: Microinjection of cultured rat embryos: A new technique for studies in chemical dysmorphogenesis. Toxicol Appl Pharmacol 100:411–416, 1989

14

DRUGS USED IN LABOR AND DELIVERY

J. CHRISTOPHER CAREY *and* CHARLOTTE S. CATZ

Many drugs are used during labor and delivery that are not routinely administered at other times in gestation or to nonpregnant women. Many of the studies addressing drug distribution between maternal and fetal organisms have taken advantage of the time of delivery as cord blood, neonatal blood, and urine samples become available. Conclusions to other periods of pregnancy have been extrapolated from these results. However, caution must be used in interpreting these data for times other than labor and delivery in view of the changing physiology of the maternal organism and of the developing fetus.

Quite often the same attention is not given to potential side effects of these drugs as that given to those administered at any other time of pregnancy. Experience has shown that consideration must be given to maternal effects as well as to consequences for the fetus and newborn infant, including those immediately observable and those of delayed appearance.

Two groups of drugs used to alter uterine contractility will be discussed in extensive detail because they are specific to problems occurring during late gestation and labor. These drugs are the *tocolytics,* which inhibit contractions in the preterm parturient, and the *oxytocics,* which are used to induce or augment labor. Another group of drugs, analgesics and anesthetics, commonly used during labor will be presented in some detail. Other drugs prescribed for acute or chronic conditions will be mentioned briefly as to their use during labor and delivery. More specific discussions can be found in the appropriate chapters.

DRUGS USED TO ALTER UTERINE CONTRACTILITY

The alteration of uterine contractility is an important component of modern obstetrics. Tocolytics are commonly used to inhibit contractions in the preterm parturient, and oxytocics are used to induce or augment labor in 15–40 percent of parturients[1] and are used in virtually all patients in the postpartum period.[2] A clear understanding of the effects of drugs used to affect labor would require a clear understanding of the physiology and pathophysiology of labor, which are poorly understood at present. The exact mechanisms leading to the initiation of labor are not known, and a diagrammatic representation of one current theory of the physiology and pathophysiology of labor is presented in Figure 14–1.

OXYTOCICS

Many drugs have an oxytocic effect, that is, the ability to produce contraction of the smooth muscle of the uterus, but only a few have a selective enough effect to be of clinical use. These are oxytocin, the ergot alkaloids, and certain prostaglandins. Each of these drugs can produce significant uterine contraction with minimal other effects in the healthy individual. Although each has other effects on multiple organs, their usefulness and their danger come primarily from their ability to effect uterine contractions. The oxytocics act in different sites on the labor cascade, as seen in Figure 14–2.

Oxytocin

Oxytocin is the prototype oxytocic drug. Because the intravenous infusion of oxytocin will bring about orderly labor in a majority of pregnant women at or near term, the compound was thought to be responsible for the initiation of labor. However, investigation revealed that there is no increase in circulating oxytocin in maternal serum in early labor and increases occur only in the second and third stages of labor.[3,4] The physiologic role of oxytocin is now thought to be action as a uterotonin in labor, postpartum constriction of uterine vessels, and milk letdown.[5]

Oxytocin occurs naturally in the posterior pituitary of most mammals. Early preparations came from animal

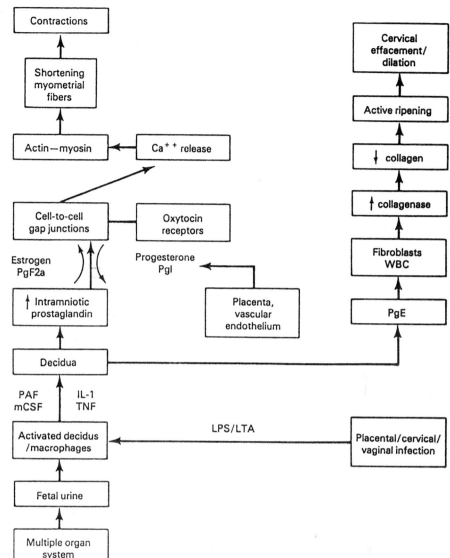

FIGURE 14–1. Diagrammatic representation of a current theory of the physiology and pathophysiology of labor.

sources and were contaminated by small but variable amounts of antidiuretic hormone. The drug is now available commercially in the United States in pure synthetic form (Pitocin, Syntocinon). One milligram of synthetic oxytocin is equal to about 500 U.S.P. units. Each milliliter of injectable oxytocin contains 10 U.S.P. units.

Oxytocin is a polypeptide whose structure is shown in Figure 14–3. It is similar to the other polypeptide hormone produced by the posterior pituitary, antidiuretic hormone, differing only in positions 3 and 8.

Effects

Oxytocin has stimulant effects on the smooth muscle of the uterus and mammary glands. The effect is very specific to these sites, and little effect is noted on other smooth muscle. Oxytocin stimulates both electrical and contractile activity in the uterine smooth muscle.[6] The responsiveness of the uterus depends on the presence of oxytocin receptors on myometrial-cell membranes.[7] The formulation of oxytocin receptors is stimulated by estrogen and prostaglandin $F_{2\alpha}$ and is inhibited by progesterone and prostacycline.[8] The promulgation of electrical activity by myometrial cells is dependent on the formation of cell–cell gap junctions, which are also stimulated by estrogen and prostaglandin $F_{2\alpha}$ and inhibited by progesterone and prostacycline.[9] Thus the effect of oxytocin is dependent on other factors, and the uterus must be "primed" to respond. The sensitivity of the uterus to oxytocin is minimal prior to puberty.[10] With increasing gestation, the uterus becomes more sensitive, with a sharper increase at parturition.[11] As little as 1 milliunit per minute of continuous infusion can induce contractions at term.

Oxytocin causes contraction of the smooth muscle surrounding the alveolar ramifications of the mammary gland in the lactating breast, leading to milk ejection.[12] Nipple stimulation of pregnant and lactating women leads to release of oxytocin by the posterior pituitary.[13] In late pregnancy, nipple stimulation is used as a clinical test to cause oxytocin release and uterine contractions as a means of fetal monitoring.[14]

Oxytocin causes a marked but transient direct relaxing effect on vascular smooth muscle when large amounts are

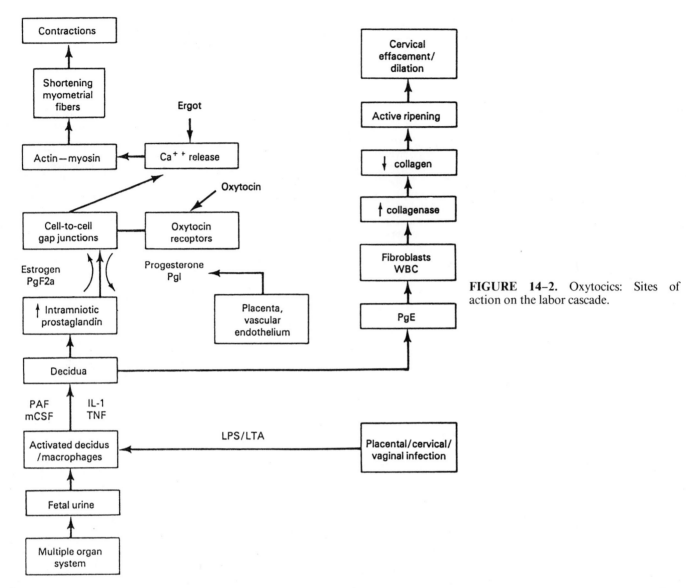

FIGURE 14–2. Oxytocics: Sites of action on the labor cascade.

given.[15] A decrease in systolic and especially diastolic blood pressures and a reflex tachycardia may be observed.[16] Doses used for induction of labor rarely lead to alterations in blood pressure, but large intravenous boluses given postpartum or in an attempt to induce abortion may do so. The avian blood vessel is particularly sensitive to oxytocin, and the hypotensive response of the chick is the basis of the U.S.P. bioassay for oxytocin.

Large doses of oxytocin can lead to water intoxication in both the mother and the fetus if the drug is administered in a large volume of electrolyte-free solution.[17] The antidiuretic effect of oxytocin is similar to that of vasopressin at doses above 45 mIU per minute.[18] We have seen systemic hyponatremia leading to convulsions with the administration of 40 units intravenously.

Absorption, Fate, and Excretion

Oxytocin is not absorbed orally. In the past, oxytocin was available as a sublingual tablet (Pitocin) and a so-called buccal pit was used to induce labor. The use was abandoned because the effect was variable, and uterine hyperstimulation was a significant risk. In current practice, oxytocin is primarily used as an intravenous infusion and occasionally as an intramuscular injection.[19]

Early *in vitro* experiments showed oxytocin to have a plasma half-life of 1–6 minutes, which was decreased in pregnancy and lactation.[20] However, these experiments used very large doses of oxytocin to achieve measurable plasma levels or used indirect methods to determine its half-life. The drug concentration at steady state and the concentration at maximal end-organ response are directly proportional to the infusion rate and inversely proportional to systemic clearance. The time to reach steady state is generally accepted as four half-lives of the drug. Recent *in vivo* experiments that employed sensitive radioimmunoassays and computer simulations demonstrated

Glu(NH2) - Asp(NH2) - Cys -- Pro -- Leu -- Gly(NH2)

Ileu --- Tyr ----- Cys

FIGURE 14–3. Structure of oxytocin.

that the time needed to reach a steady-state concentration of oxytocin in plasma is 40 to 60 minutes.[21–25] Thus the *in vivo* half-life of oxytocin is longer than previously thought—approximately 10–15 minutes.[26] Following an intramuscular injection, uterine response occurs in 3–5 minutes and persists for 2–3 hours. Following intravenous administration, uterine response occurs almost immediately and persists for approximately 1 hour. Oxytocin is bound to membrane receptors in the breast and uterus and inactivated. The drug is excreted by the liver and kidney, and a very small percentage is excreted unchanged in the urine. During pregnancy, two additional factors come into play: The drug is inactivated by a "plasma oxytocinase" and the placenta displays high oxytocinase activity.

Clinical Usage

Oxytocin is used to induce labor at term, to strengthen uterine contractions in dysfunctional labors, and to diminish blood loss in the immediate postpartum period. Although oxytocin also causes milk letdown, it does not increase the quantity or quality of breast milk and is rarely used to enhance breast-feeding.

When used to induce labor, oxytocin must be administered as a dilute infusion controlled by an infusion pump. It should be administered in an isotonic solution to avoid hyponatremia. The standard solution is obtained by mixing 10 units (1 ampule) in 1000 ml of 0.9 percent sodium chloride or lactated Ringer's solution, leading to a final dilution of 10 milliunits per milliliter. The initial dosage is 1 milliunit per minute by continuous infusion, which is equal to 6 ml/h of the dilute infusion. Some obstetrical services prefer to mix 3 ampules (30 units) in 500 ml of solution. This leads to a final dilution of 60 milliunits per milliliter, so a 1 ml/h infusion is equal to 1 milliunit per minute. Either method is acceptable. The second method has the advantage that the infusion rate in milliliters per hour equals the dosage in milliunits per minute. It has the disadvantage that the dosage must be more accurately administered, since a small variation in the volume administered leads to greater variation in the dose given.

The initial dosage should be increased arithmetically every 30 to 40 minutes with cautious observation for hyperstimulation of uterine contractions. The goal is to produce rhythmic uterine contractions that mimic those of normal labor without compromising the health of the mother or fetus. It is important to realize that a change in the sensitivity of the uterus to oxytocin may be abrupt and may occur during labor, requiring an adjustment of the dose. There is also wide individual variation in the sensitivity of the uterus to oxytocin, so dosages must be individualized and in the same individual must be carefully monitored and titrated to achieve the desired effect. The end result of titration should be rhythmic uterine contractions occurring every 3 to 4 minutes lasting 90 seconds. Hyperstimulation of the uterus, a significant risk to the health of both the mother and the fetus, has been associated with uterine rupture,[27] fetal hypoxia, and even fetal death.[28] Therefore, the parturient receiving oxytocin must be monitored continuously for both fetal heart rate abnormalities and the frequency and intensity of uterine contractions.

Oxytocin is also used to decrease postpartum hemorrhage. The prophylactic use of postpartum oxytocics reduces the risk of postpartum hemorrhage by about 40 percent.[29] The usual dosage is greater than that used to induce labor. Ten units can be given intramuscularly, or an intravenous infusion of 30 units in 1000 ml of solution can be given. The injection of oxytocin into the umbilical vein of the retained placenta has been reported by some but not all investigators[30,31] to lead to expulsion of the retained placenta and to decrease hemorrhage, postpartum anemia, and the time of the third stage.

Ergot Alkaloids

The dramatic effect of the ingestion of ergot on the pregnant uterus has been known for over 2000 years, and it was first used by physicians as an oxytocic more than 400 years ago. Ergot is the product of a fungus *(Claviceps purpurea)* that grows on rye and other grains. The consumption of grain contaminated by ergot spread death and destruction for centuries. As early as 300 B.C., the sacred books of the Parsees recorded that "among the evil things created by Angro Maynes are noxious grasses that cause pregnant women to drop the womb and die in childbed." It was mentioned as early as 1582 by Lonicer as a proven means of producing pains in the womb. In 1808, a letter by John Stearns in the Medical Repository of New York described the herb as a means of quickening childbirth.

Chemistry

Two series of alkaloids can be isolated from ergot. The L forms are pharmacologically active, whereas the D forms are not. The alkaloids fall into three groups chemically as well as pharmacologically: (1) the amino acid alkaloids, (2) the dihydrogenated amino acid alkaloids, and (3) the amine alkaloids. Their effects differ markedly between groups, but within groups, individual compounds are similar. All the ergot alkaloids increase the motor activity of the uterus, but those of group 3 are the most potent. Ergonovine maleate (Ergotrate) and methylergonovine maleate (Methergine) are the drugs from this class most commonly used in obstetrics. Since the two drugs have virtually identical effects and pharmacokinetics,[32] methylergonovine will be discussed.

Effects of Ergonovine and Methylergonovine

Methylergonovine produces marked contractions and increase in resting tone in the pregnant and puerperal uterus. High doses can cause sustained contractions. The sensitivity of the uterus to methylergonovine varies with age and with gestation, but even premenarchal uteri will respond to methylergonovine. The gravid uterus is very sensitive and will respond to doses low enough to be unaccompanied by significant side effects. The onset of action after intravenous administration is immediate; after intramuscular injection, onset is 2–3 minutes; and after oral administration, onset is 5–10 minutes. Effects last about 3 hours.[33]

Ergot alkaloids also have the ability to constrict other smooth muscle, leading to peripheral vasoconstriction. The amine alkaloids are the least potent vasoconstrictors of the ergot alkaloids and rarely cause vasoconstriction in the usual doses. However, the intravenous administration of ergonovine and methylergonovine has been associated with hypertension, nausea, vomiting, and convulsions. Blood pressure rises in 50 percent of patients given ergonovine and 20 percent of those given methylergonovine, but in only 2 percent is the rise as great as 25 mmHg systolic and 20 mmHg diastolic.[34]

The pressor effect of ergot alkaloids is particularly pronounced following administration of ephedrine or other vasopressors. In one study of 741 women, 4.6 percent had a rise in systolic blood pressure of more than 40 mmHg when given ephedrine and an ergot alkaloid 3–6 hours apart.[35] Coronary artery spasm can occur with doses as low as 0.05 mg intravenously, and the occurrence of chest pain in a woman recently given ergot alkaloids calls for immediate evaluation for myocardial ischemia.

Absorption, Fate, and Excretion

Methylergonovine is rapidly absorbed after oral, intramuscular, or intravenous injection and is rapidly distributed from plasma to peripheral tissue with an alpha-phase half-life of 2–3 minutes following intravenous injection. The beta-phase half-life is 20–30 minutes, although the clinical effects last for about 3 hours. Excretion is rapid and appears to be partially renal and partially hepatic.

Clinical Usage

Methylergonovine is primarily used for the control of postpartum hemorrhage.[36] The usual dose is 0.2 mg I.M. following delivery of the placenta, although some practitioners give the drug on delivery of the anterior shoulder or after delivery of the infant but before delivery of the placenta. The drug is also given orally 0.2 mg three or four times a day after delivery, induced abortion, or miscarriage for 3–7 days to decrease hemorrhage.

Some authorities have recommended that methylergonovine not be used prophylactically because of the risk of hypertension, but others recommend a mixture of oxytocin and ergot alkaloid as the safest and most effective means of preventing postpartum hemorrhage. It would seem wise to limit the use of ergot to those who have not received any vasopressors and who do not have risk factors for peripheral or coronary vasospasm.

Prostaglandins

Prostaglandins $F_{2\alpha}$ and E_2 have potent effects on the human uterus that make them useful oxytocic drugs.

Prostaglandins are local hormones with known effects on almost every organ system. In contrast to oxytocin and the ergot alkaloids, which can be systemically administered with relatively few side effects, prostaglandins cause a wide variety of prominent side effects. The therapeutic effects of prostaglandins are different than the other oxytocics, and different indications should be recognized for their use.

Source

Prostaglandins are available in pure synthetic forms that have been methylated at the C-15 position. PGE_2 is provided as aloprolide (Prostin) in a vaginal suppository, and $FGF_{2\alpha}$ is provided as 15(S)-15-methyl $PGF_{2\alpha}$ (Prostin/15M, Hemabate).

Effects

Prostaglandins have a wide variety of effects on virtually every organ system. Both $PGF_{2\alpha}$ and PGE_2 cause uterine contractions by increasing spike activity in the myometrial cell. $PGF_{2\alpha}$ appears to promote the appearance of oxytocin receptors on myometrial cells and the formation of cell–cell gap junctions in myometrial cells. PGE_2 seems to promote white blood cell activation in the cervix, leading to release of collagenase and consequently cervical "ripening" or dilation and effacement.

PGE_2 and $PGF_{2\alpha}$ act at any stage of gestation. The intraamniotic administration of $PGF_{2\alpha}$ leads to abortion in the second trimester of pregnancy, and vaginal application of PGE_2 leads to abortion in the first or second trimesters.[37] Currently, the vaginal administration of PGE_2 suppositories is used to effect second-trimester abortion and has virtually replaced the intraamniotic administration of $PGF_{2\alpha}$.[38] $PGF_{2\alpha}$ causes contraction of the postpartum uterus when given systemically or locally into the uterus and has been approved by the FDA for the indication of postpartum hemorrhage.

Although the use of systemic prostaglandins is accompanied by prominent side effects, these are limited with local application of the compounds. The most prominent side effects are fever, diarrhea, nausea, vomiting, and shivering. The appearance of severe vulvar edema has been reported. Other effects reported are an increase in ocular pressure, pulmonary bronchospasm, an increase in pulmonary vascular resistance, and worsening of preexisting seizures. The drugs are peripheral vasodilators and increase cardiac output as a result of reflex tachycardia.

Absorption, Fate, and Excretion

Prostaglandins are rapidly absorbed and can be given intravaginally, intraamniotically, intramuscularly, or intravenously. The compounds are rapidly metabolized to 15-keto-13,14-dihydro derivatives, and metabolites are excreted in the urine. The primary biologic inactivation of prostaglandins is dehydrogenation of the C-15 alcohol moiety. Methylization at the C-15 position leads to sustained and enhanced uterotonic potency. The 15-methylated forms are degraded more slowly and form dinor-15-methyl prostaglandins as the main metabolites.

Clinical Usage

Prostaglandins are used for three major indications: (1) the medical induction of abortion, (2) to aid in the "ripening" of the "unripe" cervix, and (3) for the control of postpartum hemorrhage. The intraamniotic administration of 20–40 mg $PGF_{2\alpha}$ will result in abortion during the second trimester of pregnancy. Approximately 25 percent of women will require more than one dose. The vaginal administration of 20-mg PGE_2 suppositories also will result in second-trimester abortions. Suppositories are administered every 3–4 hours until abortion occurs. The vaginal administration of 20-mg PGE_2 suppositories is often accompanied by nausea, vomiting, and diarrhea, and the abortion process may well last 18–24 hours.[39]

The presence of an "unripe" cervix that is neither dilated nor effaced decreases significantly the chance of a successful induction of labor with oxytocin.[40] Local administration of PGE_2 has been recognized as efficacious in "ripening" the cervix,[41] but the drug lacks FDA approval for this indication, and there is no preparation commercially available in the United States. Intracervical administration of 0.25–1 mg PGE_2 in a starch gel is efficacious in leading to cervical effacement, but there are difficulties in preparing a starch gel that will remain in the cervix. Most clinicians use a vaginal administration of 1.0–5.0 mg in a gel applied to the posterior vaginal fornix. Uterine hyperstimulation is reported in approximately 1 percent of women given PGE_2 gel to "ripen" the cervix.

$PGF_{2\alpha}$ has been approved by the FDA for the control of postpartum hemorrhage. The drug is given intramuscularly or directly into the uterine cornu in a 250-μg dose.

TOCOLYTICS

Preterm birth is the most common cause of neonatal morbidity and mortality, and the search for an effective treatment for preterm labor has occupied obstetricians for much of the past 30 years. Multiple drugs have been and are still used, but ritodrine hydrochloride (Yutopar) is the only drug currently approved by the FDA as a tocolytic. An ideal tocolytic would arrest preterm labor and prolong gestation until term with minimal side effects. No such drug exists, and all currently used tocolytics cause major side effects and have questionable efficacy. The diagnosis of true preterm labor versus false labor is difficult, and the reported efficacy of tocolytics depends on the accuracy of diagnosis of labor. Although many tocolytics have been shown to inhibit contractions and some have been shown to lengthen gestation by 48 hours to 14 days, no drug has been proven to decrease the rates of preterm birth, low birth weight, or neonatal mortality. The widespread use

of tocolytics in the United States has had little effect on the rates of preterm birth and neonatal mortality, and the search for better treatments for preterm labor continues.

Currently used tocolytics include β-mimetic agents, magnesium sulfate, and prostaglandin synthetase inhibitors. The site of action of the available tocolytics is shown in Figure 14–4.

β-Mimetic Agents

Ritodrine hydrochloride (Yutopar) is the prototypic β-mimetic agent and is the only drug approved by the FDA as a tocolytic. Other drugs of this class that have been used include isoxsuprine, salbutamol, fenoterol, and terbutaline. These drugs are all relatively selective for β_2-receptors, but all have some activity for all beta receptors. Thus the β-mimetic drugs have marked side effects and a narrow range of safety. Their use should be restricted to those practitioners who not only have a knowledge of their pharmacology and toxicity but also are qualified to recognize and manage complications of drug administration and of pregnancy. The β-mimetic drugs all have similar effects, and ritodrine will be discussed.

Effects

Stimulation of β_2-receptors inhibits contractility of smooth muscle, and ritodrine has been shown to decrease the intensity and frequency of uterine contractions.[42] The drug acts on receptors on the myometrial-cell membrane, increasing the intracellular content of cyclic AMP.[43] The increased intracellular cyclic AMP may initiate a reaction that provides more energy for calcium extrusion from the cell and reuptake of calcium by intracellular storage mechanisms, leading to a lower level of intracellular calcium.[44] Because the drug is not specific for myometrial cells, it has a wide variety of effects on other organ systems that respond to beta stimulation.

There is a marked effect on the cardiovascular system, with an increase in maternal and fetal heart rates. The tachycardia is probably due to both a direct effect on beta receptors in the heart and to a reflex response to peripheral vasodilation. Beta stimulation leads to a further increase in the cardiac output, already increased by approximately 40 percent in pregnancy. The added increase in myocardial oxygen demand from the beta stimulation can lead to myocardial ischemia, anginal pain, arrhythmias, bundle-branch block, and depression of the ST segment on the ECG. Pulmonary edema is a rare but serious complication that has led to maternal fatalities.[45] The pulmonary edema appears to be a result of ventricular failure and sodium and water retention with pulmonary vasodilation. The simultaneous administration of potent glucocorticoids to hasten fetal lung maturation may contribute to the risk of maternal pulmonary edema, but the evidence for an additive effect is not convincing. Pulmonary edema has been reported in 4–5 percent of patients in some large studies and is the most common life-threatening complication of tocolytic therapy.

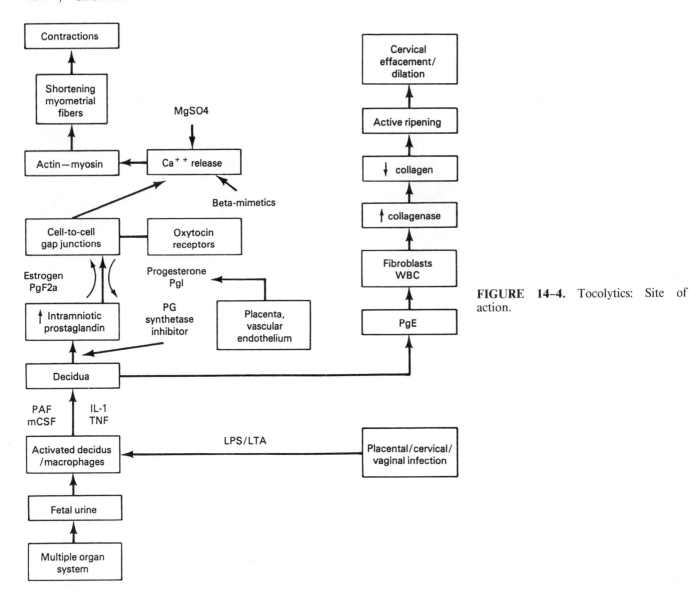

FIGURE 14–4. Tocolytics: Site of action.

Ritodrine has marked metabolic effects. An acute elevation of blood sugar is usually noted and appears to be a result of stimulation of the pancreas to secrete glucagon and insulin,[46] which in turn leads to gluconeogenesis and glycogenolysis. It is rare to see glucose levels in excess of 200 mg/100 ml. The insulin release precedes the rise in blood sugar and appears to be a result of direct pancreatic stimulation. The peak in blood glucose occurs approximately 3 hours after the infusion begins and tends to fall to normal in approximately 24 hours.

A rapid and significant fall in serum potassium occurs in most patients given ritodrine. The lowest serum potassium levels occur approximately 3 hours into the infusion. Urinary excretion of potassium is decreased, leading to the hypothesis that potassium is shifted intracellularly under the influence of glucose and insulin. Recent evidence suggests that some of the potassium shift is due to direct β-receptor stimulation.[47] Total-body potassium is not depleted by ritodrine infusion, and opinions regarding potassium replacement during infusion are divided.

β-Mimetic drugs cause marked sodium and water retention. Over 90 percent of the sodium and 80 percent of the water administered as isotonic solutions are retained when given with high-dose infusions of ritodrine.[48] The mechanism for this has been attributed to the central release of arginine vasopressin (antidiuretic hormone). Arginine vasopressin and renin are both promptly released on infusion of β-mimetic agents and lead to vasoconstriction and an increase in renal resistance with a decrease in renal plasma flow. The glomerular filtration rate is reduced, and renal tubular sodium reabsorption is increased and carries with it water. Any remaining free water is subject to reabsorption under the influence of arginine vasopressin.

Absorption, Fate, and Excretion

Ritodrine is absorbed orally and intramuscularly but is usually given as an intravenous infusion. The distribution half-life when the drug is given intravenously is 6–9 minutes, and the effective half-life 1.7–2.6 hours. Ritodrine is conjugated in the liver to sulfate and glucoronide forms. Both free drug and conjugates are excreted in the urine.[49]

Clinical Usage

Ritodrine is used to inhibit contractions in women in preterm labor. The contraindications to its use are listed in Table 14–1. The drug is given as an intravenous infusion and should be given in a salt-free solution. The usual dilution is 150 mg ritodrine hydrochloride in 500 ml of 5 percent dextrose in water. The infusion is begun at 100 μg/min and is increased by 50 μg/min every 10 minutes until the desired effect is achieved or the maximum dose of 350 μg/min is reached. The maternal pulse should be monitored, and if it is greater than 140 beats per minute, the infusion rate should be decreased. In addition, the mother should be monitored for contractions, fetal heart rate, and signs and symptoms of pulmonary edema. Once the contractions have been inhibited, the dose should be decreased by 50 μg/min every 30 minutes until the minimum effective concentration is reached. If the labor is inhibited, the infusion should be continued for 12–24 hours.

Ritodrine is available in 10-mg tablets. The use of oral ritodrine following intravenous infusion is controversial and has not been proven to be efficacious. Following a 20-mg oral dose, peak plasma concentrations are reached in 60–80 minutes but average only 10 ng/ml. Plasma concentrations needed to inhibit contractions average 20–50 ng/ml, and it has been suggested that the recommended dosage of 10 mg every 2 hours or 20 mg every 4 hours is inadequate. Further research on optimal oral dosing is being done, including testing of a high-dose sustained-release tablet. Pulmonary edema and ECG changes can occur with oral administration,[50] and the safety of high-dose oral regimens remains to be tested.

Other β-Mimetics

Of the other β-mimetic drugs, only terbutaline (Brethine) has been used to any extent in the United States. Ter-

TABLE 14–1. CONTRAINDICATIONS TO RITODRINE USE

1. Antepartum hemorrhage that demands delivery
2. Eclampsia or severe preeclampsia
3. Intrauterine fetal death
4. Chorioamnionitis
5. Maternal cardiac disease
6. Pulmonary hypertension
7. Maternal hyperthyroidism
8. Uncontrolled diabetes mellitus
9. Preexisting maternal medical conditions such as hypovolemia, cardiac arrhythmias associated with tachycardia or digitalis intoxication, uncontrolled hypertension, pheochromocytoma, and bronchial asthma already treated by β-mimetic agents and/or steroids
10. Known hypersensitivity to any of the products

butaline is not approved for the inhibition of labor, and the package insert states that "terbutaline sulfate is not indicated for tocolysis" and "terbutaline sulfate should not be used for tocolysis." However, a large body of clinical experience indicates that the safety and efficacy of terbutaline is similar to that of ritodrine. The pharmacology of terbutaline is virtually identical to ritodrine. The labor-inhibiting concentration ranges from 5–15 ng/ml of plasma. Following an oral dose of 5 mg, peak plasma levels average 4–5 ng/liter that is sustained for 1–3 hours. Because terbutaline has a more favorable oral dosing regimen and is substantially less expensive, some clinicians prefer terbutaline to ritodrine for oral administration.

Magnesium Sulfate

Magnesium sulfate is a chemical salt available as $MgSO_4 \cdot 7H_2O$. It is not approved for use as a tocolytic, but clinical experience underlines its safety and efficacy, and it has replaced β-mimetic agents in many university centers. Magnesium sulfate is primarily used for the treatment of preeclampsia/eclampsia, although its mechanism of action is unknown. It was noted that women treated with magnesium sulfate were more likely to have inadequate contractions and that sufficiently high doses could arrest labor, leading to its use as a tocolytic.

Effects

Magnesium is primarily an intracellular cation, and only a small fraction of the total magnesium is in the extracellular space. The normal serum level of magnesium is 1.8–3 mg/100 ml. The mechanism of action is not entirely known, but it is thought that magnesium may affect three aspects of muscle contraction: excitation, excitation–contraction coupling, and the contraction mechanism.[51] Magnesium affects myometrial contractions by modulating calcium uptake, binding, and distribution in smooth-muscle cells. Elevated concentrations of magnesium compete for calcium-binding sites at the cell membrane, thus preventing calcium influx. Magnesium also may interfere with intracellular calcium metabolism, possibly by increasing cyclic AMP, which depletes intracellular calcium and inhibits the action of myosin light-chain kinase. Intracellular magnesium stimulates calcium dependent ATPase, which promotes calcium uptake by the sarcoplasmic reticulum and decreases calcium availability for myosin light-chain kinase. Finally, magnesium may compete with calcium for activation of myosin light-chain kinase itself.

Magnesium is a potent peripheral vasodilator, and its infusion regularly produces sweating, warmth, and flushing. At concentrations of 6–12 mEq/liter, changes in the ECG (increases in the PR interval, widening of the QRS complex, and increases in the T-wave height) can be seen. Loss of deep tendon reflexes is seen at 8–10 mEq/liter, and respiratory paralysis occurs at levels of 12–15 mEq/liter.[52] Cardiac arrest occurs at serum concentrations of 25 mEq/liter. Acute chest pain, pulmonary edema, and shortness of breath have been reported with the use of magnesium sulfate as a tocolytic.[53]

Absorption, Fate, and Excretion

Magnesium is absorbed orally, intramuscularly, and intravenously. When given as a tocolytic, it is usually given as an intravenous infusion, although there are reports of long-term oral usage.[54] The drug is excreted by the kidney. At infusion rates of 1, 2, and 3 gm/h, the average serum magnesium concentrations are 4, 5.1, and 6.4 mg/100 ml (1.2 mg/100 ml equals 1 mEq/liter), respectively. Magnesium is widely distributed in body water and crosses the placenta, achieving fetal levels similar to maternal levels. Magnesium therapy does not usually depress the fetus, but neonatal depression has been reported with high maternal serum levels of magnesium.[55] Bolus injection of magnesium sulfate can cause decreased reactivity of the fetal heart rate.

Clinical Usage

The dosage recommendations for magnesium sulfate vary from investigator to investigator. Initial dosages from 4–8 gm I.V. have been recommended, with subsequent infusions of 1–4 gm/h. Some investigators recommend collecting serum magnesium levels every 4 hours, but others recommend following the deep tendon reflexes. The therapeutic dosage range is 5.5–7.5 mg/100 ml (4.6–6.3 mEq/liter). The infusion should be continued at a rate that ablates contractions but does not abate deep tendon reflexes.

Oral magnesium gluconate has been used as a tocolytic agent following intravenous infusion, but its safety and efficacy are not established.

Prostaglandin Synthetase Inhibitors

Because prostaglandins are thought to be necessary for uterine contractions, prostaglandin synthetase inhibitors have been used as tocolytics. Indomethacin (Indocin) has been used most frequently as a tocolytic. Indomethacin is not approved as a tocolytic, and the package insert contains the warning, "Indocin is not recommended for use in pregnant women, since safety of the drug has not been established, and because of the known effect of drugs of this class on the human fetal cardiovascular system [closure of the ductus arteriosus] during the third trimester of pregnancy." There is some evidence that the drug is an effective tocolytic, and its use has been described by several authors.

Effects

Indomethacin binds the enzyme cyclo-oxygenase. This enzyme functions to regulate the production of PGE_2

from arachidonic acid. All subsequent prostaglandins are formed from this initial step, and inhibition of cyclo-oxygenase leads to inhibition of synthesis of PGE_2 and $PGF_{2\alpha}$, which in turn leads to inhibition of uterine contractions and theoretically to the arrest of cervical effacement and dilation.

Indomethacin has a wide variety of effects on multiple organ systems. Orally administered indomethacin has been associated with gastritis and ulcerations of the esophagus, stomach, duodenum, and small intestine. Long-term administration has caused papillary necrosis of the kidney in laboratory animals, and there have been reports of interstitial nephritis in humans. Because renal prostaglandins have a role in the maintenance of renal perfusion, administration of indomethacin has resulted in a decrease in renal perfusion and renal decompensation. This effect leads to the concern that concomitant administration of β-mimetics and indomethacin could worsen the fluid retention and increase the risk of pulmonary edema.

The maintenance of the patency of the ductus arteriosus depends in part on the action of prostaglandin E_1, and administration of indomethacin to experimental animals has led to *in utero* closure of the ductus.[56] In controlled studies, there were no effects seen on the fetal cardiovascular system, but there have been anecdotal reports of neonatal pulmonary hypertension and death in neonates exposed to indomethacin *in utero*.[57] In one study specifically designed to study the effect of indomethacin on the fetal ductus arteriosus, 7 of 14 fetuses treated with indomethacin developed constriction of the ductus as measured by fetal echocardiography,[58] although no neonatal effects were seen. It should be recognized that a rare effect on neonatal mortality or morbidity might not be seen in studies with small numbers, and the risk cannot be dismissed or even accurately estimated.

Absorption, Fate, and Excretion

Indomethacin is readily absorbed orally or by rectal suppository. Following a single dose of 25 or 50 mg, peak serum levels are 1 or 2 μg/ml, respectively, at about 2 hours. The absorption from a rectal suppository is more rapid but appears to be only 80–90 percent of that absorbed orally. Indomethacin is metabolized to its desmethyl, desbenzoyl, and desmethyl–desbenzoyl forms. About 60 percent of an orally administered dose is recovered in the urine and the remainder in the feces.

Clinical Usage

Indomethacin has been given as tablets or suppositories. The most common dose for inhibition of labor is an initial dose of 50–100 mg, followed by 25 mg every 4–6 hours for 24–48 hours. The drug has been compared with placebo in two randomized clinical trials. One showed significantly more failures in the first 48 hours in the placebo group but no significant difference after 48 hours.[59] The second reported delay of delivery of 7 days in 83 percent of the treatment group and in 17 percent of controls.[60] No trials have been performed comparing indomethacin with other tocolytics.

Combination Tocolysis

In the last several years, there have been several reports of combination chemotherapy for tocolysis in an attempt to decrease side effects without decreasing efficacy. Initial reports were promising, but it appears that combination chemotherapy may lead to an increased incidence of side effects. The combination of β-mimetics and magnesium sulfate exposes the patient to an increased solute load in the presence of water retention and may worsen the risk of pulmonary edema. As discussed earlier, the combination of β-mimetics and prostaglandin synthetase inhibitors has the risk of worsening fluid retention and decreasing renal perfusion, increasing the risk of pulmonary edema. Until the efficacy and safety of combination agents can be proven, they cannot be recommended.

ANALGESICS AND ANESTHETICS

Relief of pain during labor and delivery is a complex and still-evolving science that began less than 150 years ago. Many techniques have been devised, tried, and used alone or in various combinations. The recognition that fear and anxiety also play a role in pain perception initiated the development of programs of maternal education and preparation for childbirth. In some patients, hypnosis, Lamaze, and acupuncture are successful in providing good analgesia. A recent study showed that women who expected labor to be more painful and anticipated receiving drugs for relief needed more medications than those who did not have such expectations.[61] Although psychoprophylaxis reduces the amount of pharmacologic agents used during labor, between one-third and two-thirds of patients still require supplemental analgesia.

Systemic Analgesics and Sedatives

The utilization of analgesics and sedatives has the aim of relieving pain and decreasing anxiety during labor. Sedatives and tranquilizers decrease fear and anxiety, and by depressing the central nervous system, they let the patients fall asleep. These drugs are not true analgesics.

Analgesics

Nonnarcotic analgesics and antipyretics (acetaminophen, aspirin, salicylates) and nonsteroidal anti-inflammatory agents (ibuprofen, naproxen, etc.) have a minimal role for the control of pain during labor and delivery. The use of salicylates has been associated with prolonged labor, greater blood loss during delivery, and an increase in the incidence of stillbirths. All these drugs cross the placenta and have been measured in the fetus and newborn.

Narcotic analgesics, specifically meperidine and alphaprodine, are the most popular drugs used for the relief of pain during labor. Meperidine has a half-life of 3 hours in the parturient and 23 hours in the newborn.[62] Fetal levels of meperidine are approximately 80 percent of maternal serum concentrations as measured in the newborn when meperidine was given to the mother more than 1 hour and up to 4 hours before birth. The duration of maternal analgesia lasts between 2 and 4 hours and is of shorter duration for alphaprodine. The newborn showing signs of respiratory depression must be treated with a narcotic antagonist, and the drug of choice is naloxone.

Barbiturates are used for sedation during the early stages of labor. They can be classified as ultrashort (thiopenthal), short (secobarbital–pentobarbital), intermediate (amobarbital), and long-acting (phenobarbital) based on their duration of action. Thiopental is administered intravenously for the induction of anesthesia, has an onset of action measured in seconds, and has a clinical effect ending in a few minutes. Short-acting barbiturates provide mild sedation. The intermediate and long-acting barbiturates, which start action after 1 hour or more and have a duration of effect extending from 8–12 hours, are not useful for appropriate sedation during labor and therefore are not recommended after onset of uterine contractions. In general, these drugs in appropriately prescribed oral doses have no adverse effects on the progression of labor, since they do not have an inhibitory action on uterine tone or contractility. They rapidly cross the placenta, and in the fetus they reach serum levels similar to those in the mother. With repeated use and/or high doses, the newborn may exhibit CNS depression, respiratory depression, and flaccidity.

In the past, tranquilizers were used during labor, but their utilization has markedly decreased. Benzodiazepines (diazepam, chlordiazepoxide, flurazepam) were administered for relief of maternal anxiety but were not an improvement over barbiturates. Intravenous administration of diazepam resulted in high serum levels in the fetus. Accumulation in the fetus causes CNS toxicity, loss of cardiac beat-to-beat variability, and noticeable lethargy and poor feeding in the newborn. Another group of tranquilizers, the phenothiazines (chlorpromazine, promethazine, promazine, etc.), is used in the treatment of psychiatric disorders. These drugs potentiate the effect of narcotics and are often used in conjunction with narcotics to decrease the dose needed. Their administration during labor also helps to control nausea and vomiting. Another mild sedative of rapid effect is an antihistamine hydroxyzine (Atarax). Its action is similar to that of phenothiazines when administered during labor; that is, it relieves anxiety and decreases the dose requirement for narcotics.

Local Anesthetics

Local anesthetics cause a temporary interruption of painful impulses from a specific area of the body without provoking a loss of consciousness. Both local infiltration and regional blocks can provide excellent pain relief during labor and delivery. When a local anesthetic is applied to a nerve, the anesthetic causes the cessation of impulse conduction by binding to receptor sites located on the internal surface of the cell membrane, although some other effects may take place, by a mechanism not yet totally understood, on the sodium channel of the nerve fibers. Interesting to note is that although pain is abolished, there are no changes in motor function, touch, and pressure sensations. Based on their molecular structure, local anesthetics can have an ester-type (chloroprocaine, tetracaine) or an amide linkage (lidocaine, mepivacaine, bupivacaine, etidocaine). The esters are broken down in the circulation by plasma pseudocholinesterase, and the amide agents, with longer half-lives, are metabolized in the liver. The most effective agents for epidural block are chloroprocaine, lidocaine, and bupivacaine because they cause good analgesia without excessive motor blockade. A study comparing an epidural continuous infusion technique with an intermittent top-up using bupivacaine (0.25 percent) showed no differences in pain scores, length of labor, and fetal outcomes.[63] The only differences noted were that mothers with the continuous infusion received more drug, had a lower plasma concentration of the drug, and were more likely to require outlet forceps. A randomized, double-blind study compared the analgesic efficacy of a continuous epidural infusion of 0.0625 percent bupivacaine with fentanyl (a narcotic analgesic) with an infusion of 0.125 percent bupivacaine alone.[64] The study found no significant difference between groups in duration of the second stage of labor, duration of pushing, position of the vertex before delivery, method of delivery, Apgar scores, or umbilical cord blood gas and acid–base values. For the delivery of patients with multiple gestations, lumbar epidural anesthesia has been recommended by some authors when vaginal delivery is anticipated.[65] Others have recommended the use of general anesthesia if intrauterine manipulation may be needed.[66]

The injection of a local anesthetic, its uptake, and its distribution are dependent on the site of injection, dosage, agent, and addition of a vasoconstrictor. In general, drugs that are highly lipid-soluble and strongly protein-bound will be absorbed by the target tissues and removed slowly; therefore, their concentration in blood will be low. To slow absorption even further and therefore prolong the duration of action of the drug, a vasoconstrictor may be added. However, with epidural analgesia, addition of epinephrine may interfere with uterine activity, and this is contraindicated for paracervical block because of the strong vasoconstrictive effect. Paracervical blocks, in general, have been associated with frequent fetal bradycardias. In patients in whom this complication was observed, a concomitant increase in uterine tone was detected—most likely coinciding with high concentrations of the drug in the myometrium. The most rapid rate of absorption is observed with paracervical blocks, followed in diminishing order by injection into the caudal canal, lumbar epidural space, and subarachnoid space, respectively. Local anesthetics cross the placenta, and the rate is dependent on the degree of plasma-protein binding in maternal blood and the rate of uptake by fetal tissues. The interplay of these variables plus the lipid solubility of the drug will determine its concentration in the fetus and the potential for fetal toxicity. In addition to direct effects of the drug in the fetus, indirect actions may follow when local anesthetics cause changes in maternal homeostasis or in uterine blood flow.[67]

Inhalation Agents

Although used frequently in the past, the administration of inhalation agents during labor has declined markedly. When utilized, the objective is to administer a subanesthetic level that produces analgesia in a patient who is conscious and cooperative. The most commonly used inhalation agents are nitrous oxide, which is relatively safe, has a rapid onset, and has a short duration of action; methoxyflurane, with an analgesic effect similar to that of nitrous oxide; a combination of both agents; and halothane, which causes analgesia only in anesthetic doses. Nitrous oxide is inhaled in a 50/50 percent mix with oxygen. Its effects are obtained with intermittent use prior to the onset of each contraction or in continuous administration. In the late first stage and in the second stage of labor, it can be self-administered by the patient. Methoxyflurane may cause subclinical renal toxicity and is not recommended if renal disease is present or nephrotoxic drugs are being administered. Halothane produces uterine relaxation rapidly but is known to be hepatotoxic, and its administration therefore must be carefully controlled. The use of inhalation agents for analgesia carries a substantial risk of aspiration pneumonia, and they are now predominantly used as anesthetic agents rather than as analgesic agents.

Intravenous anesthetics are utilized for induction of general anesthesia. The ultra-short-acting barbiturate thiopental sodium allows rapid induction of anesthesia. The drug crosses the placenta, but measurements in umbilical venous blood do not reach anesthetic levels.[68] A randomized study compared thiopental and propofol use, showing similar results with both drugs. However, the extensive experience with thiopental provides an advantage over other agents for obstetric anesthesia.

ANTIBIOTICS

A great number of antibiotic drugs are available for the treatment of infections. The same principles guiding antibiotic therapy in general apply during labor, delivery, and the postpartum period. When clinical symptoms point to the presence of an infection, cultures do help in identification of the organism(s) and in selection of a specific antibiotic. However, prior to bacteriologic reports, a regimen of wide coverage is instituted that is refined when the results become available. During pregnancy, labor, and delivery, preference should be given to antibiotics that have been studied and found safe for both mother and fetus. A general overview of available antibiotics follows. Penicillins are safe to use at delivery, because they are the most effective and least toxic antimicrobials. They act by inhibiting bacterial cell-wall synthesis. In general, they are well absorbed, and they bind to plasma proteins to different degrees. It is the unbound drug that exerts antibacterial activity by penetrating the microorganism or diffusing into tissues. The great variety of available penicillins can be subdivided into natural penicillins (e.g., benzylpenicillin G.), penicillinase-resistant penicillins (e.g., methicillin, nafcillin, cloxacillin, etc.), aminopenicillins (e.g., ampicillin, amoxicillin, etc.), and anti-*Pseudomonas* penicillin (e.g., carbenicillin, mezlocillin, etc.). They are excreted by the kidney, and a certain proportion of the drug is metabolized. The major adverse effects of penicillins are hypersensitive reactions. Measurements of antibiotic concentrations in amniotic fluid and neonatal plasma or tissues following maternal treatment during labor have been reported. However, no specific mention is made regarding timing of administration with regard to uterine contractions that do interfere with placental transfer. Pharmacokinetic data obtained during labor show that for methicillin and some other antimicrobial drugs, a lower concentration is reached in maternal serum than in nonpregnant female and adult male subjects.[69]

Cephalosporins are agents quite similar to penicillins with regard to structure, mechanisms of action, and general antimicrobial activity. They act by producing a defective and unstable bacterial cell wall. Cephalosporins are broad-spectrum antibiotics that are active against most gram-positive organisms and some common gram-negative bacilli: *Escherchia coli, Proteus mirabilis,* and *Klebsiella* species. The first-generation (e.g., cephalothin, cefazolin, etc.) and second-generation (e.g., cefaclor, cefuroxim, etc.) cephalosporins are considered safe to use during pregnancy. The third generation of this category has not yet been extensively studied during pregnancy. Pharmacokinetic studies have shown, as with penicillins, that at equal dosage, levels achieved during pregnancy are lower than in nonpregnant individuals. They all cross the placenta, and studies with cefuroxine administered during labor demonstrated therapeutic levels in fetal serum and amniotic fluid.[70]

Tetracycline is a broad-spectrum antimicrobial not recommended for use at any time during pregnancy and delivery. The drug crosses the placenta easily and has been associated with problems in both mother and fetus. Chloramphenicol has bacteriostatic activity and is highly active *in vitro* against all anaerobic microorganisms. The administration of this antibiotic has been associated with the "gray syndrome" caused by toxic blood levels of the drug in the newborn infant. Therefore, it is safer not to use it just prior to delivery, since it crosses the placenta easily. Erythromycin is active against most gram-positive bacteria and many anaerobes. It crosses the placenta and is considered safe during pregnancy, except for the preparations of the estolate ester, which have been associated with hepatic toxicity.

Aminoglycosides are effective against serious gram-negative infections, and as noted for other antibiotics, the serum concentrations achieved during pregnancy are lower than in nonpregnant patients. These drugs cross the placenta, and fetal blood concentrations at term are lower than in maternal samples obtained at the same time. Administration during labor is not followed by recognized toxicity in the fetus and/or newborn. The drug of choice is gentamicin, since, in these patients, gentamicin has been studied more extensively than tobramycin, amikacin, and other aminoglycosides.

ANTICONVULSANTS

The woman needing anticonvulsant therapy must be followed closely during her pregnancy to ensure that she remains free of seizures. Potential neonatal problems such as neonatal hemorrhage, depression, and hypotonia have been described in some infants exposed *in utero* to phenobarbital or primidone, which is partially metabolized to phenobarbital. Severe and even fatal hemorrhages have been observed in the first day of life, caused by a deficiency of the vitamin K–dependent coagulation factors.[71] To prevent this complication and problems during delivery, epileptic patients must be given vitamin K during the final months of pregnancy and during labor. In addition, vitamin K must be given to the neonate. A severe complication—status epilepticus—must be treated with the drug of choice: diazepam, a benzodiazepine that crosses the placenta rapidly and accumulates in the fetus. If it is to be administered intravenously during labor, an important factor to consider is the timing of the injection. If given concurrent with uterine contractions, the amount of drug reaching the fetus will be decreased.[72] Effects of this drug in the fetus have been described and include depression of short-term, beat-to-beat variability of heart rate; and in the neonate, apneic spells, hypotonia, poor suckling, and hypothermia.

ANTIHYPERTENSIVES

During labor and the immediate postpartum period, transient hypertension may develop. If there are no signs of preeclampsia, therapy with intravenous hydralazine is indicated to prevent a cerebrovascular accident. If the diastolic blood pressure is greater than 100 mmHg, an I.V. bolus of 5 mg can be administered followed by a continuous infusion. The vasodilator hydralazine reduces blood pressure through a direct effect on arterioles. Patients with a severe clinical picture of acute hypertension in pregnancy, preeclampsia, eclampsia, or pregnancy-induced hypertension should be delivered. Labor should be induced, and the fetus should be monitored with continuous electronic fetal heart-rate monitoring.

ANTICOAGULANTS AND ANTIPLATELET AGENTS

Oral Anticoagulants

Oral anticoagulants are water-soluble derivatives of coumaric acid or a synthetic relative. They act by inhibiting the generation of vitamin K–dependent coagulation factors II, VII, IX, and X. The lack of antiplatelet activity makes their usefulness in arterial disease minimal, and since they can cross the placenta, their effect on the fetus must be avoided. Therefore, oral anticoagulants should not be used during labor and delivery; instead, they should be substituted with the drug of choice: heparin.

Antiplatelet Drugs

These agents interfere with platelet aggregation at the site of vascular injury; consequently, they retard the formation and growth of arterial thrombi. Since they act mainly on arterial lesions, their role in obstetrics is limited. The most commonly used are aspirin, sulfinpyrazone, and dipyridamole. Thrombotic phenomena are a recognized obstetric complication, with thrombophlebitis recognized in the antepartum period and thromboembolic events occurring mainly in the postpartum period.

Thromboembolism may be arterial or venous, and proper diagnosis must be established to institute appropriate treatment. The arterial thrombi are a consequence of vascular injury, with platelets interacting with the damaged intima of the vessel. Venous thrombosis propagates by thrombin generation and occurs with or without injury of the intima. Patients delivered by midforceps or undergoing a cesarean birth are at risk for thromboembolic phenomena. In these cases, prophylaxis with heparin is indicated and can be obtained by two regimens known as minidose or ultralow dose. As described for nonpregnant patients, the minidose regimen consists of the administration of 5000 units of heparin subcutaneously every 12 hours and has been proved efficacious (a 75 percent reduction in deep venous thrombosis and an 86 percent reduction in pulmonary embolus have been reported).[73] However, in view of the increase in plasma volume, renal clearance, and the activity of placental heparinase during pregnancy, the dose to be administered must be higher, about 10,000 units every 12 hours, in the third trimester. In the postpartum period, the dose must be decreased to the one recommended for the nonpregnant patient. The second regimen consists of an infusion of ultra-low-dose heparin (1 unit/kg/h) and may be considered optimal for the laboring and parturient patient. This technique was shown to be efficacious in a surgical population, eliminating the risk of subcutaneous injection-site hematoma, requiring less nursing time, and reducing the incidence of infusion phlebitis.[74]

Postpartum fever not responding to appropriate antibiotic therapy may be caused by pelvic thrombophlebitis, for which full-dose heparinization is indicated. Another postpartum complication also treatable with full-dose heparinization is ovarian vein thrombosis. The treatment is required for 10–15 days, followed by low-dose heparin or oral anticoagulants for an additional 3 months.

ANTIDIABETIC AGENTS

The diabetic patient who becomes pregnant must be followed and treated carefully throughout her gestation and during labor and delivery to ensure a normal metabolic status for her and eliminate potential fetal and neonatal complications (distress, asphyxia, stillbirth, macrosomia, birth injury). Maternal hyperglycemia, in the poorly controlled patient, causes an increase in fetal endogenous insulin, which in turn may contribute to fetal macrosomia and neonatal hypoglycemia. A critical issue is to determine the timing for delivery, which under appropriate supervision can approach term without increasing risks for either the mother or the fetus.[75] During labor, frequent monitoring of blood glucose is needed to maintain maternal euglycemia, which can be achieved by a balanced regimen of dextrose solutions and regular insulin. Studies have shown that during active labor the insulin requirement drops to zero,[76] and in the first postpartum days, requirements continue to be decreased. Women with gestational diabetes should be managed like normoglycemic pregnant patients, with some restrictions in the use of glucose-containing intravenous solutions. The route of delivery must be individualized according to maternal and fetal conditions, since macrosomia was shown to be associated with the occurrence of shoulder dystocia during vaginal delivery.

The administration of insulin during pregnancy is safe and is the treatment of choice for diabetic patients, since it does not cross the placenta in any significant amount.

The use of oral hypoglycemic agents (sulfonylureas such as tolbutamide and chlorpropamide) is relatively contraindicated during pregnancy. These agents cross the placenta easily, produce increased release of endogenous insulin in both mother and fetus, and cause the development of specific pathologies. These drugs do not have a role during pregnancy nor during labor and delivery.

CONCLUSION

This review has highlighted some of the current understanding of the effects of drugs administered during labor and delivery. The issues are multiple and complex and deserve continuing interest and studies to determine the most effective and safe therapeutic regimens.

REFERENCES

1. Seitchik J, Holden AE, Castillo M: Amniotomy and the use of oxytocin in nulliparous women. Am J Obstet Gynecol 153:848–854, 1985
2. Elbourne D, Prendiville W, Chalmers I: Choice of oxytocic preparation for routine use in the management of the third stage of labour: An overview of the evidence from controlled trials. Br J Obstet Gynaecol 95:17–30, 1988
3. Leake RD: Oxytocin. Initiation of parturition: Prevention of prematurity, in Porter JC, MacDonald PC (eds): Report of the Fourth Ross Conference on Obstetric Research. Columbus, Ohio, Ross Laboratories Publications, 1983, p 43
4. Chard T: Fetal and maternal oxytocin in human parturition. Am J Perinatol 6:145–152, 1989
5. Casey ML, MacDonald PC: Biomolecular processes in the initiation of parturition: Decidual activation. Clin Obstet Gynecol 31:533–552, 1988
6. Mironneau J: Effects of oxytocin on ionic currents, underlying

rhythmic activity and contraction in uterine smooth muscle. Pfluegers Arch 363:113–118, 1976

7. Fuchs AR, Fuchs F, Husslein P, Soloff MS, Fernström MJ: Oxytocin receptors and human parturition: A dual role for oxytocin in the initiation of labor. Science 215:1396–1398, 1982

8. Garfield RE, Kannan MS, Daniel EE: Gap junction formation in myometrium: Control by estrogens, progesterone and prostaglandins. Am Physiol 238:C81–C89, 1980

9. Herman AH, Rhoads GG, Carey JC: The role of infection in initiating preterm labor: Summary of an NICHD workshop. Obstet Gynecol (submitted)

10. Caspo A: Function and regulation of the myometrium. Ann NY Acad Sci 75:790–808, 1959

11. Caldeyro-Barcia R, Poseiro JJ: Oxytocin and contractility of the pregnant human uterus. Ann NY Acad Sci 75:813–830, 1959

12. Cunningham FG, MacDonald PC, Gant NF: Williams Obstetrics, 18th ed. Norwalk, Conn: Appleton and Lange, 1989, p 150

13. McNeilly AS, Robinson IC, Houston MJ, Howie PW: Release of oxytocin and prolactin in response to suckling. Br Med J 286:257–259, 1983

14. Huddleston JF, Sutliff G, Robinson D: Contraction stress test by intermittent nipple stimulation. Obstet Gynecol 63:669–673, 1984

15. Spielman FJ, Herbert WN: Maternal cardiovascular effects of drugs that alter uterine activity. Obstet Gynecol Surv 43:516–522, 1988

16. Kitchin AH, Lloyd SM, Pickford M: Some actions of oxytocin on the cardiovascular system in man. Clin Sci 18:399–406, 1959

17. Cunningham FG, MacDonald PC, Gant NF: Williams Obstetrics, 18th ed. Norwalk, Conn: Appleton and Lange, 1989, pp 321–322

18. Abdul-Karim R, Assali NS: Renal function in human pregnancy. V. Effects of oxytocin on renal hemodynamics and water and electrolyte excretion. J Lab Clin Med 57:522–532, 1961

19. Kruse J: Oxytocin: Pharmacology and clinical application. J Fam Pract 23:473–479, 1986

20. Brindley BA, Sokol RJ: Induction and augmentation of labor: Basis and methods for current practice. Obstet Gynecol Surv 43:730–743, 1988

21. Seitchik J, Castillo M: Oxytocin augmentation of dysfunctional labor. I. Clinical data. Am J Obstet Gynecol 144:899–905, 1982

22. Seitchik J, Castillo M: Oxytocin augmentation of dysfunctional labor. II. Uterine activity data. Am J Obstet Gynecol 145:526–529, 1983

23. Seitchik J, Castillo M: Oxytocin augmentation of dysfunctional labor. III. Multiparous patients. Am J Obstet Gynecol 145:777–780, 1983

24. Seitchik J, Amico J, Robinson AG, Castillo M: Oxytocin augmentation of dysfunctional labor. IV. Oxytocin pharmacokinetics. Am J Obstet Gynecol 150:225–228, 1984

25. Seitchik J, Amico JA, Castillo M: Oxytocin augmentation of dysfunctional labor. V. An alternative oxytocin regimen. Am J Obstet Gynecol 151:757–761, 1984

26. Seitchik J: The management of functional dystocia in the first stage of labor. Clin Obstet Gynecol 30:42–49, 1987

27. Awais GM, Lebherz TB: Ruptured uterus: A complication of oxytocin induction and high parity. Obstet Gynecol 36:465–472, 1970

28. Liston WA, Campbell AJ: Dangers of oxytocin induced labour to fetuses. Br Med J 3:606–607, 1974

29. Elbourne D, Prendiville W, Chalmers I: Choice of oxytocic preparation for routine use in the management of the third stage of labour: An overview of the evidence from controlled trials. Br J Obstet Gynaecol 95:17–30, 1988

30. Reddy VV, Carey JC: Effect of umbilical vein oxytocin on puerperal blood loss and the length of the third stage of labor. Am J Obstet Gynecol 160:206–208, 1989

31. Young SB, Martelly PD, Greb L, et al: The effect of intraumbilical oxytocin on the third stage of labor. Obstet Gynecol 71:736–738, 1988

32. Kirchhof AC, Racely CA, Wilson WM, David NA: Ergonovine-like oxytocic synthesized from lysergic acid. West J Surg 52:197–208, 1944

33. Mantyla R, Katz J: Clinical pharmacokinetics of methylergometrine (methylergonovine). Int J Clin Pharmacol Ther Toxicol 19:386–391, 1981

34. Johnstone M: The cardiovascular effects of oxytocic drugs. Br J Anaesth 44:826–834, 1972

35. Casady GN, Moore DC, Bridenbaugh LD: Postpartum hypertension after use of vasoconstrictor and oxytocic drugs. Etiology, incidence, complications, and treatment. JAMA 172:1011–1015, 1960

36. Russ JS, Rayburn WF, Samuel MJ: Uterine stimulants, in Rayburn WF, Zuspan FP (eds): Drug Therapy in Obstetrics and Gynecology. Norwalk, Conn, Appleton-Century-Crofts, 1982, p 123

37. Cunningham FG, MacDonald PC, Gant NF: Williams Obstetrics, 18th ed. Norwalk, Conn: Appleton and Lange, 1989, p 197

38. Karim SM: Clinical applications of prostaglandins in obstetrics and gynaecology. Ann Acad Med Singapore 11:493–502, 1982

39. Methods of midtrimester abortion. American College of Obstetricians and Gynecologists Technical Bulletin 109. Washington, Oct 1987

40. Bishop EH: Pelvic scoring for elective induction. Obstet Gynecol 24:266–268, 1964

41. Ulmsten U, Wingerup L, Ekman G: Local application of prostaglandin E_2 for cervical ripening or induction of term labor. Clin Obstet Gynecol 26:95–105, 1983

42. Merkatz IR, Peter JB, Barden TP: Ritodrine hydrochloride: A betamimetic agent for use in preterm labor. II. Evidence of efficacy. Obstet Gynecol 56:7–12, 1980

43. Roberts JM: Receptor and transfer of information into cells. Semin Perinatol 5:203–215, 1981

44. Roberts JM: Current understanding of pharmacologic mechanisms in the prevention of preterm birth. Clin Obstet Gynecol 27:592–605, 1984

45. Benedetti TJ: Maternal complications of parenteral β-sympathomimetic therapy for premature labor. Am J Obstet Gynecol 145:1–6, 1983

46. Young DC, Toofanian A, Leveno KJ: Potassium and glucose concentrations without treatment during ritodrine tocolysis. Am J Obstet Gynecol 145:105–106, 1983

47. Cano A, Tovar I, Parilla JJ, Abad L: Metabolic disturbances during intravenous use of ritodrine: Increased insulin levels and hypokalemia. Obstet Gynecol 65:356–360, 1985

48. Hankins GD, Hauth JC: A comparison of the relative toxicities of β-sympathomimetic tocolytic agents. Am J Perinatol 2:338–346, 1985

49. Caritis SN, Darby MJ, Chan L: Pharmacologic treatment of preterm labor. Clin Obstet Gynecol 31:635–651, 1988

50. Unpublished data from the University of Oklahoma (Dr C Carey)

51. Caritis SN, Edelstone DI, Mueller-Heubach E: Pharmacologic inhibition of preterm labor. Am J Obstet Gynecol 133:557–578, 1979

52. Cunningham FG, MacDonald PC, Gant NF: Williams Obstetrics, 18th ed. Norwalk, Conn: Appleton and Lange, 1989, pp 681–683

53. Ogburn PL, Julian TM, Williams PP, Thompson TR: The use of magnesium sulfate in preterm labor complicated by twin gestation and betamimetic induced pulmonary edema. Acta Obstet Gynaecol Scand 65:793–794, 1986

54. Martin RW, Gaddy DK, Martin JN, et al: Tocolysis with oral magnesium. Am J Obstet Gynecol 156:433–434, 1987

55. Lipsitz PJ, English IC: Hypermagnesemia in the newborn infant. Pediatrics 40:856–862, 1967

56. Sideris EB, Yokochi K, Van Helder T, et al: Effects of indomethacin and prostaglandins E_2, I_2, and D_2 on the fetal circulation. Adv Prostaglandin Thromboxane Leukotriene Res 12:477–482, 1983

57. Dudley DK, Hardie MJ: Fetal and neonatal effects of indomethacin used as a tocolytic agent. Am J Obstet Gynecol 151:181–184, 1985

58. Moise KJ, Huhta JC, Sharif DS, et al: Indomethacin in the treatment of premature labor: Effects on the fetal ductus arteriosus. N Engl J Med 319:327–331, 1988

59. Niebyl JR, Blake DA, White RD, et al: The inhibition of premature labor with indomethacin. Am J Obstet Gynecol 136:1014–1019, 1980

60. Zukerman H, Reiss U, Rubenstein I: Inhibition of human pre-

mature labor by indomethacin. Obstet Gynecol 44:787–792, 1974

61. Senden IP, Van du Witering MD, Eskes TK, et al: Labor pain: A comparison of parturients in a Dutch and an American teaching hospital. Obstet Gynecol 71:541–544, 1988
62. Kuhnert BR, Kuhnert PM, Prochaska AL, Sokol RJ: Meperidine disposition in mother, neonate and nonpregnant females. Clin Pharmacol Ther 27:486–491, 1980
63. Smedstad KG, Morrison DH: A comparative study of continuous and intermittent epidural analgesia for labor and delivery. Can J Anaesth 35:234–241, 1988
64. Chestnut DH, Owen CL, Bates JN, et al: Continuous infusion epidural analgesia during labor: A randomized study. Anesthesiology 68:754–759, 1988
65. Redick LF: Anesthesia for twin delivery. Clin Perinatol 15:107–122, 1988
66. Cunningham FG, MacDonald PC, Gant NF: Williams Obstetrics, 18th ed. Norwalk, Conn: Appleton and Lange, 1989, pp 645–646
67. Vsubiaga JE: Neurologic complications following epidural analgesia. Int Anesthesiol Clin 13:1–157, 1975
68. Holdcrott A, Morgan M: Intravenous induction agents for cesarean section. Anesthesia 44:719–720, 1989
69. MacAuley MA, Molloy WB, Charles D: Placental transfer of methicillin. Am Obstet Gynecol 115:58–65, 1973
70. Bousefield RF: Use of cefuroxime in pregnant women at term. Res Clin Forums 6:53–58, 1984
71. Srinivasan G, Seeler RA, Tiruvury A, Pildes RS: Maternal anticonvulsant therapy and hemorrhagic disease of the newborn. Obstet Gynecol 59:250–252, 1982
72. Haram K, Bakke DM, Johannessen KH, Lund T: Transplacental passage of diazepam during labor: Influence of uterine contractions. Clin Pharmacol Ther 24:590–599, 1978
73. Verstraete M: The prevention of postoperative deep venous thrombosis and pulmonary embolism with low-dose subcutaneous heparin and dextran. Surg Gynecol Obstet 143:981–985, 1976
74. Stradling JR: Heparin and infusion phlebitis. Br Med J 2:1195–1196, 1978
75. Murphy J, Peters P, Morris P, et al: Conservative management of pregnancy in diabetic women. Br Med J 288:1203–1205, 1984
76. Jovanovic L, Peterson CM: Insulin and glucose requirements during the first stage of labor in insulin-dependent diabetic women. Am J Med 75:607–612, 1983

15

FETAL PHARMACOLOGY AND THERAPY: Supraventricular Arrhythmias as an Example

EVELYNE JACQZ-AIGRAIN *and* ANNABELLE AZANCOT-BENISTY

Major progress has been made in recent years in investigating fetal disorders. Echography now allows precise diagnosis of congenital malformations such as gastrointestinal, urinary tract, and cardiac abnormalities. Diagnosis of abnormal karyotype is possible with chorion villus biopsy, amniocentesis, or fetal blood sampling. Such procedures have their own complications, but their frequency is reduced in experienced hands. The therapeutic decision of whether to carry on pregnancy or to induce abortion is obviously a matter of individual decision and differences in legislation in various countries.

The evaluation of the risk-to-benefit ratio of drug administration during pregnancy remains a challenge. This is mainly due to our lack of knowledge of physiological and pharmacological changes occurring in the fetus and the mother during pregnancy. Clinicians may deal with a large variety of maternal and fetal individual situations. The human teratogenic effects of thalidomide have been clearly demonstrated, and the use of this drug is proscribed during pregnancy.[1a] In other cases, such as vitamin A and retinoic acid, the human effects are not established, but the teratogenic effects in animal strains exclude the clinical use of this drug in pregnant women.[2a] Warfarin derivatives cross the placenta during pregnancy and can induce fetal malformations and fetal hemorrhages by competing with vitamin K. Therefore, the administration of these drugs is contraindicated during pregnancy.[3a]

In fact, apart from these drastic situations, clinicians are more frequently facing compromises: between either a mandatory maternal treatment and its potential fetal effects or the maternal and fetal side-effects when fetal treatment is required. Hypertension, life-threatening maternal arrhythmias, and epilepsy are situations where maternal therapy is required, not only for maternal reasons but also for the possible fetal consequences. Most practitioners are now aware of potential fetal risks—including teratogenic effects, fetal growth retardation, and fetal and neonatal distress. Therefore, such treatments are

associated with close monitoring of the fetus. However, long term consequences can be unpredictable: The high incidence of vaginal adenocarcinoma developing in young women exposed to stilbesterol during pregnancy is a well-known example of possible delayed side-effects of drugs administered during pregnancy.[4a]

In pregnancies complicated by premature labor, deleterious effects on the fetal and maternal heart have been described with beta-sympathicomimetic agents.[5a] Nonsteroidal anti-imflammatory agents, particularly indomethacin, may induce closure of the ductus arteriosus (although reversible with drug withdrawal and major alterations of fetal and neonatal renal function). The estimation of the risk-to-benefit ratio of these drugs is still a matter of debate, but they remain formally contraindicated in late pregnancy.[6a]

Historical examples of maternal administration of drugs for fetal treatment include the administration of penicillin for the treatment of fetal syphilis or the prenatal treatment of fetal *Toxoplasma* infection with pyrimethamine and sulfonamides, which reduces the incidence of severe congenital toxoplasmosis.[7a] Other examples could be given, such as the use of maternal administered phenobarbital in late pregnancy for its inductive effects on metabolizing enzymes, reducing hyperbilirubinemia in neonates. Recently, major improvements in investigational procedures, particularly the routine use of umbilical cord taps, has increased the diagnostic and management potentials of life-threatening fetal disorders becoming accessible to fetal treatment. Administration of intravenous gamma globulins increases the fetal platelet count in fetuses with alloimmune thrombocytopenia and reduces the risk of intracranial hemorrhage.[8a] Fetal blood transfusions are performed for the treatment of severe rhesus immunization (erythroblastosis fetalis).[9a]

Applications of fetal therapy are multiple and the list just presented cannot be exhaustive. Our choice was to present in detail the pharmacology and therapy of fetal supraventricular tachyarrhythmias. Their management

143

illustrates and demonstrates recent progress in fetal diagnosis, the improvement of our understanding of pharmacokinetics during pregnancy, and a better analysis of the risk-to-benefit ratio of drugs during pregnancy.

Recent advances in Doppler echocardiography allow the visualization of fetal cardiac anatomy and the evaluation of the mechanism and tolerance of cardiac rhythm disturbances *in utero*. Antiarrhythmic drugs are usually administered to the mother for fetal treatment. Analysis of the various studies demonstrates a large discrepancy in the choice of the antiarrhythmic drugs and their efficiency *in utero*. This is due to the lack of knowledge of (1) the interactions between the state of pregnancy and the pharmacokinetics of the antiarrhythmic drugs used and (2) the factors that affect fetal response.

ANALYSIS OF FETAL SUPRAVENTRICULAR TACHYARRHYTHMIAS

The mechanism of the fetal arrhythmia can be approached by M-mode and Doppler echocardiography demonstrating the atrioventricular contraction sequence. Cardiac tolerance is evaluated by quantitative measurements according to gestational age of cardiac diameters and by the existence of effusions. Hydrops fetalis represents the usual pattern of severe cardiac failure.[1-4] Supraventricular tachycardia can be distinguished from sinus tachycardia by the higher sustained cardiac rate (generally greater than 180 beats per minute), the lack of beat-to-beat variation, the abrupt onset and termination, and in some cases the initiation and/or termination of the arrhythmia by a premature beat. Fetal arrhythmias are either intermittent or sustained. Isolated extrasystoles are frequent, supraventricular or ventricular, and usually well tolerated, although they can be the triggering factor of a sustained arrhythmia. In most cases, ultrasound examination can clarify the mechanism of a supraventricular tachyarrhythmia. During its development, the fetal conduction system is characterized by a dynamic molding of the atrioventricular node and bundle, with inhomogeneous electrophysiologic tissue pouches predisposing to reentry or ectopic foci.[5]

The most common type is fetal reentrant tachycardias either involving the A-V node or the atrium with a 1:1 A-V conduction sequence that cannot be modified without interruption of the tachycardia (Figure 15–1). A circus movement is the electrophysiologic support for a reentering mechanism, requiring a closed conduction tissue circuit with two limbs, anterograde and retrograde, of different refractoriness. This difference between the two limbs will allow the appropriately timed atrial extrasystole to be conducted first through the less refractory one (slow pathway) and then initiate the circus movement when reaching the previously refractory limb (the fast pathway with the longest refractory period). A longitudinal dissociation of conduction fibers in the A-V node is the usual anatomic support for the reentry mechanism. Accessory conduction pathways adjacent to the A-V node can be the underlying basis for reentrant tachycardias. Anatomic bridges have been reported between the fetal atrium and ventricle.[5] The predominant cholinergic control of the fetal heart, particularly on the A-V node, may enhance bypass conduction by these accessory fibers, yielding supraventricular tachycardias and neonatal preexcitation patterns.[6] However, the diagnosis of Wolff-Parkinson-White (WPW) syndrome cannot be made *in utero* at the present time.[7,8] This diagnosis was retrospectively established in the postnatal period in 29–40 percent of prena-

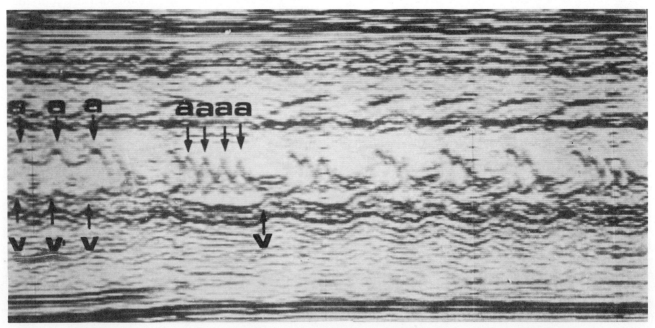

FIGURE 15–1. The atrioventricular conduction ratio is 1:1 suggesting an A-V nodal tachycardia (a, atrial systoles; v, ventricular systoles; RV, right ventricle; RA, right atrium).

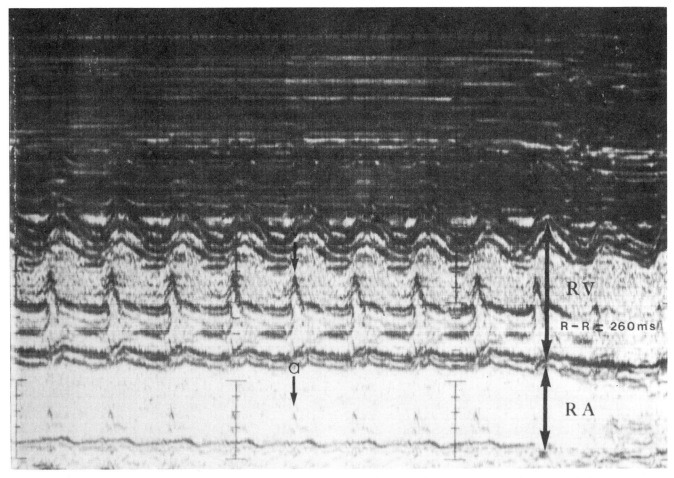

FIGURE 15–2. Atrial flutter with variable A-V conduction (a, atrial systoles; v, ventricular systoles).

tally diagnosed supraventricular tachycardias. These findings are comparable with the 50 percent reported incidence of WPW in neonatal supraventricular tachycardias.[9] Furthermore, preexcitation patterns may be a common concealed feature in normal newborns.[9] Atrial ectopic foci also can be involved, inducing atrial tachycardias with an atrioventricular 1:1 conduction ratio. Atrial fibrillation and atrial flutter according to the atrial rate are usually generated by intraatrial reentering mechanisms[10–12] (Figure 15–2). The occurrence of a second-degree A-V block either spontaneously or due to vagotonic drugs confirms the atrial origin of the tachycardia, whatever the underlying mechanism, ectopic focus or circus movement.

The actual methods of *in utero* investigations are limited, however, in their capacity to define the precise electrophysiologic mechanism of supraventricular tachyarrhythmias. An A-V nodal mechanism can be difficult or impossible to distinguish from an atrial ectopic tachycardia, a permanent reentering type from a paroxysmal. In the series reported by Maxwell et al.,[13] the diagnosis between supraventricular tachycardia and atrial flutter could not be established *in utero* in three patients. Hence diagnosis of the mechanism of the tachyarrhythmia is sometimes retrospective. Digoxin therapy or other drugs that depress the A-V node conduction may evidence a second-degree A-V block that is even transient in situa-

tions where the initial diagnosis was an A-V junctional tachycardia. Kleinman et al.[14] reported a case of 1:1 sustained tachycardia that proved, after birth, to be a ventricular tachycardia with an atrial retrograde conduction. One case of focal His-bundle tachycardia was identified postnatally.[15] Therefore, although considerable advances have been yielded by ultrasound examinations, they do not offer the diagnostic potentials of the surface electrocardiogram for identification of fetal arrhythmias. These caveats should be considered when evaluating fetal response to treatment. Cardiac malformations are present in 10–20 percent of fetuses referred for arrhythmias. In such cases, the prognosis is dependent on the severity of the underlying cardiac defect[16] and, eventually, on an abnormal karyotype.

PHYSIOLOGIC CHANGES IN PREGNANCY AND PHARMACOKINETIC CONSEQUENCES

Permanent physiologic adjustments affecting the mother, the placenta, and the fetus occur throughout pregnancy and influence the disposition of drugs. Therefore, multiple factors interfere in the fetal response to drugs during pregnancy.

Maternal Changes During Pregnancy

Pregnancy is characterized by a reduction in the rate and extent of absorption related to delayed gastric emptying and decrease mobility of the gastrointestinal tract.[17] Drug distribution is modified by the expansion of maternal fluid volumes and the increased cardiac output. In addition, significant changes in plasma composition occur during pregnancy[18]: Albumin and α_1-glycoprotein are reduced, modifying drug protein binding. The enhanced hepatic metabolism of certain drugs is related to induction of hepatic enzyme activities. Increases in renal blood flow and glomerular filtration rate were demonstrated during pregnancy. The pharmacokinetics of drugs primarily removed by renal elimination can therefore be enhanced.[19] Analysis of drug dosages during pregnancy should take into account the physiologic changes occurring during pregnancy.

Placental Transfer

The majority of drugs cross the placental barrier by simple diffusion, following their maternal-to-fetal gradient of concentration. The rate and extent of placental transfer are dependent on the physicochemical characteristics of the drug, the properties of placental tissue, and maternal and fetal parameters.[20,21]

Physicochemical Characteristics of the Drug

Molecular weight and molecular configuration influence placental transfer. Substances of molecular weight less than 600 daltons cross the placenta easily, whereas those of molecular weight between 600 and 1000 daltons have a variable and slow placental transfer and those of molecular weight over 1000 daltons do not cross the placenta at all. Lipid solubility, degree of ionization at physiologic pH, and plasma protein binding on the maternal and fetal sides of the placenta also have to be considered. Only the unbound and non-ionized drug is subjected to placental transfer. The rate of transfer is dependent on liposolubility; that is, high lipophylic substances cross the placenta readily.

Properties of Placental Tissue

The placenta undergoes major changes in thickness, surface area, and vascularization during pregnancy. In addition, the placenta is a potential organ for drug metab-

olism.[22] A variety of drug biotransformations have been observed *in vitro.* Cytochrome P-450–dependent oxidations occur at a low rate. Some of these reactions are inducible by cigarette smoking, for example. Thus the kinetics of placental drug transfer are affected by the microstructural and metabolic changes that occur throughout pregnancy.

Maternal and Fetal Parameters

Two main factors have to be considered: the plasma protein binding and the pH in the maternal and fetal compartments.[20,21] Changes in plasma protein binding influence the total concentration of a drug, whereas changes in pH affect the concentration of the free fraction of a drug. Plasma protein binding of drugs has been studied during the neonatal period. The binding of drugs, with few exceptions, is less extensive in neonates than in their mothers. During fetal life, the concentration of plasma proteins progressively increases, but it remains lower than maternal concentration in particular for glycoproteins. The fetal pH is slightly lower than the maternal pH. Therefore, the concentration of drugs with an alkaline pH will be higher in the fetal compartment. Changes in maternal or fetal pH will affect drug transfer. In addition, the maternal and fetal blood flows through the placenta determine the amount of drug locally available for placental transfer. Impaired uteroplacental blood flow is expected to alter the rapid flow-dependent transfer of highly lipophylic and non-ionized drugs.

Fetal Pharmacokinetics

Our knowledge of the factors affecting the distribution, elimination, and pharmacologic activity of a drug in the fetus is limited because such parameters are obviously difficult to study. The fetal compartment undergoes constant changes associated with growth and development. The disposition of drugs in the fetus is affected by the characteristics of the fetal circulation. Umbilical blood flow bypasses the liver in proportions ranging from 8–92 percent, the pulmonary circulation is reduced, whereas the central nervous system, the myocardium, and the placenta are vascularized preferentially. Fetal drug metabolism has been exclusively investigated *in vitro.* The enzymatic activities found in the human fetal liver are reduced and are almost insensitive to induction. Renal excretion of drugs into the amniotic fluid may lead to drug accumulation. In addition, ontogenesis of receptor binding capacities and activities is almost unknown.

Pharmacokinetic mathematical models have been designed to describe the fetal–maternal unit. They are either simple, using monocompartmental models, or complex, using multicompartmental models. They are used to simulate the pharmacokinetic disposition of drugs during pregnancy and to contribute to the interpretation of experimental data.[23]

PHARMACOKINETICS OF ANTIARRHYTHMIC DRUGS DURING PREGNANCY

The pharmacokinetic parameters of antiarrhythmic drugs during pregnancy[24] were in most cases determined during treatment for maternal cardiac diseases. Data on the effects of antiarrhythmic agents on the fetus are limited by ethical and practical considerations and thus are incomplete.

Digoxin

Digoxin is a polar digitalis glycoside. Its pharmacokinetics in adults have been extensively investigated.[25] After oral administration, digoxin is 75–85 percent absorbed, with an enterohepatic recycling of about 5 percent of the administered dose. It is 20–40 percent protein bound. The drug is mainly eliminated unchanged by the kidneys. In adults, its elimination half-life is between 1 and 2 days. Skeletal muscle receptor binding is a major determinant of digoxin blood level. Therapeutic serum levels of digoxin at steady state are 0.5–2 ng/ml, and toxic levels are over 3 ng/ml. However, overlap has been reported, with toxicity occurring at digoxin levels within the therapeutic range.[25]

The pharmacokinetics of digoxin during pregnancy were first investigated during maternal treatment. During standard maintenance therapy, the serum concentrations of digoxin were lower in pregnant than in nonpregnant women. With knowledge of the physiologic changes occurring during pregnancy, digoxin disposition should be affected by modifications of renal excretion and, if administered orally, by poor and erratic absorption.[26] Digoxin crosses readily the placenta.[27] The fetal-to-mater-nal ratio of digoxin at birth was reported to be 60–100 percent (Table 15–1). No major adverse effects of digoxin treatment during pregnancy have been reported in the fetus or newborn; in particular, digoxin is not teratogenic in humans. However, the efficacy of digoxin in the fetus, in the first half of gestation, has been questioned based on limited binding capacities to digoxin.[27] The levels of therapeutic concentrations and the placental transfer of digoxin during pregnancy should probably be reexamined in view of recent publications on endogenous digoxin-like immunoreactive substances interacting with antidigitalis antibodies.[28,29] It is possible to minimize such interferences in specific immunoassays. However, significant concentrations, reaching therapeutic levels, were described in the absence of digoxin administration in pregnant women and neonates at birth. Although recent studies outline the presence of endogenous digoxin-like immunoreactive substances in the fetal circulation, their pharmacologic activity has still to be investigated.[30] Their concentration is additive to the true digoxin levels, and their level in the maternal circulation should be determined before initiating digoxin therapy in order to allow maternal digoxin monitoring during pregnancy.

β-Adrenergic-Blocking Agents

Propranolol has been widely used during pregnancy for the treatment of maternal diseases such as hypertension, thyrotoxicosis, and subaortic stenosis.[31,32] It has been reported to be relatively safe for the mother and without teratogenic effects. Sotalol was studied during pregnancy because of its low lipid solubility and its absence of hepatic metabolism. Its pharmacokinetics are markedly altered during pregnancy: Clearance is increased, with no changes in the apparent volume of distribution. As a

TABLE 15–1. RECOMMENDED DOSES AND PLACENTAL TRANSFER OF COMMONLY USED ANTIARRHYTHMIC AGENTS

DRUG	Route	USUAL DOSES Initial (mg)	Maintenance (mg)	TRANSPLACENTAL TRANSFER Fetal–Maternal Ratio	References
Digoxin	I.V.	0.5–2	0.25/24 h	0.6–1	52,53,54,55,56
	P.O.	1–2.5	0.25–0.75/24 h	<0.4	42,53,57,58
Propranolol	P.O.	80–160 q6–8 h	40–120 q6–8 h	0.1–0.3 1	34,52,58
Sotalol	P.O.	—	300/24 h	0.8–1	34,36
Verapamil	I.V.	5–10		<0.25	59
	P.O.		80–120 q6–8 h	0.3–0.4	52
Procainamide	P.O.	—		0.8–1.3	42,52
			300 q4–6 h	<0.3	60
Quinidine	P.O.	—	800–2000/24 h	0.25–0.95	53
Amiodarone	P.O.	800–1600/24 h	200–600/24 h	0.16 0.3	15,61 62
Flecainide	P.O.	150–300/24 h	75–150/24 h	0.6–0.8	63,64

Note: The recommended doses of the antiarrhythmic drugs are presented. The transplacental data are derived from the different studies reported in the literature, as indicated in the references column.

result, its elimination half-life is shorter.[33] Both nonselective (propranolol and sotalol) and selective (metoprolol and atenolol) agents cross the placenta. Conflicting reports have been published on the placental transfer of propranolol measured at birth[34,35] (see Table 15–1). In our experience, it is less than 50 percent. Sotalol crosses the placenta readily.[34,36] Therapeutic concentrations are difficult to define because of the absence of correlation between blood concentrations and antiarrhythmic effects. A number of adverse effects on the fetus have been reported after maternal administration of propranolol. They include intrauterine growth retardation, neonatal bradycardia and hypoglycemia, and poor neonatal adaptation to stress.[32,37] Alterations in neonatal renal function were demonstrated with acebutolol and betaxolol given for maternal hypertension.

Quinidine

Quinidine is rapidly absorbed, highly protein bound, and extensively metabolized by the liver to potentially active compounds. The disposition during pregnancy may therefore be altered by changes in maternal protein concentrations and hepatic metabolism.[38] The rate of metabolism of quinidine to 3-hydroxyquinidine is subject to interindividual variations, a fast hepatic metabolism yielding a 3-hydroxyquinidine/quinidine ratio greater than 0.5. This may be associated with quinidine toxicity. Quinidine crosses the placenta; cord blood levels to maternal blood levels vary from 25–94 percent. Unexplained high concentrations in amniotic fluid have been reported.[38,40] The recommended therapeutic concentrations range from 2–5 μg/ml. Monitoring of maternal concentrations of quinidine and its major metabolite during pregnancy is necessary using adequate assays to avoid adverse effects. Fetal thrombocytopenia and intrauterine death have been reported, adding to the potential deleterious effects of the use of this drug in pregnancy.[39]

Procainamide

Procainamide is a small, weak-base molecule that is poorly protein bound and has a rapid renal elimination. Its elimination half-life is 3.5 hours, requiring high and frequent oral doses. In addition, it is metabolized to an active compound: N-acetylprocainamide. The therapeutic concentration recommended is 4–8 μg/ml for procainamide and 8–20 μg/ml for the metabolite. These drugs cross the placenta. However, conflicting reports on the amount of placental transfer have been published (see Table 15–1), suggesting the presence of a "deep fetal compartment" where the drug could accumulate as a result of lower fetal clearance.[41] Fetal–maternal concentration ratios reaching 1.4 have been reported for the drug and metabolite.[42,43] Additional studies are needed to understand the pharmacokinetics of this drug during pregnancy and to avoid fetal and neonatal adverse effects resulting from its accumulation. Procainamide should not be included in the routine protocol for fetal arrhythmias.

Verapamil

After oral administration, verapamil is submitted to a high first-past metabolism, and its bioavailability is 20 percent. The peak concentration occurs in 1–3 hours. The drug is highly protein bound. The major metabolite is an active compound: norverapamil. The elimination half-life of verapamil is 3–7 hours. Therapeutic blood levels are variable, usually 80–400 ng/ml. The I.V. route is not recommended because of the risk of maternal hypotension and sudden fetal death. Negative inotropic effects, although counterbalanced by arteriolar dilatation, have to be taken into account in the presence of fetal cardiac failure. The placental transfer is less than 50 percent (see Table 15–1). Verapamil has been extensively used as a tocolytic agent in Europe with no teratogenic effect for the newborn.[44] Verapamil may be a second-choice drug in the therapeutic management of fetal arrhythmias.

Amiodarone

Amiodarone is a lipid-soluble molecule that is highly protein bound and whose disposition is characterized by accumulation in tissues, resulting in a very large volume of distribution and a very long half-life (25–110 days).[45] Amiodarone is eliminated by the bilary tract, the skin, and the lacrimal glands. The metabolite desethylamiodarone is pharmacologically active. In addition, amiodarone contains 75 mg iodine per 200 mg and may be responsible for thyroid dysfunction.[46] Fetal–maternal concentration ratios of amiodarone and desethylamiodarone are, in our experience, less than 0.3 (see Table 15–1). Therapeutic concentration may range from 1.0–2.5 μg/ml. Neonatal hypothyroidism and goiter were reported after maternal administration of amiodarone during pregnancy.[47,48] Such pharmacokinectic parameters and potential adverse effects are limiting factors for its chronic use during pregnancy, at least as a first-choice drug.

Flecainide

The drug absorption of flecainide is rapid and extensive, with a bioavailability reaching 95 percent. Flecainide hepatic metabolism is under genetic control and yields inactive metabolites.[45] Mean elimination half-life is 12 hours in adults and shorter in children.[49,50] Recommended plasma trough levels range from 0.2–1.0 μg/ml. Arrhythmias induced by flecainide are more frequent in adults than in infants without underlying heart disease and are often related to the presence of preexisting ventricular dysfunction that can be precipitated by flecainide.[51] The use of flecainide during pregnancy was recently reported in the literature. The drug crosses the placenta, and the fetal–maternal concentration ratio at birth was greater than 0.6 (see Table 15–1). From our point of view, flecainide should not be administered for fetal arrhythmias as a first-choice drug.

Antiarrhythmic Drug Interactions

Significant drug interactions have been reported between the antiarrhythmic drugs currently used in the treatment of fetal supraventricular arrhythmias. The interaction of amiodarone and quinidine with digoxin is well established.[44,65,66] In both cases, the serum digoxin concentration rises significantly within 24 hours after administration of the second drug. Renal clearance of digoxin decreases in the presence of quinidine. The mechanism of digoxin–amiodarone interaction is only speculative and could also be related to alterations in the renal elimination of digoxin.[66] The dose of digoxin should be reduced and digoxin concentrations should be monitored when it is used in association with these drugs. Interactions between digoxin and verapamil, procainamide, and flecainide have been reported. They seem of minor clinical significance. No pharmacokinetic interactions have been described between propranolol and the other antiarrhythmic drugs.[67]

THERAPEUTIC MANAGEMENT OF FETAL SUPRAVENTRICULAR ARRHYTHMIAS

The Therapeutic Decision

The incidence of fetal tachyarrhythmias is between 1 in 10,000 and 1 in 25,000 pregnancies but is probably underestimated. The detection of a rapid or irregular rhythm or a hydrops fetalis during routine obstetrical ultrasound examination is the usual referral diagnosis. The decision to treat or not to treat is a compromise between the potential threat of the tachyarrhythmia for fetal outcome and the side effects of fetal and maternal exposure to drugs. The lack of random, double-blind studies, for obvious ethical reasons, jeopardizes our knowledge of the natural history of fetal arrhythmias. Isolated extrasystoles are often well tolerated; nonetheless, in a few reported cases, permanent arrhythmias developed.[14] Spontaneous conversion of a sustained supraventricular tachyarrhythmia to sinus rhythm may occur, as in the neonatal period, if the maturational molding of the A-V node is completed *in utero.*[9] However, we and others[14] have observed that cardiac failure can occur within hours in situations where a "wait and see" policy had been initially proposed. Hydrops fetalis, the advanced stage of fetal cardiac failure, has been found in about 70 percent of the fetal tachyarrhythmias. Whether the underlying mechanism of the arrhythmia influences the occurrence of hydrops fetalis is still a matter of dispute.

Conversely, ultrasound monitoring data suggest the potential deleterious effects of sustained and protracted tachyarrhythmias on the human fetal heart mechanics. The rate dependency of normal fetal ventricular filling is demonstrated on the A-V flow wave pattern by a predom-inant *a* wave, active filling, which will tend to disappear during the shortened diastole. Valvular regurgitations and reversal of flow in the inferior vena cava are constant findings in sustained fetal tachyarrhythmias.

Each fetal supraventricular tachyarrhythmia should be evaluated, taking into account the gestational age and lung maturity, hemodynamic status, and the mechanism of the arrhythmia. A sustained supraventricular tachyarrhythmia occurring at an early gestational age, even in the absence of hydrops fetalis, should be treated to avoid cardiac decompensation and/or the risks of prematurity. In contrast, *in utero* treatment of a hydropic fetus near term may be irrelevant, and delivery may be preferred. An incomplete therapeutic result and fetal survival are preferable to a fetal death after a successful conversion that required chronic maintenance on a myocardial depressing drug. In all cases, our policy is to begin maternal and fetal treatment as an inpatient in a specialized center that can provide continuous obstetrical and hemodynamic maternal and fetal monitoring.

The therapeutic management of fetal supraventricular tachyarrhythmias varies in the large series reported in the literature.[13,14,52,68] In addition, numerous case reports have been published. Kleinman et al.[14] reported fetal arrhythmias in 21 fetuses: 16 had supraventricular tachycardias, 3 had atrial flutter, and 2 had atrial fibrillation. Eighteen presented hydrops fetalis. The treatment *in utero* succeeded in reducing the arrhythmia in 17 cases (81 percent): 8 received digoxin alone, 2 received digoxin and propranolol, and 7 received digoxin and verapamil. One was delivered at 39 weeks' gestation, before treatment, and one was only partially controlled. Two, presenting an atrial flutter, were stillborn. The series reported by Maxwell et al.[13] included 23 fetuses: 12 had supraventricular tachycardia, 8 had atrial flutter, and 3 had supraventricular tachycardia or atrial flutter. Half of them were hydropic at the time of diagnosis. Fetal treatment was instituted in 22 patients: 7 received digoxin alone and 15 received digoxin and verapamil. Conversion to sinus rhythm was obtained in 14 cases (60 percent): 7 hydropic and 7 nonhydropic fetuses. However, Maxwell et al.[13] reported 2 deaths and 5 severe complications due to prematurity.

In our series,[62] including 14 cases of permanent supraventricular tachyarrhythmia, 7 had supraventricular tachycardias and 7 presented with atrial flutter. Heart failure or hydrops fetalis was noted in 8 cases. Treatment was instituted in all patients: 5 received digoxin alone, 5 received digoxin and amiodarone, and 2 received digoxin, propranolol, and flecainide after failure of digoxin alone. Conversion *in utero* was achieved in 10 cases (71 percent). No fetal deaths occurred, and delivery occurred at 37 weeks or more in 13 cases.

First-Choice Treatment: Administration of Digoxin

In addition to its positive inotropic properties, digoxin slows the sinus node and A-V nodal conduction and prolongs the A-V refractory period by parasympathetic activation. In junctional A-V reciprocating tachycardia, digoxin blocks the anterograde nodal conduction and prolongs the refractory period in the anterograde direction. In cases of accessory pathway with anterograde preexcitation, digoxin shortens the refractory period of the bypass tract; this effect, in conjunction with the A-V node depression, formally contraindicates the use of digoxin to avoid the potential risk of atrial fibrillation inducing ventricular fibrillation. In the majority of cases in the literature, digoxin was administered to the mother for fetal treatment as the drug of first choice. Various dosage regimens have been reported. The treatment was usually initiated using a loading dose either intravenously or orally. The doses ranged from 0.250–2 mg/day. High doses were maintained during the first days of treatment. If conversion to sinus rhythm was obtained, a maintenance dose ranging from 0.250–0.750 mg/day was administered to prevent recurrence. Otherwise, digoxin was used in association with other antiarrhythmic drugs. Conversion was obtained with digoxin administered alone in an important number of cases.[54–56,69–72]

The results obtained in our series with digoxin alone are comparable with those of the other reported series. In our population,[62] digoxin was successful alone in 5 of 14 cases (36 percent): 4 junctional tachycardias and 1 atrial flutter. Kleinman et al.[14] obtained *in utero* control with digoxin alone in 7 of 21 cases (33 percent): 6 supraventricular tachycardias and 1 atrial fibrillation. The presence of cardiac decompensation and hydrops fetalis may play a role in the therapeutic response. In particular, placental edema may modify placental transfer and fetal disposition of digoxin. The fetal–maternal concentration ratio of digoxin decreased to 0.30 in the presence of severe hydrops fetalis.[57] The modalities of digoxin administration are determinant. As previously stated, the pharmacokinetics of digoxin are markedly modified during pregnancy. Poor and erratic absorption is associated with enhanced renal elimination. We demonstrated a 50 percent increase in the plasma clearance of digoxin at 33 weeks' gestation, associated with a reduction in plasma half-life. Therefore, high loading doses of digoxin administered intravenously would rapidly achieve adequate digoxin levels. The delay for fetal response was shorter after intravenous than after oral administration of digoxin.[57] A longer duration of treatment may be necessary to achieve conversion to sinus rhythm if hydrops fetalis is present. Maternal therapeutic levels may be ineffective in the fetus. The presence and significance of digoxin-like substances have been discussed previously. In addition, fetal cardiac receptors are suspected of low sensitivity to digoxin, and neonates and fetuses may require and tolerate higher digoxin concentrations than adults. However, transplacental therapy is always limited by maternal tolerance.

Other antiarrhythmic agents were administered alone as first-choice drugs. Propranolol[58] succeeded in reducing fetal supraventricular tachycardia at 34 weeks' gestation, whereas procainamide failed[52] and toxic effects developed with quinidine.[40]

Combination of Digoxin with Another Antiarrhythmic Agent

Another antiarrhythmic drug was used in association with digoxin either at the beginning of the fetal treatment or subsequently when digoxin was estimated to be ineffective in reducing the fetal arrhythmia. In the latter situation, the delay before initiating the association therapy could be a major issue. In the case reports with partial conversion to sinus rhythm with digoxin alone, it may be possible that digoxin would have achieved control of the arrhythmia if given at higher doses or for a longer period.[60]

Association of Digoxin with β-Blockers

β-Blockers, mainly propranolol and sotalol, in association with digoxin produced discrepant results. Like digoxin, propranolol inhibits and slows A-V nodal conduction and increases the refractory period on anterograde circuit conduction. The drug was administered orally at doses ranging from 100–600 mg/day or sometimes intravenously. Conversion to sinus rhythm occurred in a few cases. In one of them, hydrops fetalis was present.[73] We observed partial conversion to sinus rhythm in two cases of supraventricular tachycardia with administration of digoxin and propranolol.[74] Limited success also was reported by others.[14,60,75,76]

Sotalol is a β-blocker with electrophysiologic properties similar to amiodarone (class III compound) that prolongs the action potential duration and thus the QT interval without modifying conduction. QT prolongation may precipitate torsades de pointes. Sotalol was administered orally at doses ranging from 160–320 mg/day. As reported with propranolol, limited successes were observed.[72,77]

Association of Digoxin with Amiodarone

Amiodarone, a class III compound, prolongs the action potential duration and thus the effective refractory period, and it is also active on the bypass tract. This drug presents a certain β-blocking and calcium-antagonist effect that inhibits A-V activity. The multiple facets of amiodarone explain its efficiency in the treatment of junctional reentrant tachycardia, WPW syndrome, paroxysmal atrial flutter, and atrial fibrillation.

Amiodarone is usually administered orally. The loading doses range from 800–1600 mg/day, and maintenance doses range from 200–600 mg/day. In rare cases, amiodarone is administered intravenously to the mother or directly to the fetus. In our experience, amiodarone was administered after failure of digoxin in five cases.[62,74] Conversion to sinus rhythm was obtained in two of the five cases. At the time of conversion, maternal toxicity (nausea, vomiting, and in one case first-degree A-V block) was associated with maternal digoxin levels over 3 ng/ml. Both the time course of drug response (5 days after initiation of therapy) and the high digoxin levels raise doubt about which drug was really responsible for the therapeutic effect.

Fetal–maternal concentration ratios of amiodarone and desethylamiodarone were consistent with previously reported values. Neonatal levels of amiodarone were about 10 percent of maternal levels (see Table 15–1). Neonatal hypothyroidism complicating maternal administration of amiodarone during pregnancy was reported in the literature. It was observed in one of our five cases and was not related to a high cumulative dose. The combination of digoxin and amiodarone has been used with success.[78] However, in most cases, amiodarone was the third[73] or fourth[79] drug administered. In view of our experience with amiodarone, it seems difficult to analyze the proper effect of amiodarone and the possible synergistic effects of the drugs administered.

Association of Digoxin with Verapamil

Verapamil is a calcium antagonist that inhibits the slow calcium channel in the A-V node, increases A-V block, and prolongs the effective refractory period of the A-V node. Verapamil also inhibits conduction of the anterograde pathway of the reentrant circuit. It is usually administered in combination with digoxin as a second-choice drug at doses of 80–360 mg/day orally. The association succeeded in reducing either supraventricular tachycardias or atrial flutters, complicated in some cases of hydrops fetalis.[13,14,59] Fetal deaths have been reported with the use of intravenous verapamil in fetuses with supraventricular tachycardias, in one case with direct cord injection.[80] The possible explanations were cardiac decompensation or complete heart block. The I.V. route should be avoided.

Association of Digoxin with Procainamide or with Quinidine

Reports on the use of type I antiarrhythmic agents for the treatment of fetal tachyarrhythmias are limited. These drugs inhibit the fast sodium channel, phase 0 of the action potential, increase the action potential duration, and slow depolarization, phase 4. They inhibit the retrograde conduction pathway (fast limb) of the A-V nodal or bypass tract WPW reentrant tachycardias. Quinidine versus procainamide demonstrates a vagolytic effect that can induce tachycardia and a more pronounced effect on the QT interval. Procainamide was used either orally[14] or intravenously.[60] Discrepancy in fetal response could be related, at least partially, to the variability of maternal procainamide levels, which were either four times higher[60] or lower[43] than fetal levels. Quinidine also succeeded in reducing fetal arrhythmias in a few reported cases.[53,81]

Flecainide

Flecainide is a class IC agent that slows His-Purkinje conduction and prolongs the QRS interval. Conduction is prolonged in the fast A-V nodal pathway and bypass tract by flecainide acetate. This powerful drug demonstrates two major drawbacks, a negative inotropic property and proarrythmic effects, which require low initial oral doses and careful monitoring of the QRS interval and serum levels. It has been introduced recently in the treatment of fetal supraventricular arrhythmias. In the first case reports, flecainide was administered after failure of first-choice drugs such as digoxin.[82,83] Recently, Allan[63] reported the use of this drug as a first-choice treatment in nine fetuses with hydrops fetalis. Flecainide was administered at a dose of 300 mg daily with a conversion to sinus rhythm in eight cases. In our experience,[74] flecainide was given in two cases of atrial tachycardia after failure of digoxin administered intravenously to the mother for 5 days. In one case complicated with pericardial effusion, low doses of digoxin were maintained. In both cases, flecainide administered orally at the dose of 150 mg daily converted the arrhythmia to sinus rhythm in less than 4 days and was maintained at the dose of 75 and 50 mg daily until the end of pregnancy[74] with favorable neonatal outcomes. From these preliminary results, flecainide may appear as a promising drug for the treatment of life-threatening fetal arrhythmias resistant to other medications. However, as stated earlier, caution should be exercised in the presence of fetal cardiac failure. Further studies are necessary to codify its use for fetal treatment.

New Issues in Fetal Therapy: Should We Use Fetal Invasive Procedures?

Fetuses with sustained supraventricular arrhythmias are in high-risk situations exposed to hydrops fetalis and fetal death. The rationale adopted by specialized centers consists of the use of a physiologic route to treat the fetus, the transplacental transfer of antiarrhythmic agents administered to the mother. The mother's consent is a preliminary for the institution of treatment. Administration of these potent drugs requires not only hospitalization for close monitoring of the fetus and the mother, but also moral and psychological support of the parents in a situation that appears to them unexpected, heavy, and compromised. When reviewing the large series in the literature, although each of us can recall one or more hydropic fetuses that failed to respond to treatment, results appear in most cases to come up to our expectations. Should we proceed to direct fetal treatment (multiple cord, intramuscular, and intraperitoneal injections[83,84]) either to correct the fetal problems or to evaluate fetal pharmacokinetics? The rationale espoused by the advocates of the invasive fetal procedures is based on the following: (1) maternal toxicity is a limiting factor that hampers drug efficiency; (2) the important flow and edematous placental changes occurring during fetal hydrops influence transplacental transfer of antiarrhythmic agents; and (3) fetal heart failure modifies fetal response to antiarrhythmic drugs. These difficulties are generally encountered during the management of fetal arrhythmias. The question is whether invasive procedures, while solving some of these difficulties (1 and 2), will not create other threats to the fetus. Cordocentesis and all invasive fetal procedures, particularly when repeated, as in this situation, can be associated with severe fetal complications, even in the most experienced hands.[85] Direct fetal injections are hazardous precisely because of the lack of knowledge about the pharmacokinetics of fetal anti-arrhythmic drugs. In fact, the choice of the adequate conditions for investigating the fetus as an "object of therapy" is an ethical issue. Diagnostic and therapeutic clinical and basic research protocols should be designed so as to conduct these studies in experienced and specialized centers where opportunities to gather data are offered, avoiding hasty conclusions from sporadically reported cases.

REFERENCES

1a. Newman CG: The thalidomide syndrome: Risks of exposure and spectrum of malformations. Clin Perinatol 3:555–573, 1986
2a. Teratology Society Position Paper: Recommendations for Vitamin A use during pregnancy. Teratology 35:269–275, 1987
3a. Holzgreve W, Carey JO, Hall BD: Warfarin induced fetal abnormalities. Lancet 2:794, 1976
4a. Herbst AL, Ulfelder H, Poskanzer DC: Adenocarcinoma of the vagina. Association of stilbestrol therapy with tumor appearance in young women. N Engl J Med 284:878–881, 1971
5a. Svenningen NW: Follow-up studies on preterm infants after maternal beta receptor agonist treatment. Acta Obstet Gynecol Scand (Suppl.) 108:67–70, 1982
6a. Niebyl JR, Witten FR: Neonatal outcome after indomethacin treatment for preterm labor. Am J Obstet Gynecol 155:747–752, 1987
7a. Hohlfeld P, Daffos F, Thulliez P, Aufrant C, Couvreur J, McAleese J, Descombey D, Forestier F: Fetal toxoplasmosis. Outcome of pregnancy and infant follow-up after in utero treatment. J Ped 115(5):765–769, 1989
8a. Rodeck CH, Nicolaides KH, Warsof SL, Fysh WJ, Gamsu HR, Kemp JR: The management of severe rhesus isoimmunisation by foetoscopic intravascular transfusions. Am J Obstet Gynecol 150:769–774, 1984
9a. Bussel JB, Berkowitz RL, McFarland JG, Lynch L, Chitkara U: Antenatal treatment of neonatal alloimmune thrombocytopenia. N Engl J Med 319:1374–1378, 1988
1. Kleinman CS, Donnerstein RL, Jaffe CC, et al: Fetal echocardiography: A tool for evaluation of in utero cardiac arrhythmias and monitoring of in utero therapy. Analysis of 71 patients. Am J Cardiol 51:237–243, 1983
2. Allan LD, Anderson RH, Sullivan ID, et al: Evaluation of fetal arrhythmias by echography. Br Heart J 50:240–245, 1983
3. Crowley DC, Dick M, Rayburn WF, Rosenthal A: Two-dimensional and M-mode echographic evaluation of fetal arrhythmias. Clin Cardiol 8:1–10, 1985
4. Kleinman CS, Donnerstein RL, Devore GR, et al: Fetal echography for evaluation of in utero congestive heart failure: A technique for study of nonimmune fetal hydrops. N Engl J Med 306:568–575, 1982
5. Swartwout JR, Campbell WE Jr, Williams LG: Observations on the fetal heart rate. Am J Obstet Gynecol 82:301–303, 1961
6. Friedman WJ, Pool PE, Jacobowitz D: Sympathetic innervation of the developing rabbit heart. Circ Res 23:25–32, 1968
7. Belhassen B, Pauzner D, Blieden L, et al: Intrauterine and postnatal atrial fibrillation in the Wolff-Parkinson-White syndrome. Circulation 66:1124–1128, 1982
8. Johnson WH, Dunnigan A, Fehr P, Woodrow Benson D Jr: Association of atrial flutter with orthodromic reciprocating fetal tachycardia. Am J Cardiol 59:374–375, 1987
9. Wolff GS, Han J, Curran J: Wolff-Parkinson-White syndrome in the Neonate. Am J Obstet Gynecol 41:559–562, 1978
10. Gillette PC: The mechanism of supraventricular tachycardia in children. Circulation 54:133–139, 1976

11. Garson A Jr: Supraventricular tachycardia, in Gillette PC, Garson A (eds): Pediatric Cardiac Dysrrhythmias. Orlando, Fla, Grune & Stratton, 1981, pp 77–120
12. Zales VR, Dunnigan A, Benson DW: Clinical and electrophysiologic features of fetal and neonatal paroxysmal atrial tachycardia resulting in congestive heart failure. Am J Cardiol 62:225–228, 1988
13. Maxwell DJ, Crawford DC, Curry PVM, et al: Obstetric importance, diagnosis and management of fetal tachycardias. Br Med J 297:107–110, 1988
14. Kleinman CS, Copel JA, Weinstein EM, et al: In utero diagnosis and treatment of fetal supraventricular tachycardia. Semin Perinatol 9:113–129, 1985
15. Fermont L: Recherche, identification, pronostic et traitement des troubles du rythme et de la conduction chez le foetus, in Doin (ed): Troubles du Rythme Cardiaque chez l'Enfant. 1987, pp 37–54
16. Kleinman CS, Hobbins JC, Jaffe CC, et al: Echocardiographic studies of the human fetus: Prenatal diagnosis of congenital heart disease and cardiac dysrrhythmias. Pediatrics 65:1059–1067, 1980
17. Prescott LF: Drug absorption interactions—Gastric emptying, in Morselli P, Cohen SN, Garattini S (eds): Drug Interactions. New York, Raven Press, 1973, pp 11–20
18. Haram K, Augensen K, Elsayed S: Serum protein pattern in normal pregnancy with special reference to acute-phase reactants. Br J Obstet Gynecol 90:139–145, 1983
19. Davidson JM: The urinary system, in Hytten FE, Chamberlain G (eds): Clinical Physiology in Obstetrics. Oxford, England, Blackwell, 1980, pp 289–327
20. McKercher HG, Radde IC: Placental transfer of drugs and fetal pharmacology, in McLeod SM, Radde IC (eds): Textbook of Pediatric Clinical Pharmacology. Littleton, Massachusetts, PSG Publishing Company, 1985, pp 293–307
21. Notarianni LJ: Plasma protein binding of drugs in pregnancy and in neonates. Clin Pharmacokinet 18:20–36, 1990
22. Juchau MR, Pedersen MG, Fantel AG, Shepard TH: Drug metabolism by the placenta. Clin Pharmacol Ther 14:673–679, 1974
23. Krauer B, Krauer F: Drug kinetics in pregnancy. Clin Pharmacokinet 2:167–181, 1977
24. Rotmensch HH, Elkayam U, Frishman W: Antiarrhythmic drug therapy during pregnancy. Ann Intern Med 98:487–497, 1983
25. Doherty JE: Digitalis glycosides: Pharmacokinetics and their clinical implications. Ann Intern Med 79:229–238, 1973
26. Rogers MC, Willerson JT, Goldblatt A, Smith TW: Serum digoxin concentrations in the fetus, neonate and infant. N Engl J Med 287:1010–1013, 1972
27. Saarikoski S: Placental transfer and fetal uptake of ³H-digoxin in humans. Br J Obstet Gynaecol 83:879–884, 1976
28. Gonzales AR, Phelps SJ, Cochran EB, Sibai BM: Digoxin-like immunoreactive substance in pregnancy. Am J Obstet Gynecol 157:660–664, 1987.
29. Guedeney X, Scherrmann JM, Chanez C, Bourre JM: Les composés digitaliques endogènes ou "digoxin-like": Impacts physiopathologiques, analytiques et pharmacocinétiques. Therapie 43:165–173, 1988
30. Weiner CP, Landas S, Persoon TJ: Digoxin-like immunoreactive substance in fetuses with and without cardiac pathology. Am J Obstet Gynecol 157:368–371, 1978
31. Ekialou DL, Silverberg DS, Reisen E, et al: Propranolol for the treatment of hypertension in pregnancy. Br J Obstet Gynaecol 85:431–436, 1978
32. Rubin PC: Beta-blockers in pregnancy. N Engl J Med 305:1323–1325, 1981
33. O'Hare MF, Leahey W, Murnaghan GA, McDevitt DG: Pharmacokinetics of sotalol during pregnancy. Eur J Clin Pharmacol 24:521–524, 1983
34. Erkkola R, Lammintausta R, Liukko P, Antiila M: Transfer of propranolol and sotalol across the human placenta: Their effect on maternal and fetal plasma renin activity. Acta Obstet Gynaecol Scand 61:31–34, 1982
35. Cottril CM, McAllister A, Gettes CG, Noonan JA: Propranolol therapy during pregnancy evidence for transplacental transfer. Pediatrics 91:812–814, 1977
36. Aujard Y, de Crepy A, Azancot-Benisty A, et al: Clinical use and

pharmacokinetics of sotalol in the fetus and newborn, in Fetal Cardiac Symposium, Paris, September 10–12, 1989

37. Gladstone GR, Hordof A, Gersony WM: Propranolol administration during pregnancy: Effects on the fetus. J Pediatr 86:962–966, 1975

38. Bowers MD, Nelson KM, Connor R, et al: Evidence supporting 3(S)-3-hydroquinidine associated cardiotoxicity. Ther Drug Monit 7:308–312, 1985

39. Hill LM, Malkasian GD: The use of quinidine sulfate throughout pregnancy. Obstet Gynecol 54:366–368, 1979

40. Killeen AA, Bowers LD: Fetal supraventricular tachycardia treated with high-dose quinidine: Toxicity associated with marked elevation of the metabolite 3(S)-3-hydroxyquinidine. Obstet Gynecol 70:445–449, 1987

41. Zapata-Diaz J, Cabrera EC, Mendez R: An experimental and clinical study on the effects on procainamide (Pronestyl) on the heart. Am Heart J 43:854–870, 1952

42. Given BD, Phillipe M, Sanders SP, Dzau VJ: Procainamide cardioversion of fetal supraventricular tachyarrhythmia. Am J Cardiol 53:1460–1461, 1984

43. Lima JJ, Kuritzky PM, Schentag JJ, Jusko WJ: Fetal uptake and neonatal disposition of procainamide and its acetylated metabolite: A case report. Pediatrics 61:491–493, 1978

44. Strigl R, Pfeiffer U, Erhardt W, Blumel G: Does the administration of the calcium antagonist verapamil in tocolysis with beta-sympathomimetics make sense? J Perinatal Med 9:235–239, 1981

45. Gillis AM, Kates RE: Clinical pharmacokinetics of the newer antiarrhythmic agents. Clin Pharmacokinet 9:375–403, 1984

46. Vrobel TR, Miller PE, Mostow ND, Rakita L: A general overview of amiodarone toxicity: Its prevention, detection, and management. Progr Cardiovasc Dis 31:393–426, 1989

47. de Wolf D, de Schepper J, Verhaaren H, et al: Congenital hypothyroid goiter and amiodarone. Acta Paediatr Scand 77:616–618, 1988

48. Laurent M, Betremieux P, Biron Y, Lehelloco A: Neonatal hypothyroidism after treatment by amiodarone during pregnancy (letter). Am J Cardiol 60:942, 1987

49. Priestley KA, Ladusans EJ, Rosenthal E, et al: Experience with flecainide for the treatment of cardiac arrhythmias in children. Eur Heart J 1284–1290, 1988

50. Perry JC, McQuinn RL, Smith RT, et al: Flecainide acetate for resistant arrhythmias in the young: Efficacy and pharmacokinetics. Am J Cardiol 14:185–191, 1989

51. Epstein AE: Flecainide for pediatric arrhythmias: Do children behave like little adults? Am J Cardiol 14:192–193, 1989

52. Kleinman CS, Copel JA, Weinstein EM, et al: Treatment of fetal supraventricular tachyarrhythmias. J Clin Ultrasound 13:365–373, 1985

53. Spinnato JA, Shaver DC, Flinn GS, et al: Fetal supraventricular tachycardia: In utero therapy with digoxin and quinidine. Obstet Gynecol 64:730–735, 1984

54. Newburger JW, Keane JF: Intrauterine supraventricular tachycardia. J Pediatr 95:780–786, 1979

55. Lingman G, Ohrlander S, Ohlin P: Intrauterine digoxin treatment of fetal paroxysmal tachycardia: Case report. Br J Obstet Gynaecol 87:340–342, 1980

56. Harrigan JT, Kangos JJ, Sikka A, et al: Successful treatment of fetal congestive heart failure secondary to tachycardia. N Engl J Med 304:1527–1529, 1981

57. Younis JS, Granat M: Insufficient transplacental digoxin transfer in severe hydrops fetalis. Am J Obstet Gynecol 157:1268–1269, 1987

58. Teuscher A, Bossi E, Imhof P, et al: Effect of propranolol on fetal tachycardia in diabetic pregnancy. Am J Cardiol 42:304–307, 1988

59. Wolff F, Breuker KH, Schlensker KH, Bolte A: Prenatal diagnosis and therapy of fetal heart rate anomalies with a contribution on the placental transfer of verapamil. J Perinatal Med 8:203–208, 1980

60. Dumesic DA, Silverman NH, Tobias S, Golbus MS: Transplacental cardioversion of fetal supraventricular tachycardia with procainamide. N Engl J Med 307:1128–1131, 1982

61. Pitcher D, Leather HM, Storey GCA, Holt DW: Amiodarone in pregnancy. Lancet 1:597–598, 1983

62. Azancot-Benisty A, Jacqz-Aigrain E: Etude des troubles du rythme supraventriculaires du foetus humain, in Biologie et Pathologie du Coeur et des Vaisseaux, Nantes, April 20–22, 1989

63. Allan L: The use of flecainide in fetal arrhythmias, in Fetal Cardiac Symposium, Paris, September 10–12, 1989

64. Wren C, Hunter S: Maternal administration of flecainide to terminate and suppress fetal tachycardia. Br Med J 296:249, 1988

65. Rodin SM, Johson BF: Pharmacokinetic interactions with digoxin. Clin Pharmacokinet 15:227–244, 1988

66. Koren G, Hesslein PS, MacLeod SM: Digoxin toxicity associated with amiodarone therapy in children. J Pediatr 104:467–470, 1984

67. Wood AJJ, Feely J: Pharmacokinetic drug interactions with propranolol. Clin Pharmacokinet 8:253–262, 1983

68. Wladimiroff JW, Stewart PA: Treatment of fetal cardiac arrhythmias. Br J Hosp Med 34:134–140, 1985

69. Abramowicz J, Jaffe R, Altaras M, Ben-Aderet N: Fetal supraventricular tachycardia: Prenatal diagnosis and pharmacological reversal of associated hydrops fetalis. Gynecol Obstet Invest 20:109–112, 1985

70. Nagashima M, Asai T, Suzuki C, et al: Intrauterine supraventricular tachyarrhythmias and transplacental digitalisation. Arch Dis Child 61:996–1000, 1986

71. Wiggins JW, Bowes W, Clewell W, et al: Echocardiographic diagnosis and intravenous digoxin management of fetal tachyarrhythmias and congestive heart failure. Am J Dis Child 140:202–204, 1986

72. Colin A, Chabaud JJ, Poinsot J, et al: Les tachycardies supraventriculaires foetales et leur traitement: A propos de 23 cas. Arch Fr Pediatr 46:335–340, 1989

73. Boutte P, Bourlon F, Tordjman C, et al: Tachycardie supraventriculaire et anasarques foetales. Arch Fr Pediatr 42:777–779, 1985

74. Azancot-Benisty A, Jacqz-Aigrain E, Guirguis NM, et al: Clinical and pharmacological study of fetal supraventricular tachyarrhythmias. (submitted)

75. Klein AM, Holzman IA, Austin EM: Fetal tachycardia prior to the development of hydrops: Attempted pharmacologic cardioversion. Case report. Am J Obstet Gynecol 134:347–348, 1979

76. Belhassen A, Vaksmann G, Francart G, et al: Intérêt de l'amiodarone dans le traitement des tachycardies supraventriculaires foetales: A propos d'une observation. J Gynecol Obstet Biol Reprod (Paris) 16:795–800, 1987

77. Auzelle MP, Mensire A, Lachassine E, et al: Traitement in utero des tachycardies foetales par l'association digitalique-béta-bloquant. J Gynecol Obstet Biol Reprod (Paris) 16:383–391, 1987

78. Vlahot N, Morvan J, Bernard AM, et al: Tachycardie supraventriculaire foetale: Traitement anténatal par l'association digoxine-amiodarone. J Gynecol Obstet Biol Reprod (Paris) 16:393–400, 1987

79. Arnoux P, Seyral P, Llurens M, et al: Amiodarone and digoxin for refractory fetal tachycardia. Am J Cardiol 56:166–167, 1987

80. Owen J, Colvin EV, Davis RO: Fetal death after successful conversion of fetal supraventricular tachycardia with digoxin and verapamil. Am J Obstet Gynecol 158:1169–1170, 1988

81. Guntheroth WG, Cyr DR, Mack LA, et al: Hydrops form reciprocating atrioventricular tachycardia in a 27-week fetus requiring quinidine for conversion. Obstet Gynecol 66:29S–33S, 1985

82. Mills MS: Fetal supraventricular tachycardia: Detection by routine auscultation and successful in utero management. Case report. Br J Obstet Gynaecol 96:501–502, 1989

83. Weiner CP, Thompson MIB: Direct treatment of fetal supraventricular tachycardia after failed transplacental therapy. Am J Obstet Gynecol 158:570–573, 1988

84. Gembruch U, Manz M, Bald R, et al: Repeated intravascular treatment with amiodarone in a fetus with refractory supraventricular tachycardia and hydrops fetalis. Am Heart J 118:1335–1338, 1989

85. Weiner CP: The role of cordocentesis in fetal diagnosis, in Pitkin RM, Scott JR (eds): Clinical Obstetrics and Gynecology. Philadelphia, JB Lippincott, 1988, pp 282–285

SECTION III

DRUGS AND THE INFANT, CHILD, AND ADOLESCENT

16

THERAPEUTIC DRUG MONITORING: Theoretical and Practical Issues

PETER GAL *and* JAMIE GILMAN

Children display unique age-related pharmacokinetic characteristics that influence drug disposition. This is complicated by wide interpatient idiosyncracies that lead to extremely diverse capacities to eliminate and respond to drugs. Although measurement of plasma drug concentrations has been useful, selection of optimal drug concentration ranges has been based on limited and sometimes misleading information in the pediatric population. Additionally, young children may be unable to verbally express symptoms of adverse effects or improvements in their disease state, eliminating valuable subjective input. Consequently, interactions among body systems, therapeutic responses, and serum drug concentrations are sometimes more difficult to interpret in children compared with adults. Therapeutic drug monitoring (TDM) in children poses some complicated challenges as well as unique opportunities for clinicians to integrate clinical skills and laboratory data. This chapter will review selected factors that have an impact on therapeutic drug monitoring in the pediatric patient as well as some clinical approaches to effective drug monitoring.

SERUM CONCENTRATION INTERPRETATION

The use of drug concentrations to guide dosing has generally been accepted as improving the safe and effective use of drugs with a narrow therapeutic range.[1-7] Despite some concerns over the validation of the commonly accepted therapeutic ranges,[1,2] clinical trials have shown TDM to provide improved patient outcomes in a cost-effective manner.[3-6]

One criterion to justify TDM is a narrow therapeutic index for a drug, usually described by a target *therapeutic drug concentration range*. In this scheme, drug concentrations above this range are considered toxic, whereas those below are subtherapeutic. The perception that drug con-

centration ranges supersede clinical responsiveness as a therapeutic endpoint is a common problem in TDM. *Therapeutic ranges* for most drugs are based on experiential reports that fail to meet either laboratory test validation criteria[1] or the necessary target-concentration strategy components.[2] In fact, identical drug concentrations can produce markedly different responses among patients and even in the same patient under different clinical conditions.[2] TDM approaches that ignore individuality may unnecessarily deny a patient adequate therapeutic drug trials if concentrations exceed the proverbial upper range limit or, conversely, induce unnecessary toxicity by increasing effective lower concentrations into the therapeutic range. Therapeutic ranges should only serve as initial drug dosing guidelines that are subject to modification based on clinical response versus the risks and benefits of altering traditionally used concentrations. There is also an increasing sense that TDM should be revised to place drug concentrations in perspective as clinical decision-making aids and not as a substitute for this process, nor as a medicolegal weapon to restrict clinicians from exercising judgment.[1,2,7-9]

Serum concentration interpretations in infants and children are largely based on extrapolations of adult therapeutic ranges.[7,8] Such extrapolations presume that (1) similar pharmacologic effects are sought, (2) protein-binding differences are adequately corrected for therapeutic ranges of unbound drug concentrations similar to adults, (3) comparable pharmacologic receptor concentrations and responses are achieved in children, and (4) active-metabolite differences in chidren are accounted for or are of minor importance.

Exceptions to all four assumptions are easily cited. For example, in the treatment of apnea of prematurity, the efficacy of theophylline is probably related to a central pharmacologic effect. The suggested therapeutic range to treat this condition, however, was based on adjusted protein-binding data using the therapeutic range for bronchodilation, a peripheral effect.[10] It is unlikely that the same pharmacologic effect is sought in these two therapies, making the validity of this theoretical therapeutic range questionable, since target organs differ.

Protein binding may be highly variable in children, especially neonates. This phenomenon obviously increases free drug fraction and, theoretically, total serum concentration responsiveness. Additionally, some drugs may demonstrate pH-dependent binding.[11] Wide daily pH fluctuations may substantially alter protein binding and, potentially, clinical response. Children also may have a variety of physiologic conditions that alter protein binding and anticipated therapeutic ranges. These include malnutrition, liver disease, renal disease, cystic fibrosis, neoplasms, .trauma,[12] and type I diabetes mellitus.[13] Although theoretical advantages for monitoring unbound drug concentrations exist, conclusive evidence that pharmacologic response differences are explained by decreased binding is lacking.[14] Nevertheless, anecdotal experiences strongly suggest a role for monitoring unbound drug concentrations in selected situations to explain pharmacologic differences.

Similar pharmacologic effects cannot be expected at similar serum concentrations, since receptor sensitivities and receptor drug concentrations may differ. Painter et al.[15] examined phenobarbital concentrations in neonatal brain tissue and plasma at autopsy. Brain/plasma concentration ratios increased with gestational age. Likewise, brain/serum phenobarbital ratios in children are reported to be lower than in adults.[16,17] The implications of such findings are unclear. However, these unknowns serve to confound our understanding of optimal therapeutic ranges.

The potential impact of active metabolites on serum drug concentration interpretation has been appreciated for some time.[14] In some cases, monitoring both parent compound and active metabolite is routine, e.g., procainamide and N-acetyl procainamide. Concurrent active metabolite concentrations are not measured, however, for most drugs.[18] Drug metabolism in children generally differs from that in adults and can result in heightened drug sensitivity or enhanced toxicity.[8] Also, for immunologically based assays, cross-reactivity of assays with metabolites may cause higher drug concentration readings, giving the appearance of decreased drug sensitivity in children. Finally, for drugs that are marketed as enantiomers, the pharmacologic activity and metabolic rates may differ.[19] This could make children appear more or less sensitive to drugs depending on which isomer is more affected. Some drugs for which this may ultimately be important in children include propranolol, verapamil, ibuprofen, and warfarin.[19]

Identification of concentrations at which the desired clinical response is achieved without toxicity, i.e., *critical drug concentrations,* is a particularly important aspect of TDM. Without this knowledge, drug concentration fluctuations may result in clinical deterioration, even though all concentrations appear to be within the recommended therapeutic range. The clinical response to this may be addition of potentially toxic agents and unnecessary and expensive laboratory testing. Thus a critical drug concentration may become one therapeutic endpoint in a situation where deteriorating disease control is associated with falling drug concentrations.

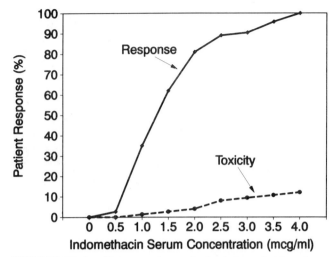

FIGURE 16–1. Pharmacodynamic depiction of risks of toxicity and likelihood of response in relation to indomethacin serum concentration in 71 neonates treated 74 times with indomethacin and furosemide for closure of patent ductus arteriosus.

Pharmacodynamic Response Curves

Pharmacodynamic response curves have been developed for several drugs and provide important descriptions of drug effects. These data can ultimately be extended to clarify relative risks and benefits of achieving similar drug concentrations in different patient populations. Powell and Jackson[20] separated severity of asthma and anticipated benefits from theophylline. It is apparent from this analysis that little benefit from theophylline can be expected in severe asthmatics, even at optimal therapeutic concentrations. Additionally, the pharmacodynamics may change with changing clinical status. Gal et al.[21] have described indomethacin pharmacodynamic curves in neonates requiring PDA closure (Figure 16–1). Such curves allow clinicians to weigh risk versus benefit across a spectrum of drug concentrations. Similar curves can be

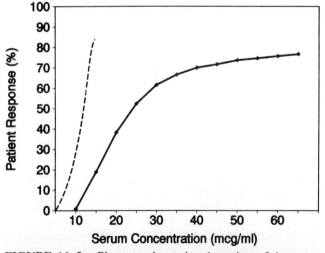

FIGURE 16–2. Pharmacodynamic adaptation of drug concentration versus percent response curves for theophylline (---) for treating neonatal apnea and bradycardia and phenobarbital (—) for neonatal seizures.

developed for other drugs for which sufficiently descriptive data are available, e.g., phenobarbital for neonatal seizures[22] and theophylline for apnea of prematurity[23] (Figure 16–2).

Unfortunately, therapeutic and toxic endpoints are not always clearly defined, and concentration–response curves may be difficult to develop. This is particularly true in outpatient pediatric settings, where obtaining reliable patient information is often unrealistic. This forces many therapeutic ranges to reflect information obtained from acute inpatient settings, where relative risks may be different. Additionally, it is important to clarify the patient group studied, since neonates, infants, children, and adolescents differ. Pharmacodynamic curves clearly delineate pharmacologic effects. In their absence, practitioners should utilize therapeutic ranges but be prepared to individualize these where pharmacologic response dictates and close clinical monitoring is employed.

Sensitivity and Specificity of Therapeutic Ranges

Laboratory tests are usually held to a standard whereby sensitivity, specificity, and false-positive and false-negative characteristics of the test are known.[1,24] *Sensitivity* of a test is used to characterize the incidence of true-positive results when applied to patients who are known to have the disease. For example, a serum phenytoin concentration of greater than 20 μg/ml has been recommended as a criterion to classify toxicity. When the serum concentrations of 100 patients with true clinical phenytoin toxicity were tested, only 80 had serum concentrations greater than 20 μg/ml. The sensitivity of this test would be 80 percent, with 20 percent false-negative results. *Specificity* describes the incidence of true-negative results when applied to healthy subjects. Thus, using the same phenytoin criteria, patients without clinical phenytoin toxicity were tested. Thirty of 100 nontoxic patients had concentrations greater than 20 μg/ml, which is considered toxic by the criterion. The test specificity is 70 percent, with 30 percent false-positive results. False negativity (involving sick patients) and false positivity (involving healthy patients) are undesirable because patients become misclassified. A good test is one that is both sensitive and specific. Calculation of sensitivity, specificity, and false-positive and false-negative values is as follows:

	TOXICITY		
	Present	**Absent**	**Total**
Test positive	a	b	a + b
Test negative	c	d	c + d
TOTAL	a + c	b + d	

$$\text{Sensitivity} = \frac{a}{a + c} \times 100 \qquad (1)$$

$$\text{Specificity} = \frac{d}{b + d} \times 100 \qquad (2)$$

$$\text{False negatives} = \frac{c}{a + c} \times 100 \qquad (3)$$

$$\text{False positives} = \frac{b}{b + d} \times 100 \qquad (4)$$

The predictive value of a laboratory test is the percentage of positive results that are true positives (e.g., truly toxic) when the test is applied to a population containing both healthy (or nontoxic) and diseased (or toxic) patients. It is the true test of the value of levels above the therapeutic range being designated as toxic. The predictive value is calculated, using the preceding example, as follows:

$$\text{Predictive value} = \frac{a}{a + b} \times 100 \qquad (5)$$

With few exceptions,[1,25] therapeutic drug monitoring has not been scrutinized in such a manner. Many therapeutic ranges may be modified as such vital studies are performed. This raises questions about such commonly accepted values as the therapeutic range cited for vancomycin[26,27] and the relationship of peak gentamicin concentrations to toxicity.[2,28] Analysis of vancomycin trough concentration relationships and nephrotoxicity can only be traced in one study where raw data are presented.[29] While other studies cite more toxicity with trough levels greater than 10 μg/ml, it is unknown if most of these levels were much higher, e.g., 30 μg/ml.[30] Downs et al.[29] studied the value of vancomycin trough concentrations greater than 10 μg/ml as a toxicity marker as follows: sensitivity = 89 percent, specificity = 31 percent, and positive predictive value = 47 percent. If trough vancomycin levels above 20 μg/ml are considered toxic, the value of this laboratory test is sensitivity = 78 percent, specificity = 23 percent, and positive predictive value = 70 percent. Since predictive value increases substantially with little sensitivity or specificity loss, perhaps vancomycin trough concentrations should be tolerated to at least 20 μg/ml. We have examined this possibility in 36 neonates treated 50 times with vancomycin (unpublished data). Only one patient exhibited renal toxicity (level 12.5 μg/ml, with concurrent gentamicin). Despite troughs greater than 20 μg/ml, 15 neonates did not have renal toxicity. Sensitivity, specificity, and predictive values for trough vancomycin levels as predictors of clinical response in neonates are 70.3, 38.5, and 76.5 percent, respectively, for troughs of 10 μg/ml or greater and 36.1, 84.6, and 86.7 percent, respectively, for troughs of 20 μg/ml or greater. Vancomycin trough limitations may be unnecessary in neonates, since higher concentrations are more predictive of response. This suggestion must be tempered by the absence of data clarifying the relationship of vancomycin levels to ototoxic risk. Clinical response, however, should not be compromised to achieve a drug concentration range with no basis. In our experience, neonates with deep line infections often respond better to trough vancomycin concentrations of 20 μg/ml.

TECHNICAL PROBLEMS

The actual acquisition of blood for therapeutic drug monitoring in children is met with numerous obstacles.

The first is sample-size limitations, particularly in newborns. Multiple phlebotomies can lead to the necessity of blood transfusions because of the relatively small blood volume in young children. Blood transfusions are usually necessary in newborns when 10 percent of the blood volume is removed. A neonate weighing 1000 gm will probably require a blood transfusion for every 8 ml of blood removed. Phlebotomy is further complicated by difficult venipuncture in children with small veins. Additionally, repeated punctures have been associated with damaged veins or heels, compromising the ability to obtain other clinically important laboratory data.[31] Fortunately, the use of microsampling has resolved some of the volume problems for the more commonly monitored agents. Also, several newer solid-phase chemistry techniques utilize fingerstick whole-blood collections to assay drugs.[32]

Another technical problem in children is the presence of endogenous compounds or drug metabolites that interfere with drug assay techniques. These substances may be absent in the adult or present only in minute concentrations with no adverse assay effects. For example, digoxin-like immunoreactive substances are present in neonates and infants and cross-react with many digoxin assay methods. The degree of interference depends on the assay method employed, resulting in falsely elevated digoxin concentrations.[8] Assay methodologies that measure parent compounds and metabolites as single entities also present a problem. Children often have a faster parent-to-metabolite conversion, which may lead to different effective ranges for such assay methods. This situation has been described with radioimmunoassay for cyclosporine and enzyme-multiplied immunoassay technique (EMIT) for carbamazepine. Cyclosporine metabolites do not possess significant immunosuppressive activity and usually represent a relatively minor contribution to total cyclosporine concentrations. Conversely, the 10,11-epoxide metabolite of carbamazepine is pharmacologically active, affecting both efficacy and toxicity. Metabolite concentrations in children, however, may approach a significant level and further add confusion to laboratory interpretation.[33,34]

Medication administration techniques in children are also a major consideration in therapeutic drug monitoring. Medications administered to children are often in small fluid volumes, which leads to the problem of precise and timely drug administration. The length and bore size of the administration tubing become a significant factor in intravenous medication delivery, causing delays as long as 4 hours in some instances.[35] The problems with intravenous infusion systems have been well documented in newborns and infants[35-37] and can have a profound effect on therapeutic drug monitoring if unrecognized. This problem also extends into the toddler age group in hospitals that use small-volume (10–15 ml) medication bags with a wide-bore secondary line connected to the primary intravenous line with a two-way adapter. The use of syringe pumps with microbore tubing can circumvent many of these delivery problems. Oral medications administered through enteral feeding tubes are also a technical concern. Medication volumes are often smaller than the tubing volume capacity and must be well flushed to ensure prompt delivery. The implication of these administration problems is that serum drug concentrations may actually be drawn during drug administration and reflect predistributive values. Pharmacokinetic parameters generated from such drug concentrations will be misleading, and consequent drug-dosing calculations will be erroneous.

PHARMACOKINETIC CONSIDERATIONS

The continual maturation of body systems in children leads to changing drug disposition over time and resultant changes in serum drug concentrations. These changes are most dramatic in newborns and infants. Progressive increases in clearance values over time in infancy have been documented for theophylline,[38,39] phenobarbital,[40,41] caffeine,[42] and phenytoin.[43] These data imply that therapeutic drug monitoring in this rapidly changing age group may best be performed by intermittent sampling over time to describe drug disposition trends, since serial sampling following a single dose may be valid only for the brief time period studied.[7] Steady state for agents with longer half-lives may virtually never be achieved in infants. Puberty represents another transitional period when drug disposition changes to an adult pattern.[44] This is particularly evident for agents with characteristically faster clearances in children. As a result, drug disposition changes can occur on a continuum from newborns to adulthood for such agents as chloramphenicol, mezlocillin, phenobarbital, theophylline, and phenytoin.[45]

Changes in medication absorption related to maturation also may have a dramatic impact on serum drug concentrations. Sustained-release products may demonstrate incomplete absorption as a result of the apparent shorter intestinal transit time in young children.[46,47] Likewise, larger oral doses of cyclosporine are required to achieve immunosuppression in infants and young children owing to the limited intestinal absorptive surface area resulting from a shorter bowel length.[48] These functional differences may be responsible for some of the idiosyncrasies found in drug absorption.[49] Impaired drug absorption in children also may occur as a result of formula and milk product consumption[50] or acute diarrheal disease.[51,52] Drug disposition in children also has been reported to be influenced by febrile illnesses.[53] Other important factors that may affect drug clearance in neonates and children include changing ventilator status,[54] dietary intake,[55] and interacting drugs.[56]

An aspect of therapeutic drug monitoring that is frequently overlooked is the rhythm-dependent changes in parameters used to characterize a drug's pharmacokinetics or bioavailability, which is referred to as *chronopharmacokinetics*.[57] Periodicity in biologic functions is displayed in all living forms. Most of these synchronize to the solar day light–dark cycle and are termed *circadian* to identify biologic phenomena that recur every 24 hours. A basic knowledge of chronopharmacokinetics in children is also important for therapeutic drug monitoring. Approximately 50 chemical agents have been identified as exhibiting chronopharmacokinetics and/or chronopharmacology.[8] It is conceivable that these rhythm-dependent changes may be more clinically significant in children because of their higher clearance rates. In children, chronopharmacokinetics for theophylline,[58,59] carbamazepine,[60] and phenytoin[61] have been substantiated. Large differences in daytime and nighttime theophylline absorption in children have been reported previously.[58,59] Studies examining this effect in children medicated with TheoDur indicate that the optimal sampling time for the absolute trough concentration is before the evening dose, whereas that for peak level is after the morning dose. Calculations based on these serum concentrations should incur a 10–15 percent overestimation error of trough levels and 10–20 percent underestimation for peak levels. Errors as high as 120 percent for trough concentration and 50 percent for peak concentration may be incurred if samples are obtained at other times during the rhythm cycle.[59] Other agents undergoing chronopharmacokinetic changes that are typically included in therapeutic drug monitoring programs include clonazepam,[60] phenobarbital,[60] valproic acid,[61] sodium salicylate,[62] indomethacin,[63] lithium,[64] cyclosporine,[65] heparin,[66] and lidocaine.[67]

Infants who sleep as much during the daytime hours as during the night have not established a circadian pattern and have resultant drug disposition differences. For example, urinary pH does not exhibit the same diurnal variations in younger children.[68] As a result, agents with pH-dependent urinary excretion display altered pharmacokinetics and resultant changes in serum concentrations. Faster elimination rates of sulfisoxazole[69] and sulfamethoxypyrazine[70] have been demonstrated in children ages 6 months to 2 years when compared with older children, who exhibit a more biphasic adult sleep pattern.[71] These differences may become important when children on chronic medication convert to a diurnal sleep pattern.

Another interesting use of therapeutic drug monitoring is in the detection of physiologic changes that may occur prior to overt disease symptomatology. Aminoglycoside monitoring may well alert the clinician of renal dysfunction through a change in drug clearance prior to a rise in serum creatinine. A marked reduction in theophylline[72] or phenobarbital[73] clearance can support the suspicion of asphyxia in the newborn. Recently, an abrupt decrease in indomethacin volume of distribution was shown to demonstrate permanent ductus arteriosus closure in neonates.[74] This "pharmacophysiologic" approach may provide important information to support or raise doubts about a suspected diagnosis and adds another important benefit to the use of therapeutic drug monitoring.

CLINICAL APPROACH

In light of the limited and often weak studies of optimal therapeutic ranges in the pediatric population, therapeutic ranges should be used as relative rather than absolute guides to drug therapy. A careful therapeutic plan identifying clinical and objective markers of therapeutic response and toxicity should be implemented. This does not diminish the importance and need for measuring drug concentrations. Effective "critical" drug concentrations

for each patient that are safe should be identified. Pharmacokinetic information generated from properly timed drug concentrations is important for maintenance dose determinations and any important physiologic data obtainable.

Timing and frequency of blood sampling depend on the situation criticality. In intensive care or hospitalized environments, frequent sampling may be necessary. For example, gentamicin maintenance dose determinations based on pharmacokinetic data generated from post-loading-dose levels have increased response and reduced mortality from gram-negative sepsis.[3] A similar dosing approach has recently been advocated to rapidly achieve therapeutic gentamicin concentrations in infants.[75] In this situation, two or three levels after an initial loading dose are necessary. Alternatively, concentrations of drugs with long half-lives may be obtained at a variety of times, depending on the pharmacokinetic system used. A discussion of the advantages and disadvantages of various pharmacokinetic approaches is presented elsewhere.[7]

Once a patient is stabilized clinically and monitored as an outpatient, the frequent sampling of drug concentrations is debatable. Obtaining drug levels periodically is probably prudent in children, however, since maturational changes alter drug disposition over time. In situations where drug interactions, changing physiology, or clinical instability are observed, measurement of drug concentrations should be more frequent. Home monitoring of drug concentrations may prove practical and provide an avenue for improved disease control and reduced health care costs in the future. Preliminary study results in this area are favorable.[76] Regardless of monitoring frequency, consistency of sample timing (e.g., trough levels) is important for proper interpretation of drug concentrations. Mixing values drawn at different times, e.g., peaks and troughs, can result in serious misinterpretation of the results with adverse clinical consequences.

SUMMARY

Therapeutic drug monitoring provides major improvements in the use of many drugs. Guidelines for therapeutic ranges in the pediatric population, however, are often based on limited and potentially flawed data. Therapeutic drug monitoring should encompass not only serum concentration monitoring but also continual assessments of drug efficacy, toxicity, and organ functions. This is especially important in children, in whom receptor drug concentration or sensitivity may be different from that seen in the adult population. Therapeutic endpoints should be identified, and serum drug concentrations should be adjusted to meet these goals.

Newborns and infants present the additional challenge of having a physiologic makeup whose degree of maturation sometimes changes on a day-to-day basis. It is this phenomenon that makes the definition of pharmacokinetic parameters following a single dose so unreliable and potentially hazardous. Therapy should be based not only on the capacity of the infant to eliminate and respond to a particular agent, but also on an understanding of the dynamic changes that will occur on an ongoing maturational basis. Serum drug concentrations also should be monitored more frequently during periods of changing clinical status.

Special consideration in children should focus on potential problems with drug administration, drug absorption, metabolite patterns, changing drug disposition, idiosyncratic reactions, receptor sensitivity, and chronopharmacokinetics. Differences in disease control often cannot be properly explained with TDM, however, and patients may undergo a multitude of expensive tests or hospitalization to resolve simple problems of changing drug disposition. Pharmacokinetic information obtained from measuring drug concentrations should be applied not only for drug dosing, but also as documentation for physiologic changes. As with other patient populations, therapeutic drug monitoring is only a small part of the clinical scenario, the total of which must be the basis for therapeutic decisions.

REFERENCES

1. Schumacher GE, Barr JT: Making serum levels more meaningful. Ther Drug Monit 11:580–584, 1989
2. Spector R, Park GD, Johnson GF, Vesell ES: Therapeutic drug monitoring. Clin Pharmacol Ther 43:345–353, 1988
3. Bootman JL, Wertheimer AI, Zaske D, Rowland C: Individualizing gentamicin dosage regimens in burn patients with gram-negative septicemia: A cost-benefit analysis. J Pharm Sci 68:267–274, 1979
4. Groce JB, Gal P, Douglas JB, Steuterman MC: Heparin dosage adjustment in patients with deep-vein thrombosis using heparin concentrations rather than activated partial thromboplastin time. Clin Pharm 6:216–222, 1987
5. Mungall D, Marshall J, Penn D, et al: Individualizing theophylline therapy: The impact of clinical pharmacokinetics on patient outcomes. Ther Drug Monit 5:95–101, 1983
6. Vozeh S: Cost-effectiveness of therapeutic drug monitoring. Clin Pharmacokinet 13:131–140, 1987
7. Gal P: Therapeutic drug monitoring in neonates: Problems and issues. Drug Intell Clin Pharm 22:317–323, 1988
8. Gilman JT: Therapeutic drug monitoring in the neonate and paediatric age group: Problems and clinical pharmacokinetic implications. Clin Pharmacokinet 19:1–10, 1990
9. Choonara IA, Rane A: Therapeutic drug monitoring of anticonvulsants: State of the art. Clin Pharmacokinet 18:318–328, 1990
10. Aranda JV, Sitar DS, Parsons WD, et al: Pharmacokinetic aspects of theophylline in premature newborns. N Engl J Med 295:413–416, 1976
11. Vallner JJ, Speir WA, Kolbeck RC, et al: Effects of pH on the binding of theophylline to serum proteins. Am Rev Respir Dis 120:83–86, 1979
12. Stewart CF, Hampton EM: Effect of maturation on drug disposition in pediatric patients. Clin Pharm 6:548–564, 1987
13. Kearns GL, Kemp SF, Turley CP, Nelson DL: Protein binding of phenytoin and lidocaine in pediatric patients with type I diabetes mellitus. Dev Pharmacol Ther 11:14–23, 1988
14. Barre J, Didey F, Delion F, Tillement JP: Problems in therapeutic drug monitoring: Free drug level monitoring. Ther Drug Monit 10:133–143, 1988
15. Painter MJ, Pippenger CE, Wasterlein C, et al: Phenobarbital and phenytoin in neonatal seizures: Metabolism and tissue distribution. Neurology 31:1107–1112, 1981
16. Onishi S, Yoshihi O, Nishimura Y, et al: Distribution of phenobarbital in serum, brain, and other organs from pediatric patients. Dev Pharmacol Ther 7:153–154, 1984
17. Houghton GW, Richens A, Toseland PA, et al: Brain concentrations of phenytoin, phenobarbital, and primidone in epileptic patients. Eur J Clin Pharmacol 9:73–78, 1975
18. Drayer DE: Pharmacologically active metabolites of drugs and other foreign compounds: Clinical, pharmacological, therapeutic, and toxicological considerations. Drugs 24:519–542, 1982
19. Matzke GR, St Peter WL: Clinical pharmacokinetics 1990. Clin Pharmacokinet 17:441–451, 1990
20. Powell JR, Jackson JE: Theophylline, in Evans WE, Schentag JJ, Jusko WJ (eds): Applied Pharmacokinetics: Principles of Therapeutic Drug Monitoring. San Francisco, Applied Therapeutics, 1980, p 141
21. Gal P, Ransom JL, Schall S, et al: Indomethacin for patent ductus arteriosus closure: Application of serum concentrations and pharmacodynamics to improve response. J Perinatol 10:20–26, 1990
22. Gilman JT, Gal P, Duchowny MS, et al: Rapid sequential phenobarbital treatment of neonatal seizures. Pediatrics 83:674–678, 1989
23. Muttitt SC, Tierney AJ, Finer NN: The dose response of theophylline in the treatment of apnea of prematurity. J Pediatr 112:115–121, 1988
24. Galen RS, Gambino SR: Beyond Normality: The Predictive Value and Efficiency of Medical Diagnoses. New York, John Wiley & Sons, 1975
25. Schumacher GE, Barr JT: Applying decision analysis in therapeutic drug monitoring: Using decision trees to interpret serum theophylline concentrations. Clin Pharm 5:325–333, 1986
26. Wenk M, Vozeh S, Follath F: Serum level monitoring of antibacterial drugs: A review. Clin Pharmacokinet 9:475–492, 1984
27. Edwards DJ, Pancorbo S: Routine monitoring of serum vancomycin concentrations: Waiting for proof of its value. Clin Pharm 6:652–654, 1987
28. Yee GC, Evans WE: Reappraisal of guidelines for pharmacokinetic monitoring of aminoglycosides. Pharmacotherapy 1:55–75, 1981
29. Downs NJ, Neihart RE, Dolezal JM, Hodges GR: Mild nephrotoxicity associated with vancomycin use. Arch Intern Med 149:1777–1781, 1989
30. Cimino MA, Rotstein C, Slaughter RL, Emrich LJ: Relationship of serum antibiotic concentrations to nephrotoxicity in cancer patients receiving concurrent aminoglycoside and vancomycin therapy. Am J Med 83:1091–1097, 1987
31. Leung AK: Cutaneous nodule resulting from blood-letting in neonates. Eur J Pediatr 145:579–580, 1986
32. Oles KS: Therapeutic drug monitoring analysis systems for the physician office laboratory. DICP 24(11):1070–1077, 1990
33. Lindholm A, Henricsson S: Comparitive analysis of cyclosporine in whole blood and plasma by radioimmunoassay, fluorescence polarization immunoassay and high performance liquid chromatography. Ther Drug Monit 12:344–352, 1990
34. Monaco F, Piredda S: Carbamazepine-10,11-epoxide determined by emit carbamazepine reagent. Epilepsia 21:475–477, 1980
35. Gould T, Roberts RJ: Therapeutic problems arising from the use of intravenous route for drug administration. J Pediatr 95:465–471, 1979
36. Nahata MC: Influence of infusion methods on therapeutic drug monitoring in pediatric patients. Drug Intell Clin Pharm 20:367–369, 1986
37. Roberts RJ: Intravenous administration of medication in pediatric patients: Problems and solutions. Pediatr Clin North Am 28:23–34, 1981
38. Gilman JT, Gal P, Levine RS, et al: Factors influencing theophylline disposition in 179 newborns. Ther Drug Monit 8:4–10, 1986
39. Nassif EG, Weinberger MM, Shannon D, et al: Theophylline disposition in infancy. J Pediatr 98:158–161, 1981
40. Painter MJ, Pippenger C, MacDonald H, Pitlick W: Phenobarbital and diphenylhydantoin levels in neonates with seizures. J Pediatr 92:315–319, 1978
41. Pitlick W, Painter M, Pippenger C: Phenobarbital pharmacokinetics in neonates. Clin Pharmacol Ther 23:346–350, 1978
42. Pearlman SA, Duran C, Wood MA, et al: Caffeine pharmacokinetics in preterm infants older than 2 weeks. Dev Pharmacol Ther 12:65–69, 1989
43. Bourgeois BF, Dodson WE: Phenytoin elimination in newborns. Neurology 23:173–178, 1983
44. Pippenger CE: Maturation of biotransformation rates, in Morselli PL, et al (eds): Antiepileptic Drug Therapy in Pediatrics. New York, Raven Press, 1984, pp 333–338

45. Milsap RL, Szetler SJ: Special pharmacokinetic considerations in children, in Evans WE, et al (eds): Applied Pharmacokinetics: Principles of Therapeutic Drug Monitoring, 2nd ed. Spokane, Wash, Applied Therapeutics, 1986, pp 294–330

46. Grand RJ, Watkins JB, Torti FM: Development of the human gastrointestinal tract: A review. Gastroenterology 70:790–810, 1976

47. Kerlin P, Zinsmeister A, Phillips S: Relationship of motility of flow of contents in the human small intestine. Gastroenterology 82:701–706, 1982

48. Whitington PF, Emon JC, Whitington SH, et al: Small-bowel length and the dose of cyclosporine in children after liver transplantation. N Engl J Med 322:733–738, 1990

49. Gilman JT, Duchowny MS, Resnick TJ, Hershorin ER: Carbamazepine malabsorption: A case report. Pediatrics 82:518–519, 1988

50. Pinkerton CR, Welshman SG, Glasgow JF, Bridges JM: Can food influence the absorption of methotrexate in children with acute lymphoblastic leukemia? Lancet 2:944–946, 1980

51. Craft JC, Holt EA, Tan SH: Malabsorption of oral antibiotics in humans and rats with giardiases. Pediatr Infect Dis J 6:832–836, 1987

52. Nelson JD, Shelton S, Kusmiesz HT, Haltalin KC: Absorption of ampicillin and nalidixic acid by infants and children with acute shigellosis. Clin Pharmacol Ther 13:879–886, 1972

53. Leppik IE, Fisher J, Kriel R, Sawchuk RJ: Altered phenytoin clearance with febrile illness. Neurology 36:1367–1370, 1986

54. Richard C, Berdeaux A, Delion F, et al: Effect of mechanical ventilation on hepatic drug pharmacokinetics. Chest 90:837–841, 1986

55. Park GD, Spector R, Kitt TM: Effect of dietary protein on renal tubular clearance of drugs in humans. Clin Pharmacokinet 18:318–328, 1990

56. Pond S: Pharmacokinetic interactions, in Benet LZ, Massoud N, Gambertoglio JG (eds): Pharmacokinetic Bases for Drug Treatment. New York, Raven Press, 1984, pp 195–220

57. Reinberg A, Smolensky MH: Circadian changes of drug disposition in man. Clin Pharmacokinet 7:401–420, 1982

58. Rogers RJ, Kalisker A, Wiener MB, Szefler SJ: Inconsistent absorption from a sustained-release theophylline preparation during continuous therapy in asthmatic children. J Pediatr 106:496–501, 1985

59. Smolensky MH, Scott PH, Kramer WG: Clinical significance of day–night differences in serum theophylline concentration with special reference to TheoDur. J Allergy Clin Immunol 78:716–722, 1986

60. Paxton JW, Aman MG, Werry JS: Fluctuation in salivary carbamazepine and carbamazepine-10,11-epoxide concentrations during the day in epileptic children. Epilepsia 24:716–724, 1983

61. Garretson LK, Jusko WJ: Diphenylhydantoin elimination kinetics in overdosed children. Clin Pharmacol Ther 17:481–491, 1971

62. Reinberg A, Zagula-Mally Z, Ghata J, Halberg F: Circadian rhythms in duration of salicylate excretion referred to phase of excretory rhythms and routine, in Proceedings of the Society for Experimental Biology, 1967, pp 826–832

63. Clench J, Reinberg A, Dziewanowska Z, et al: Circadian changes in the bioavailability and effects of indomethacin in healthy subjects. Eur J Clin Pharmacol 20:359–369, 1981

64. Lambinet I, Aymard N, Soulairac A, Reinberg A: Chronoptimization of lithium administration in five manic depressive patients: Reduction of nephrotoxicity. Int J Chronobiol 7:274, 1981

65. Bowers LD, Canafax DM, Singh J, et al: Studies of cyclosporine blood levels: Analysis, clinical utility, pharmacokinetics, metabolites, and chronopharmacology. Transplant Proc 18 (suppl 5):137–143, 1986

66. Decousus HA, Croze M, Levi FA, et al: Circadian changes in anticoagulant effect on heparin infused at a constant rate. Br Med J 290:341–344, 1985

67. Pollmann L: Etude de la chronobiologie des dents. Rev Stomatol Chir Macillo-Fac 82:201, 1981

68. Krauer B: The development of diurnal variation in drug kinetics in the human infants, in Morselli et al (eds): Basic and Therapeutic Aspects of Perinatal Pharmacology, New York, Raven Press, 1975, pp 347–356

69. Krauer B, Spring P, Dettli L: Zur pharmacokinetik der sulfonamide im ersten lebensjahr. Pharmacol Clin (Berl) 1:47–53, 1968

70. Gladtke E: Pharmacokinetics in relation to age. Boll Chim Farm (Milano) 112:333–341, 1973

71. Dettli L, Spring P: Diurnal variations in the elimination rate of a sulfonamide in man. Helv Med Acta (Basel) 4:291–306, 1966

72. Gal P, Boer HR, Toback J, et al: Effect of asphyxia on theophylline clearance in newborns. South Med J 75:836–838, 1982

73. Gal P, Toback J, Erkan NV, Boer HR: The influence of asphyxia on phenobarbital dosing requirements in neonates. Dev Pharmacol Ther 7:145–152, 1984

74. Gal P, Ransom JL, Weaver RL, et al: Indomethacin disposition in neonates: The impact of patent ductus arteriosus (PDA) closure. Pharmacotherapy 9:178, 1989

75. Gal P, Ransom JL, Weaver RL: Gentamicin in neonates: The need for loading doses. Am J Perinatol 7:254–257, 1990

76. Chandeler MHH, Clifton GD, Louis BA, et al: Home monitoring of theophylline levels: A novel therapeutic approach. Pharmacotherapy 10:294–300, 1990

77. Gal P, Ransom JL, Weaver RL, et al: Impact of concurrent furosemide on indomethacin pharmacodynamics: Efficacy for PDA closure and renal toxicity. Pharmacotherapy 10:238, 1990

17

PRINCIPLES OF NEONATAL PHARMACOLOGY

JEFFREY L. BLUMER *and* MICHAEL D. REED

The history of drug therapy is replete with examples of adverse reactions to drugs in children. Virtually all the drug-related legislation in effect in this country today stems directly from these onerous experiences.[1] Nevertheless, there continues to be no fixed rules or regulations governing the use of drugs in children or the testing and approval of new drugs for pediatric patients.

In 1956, Silverman and colleagues[2] at Columbia reported an excessive mortality rate and an increased incidence of kernicterus among premature babies receiving a sulfonamide antibiotic compared with those receiving chlortetracycline. Then, in 1959, Sutherland[3] described a syndrome of cardiovascular collapse in three newborns receiving high doses of chloramphenicol for presumed infections. Both these therapeutic misadventures serve to underscore the generally held perception that newborn infants are more likely to experience adverse reactions to drugs.

This preconception is espoused even more ardently when the xenobiotic exposure occurs during the embryonic or fetal periods of development. The thalidomide tragedy reported in 1962, in which more than 10,000 babies were born with the rare malformation phocomelia, created an international outcry and changed forever the way in which drug safety is evaluated.[4,5] More recently, issues surrounding the retinoic acid embryopathy have refocused attention on the effects of drugs on the fetus and newborn.[6]

As a result of these experiences, perinatologists, neonatologists, and pediatricians have become extremely conservative in their use of drug therapy. They have recognized that rational drug therapy for pregnant women and newborns is often confounded by a combination of unpredictable and often poorly understood pharmacokinetic and pharmacodynamic interactions.[6,7] Although this conservative approach has permitted the fulfillment of the physician's oath to "do no harm," it also has prevented the adoption of newer therapeutic modalities and their adaptation to pediatric patients.

A more specific approach to neonatal therapeutics

requires a thorough understanding of human developmental biology as well as insights regarding the dynamic ontogeny of the processes of drug absorption, drug distribution, drug metabolism, and drug excretion. In addition, there must be a rigorous appreciation of the developmental aspects of drug–receptor interactions, including the ontogenetic changes in receptor number, receptor affinity, receptor–effector coupling, and receptor modulation and regulation.

The purpose of this chapter is to attempt to develop a therapeutically relevant foundation for neonatal drug therapy based on the physiologic characteristics of extrauterine adaptation. The text will focus on the pharmacokinetic determinants of neonatal drug therapy rather than on any developmental variations in pharmacodynamics, since only the former are amenable to clinical manipulation.

DRUG ABSORPTION

Absorption refers to the translocation of a drug from its site of administration into the bloodstream. Drugs administered extravascularly, including the sublingual, buccal, oral, intramuscular, subcutaneous, rectal, and topical routes, must cross multiple membranes to reach the systemic circulation and ultimately distribute to sites of action. Absorption into the systemic circulation depends on both the physicochemical properties of a drug and a variety of host factors (Table 17–1).

Ontogeny of Gastric Acid Production

Hess[8] was the first to describe the presence of hydrochloric acid in the newborn stomach several hours after birth. At birth, gastric pH is usually between 6 and 8, but it falls rapidly to between 1.5 and 3.0 within several hours.[9] From the available data, this fall in gastric pH is

164

TABLE 17–1. FACTORS AFFECTING DRUG ABSORPTION

Physicochemical factors:
  Formulation characteristics:
    Disintegration of tablets or solid phase
    Dissolution of drug in gastric or intestinal fluid
    Release from sustained-release preparations
  Molecular weight
  pK_a and number of ionizable groups
  Degree of lipid solubility

Patient factors:
  Gastric content and gastric emptying time
  Gastric and duodenal pH
  Surface area available for absorptions
  Size of bile salt pool
  Bacterial colonization of the lower intestines
  Underlying disease states

quite variable but appears to be independent of both birth weight and gestational age. However, acid is rarely present in the fetal stomach before 32 weeks' gestation.

Extrauterine factors are most likely responsible for initiating acid production, since basal acid output correlates with postnatal but not postconceptual age. The subsequent pattern of gastric acid secretion remains controversial. Postnatally, gastric acid secretion appears to display a biphasic pattern; the highest acid concentrations occur within the first 10 days and the lowest between the 10th and 30th days of extrauterine life. Agunod et al.,[10] using betazole stimulation, essentially confirmed these early findings and found that the volume of gastric juice and acid concentration were dependent on age and that gastric acid secretions (corrected for body weight) approached the lower limit of adult values by 3 months of age. Secretion of pepsin and intrinsic factor also were found to parallel that of gastric acid.

Gastric and duodenal pH values affect drug solubility and ionization as well as gastrointestinal motility.[11] An acidic pH favors absorption of acidic drugs (low pK_a), because in such an environment the drug will be largely in an un-ionized, more lipid-soluble form. In contrast, a relatively high pH (as in states of achlorhydria) will enhance the translocation of basic drugs and retard the absorption of acidic drugs.

Gastric Emptying

Since most orally administered drugs are absorbed in the small intestine, the rate of gastric emptying is an important determinant of the rate and extent of drug absorption. If it is slowed, then the rate of intestinal drug absorption may be reduced; this will, in turn, reduce the peak serum drug concentration. On the other hand, if gastric emptying is hastened, the extent of intestinal absorption may be reduced as a result of decreased contact time with the absorptive surface. Of course, both these effects presuppose that intestinal motility remains constant.

Gastric emptying rate during the neonatal period is variable and is characterized by irregular and unpredictable peristaltic activity. It is prolonged relative to that of the adult. The rate of gastric emptying appears to be

directly affected by gestational and postnatal age, as well as the type of feeding used[9,12] (Table 17–2). Gastric emptying time appears to approach adult values within the first 6–8 months of life. Similarly, small intestinal motility in the perinatal period is variable and is influenced by the presence or absence of food.

An inverse relationship between gestational age and the amount of gastric retention 30 minutes after a 5 percent glucose in water feeding has been demonstrated. This relationship was independent of intrauterine growth. With human milk feedings, a characteristic biphasic pattern of gastric emptying in both preterm and term infants, with an initial rapid phase followed by a slower, prolonged second phase, is observed. In contrast, a linear pattern of gastric emptying was noted when infant formula was used.[12]

Gastric emptying is also affected by the composition of the meal. Slower gastric emptying times have been reported with increasing caloric density in premature infants (gestational age 25–35 weeks). Significant differences were noted between formulas containing 0 and 6.5, 6.5 and 13, and 13 and 20 calories/100 gm. These differences were significant at all times following the meal (20, 40, 60, 80, and 100 minutes). The difference in gastric emptying between a 20 and 24 calorie/oz (71.5 and 86 calories/100 gm) formula was only significant at 80 minutes. Similar findings with slower gastric emptying times have been reported in infants given a 10 percent glucose solution versus a 5 percent solution.

In contrast to the effect of caloric density on gastric emptying rates, the osmolality of the meal does not appear to be a factor. However, slower emptying is seen in feeding with long-chain fatty acids compared with medium-chain triglycerides, an important variable considering that infant formulas differ in their fatty acid content. The fat source in Portagen is mostly medium-chain triglycerides, whereas Pregestimil and several premature formulas such as Enfamil and Similac 24 LBW contain both medium-chain triglycerides and long-chain fatty acids. The fat source in the standard commercial formulas Enfamil and Similac is long-chain fatty acids.

Exocrine Pancreatic Function

The ontogeny of other physiologic processes may further influence the gastrointestinal absorption of drugs and other compounds. The rate of synthesis, character, pool size, and intestinal transport of bile acids are less in neonates than in adults.[13] At birth, pancreatic enzyme activity is low, and enzyme activities are lower in premature than

TABLE 17–2. FACTORS AFFECTING GASTRIC EMPTYING RATE

INCREASE	DECREASE	NO EFFECT
Human milk	Prematurity	Osmolality
Hypocaloric feedings	Gastroesophageal reflux	Posture
	Respiratory distress syndrome	
	Congenital heart disease	
	Long-chain fatty acids	

in full-term neonates. Interestingly, at 1 week of postnatal age, fluid output and pancreatic enzyme activity are greater in premature than in full-term neonates. Lipase activity is present by 34–36 weeks' gestation and increases fivefold during the first week and 20-fold during the first 9 months of postnatal life.[14] In contrast, amylase activity has been detected as early as 22 weeks' gestation but remains very low even after birth (approximating 10 percent of adult values). Numerous investigators have shown decreased duodenal amylase activity in both fasting and fed infants during the first year of life. Trypsin secretion in response to pancreozymin and secretin administration is blunted in term infants but develops during the first year of life.[9]

Duodenal contractions in term neonates appear to occur at rates similar to those observed in fasting adults, although the number of contractions per burst is less.[15] Fasting or interdigestive motor activity also appears to be shorter in children.[9,16] Very few studies are available, however, quantitating digestive and absorptive capacity relative to age.[9,15,16]

Additional Physiologic Processes

Colonization of the gastrointestinal tract by bacteria, a process that influences the metabolism of bile salts and drugs as well as intestinal motility, varies with age, type of delivery, type of feeding, and concurrent drug therapy. All full-term, formula-fed, vaginally delivered infants are colonized with anaerobic bacteria by 4–6 days of postnatal life. By 5–12 months of age, an adult pattern of microbial reduction products is established. Despite the description of these maturational changes, there are only limited data on the metabolic activity of the gut flora. For example, children are colonized with intestinal bacteria capable of metabolizing digoxin; the capacity to inactivate the drug appears to develop gradually with age.

The diseases that will most likely have the greatest impact on oral drug absorption are those affecting the total surface area available for absorption, such as the short-bowel syndrome (Table 17–3). This syndrome often results from massive bowel resection complicating nec-

TABLE 17–3. SELECTED DISEASE STATES AFFECTING GASTROINTESTINAL ABSORPTION OF DRUGS

Decreased surface area:
    Short-bowel syndrome
    Protein–calorie malnutrition
Delayed gastric emptying:
    Pyloric stenosis
    Congestive heart failure
    Protein–calorie malnutrition
Bile salt excretion:
    Cholestatic liver disease
    Extrahepatic biliary obstruction
Intestinal transit time:
    Protein–calorie malnutrition
    Thyroid disease
    Diarrheal disease
Gastric acid secretion:
    Proximal small-bowel resection

rotizing enterocolitis, from malrotation with volvulus, or from certain congenital anomalies of the gastrointestinal tract during the neonatal period. In addition, drug absorption may be altered during periods of protein–calorie malnutrition, a condition leading to loss of available surface area due to villous atrophy, delayed gastric emptying, and increased intestinal transit time.[17]

Extraintestinal diseases also may affect gastrointestinal drug absorption. Congestive heart failure may cause mucosal edema, or it may, by means of various hemodynamic compensations, affect drug absorption by delaying gastric emptying or by shunting blood flow away from visceral organs to accommodate the metabolic needs of the heart and brain. Additionally, hypo- or hyperthyroidism may influence drug absorption by prolonging or reducing intestinal transit time, respectively. Table 17–3 summarizes the effects of specific intestinal and extraintestinal disease states on the processes involved in oral drug absorption.

Drug Absorption Following Parenteral Administration

The parenteral route of drug administration is important when oral therapy is physiologically precluded or the bioavailability of an oral formulation is poor. The intravenous route for drug delivery is preferred over intramuscular injection; however, neonates frequently have poor intravenous access, and intramuscular injection then becomes a viable and effective alternative for the administration of many drugs. In addition to the ontogenetic factors controlling the absorption addressed previously, most extravascular routes share physicochemical and physiologic constraints (Table 17–4) that may affect the rate and/or extent of drug bioavailability. The following subsections will highlight pharmacokinetic considerations of several nonoral extravascular routes of administration.

Absorption of Drugs Given Intramuscularly

Serum concentration versus time curves following intramuscular drug administration may depend on factors germane to the drug, the site of administration, the presence of concomitant pathophysiology, and/or the developmental status of the patient. Both physicochemical and physiologic factors affect the rate of drug absorption from the injection site.[18] Lipophilicity of a drug favors rapid diffusion into the capillaries; however, the drug must retain a degree of water solubility at physiologic pH to prevent precipitation at the injection site (Table 17–5).

Another important factor influencing absorption of drugs from an intramuscular injection site is the blood flow to and from the injection site. This may be compromised in newborns with poor peripheral perfusion from low cardiac output states or the respiratory distress syndrome.[19] The rate and extent of absorption from an intramuscular injection site are also influenced by the total surface area of muscle coming into contact with the injected

TABLE 17–4. CONSIDERATIONS FOR EXTRAVASCULAR ROUTES OF DRUG ADMINISTRATION THAT MAY AFFECT DRUG ABSORPTION

Physicochemical factors:
  Molecular weight
  pK_a and degree of ionization
  Lipid–water partition coefficient
  pH and viscosity at the site(s) of membrane translocation
  Particle size
  Number and diameter of membrane pores
  Thickness and surface area of membranes at site(s) of translocation
  Relative differences in solute concentration around membranes
Physiologic factors:
  Presence or absence of facilitated or active transport mechanisms
  Relative surface area at sites of membrane translocation
  Volume of fluid at administration site
  Presence or absence of metabolic pathways and/or enzymes necessary for biotransformation
  Determinants of residence time at absorptive sites (i.e., GI motility, bulk flow of CSF, etc.)
  Blood supply to site(s) of membrane translocation
  Affinity of drug for binding to plasma and/or tissue constituents
  Concomitant pathophysiology

solution,[18] similar to the dependency of oral absorption on the total available absorptive area in the intestines. The ratio of skeletal muscle mass to body mass is less for neonates than for adults.[19]

A final consideration in intramuscular absorption is muscle activity, which may affect the rate of absorption and therefore affect the peak serum concentration. Sick, immobile neonates or those receiving a paralyzing agent such as pancuronium may show reduced absorption rates following intramuscular drug administration.

Intramuscular and intravenous dosing for a given drug may be associated with differences in both the serum concentrations and the pharmacokinetic parameter estimates (i.e., half-life and apparent volume of distribution). Consequently, these potential differences must be considered where serum concentration data following intramuscular administration are used for pharmacokinetic calculations.

Percutaneous Absorption

The skin represents an often overlooked, but important organ for systemic absorption. Chemical agents applied to the skin of a premature infant may result in inadvertent poisoning. There are numerous reports in the literature of neonatal toxicity related to the cutaneous exposure to drugs and chemicals. They include hexachlorophene,[20] pentachlorophenol-containing laundry detergents,[21] hydrocortisone,[22] and aniline-containing disinfectant solutions.[23] Therefore, extreme caution should be exercised in using topical therapy in newborn infants.

The morphologic and functional development of the skin[24] as well as the factors that influence penetration of drugs into and through the skin[25] have been reviewed recently. Basically, the percutaneous absorption of a compound is directly related to the degree of skin hydration and relative absorptive surface area and inversely related to the thickness of the stratum corneum.[26] The integument of the full-term neonate possesses intact barrier function.[27] However, the ratio of surface area to body weight of the full-term neonate is much larger than that of an adult. Theoretically, if a newborn receives the same percutaneous dose of a compound as an adult, the systemic availability per kilogram of body weight will be approximately 2.7 times greater in the neonate.

In contrast, studies in premature infants suggest the existence of an immature barrier to percutaneous absorption.[28] Nachman and Esterly[28] studied the blanching response to topical 10 percent phenylephrine in preterm and term infants. Newborn infants of 28–34 weeks' gestational age had a rapid response lasting from 30 minutes to as long as 6–8 hours. No response was apparent under the same study conditions at 21 days of postnatal age. Newborns of gestational age 35–37 weeks had a less dramatic response with a longer latency period, and term infants failed to demonstrate a blanching response.

Finally, if the integrity of the integument is compromised (denuded, burned, or inflamed skin, for example), then percutaneous translocation of compounds into the blood will be enhanced.

Rectal Absorption

Rectal administration of drugs is of potential therapeutic importance if a patient cannot take an agent orally and

TABLE 17–5. DRUGS DEMONSTRATING EFFECTIVE SYSTEMIC ABSORPTION FOLLOWING INTRAMUSCULAR ADMINISTRATION IN NEONATES

Antibacterials:
  Amikacin
  Ampicillin
  Benzathinepenicillin (penicillin G benzathine)
  Benzylpenicillin (penicillin G)
  Carbenicillin
  Cefazolin
  Cefotaxime
  Ceftazidime
  Ceftriaxone
  Clindamycin
  Gentamicin
  Kanamycin
  Latamoxef (moxalactam)
  Methicillin
  Oxacillin
  Nafcillin
  Piperacillin
  Ticarcillin
  Tobramycin
Antituberculous agents:
  Isoniazid
  Streptomycin
Anticonvulsants:
  Diazepam
  Phenobarbitone
Sedatives/tranquilizers:
  Chlorpromazine
  Promethazine

Cardiovascular drugs:
  Hydralazine
  Procainamide
  Pyridostigmine
Diuretics:
  Acetazolamide
  Fursemide (furosemide)
  Bumetanide
Endocrine:
  Corticotrophin (ACTH)
  Cortisone
  Desoxycorticosterone
  Glucagon
Pituitary:
  Vasopressin (tannate oil)
Narcotics:
  Pethidine (meperidine)
  Morphine
Vitamins:
  K
  D

Source: From Blumer JL: Therapeutic agents. In Fanaroff and Martin (eds): Neonatal-Perinatal Medicine: Diseases of the Foetus and Infant, 4th ed. St Louis, CV Mosby, 1987, p 1248.

intravenous access for drug administration is impractical. The rectal vault may serve as an important alternative site for systemic drug administration when nausea, vomiting, seizure activity, and/or preparation for surgery preclude the use of oral dosage forms. General principles regarding the physicochemical factors,[29] clinical pharmacokinetics,[30] and therapeutic use of the rectal route in children[31] have been reviewed previously.

Knowledge of the venous drainage system for the lower gastrointestinal tract is imperative in understanding the potential bioavailability of drugs administered rectally. The inferior and middle rectal veins, which drain the anus and lower rectum, respectively, drain directly into the systemic circulation by means of the inferior vena cava, whereas the superior rectal vein, which drains the upper part of the rectum, empties into the portal vein by means of the inferior mesenteric vein. Therefore, drugs administered into the superior aspect of the rectum will be subjected to the hepatic first-pass effect because portal blood enters the liver, whereas drugs administered lower into the rectum will initially bypass the liver.

The predominant mechanism for drug absorption from the rectum is probably similar to that observed in the upper gastrointestinal tract, i.e., passive diffusion. Theoretically, the physicochemical and host factors discussed earlier with respect to oral drug absorption also influence rectal drug absorption (see Table 17–1). In general, absorption from aqueous or alcoholic solutions is more rapid than from suppositories.

Lipophilic drugs with pK_a values between 7 and 8, such as barbiturates and benzodiazepines, seem to be ideally suited for rectal administration because they will be mostly in an un-ionized form and will readily cross cell membranes. Rectal administration of 0.25–0.5 mg/kg of a diazepam solution to children 2 weeks to 11 years old produced serum concentrations comparable with those observed following intravenous administration. Additionally, peak serum concentrations occurred within 6 minutes of administration. Potentially effective anticonvulsant serum concentrations were maintained for 1–3 hours. The clinical efficacy of rectal diazepam in preventing recurrent febrile seizures has been demonstrated.

Drug Administration Techniques

Certainly other routes of drug administration besides the oral, intravenous, intramuscular, percutaneous, and rectal routes may be employed when treating newborns; however, there has been little work systematically evaluating drug absorption from the endotracheal, epidural, intrathecal, and intraperitoneal routes.

An issue of equal importance to the route of administration is the actual method employed to administer the drug. For optimal therapeutics to be realized, a method of drug administration must be used that will enable the drug to reach its site of action at the desired time and in an effective concentration.[32] The technique or method of drug administration is often the most crucial factor to consider when serum concentrations are used for pharmacokinetic analysis. The lack of awareness of or attention to critical aspects of drug administration techniques can lead to therapeutic misadventures even in the face of the most sophisticated analytical and pharmacokinetic methods[33] (Table 17–6).

TABLE 17–6. POTENTIAL ERRORS IN DRUG ADMINISTRATION TECHNIQUES

Factors involving drug (dose) preparation:
 Inappropriate dilutions
 Similarity in appearance of dose units
 Loss of potentially large amounts of drug dose in the dead space of a syringe; infusion Y site, etc.
 Unsuitable drug formulations for administration
 Unlabeled or undesirable ingredients in dosage forms
 Undesirable drug concentrations and/or osmolalities
 Errors in interpreting drug orders and/or dose calculations

Factors involving I.V. drug administration:
 Loss of drug consequent to routine changing of I.V. sets
 Reduction in serum concentrations for drugs with rapid plasma clearance that are infused slowly
 Extreme increase in plasma drug concentrations consequent to rapid infusion of drugs with small central compartment volume of distribution
 Delayed infusion of total dose when I.V. line is not flushed
 Inadvertent admixture of drugs by the manual I.V. retrograde method
 Large distance between the site of drug infusion into an I.V. line and the insertion of the line into the patient
 Potential loss of large volume doses in the overflow syringe with the I.V. retrograde technique
 Possible loss of drug because of binding to I.V. tubing
 Use of large intraluminal diameter tubing for small patients
 Infiltrations not detected by pump alarms
 Infusion of multiple medications/fluids at different rates by means of a common "hub"
 Oscillations in fluid/dose rate of potent medications infused with piston-type pumps

Factors involving other routes of drug administration:
 Loss in delivery (nasogastric tube dead space) or from oral cavity
 Leakage of drug from I.M. or S.C. injection site
 Expulsion of drug from the rectum
 Misapplication to external sites (i.e., ophthalmic ointment in young infants)

Several steps can and should be taken to minimize problems with drug administration. These may include one or more of the following: standardization and documentation of complete administration times, documentation of the volume and content of the solution used to "flush" an intravenous or oral dose, tailoring of the concentrations of drug solutions for desired osmolalities, standardization of specific infusion techniques for drugs with a narrow therapeutic index, standardization of dilution and infusion volumes for drugs given by intermittent intravenous injection, avoidance of attaching lines for drug infusion to a central hub with other solutions being infused at widely disparate rates, preferential use of large-gauge Teflon cannulas, maintenance of the recommended solution head height for gravity controllers, and the use of low-volume tubing and the most distal sites for access of drug into an existing intravenous line. In every situation where monitoring of serum drug concentrations is to be employed, the method of drug administration should be noted before these data are used in pharmacokinetic calculations.

DRUG DISTRIBUTION

The movement of drugs and other compounds from the systemic circulation into various body compartments, tissues, and cells is termed *distribution*. The distribution of most drugs in the body is influenced by a variety of age-dependent factors, including protein binding, body compartment sizes, hemodynamic factors such as cardiac output and regional blood flow, and membrane permeability.[34]

The apparent volume of distribution (V_d) describes the relationship between the amount of drug in the body and its plasma concentration.[35] V_d is the volume needed to contain the total-body store of drug if the concentration throughout the whole body were the same as in plasma. This is represented by the following mathematical relationship:

$$V_d = \frac{D}{C_0} \qquad (1)$$

where D is the dose administered and C_0 is derived by extrapolating the slope of the plasma concentration versus time curve to time zero. Several factors, including plasma protein concentration and tissue binding, affect V_d. This relationship is expressed by the following equation.[36]

$$V_d = V_b + V_t \frac{f_B}{f_t} \qquad (2)$$

where V_b is blood volume, V_t is tissue volume, f_B is fraction of unbound drug in the blood, and f_t is the fraction of unbound drug in tissue. Therefore, any factor that increases the blood volume or the fraction of unbound drug in the blood or reduces the fraction of unbound drug in the tissue will increase V_d.

Developmental Aspects of Protein Binding

The binding of drugs to plasma protein is dependent on the concentration of available binding proteins, the affinity constant of the protein(s) for the drug, the number of available binding sites, and the presence of pathophysiologic conditions or endogenous compounds that may alter the drug–protein binding interaction[37–39] (Table 17–7).

The affinity of albumin for acidic drugs increases, as do total plasma protein levels, from birth into early infancy.[26] These values do not reach normal adult levels until 10–12 months of age.[40] In addition, although plasma albumin may reach adult levels shortly after birth,[41] the albumin level in blood is directly proportional to gestational age, reflecting both placental transport and fetal synthesis.[42]

Different degrees of drug–protein binding between newborn and adult plasma have been demonstrated (Table 17–8). Four mechanisms have been proposed to explain these differences: (1) displacement of drugs from binding sites by bilirubin in cord plasma, (2) different binding properties of cord and adult albumin, (3) different binding properties of globulins, and (4) decreased binding properties of albumin owing to interaction with globulins in newborns.

Albumin is not the only plasma protein that binds drugs. Basic drugs are bound by several plasma proteins, including α_1-acid glycoprotein.[39] Piafsky and Mpamugo[43] showed significant reductions in both α_1-acid glycoprotein plasma concentrations and in binding of the basic drugs lidocaine and propranolol to cord blood as compared with adult controls. When the α_1-acid glycoprotein concentration in cord blood was increased to adult values, the protein binding of lidocaine and propranolol approached adult levels, suggesting the reduced plasma concentration of α_1-acid glycoprotein as the primary reason for the decreased protein binding.

Influence of Endogenous Substances on Protein Binding

There are a number of endogenous molecules which, like drugs, may bind to plasma proteins[34] and displace drugs from these binding sites. The effect is generally transient and may increase the apparent volume of distribution of the displaced drug. More important, the increase in the fraction of free drug that occurs may result in a tran-

TABLE 17–7. PHYSIOLOGIC VARIABLES INFLUENCING DRUG–PROTEIN BINDING IN INFANCY AND CHILDHOOD*

| | PATIENT AGE GROUP | | |
PARAMETER	Neonate	Infant	Child
Total protein	Decreased	Decreased	Equivalent
Plasma albumin	Decreased	Equivalent	Equivalent
Fetal albumin	Present	Absent	Absent
Plasma globulin	Decreased	Decreased	Equivalent
Unconjugated bilirubin	Increased	Equivalent	Equivalent
Free fatty acids	Increased	Equivalent	Equivalent
Blood pH	Low	Equivalent	Equivalent
α_1-Acid glycoprotein	Decreased	Data not available	Equivalent

*Relative to adult values.
Source: Adapted from Radde.[34]

TABLE 17–8. COMPARATIVE PROTEIN BINDING OF SOME REPRESENTATIVE DRUGS

	PERCENT BOUND	
DRUG	Newborn	Adult
Ampicillin	10	18
Diazepam	84	99
Lidocaine	20	70
Phenytoin	80	90
Propranolol	60	93
Theophylline	36	56

Source: From Marx.[6]

siently intensified pharmacologic response at a given drug dose or serum total drug concentration.

Clinically significant protein binding displacement reactions will occur only when (1) a drug is more than 80–90 percent protein-bound, (2) the drug's clearance is capacity limited, (3) the drug's clearance is binding-sensitive, and (4) the V_d must be small, usually less than 0.15 liter/kg because above this value, only a small percentage of total drug in the body is found in plasma.[44]

Under these conditions, the following sequence of events may occur: The displacement reaction increases the amount of free drug, which may result in a heightened pharmacologic response if the drug's concentration–effect curve is reasonably steep. However, this intensified pharmacologic effect is only transient because the displacement reaction increases the amount of free drug available for metabolism or excretion. The net result, once steady state is achieved, is a decreased concentration of total drug in plasma accompanied by an unchanged free drug concentration.

Free Fatty Acids (FFA)

Nonesterified fatty acids are reversibly bound to albumin[45] and are present at relatively high concentrations in the plasma of newborn infants. Significant reductions in albumin binding of phenylbutazone, dicoumarol (bishydroxycoumarin), and phenytoin have been demonstrated at high serum levels of free fatty acids (FFA), approximately 2000 μEq/liter, or at an FFA/albumin molar ratio of 3.5. Although these values are rarely attained, they have been observed under certain pathophysiologic conditions such as gram-negative septicemia.

Interestingly, similar elevations in FFA levels have not been reported with gram-positive septicemia, which is common in newborns. Displacing effects of FFAs on the unbound fraction of diazepam have been reported in newborns, and a linear correlation between unbound plasma phenytoin concentrations and the ratio of serum FFA to albumin concentration in neonates has been described.

Bilirubin

Bilirubin is noncovalently bound to albumin, and this association is freely reversible.[46] The bilirubin binding affinity of albumin at birth is independent of gestational age[47,48] and is less in the newborn than in the adult.[49] The binding affinity of albumin for bilirubin increases with age[47,50] and reaches that of adult serum by approximately 5 months of age.[50] Ebbesen and Nyboe[47] found that this increased affinity, at least during the first week of life, is related to gestational age. The lower bilirubin binding affinity of albumin in neonates is believed to be a contributing factor in their susceptibility to kernicterus.[50] However, other factors, such as the effect of hypothermia, acidosis, hypoglycemia, hypoxemia, sepsis, birth asphyxia, and hypercapnia on the permeability of the blood–brain barrier and on bilirubin–albumin binding must be considered.[51]

A number of drugs are thought to be able to compete with and displace bilirubin from binding sites on the albumin molecule, thus increasing the risk of the infant's developing kernicterus[52] (Table 17–9).

Developmental Aspects of Fluid Compartment Sizes

Total-Body Water

Alterations in body water compartment sizes will affect the volume of distribution of a drug. Age-dependent changes in the various fluid compartments have been reviewed and are summarized in Table 17–10. Total-body water varies inversely with the amount of fat tissue in the body. In the young fetus, total-body water comprises nearly 92 percent of body weight, with the extracellular fluid volume responsible for 25 percent of body weight; body fat is less than 1 percent.[53]

At term, total-body water falls to approximately 75 percent of body weight, and the amount of fat increases to approximately 15 percent. By 6 months of age, total-body water and fat comprise 60 and 30 percent of body weight, respectively. In the second year of life, there is a small

TABLE 17–9. PRINCIPLES RELATED TO DRUG-INDUCED BILIRUBIN DISPLACEMENT AND THE RISK OF KERNICTERUS

1. Drugs that are administered in low doses such as hormones, cardiac glycosides, and potent loop diuretics are not dangerous because a certain molar amount of the drug is required to occupy a significant fraction of the reserve albumin.

2. Cationic drugs and most electroneutral substances, such as aminoglycosides, antihistamines, general anesthetics, and benzodiazepines, are not bound competitively to the bilirubin-binding site.

3. Sulphonamides show a highly variable effect. Sulfadiazine is the weakest competitor and is probably safe at usual doses.

4. Several analgesics and anti-inflammatory drugs are potent displacers.

5. The highest degree of displacement is observed with x-ray contrast media for cholangiography.

Source: Modified from Brodersen.[52]

TABLE 17–10. FLUID COMPARTMENT SIZE AS A FUNCTION OF AGE

AGE	TOTAL-BODY WATER*	EXTRACELLULAR FLUID*	INTRACELLULAR FLUID*
<3-month fetus	92	65	25
Term gestation	75	35–44	33
4–6 Months	60	≈23	37
12 Months		26–30	
Puberty	≈60	20	40
Adult	50–60	20	40

*As a percentage of body weight.

increase in total-body water due to a sudden increase in the intracellular fluid volume.[54] Except for a small increase prior to puberty in males, a gradual reduction in total-body water occurs in both sexes, approaching adult values of 50 to 60 percent of body weight at puberty.

Extracellular Fluid Volume

The extracellular fluid volume can be estimated from the distribution of chloride or bromide ions, since both these elements distribute primarily in extracellular fluid, entering the intracellular fluid to only a minor extent. By 40 weeks' gestation, measurements of extracellular fluid volume range from 350–440 ml/kg of body weight[54] and correlate more closely with body weight than with gestational age. By 1 year of age, the extracellular fluid volume decreases to approximately 26–30 percent of body weight, and after the first year, it decreases slowly and gradually approaches the adult value of 20 percent of body weight by puberty.

Intracellular Fluid Volume

The intracellular fluid volume cannot be measured directly, and thus it must be estimated by subtracting the extracellular fluid volume from total-body water. The intracellular fluid volume increases from 25 percent of body weight in the young fetus to 33 percent at birth to approximately 37 percent of body weight at 4 months of age.[53] Except for a sudden increase during early childhood, the intracellular fluid volume remains relatively constant, approximating 40 percent of body weight.

The clinical relevance of this gradual reduction in the size of body water compartments with age cannot be overemphasized. In order to achieve comparable plasma and tissue concentrations of drugs distributing into the extracellular fluid, higher doses per kilogram of body weight must be given to infants and children than to adults.[55]

DRUG METABOLISM

The process of drug removal from the body starts the instant a drug molecule is present within the body. The primary organ for drug metabolism is the liver, but the kidneys, intestine, lungs, and skin are also capable of biotransformation.[56] Although the metabolism of most drugs generally results in pharmacologically weaker or inactive compounds, parent compounds may be transformed into active metabolites (e.g., theophylline to caffeine or procainamide to N-acetyl procainamide). Furthermore, pharmacologically inactive compounds, or prodrugs, may be converted to their active moiety (e.g., chloramphenicol succinate or palmitate to the active chloramphenicol base) (Table 17–11).

Hepatic xenobiotic metabolism assumes an extremely important role in determining the pharmacokinetic and pharmacodynamic properties of a drug. The pharmacokinetic parameter *clearance* describes the overall rate of drug removal.[24] It can be described in terms of plasma clearance, organ clearance, or total-body clearance.[57] *Plasma clearance* is the volume of plasma from which a drug is completely removed per unit of time. Drugs can be cleared by several mechanisms, with hepatic biotransformation, renal excretion, and exhalation by the lungs representing the primary routes.[55] The clearance of a drug by an individual organ is dependent on the blood flow to the organ (Q) and the organ's extraction ratio (E) and can be described as follows[36]:

$$Cl = Q \times E \qquad (3)$$

where E is the ratio of the arteriovenous concentration difference divided by the arterial concentration, as expressed by the following relationship:

$$E = \frac{C_a - C_v}{C_a} \qquad (4)$$

where C_a and C_v are the arterial and venous concentrations, respectively. Hepatic clearance depends on hepatic blood flow, plasma free-drug concentration, cellular

TABLE 17–11. ACTIVE METABOLITES OF DRUGS USED IN NEONATES

PARENT DRUG	ACTIVE METABOLITE(S)
Diazepam	Desmethyldiazepam, oxazepam
Lidocaine	Mono- and didesethyl lignocaine
Meperidine	Normeperidine
Procainamide	N-Acetyl procainamide
Propranolol	4-Hydroxypropranolol
Theophylline	Caffeine

uptake, hepatic metabolism, and biliary excretion. The hepatic clearance of a drug can be expressed by the following equation:

$$Cl_H = Q \times \frac{f_B \times Cl_{int}}{Q + (f_B \times Cl_{int})} \qquad (5)$$

where Cl_H is hepatic clearance, Q is hepatic blood flow, f_B is the fraction of free drug, and Cl_{int} is the intrinsic clearance, which is a measure of hepatocellular metabolism. Drugs that are primarily cleared by the liver can be classified as *flow-limited* or *capacity-limited.*[36,57] If a drug displays a high Cl_{int} and E, then doubling the Cl_{int} will have little effect on Cl_H, whereas a change in blood flow will produce a proportional change in Cl_H. In other words, for drugs that are highly extracted (>80 percent) and are metabolized by the liver, Cl_H reflects the amount and rate of the drug delivered to the liver.[58]

Drugs with high extraction ratios will be subjected to the *first-pass effect* when administered orally. This term, coined by Harris and Riegelman[59] for aspirin, signifies that a drug is rapidly metabolized or altered when passing through the intestinal mucosa or liver for the first time. Therefore, the parent compound is found in lower concentrations in the systemic circulation than if the drug were administered intravenously, and conversely, metabolites that are frequently inactive are the predominant form of the parent drug found in the circulation.[60] Examples of drugs that undergo such high extraction rates include lidocaine, propranolol, acetylsalicylic acid, and isoprenaline (isoproterenol).

Capacity-limited drugs display low extraction ratios (<20 percent) and low intrinsic metabolic clearance.[36] Hepatic clearance is therefore dependent on the degree of hepatic uptake and metabolism of the drug and is independent of hepatic blood flow. Capacity-limited drugs can be further subdivided into binding-sensitive and binding-insensitive drugs. *Binding-sensitive drugs,* such as clindamycin,[36] have extraction ratios that approach the free drug concentration ($E = f_B$). Therefore, factors that increase f_B, such as decreased protein binding, will increase hepatic clearance. In contrast, other drugs may display extraction ratios that are much less than the free drug, and therefore, the hepatic clearance is only a function of the intrinsic clearance and is independent of protein binding. These drugs are referred to as *binding-insensitive* (e.g., chloramphenicol).

Developmental Aspects of Hepatic Clearance

At every level, from the ontogenetic changes in hepatic blood flow and portal oxygen tension to the developmental alterations in protein binding and xenobiotic metabolizing enzyme activities, there is the potential for age and various pathophysiologic states to have an impact on the process associated with hepatic clearance. Very little investigative effort has been expended to elucidate these effects; however, some of the important available data are discussed below.

Drug Uptake

The first step in drug metabolism is uptake of the drug by the metabolizing cell. Ligandin, or Y protein, is a basic protein that binds bilirubin and organic anions such as drugs.[61] It is present in hepatocytes, as well as proximal renal tubular cells and nongoblet, small intestinal mucosal cells.[62] The concentration of ligandin in the fetus and neonate is low but appears to approach adult values during the first 5–10 days of postnatal life.[55,61] Thus it is likely that the hepatic clearance of capacity-limited drugs will be lower in neonates than in older infants and children.

Biotransformation: Phase I Reactions

Drug biotransformation within the hepatocyte involves two primary enzymatic processes: phase I, or nonsynthetic, and phase II, or synthetic, reactions. Phase I reactions include oxidation, reduction, hydrolysis, and hydroxylation reactions, whereas phase II reactions primarily involve conjugation with glycine, glucuronide, or sulfate. Most drug-metabolizing enzymes are located in the smooth endoplasmic reticulum of cells and are recovered as the microsomal fraction on homogenation.

The ontogeny of human drug-metabolizing enzyme systems differs dramatically from that of most animal species, especially for oxidation and glucuronidation pathways.[64] Therefore, it is difficult to extrapolate data for enzyme systems capable of metabolizing drugs from animals to humans. The hepatic cytochrome P-450 mixed-function oxidase system has been studied in the most detail. It is responsible for many of the phase I reactions catalyzed in the human liver.

Yaffe et al.[65] first demonstrated drug-oxidizing enzymes in human fetal liver. During fetal life, these enzymes are present at 30–50 percent of adult activity *in vitro.* After corrections for differences in liver weight, however, the specific activity *in vitro* for many of these enzymes approaches adult levels.[66,67] Gillette and Stripp[68] correlated the appearance of these enzymes with the development of rough endoplasmic reticulum. By 7–9 weeks' gestation in humans, the rough endoplasmic reticulum is developing, and by 3 months' gestation, the smooth endoplasmic reticulum is considerably developed.[69] It appears that the increase in mono-oxygenase activity observed in the first trimester plateaus during the second trimester.[70]

Postnatally, the hepatic cytochrome P-450 mono-oxygenase system appears to mature rapidly. Phenytoin and its metabolites appear in the urine of newborns and adults in similar proportions.[71] Furthermore, the decline in serum drug concentration parallels the rate of urinary metabolite excretion, suggesting that the rate of excretion reflects the rate of hepatic metabolism of phenytoin. Several investigators have demonstrated slow elimination of phenytoin in the first 2 days of postnatal life, followed by a rapid phase thereafter. Neims et al.[70] combined the data from several studies on phenytoin kinetics in newborns and calculated the mean phenytoin plasma half-lives to be 80, 15, and 6 hours for the age groups 0–2, 3–14, and 14–150 days, respectively.

The increased rate of elimination could be explained by dose-dependent kinetics caused by saturation of the drug-metabolizing enzyme system, or it could be due to maturation of the metabolic pathway. The latter explanation is most plausible for two reasons: First, for most patients, a constant period elapsed before entrance into the rapid phase of elimination, and this period was independent of serum concentrations. Second, Elimination of other drugs, such as tolbutamide and phenobarbital, that undergo metabolic oxidation but do not display saturation kinetics follows a similar pattern of elimination.[72-74]

Neims et al.[70] calculated the elimination half-life of phenobarbital in newborns and infants based on pooled data. Half-lives of greater than 200 hours, about 100 hours, and about 50 hours for the age groups 0–5, 5–15, and 30–900 days of postnatal life, respectively, were found. This pattern supports the impressions gained from kinetic data obtained with phenytoin that certain drug-metabolizing pathways at birth have only 30–50 percent of adult activity, but shortly after birth this activity may increase to levels several times greater than are observed in adults. However, generalization about the oxidative metabolism of drugs cannot be made and thus should be avoided.

Rane et al.[75] found similar half-lives for carbamazepine in newborns and adults. However, the mothers of the infants studied were receiving the drug, and carbamazepine is known to induce its own metabolism. Other drugs given to pregnant women may induce hepatic enzymes as well. These include tricyclic antidepressants, phenytoin, diazepam, and phenobarbital.[76]

The development of other phase I enzyme systems has been studied much less extensively. Alcohol dehydrogenase activity is detectable in 2-month-old fetuses at levels no greater than 3–4 percent of adult activity.[77] Moreover, the level of activity does not approach adult values until after 5 years of age. Qualitative changes in the alcohol dehydrogenase isoenzymes also occur during fetal development, although they are poorly defined.

The ability to reduce aromatic nitro groups has been shown to be present in fetal livers by 7–8 weeks of gestation; however, the hepatic activity by midgestation remains low,[76] and no specific postnatal pattern of development had been described. Also, very few data exist on the ontogeny of hydrolytic enzymes. Ecobichon and Stephens[78] found low levels of blood esterase activity in the fetus and neonate.

Biotransformation: Phase II Reactions

Conjugation reactions, or phase II reactions, synthesize more water-soluble compounds by combining a substance with an endogenous molecule in order to enhance excretion of that substance. Glucuronide, sulfate, and glycine are the common endogenous molecules to which drugs are bound. A drug must possess a specific functional group, such as a carboxyl, hydroxyl, amino, or sulphydryl group, in order to be conjugated. Alternatively, a drug may acquire one of these functional groups by undergoing phase I reactions. Glucuronidation is the most common

conjugation pathway, owing to the availability of glucuronic acid and the variety of functional groups just listed. Sulfation mainly involves phenolic hydroxyl groups, with alcoholic hydroxyl groups with primary amino groups involved in a lesser degree. Glycine primarily combines with aromatic carboxyl groups attached to an x-amino group. Acetylation occurs at aromatic amino or hydrazino groups.[79]

Development of Conjugation Pathways

A series of reactions is necessary for glucuronidation to occur.[79] Uridine diphosphate (UDP) glucuronic acid is formed by combining UDP-glucose with NAD^+, a reaction catalyzed by UDP-glucose dehydrogenase (UDPG-D). Following this, UDP glucuronic acid combines with a substrate to form the glucuronide moiety. This reaction is catalyzed by UDP-glucuronyl transferase (UDPG-T). Felsher et al.[80] demonstrated decreased UDPG-T enzymatic activity in 2 human fetuses aged 17 and 22 weeks' gestational age, and an absence of activity in 15 fetuses aged 8–19 weeks. For UDPG-D they found the mean activity for fetuses aged 8–18 weeks to be 25 percent that of healthy adults. This confirmed earlier work by Rane et al.,[63] who found no UDPG-T activity for several substrates in human fetuses 13–22 weeks old. At birth, compounds that rely on glucuronidation for elimination have markedly prolonged half-lives or are conjugated by means of different pathways compared with children and adults.[64]

Levy et al.[81] demonstrated in 2- to 3-day-old term infants a limited ability to conjugate acetaminophen with glucuronide, which is the major conjugation pathway in adults. However, the limited ability to glucuronidate acetaminophen was compensated for by a well-developed sulfation pathway.[81] This supports the *in vitro* findings of Rollins et al.,[82] who demonstrated the capability of fetal liver at 19–22 weeks of age to conjugate acetaminophen with sulfate, and of Alam et al.,[83] who showed that rates for glucuronidation are much lower and sulfation much higher with salicylamide and paracetamol as substrates in children 7–10 years old than in adults.

Studies evaluating bilirubin and chloramphenicol as substrates for glucuronidation have described low rates at birth, with adult rates achieved by 3 years of age.[83] There is some evidence, however, that phenobarbital may induce glucuronidation in newborns. Talafant et al.[84] administered phenobarbital 10 mg/kg per day to healthy full-term infants for their first 3 days of life. One group received phenobarbital intramuscularly, one group orally, and one group served as a control. These authors described significantly higher urinary glucaric acid concentrations on day 7 in the intramuscular group than in the controls. This correlated well with a downward trend ($.05 < p < .10$) in serum bilirubin in the same group.

Other conjugating pathways in the fetus and neonate have not been studied thoroughly. The conjugation of glycine with substrates appears to occur as rapidly in fetal liver as in adults,[76] whereas certain methylation reactions, which are not clinically significant in adults, appear to be functional in the fetus and neonate. Theophylline has been shown by Aranda et al.[85] to be methylated to caffeine in 12- to 20-week-old fetal livers.

Drug Elimination

The elimination half-life ($t_{1/2B}$) of a drug is commonly used to describe its disappearance from the blood and is measured as the time required for half the amount of drug present in the blood to disappear. The following equation can be used to describe $t_{1/2B}$:[7]

$$t_{1/2B} = \frac{0.693 V_d}{Cl} \qquad (6)$$

The $t_{1/2B}$ of a drug is a parameter that may be employed clinically to devise initial drug dosing guidelines. Recognition of an unusual half-life due to pathophysiologic changes should prompt the clinician to assess the need for dosage and/or dosing interval alterations.

RENAL EXCRETION

Most drugs and/or their metabolites are excreted from the body by the kidneys. Renal excretion is dependent on glomerular filtration, tubular reabsorption, and tubular secretion[86] (Table 17–12). The amount of a drug that is filtered per unit time is influenced by the extent of protein binding and renal plasma flow.[87] If the latter is constant, the greater the extent of protein binding, the smaller will be the fraction of circulating drug that is filtered.

Renal Blood Flow

Renal blood flow and renal plasma flow increase with age as a result of an increase in cardiac output and a reduction in peripheral vascular resistance.[88] The kidneys of the neonate only receive 5–6 percent of total cardiac output compared with 15–25 percent for adults. Renal plasma flow averages 12 ml/min (0.72 liter/h) at birth and increases to 140 ml/min (8.4 liters/h) by 1 year of age. If renal plasma flow is corrected for body surface area, adult values are reached before 30 weeks of extrauterine life.[89]

TABLE 17–12. ONTOGENY OF DRUG ELIMINATION

Kidneys at birth receive only 5–6 percent of cardiac output compared with 15–25 percent in adults.

Renal plasma flow is ≈12 ml/min at birth compared with 140 ml/min in adults.

Glomerular filtration rate is directly proportional to gestational age beyond 34 weeks' gestation.

Tubular secretion increases two-fold over first week of life and 10-fold over first year of life.

Renal blood flow appears to increase in proportion to the development of the renal tubules.[89] In animals, this increase in renal blood flow is associated with intrarenal redistribution of blood flow, resulting in increased flow to the outer cortex with increasing postnatal age.[90] The clinical implications of these developmental changes in renal blood flow are unclear, but they suggest that as tubular mass and function increase, so does the blood supply to the important outer cortical nephrons.

Glomerular Filtration Rate

At birth, glomerular filtration rate (GFR) is directly proportional to gestational age. However, this linear relationship is not evident prior to 34 weeks' gestation.[91] In contrast, GFR, as measured by creatinine clearance or clearance of inulin, remains relatively constant at low rates of 1 ml/min prior to 34 weeks' gestation. The reason for this is unknown, but it appears to correlate with the ontogeny and functional organization of the glomerulus.

The GFR for full-term infants at birth ranges from 2–4 ml/min.[91,92] In the first 2–3 days of postnatal life there is a marked increase in the GFR of full-term babies to rates between 8 and 20 ml/min, compared with an increase in neonates less than 34 weeks' gestation from 1 ml/min to 2–3 ml/min.[92] The increase in GFR after birth has been shown to be dependent on postconceptual age, not on postnatal age.[91,92] Adult values for GFR are reached by 2.5–5 months of age. The postnatal increase in GFR is most likely due to the combined effects of an increase in cardiac output, a decrease in peripheral vascular resistance, an increase in mean arterial blood pressure, an increased surface area available for filtration, and an increase in membrane pore size.[26]

The clinical implications for the maturation of GFR become apparent when one considers drugs that are primarily eliminated by glomerular filtration. Several studies have investigated the pharmacokinetics of aminoglycosides in preterm and term infants.[93,94] A decreasing $t_{1/2B}$ for gentamicin with increasing gestational age in infants less than 7 days of age was found. In addition, in infants between 24 and 48 weeks postconceptual age, a much stronger correlation between gentamicin $t_{1/2B}$ and postconceptual age compared with postnatal age was noted. Since the $t_{1/2B}$ for aminoglycosides is prolonged in newborns of postconceptual age less than 34 weeks, these patients should have their dosing interval lengthened, or individual dose decreased, compared with full-term infants.

Development of Tubular Function

Proximal convoluted tubules in the normal kidney of a full-term infant are small in relation to their corresponding glomeruli. This glomerulotubular imbalance in size is reflected by functional differences in the transport capacity (secretion) of the proximal tubular cells.[88] Using the tubular transport maximum for para-aminohippurate (T_{mPAH}), a compound secreted by the proximal tubules, as

TABLE 17–13. DRUG DISPOSITION IN INFANTS COMPARED WITH ADULTS: POTENTIAL INFLUENCE OF PHARMACOKINETICS

DISPOSITION PARAMETER	NEWBORN VS. ADULT	POSSIBLE PHARMACOKINETIC RESULT	EXAMPLE DRUG
Absorption	↓	↓AUC	Penicillins, sulphonamides
Volume of distribution	↑	↓Peak	Gentamicin, digoxin
% Protein binding	↓	↑Free fraction	Clindamycin, theophylline
Metabolism	↓	↓Clearance	Chloramphenicol, theophylline
Excretion	↓	↑AUC ↑$t_{1/2}$	Gentamicin, furosemide

Abbreviations: ↓ = less than in newborns than in adults; ↑ = greater in newborns than in adults; AUC = area under the concentration versus time curve; $t_{1/2}$ = elimination half-life.

an indicator of tubular function, West et al.[89] found a 10-fold increase in T_{mPAH} in the first year of life, with adult values (corrected for body surface area) being reached by 30 weeks of life. Therefore, tubular function matures at a slower rate than glomerular function. Reasons for this reduced functional capacity include not only the small size of the tubules, but also a smaller mass of functioning tubular cells, reduced blood flow to the outer cortex, and immaturity of energy-supplying processes.[26]

Many drugs rely on either the organic anion or cation transport systems present in the proximal tubules for renal excretion. Penicillin is actively secreted by the para-aminohippurate pathway. Results of pharmacokinetic studies with ampicillin,[95] ticarcillin,[96] benzylpenicillin (penicillin G),[97] and methicillin[98] show that the $t_{1/2B}$ for the penicillins varies inversely with gestational and postnatal age.

In all studies cited above, the $t_{1/2B}$ for the penicillins was highly variable but generally decreased to 1–2 hours by 2 weeks' postnatal age. These observations may be partially explained by the findings in animals that the capacity of the secretory pathways responsible for penicillin secretion may undergo substrate stimulation. Although substrate stimulation has not been formally studied in human neonates, there is evidence that it does occur. Kaplan et al.[95] showed a reduction in $t_{1/2B}$ for ampicillin in both preterm and term infants following multiple doses compared with a single dose. Schwartz et al.[99] reported a case of a human neonate in whom they were unable to maintain therapeutic serum concentrations for dicloxacillin following parenteral penicillin therapy. Peak serum concentrations were normal, indicating normal absorption kinetics. However, the clearance was reported to be higher than that reported in older children, suggesting enhanced tubular secretion.

Furosemide is another drug secreted by the para-aminohippurate pathway in the proximal tubules. In addition to being filtered, evidence for tubular secretion is inferred from adult data describing reduced rates of plasma clearance and urinary excretion following probenecid administration.[100] Aranda et al.[101] found an 8-fold prolongation in $t_{1/2B}$ and an 8-fold reduction in the elimination rate constant for furosemide in fluid-overloaded term and pre-

term neonates with normal renal function compared with adults. Peterson et al.[102] evaluated single-dose kinetics for furosemide in preterm and term infants and found a mean $t_{1/2B}$ of 19.9 hours and 7.7 hours, respectively. This is in contrast to the $t_{1/2B}$ of 30 minutes in healthy adults. These prolonged plasma half-lives correspond with the prolonged duration of diuretic and saluretic effects seen in infants, although the response to furosemide is most likely dependent on its rate of urinary excretion.[103]

SUMMARY

There exist marked differences in drug biodisposition in the newborn compared with the adult with respect to all pharmacokinetic processes (Table 17–13). These differences and the ontogenetic changes in these processes must be considered carefully when developing therapeutic strategies for newborn and young infants.

REFERENCES

1. Shirkey H: Editorial comment: Therapeutic orphans. J Pediatr 72:119–120, 1968
2. Silverman WA, Anderson DH, Blanc WA, et al: A difference in mortality rate and incidence of kernicterus among premature infants allotted to two prophylactic antibacterial regimens. Pediatrics 18:614–624, 1956
3. Sutherland JM: Fatal cardiovascular collapse of infants receiving large amounts of chloramphenicol. Am J Dis Child 97:761–767, 1959
4. Lenz W: A study of the German outbreak of phocomelia. Lancet 2:1332, 1962
5. Taussig H: A study of the German outbreak of phocomelia. JAMA 198:1106–1114, 1962
6. Marx CM, Pope JF, Blumer JL: Developmental toxicology, in Haddad LM, Winchester JF (eds): Clinical Management of Poisoning and Drug Overdose, 2nd ed. Philadelphia, WB Saunders, 1990, pp 388–435
7. Besunder JB, Reed MD, Blumer JL: Principles of drug biodisposition in the neonate: A critical evaluation of the pharmacokinetic–pharmacodynamic interface. Clin Pharmacokinet 14:189–216, 261–286, 1988
8. Hess AF: The gastric secretion of infants at birth. Am J Dis Childs 6:264–284, 1913

9. Grand RJ, Watkins JB, Torti FM: Development of the human gastrointestinal tract: A review. Gastroenterology 70:790–810, 1976
10. Agunod M, Yomaguchi N, Lopez R, Luhby AL, Glass GBJ: Correlative study of hydrochloric acid, pepsin and intrinsic factor secretion in newborns and infants. Am J Dig Dis 14:400–414, 1969
11. Welling PG: Influence of food and diet on gastrointestinal drug absorption: A review. J Pharmacokinet Biopharm 5:291–334, 1977
12. Cavell B: Gastric emptying in infants fed human milk or infant formula. Acta Paediatr Scand 70:639–641, 1981
13. Heubi JE, Babistreri WF, Suchy FJ: Bile salt metabolism in the first year of life. J Lab Clin Med 100:127–136, 1982
14. Cavell B: Gastric emptying in preterm infants. Acta Paediatr Scand 68:725–730, 1979
15. Morriss FH Jr, Moore M, Weisbroadt NW, West NS: Ontogenetic development of gastrointestinal motility. IV. Duodenal contractions in preterm infants. Pediatrics 78:1106–1113, 1986
16. Milla PJ, Fenton TR: Small intestinal motility patterns in the perinatal period. J Pediatr Gastroenterol Nutr 2(suppl 1):5141–5144, 1983
17. Krishnaswamy K: Drug metabolism and pharmacokinetics in malnutrition. Clin Pharmacokinet 3:216–240, 1978
18. Greenblatt DJ, Koch-Weaser J: Intramuscular injection of drugs. N Engl J Med 295:542–546, 1976
19. Radde IC: Mechanisms of drug absorption and their development, in MacLeod SM, Radde IC (eds): Textbook of Pediatric Clinical Pharmacology. Littleton, Mass, PSG Publishing Company, 1985, pp 17–43
20. Tyrala EE, Hillman LS, Hillman RE, Dodson WE: Clinical pharmacology of kerochlorophene in newborn infants. J Pediatr 91:481–486, 1977
21. Armstrong RW, Eichner ER, Klein DE, et al: Pentachlorophenol poisoning in a nursery for newborn infants. II. Epidemiologic and toxicologic studies. J Pediatr 75:317–325, 1969
22. Feinblatt BI, Aceto T, Beckhorn G, Bruck E: Percutaneous absorption of hydrocortisone in children. Am J Dis Child 112:218–224, 1966
23. Fisch RO, Berglund EB, Bridge AG, et al: Methemoglobinemia in a hospital nursery. JAMA 185:760–763, 1963
24. Radde IC, McKercher HG: Transport through membranes and development of membrane transport, in MacLeod SM, Radde IC (eds): Textbook of Pediatric Clinical Pharmacology. Littleton, Mass, PSG Publishing Company, 1985, pp 1–16
25. Marks J, Rawlins MD: Skin diseases, in Speight TM (ed): Avery's Drug Treatment: Principles and Practice of Clinical Pharmacology and Therapeutics, 3rd ed. Auckland, Australia, ADIS Press, 1987, pp 439–479
26. Morselli PL, Franco-Morselli R, Bossi L: Clinical pharmacokinetics in newborns and infants: Age-related differences and therapeutic implications. Clin Pharmacokinet 5:485–527, 1980
27. Lester RS: Topical formulary for the pediatrician. Pediatr Clin North Am 30:749–765, 1983
28. Nachman RL, Esterly NB: Increased skin permeability in preterm infants. J Pediatr 96:99–103, 1980
29. Senior N: Review of rectal suppositories: Formulation and manufacture. Pharm J 203:703–706, 1969
30. de Boer AG, Moolenaar F, de Leede LGJ, Breimer DD: Rectal drug administration: Clinical pharmacokinetic considerations. Clin Pharmacokinet 7:285–311, 1982
31. Choonara IA: Giving drugs per rectum for systemic effects. Arch Dis Child 62:771–772, 1987
32. Roberts RJ: Intravenous administration of medication in pediatric patients: Problems and solutions. Pediatr Clin North Am 28:23–24, 1981
33. Roberts RJ: Pharmacologic principles in therapeutics in infants, in Roberts RJ (ed): Drug Therapy in Infants. Philadelphia, WB Saunders, 1984, pp 1–12
34. Radde IC: Drugs and protein binding, in MacLeod SM, Radde IC (eds): Textbook of Pediatric Clinical Pharmacology. Litteton, Mass, PSG Publishing Company, 1985 pp 32–43

35. Jusko WJ: Pharmacokinetic principles in pediatric pharmacology. Pediatr Clin North Am 19:81–100, 1972
36. Lesar TS, Zaske DE: Antibiotics and hepatic disease. Med Clin North Am 66:257–266, 1982
37. Meyer MC, Guttman DE: The binding of drugs by plasma proteins. J Pharm Sci 57:895–918, 1968
38. Muller WE, Wollert V: Human serum albumin as a silent receptor for drugs and endogenous substances. Pharmacology 19:59–67, 1979
39. Piafsky KM: Disease-induced changes in the plasma binding of basic drugs. Clin Pharmacokinet 5:246–262, 1980
40. Windorfer A Jr, Keunzer W, Urbanek R: The influences of age on the activity of acetylsalicylic acid esterase and protein salicylate binding. Eur J Clin Pharmacol 7:227–231, 1974
41. Gitlin D, Boesman M: Serum alpha fetoprotein, albumin, and YG-globulin in the human conceptus. J Clin Invest 45:1826–1838, 1966
42. Hyvarinen M, Zeltzer P, Oh W, Stiehm ER: Influence of gestational age on serum levels of alpha-1-fetoprotein, IgG globulin, and albumin in newborn infants. J Pediatr 82:430–437, 1973
43. Piafsky KM, Mpamugo L: Dependence of neonatal drug binding on α_1-acid glycoprotein concentration. Clin Pharmacol Ther 29:272, 1981
44. Sjoqvist F, Borga O, Orme MLE: Fundamentals of clinical pharmacology, in Speight TM (ed): Avery's Drug Treatment, 3rd ed. Auckland, Australia, ADIS Press, 1987, pp 1–64
45. Thiessen H, Jacobsen J, Brodersen R: Displacement of albumin-bound bilirubin by fatty acids. Acta Paediatr Scand 61:285–288, 1972
46. McDonagh AF, Lightner DA: Life: A shrivelled blood orange—Bilirubin, jaundice, and phototherapy. Pediatrics 75:443–455, 1985
47. Ebbesen F, Nyboe J: Postnatal changes in the ability of plasma albumin to bind bilirubin. Acta Paediatr Scand 72:665–670, 1983
48. Rittes DA, Kenny JD: Influence of gestational age on cord serum bilirubin binding studies. J Pediatr 106:118–121, 1985
49. Keenan WJ, Arnold JE, Sutherland JM: Serum bilirubin binding determined by sephadex column chromatography. J Pediatr 74:813, 1969
50. Kapitulnik J, Horner-Mboshan R, Blondheim SH, Kauffman NA, Russell A: Increase in bilirubin binding affinity of serum with age of infant. J Pediatr 86:442–445, 1975
51. Ritter DA, Kenny JD, Morton J, Rudolph AJ: A prospective study of free bilirubin and other risk factors in the development of kernicterus in premature infants. Pediatrics 69:260–266, 1982
52. Brodersen R: Bilirubin transport in the newborn infant reviewed with relation to kernicterus. J Pediatr 96:349–356, 1980
53. Friis-Hansen B: Water distribution in the fetus and newborn infant. Acta Paediatr Scand 305(suppl):7–11, 1983
54. Fink CW, Cheeck DB: The corrected bromide space (extracellular volume) in the newborn. Pediatrics 26:397–401, 1960
55. Boreus LO: Principles of pediatric pharmacology, in Azarnoff DL (ed): Monographs in Clinical Pharmacology, vol 6. New York, Churchill-Livingstore, 1982
56. Litterst CL, Minnaugh EG, Reagan RL, et al: Comparison of in vitro drug metabolism by lung, liver, and kidney of several common laboratory species. Drug Metab Disp 3:259–265, 1975
57. McLeod SM, Clinical Pharmacokinetics: A Pediatric Overview, in MacLeod SM, Radde IC (eds): Textbook of Pediatric Clinical Pharmacology. Littletown, Mass, PSG Publishing Company, 1985
58. Wilkinson GR: Pharmacokinetics of drug disposition hemodynamic considerations. Annu Rev Pharmacol Toxicol 15:11–27, 1975
59. Harris PA, Riegelman S: Influence of the route of administration on the area under the plasma concentration time curve. Pharm Sci 58:71–75, 1969
60. Routledge PA, Shand DG: Presystemic drug elimination. Annu Rev Pharmacol Toxicol 19:447–468, 1979
61. Levi AJ, Gatmaiton Z, Arias IM: Two hepatic cytoplasmic protein fractions, y and z, and their possible role in the hepatic

uptake of bilirubin, sulfobromophthalein and other anions. J Clin Invest 48:2156–2167, 1969

62. Fleischner GM, Arias IM: Structure and function of ligandin (Y protein, GSH transferase B) and Z protein in the liver: A progress report, in Popper H, Schaffner F (eds): Progress in Liver Disease, vol 5. New York, Grune & Stratton, 1976, pp 172–182

63. Rane A, Sjoqvist F, Ouenius S: Drugs and fetal metabolism. Clin Pharmacol Ther 14:666–672, 1973

64. Rane A, Tomson G: Prenatal and neonatal drug metabolism in man. Eur J Clin Pharmacol 18:9–15, 1980

65. Yaffe SJ, Rane A, Sjoqvist F, Boreus LO, Ouenuis S: The presence of a mono-oxygenase system in human fetal liver microsomes. Life Sci 9:1189–1200, 1970

66. Pelkonen O, Karki NT: Drug metabolism in human fetal tissues. Life Sci 13:1163–1180, 1973

67. Rane A, Ackermann E: Metabolism of ethylmorphine and aniline in human fetal liver. Clin Pharmacol Ther 13:663–670, 1972

68. Gillette JR, Stripp B: Pre- and postnatal enzyme capacity for drug metabolite production. Fed Proc 34:172–178, 1975

69. Zamboni L: Electron microscopic studies of blood embryogenesis in humans. J Ultrastruct Res 12:509–524, 1965

70. Neims AH, Warner M, Loughnan PM, Aranda JV: Developmental aspects of the hepatic cytochrome P-450 mono-oxygenase system. Annu Rev Pharmacol Toxicol 16:427–445, 1976

71. Leff RD, Fischer LJ, Roberts RJ: Phenytoin metabolism in infants following intravenous and oral administration. Dev Pharmacol Ther 9:217–223, 1986

72. Jalling B, Boreus LO, Kallberg N, Agurell S: Disappearance from the newborn of circulating prenatally administered phenobarbital. Eur J Clin Pharmacol 6:234–238, 1973

73. Nitowsky HM, Matz L, Berzofsky JA: Studies on oxidative drug metabolism in the fullterm infant. J Pediatr 69:1139–1149, 1966

74. Wallin A, Jalling B, Boreus LO: Plasma concentrations of phenobarbital in the neonate during prophylaxis for neonatal hyperbilirubinemia. J Pediatr 85:392–397, 1974

75. Rane A, Bertilsson L, Palmer L: Disposition of placentally transferred carbamazepine (Tegretol) in the newborn. Eur J Clin Pharmacol 8:283–284, 1975

76. Juchau MR, Chao ST, Omiecinski CJ: Drug metabolism by the human fetus. Clin Pharmacokinet 5:320–339, 1980

77. Pikkarainen PH, Raiha NCR: Development of alcohol dehydrogenase activity in the human liver. Pediatr Res 1:165–168, 1967

78. Ecobichon DJ, Stephens DS: Prenatal development of human blood esterases. Clin Pharmacol Ther 14:41–47, 1973

79. Dutton GJ: Developmental aspects of drug conjugation with special reference to glucuronidation. Annu Rev Pharmacol Toxicol 18:17–35, 1978

80. Felsher BF, Mardman JE, Capiro NM, Van Couvering K, Wooley MM: Reduced hepatic bilirubin uridine diphosphate glucose dehydrogenase activity in the human fetus. Pediatr Res 12:838–840, 1978

81. Levy G, Khanna NN, Soda DM, Tsurzuki O, Stern L: Pharmacokinetics of acetaminophen in the human neonate: Formation of acetaminophen glucuronide and sulfate in relation to plasma bilirubin concentration and D-glucaric acid excretion. Pediatrics 55:818–825, 1975

82. Rollins DE, von Bahr C, Glaumann H, Moldeus P, Rane A: Acetaminophen: Potentially toxic metabolite formed by human fetal and adult liver microsomes and isolated fetal liver cells. Science 205:1414–1416, 1979

83. Alam SN, Roberts RJ, Fischer LJ: Age-related differences in salicylamide and acetaminophen conjugation in man. J Pediatr 90:130–135, 1977

84. Talafant E, Hoskova A, Pojerova A: Glucaric acid excretion as an index of hepatic glucuronidation in neonates after phenobarbital treatment. Pediatr Res 9:480–485, 1975

85. Aranda JV, Louridas AT, Vitrillo B, et al: Metabolism of theophylline to caffeine in human fetal liver. Science 206:1319–1321, 1979

86. Brater DC: Pharmacokinetics, in Chernow BC, Lake CR (eds): The Pharmacologic Approach to the Critically Ill Patient. Baltimore, Williams & Wilkins, 1983, pp 1–21

87. Whelton A: Antibiotic pharmacokinetics and clinical application in renal insufficiency. Med Clin North Am 66:267–281, 1982

88. Hook JB, Baihe MD: Prenatal renal pharmacology. Annu Rev Pharmacol Toxicol 19:491–509, 1979

89. West JR, Smith HW, Chasis H: Glomerular filtration rate, effective renal blood flow, and maximal tubular excretory capacity in infancy. J Pediatr 32:10–18, 1948

90. Aschinberg LC, Goldsmith DI, Ohbing H, et al: Neonatal changes in renal blood flow distribution in puppies. Am J Physiol 228:1453–1461, 1975

91. Arant BS Jr: Developmental patterns of renal functional maturation compared in the human neonate. J Pediatr 92:705–712, 1978

92. Leake RD, Trygstad CW: Glomerular filtration rate during the period of adaptation to extrauterine life. Pediatr Res 11:959–962, 1977

93. Nahata MC, Powell DA, Gregoire RP, et al: Tobramycin kinetics in newborn infants. J Pediatr 103:136–138, 1983

94. Szefler SJ, Wynn RJ, Clarke DF, et al: Relationship of gentamicin serum concentrations to gestational age in preterm and term neonates. J Pediatr 97:312–315, 1980

95. Kaplan JM, McCracken GH, Horton LJ, Thomas ML, Davis N: Pharmacologic studies in neonates given large doses of ampicillin. J Pediatr 84:571–577, 1974

96. Nelson JD, Shelton S, Kusmiesz H: Clinical pharmacology of ticarcillin in the newborn infant: Relation to age, gestational age, and weight. J Pediatr 87:474–479, 1975

97. McCracken GH Jr, Ginsberg C, Chrane DF, Thomas ML, Horton LJ: Clinical pharmacology of penicillin in newborn infants. J Pediatr 82:692–698, 1973

98. Sarff LD: McCracken GH Jr, Thomas ML, Horton LJ, Thielkeld N: Clinical pharmacology of methicillin in neonates. J Pediatr 90:1005–1008, 1977

99. Schwartz GJ, Hegyi T, Spitzer A: Subtherapeutic dicloxacillin levels in a neonate: possible mechanisms. J Pediatr 89:310–312, 1976

100. Olind B, Beermann B: Renal tubular secretion and effects of furosemide. Clin Pharmacol Ther 27:784–790, 1980

101. Aranda JV, Perez J, Sitar DS, et al: Pharmacokinetic disposition and protein binding of furosemide in newborn infants. J Pediatr 93:407–511, 1978

102. Peterson RG, Simmons MA, Rumack BH, Levine RL, Brooks JG: Pharmacology of furosemide in the premature newborn infant. J Pediatr 97:139–143, 1980

103. Witte MK, Stork JE, Blumer JL: Diuretic therapeutics in the pediatric patient. Am J Cardiol 57:44A–53A, 1986

18

DRUG ADMINISTRATION IN THE NEWBORN INFANT

SHEILA JACOBSON *and* GIDEON KOREN

Infants, especially those of very low birth weight, are limited in the total volume of fluid that may be administered during parenteral nutrition or drug therapy. With increasing awareness and improved techniques of monitoring drug concentrations and their effects in neonates, it has become apparent that there is a unique set of serious problems associated with drug administration in this age group. Because the smallest infants are often the sickest, they are more vulnerable to adverse effects caused by erroneous administration of drugs.

This chapter will address the major issues in drug delivery that have been identified in the last two decades and will concentrate on those aspects which may seriously complicate the treatment of sick infants and sometimes even endanger their lives.

ISSUES OF INTRAVENOUS DRUG ADMINISTRATION

There are four methods of intravenous drug administration: rapid intravenous injection, antegrade injection, retrograde injection, and syringe pump infusion.[1-4]

RAPID INTRAVENOUS INJECTION. The medication is delivered directly into a vein, either as a *bolus* or as a *rapid infusion.* It is well acknowledged that these terms are vaguely defined and may lead to serious toxicity when applied to drugs that have rate-dependent adverse effects. Cardiovascular collapse secondary to rapid infusion of phenytoin may serve as one example; it is not confined to the neonate. Similarly, the "red man" syndrome, which is due to bolus or rapid infusion of vancomycin, has been described in adults, children, and neonates.[5] When the vancomycin is infused over a period of 45 minutes or longer, the incidence of this syndrome (which is due to histamine release) is greatly reduced.

ANTEGRADE INJECTION. When this technique is used, the drug is administered into the intravenous tubing at an injection site, such as the Y-site. The drug is then delivered to the patient at the set infusion rate. While this method obviates the risk of rapid administration of the medication, the slow infusion rates required in newborn or small infants may result in erratic and unreliable drug delivery.

RETROGRADE INJECTION. In this system, shown in Figure 18–1, an extension of tubing with stopcocks at either end is inserted between the intravenous catheter and the infusion set. The drug is injected at the stopcock closest to the patient so that it flows upstream into the extension tubing. The drug is subsequently delivered to the patient by the hydrostatic pressure of the system. The dosage volume should not exceed one-half the volume of the extension tubing in order to avoid sequestration of the drug in the overflow system. This system is also dependent on the primary infusion rate. It requires extra stopcocks and extension tubing, thus increasing the risk of contamination.

SYRINGE PUMP INFUSION. The syringe pump is by far the most effective system for precise control of drug delivery in terms of both fluid volume and drug concentration. By using this system, shown in Figure 18–2, one can control drug delivery at different rates from those dictated by the intravenous set. While the pumps are more expensive and have to be calibrated regularly, their nondisposable nature ensures their cost-effectiveness in neonatal care over time.

Several investigators have specifically addressed issues of intravenous drug delivery in the neonate. Nahata and Powell[6] have examined different infusion systems *in vivo* using serum concentrations of tobramycin in neonates. They compared an Autosyringe pump with three antegrade infusion pumps. The average interval to peak concentrations was 2.2 to 5.5 times longer with the antegrade system than with the Autosyringe. The range of times to achieve peak serum concentrations also varied considerably among the systems. With Autosyringe, times to peak varied by 0.7 hour, whereas variation was as much as 2 hours with the antegrade systems. The shortest time to

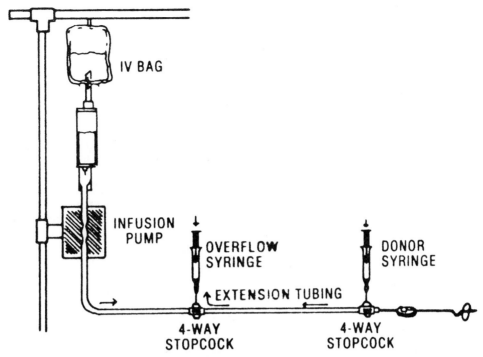

FIGURE 18–1. Retrograde infusion system.

reach peak concentration was 0.33 hour; the longest was 3 hours.

Roberts[4] has performed a considerable amount of investigation on variability of drug delivery in neonates. He noted that the rate of infusion and portal of injection are very important in determining the speed and completeness of intravenous drug administration. As one may expect, the higher the volume of fluid in which the drug is prepared, the longer is the time required to deliver the full dose. Delay in drug delivery due to low flow rates may lead to inaccurate estimation of the time needed to achieve peak and/or trough levels. Hence serum drug concentrations measured at inappropriate times may result in inappropriate changes of dosing, with the poten-

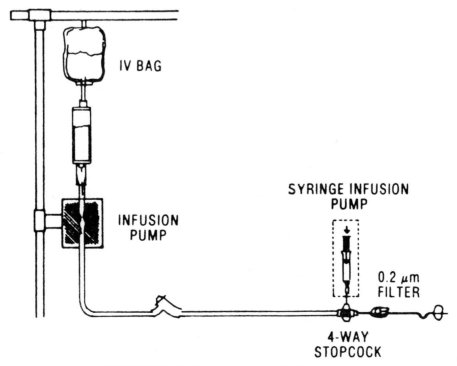

FIGURE 18–2. Syringe pump infusion system.

tial for overdosing and thus toxicity or underdosing and thus suboptimal efficacy.

In an attempt to minimize variability in drug delivery time, medications should be administered at a site as close to the infant as possible. Injections through Y- and T-type tubing should be avoided, since this may result in significant drug trapping, especially if the drug is administered in a small volume of fluid.[7]

INTRAVENOUS TUBING

Replacement of intravenous sets to prevent bacterial contamination may result in significant loss of drug. Gould and Roberts[7] have shown that as much as 38 percent of the total drug may be lost in the discarded set. It is important that physicians are aware of such losses; they may be avoided by flushing the system with an appropriate intravenous solution prior to replacement.

Polyvinyl chloride (PVC) tubing has been shown to absorb certain drugs such as insulin, diazepam, and paraldehyde.[8] Polyethylene is less likely to bind to these drugs and is therefore preferable. Paraldehyde dissolves plastics other than polyethylene or polypropylene; when paraldehyde is used intravenously, polyvinyl tubing must not be used and should be replaced by polyethylene or polypropylene.[9]

Low-volume tubing (internal diameter 0.06–0.14 cm) permits adequate mixing of drug and primary fluid because of the higher flow velocity and increased shear forces.[3] Consequently, low-volume tubing should be used to ensure optimal delivery for delivery rates of less than 10 ml/h.

FILTER DEVICES

Filters are commonly connected to intravenous tubing in an attempt to lessen contamination of intravenous fluids by bacteria and particulate matter and to clear the fluid of air bubbles. However, antimicrobial agents such as gentamicin and cloxacillin, as well as such other drugs as digoxin, amphotericin, and insulin, have been shown to bind to filter devices.[10,12] Drugs delivered at slow infusion rates tend to be sequestered in the filter according to their specific gravity; the higher the specific gravity (e.g., cloxacillin), the more likely the drug is to stay in the filter chamber. Position of the filter chamber also appears to affect accumulation of drug solution in the chamber. Drugs with high specific gravities tend to settle in dependent areas of the infusion system, whereas those with low specific gravities may float.[11] New filter chambers have been developed that permit full delivery of drugs to be infused.[12,13]

Obstruction of a filter has been demonstrated when drugs are administered in an acidic solution of dextrose. This issue can be obviated by using buffered solutions.[14]

DILUTION INTOXICATION AND INADEQUATE MIXING

One of the most obvious signs of "orphaning" infants from drug therapy is the lack of stock solutions of drugs prepared for pediatric dosages. Consequently, the very small doses of intravenous medications required by neonates often necessitate dilution of a stock solution prepared for adult use. By drawing additional fluid into a syringe, the drug in the dead space of the syringe is also drawn into the syringe. This may result in administration of significantly higher doses than intended. Berman et al.[15] have demonstrated that in the case of dilution of digoxin, the volume in the dead space would increase an intended dose of 5 μg to 12–18 μg. Roberts[16] has calculated the effect of this dilution intoxication for several medications when prepared in the routine way. Increasing the availability of drugs in pediatric dosage forms will help to alleviate this potentially serious problem.

Overdosage also may occur as a result of inadequate mixing of additives in flexible parenteral fluid containers. Williams[17] described two adults who developed probable transient hyperkalemia resulting from the addition of potassium chloride to such a container. It has been demonstrated that following injection of dye into such containers, the dye pools at the container base and then flows unmixed into the infusion tubing. Squeezing the plastic container does not effectively mix the dye with the contents of the container. Injection of the drug while the plastic container is inverted or rapid inversion of the bag following injection of dye results in more effective mixing of additives in an I.V. solution.[17,18]

Excessive drug doses also may be delivered to the patient following inadvertent flushing (with any intravenous solution) of syringes that already contain medication. Staff administering medications should be alerted to this potential error.

ADDITIVE/PRESERVATIVE TOXICITY

Certain preservatives, considered innocuous in adults, have been reported to be toxic in low-birth-weight infants. Benzyl alcohol is an antibacterial agent that is used in several injectable drugs and solutions, including bacteriostatic sodium chloride and injectable water. An increased incidence of intraventricular hemorrhage, metabolic acidosis, and mortality has been correlated with substantial benzoic acid and benzyl alcohol concentrations in low-birth-weight neonates.[19,20] It is now recommended that solutions and pharmaceutical preparations containing benzyl alcohol be avoided in neonates.

Propylene glycol is a solvent that is commonly used as a solubilizer in drug preparations. It has been shown to cause hyperosmolality in preterm infants,[21] resulting in cardiovascular and respiratory instability and seizures.[21–23] The main sources of propylene glycol–containing solutions have been intravenous multivitamin solutions (MVI-12); other drugs that contain propylene glycol include digoxin, Bactrim, phenobarbital, phenytoin, diazepam, hydralazine, and nystatin cream.

Preparations such as human albumin and calcium and phosphate salts may contain high concentrations of aluminum. There is evidence that aluminum can cause skeletal and neurologic toxicity in humans; it is likely that small infants are susceptible to such toxicity.[24] The effects of these potentially toxic additives may be cumulative, especially if multiple-drug therapy and/or prolonged hyperalimentation is required, as is common in sick neonates.

DOSAGE ERRORS

Pediatric patients, particularly infants, are vulnerable to iatrogenic administration of doses that are higher than intended. Such errors are more likely to occur in younger patients because of the small volumes of stock solution usually required to administer small drug dosages.[25] These errors are often of a tenfold magnitude owing to misplacement of the decimal point during calculation.

Perlstein and colleagues[26] tested medical personnel in a pediatric center for their ability to compute drug doses for sick newborns. One of every 12 doses computed by registered nurses contained an error that would result in administration of an amount that was 10 times higher or lower than the intended dose. Pediatricians made errors at a rate of 1 in every 26 computations attempted. Pharmacists scored better than both nurses and physicians.[26] We have found similar results in pediatric staff[25] and have identified a subgroup of nurses and physicians who tend to make substantially more calculation errors.

Misunderstanding of orders also may occur, as a result of either illegible orders or misinterpretation of appropriate orders. Errors committed by parents of a sick infant are also more likely to occur if the intended dosage is not explained clearly.[25]

Several solutions to these problems have been suggested, including a written test requirement for all personnel involved in preparation of drug doses from stock. Calculations should be checked by at least two staff members. The use of standard tables of recommended dosages and volumes of stock solutions also has been suggested. The number of errors may be lessened if clinical pharmacists prepare all solutions. However, this is expensive and impractical in emergencies.[26] Here, too, the availability of pediatric dosage forms of drugs will allow for greater accuracy and fewer errors in dosing.

We have recently documented that clinical pharmacists assigned to specific wards prevent a substantial number of medication errors committed in physician's orders. In some instances, the tenfold medication could have resulted in morbidity or even mortality in a child.[27]

PHOTOTHERAPY AND EXCHANGE TRANSFUSION

Many low-birth-weight infants will receive phototherapy for variable lengths of time. The light used during phototherapy may affect several light-sensitive compounds, including multivitamin solutions, paraldehyde, and tolazoline.[28] During delivery of such drugs, the tubing of the infusion set should be wrapped in opaque material such as aluminum foil.

In infants requiring exchange transfusion, drug concentrations should be monitored closely to assess whether replacement doses are necessary, particularly if repeat exchange transfusions are necessary. Methods of predicting or calculating drug loss have been published. In many cases, therapy will not be compromised, particularly if the exchange is conducted during a trough concentration period. In contrast, significant losses of drugs with a small distribution volume (such as theophylline) may occur.[29]

CONCLUSION

It may be difficult to achieve adequate long-term intravenous access in small infants, who are susceptible to complications associated with central and peripheral intravenous lines, such as thrombosis, infection, or extravasation. We have tried to highlight characteristics of intravenous therapy in infants that are most likely to complicate drug therapy or result in inaccurate dosing. Most of the above-mentioned problems are unique to or likely to be most deleterious in infants and neonates. It is essential that caretakers be aware of these factors in order to optimize drug treatment.

REFERENCES

1. Leff RD, Roberts RJ: Methods for intravenous drug administration in the pediatric patient. J Pediatr 98:631–635, 1982
2. Benzing G III, Loggie J: A new retrograde method for administering drugs intravenously. Pediatrics 52:420–425, 1973
3. Giacoia GP: Intravenous drug administration to low birth weight infants. Clin Pediatr 26:25–29, 1987
4. Roberts RJ: Intravenous administration of medication in pediatric patients: Problems and solutions. Pediatr Clin North Am 28:23–34, 1981
5. Levy M, Koren G: Vancomycin-induced red man syndrome. Pediatrics 86:572–580, 1990
6. Nahata MC, Powell D: Effect of infusion methods on tobramycin serum concentrations in newborn infants. J Pediatr 104:136–138, 1984
7. Gould T, Roberts RJ: Therapeutic problems arising from the use of the intravenous route for drug administration. J Pediatr 95:465–471, 1979
8. Hancock BG, Black CD: Effect of a polyethylene-lined administration set on the availability of diazepam injection. Am J Hosp Pharm 42:335–339, 1985
9. Giacoia GP, Gessner PK, Zaleska MM, et al: Pharmacokinetics of paraldehyde disposition in the neonate. J Pediatr 104:291–296, 1984
10. Wagman GH, Bailey JV, Weinstein MJ: Binding of aminoglycoside antibiotics to filtration materials. Antimicrob Agents Chemother 7:316–319, 1975
11. Rajchgot P, Radde IC, Macleod SM, et al: Influence of specific gravity on intravenous drug delivery. J Pediatr 99:658–661, 1981
12. Koren G, Rajchgot P, Good F, et al: Improved techniques for IV drug delivery in children. Am J IV Ther Nutr 10:33–38, 1983
13. Koren G, Rajchgot P, Harding E, et al: Evaluating a filter device used for intermittent intravenous drug delivery to newborn infants. Am J Hosp Pharm 46:106–108, 1985

14. Glass M, Giacoia GP: Intravenous drug therapy in premature infants. J Obstet Gynecol Neonatal Nurs 16:310–318, 1987

15. Berman WJ, Whitman V, Marks KH: Inadvertent overadministration of digoxin to low birth weight infants. J Pediatr 92:1024–1025, 1978

16. Roberts RJ: Drug Therapy in Infants. Philadelphia, WB Saunders, 1984, pp 25–35

17. Williams RHP: Potassium overdosage: A potential hazard of non-rigid parenteral fluid containers. Br Med J 1:714–715, 1973

18. Deardorff DL, Schmidt CN: Mixing additives by squeezing plastic bags. Am J Hosp Pharm 42:533–534, 1985

19. Gershanik J, Boecler B, Ensley H, et al: The gasping syndrome and benzyl alcohol poisoning. N Engl J Med 307:1384–1388, 1982

20. Committee on Drugs: "Inactive" ingredients in pharmaceutical products. Pediatrics 76:635–643, 1985

21. Glasgow AM, Boeck RL, Miller MK, et al: Hyperosmolality in small infants due to propylene glycol. Pediatrics 72:353–355, 1983

22. MacDonald MG, Getson PR, Glasgow AM, et al: Propylene glycol: Increased incidence of seizures in low birth weight infants. Pediatrics 79:622–625, 1987

23. Louis S, Ku TTM, McDowell F: The cardiocirculatory changes caused by intravenous dilantin and its solvent. Am Heart J 74:523–529, 1967

24. Sedman AB, Klein GL, Merritt RJ, et al: Evidence of aluminum loading in infants receiving intravenous therapy. N Engl J Med 312:1337–1343, 1985

25. Koren G, Barzilay Z, Greenwald M: Tenfold errors in drug administration for children: A neglected iatrogenic disease in pediatrics. Pediatrics 77:848–849, 1986

26. Perlstein PH, Callison C, White M, et al: Errors in drug computations during newborn intensive care. Am J Dis Child 133:376–379, 1979

27. Koren G, Hales B: The role of clinical pharmacists in preventing potentially fatal tenfold medication errors in children. J Pharm Technol (in press)

28. Ennever JF, Carr HS, Speck WT: Potential for genetic damage from multivitamin solutions exposed to phototherapy illumination. Pediatr Res 17:192–194, 1983

29. Lackner TE: Drug replacement following exchange transfusion. J Pediatr 100:811–814, 1982

19

ANTICONVULSANTS IN THE NEWBORN INFANT

MONIQUE ANDRE *and* PAUL VERT

Seizures commonly occur in the neonatal period, with an incidence ranging from 1.5 in 1000 term births[1] to 14 in 1000 live births,[2] and they usually require the use of anticonvulsant drugs. In the neonatal period, these drugs have pharmacologic particularities that are related to metabolic immaturity and to the circumstances of seizure occurrence.

SEIZURES IN THE NEWBORN

Seizures in the neonate are often atypical, which makes their diagnosis difficult. They occur as isolated events in 70 percent of cases, or they present as status epilepticus in the remaining 30 percent.[3]

Their prognosis initially depends on their etiology. However, seizures themselves lead to ventilatory (hypoxia, hypercapnia, or hypocapnia), circulatory[4] (increased blood pressure and cerebral blood flow), and metabolic[5] (decreased brain glucose, nucleic acids, proteins, cholesterol) disorders; these disorders also can produce harmful effects, thus modifying or aggravating the initial insult. Therefore, rapid and effective treatment should be urgently prescribed. Efficacy is usually assessed by the disappearance of clinical manifestations and, to a lesser extent, of electrical epileptiform activities.

The etiology most frequently encountered is a hypoxic–ischemic encephalopathy secondary to acute or chronic fetal distress. In these cases, other visceral injuries that alter liver, kidney, or heart functions may further compromise the metabolism and elimination of drugs.

The diseases responsible for neonatal seizures are usually acute; they rarely last more than a few days, and the treatment can rapidly be discontinued. In a small proportion of infants (5–17 percent[3,6]), recurrent convulsions need a chronic treatment, as in older epileptic children.

GENERAL PHARMACOLOGIC PRINCIPLES OF THE ANTICONVULSANT DRUGS USED IN THE NEWBORN

Peculiarities inherent to neonatal physiology account for some of the unique pharmacokinetic profiles of anticonvulsants in this age group.[7]. For instance, there is a relative biologic immaturity, such as in renal and liver functions, as well as important and rapid modifications that take place during the first days of life.[8]

Absorption

Following oral administration, absorption is slow owing to delayed gastric emptying and relative achlorhydria. However, diazepam, which is highly lipophilic, is rapidly absorbed.[9] Rectal absorption is quite efficient if an adequate pharmaceutical preparation is used.[10]

The absorption rate following intramuscular injection can be quite variable. This is so because muscular blood flow and muscular contractions are weak[8] and muscular water content is high.

Distribution

In the neonate, the contribution of total-body water to total-body weight is greater than that in the older infant. There is a higher ratio of extracellular to intracellular water. Fluid compartments undergo rapid modifications over the first few days after birth. These modifications may lead to altered volumes of distribution of different drugs. This essentially involves drugs that distribute mainly in body water (phenobarbital, phenytoin, carbamazepin, valproic acid).

In term newborns, adipose tissue accounts for only 15 percent of total-body weight, and the skeletal muscle mass accounts for 25 percent. On a body-weight basis, brain and liver volumes are greater than in the adult. Relative cerebral blood flow is lower, which should generate lower brain concentrations of lipophilic drugs such as diazepam.

Plasma protein drug binding is lower than in adults. Moreover, albumin concentration and affinity for organic anions (fetal albumin) are lower than in adults.[11] Certain albumin-bound substances, whether endogenous (unconjugated bilirubin, free fatty acids) or exogenous, compete with drugs.[12] The unbound drug fraction is increased, thus facilitating tissue distribution as well as increasing the apparent volume of distribution.

Metabolism

Hepatic drug metabolism in the newborn is deficient. This is partly due to the deficiency or absence of ligandin, which limits hepatic drug uptake, as well as to the poorly developed oxidative and hydroxylative microsomal enzymatic systems (50 percent compared to the normal adult[13]). Sulfate and glycine conjugation nearly equals that in adults, whereas glucuronide conjugation is reduced. All these processes can be increased to adult rates by the *in utero* or postnatal use of inducing agents such as phenobarbital. This induction may dramatically increase hepatic drug-metabolizing capacity over a short period of time.

Elimination

Glomerular filtration rapidly increases during the first days of life. However, since tubular function matures more slowly, renal excretion of drugs in the neonatal period remains low.

ANTICONVULSANT DRUGS

The Barbiturates

Phenobarbital (Gardenal, Luminal)

The chemical structure of the barbiturates is 5-ethyl-5-phenylbarbituric acid. Barbiturates are lipid-soluble, with a molecular weight of 232.23 daltons and a pK_a of 7.3.

Phenobarbital is sedative, hypnotic, and depressive of the nervous system and muscle. Its anticonvulsant activity is essentially due to its synaptic effects. Calcium entry into the presynaptic endings is blocked, thereby decreasing neurotransmitter release. Postsynaptic response to γ-aminobutyric acid (GABA) is enhanced, and glutamic acid activation is suppressed. Phenobarbital may activate GABA-related chloride channels.[14] Furthermore, phenobarbital is a potent inducer of the cytochrome P-450 and the UDP-glycuronyl transferase enzyme systems.

Absorption is effective by all the routes, especially orally.[15] Absorption half-lives are 7–10 hours following oral administration and 4–9 hours following intramuscular administration.[16] However, the latter should be avoided, because local resorption abnormalities, with a risk for muscular necrosis or sciatic nerve paralysis, may result after injection into the gluteal region. Distribution to all tissues is apparently equal and depends on blood pH. Tissue drug concentrations are inversely proportional to blood pH.[17]

The apparent volume of distribution (AV_d) is 0.59–0.97 liter/kg. The AV_d increases after asphyxia[18] and is independent of gestational age. Painter et al.[15] reported AV_d values of 0.96 ± 0.21 liter/kg (mean ± 1 SD) from 27–30 weeks of gestation, 0.96 ± 0.12 liter/kg from 31–36 weeks of gestation, and 0.88 ± 0.16 liter/kg after 37 weeks of gestation. The lower the plasma protein concentration, the better is the distribution in the brain. Cornford et al.,[19] however, demonstrated that larger amounts of protein-bound anticonvulsant drugs permeate the brain in newborn rabbits. This is ascribed to a capillary transit time that is longer than the drug–protein dissociation time. For phenobarbital, both free and protein-bound fractions of the drug enter the newborn brain. The brain-to-plasma concentration ratio is 0.71 ± 0.21. It increases with gestational age.[20] The distribution is the same in gray and white matters.

The most important metabolite is para-hydroxyphenobarbital, which is inactive. Para-hydroxylation is already present at birth,[21] with similar metabolic activity as the adult. Hepatic glucuronidation of the hydroxy derivative only develops in the weeks that follow birth. Phenobarbital-N-glucoside is another important metabolite in the adult; it rarely appears before 14 days of life.[22]

ELIMINATION. Phenobarbital is excreted in the urine. Following the administration of a single dose of phenobarbital, 17 percent of the product is excreted unchanged and 10 percent is excreted as para-hydroxyphenobarbital, as in the adult.[21] However, since hepatic metabolism is lower than in the adult, only 5 percent of a single dose is eliminated in the form of conjugated derivatives. The proportion of the latter in the adult is about 15 percent.

The elimination half-life ranges from 100–200 hours in term newborns (148 ± 55 hours[23]) and from 100–500 hours in preterm infants treated before 6 hours of life.[24] It often exceeds 100 hours at up to 14 days and thereafter decreases to 20 hours at 28 days of life.[15,25,26] Following hypoxia, it may be prolonged up to 400 hours.[27] Drug elimination half-life decreases with postnatal age because of the increased hepatic metabolism, as well as a probable enzymatic induction due to the drug itself. The mean clearance rate is 0.0047 ± 0.0018 liter/h/kg[18,23] (Table 19–1).

Interactions with other drugs have seldom been the object of specific studies in the newborn. As in other age groups, such interactions are probably important, especially owing to the potent inducer effects of phenobarbital.[28]

SIDE EFFECTS. Intravenous administration of phenobarbital may lead to a decrease in arterial pressure, due to a myocardial depression, and a transitory respiratory depression. On the other hand, hypotonia and hyporeactivity are often observed. However, these are more often related to the disease responsible for the seizures than to the treatment.

At therapeutic plasma concentrations (16–40 μg/ml), phenobarbital does not significantly change EEG background activity, whose prognostic value remains unchanged.[29,30]

Despite its unquestionable value in seizures treatment, phenobarbital should be used judiciously because of concerns that it may not be innocuous to the developing brain. Brain growth retardation and maturation have been observed in phenobarbital-treated newborn rats.[31–33] However, extrapolation to the human newborn is uncertain.

THERAPEUTIC USE. Effective plasma levels range from 20–40 μg/ml.[34] As in the adult, there is a relationship between plasma drug levels and pH. Plasma levels increase with alkalosis,[35] presumably due to displacement from the intracellular space. This effect at the central nervous system level could increase the risk of recurrence of the seizures.

The current loading dose is 20 mg/kg, by slow intravenous administration. Gal et al.[36] emphasize the use of monotherapy and recommend further injections of 5 mg/kg until plasma levels approach or are equal to 40 μg/ml. In the study by Donn et al.,[23] an intravenous loading dose of 30 mg/kg produced blood levels of 30.0 $\pm$ 3.2 μg/ml (mean $\pm$ 1 SD), with good cardiorespiratory tolerance.

Because of the long half-life, there is a risk of overdose when the maintenance regimen is prescribed at a dosage exceeding 4 mg/kg/day during the first week of life.[15] Most authors recommend a dose of 3 mg/kg/day, started 24 hours after the loading dose.[37] For others,[38] the daily administration of 1 mg/kg is adequate until the fifth day. Afterwards, a daily dose of 5 mg/kg can be prescribed.

Thiopental

High doses of ultra-short-acting barbiturates, such as thiopental, have been used in untractable status epilepticus.[39,40] Thiopental pharmacokinetics in the newborn following severe perinatal asphyxia were studied by Garg et al.[41] and Goldberg et al.,[42] and later by Demarquez et al.,[43] after administration of a 10–15 mg/kg loading dose. The former found a mean C $\pm$ 1 SD volume of distribution of 3.6 $\pm$ 1.7 liters/kg (range 1.1–6.7 liters/kg), an elimination half-life of 39.3 $\pm$ 15.3 hours (26–70 hours), and a clearance rate of 0.066 $\pm$ 0.040 liter/h/kg (0.031–0.172 liter/h/kg). For Demarquez et al.,[43] the respective values were 8.26 $\pm$ 3.10 liter/kg, 20.9 $\pm$ 9.6 hours, and 0.32 $\pm$ 0.09 liter/h/kg. These values approach those observed in neonates who received the drug transplacentally.

The steady-state plasma concentration is 13.4 $\pm$ 3.7 μg/ml.[41] However, this treatment did not prevent the occurrence of seizures in 76 percent of the children preventively treated by Goldberg et al.[42] after acute fetal distress (73 percent in untreated controls). Furthermore, this treatment led to a drop in arterial pressure requiring treatment. Optimal plasma concentration is unknown, and efficacy of this treatment in newborns remains questionable.

Primidone (Mysoline)

This compound, 5-ethyldihydro-5-phenyl-4,6(1H,5H)-pyrimidinedione, is in fact deoxyphenobarbital. It has a molecular weight of 218.25 daltons. It is a neutral compound that is only slightly soluble in water and most organic solvents. Its anticonvulsant properties are apparently principally due to primidone and are independent of its two main metabolites, the phenobarbital[44] and the phenylethylmalonamide (PEMA).[45] Primidone action is due to modifications in sodium and calcium ion transmembrane fluxes.

Effective therapeutic levels range from 6–15 mg/liter. Loading dose is of 15–25 mg/kg, intravenously or orally. The maintenance dose is 12–20 mg/kg/day.

Phenytoin (Dilantin)

The chemical structure of phenytoin is 5,5-diphenylhydantoin (DPH). It is a highly lipid soluble compound with a molecular weight of 252.26 daltons in acid form. Its anticonvulsant properties are free of sedative side effects. Basically, phenytoin affects synaptic transmission. It blocks the sodium membrane channels of the neurons. It decreases membrane calcium permeability and inhibits presynaptic terminal calcium uptake.

Phenytoin is also active outside the central nervous system, especially on cardiac rhythm,[46] as well as on endocrine function by inhibition of the release of certain hormones, such as insulin.[47]

ORAL ABSORPTION. Oral absorption is quite low,[15] although it is slightly better postprandially.[48] Rectal or intramuscular administration is hazardous. There is a risk of tissue necrosis by the latter route, which contraindicates its use.

DISTRIBUTION. Distribution into the brain is good. The mean brain/plasma ratio is of 1.28 $\pm$ 0.32.[15] The gray/white matter ratio ranges between 0.95 and 1.74. It is not influenced by gestational age.[20] In newborns, phenytoin binds less to plasma proteins than in the adult. The mean ($\pm$ 1 SD) unbound fraction in cord plasma is 10.6 $\pm$ 1.4 percent.[49] In icteric newborns, Rane et al.[49] demonstrated a positive correlation between the proportion of protein-unbound phenytoin and bilirubin levels. At a bilirubin concentration of 20 mg/100 ml, the unbound fraction of DPH was twice as high as in plasma of nonhyperbilirubinemic infants. The correlation is closer if the bilirubin/albumin ratio is considered. The protein binding is lower if the nonesterified fatty acid level is increased. This suggests competition between DPH and endogenous substances (bilirubin and nonesterified fatty acid) for binding sites on the albumin molecule.[50]

The volume of distribution does not change with gestational age. Painter et al.[15] found 1.20 $\pm$ 0.11 liters/kg (mean $\pm$ 1 SD) between 27 and 30 weeks, 1.17 $\pm$ 0.21 liters/kg between 31 and 36 weeks, and 1.22 $\pm$ 0.22 liters/kg after 37 weeks. For Loughnan et al.,[51] these values during the first week of life were 0.80 $\pm$ 0.22 liter/kg in term newborns and 0.80 $\pm$ 0.26 liter/kg in preterm newborns. A V_d does not seem to change with early postnatal age:

TABLE 19–1. PHARMACOKINETIC DATA OF ANTICONVULSANT DRUGS IN THE NEWBORN

DRUG	HALF-LIFE (h)	VOLUME OF DISTRIBUTION (liters/kg)	CLEARANCE (liters/h/kg)	THERAPEUTIC RANGE
Phenobarbital	First 14 days: >100* At 28 days: 20*	0.6–1.0‡	0.005*	20–40 µg/ml
Thiopental	39 ± 15† 26–70‡	3.6 ± 1.7† 1.1–6.7‡	0.07 ± 0.04† 0.03–0.17‡	
Phenytoin	First days: 140* 1 month: 2–7‡ Full-term: 21 ± 12† Preterm: 75 ± 65†	1.2*	—	15–20 µg/m
Diazepam	Preterm: 75 ± 35† Full-term: 31 ± 2†	1.3–1.8‡	—	150–700 ng/ml
Clonazepam	Before 60 hours: 140* 22–43‡	1.5–11‡	0.02–0.07‡	15–80 ng/ml
Lidocaine	3*	—	—	2–5 µg/ml
Paraldehyde	10–18‡	1.7 ± 0.2†	0.12 ± 0.02†	100–200 µg/ml
Valproic acid	26* 9–49‡	0.4* 0.36–0.47‡	14* 5.5–18.2‡	50–100 µg/ml
Carbamazepine	7–15‡	1.1–2.5‡	—	2.5–10 µg/ml

*Mean
†Mean ± 1 SD
‡Range

0.89 ± 0.35 liter/kg from 2 to 36 days[52] and 0.73 ± 0.18 liter/kg after 2 weeks of age[51] (Table 19–1).

ELIMINATION. The elimination half-life decreases with postnatal age; it falls from 140 hours (57.3 ± 48.2 hours, mean ± 1 SD) during the first days of life to 19.7 ± 1.31 hours during the fourth week.[52] It is quite variable during the first week of life, and the values decrease significantly from the third week on. These values also change with gestational age, with values of 20.7 ± 11.6 hours in six full-term newborns aged 2–4 days old and 75.4 ± 64.5 hours (range 15.6–160 hours) in five preterm infants aged between 2 and 18 postnatal days.[51] This elimination half-life is concentration-dependent, which indicates a saturation kinetics.[52] These age-related modifications and the nonlinear elimination kinetics contribute to lower phenytoin plasma levels after the first days of life.

METABOLISM. The metabolism is hepatic, by oxidation and glucuronidation.

DRUG INTERACTION. Chronic exposure to phenytoin results in decreased benzodiazepine receptor density in the rat.[53]

SIDE EFFECTS. Like phenobarbital, phenytoin inhibits cultured cortical neuron proliferation in vitro.[54] Hyperglycemia and cardiac arrhythmias may be observed during treatment.

THERAPEUTIC USE. The loading dose is 20 mg/kg intravenously. Administration should not exceed 1 mg/kg/min to avoid the risk of cardiac toxicity. The determination of an effective maintenance dose is difficult owing to the pronounced variability of pharmacokinetic parameters. However, intravenous administration of 3–4 mg/kg/day in two doses is an average dose, which is often insufficient.[55] Albani and Wernicke[48] used oral doses of 9–29 mg/kg. Blood-level monitoring should be performed regularly. Effective plasma levels are 15–20 µg/ml.

The Benzodiazepines

Benzodiazepines appear to act by facilitation of GABA-mediated synaptic transmission. They bind to specific central nervous system receptors. These benzodiazepine postsynaptic receptors are part of a neuronal mechanism acting as a GABA-ergic inhibition amplifying system. Their use in the newborn is justified because benzodiazepine receptors appear early during ontogenesis.[56]

Diazepam (Valium)

The chemical structure of diazepam is 7-chloro-1,3-dihydro-1-methyl-5-phenyl-2H-1,4-benzodiazepin-one. It has a molecular weight of 285 daltons. It is poorly water-soluble and relatively lipid-soluble. Its pK_a is 3.4.

Some of the pharmacokinetic data concerning diazepam have been obtained in neonates who received the drug transplacentally.[57] Whether or not these values are strictly identical to these observed following postnatal administration remains uncertain.

ABSORPTION. Absorption is effective, regardless of the route of administration used, intravenous, oral, intramuscular, or rectal. Intravenous administration leads to short (5–15 min), but very high peak diazepam plasma levels: 5775–10800 ng/ml after a dose of 1 mg/kg and 2750–6450 ng/ml after a dose of 0.5 mg/kg.[58] As previously shown in older children,[59] intrarectal administration allows apparent anticonvulsive plasma concentrations of 150–300 ng/ml to be reached in 5 minutes with doses of 0.5 or 1 mg/kg in children already receiving phenobarbital.[58]

Effective brain concentrations are quickly obtained, but only for a short period of time, which explains the frequent recurrence of seizures. This phenomenon is perhaps related to the redistribution of this drug to peripheral benzodiazepine-binding sites.[60] Volume of distribution is of 1.3–1.8 liters/kg.

Diazepam is bound to plasma albumin in a proportion of 85–87 percent.[61] The binding is weaker to α_1-glycoprotein acid (orosomucoid), whose concentration is low in the neonate.[62]

The mean half-life is long, 75 ± 35 hours (mean ± 1 SD) in the premature and 31 ± 2 hours in the term infant. Extreme values may reach 400 hours.[63]

METABOLISM. Metabolism is mainly hepatic and involves demethylation, followed by oxidation. The main metabolite is the N-desmethyldiazepam, which exerts both therapeutic and very depressive activity: hypotonia, cardiorespiratory depression, and sphincter disorders. After several days of treatment, the N-desmethyldiazepam concentration is higher than that of diazepam. High plasma concentrations are observed up to 7 days after diazepam discontinuation; there are risks of accumulation and adverse side effects.[58] The other metabolites (oxazepam and N-methyloxazepam) are less active. The metabolites are eliminated following glucuronidation.

THERAPEUTIC USE. Blood levels of 150–336 ng/ml are often, but not always, associated with the control of seizures.[64] Minimal plasma levels of 500–700 ng/ml are rapidly needed for acute seizure control. Maintenance of seizure control calls for levels of 150–200 ng/ml.[65] At these concentrations, EEG depression is quite transitory.[30] Gamstorp and Seden[66] used continuous infusions of 0.7–2.75 mg/h.

Rectal administration (0.5–1 mg/kg) affords rapidly effective levels and avoids the disadvantages of intravenous administration, such as high plasma concentration peaks and localized venous thrombosis. The optimal dosage for prolonged treatment in the newborn has not been documented.

SIDE EFFECTS. Diazepam by itself does not displace albumin-bound bilirubin. On the other hand, benzyl alcohol, which constitutes 2 percent of the parenteral vehicle, is capable of an *in vitro* bilirubin–albumin displacement. However, this risk might be theoretical, since the concentrations necessary to obtain this effect surpass those observed in clinical practice. Nathenson et al.[67] confirmed *in vivo* that diazepam administration did not affect bilirubin binding. A more recent study, however, has raised the possibility of such an adverse effect even at low concentrations, but without evidence of long-term consequences.[68]

Clonazepam (Rivotril, Clonopin)

The chemical structure of clonazepam is 5-(12-chlorophenyl)-1,3-dihydro-7-nitro-2H-1,4-benzodiazepin-2-one. It has a molecular weight of 315 daltons, and it is a lipid-soluble substance. The structure and effects of clonazepam are closed to those of diazepam.[69] It is a very effective drug for the control of status epilepticus in the children.[70] The binding to central benzodiazepine receptors is very specific.

Enteral absorption and bioavailability is about 80 percent of the ingested dose[71] in older children[72] and in adults, but it has not been studied in the newborn. Rectal absorption is also effective in infants.

The distribution half-life following intravenous administration of a single dose of 0.1–0.2 mg/kg in neonates presenting with seizures and already treated with phenobarbital is short: 0.16–2.10 hours.[73] This explains the fast therapeutic effect of clonazepam. The apparent volume of distribution ranges from 1.5–11 liters/kg.[73]

When administered to the mother, the protein-unbound fraction is of 17.3 ± 0.7 percent, (mean ± 1sd) at birth in umbilical venous blood and 13.9 ± 0.2 percent in the adult.[74] Therefore, clonazepam is less protein-bound than diazepam, which thereby increases its therapeutic activity. Only 47 percent is bound to albumin[75]; however, other proteins, such as α_1-acid glycoprotein, for example, could be involved.[62] Storage in adipose tissue is possible.

ELIMINATION. In most cases, the elimination half-life ranges from 22–43 hours. These values are of the same order of magnitude as those reported in older patients: 18.7–39.0 hours.[76,77] This is most likely due to exposure to the inductive effects of phenobarbital on hepatic drug-metabolizing enzyme systems.[78] Higher values (up to 140 hours) have been observed during the first 60 hours after birth, even in newborns treated with phenobarbital.[73]

The clearance rate ranges from 0.025–0.070 liter/h/kg during the first 6 days of life. Thus the clearance is lower than in the older child (0.130–0.180 liter/h/kg) and in the adult (0.08–0.240 liter/h/kg). Clearance rapidly increases with postnatal age, reaching values of 0.140–0.153 liter/h/kg between 25 and 44 days of age.

Clonazepam is metabolized in the liver to 7-amino- and 7-acetamino-clonazepam, which are inactive metabolites. They are excreted in the urine either unchanged or as conjugates, or after further biotransformation to their 3-hydroxy derivatives.

THERAPEUTIC USE. Therapeutic efficacy is usually obtained with plasma levels of 15–80 ng/ml.[72,77,79] These values are commonly observed after a single intravenous injection of 0.1 mg/kg.[73] Because of its long half-life, a single daily injection is sufficient during the first 5 days of life. Afterwards, the interval of injection should be increased to 0.1 mg/kg twice a day.

SIDE EFFECTS. Side effects such as hypotonia and apnea are difficult to assess because the treated infants suffer from neurologic disorders which themselves may bring on similar abnormalities. However, these are seemingly negligible at therapeutic levels.

In older patients, plasma levels exceeding 120–150 ng/ml have been shown to increase the frequency of the crises or modify their symptomatology.[76,78] During the first days, such values may be observed following either a single injection of 0.2 mg/kg[73] or too frequent injections.

Lorazepam (Ativan, Temesta)

Lorazepam [7-chloro-5-(2-chlorophenyl)-1,3-dihydro-3-hydroxy-2H-1,4-benzodiazepine-2-one] is recommended for the treatment of status epilepticus because of its long duration of action.[80] It has not often been used in the newborn.[81,82]

No specific pharmacologic data exist for this age group. Deshmukh et al.[81] used it in newborns who had already been treated with phenobarbital and phenytoin. They used intravenous drips of 0.05 mg/kg. The therapeutic results observed were quite good, and few adverse effects were noted (significant EEG depression during several hours). The therapeutic action of Lorazepam is fast (5 minutes) and prolonged (about 24 hours). In the adult, the drug quickly enters the central nervous system. Half-life is 13–15 hours.

As for diazepam, benzyl alcohol is used as a preservative in lorazepam solutions. However, even though it may interfere with bilirubin binding to albumin,[83] the small amounts injected (0.25 mg/kg) probably rule out the possibility of clinical importance.

Carbamazepine (Tegretol)

Carbamazepine is an iminostilbene derivative that is chemically known as 5-carbamoyl-5H-dibenz[b,f]azepine. It has a molecular weight of 236 daltons and is poorly soluble in water. Its precise mechanism of action is unknown. Like phenytoin, it blocks sodium and calcium channels, and in particular, it might stimulate the adenosine inhibitory system.

Mackintosh et al.[84] proposed its use as oral maintenance therapy. However, no clinical evaluation has been carried out to support such a proposal. Six neonates aged from 2–16 days received 5 mg/kg of carbamazepine. It should be noted that they had been treated with phenobarbital beforehand. Peak concentrations were obtained in 6.7 ± 1.4 hours on average (mean $\pm$ 1SD). Volume of distribution was of 1.1–2.5 liters/kg, which is greater than in the adult (0.8–1.4 liters/kg). Elimination half-life ranged from 7.2–15.2 hours. With this dose, therapeutic effective plasma concentrations of 2.5–10 μg/ml were obtained. They remain in this range with a maintenance dose of 5–8 mg/kg/day over 3–15 days. Rey et al.,[85] using a dose of 15–20 mg/kg, obtained concentrations of the order of 43 μg/ml, which were too high. The other pharmacokinetic parameters have not been determined in the newborn.

The main metabolite of carbamazepine is its 10,11-epoxide. It is probably active and contributes to the toxicity of the drug. Its production varies among patients. However, it should be higher in children.[86]

Carbamazepine is well tolerated. However, an increase in crises has been reported in older children presenting with atypical absences.[87] Carbamazepine also impairs cultured brain neuron growth.[88]

Sodium Valproate (Depakine)

Sodium valproate is the sodium salt of valproic acid, or 2-propylpentanoic acid. It has a molecular weight of 144 daltons and is quite water-soluble. It has two possible

mechanisms of action: an increase in the GABA concentration owing to its decreased degradation or an increase in GABA-induced postsynaptic inhibition.[89]

Few studies concerning valproate pharmacokinetics in the newborn have been undertaken. In newborns more than 5 days old already treated with phenobarbital, total valproic acid volume of distribution is of 0.40 liter/kg (0.36–0.47 liter/kg).[90] The mean clearance is 14.4 ml/h/kg (5.5–18.2 ml/h/kg), and the mean elimination half-life is 26.4 hours (8.6–48.5 hours).

The free fraction, which ranges from 11.3–31.6 percent (mean 19.2 percent), has a mean volume of distribution of 2.02 liters/kg (1.14–2.44 liters/kg), a mean clearance rate of 108.9 ml/h/kg (42.0–252.0 ml/h/kg), and a mean elimination half-life of 17.6 hours (6.7–34.2 hours). Other authors also found a longer half-life than in older age groups: 24.2 ± 6.8 hours (mean $\pm$ SD).[91,92]

Therapeutic Use. Valproic acid can be administrated orally or rectally. In the first case, absorption is rapid, occurring in less than 2 hours. A dose of 40–50 mg/day,[93] or 7.5 mg/kg every 12 hours,[91] allows for effective plasma levels of 50–100 μg/ml.

Gal et al.[91] recommend a 20–25 mg/kg loading dose, followed by a 5–10 mg/kg maintenance dose every 12 hours. Viani et al.[94] showed that, as in the adult, a 12 mg/kg dose administered rectally is rapidly absorbed and effective.

Nevertheless, valproate should be used with caution because of the risks of hepatic,[95,96] hematologic,[97] and metabolic (hyperammoniemia[90]) toxicity. These adverse side effects might be due to a disorder in the metabolism of carnitine and could be prevented by carnitine supplementation.[98]

Valproate reduces brain weight and decreases brain metabolism of glutamate and aspartate in particular in newborn mice.[99]

Progabide (Gabrene)

Progabide is a GABA-agonist drug. Its molecular weight is 335 daltons. It is rarely used in the newborn because it is available only for oral administration. Hepatic toxicity has been reported in the adult.

The administration of 20 mg/kg every 8 hours usually produces effective plasma concentrations of 800–1000 ng/ml.[100] This posology is higher than that used in older children (35–45 mg/kg/day). Newborn infants probably require higher doses because its main acid metabolite (SL 75[102]), which has significant therapeutic activity, is only present at low concentrations in the neonate. The therapeutic effect is obtained 15–20 hours after the first dose.

Lidocaine (Xylocaine)

Lidocaine, initially indicated for local anesthesia, is also a cardiac antiarrhythmic agent. It also has been used to treat certain forms of status epilepticus,[101,102] particularly in the newborn, since 1955.[103]

Chemically, it is known as 2-diethylamino-N-(2,6-

dimethylphenyl)-acetamid. Its water and lipid solubility are pH-dependent. It is largely nonionized in plasma, and it readily crosses the blood–brain barrier.

Lidocaine probably acts by stabilizing the neuronal membrane, preventing calcium uptake and blocking sodium and potassium movement.[28] However, its precise mechanism of action remains unknown.

Because of the significant metabolism that occurs during primary hepatic passage, only intravenous administration is recommended. Following administration of a single dose, the half-life is short. Values of 90–100 minutes and 3 hours, respectively, have been reported in the adult and in the newborn.[104]

Lidocaine is hydrolyzed and dealkylated by the microsomal hepatic oxidases into monoethylglycinxylidide and glycinxylidide, which are partly excreted in the urine. Both these metabolites are biologically active.

Therapeutic plasma levels are about 2–5 μg/ml. Levels exceeding 5μg/ml may induce cortical irritability and seizures. Convulsions occurring in two neonates after discontinuation of lidocaine treatment were attributed to the accumulation of the active metabolites.[105] Therapeutic efficacy can be increased with phenytoin.

For adults, Greenblatt et al.[106] recommend intravenous administration of 1.4 mg/kg and then an infusion of 29 μg/kg/min. Wilder and Bruni[28] suggest a dose of 4 mg/kg/h. In full-term and preterm neonates, Hellström-Westas et al.[107] successfully used a 2 mg/kg loading dose followed by a 2 mg/kg/h maintenance dose.

SIDE EFFECTS. The EEG is transitorily depressed. Lidocaine does not potentiate barbituric and benzodiazepine sedative effects. An overdose can produce ventricular fibrillation.

Paraldehyde

Paraldehyde is a cyclic polyester; its chemical nomenclature is 2,4,6-trimethyl-1,3,5-trioxane. It is metabolized by the liver to acetaldehyde by depolymerization. This is followed by oxidation to acetic acid, with final metabolism to H_2O and CO_2. In the adult, 20–30 percent of the drug is exhaled.

Paraldehyde volume of distribution is of 1.73 ± 0.20 liters/kg (mean ± SD), and its clearance rate is of 0.121 ± 0.023 liter/h/kg. Mean elimination half-life is 18 hours,[108] or 10.2 ± 1.0 hours.[109]

THERAPEUTIC USE. Therapeutic plasma levels range from 100–200 μg/ml.[102] Several recent studies have demonstrated its efficacy in managing intractable status epilepticus, with very few, if any, side effects.[108-110]

For Koren et al.,[108] the loading dose is 400 mg in a bolus, or 200 mg/kg/h (0.2 ml/kg in a 10 percent solution with saline). Maintenance dose is 20–50 mg/kg/h administered rectally or intravenously. Giacoia et al.[109] recommend 150 mg/kg/h of a 5 percent solution in 5 percent dextrose over a 3-hour period.

Giacoia et al.[109] underline the importance of not exceeding this concentration to prevent the risk of pulmonary precipitation. Droplets reaching the lungs may occlude capillaries, resulting in pulmonary microinfarcts,

hemorrhage, and subsequent fibrosis. This substance is extremely caustic to living tissues. Only polyethylene or polypropylene plastics can be used for administration, since other plastics are dissolved by paraldehyde.

THERAPEUTIC SCHEDULE

No controlled studies comparing the efficacies of the various therapeutic regimens proposed for the treatment of neonatal seizures have been carried out.[111] In many cases where the outcome is favorable, the distinction between the results from a given treatment and spontaneous or therapeutically induced recovery of the disorder responsible for the seizures in the first place is often difficult to make.

Initiated after a first crisis, treatment aims to prevent the recurrence of the crisis. Indications for treatment are simple when one is confronted with typical electroclinical seizures. In purely electrical crises, which are usually of short duration,[112] absolute control does not appear to be mandatory, but the aim should be to lower the frequency as much as possible. Clinically doubtful manifestations, which remain unconfirmed by EEG, are rarely of epileptic nature.[113] These should not be treated. The benefits expected from a given treatment should carefully be weighed against its possible noxious side effects.

Initial Management (Table 19–3)

Early administration of a quickly absorbed drug that easily enters the brain is called for. This is obtained by intravenous administration of a loading dose.

Phenobarbital remains the initial drug of choice.[114] It is administered at a loading dose of 20 mg/kg. If this is met with failure or is insufficient, the injection of two additional 5 mg/kg doses an hour apart, in monotherapy, appears to be the optimal solution. If necessary, a second drug may be added. Many authors recommend phenytoin. Its main disadvantage resides in the difficulty to adapt the maintenance doses to predictable pharmacokinetics.

Benzodiazepines enter the brain very quickly; therefore, their effect is nearly immediate. Unlike diazepam,

TABLE 19–2. CONVERSION OF PLASMA LEVELS OF ANTICONVULSANT DRUGS

DRUG	CONVERSION FACTOR*
Phenobarbital	4.31
Primidone	4.58
Phenytoin	3.96
Diazepam	3.51
Clonazepam	3.17
Carbamazepine	4.23
Valproate	6.94
Progabide	2.99

*Conversion: (μg/ml) × conversion factor = (μmol/liter): (μg/mol): conversion factor = (μg/mol).

TABLE 19-3. TREATMENT OF NEONATAL SEIZURES

DRUG	LOADING DOSES	MAINTENANCE DOSES
1. Phenobarbital	20 mg/kg I.V. ± additional doses of 5 mg/kg to achieve plasma concentrations of 40 μg/ml	3 mg/kg/day I.V. or P.O. 5 mg/kg/day after 1 week of age
2. Diazepam *or* Clonazepam Lorazepam*	0.5 mg/kg I.V. 0.1 mg/kg I.V. 0.05 mg/kg	0.5–1 mg/kg/day I.V. 0.1 mg/kg every 12–24 h I.V.
3. Phenytoin	20 mg/kg I.V.	3 mg/kg every 12 h I.V.
4. Or, *when they fail* Lidocaine Primidone Paraldehyde Valproic acid* Carbamazepine* Progabide	2 mg/kg I.V. or 4 mg/kg/h 20 mg/kg I.V. 400 mg I.V. or 200 mg/kg/h 20–25 mg/kg rectally	2–4 mg/kg/h I.V. 10–20 mg/kg/day I.V. 20–50 mg/kg/h I.V. or rectally 5–10 mg/kg every 12 h P.O. or rectally 5–8 mg/kg/day P.O. 20 mg/kg every 8 h P.O.

*Not enough data in the newborn.

which binds to different tissues and which has active metabolites, clonazepam selectively binds to the central nervous system and has no active metabolites. Therefore, its effects are directly and only related to plasma drug concentrations. The potent cardiorespiratory depressive effects of the benzodiazepines are not a real disadvantage in practice. At present, there are no sufficient data on the use of lorazepam in the neonate to recommend its routine use.

The decision to add a third drug (phenytoin or a benzodiazepine, depending on the choice of the second, and under extraordinary circumstances, lidocaine, paraldehyde, or valproic acid) is made after total evaluation of the infant status is performed. This evaluation concerns seizure etiology, seizure patterns, as well as EEG abnormalities. In some cases, it appears that allowing some crises to persist may be less harmful than instituting major treatment, which may multiply the risk of noxious side effects. The respiratory depression that may occur suddenly must be kept in mind in case of cumulative doses of different drugs.

Maintenance Therapy

Adequate doses of the initially prescribed drugs are called for. If insufficiently effective, orally administered drugs not normally used for initial treatment (progabide or valproic acid) may be tried.

Assessment of drug plasma concentrations is important because of the variability of the metabolism of most drugs during the first days of life (Tables 19–2 and 19–3).

Treatment Discontinuation

The possible adverse side effects of the anticonvulsant drugs warrant their discontinuation as soon as possible. Most disorders leading to convulsions disappear quickly. In such cases, all drugs are progressively stopped, beginning with the last prescribed, 2–4 days following seizure termination. Phenobarbital is usually the last to be discontinued, after several weeks Volpe [115] or Ellison et al. [116] In many cases, its discontinuation is indicated as soon as the acute period is over.[3,117]

REFERENCES

1. Eriksson M, Zetterström R: Neonatal convulsions. Incidence and causes in the Stockholm area. Acta Paediatr Scand 68:807–811, 1979
2. Brown JK, Cockburn F, Forfar JO: Clinical and chemical correlates in convulsions of the newborn. Lancet 1:135–138, 1972
3. Andre M, Matisse N, Vert P, Debruille C: Neonatal seizures: Recent aspects. Neuropediatrics 19:201–207, 1988
4. Lou HC, Friis-Hansen B: Arterial blood pressure elevations during motor activity and epileptic seizures in the newborn. Acta Paediatr Scand 68:803–806, 1979
5. Wasterlain CG: Neonatal seizures and brain growth. Neuropaediatrie 9:213–228, 1978
6. Bergman I, Painter MJ, Hirsch RP: Outcome in neonates with convulsions treated in an intensive care unit. Ann Neurol 14:642–647, 1983
7. Morselli P, Franco-Morselli R, Bossi L: Clinical pharmacokinetics in newborns and infants: Age-related differences and therapeutic implications. Clini Pharmacokinet 5:485–527, 1980
8. Guillet P, Morselli PL: Pharmacokinetics of anticonvulsants in the neonate, in Wasterlain C, Vert P (eds): Neonatal Seizures: Pathophysiology and Pharmacological Management. New York, Raven Press, 1990
9. Agurell S, Berlin A, Fengren HG, Hellstrom B: Plasma levels of diazepam after parenteral and rectal administration to children. Epilepsia 16:277–283, 1975
10. Graves NM, Kriel RL: Rectal administration of antiepileptic drugs in children. Pediatr Neurol 3:321–326, 1987
11. Wallace S: Altered plasma albumin in the newborn infant. Br J Clin Pharmacol 4:82–85, 1977
12. Hamar C, Levy G: Serum protein binding of drugs and bilirubin in newborn infants and their mothers. Clin Pharmacol Ther 28:58–63, 1980
13. Aranda JV, McLeod SM, Renton KW, Eade NR: Hepatic microsomal drug oxydation and electron transport in newborn infants. J Pediatr 85:534–542, 1974
14. McDonald RL, McClean MJ: Cellular basis of barbiturate and phenytoin anticonvulsivant drug action. Epilepsia 23:7–18, 1982
15. Painter MJ, Pippenger C, McDonald H, Pitlick W: Phenobarbital and diphenylhydantoin levels in neonates with seizures. J Pediatr 92:315–319, 1978
16. Boutroy MJ, Andre M, Vert P: Clinical pharmacology and uses of phenobarbital in the newborn, in Moss AJ (ed): Pediatrics Update. New York, Elsevier, 1981, pp 211–222

17. Wadell WJ, Butler TC: The distribution and excretion of phenobarbital. J Clin Invest 36:1217, 1957
18. Grasela TH, Donn SM: Neonatal population pharmacokinetics of phenobarbital derived from routine clinical data. Dev Pharmacol Ther 8:374–383, 1985
19. Cornford EM, Pardridge WM, Braun LD, Oldendorf WH: Increased blood–brain barrier transport of protein-bound anticonvulsant drugs in the newborn. J Cereb Blood Flow Metab 3:281–286, 1983
20. Painter MJ, Pippenger C, Wasterlain C, et al: Phenobarbital and phenytoin in neonatal seizures: Metabolism and tissue distribution. Neurology 31:1107–1112, 1981
21. Boreus LO, Jalling B, Källberg N: Phenobarbital metabolism in adults and in newborn infants. Acta Paediatr Scand 67:193–200, 1978
22. Bhargava VO, Garrettson LK: Development of phenobarbital glucosidation in the human neonate. Dev Pharmacol Ther 11:8–13, 1988
23. Donn SM, Grasela TH, Goldstein GW: Safety of a higher loading dose of phenobarbital in the term newborn. Pediatrics 75:1061–1064, 1985
24. Kossmann JC: Pharmacocinétique du phénobarbital injectable chez le prématuré: Etude à partir d'une nouvelle forme lyophilisée. Arch Fr Pediatr 42:317–320, 1985
25. Jalling B: Plasma and cerebrospinal fluid concentrations of phenobarbital in infants given single doses. Dev Med Child Neurol 16:781–793, 1974
26. Rossi LN, Nino LM, Principi N: Correlation between age and plasma level/dosage ratio for phenobarbital in infants and children. Acta Paediatr Scand 68:431–434, 1979
27. Gal P, Boer HR, Toback J: Phenobarbital dosing in neonates and asphyxia. Neurology 32:788–789, 1982
28. Wilder BJ, Bruni J: Seizure Disorders: A Pharmacological Approach to Treatment. New York, Raven Press, 1981
29. Staudt F, Scholl ML, Coen RW, Bickford RB: Phenobarbital therapy in neonatal seizures and the prognostic value of the EEG. Neuropediatrics 13:24–33, 1982
30. Couto-Sales S, Rey E, Radvanyi MF, Dreyfus-Brisac C: Essai d'évaluation des thérapeutiques (diazépam, phénobarbital) sur l'EEG néonatal pendant les premières 24 heures du traitement. Rev EEG Neurophysiol 9:26–34, 1979
31. Diaz J, Schain RJ: Phenobarbital: Effects of long-term administration on behavior and brain of artificially reared rats. Science 199:90–95, 1978
32. Yanai J, Bergman A: Neuronal deficit after exposure to phenobarbital. Exp Neurol 73:199–208, 1981
33. Daval JL, Pereira de Vasconcelos A, Lataud I: Morphological and neurochemical effects of diazepam and phenobarbital on selective culture of neurons from fetal rat brain. J Neurochem 50:665–672, 1988
34. Gilman JT, Duchowny MS, Gal P, Weaver R: Phenobarbital serum concentration and response in neonatal seizures. Ann Neurol 22:417, 1987
35. Vert P, Monin P, Morselli PL, Vibert M, Andre M: Blood gases, acid–base changes and monitoring of plasma levels of phenobarbital and clonazepam in the newborn treated for postasphyxic seizures, in Stern L (ed): Intensive Care in the Newborn, vol 2. New York, Masson, 1980, pp 313–323
36. Gal P, Toback HR, Boer HR, Erkan NV, Wells TJ: Efficacy of phenobarbital monotherapy in treatment of neonatal seizures. Relationship to blood levels. Neurology 32:1401–1404, 1982
37. Fischer JH, Lockman LA, Zaske D, Kriel R: Phenobarbital maintenance dose requirements in treating neonatal seizures. Neurology 31:1042–1044, 1981
38. Gold F, Bourin M, Chantepie E, et al: Modalités pratiques d'utilisation du phénobarbital par voie veineuse chez le nouveau-né à terme. Arch Fr Pediatr 37:613–616, 1980
39. Cloyd JC, Wright BD, Perrier D: Pharmacokinetics of thiopental in two patients treated for incontrollable seizures. Epilepsia 20:313–318, 1979
40. Young GB, Blume WT, Bolton CF: Anesthetic barbiturates and refractory status epilepticus. Can J Neurol Sci 7:291–292, 1980
41. Garg DC, Goldberg RN, Woo-Ming RB, Weidler DJ: Pharmacokinetics of thiopental in the asphyxiated neonate. Dev Pharmacol Ther 11:213–218, 1988
42. Goldberg RN, Moscoso P, Bauer CR, et al: Use of barbiturate therapy in severe perinatal asphyxia: A randomized controlled trial. J Pediatr 109:851–856, 1986
43. Demarquez JL, Galperine R, Billeaud C, Brachet-Liermain A: High-dose thiopental pharmacokinetics in brain-injured children and neonates. Dev Pharmacol Ther 10:292–300, 1987
44. Powell C, Painter MJ, Pippenger CE: Primidone therapy in refractory neonatal seizures. J Pediatr 105:651–654, 1984
45. Woodbury DM, Pippenger CE: Primidone: Mechanisms of action, in Woodbury DM, Penry JK, Pippenger CE (eds): Antiepileptic Drugs, New York, Raven Press, 1982, pp 449–452
46. Wiriyathin S, Kaojarern S, Rosenfeld CR: Dilantin toxicity in a preterm infant: Persistent bradycardia and lethargy. J Pediatr 100:146–148, 1982
47. Malherbe C, Burril KC, Larn SR, Karam JH: Effect of DPH on insulin secretion in man. N Engl J Med 286:339, 1972
48. Albani M, Wernicke I: Oral phenytoin in infancy: Dose requirement, absorption, and elimination. Pediatr Pharmacol 3:229–236, 1983
49. Rane A, Lunde PKM, Jalling B, Yaffe SJ, Sjöqvist F: Plasma protein binding of diphenylhydantoin in normal and hyperbilirubinemic infants. J Pediatr 78:877–882, 1971
50. Fredholm B, Rane A, Persson B: Diphenylhydantoin binding to plasma proteins and its dependence on free fatty acid and bilirubin concentration in dogs and newborn infants. Pediatr Res 9:26–30, 1975
51. Loughnan PM, Greenwald H, Purton WW, et al: Pharmacokinetic observations of phenytoin disposition in the newborn and young infant. Arch Dis Child 52:302–309, 1977
52. Bourgeois BFD, Dodson WE: Phenytoin elimination in newborns. Neurology 33:173–178, 1983
53. Mimaki T, Deshmukh P, Yamamura H: Decreased benzodiazepine receptor density in rat brain following chronic phenytoin administration. Ann Neurol 8:230, 1980
54. Swaiman KF, Schrier BD, Neale EA: Effects of chronic phenytoin and valproic acid exposure on fetal mouse cortical cultures. Ann Neurol 8:230, 1980
55. Whelan HT, Hendeless L, Habekern CH, Neims AH: High intravenous phenytoin dosage requirement in a newborn infant. Neurology 33:106–108, 1983
56. Aaltonen L, Erkkola R, Kanto J: Benzodiazepine receptors in the human fetus. Biol Neonate 44:54–57, 1983
57. Morselli PL, Principi N, Tognoni G, et al: Diazepam elimination in premature and full term infants and children. J Perinatal Med 1:133, 1973
58. Langslet A, Meberg A, Bredesen JE, Lunde PKM: Plasma concentrations of diazepam and N-desmethyldiazepam in newborn infants after intravenous, intramuscular, rectal, and oral administration. Acta Paediatr Scand 67:699–704, 1978
59. Dulac O, Aicardi J, Rey E, Olive G: Blood levels of diazepam after single rectal administration in infants and children. J Pediatr 93:1039–1041, 1978
60. Groh B, Muller WE: A comparison of the relative in vitro and in vivo binding affinities of various benzodiazepines and related compounds for the benzodiazepine receptor and for the peripheral benzodiazepine binding site. Res Commun Chem Pathol Pharmacol 49:463–466, 1985
61. Nau H, Kuhnz W, Egger HJ, Rating D, Helge H: Anticonvulsants during pregnancy and lactation: Transplacental maternal and neonatal kinetics. Clin Pharmacokinet 7:508–543, 1982
62. Wood M, Wood AJJ: Changes in plasma drug binding and alpha₁-acid glycoprotein in mother and newborn infant. Clin Pharmacol Ther 29:522–526, 1981
63. Mandelli M, Morselli PL, Nordio S, et al: Placental transfer of diazepam and its disposition in the neonate. Clin Pharmacol Ther 17:564–572, 1975
64. Booker HE, Celisa GB: Serum concentrations of diazepam in subjects with epilepsy. Arch Neurol 29:191, 1973
65. Schmidt D: Benzodiazepines: Diazepam, in Woodbury DM, Penry JK, Pippenger CE (eds): Antiepileptic Drugs. New York, Raven Press, 1982, pp 711–735
66. Gamstorp I, Seden G: Neonatal convulsions treated with continuous intravenous diazepam. Uppsala J Med Sci 87:143–149, 1982
67. Nathenson G, Cohen MI, McNamara H: The effect of Na ben-

zoate on serum bilirubin of the Gunn rat. J Pediatr 86:799–803, 1975

68. Jardine DS, Rogers K: Relationship of benzyl alcohol to kernicterus, intraventricular hemorrhage, and mortality in preterm infants. Pediatrics 83:153–160, 1989

69. Pinder RM, Brodgen RN, Speight TM, Avery GS: Clonazepam: A review of its pharmacological properties and therapeutic efficacy in epilepsy. Drugs 12:321–361, 1976

70. Congdon PJ, Forsythe WI: Intravenous clonazepam in the treatment of status epilepticus in children. Epilepsia 21:97–102, 1980

71. Eschenhof E: Untersuchungen über das Schicksal des Anticonvulsivums Clonazepam in Organismus der Ratte, des Hundes und Menschen. Arzneimittelforschung 23:390, 1973

72. Dreifuss FE, Penry JK, Rose SW, et al: Serum clonazepam concentrations in children with absence seizures. Neurology 25:255–258, 1975

73. Andre M, Boutroy MJ, Dubruc C, et al: Clonazepam pharmacokinetics and therapeutic efficacy in neonatal seizures. Eur J Clin Pharmacol 30:585–590, 1986

74. Pacifici GM, Taddeucci-Brunelli G, Rane A: Clonazepam serum binding during development. Clin Pharmacol Ther 35:354–359, 1984

75. Muller M, Wollert U: Characterization of the binding of benzodiazepines to human serum albumin. Arch Pharmacol 280:229–237, 1973

76. Dreifuss FE, Sato S: Benzodiazepine: Clonazepam, in Woodbury DM, Penry JK, Pippenger CE (eds): Antiepileptic Drugs. New York, Raven Press, 1982, pp 737–752

77. Knop HJ, Edmunds LC, Van Der Kleijn E: Clinical pharmacokinetics of clonazepam. Excerpta Med Int Congr Series 501:79–93, 1979

78. Morselli PL: Clinical significance of monitoring plasma levels of benzodiazepine tranquilizers and antiepileptic drugs, in Deniker P, Radouco-Thomas C, Villeneuve A (eds): Neuropsychopharmacology. Oxford, NY: Pergamon Press, 1978, pp 877–888

79. Baruzzi A, Bodo B, Bossi L, et al: Plasma levels of di-n-propylacetate and clonazepam in epileptic patient. Int J Clin Pharmacol Biopharm 15:403–408, 1977

80. Levy RJ, Krall RL: Treatment of status epilepticus with lorazepam. Arch Neurol 41:605–611, 1984

81. Deshmukh A, Wittert W, Schnitzler E, Mangurten HH: Lorazepam in the treatment of refractory neonatal seizures: A pilot study. Am J Dis Child 140:1042–1044, 1986

82. Roddy SM, McBride MC, Torres CF: Treatment of neonatal seizures with lorazepam. Ann Neurol 22:412, 1987

83. Brodersen R: Free bilirubin in blood plasma of the newborn: Effects of albumin, fatty acids, pH, displacing drugs, and phototherapy, in Stern L, Oh W, Friis-Hansen B (eds): Intensive Care of the Newborn, vol 2. New York, Masson, 1978, pp 331–345

84. Mackintosh DA, Baird-Lampert J, Buchanan N: Is carbamazepine an alternative maintenance therapy for neonatal seizures? Dev Pharmacol Ther 10:100–106, 1987

85. Rey E, d'Athis P, de Lauture D, et al: Pharmacokinetics of carbamazepine in the neonate and in the child. Int J Clin Pharmacol Biopharm 17:90–96, 1979

86. Pynnönnen S, Sillanpää M, Frey H, Iisalo E: Carbamazepine and its 10,11-epoxide in children and adults with epilepsy. Eur J Clin Pharmacol 11:129–133, 1977

87. Snead OC: Exacerbation of seizures in children by carbamazepine. N Engl J Med 313:916–200, 1985

88. Neale EA, Sher PK, Graubard BI: Differential toxicity of chronic exposure to phenytoin, phenobarbital, or carbamazepine in cerebral cortical cell cultures. Pediatr Neurol 1:143–150, 1985

89. Chapman AG, Keane PE, Meldrum BS, et al: Mechanism of action of valproate. Prog Neurobiol 19:315–359, 1982

90. Gal P, Oles KS, Gilman JT, Weaver R: Valproic acid efficacy, toxicity and pharmacokinetics in neonates with intractable seizures. Neurology 38:467–471, 1988

91. Irvine-Meek JM, Hall KW, Otten NH, et al: Pharmacokinetic study of valproic acid in a neonate. Pediatr Pharmacol 2:317–321, 1982

92. Haneda S, Takebe Y, Koide N: Pharmacokinetic study of valproic acid (VPA) in neonates with convulsions. Brain Dev 5:97, 1983

93. Brachet-Liermain A, Demarquez JL, Saint-Martin J, et al: Bases pharmacocinétiques de l'utilisation du dipropylacétate de sodium chez le nouveau-né et le jeune nourrisson. Arch Fr Pediatr 33:1010, 1976

94. Viani F, Jussi MI, Germano M, et al: Rectal administration of sodium valproate for neonatal and infantile status epilepticus. Dev Med Child Neurol 26:678–679, 1984

95. Gram L: Valproic acid and liver damage. Acta Paediatr Scand 74:796–798, 1985

96. Takeuchi T, Sugimoto T, Nishida N, Kobayashi Y: Evaluation of sodium valproate on primary cultured rat hepatocytes. Neuropediatrics 19:158–161, 1988

97. Nathan D, Guillon JL, Chevallier B, Gallet JP: Thrombopénie et érythroblastopénie chez un nourrison de un mois traité par valproate. Ann Pediatr 34:149–150, 1987

98. Nishida N, Sugimoto T, Araki A, et al: Carnitine metabolism in valproate-treated rats: The effect of L-carnitine supplementation. Pediatr Res 22:500–503, 1987

99. Thurston JH, Hauhart RE, Schulz DW, et al: Chronic valproate administration produces hepatic dysfunction and may delay brain maturation in infant mice. Neurology 31:1063–1069, 1981

100. Andre M, Boutroy MJ, Vert P, Morselli PL: Therapeutic effect of progabide in neonatal convulsions, in Proceedings of the XVIth Epilepsy International Congress, Hambourg, 1985

101. Bernhard GC, Bohm E, Höjeberg S: A new treatment of status epilepticus, intravenous injection of a local anesthesic (lidocaine). Arch Neurol Psychiatry 74:208–214, 1955

102. Browne TR: Paraldehyde, chlormethiazole and lidocaine for treatment of status epilepticus. Adv Neurol 31:509–517, 1983

103. Norell E, Garmstorp I: Neonatal seizures: Effect of lidocaine. Acta Paediatr Scand 59:97–98, 1970

104. Mihaly G, Morre G, Thomas J, et al: The pharmacokinetics and metabolism of the anilide local anesthetics in neonates. I. Lignocaine. Eur J Clin Pharmacol 13:143–152, 1978

105. Wallin A, Nergårdh A: Risks of lidocaine therapy in the neonatal period, in Proceedings of the XLII Congress of Swedish Medical Association, Stockholm, 1985

106. Greenblatt DJ, Bolognini V, Koch-Weser J, Harmatz JS: Pharmacokinetic approach to the clinical use of lidocaine intravenously. JAMA 236:273, 1976

107. Hellström-Westas L, Westgren U, Rosen I, Svenningsen NW: Lidocaine for treatment of severe seizures in newborn infants. I. Clinical effects and cerebral electrical activity monitoring. Acta Paediatr Scand 77:79–84, 1988

108. Koren G, Butt W, Rajchgot P: Intravenous paraldehyde for seizure control in newborn infants. Neurology 36:108–111, 1986

109. Giacoia GP, Gessner PK, Zaleska MM, Boutwell WC: Pharmacokinetics of paraldehyde disposition in the neonate. J Pediatr 104:291–296, 1984

110. Boutwell WC: Use of intravenous paraldehyde in neonatal status epilepticus. Pediatr Res 15:652, 1981

111. Andre M, Vert P, Wasterlain C: To treat or not to treat: A survey of medical current practice toward neonatal seizures, in Wasterlain C, Vert P (eds): Neonatal Seizures: Pathophysiology and Pharmacological Management. New York, Raven Press, 1990

112. Clancy RR, Legido A: The exact ictal and interictal duration of neonatal seizures. Epilepsia 28:537–541, 1987

113. Mizrahi EM, Kellaway P: Characterization and classification of neonatal seizures. Neurology 37:1837–1844, 1987

114. Johnston MV, Freeman JM: Pharmacologic advances in seizure control. Pediatr Clin North Am 28:179–194, 1981

115. Volpe JJ: Neurology of the Newborn. Philadelphia, WB Saunders, 1987, pp 209–235

116. Ellison PH, Horn JL, Franklin S, Jones MG: The results of checking a scoring system for neonatal seizures. Neuropediatrics 17:152–157, 1986

117. Gal P, Boer HR: Early discontinuation of anticonvulsants following neonatal seizures: A preliminary report. South Med J 75:298–300, 1982

20

DRUG TREATMENT OF NEONATAL APNEA

J. V. ARANDA, JOSE MARIA LOPES, PIERRE BLANCHARD, FABIAN EYAL, *and* GADY ALPAN

The well-modulated and well-coordinated respiratory rhythmicity exhibited by the older child and mature human is the culmination of complex developmental events involved in the control of breathing. Immaturity adversely influences the rhythmic firing of the brainstem neurons and the complex integration of the various sensory and motor inputs to the respiratory muscles, thus contributing to the development of apneic episodes. Neonatal apnea represents the most common and probably most important disorder in the control of breathing in the newborn infant.

Apnea is usually defined as the cessation of breathing for more than 20 seconds with or without bradycardia (heart rate below 100 beats/min) and/or cyanosis. It occurs in 25 percent of neonates with birth weights of less than 2500 gm. The incidence is inversely related to fetal maturity and may be as high as 84 percent in preterm neonates weighing less than 1000 gm at birth.

Considerable progress has been made in the understanding of neonatal apnea in the last decade, but the exact pathogenesis of this problem remains a matter of debate. A variety of specific factors and pathophysiologic disorders, as shown in Figure 20–1, may trigger apnea. Thus the diagnosis and management of this disorder are geared toward the treatment of these conditions. Table 20–1 enumerates some of the basic principles in the overall management of apnea. In general, identifiable and treatable causes, such as infection, hypoglycemia, hypoxia, hyperthermia, and others, should be corrected. If apnea persists despite no identifiable cause, the pharmacologic approach using respiratory stimulants should be used.

The pharmacologic approach to the management of neonatal apnea has gained universal acceptance over the past 15 years. Since the initial report of a decrease in the frequency of apneic episodes in neonates given theophylline rectally in 1973,[1] numerous studies have subsequently confirmed the usefulness of the methylated xanthines in the treatment of neonatal apnea (see later in text). Thus caffeine and theophylline, both related meth-

ylated xanthines, are now widely used in idiopathic neonatal apnea. More recently, there has been a renewed interest in the use of the respiratory stimulant doxapram hydrochloride as a potentially useful agent in some cases of apnea that are refractory to methylxanthines as well as in the facilitation of weaning babies from mechanical ventilation. Another respiratory stimulant, almitrine, holds similar promise. This chapter reviews the pharmacology of the methylated xanthines (caffeine and theophylline), doxapram, almitrine, and other agents.

METHYLXANTHINES: CAFFEINE AND THEOPHYLLINE

Pharmacologic Actions and Efficacy of Methylxanthines in Neonatal Apnea

The ability of caffeine to stimulate respiration has been known for a century, and the ability of aminophylline to regularize breathing in adult patients with Cheyne Stokes respiration was noted by Vogl in 1927. The potential role of these two drugs in the management of neonatal apnea was recognized in the last 15 years. Kuzemko and Paala[1] described the use of aminophylline in newborns in 1973, and several subsequent clinical trials have confirmed the efficacy of the xanthines in decreasing the number of apneas, cyanotic spells, and episodes of bradycardia (Table 20–2). Shannon et al.[2] described reduced numbers of severe apneas lasting more than 30 seconds and bradycardia associated with theophylline serum concentrations of 6–11 μg/ml. Peabody et al.[3] observed decreased numbers of apneas and bradycardia associated with regularization of the breathing pattern and less fluctuation in transcutaneous pO_2.

On the basis that caffeine has potent CNS stimulant properties with fewer peripheral effects compared with theophylline, we documented the efficacy of caffeine in

193

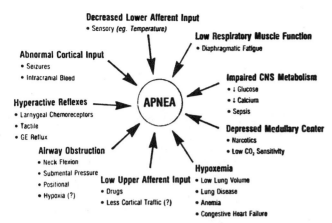

FIGURE 20–1. Factors associated with the genesis of neonatal apnea. (Reproduced with permission from Aranda JV, Trippenbach T, Turmen T, Lopes JM: Apena and control of breathing in newborn infants. In Stern L (ed) Diagnosis and Management of Respiratory Disorders in the Newborn. Addison Wesley, Menlo Park, CA, Chapter 7, pp. 134–157, 1984.)

neonatal apnea and described the same stimulatory effect of caffeine on respiration. We observed decreased episodes of apnea, regularization of the breathing pattern, and an increase in alveolar ventilation after caffeine administration. Despite relatively large doses utilized in our first study, no effects on heart rate were observed,[4] suggesting a wide therapeutic index. Subsequently, a dose–response curve for caffeine was defined and a rational approach was proposed (see later in text).[5]

Apnea can be produced by upper airway obstruction without cessation of respiratory muscle activity. The recognition of such episodes led to a reevaluation of the effect of the xanthines in decreasing apnea frequency both in infants in whom central apneas predominate and in infants in whom airway obstruction is the main pathogenetic mechanism. Roberts et al.[6] described a significant reduction in all types of apnea, suggesting that theophylline may act to improve the coordination between upper airway and respiratory muscles. This also has been observed recently in premature infants in whom diaphragmatic electromyography (EMG) and laryngeal muscle EMG were done simultaneously.[7]

Caffeine and theophylline are also effective in apnea that occurs during weaning from mechanical ventilation. Several clinical trials have suggested that the success rate

TABLE 20–1. TREATMENT OF APNEA IN PROGRESSIVE ORDER

1. Treat what is treatable
2. Monitor babies at risk
3. Prone position
4. Neutral or extended neck
5. Tactile stimulation
6. Slight increase in ambient oxygen
7. Neutral thermal zone—ambient temperature
8. Oscillating water bed (?)
9. Discontinue gavage if apnea worsens
10. Transfusion (Hct > 40)
11. Pharmacologic intervention
12. Nasal CPAP (with or without ventilation)
13. Endotracheal intubation and respirator

of extubation is improved if theophylline is preadministered.[8,9] The effect is thought to be related to improvement in respiratory muscle function and decreased pulmonary resistance.[10]

It should be noted that about 25 percent of infants, particularly very low-birth-weight infants, may not respond to the methylxanthines. Despite optimization of plasma theophylline concentrations, significant apnea reduction was observed in only about 75 percent of neonates.[39] Similarly, we observed that despite caffeine therapy, about a third of low-birth-weight neonates were ultimately intubated and ventilated as a result of apnea (Table 20–3).

Pharmacokinetics, Dose Recommendations, and Therapeutic Drug Monitoring

Several studies have shown that the plasma clearance and elimination of theophylline and caffeine are both prolonged in newborns relative to adults.[40,41] The representative kinetic profiles of these two drugs are shown in Table 20–4. The obvious difference between the two drugs is the remarkably slow elimination of caffeine relative to theophylline. The plasma half-life is about 100 hours, whereas with theophylline, the plasma half-life is about 30 hours. This difference in drug elimination indicates that caffeine can be given more sparingly (i.e., once daily) and that drug monitoring is probably not as crucial with caffeine as with theophylline. The therapeutic plasma concentrations desired for theophylline and caffeine are about 5–15 and 5–20 mg/liter, respectively. To achieve and maintain these plasma concentrations, a loading dose of 5–6 mg/kg of theophylline (active base) followed by a maintenance dose of 2–4 mg/kg/day in two to four divided doses may be required. There exists a substantial interindividual variability in the pharmacokinetic properties of theophylline; thus it is necessary to monitor plasma concentrations and adjust the dose accordingly. Similarly, caffeine has to be given as a loading dose of 10 mg/kg of active base or 20 mg/kg of caffeine citrate salt, intravenously or orally. A maintenance dose of 2.5 mg/kg/day (or 5 mg/kg/day of caffeine citrate) is usually needed to maintain plasma concentrations of 5–20 mg/liter of caffeine. Theophylline is methylated to caffeine,[42,43] with plasma theophylline/caffeine ratios sometimes reaching 0.30 to 0.40 at steady state. Thus the overall methylxanthine effect has to account for the sum of the two drugs, since both agents are pharmacologically active.

The methylxanthines are powerful CNS stimulants and may interact with anticonvulsants such as phenobarbital at a kinetic or probably pharmacodynamic level. Babies given theophylline and phenobarbital have been noted to require higher doses of theophylline to control the apnea and higher also of phenobarbital to control the seizures.[44]

Choice of Methylxanthines

Both caffeine and theophylline exert similar pharmacodynamic effects but may vary in their potency at spe-

TABLE 20–2. CLINICAL STUDIES AND DRUG REGIMENS OF METHYLXANTHINES IN NEONATAL APNEA

FIRST AUTHOR (YEAR)	N	DRUG PREPARATION	DOSE AND ROUTE
Kuzemko (1973–1974)	24	Aminophylline suppositories	5 mg q6h × 3 doses, then q6h p.r.n.
Shannon (1975)	17	Theophylline alcohol elixir (10%)	5 mg/kg q6h by nasogastric tube
Uauy (1975)	12	Theophylline 20% alcohol solution	4 mg/kg q6h orally
Bednarek (1976)	13	Aminophylline suppositories	5 mg q6h (1.7–6.4 mg/kg/day) rectally
Aranda (1977)	18	Caffeine citrate	L.D.: 20 mg/kg I.V. or orally* M.D.: 5–10 mg/kg daily or twice daily*
Peabody (1977)	4	Aminophylline	I.D.: 8 mg/kg q12h* M.D.: 4 mg/kg q12h rectally*
Davi (1978)	10	Theophylline	3 mg/kg q6h I.V. or orally
Meyers (1980)	7	Theophylline	2 mg/kg daily by nasogastric tube
Thach (1982)	10	Theophylline	6 mg/kg daily orally

*I.D. = initial dose; L.D. = loading dose; M.D. = maintenance dose.
†Apnea 5 seconds in duration.

cific organ receptors. Moreover, the differences in their kinetic properties produce a substantial difference between the dosing schedule and the need for therapeutic drug monitoring. Table 20–5 lists some of the differences between the two drugs.

Controlled comparative trials between theophylline and caffeine indicate that although both drugs are effective in the management of apnea, more adverse effects such as tachycardia are observed with theophylline.[45,46] Since caffeine has a more prolonged plasma half-life, the dosing schedule is less frequent and the need for therapeutic monitoring is less crucial. Whereas frequent monitoring is advisable for theophylline, plasma caffeine measurements once every 1 or 2 weeks is generally acceptable during the neonatal period. In cases of overdosage with caffeine, the prolonged drug elimination may result in sustained high plasma concentrations for a long period of time. However, previous observations suggest that caffeine plasma concentrations of up to 50 mg/liter may occur with no adverse effects,[4] whereas plasma concentrations of theophylline greater than 15 mg/liter may be associated with tachycardia.[2] This suggests that caffeine might have a wider therapeutic index relative to theophylline.

In practice, caffeine is preferred in infants with idiopathic apnea of prematurity. However, in instances where an added benefit of bronchodilatation is desired, such as in those babies with bronchopulmonary dysplasia, theophylline is widely used. Although bronchodilatory effects have been noted with caffeine,[31] theophylline is still preferred when airway dilatation is desired.

Mechanism of Action

Several mechanisms might be implicated in the decrease in apnea frequency after methylxanthine administration. These include the following:

1. Respiratory center stimulation

TABLE 20–3. NEONATES INTUBATED AND VENTILATED FOR APNEA, 1978–1985

BIRTH WEIGHT (gm)	NO. OF INTUBATED BABIES (TOTAL)	PERCENT
500–749	22 (34)	64.7
750–999	53 (94)	56.3
1000–1249	15 (72)	20.6
1250–1499	9 (102)	8.8
TOTAL 1500	99 (302)	32.8

Source: From Royal Victoria Hospital, McGill University, Montreal; (unpublished data by Blanchard and Usher).

TABLE 20–4. PHARMACOKINETICS OF THEOPHYLLINE AND CAFFEINE USED IN THE NEONATAL PERIOD

PHARMACOKINETIC PARAMETER	THEOPHYLLINE	CAFFEINE
Plasma half-life (hours)	30	100
Range	12–64	40–230
Mean adult value	6.7	6
Apparent volume of distribution (liters/kg)	0.69	0.9
Range	0.2–2.8	0.4–1.3
Mean adult value	0.5	0.6
Clearance (ml/kg/h)	22	8.9
Range	4.3–68	2.5–17
Adult value	66	94
Dosage (mg/kg)*		
Loading	5–6 2.5†	10
Maintenance‡	1 q8h 0.66 q8h†	2.5 q24h
Route of administration	I.V., P.O.	I.V., P.O.
Desired plasma level (mg/liter)	5–15 3–4†	5–20

*Active base.
†Low-dose regimen.
‡Adjusted according to plasma level.

TABLE 20–5. COMPARISON OF THEOPHYLLINE AND CAFFEINE IN NEONATAL APNEA

VARIABLE	THEOPHYLLINE	CAFFEINE
Efficacy	+++	+++
Peripheral side effects	+++	+/−
Drug clearance	Slow ($t_{1/2}$ = 30 h)	Very slow ($t_{1/2}$ = 100 h)
Plasma level at steady state	Fluctuating	Stable
Need for drug monitoring	+++	+/−
Dosing interval	1–3 ×/day	Once a day
Drug monitoring	HPLC/EMIT	HPLC/EMIT
Commercial preparation	+++	−

2. Adenosine blockade
3. Improvement in respiratory muscle contraction
4. Others: altered sleep states, metabolic rate, cardiac output, metabolic homeostasis, potentiation of catecholamine effect

RESPIRATORY CENTER STIMULATION. Both caffeine and theophylline produce an increase in minute ventilation, a decrease in $paCO_2$, and an increase in most indices of neural respiratory drive. Davi et al.[11] investigated the effect of theophylline on the control of breathing in newborn infants and found a decreased CO_2 threshold and an increased CO_2 sensitivity. Gerhardt et al.[12] observed a parallel shift in the slope of the CO_2 response curve after aminophylline administration. Data from our laboratory show that in both newborn infants and cats, caffeine has a potent effect on central neural drive.[4] Caffeine increases mean inspiratory flow (V_T/T_I), the pressure generated after airway occlusion, and minute ventilation. In the cat, when isocapnic conditions were maintained, ventilation was threefold greater, suggesting an interaction between caffeine and CO_2. In the newborn, doses as low as 2.5 mg/kg of caffeine increase tidal volume; however, the optimal ventilatory response is only observed with 10 mg/kg.[5]

The central respirogenic effect of the xanthines is further supported by the observation that they antagonize the depressant effects of narcotics such as codeine, morphine, and meperidine.[13–15] Whether the mechanisms of action of caffeine and theophylline on the control of breathing are the same remains to be established.

ADENOSINE RECEPTOR BLOCKADE. Over the last 5 years, a different mechanism has been proposed for the stimulatory effects of the methylxanthines on respiration. It has been shown that both caffeine and theophylline are able to bind adenosine receptors, a nucleoside now recognized as one of the possible neurotransmitters or neuromodulators.[16,17] Therefore, attention has been directed toward the role of this particular neurotransmitter in the control of breathing. Adenosine and its analogues have potent inhibitory effects on respiration. Administration of L-phenyl-isopropyl adenosine (L-PIA), a stable adenosine analogue, causes respiratory depression in laboratory animals in a dose-dependent manner.[20] This effect has already been described in several species, such as the rat, rabbit, cat, and newborn piglet. A similar effect also has been noted in the anesthetized cat, rabbit, and piglet and in the awake rat.[18–20] The inhibition of respiration can be partially or completely reversed by administration of the-

ophylline and caffeine, both of which antagonize adenosine at the receptor level.[21] Furthermore, adenosine levels in the brain increase markedly during hypoxia, which is well known to cause apnea and respiratory depression in the newborn.[18] These observations suggest that part of the efficacy of the xanthines in reducing apnea frequency in the newborn may be due to adenosine blockade with consequent CNS stimulation.

IMPROVED RESPIRATORY MUSCLE FUNCTION. The effect of caffeine and theophylline on muscle contraction has been known for many years.[22] However, it was only in the last decade that the effects of these drugs were investigated in relation to respiratory muscle function. Several reports in the literature described the effects of caffeine and theophylline on diaphragmatic contraction, both *in vivo* and *in vitro*.[23,24,26] Theophylline improved diaphragmatic efficiency and increased force production with electrical stimulation. The drug not only affected muscle contraction but also decreased the recovery time of fatigued muscles. In the newborn, fatigue of the respiratory muscles has been associated with apnea, and this is effectively treated by xanthine administration.[25] Therefore, it is possible that part of the antiapneic effect of these drugs is due to improvement in respiratory muscle function.

OTHER EFFECTS. In addition to the increase in respiratory drive, increased CO_2 sensitivity, and improvement in respiratory muscle contraction, other factors that may facilitate the action of the xanthines include increased neuromuscular transmission, catecholamine release, improved metabolic homeostasis, and changes in sleep states.[27]

The increase in metabolic rate and catecholamine levels after xanthine administration may lead to improved oxygenation and increased cardiac output. Improvement in metabolic homeostasis, such as increased blood glucose, also may lessen the frequency of apneic spells. A decrease in apnea frequency has been described at low doses of theophylline that do not alter ventilation or the CO_2 response curve.[28] Effects on the sleep–awake pattern were then implicated. Increased neuromuscular transmission may lead to improved muscle tone, a well-known *in vitro* effect of the xanthines. Improved respiratory muscle tone has been related to increased functional residual capacity and better oxygenation in the newborn.[29,30]

Other Pharmacological Effects

Besides respirogenesis, caffeine and theophylline exhibit a variety of pharmacologic actions, including CNS stimulation, smooth-muscle relaxation, diuresis, blood-vessel dilatation, cerebral vessel vasoconstriction, and cardiac stimulation[27] (Table 20–6). Bronchodilatation has now been demonstrated in premature infants with bronchopulmonary dysplasia (BPD) after the administration of both caffeine and theophylline, and the xanthines are in routine use in most centers for the care of BPD infants.[10,31] Diuresis caused by increased renal blood flow and increased glomerular filtration rate has not been shown to be significant in premature neonates treated with theophylline.[36] Neonates given theophylline and

TABLE 20–6. MAJOR PHARMACOLOGIC EFFECTS OF THE METHYLXANTHINES

Central nervous system: Stimulation of all levels
Heart: Augmentation of inotropy and chronotropy
Vascular system:
   Pulmonary: Dilatation
   Systemic: Dilatation
   Cerebral: Constriction (in adults)
Smooth muscles: Relaxation
Skeletal muscles: Stimulation
Kidneys: Increased renal blood flow and diuresis
Gastrointestinal system: Stimulation of gastric acid and fluid secretion
Endocrine system: Multiple effects
Hematologic: Mild increased clotting and shortened coagulation time
Basal metabolic rate: Augmentation

control infants not given theophylline were similar with respect to urine volume, serum osmolality and electrolytes, and urinary electrolyte excretion. Caffeine is a much weaker diuretic that appears to have no effect on renal losses of fluids and electrolytes in the neonate, as suggested by the lack of significant weight loss and increased fluid requirement.

Concern was initially raised regarding the maintenance of patency of the ductus arteriosus by the relaxant effect of the methylxanthines, presumably by increased 3',5'-cyclic AMP resulting from phosphodiesterase blockade. This should pose no problems because the concentration of xanthine required to produce relaxation *in vitro* (540–1620 mg/liter) is far greater than the plasma concentration achieved in the newborn infant (about 10 mg/liter).

Caffeine can shorten blood coagulation time resulting from increased clotting factors such as factor V, prothrombin, and fibrinogen. This aspect may be viewed as beneficial with respect to the fetus and newborn infant, since the clotting factors, particularly vitamin K–dependent factors, are deficient in the newborn infant.

A relatively important effect of the methylxanthines pertains to metabolic homeostasis. In experimental animals, in adult volunteers and patients, and in pancreatic islet-cell cultures, caffeine can stimulate insulin and glugacon release and increase catecholamine release, blood glucose, cortisol secretion, and plasma free fatty acid levels. These are potentially critical to neonatal well-being. Increased blood glucose would be beneficial to the infant with hypoglycemia but would be detrimental to the small, sick, premature infant with paradoxical hyperglycemia. The increased plasma free fatty acid could potentially compete with bilirubin in the albumin binding site, thus producing kernicterus at low levels of serum bilirubin. Previous studies suggest that there is a transient hyperglycemia following intravenous infusion of caffeine in the premature infant, with a delayed increase or no change in plasma insulin levels.

Caffeine and theophylline constrict cerebral vessels, increase cerebrovascular resistance, and decrease cerebral blood flow[37] in adults. Available evidence suggests that cerebral vasoconstriction is not a major issue at the therapeutic doses currently used. However, at doses higher than those presently recommended, the possibility of a significant cerebrovascular effect cannot be eliminated. This effect is undesirable in the fetus or newborn infant in whom adequate cerebral blood flow and oxygenation are critical. Furthermore, the decreased cerebral blood flow could be accompanied by a decrease in retinal blood flow, resulting in loss of retinal vessel caliber. This retinal vasoconstriction could potentiate the vaso-obliterative effect of oxygen, thus causing retrolental fibroplasia and consequent blindness. However, there was no increase in the incidence of cicatricial retrolental fibroplasia in babies treated with caffeine compared with a control group that did not receive caffeine.[38] Moreover, systematic studies in both newborn babies and experimental animals (i.e., newborn piglets) to determine the effect of caffeine and theophylline on cerebral blood flow suggest that cerebral blood flow alternation is not a prime concern.

Caffeine causes a slight increase in basal metabolic rate, which can be observed in the adult habitual coffee drinker. The ingestion of 0.5 gm of caffeine may increase the basal metabolic rate by an average of 10 percent and occasionally to 25 percent.[27] In the newborn, a mean increase in oxygen consumption of 25 percent has been observed after the administration of theophylline.[32] This effect could be of potential significance, especially in the tiny premature infant with limited caloric intake. Weight loss or poor weight gain (or growth) may occur if oxygen consumption and calories are mainly utilized for thermoregulation and not for growth.

Recently, some reports have suggested an association between the use of methylxanthines and necrotizing enterocolitis.[33–35] Increased incidence is reported in premature infants being treated for apnea with theophylline. However this is a very difficult association to prove based on the fact that apnea with hypoxemic episodes can per se be a risk factor for the development of necrotizing enterocolitis.

DOXAPRAM

Doxapram, a respiratory stimulant, is the subject of renewed interest in the last few years for the treatment of apnea of prematurity refractory to the methylxanthines. Although pharmacologic data are growing rapidly, adequate requisite knowledge on this medication for the newborn remains scarce. In a review article published in 1986 by our group,[64] very limited information was available on this promising drug. Over the interim, some data on kinetics and efficacy have brought new information relevant to its use in the small premature newborn. It should be noted, however, that the clinical data available are derived primarily from abstracts and letters to the editor and should be interpreted with caution pending final publication.

Doxapram and Apnea of Prematurity

Doxapram is not a new drug, despite recent enthusiasm for its use in neonatology. In 1962, the first report of its efficacy as a respiratory stimulant was published.[107] For more than a decade, its use was rather limited to adult patients, mainly as an analeptic to reverse the effects of anesthetic or sedative agents[47,83,101] or as a stimulant in adult subjects presenting different degrees of hypoventilation.[88,94,96] In 1973, Gupta and Moore[84] used doxapram in 83 full-term infants born to mothers who received narcotic analgesics or general anesthesia causing respiratory depression. The doses used varied from 0.5–3 mg/kg (as a single dose) immediately after birth. In 1978, Burnard et al.[71] used doxapram as a first-line drug in the treatment of apnea of prematurity. For some unclear reason, perhaps because of the widespread popularity of the methylxanthines over the intervening years, doxapram was used sparingly.[48] Current interest stems from Alpan's report in 1984 that showed that doxapram may be used as a second-line medication in premature newborns with apnea refractory to methylxanthines therapy. In addition to apnea of prematurity, other indications for doxapram use include central hypoventilation, weaning from mechanical ventilation, and obstructive apnea.

CENTRAL HYPOVENTILATION. Doxapram also has been used in the treatment of young children presenting with central sleep hypoventilation[87,91,108] with acceptable improvement in ventilation in isolated cases.

WEANING FROM MECHANICAL VENTILATION. Doxapram also has been used to wean babies from the respirator[78,79,81,86] with a success rate similar to that of aminophylline.[78]

OBSTRUCTIVE APNEA. Doxapram has a possible beneficial effect on obstructive apnea[62] in premature infants.

Efficacy of Doxapram

The efficacy of doxapram in the treatment of apnea of prematurity appears evident. Many studies have confirmed an improvement in the incidence of apnea of prematurity[48,52,54,60,62,63,71,77,85] with the use of doxapram given intravenously. One study thus far attests to the efficacy of doxapram in a double-blind, controlled study. Eyal et al.,[77] in a study of 26 premature infants, concluded that doxapram is at least as effective as aminophylline in abolishing apneic spells in premature infants.

Currently, because of the known safety and efficacy of the methylxanthines, and because of the uncertainty related to the side effects of doxapram, this drug is used only in cases where the methylxanthines are not effective and only before considering a more aggressive form of treatment such as mechanical ventilation.

Dosage

The dosage regimens that were initially used in 1978[71] and in 1984,[48] i.e., 2.5 mg/kg/h, were basically derived from adult data. Other studies have confirmed the efficacy of doxapram on apnea of prematurity at this dose of 2.5 mg/kg/h.[60] Recently, it was noted that some patients can respond to a dose as low as 0.25 mg/kg/h.[52] A dose–response relationship has been suggested. Barrington[62] showed that incremental doses in continuous intravenous

infusions were associated with increased response. In 18 premature infants given doxapram,[62] 47 percent responded at 0.5 mg/kg/h and up to 89 percent responded at 2.5 mg/kg/h. Hayakawa et al.,[85] in a study of 12 premature infants, reported a good correlation between dose and serum concentration and a success rate of 75 percent with infusions of 1.0–1.5 mg/kg/h.

The ideal dosage and route of administration remain to be defined, but the latest available data[58,63,90] suggest a loading dose of 2.5–3 mg/kg administered over 15 to 30 minutes followed by a continuous infusion of 1 mg/kg/h with careful surveillance of blood pressure changes. This maintenance dose may be increased if necessary by 0.5 mg/kg/h up to a maximum of 2.5 mg/kg/h.

Caution

Preparations of doxapram containing benzyl alcohol (in the United States) should be used with caution because of a possible association with the gasping syndrome,[74,82,89,92] even though the dose of benzyl alcohol that babies will receive is far below the amount associated with the gasping syndrome.[73] One preparation available in Canada contains 0.5 percent chlorobutanol as a preservative[82]; knowledge of its safety in the newborn is virtually nonexistent, but so far no side effects have been reported.[61,62] Unfortunately, there are no apparent attempts to produce a commercial preservative-free pharmaceutical formulation.[89]

MODE OF ADMINISTRATION. Because of a short duration of action despite a relatively apparent long half-life, an intermittent I.V. bolus regimen has been proposed, but continuous I.V. infusion remains the mode currently in use.

ENTERAL ROUTE. There are thus far only a few reports in animal newborns[51,67] and human newborns[53,54,103,105,108] showing that doxapram is absorbed enterally. Ideal dosage and frequency of administration still need to be defined. The oral doses used are based on bioavailability in the adult of 50–60 percent and consist of using twice the total I.V. dose divided in different intervals of administration. Limited data from six babies in our unit suggest that only about 10 percent of the oral dose is probably absorbed by the premature neonate.

THERAPEUTIC PLASMA LEVEL. The ideal plasma therapeutic concentrations still need to be defined, but available data suggest a possible therapeutic window. Those babies who responded to doxapram all had a serum level of at least 1.5 mg/liter.[62] The mean serum concentration related to this response was 2.9 mg/liter. In another study,[63] the therapeutic threshold proposed was greater than 2 mg/liter. On the other hand, adverse drug effects become more frequent at plasma levels above 5 mg/liter.[62,85]

MONITORING PLASMA LEVEL. Different techniques using gas chromatography or high-pressure liquid chromatography have been published.[50,93,97,100,102,106] Some of these techniques allow measurement not only of doxapram, but also of some of its known metabolites.

METABOLITES. Doxapram is metabolized by the human liver to at least three metabolites.[49,55] The oxidation that gives metabolites AHR-5955 (ketodoxapram) and AHR-5904 seems more active than the deethylation pathway producing AHR-0914.[55] One of the metabolites, ketodoxapram, has been shown to have strong respiratory stimulant properties[57,59] without some of the side effects reported with doxapram, i.e., increase in blood pressure and excitability,[59] at least in an animal model (lamb) and at the only dose tried, 2.5 mg/kg I.V. single-bolus dose.

Pharmacokinetics

Available data on the kinetic profile of doxapram in human infants[63,71,90] or newborn animals[51,56,67] indicate prolonged elimination relative to adults. Two recent studies on the kinetics in human infants[63,90] provided the following pharmacokinetic values:

1. Plasma $t_{1/2}$: 6.6–8.2 hours
2. Plasma clearance: 0.44–0.7 liter/kg/h
3. Apparent value of distribution (AV_d): 4.0–7.3 liters/kg

This pharmacokinetic profile suggests a first-order kinetics in premature infants[90] with substantial interpatient variability.[71,90] There is no evidence of doxapram-like or ketodoxapram-like material in the plasma of either human infants or newborn lambs or piglets.[57,59,63,65,67]

The plasma half-life has been reported to decrease with age.[67,71] In one pharmacokinetic study, there was a positive correlation between gestational age and half-life and volume of distribution.[63] A small amount of doxapram is excreted in the urine,[63] and ketodoxapram is detected in virtually every patient receiving doxapram.[63]

Side Effects

Adverse reactions to doxapram include the following.

ADVERSE DRUG REACTION (ADR) DEFINITELY RELATED TO DOXAPRAM. Increase in blood pressure, mainly at infusions of greater than 1.5 mg/kg/h or at levels greater than 5 mg/liter.[56,62,63,66]

ADR PROBABLY RELATED TO DOXAPRAM. Regurgitation,[63,84] excessive salivation,[84] increased agitation,[63,76] excessive crying,[57,63,76] disturbed sleep,[76] jitteriness,[48,85] increase in gastric residuals,[85] vomiting,[85] and irritability[85] all have been reported.

ADR POSSIBLY RELATED TO DOXAPRAM. Blood in stool,[105,108] abdominal distension,[85,108] hyperglycemia,[85] glycosuria,[85] and premature tooth buds (lower central incisors)[105] have been reported.

Usually, the adverse effects disappear rapidly (i.e., in 2–3 hours) after the infusion is stopped.[76,85] The side effects described above occur mainly when the serum concentration is 5.0 mg/liter. Aspects that have been assessed and were not shown to be affected by doxapram at therapeutic doses include the following:

1. No increase in liver enzyme activity[85] or hepatotoxicity[9] (assessed by alkaline phosphatase and light microscopy).
2. No change in hemogram, electrolyte, bilirubin, protein, or urinalysis.[63,85]
3. No clear evidence at this point for an increased incidence of intraventricular hemorrhage,[85] but this requires confirmation.
4. No clear evidence of increased EEG perturbation[62,85] or an increased incidence of seizure.[62,63]
5. No direct relationship between doxapram and an increased incidence of necrotizing enterocolitis, but patients need to be observed carefully because a few cases of necrotizing enterocolitis in babies treated with doxapram have been reported.[63,105]
6. Many studies reported no side effects at all while doxapram was being used.[77,78]

Mechanisms of Action

The exact mechanisms of action of doxapram are still a subject of debate. The data available from adult animals or adult humans seem to favor a significant involvement of the peripheral chemoreceptors mainly at low doses (<0.5 mg/kg); a stimulation of the central respiratory and nonrespiratory neurons also has been demonstrated mainly at higher doses.[68–70,72,75,80,95,98,99]

The mechanisms of action are probably similar in the newborn subject. In an animal model, our group[65] has demonstrated, using a carotid body denervated model, that the peripheral chemoreceptors play an important role in the mediation of the ventilatory response to doxapram. Barrington et al.,[60] in their study of premature human infants, have shown that doxapram seems to act by increasing the output of the respiratory centers, and they favor an effect mediated by a stimulation of the peripheral chemoreceptors. In human infants, doxapram causes a significant fall in pCO_2,[60] an increase in minute ventilation, tidal volume, and occlusion pressure,[60] but no change in respiratory rate or inspiratory and expiratory times.[60,63]

Conclusion

Available data as of 1989 suggest that doxapram can be tried as a second-line drug (until the side effects are further defined) in cases of failure with the methylxanthines and prior to a much more aggressive form of therapy, such as endotracheal intubation and mechanical ventilation. Complications from the latter therapy are significant, particularly in the very small premature infant of less than 1250 gm.

Despite the new data acquired in the last few years, considerably more information on doxapram is needed before it can be recommended for general use. Prudence dictates that the use of doxapram in neonatal apnea must be restricted to special circumstances and, ideally, in well-controlled studies.

ALMITRINE

Almitrine bismesylate is a triazine derivative that stimulates respiration through a predominant effect on peripheral arterial chemoreceptors. Unlike other analeptic agents, it does not act by stimulating the central nervous system.

Studies in animals have shown that almitrine increases the activity of the afferent fibers innervating carotid body chemoreceptors and that this effect is abolished by high concentrations of inspired oxygen[109] or transection of the 9th and 10th cranial nerves.[110] Almitrine exerts a similar sustained excitatory effect on the aortic chemoreceptors.[110,111] Microelectrode monitoring of unit discharges of respiratory neurones has shown that almitrine also stimulates breathing not only during the inspiratory phase but also during the expiratory phase of respiration.[112,113] The effect on the expiratory neurons distinguishes almitrine from other stimuli of the peripheral chemoreceptors and particularly from hypoxic stimulation. Hypoxia induces an increase in phrenic nerve discharge, but it also, contrary to almitrine, decreases the activity of the expiratory neurons of the nucleus ambiguous and of the internal intercostal nerves.

Experience with almitrine in humans is mostly limited to studies in adults, with very few reports of its use in the pediatric age group. However, it is useful to review this experience, because it provides an essential background for discussion of potential applications in neonatology. In normal human subjects, almitrine enhances the respiratory response to progressive hypoxia, whereas the ventilatory response to hypercapnia is either unchanged or increased and may depend on high serum drug levels.[114,115] In adult patients with chronic obstructive lung disease (COLD), almitrine improves gas exchange by increasing the hypoxic ventilatory response[116] and possibly by altering the pattern of breathing.[117] In these patients, the increase in ventilation seen in response to hypoxia is accompanied by shortening of both the inspiratory and the expiratory times as well as by an increase in tidal volume. Almitrine, however, caused patients to respond to hypoxia in a manner similar to that observed in normal subjects, i.e., with a greater increase in tidal volume rather than with changes in timing.[117] Almitrine also improved pulmonary gas exchange during exercise in patients with COLD[118] and decreased both the frequency and duration of hypoxemic episodes during sleep.[119]

In many patients with improved gas exchange through the use of almitrine, however, there is no measurable increase in minute ventilation,[116] or the increase in oxygenation is greater than could be accounted for by increased ventilation alone.[118,120] With the use of the multiple-inert-gas method in patients with chronic lung disease, almitrine has been shown to improve ventilation–perfusion matching.[121,122] It has been suggested that this is accomplished by enhancement of hypoxic vasoconstriction in poorly ventilated regions of the lung.[123] In this study, almitrine increased pulmonary artery pressure and pulmonary vascular resistance in healthy mongrel dogs breathing air or hypoxic gas but not in dogs breathing 100 percent oxygen. Since the animals were healthy, no changes in pulmonary gas exchange were observed before and after administration of almitrine. These results cannot be extrapolated to sick patients, however, in whom ventilation–perfusion relations are disturbed at the outset. In adults with chronic obstructive lung disease, almitrine did not cause any change in pulmonary artery pressure or pulmonary vascular resistance,[122] and similarly, pulmonary pressor effects have not been observed in isolated lungs of ferrets and rats *in vitro*.[124] However, these findings are controversial, since in one study almitrine produced a small but significant increase in pulmonary artery pressure in patients with hypoxic chronic bronchitis and emphysema and this was associated with a similarly small but significant fall in right ventricular ejection fraction.[125] Hughes et al.[126] found that although almitrine is generally a pulmonary vasoconstrictor, it can dilate vessels constricted by local hypoxia and does not enhance local hypoxic vasoconstriction in the dog. Six to 12 months of almitrine taken daily by patients with chronic lung disease does not appear to raise pulmonary artery pressure.[127] It seems that the effect of almitrine on pulmonary hemodynamics, if at all significant, depends on dosage, route of administration, and the degree of preexisting hypoxemia and pulmonary hypertension.[125] It thus appears that almitrine improves gas exchange by three mechanisms: increased hypoxic drive, change in the pattern of breathing, and improvement in ventilation–perfusion matching.

A double-blind, controlled trial in over 200 patients with chronic obstructive lung disease found that therapy with almitrine improved gas exchange, reduced dyspnea, and decreased the frequency of hospitalizations.[128] Other beneficial effects of almitrine noted in this trial were a reduction in hemoglobin concentrations in those patients in whom these were initially elevated and a decreased utilization of other conventional drugs. Almitrine also was found to improve gas exchange in patients with severe acute respiratory failure secondary to sepsis or shock but in whom there was no preexisting lung disease. The most likely mechanism was considered to be improvement in ventilation–perfusion matching.[129]

While there is thus quite extensive experience with the use of almitrine in adults with chronic lung disease, the pediatric use of this drug has been extremely limited. Almitrine was found to stimulate the carotid chemoreceptors in day-old newborn lambs and to sensitize the chemoreceptors in hypoxia. It also appeared to stimulate fetal breathing movements.[130] While some case reports have claimed the efficacy of almitrine in congenital central hypoventilation syndrome, improvement was generally not sustained and patients could not be taken off mechanical ventilatory support during sleep. A report of the largest group of patients with congenital central hypoventilation syndrome studied so far found no significant improvement in ventilation or gas exchange with almitrine,[131] but occasionally, there may be a patient who will benefit from this drug.[132] Almitrine was given to six babies with bronchopulmonary dysplasia (single oral dose of 1.5 mg/kg) and was found to improve oxygenation with a peak response 1–3 hours following administration. Although an improvement was noted in all babies, the response was highly variable, and this corresponded to wide interindividual variations in plasma levels of the

TABLE 20–7. SUGGESTED GUIDELINES FOR RESPIRATORY STIMULANTS IN NEONATAL APNEA

	THEOPHYLLINE	CAFFEINE	DOXAPRAM
Plasma $t_{1/2}$ (h)	30	100	7
Loading dose (mg/kg)	5–6	10	2.5*
Maintenance dose† (mg/kg/day)	2–4	2.5	1.0‡
Therapeutic blood level (mg/liter)	5–15	5–20	1.5–3
TDM	EMIT/HPLC	EMIT/HPLC	HPLC

*I.V. infusion only for 15 minutes.
†Adjusted according to blood level; all doses are in active base.
‡As I.V. infusion per hour.

drug. In four of these patients, repeated administration of the drug (1.5 mg/kg q12h for 9–14 days) did not produce sustained effectiveness, and it was not possible to wean any of the babies from oxygen. However, pharmacokinetic data suggested that a steady state was not achieved.[133] There were no control patients in this study, and transcutaneous pO_2 was the only variable assessed. Given the small number of patients in the study and the erratic plasma drug levels observed, these findings cannot be taken as conclusive.

Almitrine is absorbed well when given orally, and plasma concentrations peak 2–3 hours after ingestion. It is highly protein-bound and has a half-life (in adults) of about 2 days. Pharmacokinetic data in neonates are extremely limited but seem to suggest more rapid metabolization with marked interindividual variability.[133] The drug is eliminated by means of the biliary tract, which suggests that it should be given cautiously in patients with liver disease. Side effects are uncommon, mild, and reversible, but excessive levels have been associated with lethargy and anorexia and chronic administration has been implicated as a possible cause of a sensory peripheral neuropathy, although this is questionable.

Almitrine belongs to a novel therapeutic class of respiratory stimulants whose characteristic is to bring about a correction of ventilation–perfusion mismatch. It thus acts on the principal physiologic disorder underlying chronic obstructive lung disease. In view of the experience with this drug in adults with chronic lung disease and the quite extensive physiologic data available, it seems reasonable to suggest that almitrine may warrant a limited but rigorous trial in bronchopulmonary dysplasia, a disorder for which current available therapeutics are so sorely lacking. While chronic lung disease in adults is relentless, in bronchopulmonary dysplasia, an appropriate objective is to buy time for lung growth and to avoid secondary complications. Based on data derived from experiments on neonatal rabbits, almitrine also has been proposed as a possible treatment in apnea of prematurity.[134] More pharmacokinetic data are needed, however, and caution for possible side effects is warranted.

OTHER DRUGS

Naltrexone also has been used recently to treat apnea of prematurity.[135] Based on the observation that β-endorphin-like immunoreactive activity (β-ELI) is elevated in healthy newborn infants, during which respiratory drive is diminished, as well as on the finding that endorphin antagonism produces fetal breathing movement and enhances the rate of rise, amplitude, and frequency of this breathing movement and the responsiveness to carbon dioxide, MacDonald et al.[136,137] studied 11 infants with apnea but showed no effect of naltrexone, a long-acting analogue of naloxone, at a dose of 1–3 mg/kg intravenously. This contrasts with a previous observation by Burnard et al.,[138] who showed that naloxone, a competitive opiate antagonist, in doses up to 3.7 mg/kg, was effective in reversing apnea of prematurity and that this effect was additive to that of the methylxanthines. The Burnard et al. study[138] included babies receiving ventilatory support. Of 31 patients, 12 were ventilated, and an additional 10 babies were given constant distending airway pressure. The value of endorphin antagonists in the treatment of neonatal apnea other than that induced by opiates such as Demerol or morphine remains to be established.

CONCLUSIONS

Although drug therapy is a major aspect of apnea management, emphasis is placed on the multicausal nature of neonatal and infantile apnea, including metabolic, infectious and other pathophysiologic states culminating in apnea production. Treatment also should be directed toward those physiologic and biochemical perturbations illustrated in Figure 20–1. In the figure, apnea appears as a common pathway by which various noxious or other stimuli exert their effect on an immature respiratory control system not yet ready for the complex integration of various neural inputs. Whatever is the exact mechanism involved in the pathogenesis of neonatal and infantile apnea, correctible factors associated with the occurrence of apnea should be treated. In terms of pharmacologic therapy, suggested dose guidelines are shown in Table 20–7. As the survival of the very low-birth-weight infants at greatest risk for apnea increases with medical advances, the challenge for safe and effective treatment of apnea remains a primary investigative and clincial concern.

REFERENCES

1. Kuzemko JA, Paala J: Apnoeic attacks in the newborn treated with aminophylline. Archives of Disease in Childhood 48:404–406, 1973
2. Shannon DC, Gotay F, Stein IM, et al: Prevention of apnea and bradycardia in low-birth-weight infants. Pediatrics 55:589, 1975

3. Peabody J, Neese AL, Phillip AG et al: Transcutaneous oxygen monitoring in aminophylline-treated apneic infants. Pediatrics 62:698, 1978

4. Aranda JV, Gorman W, Bergsteinsson H, et al: Efficacy of caffeine in treatment of apnea in the low-birth-weight infant. J Pediatr 90:467, 1977

5. Aranda JV, Forman W, Cook C, et al: Pharmacokinetic profile of caffeine in the premature newborn infant with apnea. J Pediatr 50:467–472, 1977

6. Roberts JL, Mathew OP, Thach BT: The efficacy of theophylline in premature infants with mixed and obstructive apnea associated with pulmonary and neurologic disease. J Pediatr 100:968–970, 1982

7. Eichenwald EC, Howell GR, Leszcynski LE, Stark AR: Theophylline improves coordination of laryngeal abduction and inspiratory effort in premature infants. Ped Res (25):308A, 1989

8. Harris MC, Baumgart S, Rooklin AR et al: Successful extubation of infants with respiratory distress syndrome using aminophylline. J Pediatr 103:303, 1983

9. Viscardi RM, Faix RG, Nicks JJ, et al: Efficacy of theophylline for prevention of post-extubation respiratory failure in very low birth weight infants. J Pediatr 107:469, 1985

10. Blanchard PW, Brown TM, Coates AL: Pharmacotherapy in bronchopulmonary dysplasia. Clinics in Perinatol 14:881, 1987

11. Davi MJ, Sankaran K, Simons KJ, et al: Physiologic changes induced by theophylline in the treatment of apnea in preterm infants. J Pediatr 92:91, 1978

12. Mazzarelli M, Jaspan N, Zin WA, Aranda JV, Milic-Emili J: Dose effect of caffeine on control of breathing and respiratory response to CO_2 in cats. J Appl Physiol 60:52–59, 1986

13. Bellville JW, Escarrage LA, Wallenstein SL, et al: Antagonism by caffeine of the respiratory effects of codeine and morphine. J Pharmacol Exp Ther 136:8727, 1962

14. Lambertson CJ: Drugs and respiration. Ann. Rev. Pharmacol 6:327, 1966

15. Stroud MW, III, Lambertson CJ, Ewing JH, et al: The effects of aminophylline and meperidine alone and in combination on the respiratory response to CO_2 inhalation. J Pharmacol Exp Ther 114:461, 1955

16. Fredholm BB: On the mechanism of action of theophylline and caffeine. Acta Med Scand 217:149–153, 1985

17. Aldridge FL, Millhorm DE, Waltrop TG, Kiley JP: Mechanisms of respiratory effects of methylxanthines. Resp Physiol 53:239–261, 1983

18. Winn HR, Rubio R, Berne RM: Brain adenosine concentration during hypoxia in rats. Am J Physiol 241:H235–H242, 1981

19. Phillis JW, Wu PH: The role of adenosine and its nucleotides in central synaptic transmission. Prog Neuro 16:287–239, 1981

20. Runold M, Lagercrantz H, Fredholm BB: Ventilatory effect of an adenosine analogue in unanesthetized rabbits during development. J Appl Physiol 61:255–259, 1986

21. Darnoll RA: Aminophylline reduces hypoxic ventilatory depression: Possible role of adenosine. Pediatr Res 19:206–210, 1985

22. Huidobro F, Amenbar I: Effectiveness of caffeine (1,3,7 trimethylxanthines) against fatigue. J Pharmacol Exp Ther 84:82, 1945

23. Aubier M, Detroyer A, MacKelem PT, Roussos C: Aminophylline improves diaphragmatic contractility. N Engl J Med 305:245, 1981

24. Aubier M, Murciano D, Lecocgnic Y, et al: Diaphragmatic contractility enhanced by aminophylline: Role of extracellular calcium. J Appl Physiol 54:460–464, 1983

25. Lopes JM, Leboeuf PN, Heather MH, Bryan AC, et al: The effects of theophylline or diaphragmatic fatigue in the newborn, Ped Res 16:355A, 1982

26. Nassan-Gentina V, Parsonneau V, Rappaport SI: Fatigue and metabolism of frog muscle fibers during stimulation and in response to caffeine. Am J Physiol 241:C160–166, 1981

27. Ritchie JM: Central nervous stimulants. II. The xanthines, in Goodman LS, Gilman, A: The Pharmacological Basis of Therapeutics. Edition 5, London, Cassell and Collier, MacMillan Publishers, 1975, pp 367–378

28. Meyers RF, Milnap RL, Krauss AN, Auld PAM, et al: Low dose theophylline therapy in idiopathic apnea of prematurity. J Pediatr 96:99–104, 1980

29. Lopes J, Muller N, Bryan AC, Bryan MH: Importance of inspiratory muscle tone in maintenance of FRC in the newborn. J Appl Physiol 51:830–834, 1981

30. Davis GM, Bureau MA: Pulmonary and chest wall mechanics in the control of respiration in the newborn. Clinics in Perinatol 14:552–579, 1987

31. Davis JM, Bhutain VK, Stefano JL, Fox WW, Spitzer AR: Changes in pulmonary mechanics following caffeine administration in infants with bronchopulmonary dysplasia. Pediatr Pulmonol 6:49–52,1989

32. Gerhardt T, McCarthy J, Bancalari E: Effect of aminophylline on respiratory center activity and metabolic rate in premature infants with idiopathic apnea. Pediatrics 63:537–542, 1979

33. Miller HCA, Blackman L, Baummgart S, Pereira G: Necrotizing enterocolitis (NEC) associated with oral theophylline administration in small premature infants. Pediatr Res 25:219A, 1989

34. Davis JM, Abbasi S, Spitzer AR, Johnson L: Role of theophylline in pathogenesis of necrotizing enterocolitis. J Pediatr 109:344–347, 1986

35. Williams AJ: Xanthines and necrotizing enterocolitis. Arch Dis Child 55:973–974, 1980

36. Shannon DC, Gotay F: Effects of theophylline on serum and urine electrolytes in preterm infants with apnea. J Pediatr 94:963, 1979

37. Wechsler RL, Kleiss LM, Kety SS: Effect of intravenously administered aminophylline on cerebral circulation and metabolism in man. J Clin Invest 29:28, 1954

38. Gunn TR, Metrakos K, Riley PS, Willis D, Aranda JV: Sequelae of caffeine treatment in preterm infants with apnea. J Pediatr 94:106–110, 1979

39. Muttitt SC, Tierney AJ, Finer NN: The dose response of theophylline in the treatment of apnea of prematurity. J Pediatr 112:115–121, 1988

40. Aranda JV, Grondin D, Sasyniuk B: Pharmacologic considerations in the therapy of neonatal apnea. Pediatr Clin NA 28:113–133, 1981

41. Aranda JV: Maturational changes in theophylline and caffeine metabolism and disposition: Clinical implications. Proceedings of 2nd World Congress, Clin Pharm Ther ASPET, Rockville, Maryland, pp 868–877, 1984

42. Bory C, Baltassat P, Porthault M, Bethenod M, Frederick A, Aranda JV: Metabolism of theophylline to caffeine in premature infants. J Pediatr 94:988–993, 1979

43. Aranda JV, Louridas AT, Vitullo B, Thom P, et al: Metabolism of theophylline to caffeine in human fetal liver. Science 206:1319–1321, 1979

44. Yazdani M, Kissling GE, Tran TH, Gottschalk SK, Schuth CR: Phenobarbital increases theophylline requirement of premature infants being treated for apnea. Am J Dis Child 141:97–99,1987

45. Brouard C, Moriette G, Murat I, Flouvat B, Pajot N, Walti H, Gamarra E, Relier JP: Comparative efficacy of theophylline and caffeine in the treatment of idiopathic apnea in premature infants. Am J Dis Child 139:698–700, 1985

46. Bairam A, Boutroy MJ, Badonnel Y, Vert P: Theophylline versus caffeine: Comparative effects in treatment of idiopathic apnea in the preterm infants. J Pediatr 110:636–639, 1987

47. Allen CJ, Gough KR: Effect of doxapram on heavy sedation produced by intravenous diazepam. British Medical Journal 286:1181–2, 1983

48. Alpan G, Eyal F, Sagi E, Springer C, Patz D, Goder K: Doxapram in the treatment of idiopathic apnea of prematurity unresponsive to aminophylline. J Pediatr 104:634–638, 1984

49. Aranda JV, Mandelberg A, Beharry K, Rex J, Peleg O, Eyal F: Metabolism of doxapram in premature newborns. Pediatr Res 21:232A, 1987

50. Aranda JV, Beharry K, Rex J, Linder N, Blanchard PW: High pressure liquid chromatographic microassay for simultaneous measurement of doxapram and its metabolites in premature newborn infants. J Liq Chromatogr 11:2983–2991,1988

51. Aranda JV, Blachard PW, Beharry K, Rex J, Bairam A, Laudignon N: Doxapram bioavailability in newborns. Pediatr Res 23:254A, 1988

52. Bairam A, Vert I: Low-dose doxapram for apnea of prematurity. Lancet 1:793–4, 1986

53. Bairam A, Akramoff L, Beharry K, Rex J, Papageorgiou A,

Aranda JV: Enteral absorption of doxapram in premature newborns. Pediatr Res 23:255A, 1988

54. Bairam A, Akramoff L, Beharry K, Rex J, Papageorgiou A, Aranda JV: Oral doxapram in premature newborns: plasma levels and clinical effects. Pediatr Res 23:400A, 1988

55. Bairam A, Beharry K, Laudignon N, Rex J, Branchaud C, Papageorgiou A, Aranda JV: Metabolism of doxapram in human fetal liver organ culture. Pediatr Res 25:64A, 1989

56. Bairam A, Blanchard PW, Laudignon N, Mullahoo K, Beharry K, Aranda JV: Kinetics of doxapram and keto-doxapram in newborns. Pediatr Res 25:64A, 1989

57. Bairam A, Blanchard PW, Mullahoo K, Beharry K, Laudignon N, Aranda JV: Ventilatory effect of doxapram versus keto-doxapram. Pediatr Res 25:207A, 1989

58. Bairam A, Blanchard PW, Laudignon N, Mullahoo K, Beharry K, Rex J, Aranda JV: Interaction of doxapram and caffeine on ventilation in the newborn. Pediatr Res 25:207A, 1989

59. Bairam A, Blanchard PW, Laudignon N, Mullahoo K, Beharry K, Aranda JV: Does keto-doxapram, a metabolite of doxapram, have ventilatory stimulating properties? Pediatr Res 25:302A, 1989

60. Barrington KJ, Finer NN, Peters KL, Barton J: Physiologic effects of doxapram in idiopathic apnea of prematurity. J Pediatr 108:124–129, 1986

61. Barrington KJ, Finer NN: Doxapram for apnea of prematurity. J Pediatr 109:563, 1986

62. Barrington KJ, Finer NN, Torok-Both G, Jamali F, Coutts RT: Dose-response relationship of doxapram in the therapy for refractory idiopathic apnea of prematurity. Pediatrics 80:22–27, 1987

63. Beaudry MA, Bradley JM, Gramlich LM, Legatt D: Pharmacokinetics of doxapram in idiopathic apnea of prematurity. Dev Pharmacol Ther 11:65–72, 1988

64. Blanchard PW, Aranda JV: Drug treatment of neonatal apnea. Perinatology-Neonatology 10:21–28, 1986

65. Blanchard PW, Hobbs S, Aranda JV, Bureau MA: Ventilatory response to intravenous bolus of doxapram in newborn lambs. Pediatr Res 21:232A, 1987

66. Blanchard PW, Hobbs S, Aranda JV, Bureau MA: Blood pressure changes after bolus infusion of doxapram in newborn lambs. Pediatr Res 21:232A, 1987

67. Blanchard PW, Aranda JV, Bairam A, Beharry K, Rex J, Laudignon N: Effect of age on the kinetic of intravenous doxapram in piglets. Pediatr Res 23:255A, 1988

68. Blanchard PW, Aranda JV, Bairam A, Beharry K, Rex J, Laudignon N: Gastrointestinal absorption of doxapram in piglets. Pediatr Res 23:256A, 1988

69. Bopp P, Drummond G, Fisher J, Milic-Emili J: Effect of doxapram on control of breathing in cats. Canadian Anaesthetist Society Journal 26:191–195, 1979

70. Burki NK: Ventilatory effects of doxapram in conscious human subjects. Chest 85:600–604, 1985

71. Burnard ED, Moore RG, Nichol H: A trial of doxapram in recurrent apnea of prematurity, in Stern L, Oh W, Frus-Hansen B (eds): Intensive Care of the Newborn II. Masson Publishing, New York, pp 143–148, 1978

72. Calverley PMA, Robson RH, Wraith PK, Wescott LF, Flenley DC: The ventilatory effects of doxapram in normal man. Clinical Science 65:65–69, 1983

73. Cartaya EB, Pathak A, Hamm CR, Eyal FG: Efficacy and safety of doxapram "Made in U.S.A." in the therapy of apnea of prematurity refractory to methylxanthine treatment. Pediatr Res 25:305A, 1989

74. Cater G, Shaffer S, Hall RT: Doxapram for apnea of prematurity. J Pediatr 109:563, 1986

75. Clements JA, Robson RJ, Prescott LF: The disposition of intravenous doxapram in man. Eur J Clin Pharmacol 16:411–416, 1979

76. Dear PRF, Wheeler D: Doxapram and neonatal apnea. Arch Dis Child 59:903–904, 1984

77. Eyal F, Alpan G, Sagi E, Glick B, Peleg O, Dgani Y, Arad I: Aminophylline versus doxapram in idiopathic apnea of prematurity: A double-blind controlled study. Pediatrics 75:709–713, 1985

78. Eyal FG, Sagi EF, Alpan G, Glick B, Arad I: Aminophylline versus doxapram in weaning premature infants from mechanical

ventilation: Preliminary report. Critical Care Medicine 13:124–125, 1985

79. Fisher B, Rodarte A: Use of doxapram to increase respirations without a concomitant increase in intracranial pressure. Critical Care Medicine 15:1072–1073, 1987

80. Folgering H, Vis A, Ponte J: Ventilatory and circulatory effects of doxapram mediated by carotid body chemoreceptors. Bulletin Europeen de Physiopathologie Respiratoire 17:237–241, 1981

81. Gilbert J, Rice WH, Johnston J: Possible doxapram reversal of ventilator dependence in a brain-damaged patient. Critical Care Medicine 13:605–606, 1985

82. Golightly LK, Smolinske SS, Bennett ML, Sutherland EW, Rumack BH: Pharmaceutical excipients: Adverse effects associated with inactive ingredients in drug products (Part I). Medical Toxicol 3:128–165, 1988

83. Gupta PK, Dundee JW: Hastening of arousal after general anesthesia with doxapram hydrochloride. Br J Anaesth 45:493–496, 1973

84. Gupta PK, Moore J: The use of doxapram in the newborn. Journal of Obstetrics and Gynaecology of the British Commonwealth 80:1002–1006, 1973

85. Hayakawa F, Hakamada S, Kuno K, Nakashima T, Miyachi Y: Doxapram in the treatment of idiopathic apnea of prematurity: Desirable dosage and serum concentrations. J Pediatr 109:138–140, 1986

86. Hayakawa F: Doxapram for apnea of prematurity. J Pediatr 111:154, 1987

87. Hunt CE, Inwood RJ, Shannon DC: Respiratory and nonrespiratory effects of doxapram in congenital central hypoventilation syndrome. Am Rev Respir Dis 119:263–269, 1979

88. Hunter AR: Doxapram and idiopathic hypoventilation. Anesthesia 39:726–7, 1984

89. Jackson D: Doxapram and potential benzyl alcohol toxicity: A moratorium on clinical investigation? Pediatrics 78:541, 1986

90. Jamali F, Barrington KJ, Finer NN, Coutts RT, Torok-Both GA: Doxapram dosage regimen in apnea of prematurity based on pharmacokinetic data. Dev Pharmacol Ther 11:253–257, 1988

91. Johnston K, Newth CJL, Sheu KFR, Patel MS, Heldt GP, Schmidt KA, Packman S: Central hypoventilation syndrome in pyruvate dehydrogenase complex deficiency. Pediatrics 74:1034–1040, 1984

92. Jordan GD, Themelis JN, Messerly SO, Jarrett RV, Garcia J, Frank G: Doxapram and potential benzyl alcohol toxicity: A moratorium on clinical investigation? Pediatr 78:540–541, 1986

93. Legatt DF, Beaudry MA Bradley JM: Simultaneous determination of doxapram and 2-ketodoxapram in plasma of neonates by gas chromotography. J Chromatogr 378:478–481, 1986

94. Lugliani R, Whipp BJ, Wasserman K: Doxapram hydrochloride: A repsiratory stimulant for patients with primary alveolar hypoventilation. Chest 76:414–419, 1979

95. Mitchell RA, Herbert DA: Potencies of doxapram and hypoxia in stimulating carotid-body chemoreceptors and ventilation in anesthetized cats. Anesthesiology 42:559–566, 1975

96. Moser KM, Luchsinger PC, Adamson JS, McMahon SM, Schlueter DP, Spivack M, Weg JG: Respiratory stimulation with intravenous doxapram in respiratory failure. NEJM 288:427–431, 1973

97. Nichol J, Vine J, Thomas J: Quantitation of doxapram in blood, plasma, and urine. J Chromatogr 182:191–200, 1980

98. Nishino T, Mokashi A, Lahiri S: Stimulation of carotid chemoreceptor and ventilation by doxapram in the cat. J Appl Physiol 52:1261–1265, 1982

99. Okuho S, Konno K, Ishizaki T, Sugamima T, Takubo T, Takizawa T, Tanaka M: Serum doxapram and respiratory neuromuscular drive. Eur J Clin Pharmacol 34:55–59, 1988

100. Pitts JE, Bruce RB, Forehand JB: Identification of doxapram metabolites using high pressure exchange chromatography and mass spectroscopy. Xenobiotics 3:72–83, 1973

101. Robertson GS, MacGregor DM, Jones CJ: Evaluation of doxapram for arousal from general anaesthesia in outpatients. Br J Anaesth 49:133–139, 1977

102. Robson RH, Prescott LF: Rapid gas-liquid chromatographic estimation of doxapram in plasma. J Chromatogr 143:527–529, 1977

103. Rose SJ, Lloyd DJ, Duffty P: Doxapram for apnea of prematurity. J Pediatr 111:154, 1987

104. Sagi E, Eyal F, Alpan G, Patz D, Arad I: Idiopathic apnea of prematurity treated with doxapram and aminophylline. Arch Dis Child 59:281–283, 1984

105. Tay-Uyboco JS, Kwiatkowski K, Cates DB, Seifert B, Hasan SU, Rigatto H: Doxapram in the treatment of apnea of prematurity—a study of the clinical and physiological responses, serum concentrations and possible side effects. Pediatr Res 25:72A, 1989

106. Torok-Both GA, Coutts RT, Jamali F, Pasutto FM, Barrington KJ: Sensitive nitrogen-phosphorus capillary gas chromatographic assay of doxapram in premature infants. J Chromatogr 344:373–377, 1985

107. Ward JW, Franko BV: A new centrally acting agent (AHR-619) with marked respiratory stimulating, pressor, and "awakening" effects. Federation Proceedings 21:325, 1962

108. Weesner KM, Boyle RJ: Successful management of central sleep hypoventilation in an infant using enteral doxapram. J Pediatr 106:513–515, 1985

109. Roumy M, Leitner LM: Stimulant effect of almitrine (S2620) on the rabbit carotid chemoreceptor efferent activity. Bull Eur Physiopathol Res 1981; 17:255–259

110. Laubie M, Schmitt H: Long lasting hyperventilaton induced by almitrine; evidence for a specific effect on carotid and thoracic chemoreceptors. Eur J Pharmacol 1980; 61:125–136

111. O'Regan RG, Majcherczyk S, Przybyszewski A: Effect of Almitrine Bismesylate on activities recorded from nerves supplying the carotid bifurcation in the cat. Eur J Respir Dis 1983; 64: 197–202

112. Laubie M: Respiratory neurones in the chemoreceptor pathway activated by Almitrine Bismesylate. Europ J Respir Dis 1983; 64:191–195

113. Laubie M, Drouillat M, Schmitt H: Ventrolateral medullary respiratory neurons and peripheral chemoreceptor stimulation by Almitrine. Eur J Pharmacol 1984; 102:437–442

114. Stradling JR, Barnes P, Pride NB: The effects of almitrine on the ventilatory response to hypoxia and hypercapnia in normal subjects. Clin Sci 1982; 63:401–404

115. Stanley NN, Galloway JM, Gordon B, Pauly N: Increased respiratory chemosensitivity induced by infusing almitrine intravenously in healthy man. Thorax 1983; 38:200–204

116. Powles ACP, Tuxcen DV, Mahood CB, et al: The effect of intravenously administered almitrine, a peripheral chemoreceptor agonist, on patients with chronic air-flow obstruction. Am Rev Respir Dis 1983; 127:284–289

117. Maxwell DL, Cover D, Hughes JMB: Almitrine increases the steady-state hypoxic ventilatory response in hypoxic chronic air-flow obstruction. Am Rev Respir Dis 1985; 132:1233–1237

118. Escourrou P, Simonneau G, Ansquer JC, et al: A single orally administered dose of almitrine improves pulmonary gas exchange during exercise in patients with chronic air flow obstruction. Am Rev Respir Dis 1986; 133:562–567

119. Connaughton JJ, Douglas NJ, Morgan AD, et al. Almitrine improves oxygenation when both awake and asleep in patients with hypoxia and carbon dioxide retention caused by chronic bronchitis and emphysema. Am Rev Respir Dis 1985; 132:206–210

120. Naeije R, Mélot C, Mols P, et al: Effect of almitrine in decompensated chronic respiratory insufficiency. Bull Eur Physiopathol Respir 1981; 17:153–161

121. Melot C, Naeije R, Rothschild T, et al: Improvement in ventilation-perfusion matching by almitrine in COPD. Chest 1983; 83:528–533

122. Castaing Y, Manier G, Guenard H: Improvement in ventilation-perfusion relationships by almitrine in patients with chronic obstructive pulmonary disease during mechanical ventilation. Am Rev Respir Dis 1986; 134:910–916

123. Romaldini H, Rodriguez-Roisin R, Wagner PD, West JB: Enhancement of hypoxic pulmonary vasoconstriction by almitrine in the dog. Am Rev Respir Dis 1983; 128:288–293

124. Bee D, Gill GW, Emery CJ, et al: Action of almitrine on the pulmonary vasculature in ferrets and rats. Bull Eur Physiopath Respir 1983; 19:539–545

125. Macnee W, Connaughton JJ, Rhind BG, et al: A comparison of the effects of almitrine or oxygen breathing on pulmonary arterial pressure and right ventricular ejection fraction in hypoxic chronic bronchitis and emphysema. Am Rev Respir Dis 1986; 134:559–565

126. Hughes JMB, Allison DJ, Goatcher A, Tripathi A: Influence of alveolar hypoxia on pulmonary vasomotor responses to almitrine in the dog. Clin Sci 1986; 70:555–564

127. Paramelle B, Levy P, Priotte C: Long term follow-up of pulmonary artery pressure evaluation in COPD patients treated by almitrine bismesylate. Eur J Respir Dis 1983; 64:333–335

128. Arnand F, Bertrand A, Charpin J, et al: Long term almitrine bismesylate treatment in patients with chronic bronchitis and emphysema: A multicentre double-blind placebo controlled sutdy. Eur J Respir Dis 1983; 64:323–330

129. Reyes A, Lopez-Messa JB, Alonso P: Almitrine in acute respiratory failure. Chest 1987; 91:388–393

130. Blanco CE, Hanson MA, McCooke HB: Effects of almitrine bismesylate on chemoreceptor activity in fetal sheep and newborn lambs. Eur J Respir Dis 1983; 64:313–317

131. Oren J, Newth CJL, Hunt CE, et al: Ventilatory effects of almitrine bismesylate in congenital central hypoventilation syndrome. Am Rev Respir Dis 1986; 134:917–919

132. Fleming PJ, Levine MR, Lewis GTR, Pauly N: Almitrine bismesylate in congenital central hypoventilation. Eur J Respir Dis 1983; 64:307–312

133. Magny JF, Bromet N, Bonmarchand M, Dehan M. Study of the pharmacokinetcs and pharmacodynamic activity of almitrine bismesylate in infants during the recovery phase following bronchopulmonary dysplasia. Dev Pharmacol Ther 1987; 10:369–376

134. Weese-Mayer DE, Klemka LM, Brouillette RT, Hunt CE. Effect of almitrine on ventilaton in newborn rabbit pups. Am Rev Respir Dis 1987; 136:A177

135. MacDonald MG, Moss IR, Kefale GG, Ginzburg HM, Fink RJ, Chin L. Effect of Naltrexone on Apnea of Prematurity and Plasma B-Endorphin-Like Immunoreactivity. Dev Pharmacol Ther 9:301–309, 1986

136. Moss IR, Conner H, Yee WFH, Iorio P, Scarpelli EM. Human Beta Endorphin-like immunoreactivity in the perinatal/neonatal period. J Pediatr 101:443–446, 1982

137. Moss IR, Scarpelli EM: Generation and regulation of breathing in utero: fetal CO_2 response test. J Appl Physiol 47:527–531, 1979

138. Burnard ED: The Effect of Naloxone on recurrent apnea of prematurity: In Stern L and Bard H (eds): Intensive care in the newborn. Vol V, Masson, New York, 1987

21

THE EXCRETION OF DRUGS AND CHEMICALS IN HUMAN MILK

CHESTON M. BERLIN, JR.

During the 1960s and early 1970s, the incidence of breast-feeding reached its nadir; as recently as 1972, only 20 percent of newborns discharged from the hospital were breast-fed; only 15 percent were breast-fed at 2 months of age.[1] The last decade has seen a considerable increase in interest and enthusiasm for breast-feeding. Both medical and psychological studies have emphasized the considerable biologic and psychological benefits of breast-feeding infants. At The Milton S. Hershey Medical Center, a recent survey found 65 percent of infants breast-feeding at discharge; at 4 months, this had decreased to 40 percent. At the present time in the United States, it appears (from a number of surveys) that about 65 percent of babies are discharged from the hospital breast-fed. The American Academy of Pediatrics (among others) has published a position paper urging a return to breast-feeding as the best nutrition for infants for the first 6 months of age.[1] With both professional emphasis and lay support (by organizations such as the La Leche League), breast-feeding has become the major source of infant nutrition. Human milk has not been surpassed in its composition for feeding infants. The many advantages have been summarized in several publications.[1-5]

With this increased interest in breast-feeding, there has been a parallel increase in concern over the excretion of drugs and chemicals into breast milk. A brief review of breast function and milk synthesis will help elucidate the possible mechanisms involved in the excretion of drugs into breast milk.

It must be emphasized that virtually all work on breast function/milk secretion has been done in animal species. The difficulties and limitations of studying human lactation (anatomically and physiologically) using current methods of continuous milk collection, serial biopsy of lactation tissue, and administration of isotopic biochemical precursors are obvious. There are known biochemical differences between the milk of many species: Protein, fat, and carbohydrate content seem related to growth requirements (especially the rate of growth) of the infant of the species. Some of these differences will obviously dictate differences in drug elimination. The pH of human milk, for example, is usually 7.0 or above; in the cow (where lactation has been most extensively studied), the pH is usually 6.8 or below. However, there is no reason to suppose that the formation of human milk is qualitatively different from that in other animal species.

The lactating breast resembles a bunch of grapes, with each grape being tear-shaped and consisting of a cluster of alveolar cells in which breast milk is synthesized and secreted into a central lumen. The lumens feed into small ducts that meet each other in channels of increasing size until the nipple region is reached. With the possible exception of water transport, little alteration in the composition of the milk occurs once it leaves the alveolar lumen. Excretion of drugs most likely occurs only within this lumen.

Human milk is a suspension of fat and protein in a carbohydrate (lactose) and mineral solution. A nursing mother can easily produce 600 ml of milk per day (amount needed to provide complete nourishment for a 4-kg infant) containing 6.0 gm of protein, 22.2 gm of fat, and 42 gm of lactose with the correct amount of minerals and most vitamins. Human milk also contains immunoglobulins, macrophages, lymphocytes, transferrin, lactoferrin, interferon, complement, fibronectin, and nonprotein nitrogen. The exact composition varies with duration of lactation and may even vary within a single feeding.

Milk protein is synthesized entirely within the mammary gland. A small amount of plasma protein does enter into breast milk, presumably across the alveolar cell and/or through the extracellular space between these cells. This explains the presence of cow milk protein (β-lactoglobulin from maternal cow milk consumption) in the serum of exclusively breast-fed infants. The major human proteins are casein and lactalbumin (the latter is also needed for lactose synthesis). Synthesis is initiated by prolactin and needs insulin and hydrocortisone to continue. The proteins are very digestible and contribute to the low curd tension of human milk. Proteins are transported from the endoplasmic reticulum into the Golgi apparatus, migrate from the base of the cell toward the apex, and are discharged into the alveolar lumen by apocrine secretion. The role of these proteins in binding drugs has yet to be investigated completely. In the two reported studies that specifically measured drug (theobromine and theophylline) binding to human milk protein, it was found to vary between 0 and 24 percent.[6,7]

Short-chain fatty acids are synthesized in the mammary gland from acetate. Long-chain fatty acids are supplied by transfer from plasma. Both classes of fat are esterified in the breast with glycerol (from intracellular glucose). The lipids collect in the endoplasmic reticulum. As they ascend the cell in ever-increasing sizes of droplets, they acquire a three-layered membrane (lipoprotein) and are extruded into milk as milk fat globules.[8] It is intriguing to speculate on the possibilities of drug binding to both the protein and fat components of the milk fat globule. It is also possible that some lipid-soluble drugs may be trapped entirely within the milk fat globule.

Lactose is entirely synthesized in the breast alveolar cell. Its synthesis proceeds from UDP galactose and glucose with lactose synthetase (galactose transferase plus lactalbumin) as the enzyme. Prolactin is absolutely required. Lactose is excreted from the cell into the alveolar lumen alone and with milk protein. Electrolytes, vitamins, and water are supplied by the cell (from plasma water) to achieve the final concentration.

All the preceding elements achieve a concentration in human milk that provides the ideal nutrient supply to the infant for at least the first 6 months. After 6 months, the infant's caloric need usually requires supplemental food.

The transport of drugs into breast milk from maternal tissues and plasma may proceed by a number of routes. Figure 21–1 is a schematic drawing of the alveolar breast cell that illustrates the cellular structures a substance in maternal plasma must traverse in order to enter milk contained within the alveolar lumen. After crossing the capillary endothelium, the drug traverses the interstitial space and must cross the basement membrane (consisting mostly of mucopolysaccharides) of the alveolar breast

cell. The cell plasma membrane is trilaminar with the usual phospholipid–protein membrane structure. After reaching the cell cytoplasm, the compound travels apically and leaves the cell by diffusion, reverse pinocytosis, or apocrine secretion (apical part of cell disintegrates). This entire process is nicely detailed by Vorherr.[9] Excellent scanning electron micrographs of this process are presented in the paper by Ferguson and Anderson.[10]

The following are the most probable mechanisms of drug excretion in milk:

1. *Transcellular diffusion.* Small un-ionized molecules with lipid solubility, such as urea and ethanol, transverse the capillary epithelium, intercellular water, basal-cell membrane, alveolar cell, and its apical membrane by diffusion. This mechanism is supported by the observations that milk concentrations of such compounds mirror simultaneous plasma levels (M/P ratio = 1) and that the elimination rate constants (as calculated from the elimination phases) are very similar.[11]

2. *Intercellular diffusion.* This route avoids the breast alveolar cell entirely. Histologic studies in some animal species suggest that such a space may not exist or is very tight. It may be important functionally in the human and may explain how large molecules such as interferon, immunoglobulins, and cow milk protein enter human milk.

3. *Passive diffusion.* Small ionized molecules and small proteins may enter the basal part of the cell from interstitial water through passive diffusion in water-filled channels.

4. *Ionophore diffusion.* Polar substances may penetrate by being bound to carrier proteins within the cell membrane.

Diffusion appears to be the most common mechanism for a drug to cross a cell membrane. The distribution of a drug across a lipid biologic membrane has been shown to depend on the degree of ionization of the drug plus the assumption that a pH difference exists across the mem-

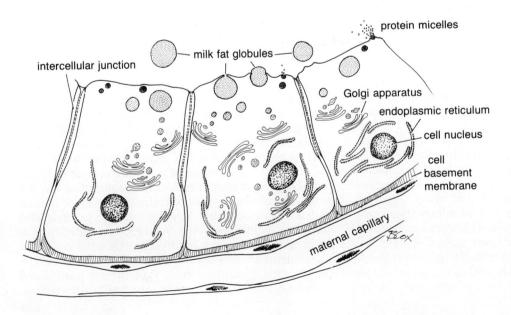

FIGURE 21–1. Schematic drawing of aveolar breast cells. All cells are actively synthesizing protein, fat, and carbohydrate. The cell on the right has discharged most of the products into the alveolar lumen as milk. Carbohydrate is secreted with protein.

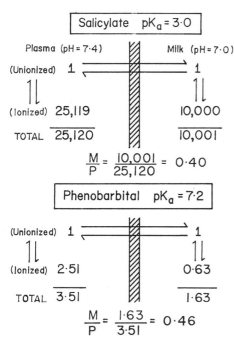

FIGURE 21–2. Theoretical distribution of weakly acidic drugs across a lipid cell membrane. Units are arbitrary for illustration.

brane; it is the un-ionized fraction that diffuses through the membrane.[12] Knowing the degree of ionization of the drug (pK$_a$) plus the pH difference, the theoretical milk/plasma (M/P) ratio can be calculated.* Figure 21–2 illustrates the situation for two weakly acidic drugs with markedly different pK$_a$ values: salicylic acid (pK$_a$ = 3.0) and phenobarbital (pK$_a$ = 7.2). Plasma pH is assumed to be 7.4, and milk pH is assumed to be 7.0 (commonly accepted for human milk). For a weak acid, the Henderson–Hasselbach equation defines the ratio of un-ionized (U) to ionized (I) drug at equilibrium as

$$\log (U/I) = pK_a - pH$$

and for a weak base as

$$\log (I/U) = pK_a - pH$$

The theoretical M/P ratio for total salicylate (un-ionized plus ionized) is 0.40; the experimental value obtained by Miller et al.[16] is 0.35. The theoretical ratio for total phenobarbital is 0.46; the experimental value is 0.7.[13,17] This difference for phenobarbital may be explained by the significant lipid solubility of this drug (chloroform/water distribution of un-ionized drug = 4.8). Thus the presence on one side of a biologic membrane of a substance rich in fat (milk) will introduce another factor in the final determination of the concentration of a drug in breast milk.

Milk also has 1.0 gm/100 ml of proteins, any one of which also may bind drugs. Little data are as yet available,

but Rasmussen[18] has demonstrated sulfonamide binding in milk to be present from 0–40 percent depending on the sulfonamide. As a general statement, weak acids (e.g., sulfanilamide, phenobarbital, salicylate, and penicillin) will have an M/P ratio (both theoretical and experimental) of less than 1.0. Weak bases (antipyrine, lincomycin, quinine, ephedrine) will have an M/P ratio greater than 1.0.[13,14] The precise experimental value will depend on factors such as maternal dosing intervals, milk pH, protein binding in plasma and milk, and lipid solubility of the drug.

The ratio of drug in the ultrafiltrate of milk to that in the ultrafiltrate of plasma was found to be independent of plasma levels (M/P ratio identical at all levels of plasma concentration). The concentration in milk also was found to be constant regardless of the volume of milk in the mammary gland. These observations support the thesis that diffusion is the major mechanism for the appearance of drugs in breast milk.[13]

A number of reviews discuss and provide tables of the concentration of drugs in breast milk.[19–24] Most of the values consist of a single measurement of the drug concentration; the period of time from maternal ingestion is usually not defined, nor is maternal dose, frequency of dose, frequency of nursing, or length of lactation. Measurement of the drug in the nursing infant's blood or urine is frequently not mentioned. Hence it is usually not possible to determine the risk to the nursling at a single isolated point. Many of the quoted references refer to data from the 1940s and 1950s, when analytical methods were primitive. The oft-quoted reference to salicylates, for example, dates from 1935 and employed a semiquantitative method (FeCl$_3$) for salicylate analysis; no quantitative values were given.[25] The discipline of pharmacokinetics was not developed when many of the drugs in breast milk were initially assayed. Hence few detailed studies employing drug measurements over a period of time in both maternal and infant body fluids are available. The availability of newer techniques (high-pressure liquid chromatography, mass spectroscopy) coupled with increased interest has resulted in the recent publication of more comprehensive studies.

Two other critical questions are what dose does the infant absorb (as measured by infant blood and urine levels), and does the breast excrete any metabolites of the parent drug? Is mammary tissue, which is so metabolically active, itself capable of drug biotransformation?

Table 21–1 is an attempt to list some drugs that appear in human milk for which some pharmacokinetic data can be found. The blank spaces in the table cannot be filled using current data. This emphasizes the gaps in current knowledge in precisely determining the risk to the nursing infant. The following general points may be made:

1. Most drugs (and environmental chemicals) with molecular weights below 200 daltons can cross from plasma to milk.
2. Concentrations in milk parallel plasma concentrations in time; milk/plasma ratios usually vary from 0.5–1.0.
3. Following a single maternal dose, $t_{1/2}$ values are similar for plasma and milk. This implies rather

---

*A complete discussion of the distribution of ionized drugs between plasma and milk is given by Rasmussen.[13] Acknowledgment must be made of the elegant experiments by Dr. Rasmussen in defining this process in the animal models of the lactating cow and goat. Equally, acknowledgment must be made to Dr. John T. Wilson et al.[14,15] for pointing out the limitations of using the M/P ratio to predict quantitation excretion of drugs into milk.

TABLE 21–1. EXCRETION OF DRUGS IN HUMAN MILK

DRUG	MATERNAL DOSE	PEAK CONCENTRATION IN MILK	M/P RATIO AT PEAK	TIME OF PEAK CONCENTRATION IN MILK	$t_{1/2}$ IN MILK*	AMOUNT SECRETED IN MILK 24 H AFTER SINGLE DOSE†	MATERNAL DOSE (%)‡
Acetaminophen[26]	650 mg P.O.	10–15 μg/ml	0.8	1–2 h	2.3 h	0.88 mg	0.14
Antipyrine[27]	18 mg/kg P.O.	20–30 μg/ml	1.0	10 min	6–22 h	7–25 mg	0.5–2.4
Caffeine[28]	35–336 mg P.O. as beverage	2–7 μg/ml	0.6–0.8	½–1 h	6.1 h	0.57 mg	0.53
Cefazolin[29]	2 gm I.V.	1.51 μg/ml	0.023	3 h		1.5 mg	0.075
	500 mg I.M. t.i.d.	0		Not detected in milk		0	
Chlorothiazide[30]	500 mg P.O.	0		Not detected in milk		<1 mg/day	
Diazepam[31]	Not stated	0.27 μg/ml	0.68	3 days	3 days	0.27 mg (peak) on day 3	
Digoxin[32]	0.25 mg P.O.	0.6–1.0 ng/ml	0.8–0.9	4 h	12 h	0.18–0.36 μg/day	0.07–0.14
Ethanol[11]	0.6 gm/kg P.O.	777 μg/ml	0.93	90 min	2.9 h	300 mg	1
Isoniazid[33]	300 mg P.O.	16.6 μg/ml	1.6	3 h	5.9 h	7 mg	2.3
Lithium[34]	Chronic: dose not specified P.O.	0.1–0.6 mmol/liter	0.5	Levels fairly constant			
Methadone[35]	70 mg/day P.O.	0.36 μg/ml	0.83			300 μg	0.4
		0.51 μg/ml	1.89				
Metronidazole[36]	2.0 gm P.O.	50–57 μg/ml		2–4 h	9 h	21.8 mg	1.1
Nicotine[37]	1 pack/day (400 mg)	91 ng/ml Range: 20–512 ng/ml		No correlation		0.68 mg	0.17
Prednisolone[38]	5 mg P.O.	26 ng/ml		1 h	8.2 h	6 μg	0.12
Prednisone[39]	120 mg P.O.	154 ng/ml (prednisone)		2 h	1.8 h	47 μg (as both prednisone and prednisolone)	0.04
		473 ng/ml (prednisolone)		2 h	1.1 h		
Propranolol[40]	20 mg	10 ng/ml	0.56	3 h		0.6 μg	0.03
	160 mg	150 ng/ml	0.65	3 h		90 μg	0.05
Salicylate[41]	20 mg/kg						0.18–0.36
Sulfasalazine[42]	2 gm/day P.O.	9–15 mg/ml	0.6	Constant		1.4–2.1 mg	0.16
Sulphone[43]	5 gm I.M. sulphetrone or 500 mg P.O. dapsone	14 μg/ml	0.16	4–6 h		10 mg	2
Theophylline[7]	4.25 mg/kg	4 μg/ml	0.7	2 h	4.0 h	8 mg	4
Verapamil[44]	80 mg P.O. t.i.d.		0.6	1–2 h	4.3	31 μg	0.01

*$t_{1/2}$ is calculated from the elimination (β) phase.
†Amount excreted in 24 hours is estimated by assuming the infant ingests 90 ml of milk every 4 hours.
‡The percentage of maternal dose is calculated by dividing the amount secreted in 24 hours by the maternal dose (single dose or 24-hour total maternal dose).

rapid transport from plasma to milk (according to M/P ratios).

4. The total amount available for infant absorption is usually less than 1 percent of maternal dose. This amount may be minimized by planning nursing periods at times of low maternal plasma levels (e.g., just before a maternal dose).

5. There are little data about the situation with repetitive maternal doses over days or weeks. One infant became salicylate-toxic after nursing for 2 weeks from a mother ingesting 650 mg of aspirin four times per day.[45]

6. For most drugs, even those with potent pharmacologic actions, the risk to the infant (with attention to proper nursing scheduling to minimize drug exposure of the infant) is negligible.

Table 21–2 lists those few drugs which are contraindicated (or during therapy, nursing is contraindicated) during lactation. The number is small; no doubt it might be increased as more data are collected and with the introduction of new drugs.

The use of radioactive isotopes for diagnostic purposes is very common; all women of childbearing age should be asked whether they are nursing before an isotope is given.

TABLE 21–2. DRUGS CONTRAINDICATED IN THE NURSING MOTHER

DRUG	REASON
Bromocriptine[46]	Suppresses lactation
Cocaine[47,48]	Cocaine poisoning in infant
Cyclophosphamide[49,50]	Anticancer drug; neutropenia
Cyclosporine[51]	Possible immune suppressive
Doxorubicin[52]	Anticancer drug
Ergotamine[53] (as used in migraine medication)	Vomiting, diarrhea, convulsions
Lithium[34]	Significant blood concentrations in the infant (one-third to one-half maternal levels)
Methotrexate[54]	Anticancer drug
Phencyclidine (PCP)[55]	Potent hallucinogen
Phenindione[56]	Anticoagulant; bleeding in one case report with ↑PT and ↑PTT, not used in United States

TABLE 21–3. SECRETION OF RADIOACTIVE ISOTOPES IN MILK

ISOTOPE	MATERNAL DOSE	$t_{1/2}$ (h)	AMOUNT IN MILK (μCi/ml)	INFANT DOSE* ON DAY 1 (μCi/day)	CUMULATIVE DOSE TO INFANT* (μCi)
Gallium-67[57]	3 mCi I.V.	78	3 days: 0.15	75	350 (if nursed from day 3 on)
			7 days: 0.045	23	108 (if nursed from day 7 on)
			14 days: 0.010	5	23 (if nursed from day 14 on)
Indium-111[58]	0.32 mCi I.V.		6 h: 0.028	0.1	
			20 h: 0.06		
Iodine-131[59]	200 μCi I.V.	24	25 h: 0.028	6	15 (if nursed through day 5)
					7.5% of maternal dose
Sodium-123 iodide[60]	183 mCi I.V.	5.8	6 h: 0.0128	2.8	2.6% of maternal dose
Technetium-99[61]	15 mCi I.V.	4	8.5 h: 0.1	95	0.63% of maternal dose
			20 h: 0.02		
			60 h: 0.006		

*Data are calculated by assuming the infant takes 3 ounces of breast milk every 4 hours.

It may be possible to delay the test, employ an alternate test, or give specific instructions about how long to avoid nursing to ensure the disappearance from the milk of all significant radioactivity. Table 21–3 summarizes the excretion of the more commonly used radiopharmaceuticals in human milk. For technetium-99, it is safe to resume nursing 48 hours after maternal injection. For gallium-67 or iodine-131, nursing will usually have to be terminated, since it is unlikely for the mother to continue to hand express (or by breast pump) much for the 7–14 days necessary to achieve a low radiation level in breast milk.

ENVIRONMENTAL CHEMICALS

In 1951, Laug et al.[62] published a report of DDT excretion in human milk samples collected in the United States (Washington, D.C.). They found DDT present in 94 percent of samples, with a mean level of 0.13 ppm (mg/kg milk). This is in excess of the level permitted by WHO[63] and the *U.S. Code of Federal Regulations* (Title 21, 120.147C) of 0.050 ppm. Similar numbers have been reported from other parts of the world, including Norway,[64,65] Australia,[66] The Netherlands,[67] and Canada.[68] Within the United States, similar concentrations of DDT are present in human milk regardless of geographic location or population size.[69] In 1951 in the United States, the amount of DDT found by Laug et al.[62] was 0.13 ppm. In 1965, Quinby et al.[69] found levels of 0.12 ppm, and in 1972, Kroger[70] found levels of 0.10 ppm from six areas throughout the United States. Mean control of DDT was 0.17 ppm. Thus, in the United States, there has been no change in content over 20 years. In Norway, 7 years after the total ban of DDT (1969–1970), the level in milk in Oslo had fallen from a mean of 0.082 ppm in 1969 to 0.050 ppm in 1976.[65] Other areas of Norway showed similar decreases. There has been no change in the content of other organochlorine compounds (polychlorinated biphenyls, hexachlorobenzene); in fact, there was a significant increase (doubling) in the content of PCBs from 0.011 ppm in 1969 to 0.024 ppm in 1976.[65] There is no evidence that the organochlorines in these concentrations adversely affect nursing infants.

These studies present the following information that suggests that these highly lipid-soluble chemicals are stored in body fat and that milk may be the only route of elimination from the body:

1. DDT concentrations are 11-fold higher in fat samples than in milk.
2. DDT concentrations decrease with numbers of infants nursed by the same mother.
3. DDT concentrations decrease during increasing numbers of months nursed.
4. DDT concentrations are significantly lower at the end of a single feed.

The unfortunate contamination of cattle feed with polybrominated biphenyls (PBBs) on Michigan cattle farms in 1973–1974 resulted in detectable levels of PBBs in human milk. For samples from the lower Michigan peninsula (site of heaviest contamination), 96 percent were positive for PBBs in the range 0.02–1.0 ppm. The upper-peninsula samples were positive for PBB in 43 percent of samples in a range from 0.02–0.5 ppm, with most samples below 0.1.[71] There was a high degree of correlation between values in paired samples of milk and adipose tissue. The degree of risk even at these levels is not known.[72]

Other highly lipid-soluble chemicals (e.g., tetrahydrocannibol[73]) may be expected to act in a similar fashion. For women known to have had high exposure (by occupation or food ingestion), it is reasonable to assay milk samples to determine exact risk.

ORAL CONTRACEPTIVES

The postpartum use of oral contraceptives by nursing mothers represents a common drug exposure. Vorherr[74] has summarized 18 separate papers published over 10 years dealing with this problem. Others have more recently published similar series.[75–78] It does not appear, using this information, that these compounds significantly interfere with milk production, especially if the oral contraceptive is withheld for several weeks until lactation is firmly established. Except for very rare reports,[79] nursing infants do not appear to be hormonally affected. Most recently, oral contraceptives have been reformulated with smaller amounts of estrogen. The amount of estrogen excreted is, in most cases, not any greater than that naturally excreted by ovulating women.[78]

DRUG METABOLISM IN BREAST TISSUE

Little evidence is available concerning the actual drug-metabolizing activity of breast tissue. Rasmussen and Linzell[80] have described the acetylation of sulfanilamide by the mammary tissue of the lactating goat. Dao[81] was unable to demonstrate metabolism of the carcinogen 3-methylcholanthrene in mammary tissue. Bruder et al.[82] have described cytochrome P-420 and cytochrome b_5 in the membranes of the milk fat globule of human milk; the same cytochromes were identified in the rough endoplasmic reticulum of lactating bovine and rat mammary epithelial cells. No cytochrome P-450 was identified in human, bovine, or rat milk or mammary tissue. Liu et al.[83] have identified a calcium-stimulated ribonuclease in rat milk and mammary tissue. A reverse transcriptase has been observed in human milk.[84] It is intriguing to speculate on its role in light of the observation by Scholm et al.[85] that human milk contains high-molecular-weight RNA particles.

SUMMARY

Nearly all drugs (or environmental chemicals) may be found in breast milk after maternal ingestion. It is prudent to minimize maternal exposure, although very few are known to be hazardous to the nursing infant (see Tables 21–2 and 21–3). Chronic maternal drug administration and exposure to environmental chemicals are areas that need further exploration. More sensitive analytical techniques are being used to detect metabolites that may present a greater risk than the parent compound. Nursing mothers should avoid all chemicals. If maternal medication is necessary, drug exposure to the nursing infant can be minimized by the timing of a maternal dose just after nursing and/or at least 1 half-life of the drug prior to another nursing period. In the older infant who sleeps through the night, medication prescribed on a once-daily frequency would best be taken after the last evening feeding of the baby. Breast milk, the ideal infant food, must be made as safe as possible.

REFERENCES

1. Nutrition Committee of the Canadian Paediatric Society and the Committee on Nutrition of the American Academy of Pediatrics: Breast feeding. Pediatrics 62:591–601, 1978
2. Fomon SJ: Infant Nutrition, 2nd ed. Philadelphia, WB Saunders, 1974, pp 360–370
3. Jelliffe DB, Jelliffe EFP: Breast is best: Modern meanings. N Engl J Med 297:912–915, 1977
4. Applebaum RM: The obstetrician's approach to the breasts and breast feeding. J Reprod Med 14:98–116, 1975
5. Lawrence RA: Breast feeding: A Guide for the Medical Profession, 2nd ed. St Louis, CV Mosby, 1985
6. Resman BH, Blumenthal HP, Jusko WJ: Breast milk distribution of theobromine from chocolate. J Pediatr 91:477–480, 1977
7. Yurchak AM, Jusko WJ: Theophylline secretion into breast milk. Pediatrics 57:518–520, 1976
8. Patton S, Keenan TW: The milk fat globule membrane. Biochem Biophys Acta 415:273–309, 1975
9. Vorherr H: The Breast. New York, Academic Press, 1974, pp 107–124
10. Ferguson DJP, Anderson TJ: An ultrastructural study of lactation in the human breast. Anat Embryol 168:349–359, 1983
11. Kesaniemi YA: Ethanol and acetaldehyde in the milk and peripheral blood of lactating women after ethanol administration. J Obstet Gynaecol Br Commonw 81:84–86, 1974
12. Schanker LS: Passage of drugs across body membranes. Pharmacol Rev 14:501–530, 1962
13. Rasmussen F: Excretion of drugs by milk, in Brodie BB, Gilette JR (eds): Handbook of Experimental Pharmacology, vol 28. New York, Springer-Verlag, 1971, pp 390–402
14. Wilson JT, Brown RD, Cherek DR, et al: Drug excretion in human breast milk. Clin Pharmacokinet 5:1–66, 1980
15. Wilson JT, Brown RD, Hinson JL, et al: Pharmacokinetic pitfalls in the estimation of the breast milk/plasma ratio for drugs. Annu Rev Pharmacol Toxicol 25:667–689, 1985
16. Miller GE, Banejee NC, Stowie CM Jr: Drug movement between bovine milk and plasma as affected by milk pH. J Dairy Sci 50:1395–1403, 1967
17. Rasmussen F: Studies on the Mammary Excretion and Absorption of Drugs. Copenhagen, Martenson, 1966
18. Rasmussen F: The mechanisms of drug secretion into milk, in Galli G, Jacini G, Pecile A (eds): Dietary Lipids and Postnatal Development. New York, Raven Press, 1973, pp 231–245
19. Committee on Drugs, American Academy of Pediatrics: Psychotropic drugs in pregnancy and lactation. Pediatrics 69:241–244, 1982
20. Nation RL, Hotham N: Drugs and breast-feeding. Med J Aust 146:308–313, 1987
21. Reisner SH, Eisenberg NH, Stahl B, et al: Maternal medications and breast-feeding. Dev Pharmacol Ther 6:285–304, 1983
22. Committee on Drugs, American Academy of Pediatrics: The transfer of drugs and other chemicals in human breast milk. Pediatrics 72:375–380, 1983
23. Berglund F, Flodh H, Lundborg P, et al: Drug use during pregnancy and breast-feeding. Acta Obstet Gynaecol Scand Suppl 126:1–55, 1984
24. Briggs GG, Freeman RK, Yaffe SJ: Drugs in Pregnancy and Lactation, 2nd ed. Baltimore, Williams & Wilkins, 1986
25. Kwit NT, Hatcher RA: Excretion of drugs in milk. Am J Dis Child 49:900–904, 1935
26. Berlin CM, Yaffe SJ, Ragni M: Disposition of acetaminophen in milk, saliva, and plasma of lactating women. Pediatr Pharmacol 1:135–141, 1980
27. Berlin CM, Vesell ES: Antipyrine disposition in milk or saliva of lactating women. Clin Pharmacol Ther 31:38–44, 1982
28. Berlin CM, Denson HM, Daniel CH, et al: Disposition of dietary caffeine in milk, saliva and plasma of lactating women. Pediatrics 73:59–63, 1984
29. Yoshioka H, Cho K, Takimoto M, et al: Transfer of cefazolin into human milk. J Pediatr 94:151–152, 1979
30. Werthmann MW, Krees SV: Excretion of chlorothiazide in human breast milk. J Pediatr 81:781–783, 1972
31. Cole AP, Hailey DM: Diazepam and active metabolite in breast milk and their transfer to the neonate. Arch Dis Child 50:741–742, 1975
32. Loughnan PM: Digoxin excretion in human breast milk. J Pediatr 92:1019–1020, 1978
33. Berlin CM, Lee C: Isoniazid and acetylisoniazid disposition in human milk, saliva and plasma. Fed Proc 38:426, 1979
34. Schou M, Amdisen A: Lithium and pregnancy. III. Lithium ingestion by children breast fed by women on lithium treatment. Br Med J 2:138, 1973
35. Blinick G, Inturrisi CE, Jerez E, et al: Methadone assays in preg-

nant women and progeny. Am J Obstet Gynecol 121:617–621, 1975

36. Erickson SH, Oppenheim GL, Smith GH: Metronidazole in breast milk. Obstet Gynecol 57:48–50, 1981
37. Ferguson BB, Wilson DJ, Schaffner W: Determination of nicotine concentrations in human milk. Am J Dis Child 130:837–839, 1976
38. McKenzie SA, Selley JA, Agnew JE: Secretion of prednisolone into breast milk. Arch Dis Child 50:894–896, 1975
39. Berlin CM, Demers L, Kaiser D: Prednisone and prednisolone in human milk after large oral dose of prednisone. Pharmacologist 13:396, 1979
40. Karlberg B, Lindberg D, Aberg H: Excretion of propranolol in human breast milk. Acta Pharmacol Toxicol 34:222–224, 1974
41. Levy G: Salicylate pharmacokinetics in the human neonate, in Morselli PL, Garactini G, Sereni F (eds): Basic and Therapeutic Aspects of Perinatal Pharmacology. New York, Raven Press, 1975, pp 319–330
42. Berlin CM, Yaffe SJ: Disposition of sulfasalazine (Azulfidine) in human breast milk, plasma, and saliva. Dev Pharmacol Ther 1:31–39, 1980
43. Dreisbach JA: Sulphone levels in breast milk of mothers on sulphone therapy. Leprosy Rev 23:101–106, 1952
44. Anderson P, Bondesson U, Mattiasson I, et al: Verapamil and norverapamil in plasma and breast milk during breast-feeding. Eur J Clin Pharmacol 31:625–627, 1987
45. Clark JH, Wilson WG: A 16-day-old breast-fed infant with metabolic acidosis caused by salicylate. Clin Pediatr 20:53–54, 1981
46. Kulski JK, Hartmann PE, Martin JD, et al: Effects of bromocriptine mesylate on the composition of the mammary secretion in non-breast-feeding women. Obstet Gynecol 52:38–42, 1978
47. Chasnoff IJ, Lewis DE, Squires L: Cocaine intoxication in a breast-fed infant. Pediatrics 80:836–838, 1978
48. Chaney NE, Franke J, Wadlington WB: Cocaine convulsions in a breast-feeding baby. J Pediatr 112:134–135, 1988
49. Wienick PH, Duncan JH: Cyclophosphamide in human milk. Lancet 1:912, 1971
50. Amato D, Niblett JS: Neutropenia from cyclophosphamide in breast milk. Med J Aust 1:383–384, 1977
51. Fletcher SM, Katz AR, Rogers AJ, et al: The presence of cyclosporine in body tissue and fluids during pregnancy. Am J Kidney Dis 5:60–63, 1985
52. Egan PC, Costanza ME, Dodion P, et al: Doxorubicin and cisplatin excretion into human milk. Cancer Treat Rep 69:1387–1389, 1985
53. Fomina PL: Untersuchungen uber den Ubergang des aktiven agens des Mutterkorns in die milch stillender Mutter. Arch Gynecol Obstet 157:275–285, 1934
54. Johns DG, Rutherford LD, Leighton PC, et al: Secretion of methotrexate into human milk. Am J Obstet Gynecol 113:978–980, 1972
55. Kaufman KR, Petrucha RA, Pitts FN Jr, et al: PCP in aminiotic fluid and breast milk: Case report. J Clin Psychiatry 44:269–270, 1983
56. Eckstein HB, Jack B: Breast-feeding and anticoagulant therapy. Lancet 1:672, 1970
57. Tobin RE, Schneider PB: Uptake of ^{67}Ga in the lactating breast and its persistence in milk: Case report. J Nucl Med 17:1055–1056, 1976
58. Butt D, Szaz KF: Indium-111 radioactivity in breast milk. Br J Radiol 59:80–82, 1986
59. Wyburn JR: Human breast milk excretion of radionuclides following administration of radiopharmaceuticals. J Nucl Med 14:115–117, 1973
60. Hedrick WR, DiSimone RN, Keen RL: Radiation dosimetry from breast milk excretion of radioiodine and pertechnetate. J Nucl Med 27:1569–1571, 1986
61. Rumble WF, Aamodt RL, Jones AE, et al: Accidental ingestion of Tc-99m in breast milk by a 10-week-old child. J Nucl Med 19:913–915, 1978
62. Laug EP, Kunze FM, Prickett CS: Occurrence of DDT in human fat and milk. Arch Ind Hyg Occup Med 3:245–246, 1951
63. WHO/FAO: Pesticide Residues in Food. Geneva, Technical Report Series No. 417, 1969
64. Brenik EM, Bjerk JE: Organochlorine compounds in Norwegian human fat and milk. Acta Pharmacol Toxicol 43:59–63, 1978
65. Bakken Arne F, Seip M: Insecticides in human breast milk. Acta Paediatr Scand 65:535–539, 1976
66. Siyali DS: Polychlorinated biphenyls, hexachlorobenzene and other organochlorine pesticides in human milk. Med J Aust 2:815–818, 1973
67. Turistra LGMT: Organochlorine insecticide residues in human milk in one Leiden region. Neth Milk Dairy J 25:24–32, 1971
68. Holdrinet MVH, Braun HE, Frank R, et al: Organochlorine residues in human adipose tissue and milk from Ontario residents 1969–1974. Can J Public Health 68:74–80, 1977
69. Quinby GE, Armstrong JF, Durham WF: DDT in human milk. Nature 207:726–728, 1965
70. Kroger M: Insecticide residues in human milk. J Pediatr 80:401–405, 1972
71. Brilliant LB, Amburg GV, Isbister J, et al: Breast-milk monitoring to measure Michigan's contamination with polybrominated biphenyls. Lancet 2:643–646, 1978
72. Wolff MS: Occupationally derived chemicals in breast milk. Am J Ind Med 4:259–281, 1983
73. Perez-Reyes M, Wall EM: Presence of tetrahydrocannabinol in human milk. N Engl J Med 307:819, 1982
74. Vorherr H: The Breast. New York, Academic Press, 1974, pp 118–123
75. Zacharias S, Aguillern E, Assenzo JR, et al: Effects of hormonal and nonhormonal contraceptives on lactation and incidence of pregnancy. Contraception 33:203–213, 1986
76. Nilsson S, Mellbin T, Hofvander Y, et al: Long-term followup of children breast-fed by mothers using oral contraceptives. Contraception 34:443–457, 1986
77. Nilsson S, Nygren KG: Transfer of contraceptive steroids to human milk. Res Reprod 11:1–2, 1979
78. Committee on Drugs, American Academy of Pediatrics: Breast-feeding and contraception. Pediatrics 68:138–140, 1981
79. Curtis EM: Oral-contraceptive feminization of a normal male infant: Report of a case. Obstet Gynecol 23:295–296, 1964
80. Rasmussen F, Linzell JL: The acetylation of sulphanilamide by mammary tissue of lactating goats. Biochem Pharmacol 16:918–919, 1967
81. Dao TL: Studies on mechanism of carcinogenesis in mammary gland. Prog Exp Tumor Res 11:235–261, 1969
82. Bruder G, Fink A, Jarasch E-D: The B-type cytochrome in endoplasmic reticulum of mammary gland epithelium and milk fat globule membranes consists of two components, cytochrome b_5 and cytochrome P-420. Exp Cell Res 117:207–217, 1978
83. Liu DK, Kulick D, Williams GH: Ca^{2+}-stimulated ribonuclease. Biochem J 178:241–244, 1979
84. McCormick JJ, Larson LJ, Rich MA: RNAse inhibition of reverse transcriptase activity in human milk. Nature 251:737–740, 1974
85. Scholm J, Spiegelman S, Moore DH: Detection of high-molecular-weight RNA in particles from human milk. Science 175:542–544, 1972

22

DRUG THERAPEUTICS IN THE INFANT AND CHILD

RALPH E. KAUFFMAN

Infancy and childhood extend from 2 months of age to the onset of puberty, which typically occurs at approximately 10–12 years in females and 12–14 years in males. The first 2–3 years of life is a period of particularly rapid growth and development. Body weight doubles by 5 months and triples by the first birthday. Body length increases by 50 percent during the first year. Body surface area doubles by the first birthday. Caloric expenditure increases threefold to fourfold during the first year. The child becomes ambulatory, develops socialization, and learns verbal language.

Substantial changes in body proportions and composition accompany growth and development. Major organ systems differentiate, grow, and mature throughout infancy and childhood. Although growth and development are most rapid during the first several years of life, maturation continues at a slower pace throughout middle and later childhood. This dynamic process of growth, differentiation, and maturation is what sets the infant and child apart from adults, both physiologically and pharmacologically. It should be no surprise, then, that important changes in response to and biodisposition of drugs occur during infancy and childhood. These changes influence the response to, toxicity of, and dosing regimens for drugs.

This chapter will focus on the impact of growth and development on drug actions and biodisposition and the resultant practical implications for pharmacotherapy in children. Comparative pharmacologic data in children and adults will be used to illustrate general principles.

DEVELOPMENTAL CHANGES IN BODY COMPOSITION AND PROPORTION

Developmental changes in body composition, body proportions, and relative mass of the liver and kidneys affect pharmacokinetic characteristics of drugs at different ages. It is therefore important to review the relevant

changes that take place between early infancy and pubescence.

The proportions of body weight contributed by fat, protein, intracellular water, and extracellular water, respectively, change significantly during infancy and childhood (Figure 22–1). Total-body water comprises approximately 75–80 percent of body weight in the full-term newborn. This decreases to approximately 60 percent by 5 months of age and remains relatively constant thereafter. Although the percentage of total-body weight comprised by total-body water does not change significantly after late infancy, there is a progressive decrease in extracellular water from infancy to young adulthood. In addition, the percentage of body weight contributed by fat doubles by 4–5 months of age, primarily at the expense of total-body water. During the second year of life, protein mass increases, with a compensatory reduction in fat. This corresponds to ambulation and loss of "baby fat" during the transition from infancy to childhood.

Liver and kidney size, relative to body weight, also change during growth and development[1] (Figure 22–2). These two organs reach maximum relative weight in the 1- to 2-year-old child, the period of life when capacity for drug metabolism and elimination also tends to be great-

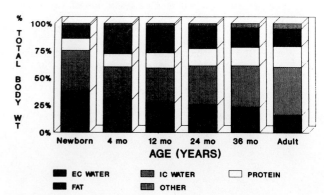

FIGURE 22–1. Schematic of change in proportional body composition with age. (Adapted from Habersang.[81])

212

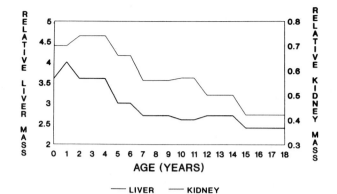

FIGURE 22–2. Change in relative liver and kidney mass expressed as percent of body weight from infancy to young adulthood. (Data from Maxwell.[1])

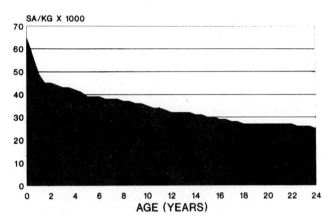

FIGURE 22–3. Change in the ratio of body surface area to body mass from infancy to young adulthood. (Data from Maxwell[1] and Spino.[2])

est. Likewise, body surface area is greatest relative to body mass in the infant and young child compared with the older child and young adult[1,2] (Figure 22–3).

DEVELOPMENTAL CHANGES IN ORGAN FUNCTION

Gastrointestinal Tract

Various functional aspects of the gastrointestinal (GI) tract mature at different rates and times. Immaturity of esophageal and gastric motility predisposes the young infant to reflux of gastric contents.[3] Slower gastric emptying in infants also may contribute to reflux. This problem resolves by the first birthday in most infants, along with maturation of esophageal and gastric function.

Although gastric acid production is temporarily decreased during the neonatal period, acid production approaches adult values by 3 months of age.[4] Exocrine pancreatic function also matures during the first year of life.[4]

The absorptive surface of the small gut is proportionately greater and gastrointestinal transit time may be

shorter in infants and younger children compared with adults.

Organs of Elimination

The liver and kidney are the primary organs of metabolism and elimination. Although a great deal has been written about immaturity of hepatic and renal function in the neonate, relatively less emphasis has been placed on maturation of the liver and kidney during childhood and the impact on drug disposition.

Hepatic function is complex, and metabolic pathways for various substrates develop at different rates. Bromsulphalein (BSP) has been used as a substrate to evaluate maturation of hepatic clearance during infancy and childhood.[5,6] BSP clearance, normalized for body surface area, increases rapidly during the first 3 months of life, significantly exceeds adult clearance in the preschool child, and declines to adult levels during adolescence (Figure 22–4).

Glomerular filtration rate, as reflected by endogenous creatinine clearance, also increases rapidly during the first year of life. Creatinine clearance, normalized for body surface area, equals adult clearance by 1 year of life, and there is some evidence that average clearance in prepubescent children exceeds clearance in adults[6] (Figure 22–5). Tubular function matures later than glomerular function. However, tubular function is essentially mature by 1 year of age.[4]

It is important to recognize, then, that both hepatic and renal function not only equals, but in some cases exceeds normal adult function between 1 year of age and puberty.

INFLUENCE OF DEVELOPMENT ON DRUG BIODISPOSITION

Drug Absorption

Developmental changes in the GI tract are important, because medications are commonly administered to chil-

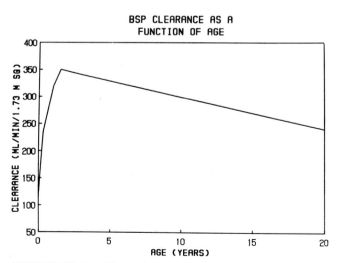

FIGURE 22–4. Change in hepatic clearance (expressed as ml/min/1.73 m²) of Bromsulphalein during childhood. (Adapted from Habersang.[81])

DEVELOPMENT OF RENAL CLEARANCE

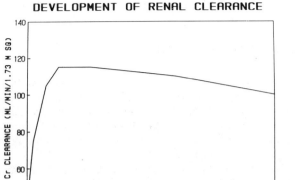

FIGURE 22–5. Change in endogenous creatinine clearance during childhood. (Adapted from Habersang.[81])

dren by mouth and maturational changes may influence drug absorption. It is difficult to generalize, however, because differences in absorption of orally administered drugs associated with growth and maturation are unpredictable and inconsistent. Nevertheless, it is important to be aware of those aspects of GI tract development which may influence drug absorption.

Reflux of gastric contents retrograde into the esophagus is very common during the first year of life.[3] Excessive gastroesophageal reflux may result in regurgitation of medication, resulting in variable and unpredictable loss of an orally administered dose.

Gastric emptying is an important determinant of rate of absorption, since most drug absorption takes place in the duodenum. Delayed gastric emptying in infants not only contributes to gastroesophageal reflux, but also may result in delayed drug absorption.[7–9] On the other hand, gastric emptying in prepubescent children is equal to or exceeds that in adults. This tends to facilitate more rapid drug absorption, other factors being equal.[4,8] Administration of medication in liquid as opposed to solid dosage forms, as is commonly the case for children, also increases the rate of absorption. In contrast, shorter gastrointestinal transit time in young children may actually reduce the fraction of dose absorbed when drugs are administered in sustained-release formulations.[10,11]

Decreased gastric acid production in the younger infant may result in increased bioavailability of acid-labile drugs such as the penicillins.[9] For example, increased absorption of penicillin G, ampicillin, and nafcillin in infants compared with older children and adults has been reported.[7] However, perturbation of drug absorption due to reduction in gastric acidity is negligible beyond infancy.

Rate and extent of drug absorption are determined to a significant degree by the absorptive surface area of the duodenum. Greater relative small gut surface area in young children tends to enhance drug absorption.

Drugs absorbed from the intestine into the portal circulation are delivered to the liver prior to entering the systemic circulation. High hepatic extraction of some drugs on the first pass through the liver results in removal of a large fraction of the absorbed drug by the liver, resulting in decreased systemic bioavailability. Little is known about the effect of intestinal and hepatic maturation on first-pass uptake of drugs. However, one would predict, based on increased hepatic clearance in children, that first-pass processes in children would be equal to or exceed uptake in adults. Wilson et al.[12] described wide intersubject variability and low serum concentrations of two high-uptake drugs, propoxyphene and propanolol, when administered orally to children 2–13 years of age. This is consistent with extensive first-pass uptake.

Maturation of gut flora during childhood modifies digoxin metabolism. Reduction of digoxin to inactive metabolites by anaerobic gastrointestinal bacteria accounts for a significant fraction of digoxin clearance in approximately 10 percent of adult patients.[13] Reduction metabolites are not detected in children until after 16 months of age, and the adult metabolite pattern is not found until 9 years of age.[14]

The rectum is an alternative route of enteral drug administration in children that may be used when vomiting or other intervening conditions preclude oral dosing. Drugs administered rectally are absorbed into the hemorrhoidal veins, which are part of the systemic rather than the portal circulation. First-pass uptake, therefore, is not a consideration with rectal administration. However, rectal dosing is less than satisfactory in many cases for other reasons. Absorption of drugs administered in suppository form is typically erratic and incomplete. Furthermore, presence of feces in the rectal vault impedes absorption. In younger children and infants, the dose may be expelled before absorption is complete, thereby reducing bioavailability to a variable extent. Nevertheless, some medications may be successfully administered rectally in solution.[15] These include diazepam and valproic acid for seizures and phenobarbital for seizures, sedation, or preanesthesia.[16,17] In addition, rectal corticosteroids are routinely used in the treatment of inflammatory bowel disease.

Absorption of drugs from intramuscular or subcutaneous injection sites is influenced by characteristics of the patient as well as properties of the injected drug. Blood flow to the injection site, muscle mass, quantity of adipose tissue, and muscle activity are patient characteristics that determine rate and extent of absorption. Solubility of the drug at the pH of extracellular fluid, ease with which the drug diffuses across capillary membranes, and surface area over which the injection volume spreads also determine absorption.[8,9,15,16,18] Extravascular injection is not an optimal route of administration in the presence of hypoperfusion syndromes, dehydration, vasomotor instability, starvation, or cachexia, since all these conditions impede absorption. Some drugs, such as erythromycin and certain cephalosporin antibiotics, are not usually administered intramuscularly because they cause unacceptable pain and tissue reaction. However, many drugs, including most aminoglycoside and penicillin antibiotics, may be administered intramuscularly with resulting plasma concentrations comparable with those achieved with intravenous administration. Conversely, highly hydrophobic drugs such as diazepam and phenytoin are not absorbed well following intramuscular injection and should not be given by this route. Furthermore, phenytoin forms insoluble crystals in intramuscular injection sites associated with local hemorrhage, muscle necrosis, and minimal systemic absorption.[19]

Drug Distribution

The distribution of a drug throughout the body is influenced by binding affinity of the drug for plasma and tissue proteins, lipid/water solubility partition of the drug, molecular weight of the drug, and degree of ionization of the drug at physiologic pH. Age-dependent changes in body composition (see earlier in text) may influence drug distribution in the developing child. Highly lipid-soluble compounds such as inhalation anesthetics and lipophilic sedative/hypnotic agents typically exhibit relatively larger distribution volumes in infants during the first year of life compared with older children because of the relatively larger proportion of body fat in infants. Likewise, the apparent distribution volume of drugs such as penicillin, aminoglycoside, and cephalosporin antibiotics, which distribute primarily in extracellular water, tends to be greater in infants and decrease during maturation coincident with the progressive relative decrease in extracellular water.[4,8,18]

In general, the apparent volume of distribution of drugs tends to be greater in infants and decreases toward adult values during childhood. However, there is a great deal of interindividual variation, and important exceptions to this general rule exist. Examples of such exceptions are theophylline[20] and phenobarbital,[21] which show little consistent age-related change in distribution volume.

Although the plasma protein binding of many drugs is decreased in the fetus and newborn infant relative to adults, age-related differences in plasma protein binding are not clinically significant beyond the newborn period.[22] However, maturational changes in tissue binding can significantly affect drug distribution. The myocardial-to-plasma digoxin concentration in infants and children up to 36 months of age is two to three times that of adults.[23–25] Increased myocardial digoxin concentrations relative to adults have been demonstrated in children using specific assay methods and do not appear to be due to assay interference by endogenous digoxin-like substances.[26] In addition, erythrocytes from infants bind three times the quantity of digoxin of adult erythrocytes.[25] The increased myocardial and erythrocyte binding of digoxin is associated with a significantly greater volume of distribution of digoxin in infants and children compared with adults.

Metabolism and Elimination

Clearance of many drugs is primarily dependent on hepatic metabolism, followed by excretion of parent drug and metabolites by the liver and kidney. Nonpolar, lipid-soluble drugs typically are metabolized to more polar and water-soluble compounds prior to excretion, whereas water-soluble drugs usually are excreted unchanged by glomerular filtration and/or renal tubular secretion.

Phase I metabolic processes involve oxidative, reductive, or hydrolytic reactions that most often are catalyzed by the mixed-function oxidase enzyme systems located in the microsomes. Less commonly, such reactions may be mediated by mitochondrial or cytosolic enzymes. Phase II, or synthetic, metabolism involves conjugation of the substrate to a polar compound such as glucuronic acid, sulfate, or glycine. This usually results in a polar, water-soluble compound that is readily excreted.

Although the capacity to metabolize a number of drug substrates is decreased during the newborn period, with few exceptions, maturation of the various pathways occurs during the first year of life.[4,7] The various pathways mature at different times, and there is considerable interindividual variation in rate of maturation of specific pathways.[8,9] This should not be surprising, since other aspects of development proceed at varying rates in different individuals; i.e., the chronologic age at which infants sit, crawl, walk, and talk is quite variable.

In some cases, the dominant metabolic pathway in infants and children is different from adults. For example, N_7-methylation of theophylline to produce caffeine is well developed in the newborn infant, whereas oxidative demethylation is deficient.[27] Therefore, in contrast to older infants and children, theophylline is metabolized to caffeine, which accumulates to pharmacologically active concentrations as a result of its long half-life when theophylline is administered to newborn infants for longer than 10 days. This pathway is important until 4–6 months of age, when the oxidative pathways mature, caffeine clearance increases, and caffeine accumulation no longer occurs. Interestingly, the clearances of theophylline and caffeine increase dramatically coincident with maturation of oxidative N_3-demethylase activity.[28] The metabolic profile of acetaminophen also differs in children compared with adults. The dominant metabolic pathway in infants and children less than 12 years of age is sulfate conjugation, whereas glucuronidation is the major pathway in adolescents and adults.[29] Although the major metabolic pathways differ with age, there is not an age-related difference in clearance.

Maturation of renal clearance of drugs and their metabolites occurs coincident with maturation of renal function during the first year. With maturation of hepatic and renal function, the clearance of many drugs in young children, when corrected for body surface area, equals or exceeds that in adults after 1 year of age. Table 22–1 compares reported elimination half-lives for a number of drugs among newborns, infants, children, and adults. Typically, the half-life is prolonged in the newborn, decreases during infancy, is shortest in the prepubescent child, and is somewhat longer in adults than in children. With rare exception, a shorter half-life reflects greater clearance. The changes in drug disposition during growth and development reflect the changes in hepatic and renal function described earlier.

TABLE 22–1. CHANGE IN ELIMINATION HALF-LIFE (HOURS) DURING DEVELOPMENT

DRUG	NEWBORN	INFANT	CHILD	ADULT	REFERENCE
Acetaminophen	4.9		4.5	3.6	29
Amikacin	5.0–6.5		1.6	2.3	30–32
Ampicillin	4.0	1.7		1.0–1.5	33
Amoxicillin	3.7		0.9–1.9	0.6–1.5	9
Carbamazepine			8–25	10–20	34
Cefazolin			1.7	2.0	35
Cefotaxime	4.0	0.8	1.0	1.1	35
Cefoxitin	3.8	1.4	0.8	0.8	35
Ceftazidime	4.5	4.5	2.0	1.8	35
Ceftriaxone	17.0	5.9	4.7	7.8	35
Cefuroxime	5.5	3.5	1.2	1.5	35
Cephalothin			0.3	0.6	35
Clindamycin	3.6	3.0	2.4	4.5	36,37
Clonazepam			22–33	20–60	38
Cyclosporine			4.8	5.5	4
Diazepam	30	10	25	30	39
Digoxin		18–33	37	30–50	4
Ethosuximide			30	52–56	38
Gentamicin	4.0	2.6	1.2	2–3	40–43
Ibuprofen	.		1.0–2.0	2.0–3.0	44–46
Isoniazid			2.9	2.8	47
				(Slow acetylators)	
Mezlocillin	3.7		0.8	1.0	7
Moxalactam	5.4	1.7	1.6	2.2	35
Naproxen			11–13	10–17	48,49
Phenobarbital	67–99		36–72	48–120	7,38
Primidone			5–11	12–15	50,51
Piperacillin	0.8	0.5	0.4	0.9	52
Quinidine			4.0	5–7	53
Rifampin			2.9	3.3–3.9	54
Sulfadiazine	40	10		10–15	55
Sulfamethoxypyridazine	280	50	50	50	55
Sulfisoxizole	18	8	8	8	55
Theophylline	30	6.9	3.4	8.1	20,56
Ticarcillin	5–6		0.9	1.3	57
Tobramycin	4.6		1–2	2–3	40,58
Valproate			7.0	6–12	59,60
Vancomycin	4.1–9.1		2.2–2.4	5–6	40,61
Zidovudine			1.0–1.5	1.6	62,63

THERAPEUTIC IMPLICATIONS OF DEVELOPMENTAL CHANGES

The onset and intensity of effect of most drugs are related to the drug concentration at the site of action, which, in turn, is assumed to be reflected by the plasma concentration. The drug concentration at any point in time after a dose is determined by the dose and the pharmacokinetic characteristics of the drug in a particular patient. As described earlier, developmental changes in drug disposition result in significant changes in the pharmacokinetics of many drugs, which must be considered when calculating doses for children of different ages. Dose requirements vary with age as volume of distribution, half-life, and clearance change during development. The dose of many drugs must be adjusted not only for increased body mass, but also to compensate for increased clearance and shorter half-life. This is particularly important for drugs that are administered chronically, such as anticonvulsants, cardiovascular agents, and bronchodilators. The loading dose of a drug is primarily determined by its volume of distribution, whereas the maintenance dose is determined by the clearance. In addition, the dos-

ing interval relative to the half-life determines the degree of fluctuation of drug concentration between doses. Several key examples follow.

Recommended loading and maintenance doses for digoxin reflect changes in volume of distribution and clearance with age. The digitalizing dose for premature infants is 20 μg/kg; for full-term newborns, 30 μg/kg; for infants less than 2 years, 40–50 μg/kg; and for children greater than 2 years, 30–40 μg/kg. Likewise, the maintenance dose for premature infants is 5 μg/kg; for full-term newborns, 8–10 μg/kg; for infants less than 2 years, 10–12 μg/kg; and for children greater than 2 years, 8–10 μg/kg.[65]

Theophylline dose requirements mirror changes in clearance from infancy to adulthood. Recommended initial infusion rates for intravenous theophylline are 0.3–0.6 mg/kg/h for infants less than 12 months old, 0.8 mg/kg/h for children 1–9 years old, 0.7 mg/kg/h for children 9–12 years old, and 0.5 mg/kg/h for nonsmoking adolescents.[20]

The dose of aminoglycoside antibiotics in children required to achieve equivalent plasma concentrations typically is 50–100 percent greater than that in adults

TABLE 22–2. CHANGES IN PHENYTOIN METABOLISM WITH DEVELOPMENT

AGE (years)	K_m (mg/liter)	V_{max} (mg/kg/day)
≤1	4.54	17.9
1–4	5.23	12.0
4–8	3.85	10.4
8–12	5.69	11.1
12–16	5.14	7.85
16–22	7.15	9.57

Source: From Dodson.[82]

because of the greater renal clearance in children.[32] The dosing interval in children also may need to be shorter, e.g., every 6 hours versus every 8 hours. Likewise, dosage requirements of the anticonvulsants carbamazepine, ethosuximide, phenobarbital, and phenytoin also are significantly greater on a milligram per kilogram basis in prepubescent children compared with adults[39,66] because of the greater metabolic capacity in children (Table 22–2). In contrast to newborn patients, there is greater risk of underdosing than overdosing older infants and children unless age-related changes in clearance are considered.

Use of sustained-release oral dosage formulations presents unique problems in young children. Absorption may be unpredictable and incomplete, leading to therapeutic failures. In addition, even though the formulation is designed for slow absorption, concentrations may exhibit greater fluctuations between doses than in adults because of the greater clearance in children. For example, sustained-release theophylline products, which provide satisfactory concentrations when given every 12 hours to adults, frequently must be given every 8 hours to children to avoid excessive fluctuation in concentration during the dosing interval.[20]

GROWTH, DEVELOPMENT, AND DRUG TOXICITY

Examples of Increased Toxicity

The complex processes involved in growth and development frequently make the child uniquely vulnerable to mechanisms of toxicity that are not present in mature individuals. Chronic treatment with adrenocorticosteroids,[67] amphetamine, and methylphenidate[68] impede linear growth, an adverse effect that obviously occurs only in the growing individual. Tetracycline antibiotics are not recommended for children less than 9 years of age because they cause enamel dysplasia in developing teeth.[69] Use of the fluoroquinolone antibiotics in children is contraindicated because of toxicity to growing cartilage.[70]

Metoclopramide and prochlorperazine are commonly used as antiemetic agents during cancer chemotherapy, and metoclopramide is used as a prokinetic agent to treat gastroesophareal reflux. Both these drugs are dopamine-2 antagonists and in excessive dose can produce acute dystonic reactions.[15] Haloperidol also shares this adverse side

effect. Younger children seem to be more susceptible to dystonic reactions than adults. This may be related to greater concentration of dopamine-2 receptors in the brain of young patients.[71]

Infants and young children are more prone than adults to acute central nervous system and hyperpyrexic reactions to anticholinergic drugs such as atropine and scopolamine.[72] Toxicity associated with topical ocular administration has been described.

Children less than 1 year of age are more susceptible to respiratory depression from weight-adjusted doses of opioid drugs, which are generally safe in older children and adults. For this reason, opioid antitussive agents such as codeine and dextromethorphan are not recommended for use in this age group.[73]

Verapamil is a drug of choice for the treatment of supraventricular arrhythmias in older children and adult patients. However, infants with supraventricular tachyarrhythmias appear to be at increased risk of sudden cardiac arrest. The mechanism for this increased risk is poorly understood. Verapamil is not recommended for treatment of acute arrhythmias in infants less than 1 year of age.[74]

Valproic acid is one of the anticonvulsants most commonly used in children. In rare cases, it can cause acute hyperammonemia associated with hepatoencephalopathy. Children under 5 years of age are at greatest risk for developing this life-threatening adverse reaction, particularly if they are receiving concurrent therapy with other anticonvulsant drugs.[75]

Examples of Decreased Toxicity

Immaturity does not invariably predispose to increased risk of toxicity. Although infants and children may be more susceptible than adults to certain types of drug toxicity, there are important examples in which differences in drug disposition appear to result in decreased risk of toxicity in immature individuals.

Infants and young children appear to be less susceptible to ototoxicity and renal toxicity from aminoglycoside antibiotics[76] compared with older adult patients. This may be due, in part, to reduced intracellular accumulation of the aminoglycoside in renal tubular epithelial cells.[77]

Children tend to experience relatively mild liver toxicity from acute acetaminophen overdose. Weight-adjusted doses and serum concentrations that invariably are associated with severe hepatotoxicity in young adults produce much less hepatocellular damage in preschool children.[78] There is evidence that this is due to a greater capacity of children to metabolize acetaminophen by nontoxic pathways.[79]

Hepatotoxicity from halothane is relatively rare in children, even following multiple exposures, whereas it is not that uncommon in adults. The mechanism of reduced hepatotoxicity in children is not known.[80]

The risk of isoniazid-induced hepatitis is age-related. An incidence of 0 per 1000 patients less than 20 years of age was reported by the Food and Drug Administration, whereas the incidence was 23 per 1000 in patients 50–65 years old.[80] It is usually unnecessary to routinely check liver function tests in children receiving isoniazid.

SUMMARY

The prepubescent child is clearly different from the newborn infant and the adolescent. From a pharmacotherapy perspective, the dynamic processes of growth and development create a moving target for the physician. It is important to remember that, in contrast with newborn infants, young children typically have a greater capacity to metabolize and excrete drugs than at any other time during their life. This, in turn, requires that appropriate dosage regimens be designed to compensate for developmental changes. It also is important to keep in mind that developing human beings may be uniquely susceptible to some types of drug toxicity while being protected from other toxic mechanisms by their immaturity. A knowledge of the developmental changes in drug disposition that influence therapeutic response and toxicity is essential to optimize therapy at different stages of childhood.

REFERENCES

1. Maxwell GM: Principles of Paediatric Pharmacology. New York, Oxford University Press, 1984, p 96
2. Spino M: Pediatric dosing rules and nomograms, in MacLeod SM, Radde IC (eds): Textbook of Pediatric Clinical Pharmacology. Littleton, Mass, PSG, 1985, pp 118–128
3. Sondheimer JM: Gastroesophageal reflux: Update on pathogenesis and diagnosis. Pediatr Clin North Am 35:103–116, 1988
4. Kearns GL, Reed MD: Clinical pharmacokinetics in infants and children: A reappraisal. Clin Pharmacokinet 17(suppl 1):29–67, 1989
5. Wichmann HM, Rind H, Gladtke E: Die elimination von bromsulphalein beim kind. Z Kinderheilk 103:262–276, 1968
6. Habersang R, Kauffman RE: Drug doses for children: A rational approach to an old problem. J Kans Med Soc 75:98–103, 1974
7. Milsap RL, Szefler SJ: Special pharmacokinetic considerations in children, in Evans WE, Schentag JJ, Jusko WJ (eds): Applied Pharmacokinetics: Principles of Therapeutic Drug Monitoring. Spokane, Wash, Applied Therapeutics, 1986, pp 294–328
8. Green TP, Mirkin BL: Clinical pharmacokinetics: Pediatric considerations, in Benet LZ, et al (eds): Pharmacokinetic Basis for Drug Treatment. New York, Raven Press, 1984, pp 269–282
9. Morselli PL, Franco-Morselli R, Bossi L: Clinical pharmacokinetics in newborns and infants: Age-related differences and therapeutic implications. Clin Pharmacokinet 5:485–527, 1980
10. Pedersen S, Moller-Petersen J: Erratic absorption of a slow-release theophylline spinkle product. Pediatrics 74:534–538, 1984
11. Rogers RJ, Kalisker A, Wiener MB, et al.: Inconsistent absorption from a sustained-release theophylline preparation during continuous therapy in asthmatic children. J Pediatr 106:496–501, 1985
12. Wilson JT, Atwood GF, Shand DG: Disposition of propoxyphene and propranolol in children. Clin Pharmacol Ther 19:264–270, 1976
13. Lindenbaum J, Rund DG, Butler VP Jr, et al: Inactivation of digoxin by the gut flora: Reversal by antibiotic therapy. N Engl J Med 305:789–827, 1981
14. Linday L, Dobkin JF, Wang TC, et al: Digoxin inactivation by the gut flora in infancy and childhood. Pediatrics 79:544–548, 1987
15. Notterman DA: Pediatric pharmacotherapy, in Chernow B (ed): The Pharmacologic Approach to the Critically Ill Patient, 2nd ed. Baltimore, Williams & Wilkins, 1988, pp 131–155
16. Radde IC: Mechanisms of drug absorption and their development, in MacLeod SM, Radde IC (eds): Textbook of Pediatric Clinical Pharmacology. Littleton, Mass, PSG, 1985, pp 25–26
17. Steward DJ: Anaesthesia in childhood, in MacLeod SM, Radde IC (eds): Textbook of Pediatric Clinical Pharmacology. Littleton, Mass, PSG, 1985, pp 365–378
18. Koren G: Clinical pharmacology of antimicrobial drugs during development: How are infants and children different? in Koren G, Prober CG, Gold R (eds): Antimicrobial Therapy in Infants and Children. New York, Marcel Dekker, 1988, pp 47–52
19. Dill WA, Kazenko A, Wolf LM, et al: Studies on 5,5-diphenylhydantoin (Dilantin) in animals and man. J Pharmacol Exp Ther 118:270–276, 1956
20. Hendeles L, Weinberger M: Theophylline: A state of the art review. Pharmacotherapy 3:2–44, 1983
21. Heimann G, Gladtke E: Pharmacokinetics of phenobarbital in childhood. Eur J Clin Pharmacol 12:305–310, 1977
22. Pacifici GM, Viani A, Teddencci-Brunelli G, et al: Effects of development, aging and renal and hepatic insufficiency as well as hemodialysis on the plasma concentrations of albumin and alpha$_1$ acid glycoprotein: Implications for binding of drugs. Ther Drug Monit 8:259–263, 1986
23. Andersson KE, Bertler A, Wettrell G: Post-mortem distribution and tissue concentrations of digoxin in infants and adults. Acta Paediatr Scand 64:497–504, 1975
24. Park MK, Ludden T, Arom KV, et al: Myocardial vs serum digoxin concentrations in infants and adults. Am J Dis Child 136:418–420, 1982
25. Gorodischer R, Jusko WJ, Jaffe SJ: Tissue and erythrocyte distribution of digoxin in infants. Clin Pharmacol Ther 19:256–263, 1976
26. Wagner JG, Dick M, Behrendt DM, et al: Determination of myocardial and serum digoxin concentrations in children by specific and nonspecific assay methods. Clin Pharmacol Ther 33:577–583, 1983
27. Brazier JL, Salle B, Ribon B, et al: In vivo N$_7$-methylation of theophylline to caffeine in premature infants. Dev Pharmacol Ther 2:137–144, 1981
28. Aranda JV, Scalais E, Papageorgiou A, Beharry K: Ontogeny of human caffeine and theophylline metabolism. Dev Pharmacol Ther 7(suppl 1):18–25, 1984
29. Miller RP, Roberts RJ, Fischer LJ. Acetaminophen elimination kinetics in neonates, children and adults. Clin Pharmacol Ther 19:284–294, 1976
30. Clarke JT, Libke RD, Regamey C, Kirby WMM: Comparative pharmacokinetics of amikacin and kanamycin. Clin Pharmacol Ther 15:610–616, 1974
31. Howard JB, McCracken GH Jr: Pharmacological evaluation of amikacin in neonates. Antimicrob Agents Chemother 8:86–90, 1975
32. Vogelstein B, Kowarski A, Lietman PS: The pharmacokinetics of amikacin in children. J Pediatr 91:333–339, 1977
33. Brown RD, Campoli-Richards DM: Antimicrobial therapy in neonates, infants, and children. Clin Pharmacokinet 17(suppl 1):105–115, 1989
34. Riva R, Contin M, Albani F, et al: Free concentration of carbamazepine and carbamazepine-10,11-epoxide in children and adults: Influence of age and phenobarbitone cometabolism. Clin Pharmacokinet 10:524–531, 1985
35. Leeder JS, Gold R: Cephalosporins, in Koren G, Prober CG, Gold R (eds): Antimicrobial Therapy in Infants and Children. New York, Marcel Dekker, 1988, pp 173–235
36. Bell MJ, Shackelford P, Smith R, Schroeder K: Pharmacokinetics of clindamycin phosphate in the first year of life. J Pediatr 105:482–486, 1984
37. Kauffman RE, Shoeman DW, Wan SH, Azarnoff DL: Absorption and excretion of clindamycin———phosphate in children after intramuscular injection. Clin Pharmacol Ther 13:704–709, 1973
38. Morrow JI, Richens A: Disposition of anticonvulsants in childhood. Clin Pharmacokinet 17(suppl 1):89–104, 1989
39. Rowland M, Tozer TN: Age and weight, in Rowland M, Tozer TN (eds): Clinical Pharmacokinetics Concepts and Applications. Philadelphia, Lea & Febiger, 1980, p 224
40. Benet LZ, Massoud N, Gambertoglio JG (eds): Pharmacokinetic

Basis for Drug Treatment. New York, Raven Press, 1984, pp 435–438

41. Evans WE, Feldman S, Ossi M, et al: Gentamicin dosage in children: A randomized prospective comparison of body weight and body surface area as dose determinants. J Pediatr 94:139–143, 1979

42. McCracken GH: Clinical pharmacology of gentamicin in infants 2 to 24 months of age. Am J Dis Child 124:884–887, 1972

43. Paisley JW, Smith AL, Smith DH: Gentamicin in new born infants. Am J Dis Child 126:473–477, 1973

44. Kauffman RE, Fox B, Gupta N: Ibuprofen antipyresis and pharmacokinetics in children (abstract). Pediatr Res 25:67A, 1989

45. Walson PD, Galletta G, Braden NJ, Alexander L: Ibuprofen, acetaminophen, and placebo treatment of febrile children. Clin Pharmacol Ther 46:9–17, 1989

46. Benvenuti C, Cancellieri V, Gambaro V, et al: Pharmacokinetics of two new oral formulations of ibuprofen. Int J Clin Pharmacol Ther Toxicol 24:308–312, 1986

47. Kergueris MF, Bourin M, Laroussec: Pharmacokinetics of isoniazid: Influence of age. Eur J Clin Pharmacol 30:335–340, 1986

48. Brogden RN, Pinder RM, Sower PR, et al: Naproxen: A review of its pharmacological properties and therapeutic efficacy and use. Drugs 9:326–363, 1975

49. Kauffman RE, Bolinger RO, Wan SH, Oren J: Pharmacokinetics and metabolism of naproxen in children. Dev Pharmacol Ther 5:143–150, 1982

50. Cloyd JC, Leppik IE: Primidone absorption, distribution, and excretion, in Levy RH, et al (eds): Antiepileptic Drugs, 3rd ed. New York, Raven Press, 1989, pp 391–400

51. Kauffman RE, Habersang R, Lansky L: Kinetics of primidone metabolism and excretion in children. Clin Pharmacol Ther 22:200–205, 1977

52. Thirumoorthi MC, Asmar BI, Buckley JA, et al: Pharmacokinetics of intravenously administered piperacillin in preadolescent children. J Pediatr 102:941–946, 1983

53. Szefler SJ, Pieroni DR, Gingell RL, Shen DD: Rapid elimination of quinidine in pediatric patients. Pediatrics 70:370–375, 1982

54. Shalit I: Rifampin, in Koren G, Prober CG, Gold R (eds): Antimicrobial Therapy in Infants and Children. New York, Marcel Dekker, 1988, pp 373–403

55. Vree TB, Hekster YA, Lippens RJJ: Clinical pharmacokinetics of sulfonamides in children: Relationship between maturing kidney function and renal clearance of sulfonamides. Ther Drug Monit 7:130–147, 1985

56. Aranda JV, Grondin D, Sasyniuk BI: Pharmacologic considerations in the therapy of neonatal apnea. Pediatr Clin North Am 28:113–133, 1981

57. Lisby SM, Nahata M: Penicillins, in Koren G, Prober CG, Gold R (eds): Antimicrobial Therapy in Infants and Children. New York, Marcel Dekker, 1988, pp 117–152

58. Kaplan JM, McCrackin GH, Thomas ML, et al: Clinical pharmacology of tobramycin in newborns. Am J Dis Child 125:656–660, 1973

59. Bruni J, Wilder BJ, Willmore LJ, et al: Steady-state kinetics of valproic acid in epileptic patients. Clin Pharmacol Ther 24:324–332, 1978

60. Hall K, Otten N, Irvine-Meek J, et al: First-dose and steady-state pharmacokinetics of valproic acid in children with seizures. Clin Pharmacokinet 8:447–455, 1983

61. Milliken JF: Vancomycin, in Koren G, Prober CG, Gold R (eds): Antimicrobial Therapy in Infants and Children. New York, Marcel Dekker, 1988, pp 265–285

62. Balis FM, Pizzo PA, Eddy J, et al: Pharmacokinetics of zidovudine administered intravenously and orally in children with human immunodeficiency virus infection. J Pediatr 114:880–884, 1989

63. Langtry HD, Campoli-Richards DM: Zidovudine: A review of its pharmacodynamic and pharmacokinetic properties and therapeutic efficacy. Drugs 37:408–450, 1989

64. Park MK: Use of digoxin in infants and children with specific emphasis on dosage. J Pediatr 108:871–877, 1986

65. Wilder BJ, Rangel RJ: Phenytoin clinical use, in Levy RH, et al (eds): Antiepileptic Drugs, 3rd ed. New York, Raven Press, 1989, pp 233–239

66. Elders MJ, Wingfield BS, McNatt ML, et al: Glucocorticoid therapy in children. Am J Dis Child 129:1393–1396, 1975

67. Mattes J, Gittleman R: Growth of hyperactive children on maintenance regimen of methylphenidate. Arch Gen Psychiatry 4:317–322, 1983

68. Stewart DJ: Prevalence of tetracyclines in children's teeth. II. Resurvey after five years. Br Med J 3:320–322, 1973

69. Muszynski MJ, Christenson JC, Scribner RK: DNA-gyrase inhibitors: Nalidixic acid, quinolones, and novobiocin, in Koren G, Prober CG, Gold R (eds): Antimicrobial Therapy in Infants and Children. New York, Marcel Dekker, 1988, pp 433–463

70. Wong DF, Wagner HN, Dannals RF, et al: Effects of age on dopamine and serotonin receptors measured by positron tomography of the living human brain. Science 226:1393, 1984

71. Morton HG: Atropine intoxication its manifestations in infants and children. J Pediatr 14:755–760, 1939

72. American Academy of Pediatrics: Use of codeine and dextromethorphan-containing cough syrups in pediatrics. Pediatrics 62:118–122, 1978

73. Garson A Jr: Medicolegal problems in the management of cardiac arrhythmias in children. Pediatrics 79:84–88, 1987

74. American Academy of Pediatrics: Valproic acid: Benefits and risks. Pediatrics 70:316–319, 1982

75. McCraken GH Jr: Aminoglycoside toxicity in infants and children. Am J Med 8:172–175, 1986

76. Hermann G: Renal toxicity of aminoglycosides in the neonatal period. Pediatr Pharmacol 3:251–254, 1983

77. Peterson RG, Rumack GH: Age as a variable in acetaminophen overdose. Arch Intern Med 141:390–398, 1981

78. Lieh-lai MW, Sarnaik AP, Newton JF, et al: Metabolism and pharmacokinetics of acetaminophen in a severely poisoned young child. J Pediatr 105:125–128, 1984

79. Warner LO, Beach TP, Garvin JP: Halothane and children: The first quarter century. Anesth Analg 63:838–842, 1984

80. Food and Drug Administration: Hepatitis associated with isoniazid—warning. FDA Drug Bull 8:11, 1978

81. Habersang RWO: Dosage, in Shirkey HC (ed): Pediatric Therapy, 6th ed. St Louis, CV Mosby, 1980, pp 17–20

82. Dodson WE: Nonlinear kinetics of phenytoin in children. Neurology 32:42–48, 1982

23

DRUG THERAPEUTICS IN THE ADOLESCENT

KAREN HEIN

The reasons for including a special review on therapeutics in adolescence are as follows. Growth during puberty of body tissues and organs that absorb, distribute, metabolize, and excrete drugs affects the amount of drug needed and the frequency of drug administration.[1] Behavioral and psychological changes in adolescence require a different "contract" between patient and health provider.[2] Certain biochemical properties of a drug may have special importance during the teenage years. Examples include the lipid solubility of a compound, the extent of protein binding, and the degree of competition with endogenous substances (e.g., sex steroids) for common metabolizing enzyme systems.

A review of the changes in the body and environment of the adolescent that have particular relevance for the type, amount, and frequency of drug use is provided. For most classes of drugs, the dose and dose interval differ between childhood and adulthood. When one considers the total amount of medication that is prescribed or taken therapeutically plus the nontherapeutic or illegal substances consumed, it behooves the health care provider to know the action and interaction of these agents in order to provide optimal care for teenagers.

Virtually all youngsters will use a prescribed, over-the-counter (OTC), and/or illicit drug during their teenage years. The dose, response, and side effects of these medications when taken by teenagers may be very different from those noted in children and adults. Even among different teenagers, a wide range of doses is required. Some of the factors that are known to influence the dose–response relationship are reviewed.[3] More important, some of the special factors that must be considered in caring for adolescent patients are highlighted.

TYPES OF DRUGS

Teenagers certainly take much more medication than that prescribed by a physician. Rarely do we consider the

effects of the interaction of OTC drugs or illicit drugs on the adolescent. The exact amounts of medications consumed by American adolescents over the decade of the teenager years is unknown.[4] Most surveys focus on illicit drug use by young people. There are no comparable data about the extent of use of OTC and prescribed medications.

Prescribed and Over-the-Counter Medications

There are only two surveys of the use of OTC and prescribed medication by youngsters under the age of 17. An annual survey of high school students includes the use of psychoactive medications among high school students.[5] In the other survey of OTC and prescribed medications other than psychoactive medications,[6] the authors grouped children and adolescents under the age of 17 years together. Nonetheless, there is some information about the extent of OTC use by youngsters in the community who are not necessarily seeking health care in a doctor's office. During the 2-week period of the survey, 13 percent had taken one prescribed medication and 21.5 percent had taken one OTC medication. The most frequently used OTC categories were analgesics (29.4 percent), cold/cough remedies (19.2 percent), vitamins (15.7 percent), and anti-infectious agents (12.4 percent). These four categories accounted for three-fourths of the instances of drug use. Although most of the prescribed medications taken were new prescriptions as opposed to refills, the majority (63 percent) of the OTC medications taken were already in the household. It is not known if the amount, types, and frequency of use of prescribed or OTC medications differ between childhood and adolescence. If these data are used to estimate yearly consumption of medications by youngsters under the age of 17 years, an average of three prescriptions and five OTC medications would be consumed per child per year.

TABLE 23-1. PRINCIPAL DRUGS MISUSED BY ADOLESCENT ATHLETES

DRUGS	ERGOGENIC?	MAIN TOXIC EFFECTS
Amphetamines	Yes	Tachycardia, hypertension, hyperactivity, insomnia, tremor, palpitations, aggressiveness, increased number of injuries
Caffeine	Yes	Tremor, hyperactivity, diuresis
Anabolic/androgenic steroids	Yes	Azospermia, testicular atrophy, hepatocellular carcinoma, atherogenic cholesterol profile, gynecomastia (in males), hirsutism (in females)
Vitamins	No	None in moderate doses
Protein supplements	No	None

Source: Reprinted by permission of Elsevier Science Publishing Co., Inc., from Dyment P: The adolescent athlete and ergogenic aids. J Adolesc Health Care 8:68–73, 1987. Copyright 1987 by the Society for Adolescent Medicine.

Ergogenic Aids

Ergogenic aids are substances used by adolescents to improve their athletic performance. Some examples of such drugs include psychomotor stimulants, anabolic steroids, nutritional aids, narcotic analgesics, local anesthetics, illicit drugs, and anti-inflammatory agents.

These drugs are commonly used and are available outside the health care delivery network. The balance of benefits versus risks, side effects, and drug interactions are rarely considered by the teenage athlete because the consensus among young people is that these agents are safe and effective.[7]

The principal drugs misused by adolescent athletes are shown on Table 23-1. Since most teenage athletes know that the use of some of the ergogenic aids such as amphetamines and anabolic steroids is not permitted, adolescents will not reveal use to a physician unless confidentiality is ensured. Despite the fact that the use of over 50 specific stimulants, sympathomimetic amines, narcotic analgesics, and anabolic steroids was banned at the Olympics and by other competitive athletic organizations for youth, nonetheless, use of ergogenic aids continues to be common among teenage athletes.

Illicit Drugs

Current data regarding illicit drug use by high school students are provided in Figure 23-1.[5] The epidemic of illicit drug use in the 1960s and 1970s has declined among American high school students. The proportion of students reporting any illicit drug use declined by approximately one-fourth between 1979 and 1984. However, the rates are still the highest among all industrialized nations. In 1987, over half (57 percent) of seniors had tried an illicit drug and over a third had tried a drug other than marijuana.

The vast majority of students had tried alcohol (over 90 percent) and cigarettes (over 60 percent) by their senior year. Of concern is the persistence of a small subgroup of heavy users over the last 5 of the 13 years of the annual survey. For cigarettes, there is a higher percentage of female daily users (>20 percent) and ½ pack per day smokers (about 15 percent) than males. In addition, roughly 10 percent of males and 5 percent of females reported daily use of alcohol, and 3.3 percent report daily use of marijuana. Cocaine use had risen to nearly 13 percent of students in 1986. However, the most recent survey, in 1987, showed a decline by one-fifth in "ever use" as well as "frequent use" among students in the past year. The principal investigators of the Monitoring the Future project concluded that "the kinds of young people most at risk remain much the same, although the types and amounts of substances they use shift somewhat from year to year."[5]

The longitudinal studies provide invaluable information about trends among high school students. However, a subgroup of adolescents who are not living at home and are not attending school accounts for some of the heavier drug users and abusers during adolescence. Trends in substance use by one group of inner-city institutionalized youngsters with a high percentage of teenage runaways and truants help complete the picture of the usage pattern of teenagers in the past two decades.[8] Opiate use peaked in the early 1970s and was replaced by marijuana as the most common illicit drug reported by 80,000 teenagers admitted to New York City's only detention facility for adolescents between 1968 and 1978. Although no system-

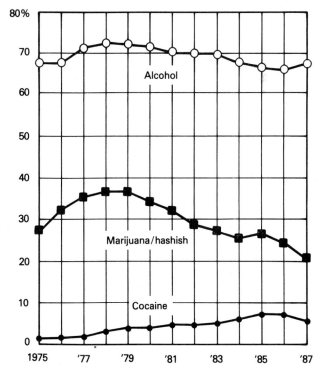

FIGURE 23-1. Drug and alcohol use among high school seniors. (From Johnston L, O'Malley P, Bachman J: Illicit Drug Use, Smoking and Drinking by America's High School Students, College Students and Young Adults, 1975–1987. Washington, National Institute on Drug Abuse, 1988, by permission.)

atic surveys of cocaine use by disenfranchised youth (runaways, incarcerated youth, or school dropouts) have been conducted, nonetheless, it is evident that many of the more troubled youth are now heavy users of "crack," the smokable form of cocaine.

Census estimates are that there are approximately 1 million teenage runaways per year and 250,000 youths living in institutions in the United States. We must include this "hidden population" in our review of national drug use patterns.

Brunswick and Josefson[9] surveyed a representative sample of Harlem youths twice, first when they were 12–17 years old and again when they were 18–23 years old. Although this was a household survey, the data are helpful because they were gathered from a population whose truancy rate is higher than average. Lifetime prevalence for three or more episodes of the use of alcohol (80 percent), marijuana (79 percent), cocaine (33 percent), and heroin (15 percent) were higher than those reported in a national probability sample in 1977.

Finally, the nontherapeutic use of psychoactive drugs has increased dramatically in the past decades.[10] In summary, four categories of medications are consumed by American youths: prescribed, over-the-counter, ergogenic, and illicit. An appropriate evaluation of the teenager means that each category must be considered by the health professional at all stages of evaluation and treatment of an adolescent.

DETECTING DRUGS OF ABUSE BY LABORATORY TECHNIQUES

Until recently, a history of illicit drug use was the only method of determining actual use. However, with the increased availability of relatively inexpensive enzyme-multiplied immunoassay tests (EMIT), thin-layer chromatography (TLC), and radioimmunoassay (RIA), and the more expensive, but more definitive gas chromatography/mass spectrometry (GS/MS), testing body fluids for the presence of illicit drugs has become a widely available, albeit controversial, resource.

Despite the widespread use of laboratory testing for adults, there are special considerations in applying these technical capabilities to adolescents:

1. Are the standards developed for adults appropriate for adolescents?
2. Does the use of these methods of detection further or hinder the development of a trusting relationship between physician and teenager that will result in the ability to achieve longer-term objectives of care?
3. Are the specific characteristics of drug metabolism, distribution, storage, and release sufficiently well delineated in adolescents to ensure proper interpretation of results?
4. Do the circumstances under which laboratory detection of drugs of abuse occur take into consideration the legal and ethical rights of the adolescent? Is the adolescent aware that these tests are

being performed and what the possible consequences are? When dealing with minors, what degree of confidentiality exists concerning notification of parents or other authorities?

In cases of overdose, where knowledge of the etiologic agent may be lifesaving, laboratory testing for illicit substances is often indicated. However, routine or mandatory screening for job or school entry or periodic random testing are areas of greater controversy. If the purpose is to identify individuals in need of counseling, laboratory detection may deter rather than encourage teenagers to engage in the long-term process of behavioral change.

Technical Aspects of Determining Agents of Abuse[11]

EMIT techniques have been modified to permit semiquantitative determination of some substances. For example, the EMIT-dau system can be used to differentiate low-positive (20–75 ng/ml) from high-positive results (>75 ng/ml) for marijuana metabolites. EMIT can be used for most common drugs of abuse except LSD. Urine specimens used for LSD detection must be shielded from light because metabolites decompose on exposure to light or heat. RIA techniques can detect cocaine, PCP, amphetamines, barbiturates, LSD, and heroin. TLC enables quantitative evaluation of metabolites, including the most common marijuana metabolite as well as other common drugs of abuse. GC/MS is highly sensitive and specific but is not as widely available. The equipment and personnel costs result in this technique being used for confirmation rather than initial screening. Alternative techniques employing HPLC and GLC are rarely used because of high cost and necessity for highly trained personnel. There are also commercially available tests promoted as being particularly easy and quick to perform. The Federal Drug Administration's Bureau of Medical Devices can be used as a source of information for the reliability of these methods, which can vary enormously. Therefore, such methods should not be used unless approved by this agency.

Because the consequences of the results of laboratory detection can be considerable, the decision to test (except in the case of an overdose) is optimally made by the adolescent in conjunction with the physician, not merely at the request of the parent. The degree of confidentiality about the tests being done, the results, and the recording of the information for current and future use are all items that require careful and thorough discussion with the adolescent prior to obtaining body fluid samples for drug determination (except, of course, in a life-threatening situation).

Marijuana metabolites can be detected in blood for only a few hours. However, given the lipophilic nature of the compounds, delta 9-THC, a common major cannabinoid metabolite can be detected in urine for days after last use. Repeated marijuana use can result in storage of metabolites in adipose tissue that can be released for a month or more after last use. Similarly, PCP, another lipophilic substance, can be detected in urine for more than a week after last exposure. Therefore, the selection of body fluid for testing and the interpretation of the results require knowledge of the characteristics of the specific drug, the limitations and strengths of the particular method of detection, and possible sources of variation in drug disposition in a given teenager. These three factors necessitate a close working relationship between the primary care physician and a knowledgeable clinical pharmacologist or laboratory staff.

AGE-RELATED CHANGES IN DRUG DISPOSITION

Variation in drug disposition between subjects ranges from 3- to 40-fold. Factors accounting for the variation include age, sex, and genetic constitution, as well as environmental influences.[12] Reviews of age-related differences in dose requirements, toxicity, and effectiveness of many therapeutic agents have elucidated changes in drug absorption, distribution, metabolism, and excretion principally during four stages of development: neonates, children, adults, and the elderly.[13] Studies of sex-related differences in drug metabolism for many classes of drugs[14] (anesthetics, narcotics, alcohol, analgesics, anticonvulsants, and stimulants) demonstrate that the drug effect may be more pronounced or may persist longer in adult females as compared with males or younger children.[15] It is assumed that puberty is a time when certain alterations in drug-utilization patterns appear. Few studies have determined the exact time or nature of the alterations in adolescence.[16,17]

Definition of Age-Related Changes

Three ways of defining the age-related changes between childhood and adulthood that occur mainly in adolescence are (1) the decrease in dose (mg/kg), (2) the increase in half-life of elimination (minutes or hours), and (3) the increase in the ratio of concentration to dose. These three age-related changes are graphically displayed in Figure 23–2. These changes appear mostly to be due to the effects of somatic growth and changes in organ function, such as the liver, that occur within the growing adolescent's body.

Effect of Pubertal Hormonal Changes

CHANGES IN BODY COMPOSITION. Because drugs are differentially distributed into body tissues depending on their solubility characteristics, knowing the amount of fat or water in a given patient may be a key factor in understanding why that patient requires a certain amount of a given drug. As an individual enters puberty, the amounts of fat, water, and lean body mass change. Drugs will be distributed in a new way based on these body compositional factors.[18]

During adolescence, height is increased by approximately 25 percent, and weight is nearly doubled.[19] Lean body mass, skeletal mass, and body fat are equal per unit of body weight in prepubertal boys and girls, but by maturity, women have twice as much fat relative to total-body weight as adult men.[20] The peak lean body mass growth velocity in males occurs 2 years later than in females on average and coincides with peak height velocity.[21] Total-body water and extracellular water decrease with age.[22] Nomograms[23] and formulas have been developed for predicting body density and total-body fat from combinations of anthropometric measures, including skin-fold thickness and limb and girth circumferences.[24-27] These relationships are based on direct measurements of body composition by either underwater weighing, potassium (^{40}K) counting techniques, or chloride space measurements.

The effect of puberty on drug disposition is graphically displayed in Figures 23–3 and 23–4. In Figure 23–3, the teenager's body is viewed as a "tank" with various compartments. Drugs that are put into the tank exit by one of two outflow tracts, either metabolism or excretion. During puberty, the rise in sex steroids predominantly affects two parts of this system. First, it affects the composition of the tank by influencing body composition. Second, it affects metabolism largely through alterations in liver function.

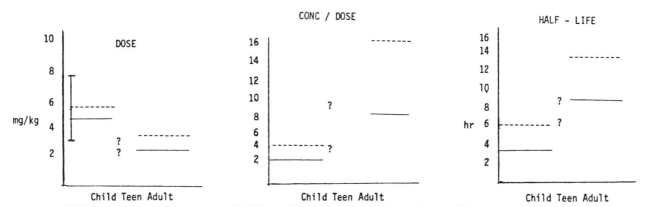

FIGURE 23–2. Comparison of children, adolescents, and adults in dose, half-life, and ratio of concentration to dose for two model drugs, theophylline (———) and imipramine (---------). (From Hein K: Use of therapeutics in adolescence. J Adolesc Health Care 8: 8–35, 1987, by permission.)

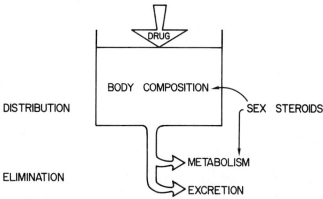

FIGURE 23–3. Schematic representation of the effect of pubertal development on drug disposition showing the potential effects of the rise in sex steroids on body composition and organ function. (From Hein K: Use of therapeutics in adolescence. J Adolesc Health Care 8: 8–35, 1987, by permission.)

In Figure 23–3, the schematic diagram shows a simplified version of the potential effect of the rise in sex steroids on drug disposition. As a drug or medication enters the adolescent's body, it is distributed according to its solubility characteristics and transport features into various body compartments. The composition of the tank will influence the distribution and extent of storage in each compartment. For example, a given dose of a water-soluble drug will be distributed very differently into the tissues of two normal 14-year-old teenagers if one is a male (Tanner V) with 60 percent of his body weight composed of water and the other is a female (Tanner V) with only 45 percent of her total body weight composed of water. Once distributed, there may be a difference in rates of metabolism and excretion. These differences are, to a large extent, due to genetic factors. However, differences also have been documented in rates of elimination between males and females.

In Figure 23–4, the system is translated into simplified pharmacologic terms. The size of the tank into which the drug is distributed is described by the volume of distribution. The process of drug elimination, simply stated, is

a combination of drug metabolism and excretion. These processes are described by drug half-life. Clearance is a function of both volume of distribution and the effect of changes in organs (such as the liver) on subsequent changes in drug metabolism. By investigating these two aspects of drug disposition, a clearer understanding of the differences in drug clearance between childhood and adulthood will emerge and can form the basis of a more rational dose schedule for rapidly growing teenagers.

CHANGES IN ORGAN FUNCTION. Understanding hepatic changes is key to explaining the alterations in drug utilization that occur during puberty.[28] Several structural and functional changes occur during puberty. The rate of enzyme activity is usually low in the fetus, higher in the neonate, and in some cases, peak in preadolescence.[29] Liver cells are predominantly of a higher nuclear class and are multinuclear by the time sexual maturation is established in animals and humans.[30] The activity of liver microsomal enzyme systems changes with age and differs between males and females by adulthood.[31] Steroid hormones are metabolized by the same enzymes that metabolize many drugs. Sex differences in the oxidation of drugs by liver enzymes appear mainly to be due to higher binding capacity of the cytochrome P-450 system in males as compared with females. In addition, a slight sex difference in the activity of microsomal NADPH-linked electron transport systems may be a contributory factor.[32] Studies of hepatic fine structure in rodents have delineated changes in the surface area of smooth endoplasmic reticulum (SER) in the portal and central lobar areas. The presence of higher amounts of androgens is believed to play an important role in the changes in oxidative enzyme systems and the resultant changes in SER.

In summary, the changes in body composition affect the way a given drug is distributed within the body. Changes in organ structure and function, specifically those in the liver, affect the rate of metabolism and, therefore, the excretion of a drug. These two factors may account for some of the variability in drug dose and response noted among pubertal individuals and between children and adults for almost all classes of drugs.

PHARMACOLOGIC PRINCIPLES

Dose–Response Relationship

When a teenager takes a medication, the response depends on three things: how much is taken, what happens once it has entered the body, and how quickly and completely it is eliminated.

In the remainder of this section, selected pharmacokinetic principles will be reviewed, emphasizing those features of greatest importance in caring for the teenager. If a different age group, i.e., the neonate, were the focus of discussion, then other factors would be given greater importance. As an example, changes in absorption of drugs are key to understanding pharmacokinetics in the neonate, whereas there appears to be little difference in absorption of many drug medications between children and adolescents.

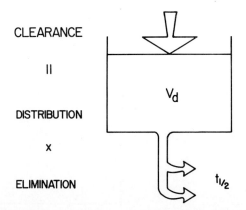

FIGURE 23–4. Schematic representation of the effect of pubertal development on drug disposition translated into pharmacologic terms. (From Hein K: Use of therapeutics in adolescence. J Adolesc Health Care 8: 8–35, 1987, by permission.)

Step 1

DRUG DOSE. Doses for children that are based on a proportion of the adult dose tend to underestimate required dose. For young children, the doses based on weight (mg/kg) required by most children are a reflection of their higher metabolic rate and different organ/body tissue proportions.[12] At some point, adult dose ranges are needed to achieve therapeutic or desired response. The point of conversion from the higher childhood dose to the lower adult dose differs depending on the drug and the stage of development of the teenager. For only a few compounds is the precise time of changeover in dose known.[33] Studies are currently underway to define this change in dose as a function of Tanner staging and body composition so that in the future we will be better able to predict the proper dose for a rapidly growing teenager.

TYPE OF PREPARATION AND ROUTE. Tablets and capsules are acceptable to most teenagers. Because they are more easily transported than liquids and are more "adult appearing," adolescents may be more likely to be compliant with a pill and capsule regimen than with a regimen involving liquid preparations. Rectal administration is particularly objectionable to most adolescents.

Step 2

ABSORPTION. The amount of drug absorbed is a function of properties of the drug itself (biochemical properties, e.g., lipid solubility), the formulation (capsule versus liquid), preferred absorption site (stomach, duodenum, jejunum, etc.), and the means of absorption (passive diffusion versus active transport). Knowing the site of absorption is important. For example, alcohol is absorbed from the stomach. A rapid, fairly predictable clinical effect is noted when alcohol is consumed without food. Marijuana, a very lipid-soluble compound, has greatly variable absorption that is often delayed and is highly unpredictable when consumed by mouth, particularly in the presence of food.[34] Theophylline can be formulated in a variety of slow-release products with resulting differences in rate of absorption.[35] These common examples emphasize the importance of knowing where the drug is absorbed and what other factors are likely to affect absorption.

Few studies have compared absorption differences between children and adolescents. In one study, adolescents aged 13 years had slower absorption of anticonvulsants (ethosuximide, phenobarbital, clonazepam, and diazepam) than children.[36]

Malabsorption may be present in teenagers with chronic inflammatory bowel disease or in patients with prolonged severe eating disorders (anorexia nervosa or bulimia), which can affect gastrointestinal morphology, pH, and motility. Generally speaking, a higher dose is required if malabsorption is present.[37]

DISTRIBUTION. Drugs are absorbed from the gastrointestinal tract when given by mouth or rectum or are deposited directly into the plasma compartment when given parenterally. Most drugs are bound to plasma proteins, yet only free drug is available for diffusion into cells or other compartments. An equilibrium is created between bound and free drug. Factors that influence binding, therefore, are important in determining how much free drug reaches cells, the true site of drug action.[38] Drugs differ in their affinity for plasma proteins and the type of protein that binds the drug.[39] A drug with a greater affinity for plasma proteins can displace a weakly bound drug.

Decreased levels of plasma proteins can result in increased levels of free drug. Certain disease states (chronic inflammatory bowel disease, renal failure, severe or extreme starvation, hepatic disease) in which total-body protein and albumin are diminished may produce drug toxicity in patients taking the usual dosage if the serum proteins are not available for binding, causing higher free-drug levels.

TISSUE DISTRIBUTION. The amount of drug distribution into a given body compartment will depend on the biochemical properties of the drug (e.g., lipid solubility) and the amount of each tissue in a given patient's body.[40] For example, after a drug is absorbed or injected into the bloodstream, it is distributed to interstitial and cellular fluid according to two factors. The initial phase of distribution is most dependent on cardiac output and regional blood flow to certain organs that are highly perfused. During the first few minutes, the liver, heart, brain, and kidney receive most of the drug. The ratio between the size of these organs and the total body weight with a smaller proportion of total body weight represented by these organs as age increases.

The second phase of distribution is distinguished by the longer time period required for penetration to the remaining compartments, which are less highly perfused. This second phase includes distribution to muscle, fat, skin, and most viscera. For some drugs, the equilibrium between various body compartments is reached in minutes, whereas for others, the tissue distribution equilibrium takes several hours.

As with absorption, factors that account for accumulation of drug in tissues in higher amounts than would be explained by simple diffusion equilibrium include pH differences, binding to intracellular components, and once again, degree of fat solubility. Lipid-soluble substances obviously diffuse more quickly and completely through lipid membranes and can be stored in vast amounts in fatty tissues. For example, marijuana, a highly lipid-soluble compound, can be stored for weeks or, theoretically, longer in fat depots. Adolescent females who are Tanner IV or V may have twice as much fat relative to total body weight as Tanner IV or V males. Therefore, the duration of marijuana effect may be much longer in some teenage females. The range of fat as a percentage of total body weight between very thin and very obese teenagers is 7–50 percent. Because fat is relatively poorly perfused, it is a stable reservoir for drugs with a high partition coefficient (i.e., very fat soluble).

In contradistinction to marijuana, theophylline is an example of a drug with poor lipid solubility. It is largely distributed, therefore, in proportion to body water.[41] Dose should be based on lean body mass that contains approximately 73 percent water. The amount of fat, a relatively anhydrous tissue, is not a major factor in theophylline distribution. In obese adolescents or in females with a higher percent of fat, doses based on total body weight would tend to overestimate the amount needed to reach therapeutic levels.

Bone can become a reservoir for slow release of potentially toxic agents such as lead into the blood, a principle well known to health providers caring for younger children. Other agents can similarly be stored in bone for long periods of time. Tetracycline, frequently used to treat acne, bronchitis, or genitourinary tract infections in teenagers, as well as divalent metal ion chelating agents and other heavy metals accumulate in bone by absorption to bone surfaces and eventual incorporation into bone crystal itself.

The increase in the rate of long bone growth during the adolescent growth spurt results in greater surface area for drug absorption and incorporation. Some drugs influence bone growth by their effects on vitamin D metabolism. For example, anticonvulsants (phenytoin and phenobarbital) have been associated with the development of rickets in rapidly growing patients and/or in patients who had prolonged use of the drugs in childhood.[42] Some drugs are distributed differently into gonadal tissue. The use of more effective antineoplastic agents in children and adolescents has now led to long-term survivors of childhood cancer. Only recently have studies begun to focus on the effects of chemotherapy on reproductive capacity. Some agents are known to affect gonadal function. For example, cyclophosphamide can produce amenorrhea in females and testicular atrophy in some males.

Drugs that are bound to red blood cells or metabolized in red blood cells may be affected by hemoglobin concentration or hematocrit changes. For example, gentamicin levels vary inversely with hematocrit. A difference of 5 percent in hematocrit can lead to changes of 2 gm/ml. The normal rise in hemoglobin concentration that occurs during puberty, particularly in males, is likely to be important in predicting gentamicin levels.

Step 3: Biotransformation of Drugs

METABOLISM. Some of the metabolites may possess biologic activity that is more potent or toxic than the parent compound.[43] Hence the rate of formation of metabolites is a factor that may account for some of the age-related and sex-related differences in drug effect and toxicity.

Biotransformation of most drugs is accomplished by the liver microsomal enzyme systems.[44] Drugs absorbed by the gastrointestinal tract pass through the liver before entering the general circulation. Therefore, the liver enzyme systems have an opportunity to transform a drug before distribution to other body tissues. This *first-pass effect* is important in many drugs, such as imipramine, where up to 75 percent of the parent compound is metabolized during the first pass through the liver.[45]

Microsomal enzymes are responsible for glucuronide conjugation and most oxidative reactions involving drugs.[46] Processes of reduction and hydrolysis of drugs occur in both microsomal and nonmicrosomal systems. The degree of lipid solubility of a drug determines the ease

of penetration into the endoplasmic reticulum and also the degree of binding to cytochrome P-450, an important component of the oxidative enzyme system.

Some endogenous substances are also transformed by the same microsomal enzyme systems as drugs. For example, steroid hormones, fatty acids, and bilirubin compete for many of the same microsomal enzymes as drugs.

The rate of biotransformation of drugs can vary sixfold among individual patients. Both the rate and the susceptibility to induction of enzyme systems is genetically determined. However, clinical manifestations appear at different times in the life cycle. Activity of microsomal enzyme systems is low in the neonate, as is the ability to conjugate. The structural and functional changes in the liver that occur at puberty influence the rate of drug biotransformation. Before puberty, there are no functional differences between the male and female liver in rates of biotransformation. This is particularly true for those enzyme systems (oxidation and hydroxylation) which compete with the sex steroids themselves.

Volume of Distribution

The apparent V_d of a drug is that volume in which it appears to be distributed. If a drug is well distributed into both body water and fat, then the apparent V_d would be many times larger than body water itself.

The concept of volume of distribution is of utmost importance during adolescence because the pool or compartment into which a drug is distributed changes at this age. Total-body water (TBW), highest in the neonate (80 percent of body weight), decreases throughout childhood and is similar between girls and boys before puberty. In adulthood, men have a higher TBW (50–60 percent body weight). Once again, women usually have twice as much fat per unit of body weight as compared with men. Therefore, the volume of distribution of a drug changes as body composition changes. This is a predictable and important event in the course of development and will affect the dose of a drug needed to achieve a certain concentration. If the drug is distributed largely in body water, the dose for males may be higher than that for females after puberty but similar before puberty. If the drug is fat soluble, mature females may require a higher dose than younger females or mature males.

Half-Life

Drug half-life (elimination) may change during childhood and adolescence if the rate of metabolism or excretion changes. Differences in drug $t_{1/2}$ occur during the transition from neonate to child or adult to elderly. Adolescence is also a time when sex steroid–induced changes in organs that eliminate drugs occur. Therefore, changes in liver structure and function or renal function during puberty are likely to influence drug $t_{1/2}$. In general, children have a shorter $t_{1/2}$ than adults, whereas neonates and the elderly tend to have longer $t_{1/2}$ values.[47] Mature males may have a shorter $t_{1/2}$ for some drugs as compared with females because of the differences in function of drug excretory organs that occur during puberty.

Important examples of dose-dependent kinetics include ethanol, aspirin, phenytoin,[48] theophylline,[49,50] and imipramine. These drugs are commonly ingested by adolescents. In some cases, children or younger teenagers (early stages of development) may exhibit dose-dependent kinetics, whereas older teens and adults may not. Because $t_{1/2}$ and the time required to reach a plateau state can change if dose-dependent kinetics are operant, the clinician should be aware of which drugs are likely to exhibit this saturation effect, where increasing dose above a certain point will rapidly produce high concentrations and therefore toxic levels.

Clearance

Total-body clearance of a drug is the product of distribution (V_d) and the elimination rate constant (K_e). Generally speaking, clearance is lowest in the newborn. The elderly, adult, and child have increasing rates of drug clearance, respectively. Once again, the adolescent, depending on his or her degree of physical maturity, may demonstrate a higher or lower drug clearance than the child or adult depending on such factors as body composition (which determines volume of distribution) and liver renal function (which determines metabolic and excretory rates).

SPECIAL IMPLICATIONS FOR CERTAIN CLASSES OF MEDICATIONS

There are some conditions that are more common in adolescents than in children; therefore, the physician caring for teenagers should be familiar with the indications, side effects, and modifications in dose or frequency for teenagers. A few examples have been selected.

Drugs That Cause Sexual Dysfunction

Physical, psychological, and social changes are the major hallmarks of adolescent development. One's sense as a sexual being is profoundly affected by puberty and the social experiences that accompany this phase of life.

Medications that are associated with sexual dysfunction are sometimes required for treating conditions occurring during adolescence. It is important for physicians caring for adolescents to be knowledgeable about this aspect of medicating adolescents, and therefore, a special section of this chapter is dedicated to this topic. Pediatricians may not be as aware of these particular side effects because the medications are often used in treating adults. Also, anticipatory guidance is an important aspect of adolescent care, since sexual function and dysfunction are not topics that teenagers are likely to discuss unless the physician sets the stage for a nonjudgmental, confidential dialogue.

Some of the medications that are both linked to sexual dysfunction[51] and are more likely to be used by teenagers are as follows:

1. *Antihypertensive agents.* Thiazide diuretics are associated with impotence. Agents acting by means of peripheral sympatholytic action can additionally cause ejaculatory failure as opposed to centrally acting sympatholytics, where impotence is more common. Propranolol and other β-adrenergic-receptor blocking agents are associated with loss of libido and impotence. Medications not generally associated with sexual dysfunction include the angiotensin-converting enzyme inhibitors, calcium-channel blockers, and arteriolar dilators such as hydralazine, but the latter are less likely to be selected for use in adolescents for other reasons.

2. *Cimetidine.* Because of its antiandrogen activity and effect on prolactin, both loss of libido and/or impotence and galactorrhea are potential problems with cimetidine use.

3. *Antidepressant and antipsychotic agents.* Tricyclic antidepressants and monoamine oxidase inhibitors may affect sexual function in both males and females causing anorgasmia in some individuals.

4. *CNS depressants in large doses.* Medications that cause central nervous system depression in general, such as sedatives, antianxiety agents, and such illicit drugs as alcohol, opiates, and marijuana, can affect libido, impair erection, and delay or inhibit ejaculation.

5. *Anticancer agents.* As a result of the gonadal damage associated with some cancer chemotherapy, there may be a progressive loss of libido in both male and female patients as well as alterations in the timing and progress of puberty and, ultimately, reproductive capability.

Research in the area of sexual dysfunction related to medication use has focused almost entirely on adults, usually adult men. Therefore, some of the side effects mentioned are only assumed to occur in adolescents. However, there is no reason to believe that these side effects do not occur after puberty. Therefore, it is the responsibility of the physician to be able to initiate discussion of the possible side effects of prescribed medications, including the possibility of sexual dysfunction, when appropriate.

Antiepileptic Medications

Guidelines for some of the more commonly used antiepileptic medications are provided in Table 23–2.[33] Comparisons between children and adults of dose and half-life are provided.

Oral Contraceptives

Some of the positive and negative considerations for oral contraceptives as a choice for adolescents are given in Table 23–3.[54]

TABLE 23–2. DOSAGE OF COMMONLY USED ANTIEPILEPTIC DRUGS IN ADOLESCENTS

DRUG	ADOLESCENTS Dosage Range* (mg/day)	Therapeutic Range (μg/ml)	CHILDREN Dosage (mg/kg/day)	Half-Life (h)	ADULTS Dosage (mg/kg/day)	Half-Life (h)
Carbamazepine	600–1400	4–12	10–30	14–27	10–20	14–27
Clonazepam	2–8	0.005–0.070	0.05–0.2	20–40	0.05–0.2	20–40
Ethosuximide	750–1500	40–100	15–40	20–60	10–30	20–60
Phenobarbital	90–180	15–40	4–8	37–73	1.5–2	46–136
Phenytoin	200–500	10–20	5–10	5–14	4–6	10–34
Primidone	500–1500	5–12	10–25	5–11	10–20	6–18
Phenobarbital (derived)	—	15–40	—	37–73	—	46–136
Valproic acid	750–3000	40–150	15–60	8–15	15–60	6–15

*These dosage ranges are guidelines only. Individual patients may require more or less medication depending on the severity of their seizure disorder, the individual metabolic rate and clearance of the drug, and the presence of clinical toxicity.

Source: Reprinted by permission of Elsevier Science Publishing Co., Inc. from Shinnar S: Antiepileptic drugs in adolescents. J Adolesc Health Care 8:105–112, 1987. Copyright 1987 by the Society for Adolescent Medicine.

TABLE 23–3. POSITIVE AND NEGATIVE CONSIDERATIONS FOR ORAL CONTRACEPTIVES AS A CHOICE FOR ADOLESCENTS

POSITIVE	NEGATIVE
Highly effective	Must be taken daily
Protection against pelvic inflammatory disease	
Decreased incidence of anemia and benign ovarian cyst	Increased risk of thromboembolic disease
Decreased incidence of ovarian and endometrial cancer	Increased insulin resistance Increased gallbladder disease
Improvement in acne	Small risk of hepatocellular adenoma
Treatment of amenorrhea and oligoamenorrhea of known etiology	Occasional development of hypertension

Source: Reprinted by permission of Elsevier Science Publishing Co., Inc. from Cholst I, Carlon A: Oral contraceptives and dysmenorrhea. J Adolesc Health Care 8:121–128, 1987. Copyright 1987 by the Society for Adolescent Medicine.

Dysmenorrhea

Dysmenorrhea is the leading cause of school absence among adolescent females. This condition is more prevalent in young females after menarche than it is among older women. Some of the more frequently used medications for this common problem in adolescence are provided in Table 23–4.[52]

Common Genital Infections

A variety of organisms produce symptomatic and asymptomatic genital infections in adolescents. Many are transmitted sexually. The most common genital infections, the medications commonly used to treat them with the dosage schedules, and average wholesale price are provided in Table 23–5.[53]

Common Drug Interactions

Some medications are used alone or in combination more commonly in adolescence than during childhood. Therefore, a summary of the major interactions is provided in Table 23–6.

TABLE 23–4. RECOMMENDED DOSAGES OF DRUGS MOST FREQUENTLY USED TO TREAT DYSMENORRHEA*

CATEGORY	GENERIC NAME	COMMON TRADE NAME	DOSAGE
Salicylates	Aspirin		650 mg q4h
Acetic acid analogues	Indomethicin	Indocin	25 mg t.i.d.
Propionic acids	Ibuprofen	Motrin	400 mg q.i.d.
	Naproxen sodium	Anaprox	275 mg q6h (double first dose)
Fenamates	Metenamic acid	Ponstel	250 mg q6h (double first dose)

*Dosages may be adjusted. Consult package insert of *Physicians Desk Reference.*
Source: Reprinted by permission of Elsevier Science Publishing Co., Inc. from Cholst I, Carlon A: Oral contraceptives and dysmenorrhea. J Adolesc Health Care 8:121–128, 1987. Copyright 1987 by the Society for Adolescent Medicine.

TABLE 23–5. COMMONLY USED THERAPIES FOR TREATMENT OF ADOLESCENT GENITAL INFECTIONS

INFECTION	DRUG	DOSAGE SCHEDULE	AVERAGE WHOLESALE PRICE ($)
Trichomonas	Metronidazole (generic), Flagyl	2 gm × 1 day	1.60
			5.92
Candida	Nystatin (generic), Mycostatin	1 app. × 7 days	
			2.00
			7.95
	Clotrimazole	500 mg × 1	7.92
		200 mg × 3	9.49
Gardnerella vaginalis (NSV)	Metronidazole (generic), Flagyl	500 mg b.i.d. × 7 days	
			5.60
			20.72
N. gonorrhoeae	Procaine	4.8 × 10⁶ U	10.60
	Pen G +	I.M.	
	Probenecid	+ 1 gm	0.38
	Amoxicillin	3 gm × 1	2.52
	Tetracycline	500 mg q.i.d. × 7 days	2.80
	Doxycycline (generic), Vibramycin	100 mg b.i.d. × 7 days	
			9.10
			23.10
	Spectinomycin	2 gm I.M.	10.04
	Ceftriaxone	250 mg I.M.	8.70
C. trachomatis	see Tetracycline Doxycycline		
Herpes simplex	Acyclovir, topical ointment	15 gm	17.46
	Acyclovir, oral	200 mg 5×/day × 7 days	18.02

Source: Reprinted by permission of Elsevier Science Publishing Co., Inc. from Martien, K, Emans SJ: Treatment of common genital infections in adolescents. J Adolesc Health Care 8:129–136, 1987. Copyright 1987 by the Society for Adolescent Medicine.

TABLE 23–6. DRUG INTERACTIONS AMONG MEDICATIONS COMMONLY USED BY TEENAGERS

Alcohol

Despite the fact that alcohol is often considered a beverage, it is actually a drug with potent central nervous system depressant activity. Alcohol has a number of effects when taken concomitantly with other drugs.

Central nervous system depressants, sedatives, hypnotics, etc.: Tranquilizers, neuroleptics, hypnotics, antidepressants, antihistamines, antinauseants, analgesics are effect additive.
Beta blockers: Propranolol may enhance effects.
Caffeine: Despite commonly held opinion, caffeine does not reverse or counteract effects of alcohol.
INH: Small potential risk of increased hazards of driving (demonstration in driving-simulator tests).
Metronidazole: Has a disulfiramlike reaction.

Naproxen

Antacids: May reduce absorption.
Probenecid: Serum levels of naproxen raised.

Isoniazid

Antacids: Absorption of isoniazid is reduced by aluminum hydroxide.
Cheese or fish: Occasional reports of flushing reaction (headache, tachycardia, hypertension).
Rifampin: May increase incidence of hepatoxicity.

Tetracycline

Antacids: Markedly reduce absorption if taken with aluminum-containing antacids.
Iron preparations: Absorption of both markedly reduced.
Milk and dairy products: Reduced absorption due to tetracycline-calcium chelates.

Anticonvulsants

Barbiturates and caffeine: Hypnotic effects of pentobarbital antagonized by caffeine.
Rifampin: Increases metabolism of hexobarbital threefold.
Carbamazepine and dextropropoxyphene: Level of carbamazepine can be raised into toxic range.
Phenytoin and INH: Rise in phenytoin levels; particularly at risk are slow isoniazid metabolizers.
Phenytoin and theophylline: Phenytoin levels lowered.

Antihypertensives.

Phenothiazines: With exception of guanethidine-like drugs, hypotension can be precipitated by some phenothiazines.
Guanethidine and related drugs and alcohol: Orthostatic hypotension exaggerated by alcohol.

Oral Contraceptives

Antacids: Reduced *(in vitro)* reliability if taken with magnesium trisilicate.
Antiasthmatic preparations: Oral contraceptives may improve or worsen asthma; therefore, asthma medications may need to be altered.
Antibiotics: Case reports of pregnancy with use of chloramphenicol, erythromycin, cephalexin, rifampin, tetracycline, clindamycin, nitrofurantoin, clotrimazole, and more commonly, ampicillin (sometimes preceded by breakthrough bleeding indicating possible insufficient oral contraceptive hormonal levels).
Anticonvulsant: Contraceptive failure reported with phenytoin, primidone, barbiturates, and possibly carbamazepine. Also, epileptic control may be disturbed.
Antihypertensive agents: Because oral contraceptives are associated with a rise in blood pressure, probably by means of the renin-angiotensin mechanism, antihypertensive agents that affect the sympathetic system may not be effective in lowering blood pressure (guanethidine, methyldopa).
Tobacco: Increased risk of coronary heart disease (particularly in older women).
Vitamins: May raise levels of vitamin A and lower levels of pyridoxine, folic acid, ascorbic acid.

MAO Inhibitors

Tyramine: Hypertensive reaction with headache, flushing, nausea, etc., sometimes severe. Tyramine is contained in certain foods, such as cheese, yeast extracts, pickled herring, hydrolyzed soups, chicken and beef, certain sausages, liver, and alcohol-containing beverages (particularly ale, beer, chianti, and certain sherries).
Tricyclic antidepressants: Severe toxic, potentially fatal reactions occasionally. Extreme caution and limited combined use in only most refractory patients advised.

Neuroleptic and Tranquilizing Drugs

Phenothiazines or butryophenones and alcohol: Enhanced central nervous system depression or extrapyramidal side effects.
Phenothiazines and antacids: Reduced levels.
Phenothiazines and propranolol: Rise in levels of both.
Phenothiazines and tricyclic antidepressants: Can lead, in some combinations, to increased levels of both and increased incidences of tardive dyskinesia.

Sympathomimetics

Amphetamines and chlorpromazine: Anorectic effects antagonized by chlorpromazine; antipsychotic effects antagonized by amphetamines.
Amphetamines and nasal decongestants: Case report in one adolescent describing antagonism.

Tricyclic Antidepressants

Methylphenidate: May cause marked rise in imipramine level.

Corticosteroids

Barbiturates: Therapeutic effects of steroids may be reduced (clearance increased by more than 100 percent and half-life reduced by as much as 50 percent depending on specific drugs.)
Diuretics (thiazides, ethacrynic acid, furosemide): Potassium depletion may be pronounced.
Ephedrine: Increases clearance of dexamethasone.
Phenytoin: Steroid effectiveness reduced.
Vaccines: Some live vaccines should not be administered with corticosteroids. The immune response may be diminished due to a reduction in the number of circulating lymphocytes.

Theophylline

Corticosteroids: Case reports of theophylline concentration doubling with addition of hydrocortisone.
Ephedrine: Increase in adverse side effects with no improvement in lung function.
Erythromycin: Increased theophylline levels.
Tobacco smoking: Reduced effectiveness and half-life of theophylline.

Source: From Stockley IH: Drug Interactions: A Source Book of Adverse Interactions, Their Mechanisms, Clinical Importance and Management. New York, Blackwell Scientific, 1981.

ENVIRONMENTAL INFLUENCES ON DRUG DISPOSITION

Altered Internal Environment: Changing Physiologic Status

ELIMINATION ORGAN FAILURE. Acute or chronic liver or renal disease causing failure of organs that transform or excrete drugs tends to prolong drug half-life or clearance. In such situations, a reduction in drug and dose interval is necessary to avoid toxicity. During adolescence, symptomatic or asymptomatic hepatitis is a common disorder. Regardless of etiology (drug-related, viral, or toxic), hepatic dysfunction can impair drug metabolism and therefore drug elimination. Of particular danger is combining illicit drug use (alcohol ingestion) with prescribed or OTC drugs transformed by the liver in the presence of hepatic dysfunction in the unsuspecting teenager. Acute behavioral changes or a change in the level of consciousness may be produced rapidly under these circumstances.

THYROID DISEASE.   Thyroid dysfunction is a common endocrine disorder that appears during adolescence. Hyperthyroidism is associated with tolerance of large doses of opiates. Conversely, hypothyroid patients are exquisitely sensitive to low doses of ephedrine commonly contained in OTC cold remedies.

Pregnancy

Over a million teenagers become pregnant each year. Eighty-five percent of these pregnancies are unintended. Teenagers tend to have less prenatal care and start care later in pregnancy compared with adults. Therefore, more teenagers than adult women are likely to ingest medications or substances that may adversely affect them or their fetuses without knowing it. Those who continue pregnancy put their fetuses at risk of drug effects during gestation.

There is still considerable debate about the physiologic differences between the pregnant teenager and the pregnant adult female. By the time of menarche, most girls have already experienced their growth spurt. In the 2 years after menarche, most girls grow about 2 more inches in height. By menarche, body composition has usually changed from the prepubertal proportions to those more closely resembling the adult female, but the percentage of fat continues to rise throughout adolescence and adulthood in most females.

Pregnancy, whether in the adult or adolescent, produces marked changes in body composition and therefore has a direct effect on drug disposition.[54] The effects of smoking cigarettes and marijuana and drinking alcohol during pregnancy have been well publicized recently. We do not know if the pregnant adolescent is at greater or less risk than her adult female counterpart regarding the effects of alcohol and tobacco on the fetus. Clearly, however there is a higher rate of marijuana use among some adolescent females who also became pregnant than among adults. However, because many teenagers are not aware or do not seek medical care during the first trimester, they may continue to expose their fetuses to these substances unwittingly.[55]

TREATMENT OF ACUTE DRUG ABUSE REACTIONS

Adolescence is often a time of experimentation with licit and illicit drugs. With little previous experience, adolescents often exceed limits, causing them to seek medical help while acutely intoxicated. In addition, suicide attempts may involve overdoses of both prescribed and illicit substances. For both these reasons, investigating the underlying cause of the overdose is as important as diagnosing the particular substances and providing medical treatment.

A brief review of some of the main aspects of treating acute reactions to commonly abused substances is therefore provided.[56]

Cocaine and Other CNS Stimulants

Cocaine use has been associated with a variety of cardiac dysfunctional states, including arrhythmias, myocarditis, and myocardial infarction, occasionally resulting in sudden death in otherwise healthy young people. These conditions have resulted from intravenous use as well as smoking "crack" or ingesting or sniffing cocaine. Mental status changes include euphoria, paranoia, and seizures. Systemic effects include hypertension and hyperpyrexia. Withdrawal syndromes from cocaine, amphetamines, and other stimulants are characterized by depression and irritability.

Opioids

Many of the disease states associated with intravenous opiate use are due to the presence of contaminants or substances used to adulterate illegal opioids. Some of these substances include quinine, lactose, and mannitol, as well as "cocktails" made by combinations of illicit drugs. Inadvertent injection of viruses (e.g., hepatitis, human immunodeficiency virus), bacteria, fungi, and particulate matter are not infrequent concomitants of I.V. opiate use. Therefore, the disease states are manifold. Naloxone can reverse the coma and apnea associated with severe opiate overdose and is also useful in propoxyphene intoxication. However, the pulmonary edema seen in acute overdoses is not reversed with naloxone. Symptoms of withdrawal for opioid-dependent teenagers can be treated with methadone orally (10 mg three or four times per day with decreasing doses after 24 hours). There are few methadone maintenance programs that accept adolescents under the age of 18 years; therefore, plans for long-term rehabilitation of the opiate-dependent teenager should be fully explored while the youngster is being treated for intoxication or withdrawal. Drug-free ambulatory or residential treatment programs are options for adolescents.

Other CNS Depressants

Diazepam and other benzodiazepines are frequently used by adolescents as part of a suicide attempt. Combinations with alcohol or other depressants add to the likelihood of significant respiratory depression. Depressants, including glutethimide and methaqualone (which is no longer manufactured in the United States but is available in other countries, including Mexico and Canada), are other medications associated with overdoses in teenagers. Barbiturate addiction is not common among adolescents in the 1980s; however, acute withdrawal as well as severe overdose, when either does occur, can be life-threatening.

Hallucinogens

Use of hallucinogens has decreased over the past decade. However, some youngsters still include LSD, mescaline, and particularly phencyclidine (PCP) among substances they experiment with. PCP is not infrequently combined with marijuana, either with or without the knowledge of the smoker. The associated agitation often responds to being in a quiet setting with reassurance and verbal support; however, diazepam or haloperidol can be used if necessary. Periodic prolonged states of anxiety, panic attacks, or "flashbacks" are described by some users. Reassurance and occasional use of benzodiazepine are often sufficient to treat these reoccurrences.

Cannabis

Acute reactions usually respond to reassurance and a quiet setting, but if the cannabis is orally ingested and the overdose causes a great deal of anxiety or dysphoria, then emetics and gastric lavage may reduce the amount of unabsorbed drug.

Volatile Inhalants

Over the past few decades, inhalation of a variety of substances has been part of the teen as well as adult drug use scene. Inhaling gasoline fumes, glue, and hydrocarbon solvents was more prominent among youth than in the 1960s and 1970s. However, occasional youngsters do present for treatment of overdoses. Acute as well as long-term consequences can be severe, so a careful history of the exact type of inhalant is essential. More commonly inhaled substances in the 1980s include nitrous oxide and amyl, butyl, or isobutyl nitrites. These can cause dizziness, headache, tachycardia, syncope, hypotension, acute psychosis, increased ocular pressure, neurologic manifestations including coma, methemoglobinemia, and on occasion, sudden death.

CONCLUSION

Despite growing interest in developmental pharmacology, specific information about adolescence is relatively scanty. Studies of the dose–concentration–effect relationship over the life cycle tend to emphasize the neonate, child, adult, or elderly patient, excluding specific information about teenagers. In many cases, errors in management would be made if physicians were to treat teenagers as big children requiring a high milligram per kilogram dose or as little adults.

UNEXPECTED TOXICITY OR INEFFECTIVENESS. Low blood levels in adolescents should not necessarily be equated with noncompliance. Many factors work synergistically to raise levels or antagonistically to lower levels so that the net effect may be difficult to predict for a given teenager taking a given drug at a given time. Therefore, if an unexpected clinical finding is observed, multiple blood levels are necessary in addition to knowledge of the dose to understand the balance of individual dispositional factors.

When range and dose requirements vary widely among individuals, therapeutic drug monitoring is usually indicated. For example, a phenobarbital dose of 1 mg/kg may be sufficient for providing hypnotic effects in adults, whereas in very young children, 5, 8, or 10 mg/kg may be required. Similarly, the imipramine dose in adults may be 1 mg/kg, whereas for children, 7 mg/kg may be required (FDA current recommendation for children is not to exceed 5 mg/kg). For a given teenager, it is sometimes imperative to monitor level to know how the majority of factors (genetic, distributional, excretory, etc.) will balance out.

Information about drug safety and efficacy in children is still quite limited. In 1975, 70 percent of the drugs listed in the *Physicians' Desk Reference* contained some form of disclaimer or lacked specific dose information for youth and children at all. The term *therapeutic orphans* refers not only to children, but also to adolescents. Adolescence is a time of exposure to illicit, nontherapeutic, and environmental chemical agents as well as prescribed and OTC medications. Studies of the pharmacodynamics of alcohol, marijuana, methaqualone, etc. are usually based on adults as the study population. Understanding the dose–response relationship of these agents in teenagers requires knowledge of the chemical properties of the drugs and physiologic changes in body composition and organ function. Finally, the clinician must possess a balanced view between those behavioral factors likely to affect compliance and the physiologic factors which have been described in this review.

EMERGING ISSUES IN MEDICATION USE FOR ADOLESCENTS. Adolescents are not big children, nor are they small adults. Their unique physical, psychological, and social status renders extrapolation from younger or older age groups inappropriate. One of the latest examples of adolescents "falling through the cracks" has been the history of the clinical trials program for the development and evaluation of treatments for HIV infection and AIDS. After the first protocols were developed for adults, special protocols for children under the age of 13 followed. However, adults were defined as persons over the age of 18 years. Therefore, teenagers 13–17 years of age were initially excluded. As discussion ensued about the appropriate place to include teenagers, it became evident that the unique physiologic status of the adolescent made inclusion in either age group inappropriate without some modification to take into account the diversity in body size and organ function, the effect of endocrinologic changes during puberty, and the cofactors that would influence the natural history of HIV infection or drug disposition in this age group. This most recent example epitomizes the special needs of adolescents regarding the use of medications.

REFERENCES

1. Hein K: Use of therapeutics in adolescence. J Adolesc Health Care 8:8–35, 1987

2. Friedman I, Litt I: Adolescents' compliance with therapeutic regimens. J Adolesc Health Care 8:52–67, 1987
3. Vessell ES: Why are toxic reactions to drugs so often undetected initially? N Engl J Med 303:1027–1029, 1980
4. Pente P: Toxicity of over-the-counter stimulants. JAMA 252:1898–1903, 1984
5. Johnston L, O'Malley P, Bachman J: Illicit Drug Use, Smoking and Drinking by America's High School Students, College Students and Young Adults, 1975–1987. Washington, National Institute on Drug Abuse, 1988
6. Sharpe TR, Smith MC: Patterns of medication use among children in households enrolled in the Aid of Families with Dependent Children Program. Pediatr Res 17:617–619, 1983
7. Dyment PG: The adolescent athlete and ergogenic aids. J Adolesc Health Care 8:68–73, 1987
8. Hein K, Cohen MI, Litt I: Illicit drug use among urban adolescents. Am J Dis Child 133:38–40, 1979
9. Brunswick A, Josefson E: Adolescent health in Harlem. Am J Public Health (suppl) 1972
10. Nicholi AM Jr: The nontherapeutic use of psychoactive drugs: A modern epidemic. N Engl J Med 308:925–933, 1983
11. Schwartz RH: Laboratory detection of drugs of abuse. Am Acad Pediatr Sec Adolesc Health Newsletter 8:17–26, 1987
12. Aranda JV, Stern L: Clinical aspects of developmental pharmacology and toxicology. Pharmacol Ther 20:1–51, 1983
13. Morselli PL: Drug Disposition During Development. Spectrum, New York, 1979
14. Goble FA: Sex as a factor in metabolism, toxicity, and efficacy of pharmacodynamic and chemotherapeutic agents. Adv Pharmacol Chemother 13:173–252, 1975
15. Steger RW: Age-dependent changes in the responsiveness of the reproductive system to pharmacological agents. Pharmacol Ther 17:1–64, 1982
16. Hein K, Dell R, Puig-Antich K, Cooper T: Effect of adolescent development on imipramine disposition. Pediatr Res 17:89A, 1983
17. Hein K, Dell R, Pesce M, Copoulos E, Miller M: Effects of adolescent development on theophylline half-life. Pediatr Res 19:173, 1985
18. Butler A, Richie R: Simplification and improvement in estimating drug dosage and fluid and dietary allowances for patients of varying sizes. N Engl J Med 262:903–908, 1960
19. Tanner JM: Growth at Adolescence, 2nd ed. New York, Blackwell Scientific, 1962
20. Forbes G: Growth of the lean body mass in man. Growth 36:325–338, 1972
21. Styne D, Grumbach M: Puberty in the male and female, in Reproductive Endocrinology. Philadelphia, Saunders, 1978, pp 189–240
22. Cheek D, Talbert JL: Extracellular volume and body water in infants, in Cheek D (ed): Human Growth. Philadelphia, Lea & Febiger, 1986, pp 118–196
23. Dubois D, Dubois E: Clinical calorimetry: A formula to estimate the appropriate surface area if height and weight be known. Arch Intern Med 17:863–871, 1916
24. Sloan A, de Weir JB: Nomograms for prediction of body density and total body fat from skin fold measurements. J Appl Physiol 28:221–222, 1970
25. Forbes G, Amikhakimi G: Skin-fold thickness and body fat in children. Hum Biol 42:401–418, 1970
26. Lohman T, Bioleau R, Rassey B: Prediction of lean body mass in young boys from skin-fold thickness and body weight. Hum Biol 47:345–362, 1975
27. Lohman T: Skin folds and body density and their relationship to body fatness. Hum Biol 53:181–225, 1981
28. Blizzard RM: Differentiation, morphogenesis, and growth, in Cheek D (ed): Human growth. Philadelphia, Lea & Febiger, 1968, pp 48–50
29. Schmucker D, Mooney J, Jones A: Age-related changes in the hepatic endoplasmic reticulum: A quantitive analysis. Science 197:1005–1008, 1977
30. Schmucker D, Mooney J, Jones A: Stereological analysis of hepatic fine structure in the Fischer 344 rat: Influence of sublobular location and animal age. J Cell Biol 78:31–37, 1978
31. Kato R, Takanaka A, Takayanagie M: Studies on mechanism of sex differences in drug oxidizing activity of liver microsomes. Jpn J Pharmacol 18:482–489, 1968
32. Kato R: Sex-related differences in drug metabolism. Drug Metab Rev 1:1–32, 1974
33. Shinnar S: Antiepileptic drugs in adolescence. J Adolesc Health Care 8:105–112, 1987
34. Institute of Medicine: Marijuana and Health. Washington, National Academy Press, 1982
35. Weinberger M, Hendeles L, Bigley L: Relation of product formulation to absorption of oral theophylline. N Engl J Med 299:852–857, 1978
36. Buchthal F, Lennon-Buchthal M: Diphenylhydantoin: Relation of anticonvulsant effect of concentration in serum, in Woodbury DM, Penry JK, Schmidt, (eds): Antiepileptic Drugs. New York, Raven Press, 1972, pp 193–209
37. Sonawane B, Catz C: Nutritional status and drug metabolism during development, in Soyka L, Redmond GP (eds): Drug Metabolism in the Immature Human. New York, Raven Press, 1981, pp 87–100
38. Greenblatt DJ, Sellers EM, Koch-Weser J: Importance of protein binding for the interpretation of serum of plasma drug concentrations. J Clin Pharmacol 22:259–263, 1982
39. Wiegand VW, Hintze KL, Slattery J, et al: Protein binding of several drugs in serum and plasma of healthy subjects. Clin Pharmacol Ther 27:297–300, 1980
40. Abernethy DR, Greenblatt J: Pharmacokinetics of drugs in obesity. Clin Pharmacokinet 7:108–124, 1982
41. Rohrbaugh T, Danish M, Ragni M, Taffe S: The effect of obesity on apparent volume of distribution of theophylline. Pediatr Pharmacol 2:75–83, 1982
42. Johnson MV, Freeman JM: Pharmacologic advances in seizure control: Symposium on progress in drug therapy for children. Pediatr Clin North Am 28:179–193, 1981
43. Potter, Calil H, Sutfin T, et al: Active metabolites of imipramine and desipramine in man. Clin Pharmacol Ther 31:393–401, 1982
44. Lu AYH: Multiplicity of liver drug metabolizing enzymes. Drug Metab Rev 10:187–208, 1979
45. Winsberg B, Perel J, Hurwic M, et al: Imipramine protein binding and pharmacokinetics in children, in Forrest C, Carr J (eds): Phenothiazines and Structurally Related Drugs. New York, Raven Press, 1974, pp 425–431
46. Davies DS, Thorgeirsson SS: Mechanism of hepatic drug oxidation and its relationship to individual differences in rates of oxidation in man. Ann NY Acad Sci 179: 411–420, 1971
47. Morselli PL (ed): Drug Disposition During Development. Spectrum, New York, 1977
48. Chiba K, Ishizaki T, Miura H, et al: Michaelis–Menten pharmacokinetics of diphenylhydantoin and application in the pediatric age patient. J Pediatr 96:479–484, 1980
49. Sarrazin E, Hendesles L, Winberger M, et al: Dose-dependent kinetics for theophylline: Observations among ambulatory asthmatic children. J Pediatr 97:825–828, 1980
50. Tang-Lui D, Williams R, Riegelman S: Nonlinear theophylline elimination. Clin Pharmacol Ther 31:358–369, 1982
51. Drugs that cause sexual dysfunction. Med Lett Drugs and Ther 29:65–73, 1987
52. Cholst I, Carlon A: Oral contraceptives and dysmenorrhea. J Adolesc Health Care 8:121–128, 1987
53. Martien K, Emans SJ: Treatment of common genital infections in adolescents. J Adolesc Health Care 8:129–136, 1987
54. Jacobson HN: Nutritional risk of pregnancy during adolescence. Birth Defects 17:69–83, 1981
55. Fried PA: Marijuana use by pregnant women and effects on offspring: An update. Neurobehav Toxicol Teratol 4:451–454, 1982
56. Treatment of acute drug abuse reactions. Med Lett Drugs Ther 29:83–86, 1987

SECTION IV

SPECIFIC DRUGS

24

THE PENICILLINS

JANAK A. PATEL *and* WAYNE R. SNODGRASS

HISTORICAL PERSPECTIVE ON THE DEVELOPMENT OF PENICILLINS

The discovery of penicillin G in 1929 heralded the modern antibiotic era and has served as a model for the development of future antimicrobial agents. In clinical practice, the use of penicillins was delayed until the early 1940s, at which time they were found to be very effective against gram-positive and gram-negative cocci. However, within a few years of widespread use, up to 50 percent of hospital isolates of *Staphylococcus aureus* were found to be resistant to the penicillins. The increasing level of resistance of up to 80 percent by 1957 lead to the development of other penicillin derivatives that would be stable against inactivation by the penicillinase enzymes elaborated by bacteria.

In 1957, the 6-aminopenicillenic acid (6-APA) nucleus of penicillin was identified, and this served as the basis for development of newer semisynthetic compounds with different side chains.[1] In 1961, ampicillin was introduced, which was effective against many enteric bacilli and *Haemophilus influenzae.* However, ampicillin was not stable against penicillinases. Other efforts lead to the development of methicillin, oxacillin, nafcillin, and cloxacillin, which were stable against penicillinases produced by staphylocci. With an expanded spectrum against gram-negative bacteria such as *Pseudomonas aeruginosa,* carbenicillin was introduced in 1967, followed by ticarcillin. Later, more potent antipseudomonal penicillins such as azlocillin, mezlocillin, and piperacillin were introduced in the late 1970s.

HISTORICAL PERSPECTIVE ON THE USE OF PENICILLINS IN PEDIATRICS

Although penicillins were introduced in clinical practice in the early 1940s, it is not clear when their use began in children. In 1949, Barnett et al.[2] published their observations on renal clearance of intramuscular preparations of penicillins in premature infants and children. That same year, Levine et al.[3] demonstrated the efficacy of orally administered penicillin in the treatment of neonatal infections. In 1953, Haung et al.[4] made further observations on oral and injectable penicillin G and procaine penicillin in the neonate. With the increasing incidence of penicillin-resistant staphylococcal epidemics in the newborn nurseries, O'Connor et al.[5] (1964) and Grossman et al.[6] (1965) studied pharmacokinetics of nafcillin in the neonate. Meanwhile, development of ampicillin lead to its applications in gram-negative bacterial infections. Studies on pharmacokinetics of ampicillin were published by Grossman et al.[6] (1965), Boe et al.[7] (1967), and Axline et al.[8] (1967). Later, to combat infections with *Proteus* and *Pseudomonas,* pharmacokinetic data were obtained for carbenicillin in the neonate by Morehead et al.[9] (1972) and Nelson et al.[10] (1973). As other penicillins with more antipseudomonal activity became available, they also were tested in the young pediatric patient. These agents included ticarcillin (Nelson et al.,[11] 1976), mezlocillin (Gladtke et al.,[12] 1980), and piperacillin (Wilson et al.,[13] 1982). Simultaneously, amoxicillin, an analogue of ampicillin was introduced in the mid-1970s, and this was studied in children by Marks et al.[14] (1978). The availability of this drug with broad-spectrum activity and excellent oral bioavailability revolutionized the outpatient management of common childhood infections. The problem of degradation of amoxicillin by β-lactamase was overcome by the incorporation of the clavulanate molecule, a β-lactamase inhibitor. The pharmacokinetics of the amoxicillin/clavulanate product was evaluated in children by Nelson et al.[15] (1982).

A similar approach has been used in the development of intravenous preparations of ampicillin and ticarcillin combined with the sulbactam, also a β-lactamase inhibitor, or clavulanate, respectively. These conjugates also have been evaluated in infants and children by Rodriguez et al.[16] (1986) and Begue et al.[17] (1986). Thus, from the

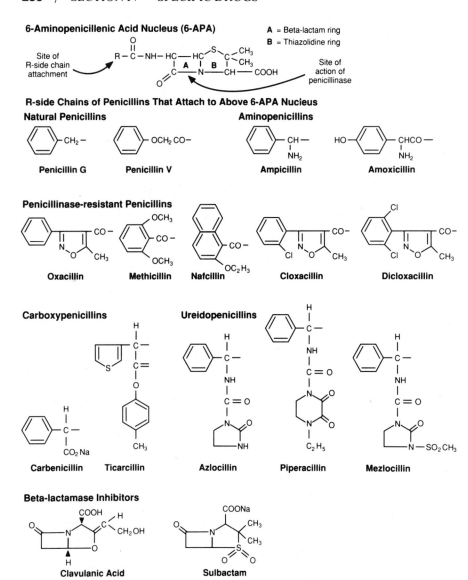

FIGURE 24–1. Structural formulas of 6-aminopenicillenic acid nucleus, *R* side chains of commonly used penicillins, and β-lactamase inhibitors.

early era of antibiotics to the present time, penicillins remain as much the backbone of antimicrobial therapy of pediatric patients as in other age groups.

STRUCTURE AND MODE OF ACTION OF PENICILLINS

To be effective, the penicillins must pass through the cell wall of bacteria and bind with the penicillin-binding proteins (PBPs) located on the cytoplasmic membrane. The PBPs, such as transpeptidases, carboxypeptidases, and endopeptidases, are bacterial enzymes involved in cell-wall synthesis. The chief structural requirement for biologic activity of penicillins resides in the 6-aminopenicillenic acid (6-APA) nucleus. The exact molecular interaction between the 6-APA nucleus and the PBPs is not clear; however, it ultimately leads to the decreased biosynthesis of cell-wall peptidoglycans.

The PBPs differ in number and size among different bacteria species and strains and have varying degrees of affinity for different penicillins and other β-lactam antibiotics. However, the attachment of various penicillins to the PBPs depends on factors other than just binding affinity. Bacterial enzymes such as penicillinases may inactivate the antibiotic before it reaches the receptor site on the PBPs. In addition, even though penicillins may easily pass through the simple cell wall of gram-positive bacteria, for gram-negative bacteria, the size (molecular weight) and charge characteristics of a penicillin may determine its passage through the porin–protein channels in the gram-negative cell wall.

The stability, penetration, and binding activity of various penicillins against a broad spectrum of bacteria have been enhanced by altering the side chains on the basic 6-APA nucleus (Figure 24–1). The phenyl group on the acyl (*R'*) side chain of penicillin G gives it high affinity for PBPs of gram-positive anaerobes, cocci, and bacilli, gram-negative cocci, and most spirochetes. The aminopenicillins, such as ampicillin, have an amino acid group on the acyl (*R'*) side chain that increases the antibacterial spectrum by enhancing the permeability of aminopenicillins through the outer membrane of gram-negative bacteria.

However, aminopenicillins, similar to the natural penicillins, are not penicillinase stable. The stability of natural penicillins against the penicillinases is improved by substitution of side chains that act by steric hinderance at the site of penicillinase attachment. Unfortunately, these penicillinase-resistant penicillins, namely, methicillin, oxacillin, and nafcillin, are becoming less useful by virtue of increasing intrinsic resistance in staphylococci. The mechanism of methicillin resistance involves the expression of PBP 2a, which has a lowered affinity for methicillin and other β-lactams.

The gram-negative coverage of penicillins has been further extended to include *Pseudomonas aeruginosa* by substituting carboxy and thienyl groups on the R' side chain to produce carbenicillin and ticarcillin, respectively (carboxypenicillins). Further modification by attaching a complex acyl moiety (a ureido group) onto the alpha amino carbon atom of ampicillin has produced the ureidopenicillins—mezlocillin, azlocillin, and pipercillin—

with better coverage against gram-negative bacilli and anaerobes while maintaining coverage against many gram-positive bacteria. Nonetheless, all the amino-, carboxy-, and ureidopenicillins are typically penicillinase susceptible. A new approach to resist hydrolysis by the penicillinases has been to develop combinations of penicillins with inhibitors of penicillinases. Clavulanic acid and sulbactam are the β-lactam inhibitors that bind and inactivate penicillinases, thereby protecting the "partner" penicillin. They also may potentiate the activity of the penicillins by binding directly with the PBPs.

PHARMACOKINETICS OF THE PENICILLINS

The various pharmacokinetic aspects of penicillins in the neonate have been summarized in Table 24–1. For

TABLE 24–1. PHARMACOKINETIC STUDIES OF PENICILLIN IN THE NEONATE

DRUG	AGE (days)	WEIGHT (gm)	DOSE (mg/kg)	ROUTE	C_{max}*	$t_{1/2}$† (h)	REFERENCE
Penicillin G	<8	<2001	25,000 U‡ q12h	I.M.	24	4.9	18
	<8	>2000	25,000 U q12h	I.M.	22	2.6	18
	8–14	<2001	25,000 U q12h	I.M.	24	2.6	18
	8–14	>2000	25,000 U q12h	I.M.	21	2.1	18
	<28	680–4400	25,000 U q6h	I.V.	32	3.8	19
				I.M.	22	3.2	19
Benzathine penicillin G			50,000 U	I.M.	1.05		20
Procaine penicillin G	<7	Full term	50,000 U	I.M.	17	6.6	21
	<8	>2000	50	I.M.	81	4.9	18
	<8	<2000	50	I.M.	104	6.4	18
	>8	Full term	50,000 U	I.M.	6.2	5.4	18
	>8	>2000	50	I.M.	84	2.3	18
Methicillin	<8	<2000	25	I.M.	58	2.8	18
	<8	>2000	25	I.M.	48	2.2	18
	>8	<2000	25	I.M.	58	3.1	18
	>8	>2000	25	I.M.	45	1.8	18
Nafcillin	<28	<2300	100/day	I.V.	>80	3	22
	<25		25	I.V.	88	5.9	23
Oxacillin	>8	<2300	20	I.M.	47–52	1.4	8
Carbenicillin	<8	<2001	100	I.M.	180	5.7	18
	<8	>2000	100	I.M.	185	4.2	18
	>8	<2001	100	I.M.	186	3.6	18
	>8	>2000	100	I.M.	143	2.1	18
Ticarcillin	<7	<2000	75 q8h	I.M.	189	5.6	24
		>2000	75 q6h	I.M.	159	4.9	24
			100 q4h	I.M.	125	2.2	24
Ticarcillin/ clavulanate	<9	<3501	54–62/2–2.3	I.V.	185/5	4/3.5	17
		895–3900	75/5	I.V.	183/2.4	4.5/2	25
Azlocillin		<2000	50	I.V.	144	2.1	26
		>2500	50	I.V.	153	2.6	26
Mezlocillin	<8	<2001	75–100	I.M.	139	4.3	27
	<8	>2001	75–100	I.M.	136	4.4	27
	>7	<2001	75–100	I.M.	140	2.6	27
	>7	>2000	75–100	I.M.	147	2.4	27
Piperacillin		Mean 1625	100–200 q12h	I.V.	130–300	6.5	28

*C_{max} = peak serum concentration.
†$t_{1/2}$ = serum half-life.
‡U = units; for penicillin G 1.0 mg/kg = 1600 U/kg, 0.6 mg = 1000 U.

TABLE 24–2. PHARMACOKINETIC PROPERTIES OF AMINOPENICILLINS IN OLDER INFANTS AND CHILDREN

DRUG	DOSE (mg/kg)	ROUTE	C_{max}	$t_{1/2}$ (h)	REFERENCE
Ampicillin	25	P.O.	5	1.1	29
	25	I.V.	36	1.5	29
Amoxicillin	25	P.O.	8.9	1.2	29
	15	P.O.	5.4	1.1	29
Amoxicillin/clavulanate	13.2/3.3	P.O.	4.7/1.5	1.5/1.2	29

older infants and children, the pharmacokinetic parameters are very similar to those of adults; hence they are not presented here. However, data relating to the commonly used aminopenicillins are shown in Table 24–2.

A number of factors affect the pharmacokinetic properties and bioavailability of penicillins that relate to age and growth of children.

Absorption

Gut absorption of penicillins occurs mainly in the duodenum and upper jejunum. The acidic pH of the stomach can hydrolyze certain penicillins such as penicillin G and methicillin. However, the aminopenicillins (e.g., amoxicillin and ampicillin) and, to a lesser extent, penicillin V and dicloxacillin are resistant to acid hydrolysis and are therefore better absorbed. In neonates, reduced gastric acid secretion results in better absorption of penicillin V, but owing to unknown reasons, the absorption of aminopenicillins is delayed. The basal gastric acid secretion appears to correlate with postnatal although not postconceptual age.[30] Other factors that lead to decreased gut absorption of the penicillins include the molecular configuration of the penicillin derivative (e.g., ureidopenicillins), presence of food in the GI tract, and states of malabsorption and diarrheal diseases. Interestingly, absorption of amoxicillin has been noted to be greater in patients with shigellosis than in infants without gastrointestinal disease.[31]

After intramuscular administration, the systemic absorption of penicillins has been considered to be therapeutically equivalent to intravenous administration in neonates who are hemodynamically stable.[19] However, the absorption may be compromised in disease states, and therefore, intramuscular administration should be reserved for neonates with difficult intravenous access. In older children and adults, penicillin G also attains prompt peak serum levels following intramuscular administration; however, with other forms of penicillins, the peak levels are lower and delayed.

The benzathine and procaine salts of penicillin G are insoluble and require hydrolysis to free the penicillin G moiety; hence their absorption from an intramuscular site is slow, prolonged, and with lower serum peak levels. This effect is more pronounced with the benzathine than with the procaine salts.

Distribution

Compared with adults, drug distribution of water-soluble antibiotics such as penicillin is larger in infants, particularly premature neonates, because of the higher extracellular fluid volume, greater total-body water, and reduced fat content.[32] These differences imply the possible need for larger dosages for the penicillins on a milligram per kilogram body-weight basis relative to adult dosages.

Plasma protein binding of the penicillins is decreased in the neonatal period when compared with the adult values.[33] However, the clinical significance of the availability of unbound penicillins on therapeutic efficacy has not been determined. An important consideration in the newborn is that the penicillins do not cause significant displacement of bilirubin from albumin binding sites.[33] Hence the risk of kernicterus as a result of entry into brain of free, displaced bilirubin is low.

Penicillins are widely distributed into the various body tissues and fluids. The highest concentrations are attained in the kidneys, liver, lungs, skin, intestines, muscle, and erythrocytes. Only minimal amounts are generally attained in avascular areas, abscesses, aqueous humor, sweat, tears, bone (except with penicillanase-resistant penicillins), and cerebrospinal fluid (CSF). With inflamed meninges, higher concentrations of penicillins are attained in CSF because of increased vascular permeability and partial inhibition of the organic acid transport mechanism. With the use of benzathine and procaine salts of penicillin G, very low levels are attained in CSF.[20,21] The distribution of clavulanic acid and sulbactam is very similar to the penicillins with which they are mixed in the combination products.[34]

Disposition

The penicillins are metabolized in the liver to varying extents by hydrolysis of the β-lactam ring to penicilloic acids, which are microbiologically inactive. However, elimination of the penicillins does not necessarily require metabolic degradation. Renal excretion is the major route of elimination for the penicillins and their metabolites and correlates well with creatinine clearance. Smaller amounts of penicillins are secreted into bile. A notable exception to this rule is nafcillin, which is mostly metabolized by the liver and excreted in bile.

In premature infants, neonates, and patients with impaired renal function, the half-life of penicillins is prolonged. In neonates, it is suggested that glomerular filtration rather than tubular secretion is primarily responsible for most of the renal elimination of penicillin.[18] As the renal tubular function matures, most of the drug is excreted by tubular secretion and is similar to adults by 3 months of age. Oral probenecid competitively inhibits renal tubular secretion and produces higher and prolonged serum concentrations of the penicillins.

The clavulanic acid and sulbactam molecules are excreted by kidneys and show comparable serum half-lives with those of the penicillins with which they are mixed in the combination products. Their levels also are higher and prolonged with the concurrent administration of probenecid.

Major renal impairment requires modification of the dosage schedule. All the penicillins and the clavulanic acid and sulbactam conjugates are hemodialyzable to various degrees.

In cystic fibrosis patients, the rate of penicillin elimination is increased, probably due to enhanced tubular secretion, abnormal hepatic function, and cachexia. For example, the penicillinase-resistant penicillins are eliminated up to three times more rapidly in children with cystic fibrosis than in control subjects.[35,36]

TOXICITY AND ADVERSE REACTIONS

Penicillins cause both local and systemic adverse reactions. Most frequent local reactions are gastrointestinal, i.e., nausea, vomiting, epigastric pain, and diarrhea. Other effects include pseudomembranous colitis with penicillinase-resistant *Clostridium deficile,* which is more frequent with the use of aminopenicillins.

A peculiar, nonallergic rash called *ampicillin rash* also occurs, particularly with the use of aminopenicillins in children. It is a generalized maculopapular, erythematous rash that begins on the trunk and spreads peripherally. It generally appears 3–14 days after beginning therapy and resolves in 6–14 days despite continuing therapy. A high incidence (65–100 percent) of this rash occurs in patients with infectious mononucleosis. It also occurs fairly frequently with other viral respiratory tract infections, cytomegalovirus infections, leukemias, and lymphomas.

Acute interstitial nephritis, manifested by fever, rash, eosinophilia, azotemia, hematuria, proteinuria, and cylindruria, occurs with the use of penicillinase-resistant penicillins, particularly with I.V. methicillin. It is reversible on cessation of penicillin therapy.

Hepatic dysfunction, manifested by elevations in serum levels of alkaline phosphatase, AST, ALT, and LDH occurs particularly during therapy with I.V. oxacillin.

Neurotoxicity with seizures, clonus, hallucinations, confusion, lethargy, coma, and even fatal encephalopathy has been reported rarely with the high-dose use of parenteral penicillin G.

Transient hematologic effects, including neutropenia, leukopenia, thrombocytopenia, eosinophilia, and anemia, have been reported with all penicillins. Agranulocytosis has been reported particularly with I.V. methicillin, nafcillin, and oxacillin and oral cloxacillin. Abnormal clotting profiles have been reported with broad-spectrum penicillins.

Despite the numerous adverse reactions just discussed, one of the most important reasons for nonuse of penicillins in patients is the history of allergic reactions to penicillins, even though they actually are rare. Allergic reactions to penicillins may be of (1) immediate or anaphylactic type, (2) accelerated type, and (3) late type.

The *anaphylactic reactions* occur within 30 minutes of administration. The characteristic angioedema, urticaria, and shock are considered to be due to IgE antibodies to penicillin and its metabolites. Fortunately, this form of reaction is rare (1 case per 20,000 courses in adults). Although the exact incidence is not known in children, it is believed to occur much less frequently, presumably because of less previous exposure to penicillin antigens. Such reactions are less frequent with oral preparations than with parenteral forms. The *accelerated reactions* are similar to those of the immediate reaction but occur 1–72 hours after administration, and the symptoms are less severe. The *late reactions,* characterized by serum sickness, hemolytic anemia, and drug fever, are caused by complexes of penicillin with IgG antibodies.

Determination of penicillin allergy requires careful

TABLE 24–3. SUGGESTED DAILY DOSAGE (MG/KG) SCHEDULES FOR MODERATE INFECTIONS WITH PENICILLIN-SUSCEPTIBLE ORGANISMS IN THE NEWBORN

ANTIBIOTIC	ROUTE	BODY WEIGHT < 2000 gm		BODY WEIGHT > 2000 gm	
		Age 0–7 Days	>7 Days	Age 0–7 Days	>7 Days
Ampicillin	I.V., I.M.	50 q12h	75 q12h	75 q8h	100 q6h
Penicillin G	I.V., I.M.	50,000 U/kg q12h	75,000 U/kg 75 q8h	50,000 U/kg q8h	100,000 U/kg q6h
Methicillin	I.V.	50 q12h	75 q8h	75 q8h	100 q6h
Oxacillin	I.V.	50 q12h	100 q8h	75 q8h	150 q6h
Nafcillin	I.V.	50 q12h	75 q8h	50 q8h	75 q6h
Ticarcillin	I.V.	150 q12h	225 q8h	225 q8h	300 q6h
Mezlocillin	I.V.	150 q8h	225 q8h	150 q12h	225 q6h

Note: For severe infections (meningitis, septic shock, etc.), double dosage.

TABLE 24–4. SUGGESTED DAILY DOSAGE (MG/KG) SCHEDULES FOR INFECTIONS WITH PENICILLIN-SUSCEPTIBLE ORGANISMS IN INFANTS AND OLDER CHILDREN

ANTIBIOTIC	MILD INFECTIONS (OUTPATIENT)	MODERATE INFECTIONS	SEVERE INFECTIONS AND MENINGITIS
Penicillin G, crystalline		25,000–50,000 U/kg q6h, I.M. or I.V.	100,000–300,000 q4–6h
Penicillin G, procaine	25,000–50,000 U/kg q24h, I.M.	25,000–50,000 U/kg q6h, I.M. or I.V.	
Penicillin G, benzathine	50,000 U/kg, I.M.		
Penicillin, V	25–50 q6h, P.O.		
Ampicillin	50 q6h, P.O.	100–200 q6h, I.V. or I.M.	200–400 q4–6h, I.V.
Ampicillin + sulbactam		100–200 q6h, I.V.	200–400 q4–6h, I.V.*
Amoxicillin	40 q8h, P.O.		
Amoxicillin + clavulanate	40 q8h, P.O.		
Cloxacillin	50–100 q6h, P.O.		
Dicloxacillin	12–25 q6h, P.O.		
Nafcillin		50–150 q6h, I.M. or I.V.	100–200 q4–6h, I.V.
Oxacillin		50–100 q6h, I.M. or I.V.	100–200 q4–6h, I.V.
Methicillin		50–100 q6h, I.M. or I.V.	200–300 q4–6h, I.V.
Ticarcillin		100–200 q4–6h, I.V.	200–300 q4–6h, I.V.
Ticarcillin clavulanate		100–200 q4–6h, I.V.	200–300 q4–6h, I.V.
Mezlocillin		200–300 q6h, I.V.	200–300 q6h
Azlocillin		200–450 q4–6h, I.V.	200–450 q6h
Piperacillin		200–300 q4–6h, I.V.	300–400 q4–6h

*Do not use in meningitis.

review of history, laboratory evaluations, and skin tests. If necessary, desensitization to penicillin allergy can be undertaken.

CLINICAL USES OF PENICILLINS

A discussion on various clinical conditions in which the penicillins are used in the pediatric population is beyond the scope of this chapter. The dosage guidelines of penicillin use in pediatric population are summarized in Tables 24–3 and 24–4.

The following is a list of the various classes of penicillins and pathogenetic organisms for which they are commonly used:

- The *natural penicillins:* Streptococci (groups A, B, C, G, H, L, and M), pneumococci, anthrax, actinomyces, anaerobic flora of mouth, clostridia (including tetanus), *Listeria, Pasteurella, N. gonorrhoea, T. pallidum* (syphilis), meningococci, corynebacteria, and *B. burgdorferi* (Lyme disease). Penicillin G procaine can be used for mild to moderately severe infections due to these organisms. Penicillin G benzathine is indicated for streptococcal infections of the upper respiratory tract, syphilis, and prophylaxis in rheumatic fever.

- The *penicillinase-resistant penicillins:* Susceptible strains of staphylococci. As empiric treatment, they

also provide adequate coverage for β-hemolytic streptococci and pneumococci.

- The *aminopenicillins:* Streptococci (groups A, B, C, G, H, L, and M), pneumococci, *Listeria, N. gonorrhoea,* actinomyces, corynebacteria, and *B. burgdorferi.* Also, susceptible strains of gram-negative organisms such as *Haemophilus influenzae* (typable and nontypable), *E. coli,* and *Shigella.* Oral ampicillin is preferable to amoxicillin in the treatment of *Shigella* enteritis. The combination of amoxicillin with clavulanate and ampicillin with sulbactam increases the spectrum of these aminopenicillins against β-lactamase–producing strains of the previously listed organisms, including staphylococci.

- The *extended-spectrum penicillins* (carboxy- and ureidopenicillins): Gram-negative coverage similar to ampicillin, in addition to many strains of *Pseudomonas, Enterobacter, Morganella,* and *Proteus providencia, Serratia, B. fragilis,* and *Klebsiella.* Azlocillin and piperacillin are also active against streptococci. The combination of ticarcillin with clavulanate increases the spectrum of ticarcillin against β-lactmase–producing strains of staphylococci and gram-negative bacteria.

REFERENCES

1. Robinson GN: 6-APA and the development of the beta-lactam antibiotics. J Antimicrob Chemother 5:7–13, 1979

2. Barnett HL, McNamara H, Shultz S, Tompsett R: Renal clearances of sodium penicillin G, procaine penicillin G, and inulin in infants and children. Pediatrics 3:418–422, 1949

3. Levin B, Neill CA: Oral penicillin in the newborn. Arch Dis Child 24:171–175, 1949

4. Huang NN, High RH: Comparison of serum levels following the administration of oral and parenteral preparations of penicillin to infants and children of various age groups. J Pediatr 42:657–668, 1953

5. O'Connor WJ, Warren GH, Mandala PS, et al: Serum concentrations of nafcillin in newborn infants and children. Antimicrob Agents Chemother 188–191, 1964

6. Grossman M, Ticknor W: Serum levels of ampicillin, cephalothin, cloxacillin, and nafcillin in the newborn infant. Antimicrob Agents Chemother 214–219, 1965

7. Boe RW, Williams CP, Bennett JV, Oliver TK: Serum levels of methicillin and ampicillin in newborn and premature infants in relation to postnatal age. Pediatrics 39:194–201, 1967

8. Axline SG, Yaffe SJ, Simon HJ: Clinical pharmacology of antimicrobials in premature infants. II. Ampicillin, methicillin, oxacillin, neomycin, and colistin. Pediatrics 39:97–107, 1967

9. Morehead CD, Shelton S, Kusmiesz H, Nelson JD: Pharmacokinetics of carbenicillin in neonates of normal and low birth weight. Antimicrob Agents Chemother 2:267–271, 1972

10. Nelson JD, McCracken GH: Clinical pharmacology of carbenicillin and gentamicin in the neonate and comparative efficacy with ampicillin and gentamicin. Pediatrics 52:801–812, 1973

11. Nelson JD, Shelton S, Kusmeisz H: Clinical pharmacology of ticarcillin in the newborn infant: Relation to age, gestational age, and weight. J Pediatr 87:474–479, 1976

12. Gladtke E, Sanchez-deReutus A, Heimann C: Pharmacokinetics of acyl ureido penicillins in premature and newborn infants, in Proceedings of 11th Interscience Conference on Antimicrobial Agents and Chemotherapy, 1987

13. Wilson C, Koup JR, Opheim KE: Piperacillin pharmacokinetics in pediatric patients. Antimicrob Agents Chemother 22:442–447, 1982

14. Marks MI, Vose AD: Evaluation of amoxicillin therapy in all children. J Clin Pharmacol 18:61–66, 1978

15. Nelson JD, Kusmiesz H, Shelton S: Pharmacokinetics of potassium clavulanate in combination with amoxicillin in pediatric patients. Antimicrob Agents Chemother 21:681–682, 1982

16. Rodriguez WJ, Khan WN, Puig J, et al: Sulbactam/ampicillin vs chloramphenicol/ampicillin for the treatment of meningitis in infants and children. Rev Infect Dis (suppl 8):S620–629, 1986

17. Begue P, Quinou F, Quinet B: Efficacy and pharmacokinetics of timentin in pediatric infections. J Antimicrob Chemother 17(suppl C):81–91, 1986

18. McCracken GH, Ginsberg C, Chrane DF, et al: Clinical pharmacology of penicillin in newborn infants. J Pediatr 82:692–698, 1973

19. Mulhall A: Antibiotic treatment of neonates—Does route of administration matter? Dev Pharmacol Ther 8:1–8, 1985

20. Kaplan JM, McCracken GH: Clinical pharmacology of benzathine penicillin G in neonates with regard to its recommended use in congenital syphilis. J Pediatr 82:1069–1072, 1973

21. Speer ME, Mason EO, Scharnberg JT: Cerebrospinal fluid concentrations of aqueous procaine penicillin G in the neonate. Pediatrics 67:387–388, 1981

22. Banner W, Gooch WM, Burckart G, Korones SB: Pharmacokinetics of nafcillin in infants with low birth weights. Antimicrob Agents Chemother 17:691–694, 1980

23. Sarff LD, Deitch MW, Chiang ST: Nafcillin pharmacokinetics in neonates: Dosage recommendations, in Nelson JD, Grassi C (eds): Current Chemotherapy and Infectious Disease, vol 2. Washington, American Society for Microbiology, 1980, p 1154–1155

24. Nelson JD, Kusmiesz H, Shelton S, Woodman E: Clinical pharmacology and efficacy of ticarcillin in infants and children. Pediatrics 61:858–863, 1978

25. Fayed SB, Sutton AM, Turner TL, McAllister TA: The prophylactic use of ticarcillin/clavulante in the neonate. J Antimicrob Chemother 19:113–118, 1987

26. Heimann G: Pharmacokinetics and clinical aspects of azlocillin in pediatrics. J Antimicrob Chemother 11(suppl B):127–135, 1983

27. Rubio T, Wirth F, Karotkin E: Pharmacokinetic studies of mezlocillin in newborn infants. J Antimicrob Chemother 9(suppl A):241–244, 1982

28. Reed MD, Myers CM, Yamashita TS, Blumer JL: Developmental pharmacology and therapeutics of piperacillin in gram-negative infections. Dev Pharmacol Ther 9:102–114, 1986

29. McCracken GH: Comparative evaluation of aminopenicillins for oral use, in Nelson JD, McCracken GH (eds): Clinical Reviews in Pediatric Infectious Disease. Toronto, BC Decker, 1985, pp 73–77

30. Hyman PE, Feldman EJ, Ament ME, et al: Effect of external feeding on the maintenance of gastric acid secretory function. Gastroenterology 84:341–345, 1983

31. Nelson JD, Haltalin KC: Amoxicillin is less effective than ampicillin against Shigella in vitro and in vivo. J Infect Dis 129:S222–227, 1974

32. Friis-Hansen B: Water distribution in the fetus and newborn infant. Acta Paediatr Scand (suppl 305):7–11, 1983

33. Fink S, Karp W, Robertson A: Effect of penicillins on bilirubin-albumin binding. J Pediatr 113:556–563, 1988

34. Yogev R: The role of beta-lactamase inhibitors in pediatrics, in Arnoff SC, et al (eds): Advances in Pediatric Infectious Diseases. Chicago, Year Book Medical Publishers, 1988, pp 181–205

35. Jusko WJ, Mosovich LL, Gerbracht, LM, et al: Enhanced renal excretion of dicloxacillin in patients with cystic fibrosis. Pediatrics 56:1038–1044, 1975

36. Nelson JD: Antimicrobial drugs, in Yaffe ST (ed): Pediatric Pharmacology: Therapeutic Principles in Practice. Philadelphia, Grune & Stratton, 1980, pp 167–193

25

AMINOGLYCOSIDE ANTIBIOTICS

B. M. ASSAEL *and* F. RUSCONI

Aminoglycoside antibiotics are structurally related compounds with common chemical and pharmacologic properties. Several aminoglycosides are currently available for clinical use, the most common being streptomycin, neomycin, kanamycin, gentamicin, amikacin, tobramycin, sisomicin, and netilmicin. Amikacin and netilmicin are semisynthetic compounds obtained, respectively, from kanamycin and sisomicin.

The aminoglycosides are bactericidal antibiotics. Their lethal effects are activated by irreversible binding to ribosomes and disruption of normal protein synthesis. Bacterial resistance to aminoglycosides may occur through various mechanisms. The most common is the plasmid-mediated synthesis of enzymes that acetylate, phosphorylate, and adenylate the molecule at different sites. This retards penetration of the aminoglycosides into the bacteria. Differences in resistance levels between (apparently) similar aminoglycoside antibiotics are the result of differences in affinity of the modifying enzyme for the different antibiotic substrates. Other known mechanisms of resistance involve changes in the ribosomal proteins that lower their affinity for the antibiotic and mutations that affect the active incorporating system of the drug into the bacteria.[1]

The pattern of bacterial resistance may differ from institution to institution, and *in vitro* sensitivity testing should be performed on all clinical isolates. Extensive use of an aminoglycoside in a closed unit can be followed by the emergence of resistant organisms. This was clearly demonstrated when kanamycin and then gentamicin were used extensively in neonatal intensive care units[2,3] and was confirmed in other studies in adults treated with different aminoglycosides. Nevertheless, more recently, several investigators reported that the extensive use of amikacin both in neonatal units and in adult general hospitals did not result in an increase of amikacin-resistant gram-negative bacteria. These observations might be accounted for by the fact that amikacin is only susceptible to a single aminoglycoside-inactivating enzyme.[4,5]

SPECTRUM OF ACTIVITY

Aminoglycosides are primarily active against aerobic gram-negative bacilli. They have good *in vitro* and *in vivo* activity against Enterobacteriaceae, in particular *E. coli, Klebsiella* spp., *Enterobacter* spp., and *Proteus* spp. Despite some differences in their *in vitro* activity toward these bacteria, aminoglycosides, with the exception of those first discovered, streptomycin and kanamycin, generally have similar spectra of activity. Aminoglycosides activity toward *Pseudomonas aeruginosa* may vary, and only since the discovery of gentamicin has a substantial improvement in activity against this pathogen been obtained.

These antibiotics usually have significant *in vitro* activity against *Staphylococcus aureus* and *epidermidis* but are less effective against other clinically important gram-positive bacteria such as group A and B streptococci, *S. pneumoniae,* and *S. faecalis.*[6] Streptomycin is a drug of choice in tuberculosis, but this will not be discussed in the present chapter.

The *in vitro* activity of aminoglycosides may be enhanced by combination with antibiotics (e.g., β-lactams) acting on the bacteria cell wall and thus augmenting the entry of aminoglycosides. Synergism with penicillins and cephalosporins has been documented against streptococci, *Pseudomonas,* and Enterobacteriaceae. On the other hand, several studies have demonstrated *in vitro* and *in vivo* antagonism of aminoglycosides and chloramphenicol against Enterobacteriaceae.[7]

Aminoglycosides can be inactivated by a physicochemical interaction with β-lactam compounds. When mixed together at administration, a clinically significant inactivation will occur in patients with severe renal insufficiency who may have elevated serum levels of both drugs.[8]

PHARMACOKINETICS

Aminoglycosides are polar agents that pass with difficulty through the skin and gastrointestinal membranes. This allows the local use of neomycin, which would be too toxic if absorbed.[9] Caution should always be used, since cases of toxic reactions to orally administered neomycin have been reported.[10] A certain absorption of gentamicin following oral administration has been observed in neonates treated for necrotizing enterocolitis, and deafness also has occurred in burned infants as a consequence of excessive absorption of neomycin through the skin.[11] After intramuscular administration, serum peak concentrations are usually reached in 15–60 minutes, although the rate of absorption may vary.

Aminoglycosides are bound minimally to proteins. They diffuse rapidly to interstitial fluid, and their volume of distribution is about 25–30 percent of total body weight in adults,[12,13] but higher in neonates, infants, and children owing to the larger extracellular fluid compartment.[14,15,16]

The concentrations in peritoneal fluid during infections are satisfactory in most cases, although lower and slightly delayed with respect to serum.[17] Penetration of aminoglycosides into bronchial secretions is poor and often fails to reach therapeutic levels.[18] Aerosol administration in children with cystic fibrosis results in higher concentrations of aminoglycosides in the sputum. This does not, however, lead to substantial clinical improvement.[19,20]

In joint fluids, adequate levels have been found in some studies, but available information is scanty.[21] Penetration of aminoglycosides in the central nervous system is highly variable; even when meninges are inflamed, concentrations that greatly exceed the *in vitro* minimal bactericidal concentrations of bacteria are seldom obtained.[3,22,23] Studies of aminoglycoside administration in the lumbar subarachnoid space indicate that high levels can be achieved in the lumbar CSF, but little drug enters the ventricular fluid.[22,24] Intraventricular administration of aminoglycosides by means of reservoirs can produce therapeutic ventricular levels for more than 24 hours.[25] This route of administration, however, involves invasive procedures.

Penetration of aminoglycosides in the eye is low, and in intraocular infections, subconjunctival administration is needed.[26] Aminoglycosides penetrate poorly into fat. This explains the need to adjust dosage according to lean body weight or to take into account only a part of the mass in order to avoid overdosage in obese patients.[27]

Maternofetal distribution of aminoglycosides has been studied in humans and in experimental animals.[28] In humans, drug levels were found in the amniotic fluid and in fetal urine as early as 12–13 weeks' gestational age. The fetal kidneys show high concentrations of aminoglycosides, demonstrating that active uptake of these antibiotics by the developing tubule is an early function.[29] Knowledge of the mechanisms determining the penetration of aminoglycosides into the kidney and inner ear is relevant because these drugs exhibit their toxicity at these sites.

Elevated concentrations are found especially in the renal cortex. This is due to active uptake and storage of these drugs in the proximal tubular cells. This process is not linear, however, and relatively less drug is accumulated in the kidney at higher dosages.[30]

Several studies have been performed on the kinetics of aminoglycosides in the inner ear in experimental animals, but very few data have been obtained in humans. Higher perilymph levels have been related to longer duration of treatment and the presence of abnormal renal function.[31]

Aminoglycosides are eliminated almost exclusively through the kidney. Following I.V. administration, their serum concentrations follow a multiexponential decay. The first phase occurs rapidly and is accounted for by distribution processes. It is followed by an elimination phase with a half-life directly related to the rate of glomerular filtration. Slow release from the kidney, where the drug has been accumulated, accounts, however, for the persistent presence of the drug in the urine. During this late phase, serum concentrations are minimal and only measurable by sensitive analytical methods. Urinary concentrations may be detected over a period longer than 10 days after suspension of treatment. Such persistence of the antibiotic in the urine may have clinical relevance in infections of the urinary tract, since the amount of antibiotic eliminated may exceed the minimal inhibiting concentration of various urinary pathogens even a week after the end of the treatment.[32]

AGE-RELATED DIFFERENCES IN AMINOGLYCOSIDE KINETICS

Age is a major determinant in aminoglycoside kinetics, as can be expected, since important changes in body composition and kidney function take place during growth and can directly affect both the distribution and elimination processes involved in aminoglycoside disposition.

Neonates exhibit a larger volume of distribution for all aminoglycosides together with a low clearance of the drug from the body.[14,16,33,34,35] These two phenomena result in a prolonged elimination half-life and thus increase the risk of drug accumulation during treatment. Various studies have demonstrated that the more immature the neonate, the greater are the chances of achieving high blood levels, both peaks and troughs. This has led to the recommendation to prolong the time interval between administrations. Some studies have suggested that it might be correct to start the treatment with a loading dose followed by smaller subsequent doses at times and in amounts depending on postnatal and gestational age.[14,15,33,34,36,37]

Other factors may be worth considering. Hypoxemia and low Apgar score at birth may prolong the elimination half-life of aminoglycosides in small preterm neonates presumably by depressing the glomerular filtration rate.[38] This may lead to unexpectedly high blood levels. By a similar mechanism, the use of indomethacin also may slow the elimination of aminoglycosides with increasing risk of drug accumulation.[39]

Premature neonates with patent ductus arteriosus show a larger volume of distribution for aminoglycosides, longer serum half-life, but no change in total-body clearance. This has been attributed to the fact that patent ductus increases extracellular fluid volume while not affecting glomerular filtration rate adversely.[40]

It is not known whether the high serum levels often found in the neonate are paralleled by a similar increased risk of drug accumulation in the tissue. This is important to know, since renal and ototoxicity are at least partly related to high tissue accumulation of aminoglycosides. Direct data have been obtained experimentally indicating that immaturity influences the degree of renal accumulation of aminoglycosides. Lower renal levels have been found in young animals. This could be attributable to various factors, such as the lower blood perfusion, reduced uptake by proximal tubular cells, and larger kidney volume/body volume ratio, and has been related to a reduced toxicity of the drugs.[41,42] Direct tissue measurements in human neonates have been performed only by Edwards et al.,[43] who found low kidney concentrations of amikacin in one neonate compared with adults. In human fetuses, kidney tobramycin concentrations have been directly related to gestational age.[23] Pharmacokinetic studies also have provided indirect evidence that the degree of accumulation of aminoglycosides in the immature neonate might be lower than in term neonates or in older children.[14,34]

After the first month of life, the elimination half-life of aminoglycosides shortens rapidly, and in infants and children with normal renal function, usually no accumulation of serum levels is seen even after prolonged treatment. The volume of distribution relative to body weight decreases progressively from infancy to adulthood.[16,44] Correspondingly, higher dosages per unit of body weight are needed in infants and young patients in order to achieve serum levels comparable with those obtained in adults.[44] These differences diminish when dosages are based on body surface area.[16]

CLINICAL PHARMACOLOGY OF AMINOGLYCOSIDES IN VARIOUS DISEASES

A number of pathologic conditions have been found to influence aminoglycoside kinetics. They are mentioned here, although their practical clinical relevance is not always evident. Low serum levels have been reported in extensively burned children and adults due possibly to elimination of the drug with the exudate.[45] Problems related to obesity have already been discussed (see above). In ascitic patients, higher volumes of distribution have been found[46] that can produce lower than expected peak levels with standard dosage.

Renal failure is certainly the main clinically important factor influencing aminoglycoside disposition. Prediction of accumulation is critical, since ototoxicity is likely to develop in patients with low glomerular filtration rates, eventually leading to total and irreversible deafness. Several studies have been performed on aminoglycoside kinetics in adults with various degrees of renal insufficiency or on hemodialysis, whereas only few concern infants and children.

If serum creatinine is in a steady state, it may be considered to be an indicator of renal function for the purpose of developing nomograms or equations intended to optimize dosages. These aspects have been reviewed by Péchére and Dugal.[47] In order to maintain serum levels between predetermined ranges in patients with low glomerular filtration rates, dosages may be kept constant while increasing the interval between administrations. Conversely, it is also possible to keep the time interval constant while reducing dosages. The first formula produces greater fluctuations between doses, and the second one produces higher and steadier levels. For aminoglycosides it has not been established whether one of these methods offers therapeutic efficacy and/or reduces the risk of toxicity.

Nomograms for establishing dosages should be considered only as general guidelines, and treatments should be individualized based on drug monitoring. Dosage adjustment is also needed when patients undergo hemodialysis. The elimination half-life during interdialysis periods is extremely low, the reduced serum levels in these periods also reflecting fluid retention and expansion of volume of distribution. Elimination during dialysis is rapid but is influenced by the technique.[48] In contrast, peritoneal dialysis is much less efficient in clearing aminoglycosides from the body.[49] Studies in children with renal failure are available[50,51] and substantially confirm the findings in adults.

Altered kinetics of several antibiotics have been reported in cystic fibrosis.[52] The need for larger dosages of aminoglycosides has been suggested.[52-54] Hsu et al.[53] have shown that cystic fibrosis patients may need dosages of tobramycin as high as 12 mg/kg at intervals of 4–6 hours in order to maintain serum levels exceeding the minimal inhibiting concentrations against *Pseudomonas* for at least 75 percent of the dosing interval without reaching potentially toxic serum levels. While rational from a pharmacokinetic point of view, it is not known whether this approach ensures better clinical results than conventional dosages.

TOXICITY

Oto- and nephrotoxicity are the most serious adverse reactions caused by aminoglycosides. These drugs also may cause other negative side effects, such as neuromuscular blockade, neuropathies, malabsorption following oral administration, elevation of serum transaminases, hypomagnesemia, and eosinophilia.[6] Some of these reactions also have been observed in pediatric patients.

Nephrotoxicity

Aminoglycosides do not differ qualitatively as far as their mechanism of nephrotoxicity is concerned. Tubular damage occurs early and may be seen during treatment as an increase in tubular-cell enzyme (N-acetylglucosaminidase) excretion or as an increased excretion of low-molecular-weight protein (β_2-microglobulin) reflecting reduced reabsorption by proximal tubular cells.[55] Although these indexes may be sensitive and specific, they may not be clinically important.[56] In some patients, however, tubular damage may progress and lead to electrolyte-handling disturbances that may be of clinical concern.[57] A reduction in glomerular filtration rate also may follow after some days of treatment.[58]

The series of events leading from early tubular damage to reduction of glomerular filtration rate need clarification. They may involve the tubuloglomerular feedback mechanism. Evidence of the role of the renin-angiotensin system is conflicting.[59] When glomerular filtration rate is depressed, it usually parallels the severity and extent of proximal tubular necrosis. However, early pathologic changes in the glomerulus have been found.[60]

In most patients who manifest an increase in serum creatinine during treatment with aminoglycosides, the changes are mild and reversible on suspension of administration. In adults it may be estimated that the incidence of clinically important renal damage (increased serum creatinine associated with reduced glomerular filtration rate) is between 5 and 15 percent if critically ill patients are excluded.[61-63]

Of the various factors suggested as relevant in the development of renal toxicity, some seem of importance, such as dose regimen, total dose, duration of therapy, trough serum levels, sodium balance, state of hydration, administration of other nephrotoxic drugs, and concomitant liver disease.[64] A bedside scoring system using some of these factors identifies high-risk adult patients accurately.[65]

Differences in nephrotoxicity of the various aminoglycosides in experimental animal models have been claimed by several authors.[60,66,67] Extrapolation of these results to the clinical setting is difficult. Large comparative studies indicating relatively minor differences in nephrotoxicity in adults with different aminoglycosides have been published. In some studies, gentamicin seems a more frequent cause of nephrotoxicity than tobramycin and netilmicin.[62,63] These differences, however, were not confirmed in other studies conducted under similar rigorous criteria.[61,68] No comparative data are available for children.

There is a considerable lack of information on aminoglycoside nephrotoxicity in infancy. Prospective studies with frequent monitoring of serum creatinine have not been done on children. Some studies have failed to demonstrate any significant change in serum creatinine in neonates receiving aminoglycosides compared with control groups of patients.[35,69] This does not mean that aminoglycosides are not nephrotoxic in human neonates or infants. Such studies are difficult to perform. In the first days of life, serum creatinine decreases rapidly, and slight deviations from normal values are difficult to interpret. In a randomized, controlled study, treatment of neonates with amikacin plus ampicillin, in contrast with mezlocillin, led to a delayed postnatal maturation in glomerular filtration rate, suggesting aminoglycoside toxicity in the neonatal period.[70]

In other studies, slight but reversible increases in serum creatinine have been reported in neonates and infants,[71,72] particularly in connection with prolonged therapy[73] or when aminoglycosides were combined with other potentially nephrotoxic drugs, such as vancomycin or indomethacin.[39,74] Increases in enzymuria and in β_2-microglobulin excretion have been found in neonates and children receiving aminoglycosides.[35,69,71,75-77] These changes were transient and not predictive of glomerular function impairment.

We have already discussed the lower accumulation found in the kidney of immature animals. In general, this has been related also to a lower nephrotoxicity in the young animal compared with the adult one. Whether this can be confidently extrapolated to human beings is unknown.

Ototoxicity

The biochemical mechanisms involved in the genesis of aminoglycoside ototoxic reactions have been studied by various authors.[9,78] Mild intoxication selectively damages type 1 vestibular sensory cells and outer hair cells of the basal cochlear turn. This accounts for higher-frequency cochlear potentials being primarily affected. Increasing intoxication progressively affects other sensory cells and cochlear structures. These changes are irreversible and progress to focal and general cell destruction. Among the clinically used aminoglycosides, streptomycin is predominantly vestibulotoxic, whereas neomycin, kanamycin, and amikacin are primarily toxic to the cochlea. Gentamicin, tobramycin, and sisomicin have both cochlear and vestibular toxicity, with more frequent vestibular toxicity. Netilmicin causes very low 8th nerve toxicity.[80]

Clinically, ototoxicity is manifested by a feeling of fullness in the ear and tinnitus followed by varying degrees of hearing loss, especially of high tones. Vestibular impairment results in loss of equilibrium, nystagmus, nausea, and vertigo. Ototoxicity is usually reversible and may be unilateral; however, hearing loss can progress to total deafness. Cases of delayed ototoxicity may occur some days after discontinuation of the treatment.[81,82] The incidence of hearing loss in adults has been found to be between 2 and 40 percent of the treated subjects.[62,81-84]

Several factors have been claimed to influence the ototoxicity of aminoglycosides in human studies. Peak and trough serum levels, total dose, renal functional impairment, and previous or concomitant administration of other aminoglycosides or ototoxic drugs have all been considered.[81-83] More recently, the records of large numbers of patients enrolled in prospective, randomized trials comparing the toxicity of gentamicin, tobramycin, amikacin, and netilmicin were analyzed by a multivariate statistical analysis (adjustments for confounding factors).[85,86]

In the study of Moore et al.,[85] patients with auditory toxicity underwent therapy for a longer period and were more likely to be bacteremic, dehydrated, or have an underlying liver dysfunction. Conversely, in the study of Gatell et al.,[86] only older age was identified as a predisposing factor for the development of auditory toxicity. Comparative studies in humans failed to reveal differences in ototoxicity among amikacin, gentamicin, and tobramycin,[62,84] whereas a trend toward lower ototoxic potential for netilmicin has been confirmed in several randomized, prospective studies.[61,63,86]

Among pediatric patients, aminoglycoside ototoxicity has been studied mainly in the neonatal period. Only in the last years, however, has brain stem evoked audiometry been used, enabling infants to be tested soon after the suspension of the treatment. Most previous studies tested infants by behavioral audiometry, which only allows examination of older infants. Studies in the neonate are often difficult to interpret. The role of various potential ototoxic factors has to be ruled out: meningitis, prematurity per se, endocranial hemorrhages, and otitis, among others. Nevertheless, well-conducted studies have detected only a few cases of permanent injury in neonates and children receiving treatments with high dosages of these drugs.[35,69,87,88] This suggests that aminoglycosides may be used in the pediatric population with more confidence than in the elderly. The reason why younger patients can better tolerate these drugs is not clear. It should be considered that in animals, on the contrary, the newly born seem more susceptible to the ototoxic effects of aminoglycosides.[89]

CLINICAL USE OF AMINOGLYCOSIDES IN PEDIATRIC PRACTICE

The major use of aminoglycosides in pediatric practice is in the treatment of infections caused by gram-negative enteric bacilli. In addition, they are used in combination with other antibiotics when synergistic antibacterial effect has been proven. This is the case, for example, in infections sustained by methicillin-resistant *Staphylococcus*, *Listeria monocytogenes,* group B and D streptococci, and *Streptococcus viridans.*

The clinical conditions where the use of aminoglycoside alone or in combination is recommended are reported in Table 25-1.[90] Three conditions deserve more detailed consideration: neonatal sepsis and meningitis, cystic fibrosis, and urinary tract infections.

Neonatal Sepsis

The spectrum of bacteria responsible for neonatal sepsis has changed in the last two decades, gram-negative bacilli, mainly *E. coli,* being the most frequently isolated germ until the early seventies. In several institutions, however, group B streptococci are now the most frequent single agent isolated. This, together with the possibility

that *Listeria monocytogenes* could cause neonatal meningitis, prevents the use of aminoglycosides as single agents in empirical treatment of severely ill neonates.

The recommended treatment is therefore a combination of an aminoglycoside and ampicillin. This treatment does not always afford good protection against meningitis caused by gram-negative bacteria. CSF sterilization is slow, and the outcome is not improved by intrathecal administration of the aminoglycoside.[22] The possible benefit of direct intraventricular injection of aminoglycosides is still controversial.[23,25,91,92] In the last few years, no further clinical trials have been performed, and attention has shifted toward a possible alternative, the new β-lactam antibiotics. Only one comparative study has been published, and this has failed to demonstrate any superiority of moxalactam over amikacin in the treatment of this condition, which still has a high mortality and long-term sequelae rate.[93]

TABLE 25–1. CLINICAL USE OF AMINOGLYCOSIDE ANTIBIOTICS IN PEDIATRIC PRACTICE

CLINICAL CONDITION (PATHOGEN)	COMBINED THERAPY
Newborns	
Necrotizing enterocolitis, peritonitis	Ticarcillin or mezlocillin
Aspiration pneumonia	Nafcillin or oxacillin
Sepsis and meningitis	
Pseudomonas	Ticarcillin or mezlocillin
Gram-negative enteric bacteria	Ampicillin
Group B streptococcus	Ampicillin or penicillin G (synergy against penicillin-tolerant streptococci)
Osteomyelitis, septic arthritis, skin soft-tissue infection, urinary tract infection	
Pseudomonas	
Gram-negative enteric bacteria	
Infants and Children	
Pneumonia	
Gram-negative enteric bacteria	
Pulmonary acute exacerbations in cystic fibrosis	Ticarcillin or other anti-*Pseudomonas* β-lactam
Endocarditis	
Enterococcus	Ampicillin or penicillin
Streptococcus viridans	Penicillin
Peritonitis secondary to bowel perforation	Clindamicin
Peritonitis secondary to peritoneal dyalisis	
Pseudomonas and gram-negative enteric bacteria*	
Gastroenteritis	
Enteroinvasive *E. coli*	
Febrile neutropenic patient	Anti-*Pseudomonas* β-lactam
CNS shunt infections	
S. aureus or *epidermidis*	Vancomycin (synergy against penicillin-tolerant staphylococci)
Brain abscess	Nafcillin and metronidazole

*Aminoglycosides are added to perfusate.

TABLE 25–2. DOSAGES AND SUITABLE PEAK AND TROUGH CONCENTRATIONS FOR SEVERAL AMINOGLYCOSIDES

AMINOGLYCOSIDE		DOSAGE (mg/kg/dose)	ACCEPTABLE SERUM CONCENTRATIONS (μg/ml)	
			Peak	Trough
Amikacin	Adult	5–7.5 (8–12 hourly)	20–30	10
	Child	5–7.5 (8–12 hourly)		
	Neonate	7.5 (12 hourly)*		
Tobramycin, Gentamicin, Netilmicin	Adult	1.5–2.0 (8–12 hourly)	8–12†	2
	Child	1.5–2.5 (8 hourly)		
	Neonate	2.5 (12 hourly)*		

*Premature neonates less than 34 weeks of gestation and in the first 10 days of life may need more prolonged intervals between dosages.
†For netilmicin, the manufacturer's indication is 16 μg/ml.

Cystic Fibrosis

High dosages of aminoglycosides are commonly used in the treatment of acute exacerbation in children with cystic fibrosis.[52–54] The efficacy of single courses of antibiotics in ameliorating acute symptoms as well as reducing the number of *Pseudomonas* bacteria in the sputum is documented. Studies comparing the use of aminoglycosides and third-generation cephalosporin or anti-*Pseudomonas* penicillins have shown similar clinical effects.[94,95] As already mentioned, the benefit of administering aminoglycosides by areosol to patients with cystic fibrosis is still unproven.[19,20]

Urinary Tract Infections

Aminoglycosides reach elevated concentrations in the renal parenchyma and are the drug of choice in the treatment of small infants with acute pyelonephritis. In older children with cystitis, with or without urinary tract abnormalities, their administration as single agents and in single doses has been proven useful. The peculiar urinary kinetics of aminoglycosides allow high concentrations of these drugs to be achieved in the urine and therapeutically active concentrations to be maintained for prolonged periods even following a single dose.[96–98]

MONITORING SERUM LEVELS

Several of the conditions requiring treatment with an aminoglycoside are severe and life threatening. In these cases, fluid and electrolyte imbalance, reduction in renal function or cardiac output, and acidosis may easily develop and account for unexpected variations of the pharmacokinetics of the antibiotic. This may lead to lower than desirable serum concentrations and thus undertreatment or, on the other hand, to excessive increases in blood levels and thus toxicity.

Monitoring aminoglycoside serum concentrations is recommended. This may allow individualization of treatment schedules. A variety of rapid and accurate methods

are available in most hospital laboratories. The desirable serum concentrations are listed in Table 25–2.

REFERENCES

1. Davies JE: Aminoglycoside-aminocyclitol antibiotics and their modifying enzymes, in Lorian V (ed): Antibiotics in Laboratory Medecine. Baltimore, Williams & Wilkins, 1986, pp 790–809
2. Maver GE, Ahmad R, Dobbs SM, McGough JM: Prescribing aids for gentamicin. Br J Clin Pharmacol 1:45–50, 1974
3. Howard JB, McCracken GH Jr: Reappraisal of kanamycin usage in neonates. J Pediatr 86:949–956, 1975
4. Powell KR, Pincus PH: Five years of experience with the exclusive use of amikacin in a neonatal intensive care unit. Pediatr Infect Dis J 6:461–466, 1987
5. Gerding D, Larson TA: Aminoglycoside resistance in gram-negative bacilli during increased amikacin use. Am J Med 79:(suppl 1A):1–7, 1985
6. Sande MA, Mandell GL: Antimicrobial agents: The aminoglycosides, in Goodman A, Gilman AG, et al (eds): The Pharmacological Basis of Therapeutics. New York, MacMillan Pub Co., 1985, pp 1150–1169
7. Krogstad DJ, Moellering RC: Antimicrobial combinations, in Lorian V (ed): Antibiotics in Laboratory Medicine. Baltimore, Williams & Wilkins, 1986, pp 537–595
8. Weibert R, Keane W, Shapiro F: Carbenicillin inactivation of aminoglycosides in patients with severe renal failure. Trans Soc Artif Intern Organs 22:439–443, 1976
9. Greenberg LH, Momary H: Audiotoxicity and nephrotoxicity due to orally administered neomycin. JAMA 194:237–238, 1975
10. Miranda JC, Schimmel MS, Himms GM, et al: Gentamicin absorption during prophylactic use for necrotizing enterocolitis. Dev Pharmacol Ther 7:303–306, 1984
11. Bamfort MFM, Jones LF: Deafness and biochemical imbalance after burns treatment with topical antibiotics in young children. Arch Dis Child 53:326–329, 1978
12. Clark JT, Libke RD, Regamey C, Kirby WMM: Comparative pharmacokinetics of amikacin and kanamycin. Clin Pharmacol Ther 15:610–616, 1974
13. Jahre JA, Fu KP, Neu HC: Kinetics of netilmicin and gentamicin. Clin Pharmacol Ther 23:591–597, 1978
14. Assael BM, Cavanna G, Jusko WJ, et al: Multiexponential elimination of gentamicin: A kinetic study during development. Dev Pharmacol Ther 1:171–181, 1980
15. Howard JB, McCracken GH Jr, Trujillo H, Mohs E: Amikacin in newborn infants: Comparative pharmacology with kanamicin and clinical efficacy in 45 neonates with bacterial diseases. Antimicrob Agents Chemother 10:205–210, 1976
16. Vogelstein B, Kowarski AA, Lietman PS: The pharmacokinetics of amikacin in children. J Pediatr 91:333–339, 1977
17. Dale Richey G, Scholeopoer CJ: Peritoneal fluid concentration of gentamicin in patients with spontaneous bacterial peritonitis. Antimicrob Agents Chemother 19:312–315, 1981

18. Mombelli G, Coppens L, Thys JP, Klastersky J: Anti-Pseudomonas activity in bronchial secretions of patients receiving amikacin or tobramycin as a continuous infusion. Antimicrob Agents Chemother 19:72–75, 1981

19. MacLusky I, Levison H, Gold R, MacLaughlin FJ: Inhaled antibiotics in cystic fibrosis: Is there a therapeutic effect? J Pediatr 108:861–865, 1986

20. Schaad UB, Wedgwood-Krucko J, Suter S, Kraemer R: Efficacy of inhaled amikacin as adjunct to intravenous combination therapy (ceftazidime and amikacin) in cystic fibrosis. J Pediatr 111:599–605, 1987

21. Chow A, Hecht R, Winters R: Gentamicin and carbenicillin penetration into septic joint. N Engl J Med 285:178–179, 1971

22. McCracken GH Jr, Mize SG: A controlled study of intratechal antibiotic therapy in gram-negative enteric meningitis of infancy: Report of the Neonatal Meningitis Cooperative Study Group. J Pediatr 89:66–72, 1976

23. Swartz MN: Intraventricular use of aminoglycosides in the treatment of gram-negative bacillary meningitis: Conflicting views. J Infect Dis 143:293–295, 1981

24. Kaiser AB, McGee ZA: Aminoglycoside therapy of gram-negative bacillary meningitis. N Engl J Med 293:1215–1220, 1975

25. Wright PF, Kaiser AB, Bowman CM, et al: The pharmacokinetics and efficacy of an aminoglycoside administered into the cerebral ventricles in neonates: Implication for further evaluation of this route of therapy in meningitis. J Infect Dis 143:141–147, 1981

26. Golden B: Subtenon injection of gentamicin for bacterial infections of the eye. J Infect Dis 124(suppl 1):271–274, 1971

27. Hull JH, Sarubbi FA: Gentamicin serum concentrations: Pharmacokinetic predictions. Ann Intern Med 85:183–189, 1979

28. Bernard B, Garcia-Cazares SJ, Ballard CA, et al: Tobramycin: Maternal-fetal pharmacology. Antimicrob Agents Chemother 11:688–694, 1977

29. Labierne-Pegorier M, Gilbert T, Sackly R, et al: Effect of fetal exposure to gentamicin on kidney of young guinea pigs. Antimcrob Agents Chemother 31:88–92, 1987

30. Giuliano RA, Verpooten GA, De Broe ME: The effect of dosing strategy on kidney cortical accumulation of aminoglycosides in rats. Am J Kidney Dis 8:297–303, 1986

31. Lerner SA, Seligsohn R, Bhattacharya I, et al: Pharmacokinetic of gentamicin in the inner ear perilymph of man, in Lerner SA, Matz GJ, Hawkins JE (eds): Aminoglycosides Ototoxicity. Boston, Little, Brown, 1981, pp 357–369

32. Schentag JJ, Jusko WJ, Vance JW, et al: Gentamicin disposition and tissue accumulation on multiple dosing. J Pharmacol Biopharm 5:559–577, 1977

33. Assael BM, Gianni V, Marini A, et al: Gentamicin dosage in preterm and term neonates. Arch Dis Child 52:883–886, 1977

34. Assael BM, Parini R, Rusconi F, Cavanna G: Influence of intrauterine maturation on the pharmacokinetics of amikacin in the neonatal period. Pediatr Res 16:810–815, 1982

35. Granati B, Assael BM, Chung M, et al: Clinical pharmacology of netilmicin in preterm and term newborn infants. J Pediatr 106:664–669, 1985

36. Szefler SJ, Wynn RJ, Clarke DF, et al: Relationship of gentamicin serum concentrations to gestational age in preterm and term neonates. J Pediatr 97:312–315, 1980

37. Thomson AH, Way S, Bryson SM, et al: Population pharmacokinetics of gentamicin in neonates. Dev Pharmacol Ther 11:173–179, 1988

38. Rusconi F, Parini R, Cavanna G, Assael BM: Monitoring of amikacin in the neonate. Ther Drug Monit 5:179–183, 1983

39. Zarfin J, Koren G, Maresky D, et al: Possible indomethacin aminoglycoside interaction in preterm infants. J Pediatr 106:511–513, 1985

40. Watterberg KL, Kelly HW, Johnson JD, et al: Effect of patent ductus arteriosus on gentamicin pharmacokinetics in very low birth weight (<1500 gm) babies. Dev Pharmacol Ther 10:107–117, 1987

41. Cowan RH, Jukkola AF, Arant BS: Pathophysiologic evidence of gentamicin nephrotoxicity in neonatal puppies. Pediatr Res 14:1204–1211, 1980

42. Marre R, Tarara M, Louton T, Sack K: Age-dependent nephrotoxicity and the pharmacokinetics of gentamicin in rats. Eur J Pediatr 133:25–29, 1980

43. Edwards GQ, Smith CR, Baughman KL, et al: Concentrations of gentamicin and amikacin in human kidney. Antimicrob Agents Chemother 9:925–927, 1976

44. Echeverria P, Siber GR, Paisley J, et al: Age-dependent dose–response to gentamicin. J Pediatr 87:805–808, 1975

45. Loirat P, Rohan J, Baillet A, et al: Increased glomerular filtration rate in patients with major burns and its effect on the pharmacokinetics of tobramycin. N Engl J Med 299:915–919, 1978

46. Gill MA, Kern JW: Altered gentamicin distribution in ascitic patients. Am J Hosp Pharm 36:1704–1706, 1979

47. Péchére JC, Dugal R: Clinical pharmacokinetics of aminoglycoside antibiotics. Clin Pharmacokinet 4:170–199, 1979

48. Halpren BA, Axline SF, Coplon NS, Brown DM: Clearance of gentamicin during hemodialysis: Comparison of four artificial kidneys. J Infect Dis 133:627–636, 1976

49. Regeur L, Colding H, Jensen H, Kampmann JP: Pharmacokinetics of amikacin during hemodialysis and peritoneal dialysis. Antimicrob Agents Chemother 11:214–218, 1977

50. Sirinavin S, McCracken GH Jr, Nelson JD: Determining gentamicin dosage in infants and children with renal failure. J Pediatr 96:331–334, 1980

51. Yoshioka H, Takimoto M, Matsuda I, Hattori S: Dosage schedule of gentamicin for chronic renal insufficiency in children. Arch Dis Child 53:334–337, 1978

52. Nelson JD: Management of acute pulmonary exacerbations in cystic fibrosis: A critical appraisal. J Pediatr 106:1030–1033, 1985

53. Hsu MC, Agula HA, Schmidt VL, et al: Individualization of tobramycin dosage in patients with cystic fibrosis. Pediatr Infect Dis 3:526–529, 1984

54. Kearns GL, Hilman B, Wilson JT: Dosing implications of altered gentamicin disposition in patients with cystic fibrosis. J Pediatr 100:312–318, 1982

55. Mondorf AW, Breier J, Hendus J, et al: Effect of aminoglycosides on proximal tubular membranes of the human kidney. Eur J Clin Pharmacol 13:113–142, 1978

56. Trollfors B, Alestig K, Krantz I: Quantitative nephrotoxicity of gentamicin in nontoxic doses. J Infect Dis 141:306–309, 1980

57. Russo JC, Adelman RD: Gentamicin induced Fanconi syndrome. J Pediatr 96:151–153, 1980

58. Gary EN, Buzzeo L, Salaki J, Eisinger RP: Gentamicin-associated acute renal failure. Arch Intern Med 136:1101–1104, 1976

59. Luft FC, Azonoff GR, Evan AP, et al: The renin-angiotensin system in aminoglycoside-induced acute renal failure. J Pharmacol Exp Ther 220:433–439, 1982

60. Luft FC, Evan AP: Comparative effects of tobramycin and gentamicin on glomerular ultrastructure. J Infect Dis 142:910–914, 1980

61. Gatell JM, San Miguel JG, Aranjo V, et al: Prospective randomized double-blind comparison of nephrotoxicity and auditory toxicity of tobramycin and netilmicin. Antimicrob Agents Chemother 26:766–769, 1984

62. Smith CR, Lipsky JJ, Laskin OL, et al: Double-blind comparison of the nephrotoxicity and auditory toxicity of gentamicin and tobramycin. N Engl J Med 302:1106–1109, 1980

63. Lerner AM, Reyes MP, Cone LA, et al: Randomized controlled trial of the comparative efficacy, auditory toxicity and nephrotoxicity of tobramycin and netilmicin. Lancet 1:1123–1126, 1983

64. Moore RD, Smith CR, Lipsky JJ, Mellits ED, Lietman PS: Risk factors for nephrotoxicity in patients treated with aminoglycoside. Ann Int Med 100:352–357, 1984

65. Sawyers CL, Moore RD, Lerner SA, Smith CR: A model for predicting nephrotoxicity in patients treated with aminoglycosides. J Infect Dis 153:1062–1068, 1986

66. Laurent G, Carlier MB, Rollman B, et al: Mechanisms of aminoglycoside-induced lysosomal phospholipidosis: In vitro and in vivo studies with gentamicin and amikacin. Biochem Pharmacol 31:3861–3870, 1982

67. Soberon L, Bowman RL, Pastoriza-Munez E, Kaloyanides GI: Comparative nephrotoxicities of gentamicin, netilmicin and tobramycin in the rat. J Pharmacol Exp Ther 210:334–343, 1979

68. Fong JW, Fenton RS, Bird R: Comparative toxicity of gentamicin versus tobramycin: A randomized prospspective study. J Antimicrob Chemother 7:81–88, 1981

69. Parini R, Rusconi F, Cavanna G, et al: Evaluation of the auditory

and renal function of neonates treated with amikacin. Dev Pharmacol Ther 5:33–40, 1982

70. Adelman RD, Wirth F, Rubio T: A controlled study of the nephrotoxicity of mezlocillin and amikacin in the neonate. Am J Dis Child 141:1175–1178, 1987

71. Elinder G, Aperia A: Development of glomerular filtration rate and excretion of beta-2-microglobulin in neonates during gentamicin treatment. Acta Paediatr Scand 72:219–223, 1983

72. Feldman H, Guignard JP: Plasma creatinine in the first month of life. Arch Dis Child 57:123–126, 1982

73. Marks MI, Vose A, Hammerberg S, Dugal R: Clinicopharmacological studies of sisomicin in ill children. Antimicrob Agents Chemother 13:753–758, 1978

74. Odio C, McCracken GH Jr, Nelson JD: Nephrotoxicity associated with vancomicin-aminoglycoside therapy in four children. J Pediatr 105:491–493, 1984

75. Adelman RD, Zakauddin S: Urinary enzyme activities in children and neonates receiving gentamicin therapy. Dev Pharmacol Ther 1:325–332, 1980

76. Reed MD, Vermeulen MW, Stern RC, et al: Are measurements of urine enzymes useful during aminoglycoside therapy? Pediatr Res 15:1234–1239, 1981

77. Rajchgot P, Prober CG, Soldin S, et al: Aminoglycoside-related nephrotoxicity in the premature newborn. Clin Pharmacol Ther 35:394–401, 1984

78. Hawkins E Jr: Ototoxic mechanisms. Audiology 12:383–393, 1973

79. Assael BM, Parini R, Rusconi F: Ototoxicity of aminoglycosides antibiotics in infants and children, in Nelson JD, McCracken GH Jr (eds): Clinical Review in Pediatrics Infectious Diseases. Toronto, BC Decker, Inc, 1985, pp 107–116

80. Arpini A, Cornacchia L, Albiero L, et al: Auditory function in guinea pigs treated with netilmicin and other aminoglycoside antibiotics. Arch Otolaryngol 224:137–142, 1979

81. Black RE, Lau WK, Weinstein RJ, et al: Ototoxicity of amikacin. Antimicrob Agents Chemother 9:956–961, 1976

82. Neu HC, Bendush CL: Ototoxicity of tobramycin: A clinical overview. J Infect Dis 134(suppl 2):206–218, 1976

83. Lane AZ, Wright GE, Blair DC: Ototoxicity and nephrotoxicity of amikacin: An overview of phase II and phase III experience in the United States. Am J Med 62:911–923, 1977

84. Smith CR, Baughman KL, Edwards CQ, et al: Controlled comparison of amikacin and gentamicin. N Engl J Med 296:349–353, 1977

85. Moore RD, Smith CR, Lietman PS: Risk factors for the development of auditory toxicity in patients receiving aminoglycosides. J Infect Dis 149:23–29, 1984

86. Gatell JM, Ferran F, Araujo V, et al: Univariate and multivariate analysis of risk factors predisposing to auditory toxicity in patients receiving aminoglycosides. Antimicrob Agents Chemother 31:1383–1387, 1987

87. Finitzo-Hieber T, McCracken GH Jr, Clinton Brown K: Prospective, controlled evaluation of auditory function in neonates given netilmicin or amikacin. J Pediatr 106:129–136, 1985

88. Gianni V, Vigliani E, Assael BM, et al: Valutazione della funzione uditiva in bambini trattati con gentamicina in periodo neonatale. Riv Ital Ped (IJP)7:17–20, 1981

89. Henry KR, Chole RA, McGinn MD, Frush DP: Increased ototoxicity in both young and old mice. Arch Otolaryngol 107:92–95, 1981

90. Nelson JD: Pocketbook of Pediatric Antimicrobial Therapy, 7th ed. Baltimore, Williams & Wilkins, 1987

91. Lee EL, Robinson MJ, Thong ML, et al: Intraventricular chemotherapy in neonatal meningitis. J Pediatr 91:991–995, 1977

92. McCracken GH Jr, Mize SG, Threlkeld N: Intraventricular gentamicin therapy in gram-negative bacillary meningitis of infancy: Report of the Second Neonatal Meningitis Cooperative Study Group. Lancet 1:787–791, 1980

93. McCracken GH Jr, Threlkeld N, Mize S, et al: The Neonatal Meningitis Cooperative Study Group: Moxalactam therapy for neonatal meningitis due to gramnegative enteric bacilli. JAMA 252:1427–1432, 1984

94. Padoan R, Cambisano W, Costantini D, et al: Ceftazidime monotherapy vs combined therapy in Pseudomonas pulmonary infections in cystic fibrosis. Pediatr Infect Dis J 6:648–653, 1987

95. Bosso JR, Black PG: Controlled trial of aztreonam vs tobramycin and azlocillin for acute pulmonary exacerbations of cystic fibrosis. Pediatr Infect Dis J 7:171–176, 1987

96. Viganò A, Dalla Villa A, Bianchi C, et al: Single dose netilmicin therapy of complicated and uncomplicated lower urinary tract infections in children. Acta Paediatr Scand 74:584–588, 1985

97. Kahn AJ, Kumar K, Evans HE: Single-dose gentamicin therapy for recurrent urinary tract infections in patients with normal urinary tract. J Pediatr 110:131–135, 1987

98. Wallen L, Zeller WP, Goessler H, et al: Single-dose amikacin treatment of first childhood E. coli lower urinary tract infections. J Pediatr 103:316–317, 1983

26

CEPHALOSPORINS

HARRIS R. STUTMAN *and* MELVIN I. MARKS

Any review of cephalosporin pharmacology must contend with the multiplicity of new antimicrobial agents that have been developed and marketed in the past decade. These have generally been categorized into first-, second-, and third-generation drugs dependent on their antimicrobial activity.[1] Because of its common usage, this classification scheme will be used in this chapter (Table 26–1). First-generation compounds generally have high activity against gram-positive cocci, with the exception of *Streptococcus faecalis* (enterococcus). Second-generation compounds have enhanced activity against Enterobacteriaceae and often against fastidious bacteria, such as *Haemophilus influenzae* and *Neisseria meningitidis.* They have increased stability to β-lactamase–induced hydrolysis. Third-generation compounds have even further enhanced activity against gram-negative bacilli, usually at the expense of diminished activity against gram-positive cocci. Several cephalosporins do not easily fit into this categorization scheme, including those with enhanced activity against anaerobic bacteria, including *Bacteroides fragilis* (e.g., cefoxitin), and those with augmented activity against *Pseudomonas aeruginosa* and related nonfermenting bacteria (e.g., ceftazidime).

Unfortunately, pharmacologic properties do not necessarily vary along the same lines as antimicrobial activity. The typical cephalosporin compound is parenterally administered and has a serum half-life of some 1–2 hours, with the majority of drug (75–90 percent) being excreted in unchanged form by renal mechanisms.[2] In reviewing aspects of pediatric pharmacology, reference will be made to this typical pharmacologic profile while pointing out those compounds which vary from this pattern. These include orally bioavailable compounds, those with a prolonged serum half-life (often related to markedly increased protein binding), those excreted by routes other than the kidney, and those compounds which are metabolized *in vivo* to active or inactive compounds prior to excretion.

The field of pediatric antimicrobial pharmacology must contend with additional problems. Children may not volunteer for the study of the basic pharmacology or pharmacokinetics of antibiotics, and therefore, available data are derived from ill children with underlying disease. This creates problems in the interpretation of metabolic processes and adverse effects. Information on excretory patterns is difficult to obtain because of the problem of collecting specimens from infants and small children. Because of the small numbers of children who are involved in clinical trials, available data are often subject to change as additional studies are reported. This is especially true for adverse reactions. Nevertheless, the field of pediatric pharmacology, including the cephalosporins, has advanced markedly over the past few years. Clinical investigators and clinicians alike are increasingly cognizant of the need to demonstrate pharmacologic and pharmacokinetic patterns for each new antimicrobial agent before introduction into common clinical use, regardless of its *in vitro* advantages.

CEPHALOSPORIN ABSORPTION, DISTRIBUTION, METABOLISM, AND EXCRETION

Because of the wide variability in renal function in newborns, particularly premature infants, as compared with older infants and children, there is wide variability in pharmacologic handling of compounds like the cephalosporins, which are generally excreted by renal mechanisms. The decreased glomerular filtration rate and renal tubular function characteristic of younger infants may increase elimination half-life and hence serum concentrations.[3] In addition, the larger extracellular fluid volumes found in infants cause an apparent increase in volume of distribution, adding complexity to the assessment of cephalosporin metabolism. Changes occurring over the first few days of life during physiologic diuresis enhance this problem.

TABLE 26–1. CLASSIFICATION OF CEPHALOSPORIN ANTIBIOTICS

PEDIATRIC USEFULNESS	FIRST GENERATION	SECOND GENERATION	THIRD-GENERATION EXTENDED SPECTRUM
Common	Cefazolin Cephradine Cephapirin Cephalexin Cefadroxil	Cefuroxime Cefaclor Cefoxitin	Cefotaxime Ceftriaxone Ceftazidime
Uncommon	Cephalothin	Cefamandole Cefonicid Cefotetan	Ceftizoxime Cefoperazone Moxalactam

Representative examples of pharmacologic parameters for the newer cephalosporins in neonates are given (Table 26–2). These data are generally not available for oral cephalosporins and older agents that have limited neonatal application. The diminished creatinine clearance and renal tubular secretion rates in newborns result in decreased total serum clearance and increased elimination half-life compared with older infants and children.[3] These pharmacokinetic variables usually correlate well with gestational age and to a lesser degree with birth weight. Increasing postnatal age results in improved clearance and diminished half-life until values corresponding with those of infants and children are reached by 1–2 months of age.[4] The only exception is cefoperazone, which, perhaps related to its primary biliary excretion, shows no correlation of clearance with gestational age or birth weight.[5]

Because of the inapplicability of volunteer studies, there are relatively few data on the influence of hepatic or renal dysfunction or common disease states on the pharmacology of cephalosporins. In most cases, this is not a serious problem because of the lack of toxicity of these agents. However, most cephalosporins are excreted by renal mechanisms, and standard dosing regimens may result in drug accumulation over time. The exceptions are likely to be cefoperazone and ceftriaxone, which are 75 and 35 percent, respectively, excreted by biliary mechanisms.[6,7] A study of cefotaxime and ceftazidime in liver transplant patients showed normal kinetics in those children with normal renal function.[8]

Cystic fibrosis (CF) is a common childhood condition associated with altered drug handling. Many children show increased volumes of distribution or total serum clearance with a variety of antimicrobial agents, including cephalosporins.[9] Although systematic studies are often lacking, data for ceftazidime seem to confirm this observation, with a shorter elimination half-life (1.7 versus 2.5 hours) and a larger volume of distribution (725 versus 485 ml/kg) in CF versus non-CF patients.[10] Although these differences are most relevant to the aminoglycosides with their toxic potential, their clinical relevance to cephalosporin therapy in cystic fibrosis is less clear. Nevertheless, this possibility must be considered in constructing appropriate treatment regimens and evaluating responses to therapy. A separate issue is the administration of oral cephalosporins to children with CF concurrently receiving pancreatic enzyme supplements. Although an early study suggested diminished absorption with concurrent administration,[11] our own data indicate that serum concentrations under such conditions are similar to those obtained in fasting, non-CF patients.[12]

ORAL AND PARENTERAL ADMINISTRATION

Five oral cephalosporins are currently available in the United States. They are cephalexin, cephradine, cefadroxil, cefaclor, and cefuroxime axetil. Although cefurox-

TABLE 26–2. PHARMACOKINETIC FEATURES OF PARENTERAL CEPHALOSPORINS IN NEONATES

DRUG (DOSAGE)	AGE	PEAK SERUM CONCENTRATION (mg/liter)	ELIMINATION HALF-LIFE (h)	VOLUME OF DISTRIBUTION (ml/kg)	TOTAL SERUM CLEARANCE (ml/min/kg)
Cefotaxime[26] (50 mg/kg)	<1500 gm >1500 gm	96 106	4.6 3.4	510 440	0.36 0.63
Cefoperazone[4] (100 mg/kg)	2–5 days	352	6.5	410	0.78
Ceftriaxone[67] (50 mg/kg)	<1 week >1 week	124 108	16.2 9.2	450 480	0.37 0.77
Ceftazidime[68] (50 mg/kg)	<32 weeks* 33–37 weeks ≥38 weeks	121 101 95	3.7 2.9 3.5	423 425 546	1.58 1.75 1.77

*Gestational age.

TABLE 26–3. EFFECTS OF FEEDING ON ABSORPTION OF ORAL CEPHALOSPORINS

DRUG (DOSAGE)	FEEDING	TIME TO PEAK CONCENTRATION (h)	PEAK SERUM CONCENTRATION (mg/liter)	PERCENT ABSORBED
Liquid				
Cephalexin[13] (15 mg/kg)	Fasting	0.5	23.4	90
	Food	1.0	9.0	35
Cephradine[13] (15 mg/kg)	Fasting	0.5	21.3	90
	Food	0.5	9.9	43
Capsules				
Cephalexin[14] (25 mg/kg)	Fasting	2.0	19.5	86
	Food	2.0	20.5	90
Cefuroxime[15] (500 mg)	Fasting	2.0	4.8	36
	Food	3.0	7.2	52

ime has a parenteral counterpart, its absorption does not suggest therapeutic interchangeability. Cefaclor and cefuroxime are 40–50 percent bioavailable, whereas the other oral cephalosporins are 80–95 percent absorbed.[13] With the exception of cefuroxime, all are available in both liquid and tablet (or capsule) form.

Again, with the exception of cefuroxime axetil, each of the oral cephalosporins is best absorbed on an empty stomach,[14] although the effect of feeding on the absorption of capsule formulations is probably not clinically significant (Table 26–3). Cefuroxime's absorption increases from 36 to 52 percent when administered with food or milk.[15] Milk, particularly, interferes with the absorption of liquid cephalexin and cephradine, and concomitant administration should be avoided.[14]

Parenteral cephalosporins are generally well absorbed after either intramuscular or intravenous administration, with similar areas under the time concentration curve by either route.[16] The only exception is cephapirin, which is only 50 percent bioavailable when given intramuscularly. A traditional limiting factor in the use of cephalosporins in pediatrics has been their irritating properties. Indeed, cephalothin and cefoxitin are so painful that they should not be used intramuscularly in children (and only when mixed with lidocaine in adults).[17] The newer second- and third-generation cephalosporins have largely circumvented this problem and are well tolerated, without significant pain on local injection and with minimal risk of phlebitis on intravenous infusion.[18] The development of drugs, such as ceftriaxone and cefonicid, with long half-lives and good intramuscular tolerance and absorption markedly enhances our therapeutic options. However, erratic absorption in seriously ill patients and inadequate muscle mass in small infants may mandate intravenous therapy.[19]

Cephalosporins are generally physically and chemically compatible with most diluents and drugs that are likely to be coadministered. Exceptions are the incompatibility of cephradine with saline, ceftazidime with bicarbonate, and cephalothin with calcium compounds, erythromycin, and tetracycline.[20] In addition, β-lactams, including cephalosporins, should not generally be mixed in the same solution with aminoglycosides, lest the latter compounds be inactivated.[21]

TABLE 26–4. SELECTED PHARMACOKINETIC FEATURES FOR PARENTERAL CEPHALOSPORINS USED IN CHILDREN

DRUG	DOSE (mg/kg)	PEAK SERUM CONCENTRATION (mg/liter)	ELIMINATION HALF-LIFE (h)	VOLUME OF DISTRIBUTION (ml/kg)	EXCRETORY MECHANISMS*	SERUM CLEARANCE (ml/min/kg)
Cephalothin	25	30	0.6	930	70% R 30% RM	6.4
Cefazolin	25	60	1.6		65% R	0.7
Cefoxitin	37.5	80	0.7		80% R	3.5
Cefuroxime	50	130	1.5	600	95% R	2.0
Cefotaxime	50	124	1.2	360	65% R 20% RM	4.8
Ceftizoxime	50	101	1.5		>90% R	
Cefoperazone	50	320	1.8	200	75% B	
Ceftriaxone	50	170–240	4–6.5	350	35% B 60% R	0.8
Ceftazidime	50	150	1.5	310	75% R	1.5

*R = renal, RM = renal (metabolized form), B = biliary.

TABLE 26–5. SELECTED PHARMACOKINETIC FEATURES FOR ORAL CEPHALOSPORINS USED IN CHILDREN

DRUG	DOSAGE (mg/kg)	PEAK SERUM CONCENTRATION (mg/liter)	ELIMINATION HALF-LIFE (h)	CLEARANCE TOTAL (ml/min/kg)	ORAL ABSORPTION (%)
Cephalexin	25	19.4	1.4	380	90
Cefaclor	15	13	0.7	400	50
Cephradine	15	10	1.0	500	95
Cefadroxil	15	13	1.5	300	85
Cefuroxime	20	10	1.4	150	52

PHARMACOKINETICS

Pharmacokinetic studies in normal children are rarely available, and data are usually derived from small numbers of hospitalized children. Therefore, this information must be interpreted cautiously. Selected pharmacokinetic data are presented for oral and parenteral cephalosporin antibiotics (Tables 26–4 and 26–5). The concepts of elimination half-life, volume of distribution, and clearance are discussed in detail elsewhere in this text. The typical cephalosporin has an elimination half-life of 1–2 hours and undergoes primarily unmetabolized excretion by renal mechanisms.[2] Parenteral agents are best administered intravenously because of tissue irritation. When given intravenously, rapid infusions (20–30 minutes) are usually appropriate.

Exceptions to the preceding general characteristics deserve mention. Ceftriaxone is a recently marketed cephalosporin with a prolonged half-life of 4–7 hours in children and 6–18 hours in neonates.[22] This fact, combined with tolerance on intramuscular injection, suggests increased opportunities for ambulatory treatment of some serious pediatric infections.[23] Cefoperazone is the only cephalosporin developed to date that is primarily excreted by means of biliary mechanisms (75 percent), although minor portions of ceftriaxone (35 percent) and cefoxitin (20 percent) are excreted by this route.[6,7] Although other factors must be considered, cefoperazone and, to a lesser extent, ceftriaxone may merit consideration in the treatment of patients with preexisting renal disease and those with cholangitic infections.

The oral cephalosporins are generally better absorbed when fasting. The only exception is cefuroxime axetil, which has higher serum concentrations when given with food.[15] This does not appear to be related to altered intestinal motility or meal composition (milk versus solids). Otherwise, the pharmacokinetic behavior of oral agents is reasonably similar, and drug selection would ordinarily be based on other factors (antibacterial activity, tolerance, cost).

Although most cephalosporins are excreted in unchanged form, cephalothin and cefotaxime undergo transformation to bioactive desacetyl metabolites.[24,25] Desacetyl cephalothin retains 25–50 percent and desacetyl cefotaxime retains 15–25 percent of the antibacterial activity of the parent antibiotic. However, the cefotaxime metabolite achieves better concentrations in many body fluids (e.g., CSF) than the parent compound,[26] and the combination often displays synergistic antibacterial activity as well.[27] Therefore, some caution is required in assessing the bioactivity of these compounds based solely on concentrations of the original drug in infected body fluids.[24] Other compounds less commonly used in children that are desacetylated are cefapirin and cefotiam.[2] Cefoxitin is metabolized to a descarbamyl derivative, but this inactive metabolite makes up less than 5 percent of amounts recovered in urine.

Dosages of cephalosporins for serious infections are summarized in Table 26–6. These recommendations are empiric and based on antibacterial activity, penetration into sites of infection, and the large therapeutic/toxic ratios characteristic of cephalosporins.

TABLE 26–6. RECOMMENDED DOSAGES OF PARENTERAL CEPHALOSPORINS FOR SERIOUS PEDIATRIC INFECTIONS*

DRUG	NEONATES† mg/kg/day	NEONATES† Daily Doses	CHILDREN mg/kg/day	CHILDREN Daily Doses
Cephalothin	50–100	2–3	110–150	4–6
Cefazolin	40–50	2	50–100	3–4
Cefoxitin	N.A.‡		150	4–6
Cefuroxime	N.A.		150–225	3
Cefotaxime	100–150	2–3	180–200	4
Ceftizoxime	N.A.		150–200	2–3
Ceftriaxone	50	1	50–100	1–2
Ceftazidime	50–100	2–3	100–150	3
Cefoperazone	N.A.		150	2–3

*Lower doses may be appropriate for nonmeningeal infections.
†Many of the listed agents have limited neonatal indications.
‡N.A. = not available.

TISSUE CONCENTRATIONS

The maximum concentrations of cephalosporins achieved in body fluids during inflammation are given in Table 26–7. In most cases, these are based on limited pediatric data. In serious infections, confirmation of bactericidal activity at the site of infection is always helpful. With the exception of liver and biliary concentrations, obviously influenced by route of excretion, relative concentrations at other sites are similar for most cephalosporins. The therapeutic value of third-generation cephalosporins in pediatric meningitis, for example, rests not with enhanced CSF penetration but with higher serum concentrations and markedly greater bactericidal activity.[28] Certain cephalosporins, e.g., cefamandole, have such erratic CSF penetration, however, that breakthrough meningitis has sharply limited their pediatric usefulness.[29] As with other β-lactams, the best CSF concentrations are found with acute inflammation, and much lower values occur late in the course of treatment and in patients without meningeal inflammation.[30] This results primarily from the relatively low lipid solubility of ionized substances such as the cephalosporins.

Sputum and bronchial concentrations, although variable, are generally low but sufficient to be effective therapeutically.[31] Lung tissue concentrations for cefuroxime and ceftazidime are apparently greater (12–17 μg/gm) than values in sputum, however.[32] Concentrations in synovium and bone are somewhat better for the second- and third-generation compounds,[33] suggesting a therapeutic role that is equivocal for the older cephalosporins, which have lesser antibacterial activity.

A problem in interpreting tissue concentration data often arises from the presentation of serum/tissue ratios. Simultaneous measurements produce much greater values than the comparison of peak concentrations owing to the rapid falloff in serum concentrations over time. This difference needs to be considered in comparing data from different studies and between different cephalosporins.

RENAL AND HEPATIC DYSFUNCTION

There are relatively few data derived directly from pediatric patients, and extrapolation from adult studies is required. However, in those instances where pediatric data do exist, they corroborate this correlation. Most cephalosporins are eliminated by a combination of glomerular filtration and active renal tubular secretion.[2] Cefoperazone, ceftriaxone, and ceftazidime are the only cephalosporins commonly used in children that undergo little or no tubular filtration.[6,7,34] Probenecid, a drug that interferes with renal tubular secretion, therefore, prolongs the elimination half-life of all cephalosporins except for these three drugs. The high protein binding (with decreased glomerular filtration), lack of in vivo metabolism, and minimal tubular secretion are responsible for the long half-life of ceftriaxone.[23] Compounds such as cefotaxime with low protein binding and enhanced tubu-

TABLE 26–7. CONCENTRATIONS (mg/liter) OF CEPHALOSPORINS IN BODY FLUIDS DURING ACUTE INFECTION

DRUG	CSF	BILE	SPUTUM	BONE
Cephalothin	L*	12	0–1	L
Cefazolin	L	4.6	2–3	7.5
Cefoxitin	2–5 (10–15%)†	50–400	2–3	1–25
Cefuroxime	2–20 (6–10%)	43	2–3	14
Cefotaxime	2–12 (5–15%)	10–20	1–2	15
Ceftriaxone	2–35 (2–6%)	500	2–5	25
Ceftazidime	2–8 (2–5%)	40	2–4	30
Cefoperazone	2–8 (<5%)	60–6000	4–6	40

*L = very low concentrations.
†Percent of peak serum concentrations.

lar secretion have much shorter half-lives (1–1.2 hours), mandating more frequent dosing.[26]

The primarily renal excretion of most cephalosporins results in prolonged elimination half-lives for patients with renal dysfunction.[35] Although this is often moot because of favorable safety profiles (even with high serum concentrations), it must not be overlooked. Drugs that are primarily excreted by biliary mechanism (e.g., cefoperazone) or are metabolized in vivo (e.g., cephalothin and cefotaxime) may be preferable in these circumstances. Similarly, those cephalosporins which are most protein bound (see Table 26–8) are not readily dialyzed. This would include ceftriaxone, cefonicid, and cefazolin, among others.

Because less than 5 percent of the dose of most cephalosporins is metabolized in the liver or excreted in the bile, dosage modifications in hepatic disease are seldom necessary. An exception is cefoperazone, largely excreted in bile, whose half-life in adult cirrhotics is prolonged 2.5-fold.[36] None of the cephalosporins, including cefoperazone, manifests hepatic toxicity as a major adverse effect, although ceftriaxone is associated with reversible biliary pseudolithiasis (sludging) in up to 50 percent of children with meningitis treated with this drug.[37] This is rarely associated with symptomatic gallbladder disease, however.

PROTEIN BINDING AND BILIRUBIN DISPLACEMENT

Cephalosporins exhibit a very wide range of affinity for serum proteins, from 10 (ceftazidime) to 95 percent (cefonicid) (Table 26–8). The clinical significance of protein binding remains unclear. Logically, highly bound antibiotics should be less likely to leave the intravascular space to reach extravascular sites of infection. However, there are numerous exceptions, with ceftriaxone (85 percent bound) reaching higher concentrations in breast milk and cerebrospinal fluid than many antibiotics with much lower degrees of affinity.[38,39] Hence protein binding should be considered as only one of several factors influencing tissue diffusion of cephalosporins.

One important consideration in pediatrics has been the degree to which administered drugs are likely to compete

TABLE 26–8. PROTEIN BINDING OF CEPHALOSPORIN ANTIBIOTICS

CLASS	LOW (<25%)	MODERATE (25–50%)	HIGH (50–75%)	VERY HIGH (>75%)
First generation	Cephalexin* Cephradine* Cephadroxil*	Cephapirin*	Cephalothin	Cefazolin
Second generation	Cefaclor*	Cefuroxime*	Cefamandole Cefoxitin	Cefonicid Cefotetan
Third generation (extended spectrum)	Ceftazidime Cefotaxime	Ceftizoxime		Cefoperazone Ceftriaxone

*Orally bioavailable.

with and displace bilirubin from binding sites on albumin and other serum proteins. This is so because of the unfortunate experience with sulfonamides producing kernicterus when administered to jaundiced newborns. With the development of cephalosporins potentially useful in neonatal infections, this has become a more relevant consideration.

The degree of protein binding provides some guidelines, but with exceptions. Our own data and those of others suggest that (1) moxalactam has a particular capacity to increase unbound bilirubin,[40] (2) ceftriaxone and cefoperazone have a lesser but not insignificant capability to displace bilirubin from albumin in neonatal sera,[40,41] and (3) cefotaxime, ceftazidime, and other cephalosporins appear, to date, to have little or no effect on unbound bilirubin concentrations.[41] These results should caution the clinician concerning the use of moxalactam, ceftriaxone, and cefoperazone in jaundiced newborns. Their use in nonjaundiced neonates is probably safe, pending additional clinical studies.[42]

ANTIBIOTIC CONCENTRATIONS IN THE FETUS AND IN BREAST MILK

For obvious reasons, there is a paucity of information about the degree of transplacental passage of most antibiotics. The transit of cephalosporins from maternal serum to fetus is quite variable and not well correlated with characteristics such as protein binding.[41] For example, ceftriaxone, a highly protein bound drug (85–95 percent), achieves peak concentrations in cord serum, amniotic fluid, and placenta equal to 20–30 percent of maternal concentrations.[39] Furthermore, elimination rates from fetal tissues are often the same or slower than maternal rates. This has been shown to be true for cefazolin, cephaloridine, and cefotaxime, as well as for ceftriaxone. Therefore, with chronic maternal dosing, e.g., in the treatment of amnionitis, fetal concentrations could well be clinically relevant. The safety profile of most cephalosporins may make this moot, but potential problems such as bilirubin displacement in the infant exposed to these agents *in utero* must still be considered.[44]

The increasing use of cephalosporins to treat postpartum endometritis entails the measurement of transfer into breast milk. The concentrations of antibiotic in breast milk are affected by a variety of factors, including protein binding, lipid solubility, and molecular weight. Although ceftazidime, among the least protein bound cephalosporins, achieved the highest breast milk concentrations in one multiple-dose study,[45] in other studies, cephalosporins show minimal transfer, regardless of binding percentage (Table 26–9). In the cited study, however, there was no accumulation of ceftazidime in breast milk over a 4-day period.[45] The concentrations of cephalosporins found in breast milk do not suggest the possibility of dose-related problems, but other effects, including bilirubin displacement, hypersensitivity reactions, and alterations in infant's emerging flora, cannot be ignored.

ADVERSE REACTIONS TO CEPHALOSPORINS

It is often difficult to exclude the possibility of any antibiotic causing a coincidentally occurring reaction. Furthermore, since antibiotics are almost always given to patients with infection, the ascertainment of those effects caused by disease and those caused by therapy can be problematic. Those reactions most commonly associated with cephalosporin therapy are summarized in Table 26–10. There are few, if any, differences between these adverse reactions described in adults and children. Because dose-related reactions are rare, routine monitoring of serum concentrations, in an attempt to diminish toxicity, is not recommended. It is important to note that uncommon, but serious side effects may not be detected during early clinical trials with relatively small numbers of patients. This is especially true for the newer parenteral cephalosporins, which are often not given to large numbers of children until after they are licensed. The typical delay in pediatric licensure gives the clinician additional information on uncommon side effects, but a high index of suspicion and a willingness to consider the possibility that an unexpected clinical course might be due to iatrogenic factors is always helpful.

Local reactions to cephalosporins have been a traditional pediatric problem owing to the smaller muscle mass and intravascular caliber of these patients. This is especially true for the older cephalosporins. Cephalothin and cefoxitin should never be administered intramuscularly because of severe pain.[17] Phlebitis is also occasionally seen with intravenous use of these drugs. Cefazolin is

TABLE 26–9. CEPHALOSPORIN CONCENTRATIONS IN BREAST MILK

ANTIBIOTIC	SINGLE/MULTIPLE DOSE	BREAST MILK CONCENTRATION (mg/liter)	MILK/PLASMA RATIO* (%)	PROTEIN BINDING (%)
Cefazolin[69]	M	1.5	2.5	75
Cefoxitin[70]	S	<0.5	<2	70
Cefotaxime[71]	S	0.3	<1	25
Cephalothin[70]	S	0.8	2.2	65
Ceftriaxone[39]	S	0.7	3	90
Ceftazidime[45]	M	5.2	7	17
Cefoperazone	S	0.3	<2	85

*Peak milk concentration/peak plasma concentration.

much better tolerated than cephalothin (5–10 percent incidence phlebitis) and should ordinarily be used when a first-generation parenteral drug is indicated.[46] The newer cephalosporins, such as cefuroxime, cefotaxime, and ceftriaxone, are associated with a much lower frequency (<1 percent) of phlebitis and are reasonably well tolerated intramuscularly on the rare occasions when this route is necessary.[47]

A variety of "immunologic" reactions have been described with the cephalosporins with relatively small differences in frequency among the many compounds. Because they are not dose or duration related, these reactions are considered hypersensitivity phenomena, although evidence is often circumstantial. Almost all these reactions are uncommon, occurring in less than 2 percent of treated patients.[47] Drug fever is less common with cephalosporins than with penicillins. In a study in CF patients, fever occurred in 10 percent of penicillin-treated children[48] and only 2 percent of those receiving a cephalosporin. On the other hand, serum sickness-like reactions (fever, rash, arthralgia, myalgia) appear more commonly with cephalosporins, especially first-generation compounds. Cephalothin and cephapirin will produce serum sickness-like illnesses in healthy volunteers,[49] and a large comparative study in children with otitis media found erythema multiforme or serum sickness in 11 (1.1 percent) of cefaclor-treated patients versus 0 percent of those given amoxicillin.[50] Rashes of various types (maculopapular, urticarial, morbilliform) are among the more common reactions, occurring in 1–3 percent of treated patients regardless of the individual cephalosporin used. Severe rashes such as Stevens-Johnson syndrome are distinctly unusual, as are life-threatening conditions, such as anaphylaxis.

Cephalosporin and penicillin cross-allergenicity remains a debated topic. Many of these patients show sensitivity to non-β-lactams as well, and a direct relationship is often unclear. In a large review of some 16,000 patients, cephalosporin reactions were seen in 8 percent of penicillin-allergic and 1.9 percent of non-penicillin-allergic adults.[51] However, many of these reactions (rash, fever, etc.) may not be immunologically based. A recent detailed review suggests that a "history" of penicillin reaction is associated with a risk of cephalosporin reaction of 1–2 percent.[52] Children with a positive history and positive skin tests have much higher cross-allergenicity (up to 50 percent), and both drug classes are best avoided.

Eosinophilia and thrombocytosis are found in 4–10 percent[53] of treated children, but these abnormalities may be due to infection as well as drug therapy. Neutropenia of moderate degree has been reported in 0.1–1.0 percent of children receiving parenteral cephalosporins. Kaplan and colleagues[54] reported that 42 percent of children receiving moxalactam for bacterial meningitis had moderate neutropenia, but only 2 of 47 had counts of less than 500/mm³; and all were reversible on cessation of therapy. Although thrombocytopenia occurs rarely with cephalosporin therapy, other coagulopathies have been reported more frequently. The methylthiotetrazole side chain of cefoperazone, moxalactam, cefamandole, cefotetan, and ceftriaxone can inhibit conversion of vitamin K–dependent factors to their active forms and has been associated with abnormal hemostasis in treated adults.[55] Descriptions of this reaction in children are uncommon, however. Similarly, cephalothin and moxalactam have been associated with defective platelet aggregation in adults,[56] although documentation in children is lacking. Coombs-positive hemolytic anemias (of a mild degree) have been

TABLE 26–10. ADVERSE REACTIONS TO CEPHALOSPORINS

LOCAL	HYPERSENSITIVITY	DOSE RELATED (?)	OTHER
Pain	Rash	Neurotoxicity	Coagulopathy
	Fever	Renal dysfunction (?)	Nonspecific diarrhea
Phlebitis	Serum sickness	Platelet dysfunction	Antibiotic-associated colitis
	Anaphylaxis	Electrolyte excess	Interactions with:
	Neutropenia		Diagnostic tests
	Eosinophilia		Other drugs
	Liver toxicity		
	Interstitial nephritis		

reported rarely with all β-lactams, including cephalosporins. The Coombs antibody may occasionally confuse crossmatching in children requiring transfusion.

Other uncommon targets for immunologic reactions include the liver and kidney. Although 1–10 percent of cephalosporin-treated patients have increased serum transaminase concentrations, significant hepatic toxicity is uncommon, and most abnormalities are readily reversible. High biliary concentrations of ceftriaxone have been associated frequently with reversible bile "sludging" (pseudolithiasis) in children receiving this drug,[37] but biliary colic is uncommon. Nephrotoxicity is also uncommon with the currently used cephalosporins. Interstitial (tubular) nephritis can occur very rarely with any cephalosporin. Ceftazidime has been shown to cause a slight decrease in glomerular function, although the clinical significance of this observation is uncertain.[57] Cephalosporin antibiotics have potentiated the nephrotoxicity of diuretics and aminoglycosides in some adult patients. Since these drugs are themselves nephrotoxic, causality is unclear, and these observations have not generally been made in children.

Vomiting has been associated with the oral cephalosporins but appears to be less frequent (<5 percent) than with many other oral antibiotics. Nonspecific diarrhea is not a common problem with oral or parenteral cephalosporins, with the exception of those which achieve significant biliary concentrations—cefoperazone, ceftriaxone, moxalactam, and cefoxitin.[58] For example, Mastella et al.[48] noted diarrhea in 25 percent of CF patients receiving cefoperazone and 0 of 32 CF children given ceftazidime, a drug excreted almost entirely by renal mechanisms. Similar reports have described diarrhea occurring in 10–30 percent of children receiving ceftriaxone or moxalactam.[59] Diarrhea is occasionally (5–10 percent) seen in children receiving large doses of other extended-spectrum cephalosporins such as cefuroxime or cefoxitin.

Antibiotic-associated colitis is a more ominous diarrheal condition associated with cytotoxin-producing *Clostridium difficile*. This has been associated with almost all antibiotics, although its association with cephalosporins is not frequent. Because oral cephalosporins are well absorbed and parenteral forms generally do not cause significant changes in flora (probably due to lack of anaerobic and enterococcal activity), this is not likely to be a problem. A potential exception is cefoperazone, which is excreted in bile (75 percent) and has some anaerobic activity. In one study, 8 of 52 patients (15 percent) given cefoperazone developed diarrhea associated with *C. difficile* toxin in stools.[60]

Other adverse effects are very rare or undescribed in pediatric patients. Neurotoxicity has been described rarely with intrathecal or intraventricular administration of cephalothin and cephaloridine, but not with intravenous use.[61] In addition, Schaad and colleagues[62] recently showed that cefuroxime and ceftazidime may interfere with cerebral enzyme activity at concentrations conceivably achievable with intraventricular dosing. Superinfections, often due to enterococci or *Candida,* have occasionally occurred with third-generation agents administered for extended periods. Cephalosporins also can interfere with diagnostic tests. Cephalothin and cefoxitin may interfere with creatinine measurements, and serum or urinary concentrations of this compound must be interpreted with caution.[63] These same two antibiotics interfere with the measurement of urinary 17-hydroxycorticosteroids.[64] Cefotaxime may interfere with HPLC measurements of theophylline,[65] and most cephalosporins will falsely elevate urinary glucose concentrations assessed by the copper-reduction method (Clinitest). Cefotaxime (and presumably other cephalosporins of similar spectrum) can produce falsely positive results in newborn screening for galactosemia if the Guthrie metabolite inhibition test is used.[66]

With the exception of probenecid, which interferes with the excretion of most cephalosporins, drug–drug interactions are uncommon. As noted earlier, interactions with aminoglycosides and diuretics to enhance nephrotoxicity are possibilities that have not been well described in children.

REFERENCES

1. Williams JD: Classification of cephalosporins. Drugs 34:15–22, 1987
2. Bergan T: Pharmacokinetic properties of the cephalosporins. Drugs (suppl 2): 34:89–104, 1987
3. McCracken GH Jr, Freij BJ: Clinical pharmacology of antimicrobial agents, in Remington JS, Klein JO (eds): Infectious Diseases, of the Fetus and Newborn Infant. Philadelphia, WB Saunders, 1990, pp 1020–1078
4. Phillips JB III, Braune K, Ravis W, et al: Pharmacokinetics of cefoperazone in newborn infants. Pediatr Pharmacol 4:193–197, 1984
5. Varghese M, Khan AJ, Kumar K, et al: Pharmacokinetic evaluation of cefoperazone in infants. Antimicrob Agents Chemother 28:149–150, 1985
6. Brogden RN, Carmine A, Heel RC, et al: Cefoperazone: A review of its in vitro antimicrobial activity, pharmacological properties and therapeutic efficacy. Drugs 22:423–460, 1981
7. Richards DM, Heel RC, Brogden RN, et al: Ceftriaxone: A review of its antibacterial activity, pharmacological properties and therapeutic use. Drugs 27:469–517, 1984
8. Burckart GJ, Jones D, Ptachcinski R, et al: Ceftizoxime and cefotaxime pharmacokinetics in pediatric liver transplant patients. Drug Intell Clin Pharmacol 19:450–451, 1985
9. Prandota J: Drug disposition in cystic fibrosis: Progress in understanding pathophysiology and pharmacokinetics. Pediatr Infect Dis J 6:1111–1126, 1987
10. Berthelot G, Lenoir G, Grenier B, et al: Etude de la penetration de la ceftazidime chez les patients atteints de mucoviscidose. Pathol Biol 33:430–434, 1985
11. Hoiby N, Birgitte F, Jensen K, et al: Antimicrobial chemotherapy in cystic fibrosis patients. Acta Paediatr Scand Suppl 301:75–100, 1982
12. Harrison CJ, Marks MI, Welch DF, et al: A multicenter comparison of related pharmacologic features of cephalexin and dicloxacillin given for two months to young children with cystic fibrosis. Pediatr Pharmacol 5:7–16, 1985
13. McCracken GH Jr, Ginsburg CM, Clahsen JC, et al: Pharmacologic evaluation of orally administered antibiotics in infants and children: Effect of feeding on bioavailability. Pediatrics 62:738–743, 1978
14. Tetzlaff TR, McCracken GH Jr, Thomas ML: Bioavailability of cephalexin in children: Relationship to drug formulations and meals. J Pediatr 92:292–294, 1978
15. Emmerson AM: Cefuroxime axetil. J Antimicrob Chemother 22(2):101–104, 1988
16. Geddes AM: Antibiotic therapy: A resumé. Lancet 1:286–289, 1988
17. Moellering RC Jr, Swartz MN: The newer cephalosporins. N Engl J Med 294:24–28, 1976

18. Fried JS, Hinthorn DR: The cephalosporins. Dis Mon 31:1–60, 1985

19. Abraham EP: Cephalosporins, 1945–1986. Drugs 34:1–14, 1987

20. Norrby SR: Side effects of cephalosporins. Drugs 34:105–120, 1987

21. Donowitz GR, Mandell GL: Beta-lactam antibiotics. N Engl J Med 318:490–496, 1988

22. Schaad UB, Stoeckel K: Single-dose pharmacokinetics of ceftriaxone in infants and young children. Antimicrob Agents Chemother 21:248–253, 1982

23. Steele RW: Ceftriaxone: Increasing the half-life and activity of third generation cephalosporins. Pediatr Infect Dis 4:188–191, 1985

24. Rolewicz TF, Mirkin BL, Cooper MJ, et al: Metabolic disposition of cephalothin and deacetylcephalothin in children and adults: Comparison of high-performance liquid chromatographic and microbial assay procedures. Clin Pharmacol Ther 22:928–935, 1977

25. Trang JM, Jacobs RF, Kearns GL, et al: Cefotaxime and desacetylcefotaxime pharmacokinetics in infants and children with meningitis. Antimicrob Agents Chemother 28:791–795, 1985

26. McCracken GH Jr, Threlkeld NE, Thomas ML: Pharmacokinetics of cefotaxime in newborn infants. Antimicrob Agents Chemother 21:683–684, 1982

27. Jones RN: A review of cephalosporin metabolism: A lesson to be learned for future chemotherapy. Diagn Microbiol Infect Dis 12:25–31, 1989

28. Cherubin CE, Eng RH, Norrby R, et al: Penetration of newer cephalosporins into cerebrospinal fluid. Rev Infect Dis 11:526–548, 1989

29. Sanders CV, Greenberg RN, Marier RL: Cefamandole and cefoxitin. Ann Intern Med 103:70–78, 1985

30. Begue P, Safran C, Quiniou F, et al: Comparative pharmacokinetics of four new cephalosporins: moxalactam, cefotaxime, cefoperazone and ceftazidime in neonates. Dev Pharmacol Ther (suppl 1) 7:105–108, 1984

31. Finch R: Treatment of respiratory tract infections with cephalosporin antibiotics. Drugs 34:180–204, 1987

32. Perea EJ, Ayarre J, Garcia Iglesias MC, et al: Penetration of cefuroxime and ceftazidime into human lungs. Chemotherapy 34:1–7, 1988

33. Bertino JS Jr, Speck WT: The cephalosporin antibiotics. Pediatr Clin North Am 30:17–26, 1983

34. Moellering RC Jr: Ceftazidime: A new broad spectrum cephalosporin. Pediatr Infect Dis 4:390–393, 1985

35. Patel IH, Sugihara JG, Weinfeld RE, et al: Ceftriaxone pharmacokinetics in patients with various degrees of renal impairment. Antimicrob Agents Chemother 25:438–442, 1984

36. Cochet B, Belaieff J, Allaz AF, et al: Decreased extrarenal clearance of cefoperazone in hepatocellular diseases. Br J Clin Pharmacol 11:389–390, 1981

37. Schaad UB, Cianella-Borradori A, Suter S, et al: A comparison of ceftriaxone and cefuroxime for the treatment of bacterial meningitis in children. N Engl J Med 322:141–147, 1990

38. Steele RW, Eyre LB, Bradsher RW, et al: Pharmacokinetics of ceftriaxone in pediatric patients with meningitis. Antimicrob Agents Chemother 23:191–194, 1983

39. Kafetzis DA, Brater DC, Fanourgakis JE, et al: Ceftriaxone distribution between maternal blood and fetal blood and tissues at parturition and between blood and milk postpartum. Antimicrob Agents Chemother 23:870–873, 1983

40. Stutman HR, Parker KM, Marks MI: Potential of moxalactam and other new antimicrobial agents for bilirubin-albumin displacement in neonates. Pediatrics 75:294–298, 1985

41. Fink S, Karp W, Robertson A: Ceftriaxone effect on bilirubin-albumin binding. Pediatrics 80:873–875, 1987

42. Mulhall A, De Louvois J: The pharmacokinetics and safety of ceftazidime in the neonate. J Antimicrob Chemother 15:97–103, 1985

43. Philipson A: Pharmacokinetics of antibiotics in pregnancy and labor. Clin Pharmacokinet 4:297–309, 1979

44. Robinson PJ, Rapoport SI: Binding effect of albumin on uptake of bilirubin by brain. Pediatrics 79:553–558, 1987

45. Blanco JD, Jorgensen JH, Casteneda YS, et al: Ceftazidime levels in human breast milk. Antimicrob Agents Chemother 23:479–480, 1983

46. Quintiliani R: The use of beta-lactam antibiotics in infections: An overview. Scand J Infect Dis Suppl 42:99–109, 1984

47. Smith CR: Cefotaxime and cephalosporins: Adverse reactions in perspective. Rev Infect Dis 4:S481–488, 1982

48. Mastella G, Agostini M, Barlocco G, et al: Alternative antibiotics for treatment of Pseudomonas infections in cystic fibrosis. J Antimicrob Chemother 12:297–311, 1983

49. Sanders EW, Johnson JE, Taggart JG: Adverse reactions to cephalothin and cephapirin: Uniform occurrence on prolonged intravenous administration of high doses. N Engl J Med 290:424–429, 1974

50. Levine LR: Quantitative comparison of adverse reactions to cefaclor vs amoxicillin in a surveillance study. Pediatr Infect Dis 4:358–361, 1985

51. Petz LD: Immunologic cross-reactivity between penicillins and cephalosporins: A review. J Infect Dis 137:574–579, 1978

52. Anderson JA: Cross-sensitivity to cephalosporins in patients allergic to penicillin. Pediatric Infect Dis 5:557–561, 1986

53. Mouallem R: Comparative efficacy and safety of cephradine and cephalexin in children. J Intl Med Res 4:265–271, 1976

54. Kaplan SL, Mason EO Jr, Kvernland SJ, et al: Moxalactam treatment of serious infections primarily due to Haemophilus influenzae type b in children. Pediatrics 71:187–191, 1983

55. Agnelli G, Del Favero A, Parise P, et al: Cephalosporin-induced hypoprothrombinemia: Is the N-methylthiotetrazole side chain the culprit? Antimicrob Agents Chemother 29:1108–1109, 1986

56. Weitekamp MR, Caputo GM, Al-Mondhiry HA, et al: The effect of latamoxef, cefotaxime, and cefoperazone on platelet function and coagulation in normal volunteers. J Antimicrob Chemother 16:95–101, 1985

57. Alestig K, Trollfors B, Andersson R, et al: Ceftazidime and renal function. J Antimicrob Chemother 13:177–181, 1984

58. Platt R: Adverse effects of third-generation cephalosporins. J Antimicrob Chemother (suppl C) 10:135–140, 1982

59. Harrison CJ, Welch D, Marks MI: Ceftriaxone therapy in pediatric patients. Am J Dis Child 137:1048–1051, 1983

60. Carlberg H, Alestig K, Nord CE, et al: Intestinal side effects of cefoperazone. J Antimicrob Chemother 10:483–487, 1982

61. Snavely SR, Hodges GR: The neurotoxicity of antibacterial agents. Ann Intern Med 101:92–104, 1984

62. Schaad UB, Guenin K, Steffen C, et al: Effects of antimicrobial agents used for therapy of CNS infections on dissociated brain cell cultures. Pediatr Res 24:367–372, 1988

63. Saah AJ, Koch TR, Drusano GL: Cefoxitin falsely elevates creatinine levels. JAMA 247:205–206, 1982

64. Faas FH, Norman J, Carter WJ: Cefoxitin interference with urinary 17-hydroxycorticosteroid determination. Clin Chem 29:1311–1313, 1983

65. Gannon RH, Levy RM: Interference of third-generation cephalosporins with theophylline assay by high-performance liquid chromatography. Am J Hosp Pharm 41:1185–1186, 1984

66. Clemens P, Voltmer C, Plettner C: Interference by antibiotics with neonatal screening for galactosemia. J Pediatr 109:713–714, 1986

67. Martin E, Koup JR, Paravicini U, et al: Pharmacokinetics of ceftriaxone in neonates and infants with meningitis. J Pediatr 105:475–481, 1984

68. McCracken GH Jr, Threlkeld N, Thomas ML: Pharmacokinetics of ceftazidime in newborn infants. Antimicrob Agents Chemother 26:583–584, 1984

69. Yoshioka H, Cho K, Takimoto M, et al: Transfer of cefazolin into human milk. J Pediatr 94:151–152, 1979

70. Kapetzis DA, Siafas CA, Georgakopoulos PA, et al: Passage of cephalosporins and amoxicillin into the breast milk. Acta Paediatr Scand 70:285–288, 1981

71. Kapetzis DA, Lazarides CV, Siafas CA, et al: Transfer of cefotaxime in human milk and from mother to fetus. J Antimicrob Chemother 6:135–141, 1980

27

ANTIFUNGAL AGENTS FOR SYSTEMIC MYCOTIC INFECTIONS

MARC H. LEBEL, PIERRE LEBEL, *and* ELAINE L. MILLS

During the last decade invasive fungal infections have been recognized more frequently in infants and children and represent a significant cause of morbidity and mortality in immunocompromised patients. This chapter will focus on antifungal therapy for systemic fungal infections. The antimycotic drugs can be divided into three groups: amphotericin B, flucytosine, and the imidazole derivatives. Amphotericin B has the widest spectrum of activity but is also the most toxic. In the coming years, liposomal amphotericin B may prove to be as efficacious as, and less toxic than, the original compound. Flucytosine has a narrow spectrum of activity and is most often used in combination with amphotericin B for cryptococcal or disseminated candidal infections. Two new imidazole derivatives have been recently approved for clinical use: fluconazole in the United States and itraconazole in Europe.

AMPHOTERICIN B

Even after more than 30 years of use and despite its toxicity, amphotericin B (Fungizone) remains the drug of choice for therapy of most severe fungal infections.[1] No other agent has yet been found to be as effective for most of the systemic fungal diseases.

Mechanism of Action

Amphotericin B binds with ergosterol, fungisterol, and other sterols of the fungal cell membrane and produces a disruption of its integrity and transport characteristics in susceptible organisms.[1-3] Amphotericin resistance develops very slowly and may result from a decrease in membrane concentration of ergosterol.

Spectrum of Activity

Amphotericin B has a wide spectrum of activity (Table 27-1). It is active against *Aspergillus fumigatus* and *Aspergillus* sp., *Blastomyces dermatitidis*, *Candida albicans* and other *Candida* sp., *Coccidioides immitis*, *Cryptococcus neoformans*, *Histoplasma capsulatum*, *Mucor* sp., *Paracoccidioides brasiliensis*, and *Sporothrix schenckii*. Some *Pseudoallescheria*, *C. immitis*, and *Candida* strains are resistant.[22-27] Amphotericin B demonstrates *in vitro* synergy with flucytosine against *C. neoformans* and certain strains of *Candida*.[28-31] Rifampin or tetracycline may be synergistic *in vitro* with amphotericin for certain fungal infections. There is possible *in vitro* antagonism between amphotericin B and ketoconazole or miconazole.[32-34]

Formulation

Amphotericin B is available in 20-ml vials containing 50 mg of amphotericin B, 41 mg of deoxycholate, and 25 mg of sodium phosphate buffer.

Pharmacology

Amphotericin B is a water-insoluble polyene antibiotic which is not absorbed significantly after oral administration.[35-37] After intravenous administration, amphotericin B separates from deoxycholate.[38] The drug is 95 percent protein-bound, mainly to β-lipoproteins.[39,40] More than 90 percent of the drug leaves the circulation rapidly, perhaps bound to cholesterol-containing cytoplasmic membranes. Amphotericin B is stored in different organs and reenters the circulation slowly.[41]

In infants peak serum concentrations ranging from 0.2

to 0.5 μg/ml and from 0.31 to 2.08 μg/ml are obtained after doses of 0.5 and 1.0 mg/kg, respectively.[42-45] Trough levels range from 0.08 to 0.55 μg/ml.[45] In children a dose of 1 mg/kg produces a mean peak concentration of 2.9 μg/ml (range: 0.78–10.02 μg/ml), with a wide variation between patients.[46] After the same dose of 1 mg/kg, serum concentrations over a 24-hour period are greater than 0.5 μg/ml in the majority of children.[47,48] The mean serum concentration is proportional to the dose of amphotericin B per kilogram.[47] Many authors have suggested monitoring amphotericin B concentrations,[42,49] but the clinical usefulness and validity of such determinations remain to be proven, as outcome does not seem to be related to plasma drug levels.[21] Amphotericin B levels are difficult to measure and can be determined by high-performance liquid chromatography (HPLC) or by biologic assays.

There is a significant inverse correlation between patient age and clearance of the drug.[46,48] In children 8 months to 9 years, the mean total clearance is 0.57 ml/kg/min, and it is 0.24 ml/kg/min in those older than 9 years.[46] Benson and Nahata[46] reported a mean elimination half-life of 18.1 hours (range: 11.9–40.3) with a volume of distribution of 0.76 liters/kg, whereas Koren et al.[48] reported a half-life of 9.9 hours (range: 5.5–20.9) with a volume of distribution of 0.38 liters/kg. Half-life is markedly increased in small neonates and younger infants.[45,46,48] In adult patients the terminal half-life is approximately 15 days.

Concentrations of amphotericin B in body fluids are 50–67 percent of that in serum except for cerebrospinal fluid, into which penetration is poor. In the organs, 27.5 percent of the dose is recovered in the liver, 5.2 percent in the spleen, 3.2 percent in the lungs, and 1.5 percent in the kidneys.[50] Only 3 percent of the dose is excreted in the urine, although excretion may continue for several weeks.[41,51,52] Biliary excretion accounts for 1–15 percent of the daily dose.[50] Renal or hepatic failure does not alter the blood concentration. Amphotericin B is not significantly removed by hemodialysis.[39,52,53]

Clinical Studies

Candidiasis

Amphotericin B is the drug of choice for systemic *Candida* infections.[1,50,54-59] In disseminated neonatal candidiasis, arthritis, osteomyelitis, meningitis, endocarditis, and peritonitis, amphotericin B alone has been shown to be efficacious therapy.[43-45,57-62] The addition of flucytosine to amphotericin B has been suggested for the treatment of meningitis, endocarditis, endophthalmitis, and sepsis caused by flucytosine-susceptible strains.[58,63-65] However, there are no controlled studies demonstrating that this combination is more efficacious or less toxic than amphotericin B alone. Some authors have reported that a daily dose of 0.5 mg/kg is an adequate regimen for disseminated neonatal candidiasis and decreases the incidence of toxic side effects compared to larger doses.[45,63] The total dose or duration of therapy for fungal infections in the neonate is unknown, but good results have been

obtained with 20–40 mg/kg.[45,55,63] There are reports of clinical cure with short-course (7 days) amphotericin B therapy for treatment of mucocutaneous, esophageal, and bladder infections caused by *Candida*.[31,66] In catheterized patients continuous bladder washout of amphotericin B (50 μg/ml at 40 ml/h) is efficacious for treatment of lower urinary tract infections caused by *Candida albicans*.[67]

Cryptococcosis

In two large multicenter studies, the combination of low-dose amphotericin B (0.3 mg/kg/day) and a high dose of flucytosine (150 mg/kg/day) for a 6-week course has been demonstrated to be as effective as and less nephrotoxic than treatment with high-dose amphotericin B alone.[28,68] Intrathecal or intraventricular administration of amphotericin B has been advocated for patients who are severely ill or who fail to respond to intravenous therapy.[55,61,69] Relapse of meningitis may occur in immunocompromised patients (especially HIV-infected patients), and intermittent doses of amphotericin B have been used for prophylaxis after completion of therapy.[1,70] However, daily fluconazole therapy represents an efficacious and less toxic alternative to amphotericin B.[70,71]

Aspergillosis

Amphotericin B (1 mg/kg/day for prolonged periods of time) is of benefit for pulmonary or disseminated *Aspergillosis*.[1,72,73] However, treatment of invasive aspergillosis is often difficult, as it usually occurs in compromised hosts. The drug is not efficacious for aspergillomas, and surgical resection is often indicated for this condition. *Aspergillus* endocarditis requires in many cases a combination of surgery and amphotericin B therapy.[63]

Histoplasmosis, Blastomycosis, and Coccidioidomycosis

Some patients have spontaneous resolution of their infections. Oral imidazole therapy is frequently used for treatment of these conditions.[74-78] Amphotericin B can be considered for the normal or immunocompromised patient with progressive or extrapulmonary disease.[72,73]

Peritonitis

Amphotericin B has been administered intraperitoneally to some patients,[60,79] but the administration can cause abdominal pain and predispose to peritoneal fibrosis.[80] In patients with continuous ambulatory peritoneal dialysis peritonitis, the optimal therapy consists of early removal of the catheter along with 1–4 weeks of intravenous amphotericin B.[80]

TABLE 27–1. *IN VITRO* **SUSCEPTIBILITIES OF FUNGI TO SYSTEMIC ANTIFUNGAL AGENTS***

PATHOGEN	MINIMAL INHIBITORY CONCENTRATIONS (μg/ml)—RANGE†					
	Amphotericin B	Flucytosine	Ketoconazole	Miconazole	Itraconazole	Fluconazole
Candida albicans	0.05–4.0	0.016–>100	0.01–>100	0.016–100	0.063–128	0.063–100
Candida krusei	0.05–>6.25	0.1–>25.0	0.1–10	<0.063–6.25	0.01–0.1	100
Candida parapsilosis	0.025–>6.25	<0.025–>100	<0.125–>64.0	0.016–32	0.063–>128	–
Candida tropicalis	0.04–16.0	0.016–>100	<0.125–>64.0	0.016–33.0	0.13–>128	100
Cryptococcus neoformans	0.03–2.8	0.46–3.9	0.063–32.0	0.063–25.0	0.01–0.13	3.12–6.25
Sporothrix schenckii	0.07–>100	1.6–3.12	0.1–16.0	0.5–16.0	0.1–4.0	–
Blastomyces dermatitidis	0.05–0.78	–	0.005–2.0	0.001–2.0	0.001–0.13	6.0
Histoplasma capsulatum	0.04–>100	–	0.063–3.12	0.05–2.0	0.01–>128	16–250
Coccidioides immitis	0.15–96	>97	0.05–0.8	0.063–6.0	–	–
Aspergillus fumigatus	0.14–>25	0.5–>100	0.12–100	0.5–64.0	0.01–10.0	>50.0
Aspergillus sp.	0.14–>25	0.48–500	0.5–100	0.39–>4.0	0.01–100.0	>50.0

*Compiled from references 4–20.

†Interpretation of the *in vitro* data must be made with caution, as the minimal inhibitory concentrations vary with testing conditions.[21]

Liposomal Amphotericin B

In animals, amphotericin B incorporated in liposomes seems to be less toxic than and as efficacious as, if not more efficacious than, conventional amphotericin B therapy.[81,82] Liposomal amphotericin B has cured some patients who failed to respond to conventional amphotericin B; the incidence of adverse effects such as fever, chills, and potassium loss was less than for conventional therapy.[27,82–85] No chronic renal, hematologic, or central nervous system side effects were observed in one study.[84]

Aerosolized Amphotericin B

In a rat model, aerosolized amphotericin B produced high concentrations in the lungs and delayed the progression of pulmonary aspergillosis by killing inhaled spores and inhibiting mycelial proliferation.[86,87] There are no published data on this mode of therapy in humans.

Clinical Indications and Posology

The principal indications for amphotericin B are summarized in Table 27–2. The appropriate daily dose and duration of therapy are not precisely known for infants and children or for a given fungal infection. Doses of 0.3–1.0 mg/kg/day seem adequate for the majority of patients, but therapy should be individualized. In the neonatal period, some authors have recommended a daily dose of 0.5 mg/kg.[44,63]

Flucytosine (150 mg/kg/day) should be combined with amphotericin B (0.3 mg/kg/day) for patients with cryptococcal meningitis. Dosages greater than 0.3 mg/kg/day do not increase the cure rates for patients with cryptococcal meningitis. Flucytosine might be considered in patients with neonatal candidiasis, fungal meningitis, or endocarditis. Intrathecal administration of amphotericin B is useful for some patients with cryptococcal or coccidioidal meningitis that do not respond to intravenous amphotericin B. The drug should be administered through an Ommaya reservoir that drains into the lateral ventricle.[69,88] In children the initial dose should be 0.01 mg gradually increased to 0.1 mg every 2 or 3 days.[55,61] Amphotericin B should be diluted in water with a maximal concentration of 0.25 mg/ml.

Amphotericin B can be injected intraarticularly in patients with sporotrichosis or coccidioidomycosis of the joint; the exact dosage in children for this form of therapy is not known. Bladder irrigation with amphotericin B (50 μg/ml diluted in distilled water) is an alternative therapy for lower urinary tract infections caused by *Candida albicans* in the catheterized patient.

Administration

Amphotericin B should be dissolved in 5% glucose in water at a concentration of not more than 0.1 mg/ml. The preparation should not be used if cloudy. Amphotericin B is incompatible with electrolyte solutions and preservatives. The final solution is stable for the duration of infusion and is not denatured by light.[89] A test dose of 1 mg (0.05 mg/kg) of amphotericin is infused over a period of 30–60 minutes. During the administration, vital signs should be closely monitored to detect hypotension and arrhythmias. If no severe reactions occur, then the first daily dose is completed to 0.25 mg/kg given in a 2- to 4-hour infusion. Some authors prefer a 1-hour infusion if the vital signs are stable, because this method of administration seems to be associated with fewer side effects such as fever, chills, and nausea.[90,91] However, the duration of administration should not be less than 1 hour because of the increased risk of developing serious side effects such as cardiac arrest or arrhythmias.[92–94] The dose is increased by 0.25 mg/kg/day to the total daily dose desired until 1.0 mg/kg/day is reached. In severe disease, a dose of 0.3 mg/kg the first day, 0.6 mg/kg the second day, and 1.0 mg/kg the third day can be given.[95] The regimen is then continued with 1 mg/kg/day unless signs of toxicity occur. When the patient's clinical condition has stabilized and improvement has been noted (usually after 1 to 2 weeks), the dose may be given every other day (maximum of 1.5 mg/kg/dose/48 h). This therapy is effective

TABLE 27–2. CLINICAL INDICATIONS OF AMPHOTERICIN B

TYPE OF INFECTION	ROUTE OF ADMINISTRATION*	COMMENTS
Candidiasis		
Systemic	I.V.	Possible synergism with flucytosine
		A dose of 0.5 mg/kg/day may be sufficient in the neonatal period
		Fluconazole as alternative
Central line infection	I.V.	Catheter must be removed
Meningitis	I.V.	Possible synergism with flucytosine
		Intrathecal administration may be considered in patients whose cerebrospinal fluid is not sterilized by I.V. amphotericin B
Osteoarticular	I.V.	No benefit from intraarticular injection
Lower urinary tract	I.V.	Short course I.V.
(localized infection)	I.VES.	Bladder irrigation 50 µg/ml effective
CAPD peritonitis†	I.V.	Intraperitoneal administration may produce peritoneal adhesions and fibrosis
Esophagitis	I.V., P.O.	Immunocompromised patients
Endocarditis	I.V.	Surgery may be required
		Possible synergism with flucytosine
Aspergillosis		
Invasive disease	I.V.	Prognosis depends on underlying condition
Histoplasmosis, blastomycosis		
Invasive	I.V.	Imidazoles as alternatives
Coccidioidomycosis		
Invasive	I.V.	Imidazoles as alternatives
Meningitis	I.V.	Intrathecal administration advocated by some authors
Cryptococcosis		
		Proved synergy with flucytosine for meningitis
Meningitis or disseminated	I.V.	Fluconazole for prophylaxis of recurrences
Mucormycosis		
Invasive disease	I.V.	Surgical debridement

*I.V., intravenous; I.VES., intravesicular; P.O., orally.
†CAPD, continuous ambulatory peritoneal dialysis.

and allows outpatient administration of the drug, but there is no significant reduction in the degree of nephrotoxicity of the alternate-day dose is doubled.

Premedication consisting of acetaminophen (10 mg/kg orally) and diphenhydramine hydrochloride (1.25 mg/kg orally) can be given 30 minutes before the infusion for patients who experience mild adverse reactions. Meperidine (0.5–1 mg/kg intravenously) has been advocated for treatment of rigors that occur during administration of the drug.[96] Hydrocortisone (0.5–0.7 mg/kg intravenously) can be given before the infusion for patients with more severe symptoms. Tolerance to the febrile reactions may develop with time, allowing a decrease or discontinuation of the premedication.

Monitoring

During therapy with amphotericin B, potassium and other serum electrolytes, creatinine, urea, and hematocrit should be closely followed, especially if other nephrotoxic drugs are given at the same time. Potassium and bicarbonate supplements are given as needed. If the serum creatinine rises to more than three times the normal value or above 3 mg/dl (273 µmol/liter), the dosage is decreased until a significant improvement in renal function occurs. Further reduction in dosage or discontinuation of therapy might be necessary in some patients. However, renal insufficiency is not a contraindication for amphotericin use, as it is not metabolized by the kidneys.

Adverse Effects

During amphotericin B infusion, patients may experience fever, shaking chills, rigors, nausea, vomiting, diarrhea, epigastric pain, and muscle and joint pain.[1] The fever may be mediated through release of tumor necrosis factor, interleukin-1, or prostaglandin E_2.[97,98] Slowing the speed of infusion and the use of premedication may decrease the incidence of side effects. Some patients develop shock or cardiac arrhythmias, especially when the drug is infused rapidly.[92–94,99]

There are reports of acute pulmonary deterioration in patients receiving granulocyte transfusions during amphotericin B therapy.[100–103] Rare side effects include anaphylaxis, phlebitis, bitter taste in the mouth, and motor or sensory neuropathy.[104–106] Intrathecal administration of amphotericin B has been associated with arachnoiditis, transient radiculitis, sensory loss, headaches, and seizures. Intraperitoneal administration of the drug can cause peritoneal fibrosis.[80]

A vast majority of patients develop nephrotoxicity, the major cause of discontinuation of the drug. Amphotericin B damages the renal tubules, producing azotemia, hypokalemia, renal tubular acidosis, cylindruria, and impaired urinary concentrating ability.[107–109] The renal damage seems to correlate with the total dose of the drug,[110] and the pharmacokinetics of concomitantly administered drugs may be altered. The hypokalemia may cause muscle weakness and rhabdomyolysis.[111] Amiloride and salt repletion have been reported to decrease the nephrotoxicity and hypokalemia associated with amphotericin B therapy.[112,113] Anemia, neutropenia, thrombocytopenia, and hypomagnesemia can also occur.[114,115]

Toxicity in infants and children has not been well studied, but it seems to be similar to that found in adults.[42,46,48] There are contradictory reports regarding the toxicity of amphotericin B in the neonatal period. In two studies the drug was well tolerated,[58,59] but in two others there was an increased incidence of adverse reactions.[57,63] In very-low-birth-weight infants, one study reported that thrombocytopenia occurred in 69 percent of patients, alteration of renal function tests in 54 percent, and alterations of hepatic function tests in 50 percent.[57] In older children azotemia is the most frequent laboratory complication (96 percent), followed by anemia (71 percent), hypokalemia (46 percent), thrombocytopenia (38 percent), and neutropenia (25 percent).[56] Drug-related fever occurs in 92 percent of patients, chills in 75 percent, nausea in 58 percent, and tachycardia in 4 percent.[56]

Amphotericin B has been shown to pass from the maternal to the fetal circulation.[116,117] There is no known toxicity or teratogenicity for the fetus when the mother is treated with amphotericin B. In several reports it appeared to be safe.[116,118–131] Caution is advised when making the decision to use the drug during pregnancy.[132] Amphotericin B is recommended for use in patients who would clearly benefit from the drug.[133]

Drug Interactions

Under certain conditions there is synergism between amphotericin B and flucytosine, rifampin, tetracycline, or antineoplastic agents.[28–31,134] There is possible antagonism between amphotericin B and ketoconazole or miconazole.[32–34,135] Aminoglycosides, cyclosporine, and pentamidine may increase the nephrotoxicity of amphotericin B.[81,136–139] The half-life of aminoglycosides is significantly increased (>50 percent) in approximately 75 percent of children receiving amphotericin B, even without a significant rise in serum creatinine concentration.[136] Because of amphotericin B–induced hypokalemia, there is an increased risk of digitalis toxicity and prolonged curariform effect.

FLUCYTOSINE (5-FLUOROCYTOSINE; 5-FC)

Flucytosine (Ancobon) is an orally absorbable fluoropyrimidine drug. It is usually combined with amphotericin B for the treatment of certain deep-seated fungal infections.

Mechanism of Action

Flucytosine is a fluorine analogue of cytosine, a normal body constituent. The drug is transformed to 5-fluoroura-cil after deamination in the fungal cell.[140] 5-Fluorouracil acts as an inactive pyrimidine substitute and also inhibits thymidylate synthetase; these two mechanisms interfere with DNA synthesis and cell growth.[140] Development of resistance (through loss of deaminase or decreased permeability to the drug) has been demonstrated *in vitro* and can occur during therapy.[64]

Spectrum of Activity

Flucytosine has a narrow spectrum of activity but is active against many fungi, including *Candida albicans, some Candida* sp., and *Cryptococcus neoformans* (Table 27–1). Most isolates of *Aspergillus* are resistant to flucytosine. Strains of *Histoplasma* and *Blastomyces* are often resistant to the drug. There are *in vitro* data that suggest that synergism with amphotericin B occurs, resulting in an enhanced antifungal effect against *Candida* and *Cryptococcus*.[141,142]

Formulation

Flucytosine is available in 250-mg and 500-mg capsules. A 1 percent injectable formulation (2.5 gm in 250 ml of normal saline) is not commercially available but can be obtained from the company (Hoffman-LaRoche Company) on a compassionate use basis.

Pharmacology

Absorption from the gastrointestinal tract is rapid, with a bioavailability of 76 to 89 percent.[143,144] Antacids and food decrease the rate of absorption of the drug.[144] Bioavailability is decreased in patients with end-stage renal disease.[145]

In adults peak serum concentrations are 16–56 μg/ml after a dose of 25 mg/kg and 23–86 μg/ml after a dose of 37.5 mg/kg.[143] In children peak serum concentrations are $\geq$ 20 μg/ml after a dose of 25 mg/kg.[146] In a premature infant a dose of 25 mg/kg produced serum levels of 40 μg/ml at 2 hours and 27 μg/ml at 4 and 6 hours.[54] The half-life is about 4–6 hours in the adult and is increased in the neonate.[147] Decreased renal function can prolong the half-life to beyond 24 hours.[144]

Flucytosine is minimally protein-bound and is distributed to most tissues in a volume of 0.6 liter/kg.[39,144] Cerebrospinal fluid concentrations are 60–80 percent of simultaneous serum concentrations.[148] Less than 4 percent of flucytosine is metabolized, and the drug is excreted unchanged by glomerular filtration.[143,149] Concentrations in the urine reach 10 times or more the concentrations in serum.[143,149] From 0.5 to 11 percent of flucytosine is excreted in the feces.[150]

Peritoneal dialysis and hemodialysis decrease plasma concentrations, and a supplementary dose is recommended after dialysis.[39,144,145] The presence of hepatic dysfunction does not alter flucytosine pharmacokinetics.

Clinical Studies

Flucytosine monotherapy has been used in patients with lower urinary tract infection caused by sensitive strains of *Candida* and in cutaneous chromomycosis.[151-153] For cryptococcal meningitis the combination of low-dose amphotericin B (0.3 mg/kg/day) and a high dose of flucytosine (150 mg/kg/day) is more effective and less nephrotoxic than treatment with high-dose amphotericin B therapy alone.[28,68] The combination of amphotericin B and flucytosine has been shown effective in patients with *Candida* endophthalmitis, endocarditis, and meningitis as well as neonatal candidiasis.[29,58,63-65] However, with the exception of cryptococcal meningitis, there are no studies demonstrating a clear benefit of the combined therapy over amphotericin B therapy alone.[57,63-65,154-156]

In a report of 304 critically ill patients (including 55 neonates) who received flucytosine intravenously (because the oral form could not be administered) in addition to amphotericin B, the tolerance to the drug was good.[157] For the neonates microbiologic cure occurred in 88 percent of the patients and clinical cure in 65 percent of the patients.[157]

Clinical Indications and Posology

Flucytosine is recommended as an adjunctive therapy to amphotericin B for treatment of cryptococcal meningitis. Some authors have recommended this combination for patients with *Candida* meningitis or neonatal candidiasis.[29,58] Susceptibilities to flucytosine should preferably be determined before using the drug because many strains of *Candida* and other fungi are resistant. In patients with impaired renal function, the dose should be reduced. It is recommended to routinely monitor peak serum concentrations and to maintain them between 50 and 100 μg/ml.

Side Effects

When properly used and monitored, flucytosine is a relatively safe drug. Side effects of flucytosine have been attributed to transformation to 5-fluorouracil in the body.[149,158] The most common clinical side effects are gastrointestinal (6 percent), including nausea, vomiting, and diarrhea.[151,152,159] Erosive enteritis of the small bowel and intestinal perforation have been reported.[160] Uncommon side effects include rashes, headaches, and hallucinations.[143]

Bone marrow suppression with leukopenia and thrombocytopenia occurs in 5–30 percent of patients and seems to be more frequent when flucytosine blood levels exceed 100–125 μg/ml.[68,145,161] Hepatic dysfunction occurs in 5–10 percent of patients.[143,159]

Flucytosine has been shown to be teratogenic in animals. No defects were observed in three infants born to pregnant women treated in the 2nd and 3rd trimesters of gestation.[131,162,163] Caution is advised for its use in pregnant women.[132] No data are available for its passage into breast milk.

False elevation of the serum creatinine level has been reported,[164] resulting from interference by flucytosine with the method of measurement used by the Kodak Ektachem analyzer.[164,165] Physicians should be aware of this phenomenon and be cautious when interpreting serum creatinine levels in patients receiving flucytosine.

Drug Interactions

Antacids decrease the rate of absorption of flucytosine but not its total bioavailability.

KETOCONAZOLE

Ketoconazole (Nizoral) is an orally formulated antifungal drug with broad-spectrum activity and low toxicity.[166] Ketoconazole is an imidazole derivative that is chemically related to miconazole.

Mechanism of Action

Ketoconazole inhibits 14-α-demethylation of lanosterol by binding to one of the cytochrome P-450 enzymes.[167] This impairs the synthesis of ergosterol and interferes with the formation of other cell membrane lipids.[167]

Spectrum of Activity

Ketoconazole is effective *in vitro* against *Candida* sp., *Histoplasma capsulatum, Coccidioides immitis, Blastomyces dermatitidis, Paracoccidioides brasiliensis, Cryptococcus neoformans, Phialophora* sp., and most dermatophytes (Table 27–1).[4,168]

Formulation

Ketoconazole is available in 200-mg tablets (stable for 2 years under normal room temperature[33]). A 20 mg/ml suspension is available in several countries but not in the United States.

Pharmacology

Ketoconazole requires an acid pH in the stomach for optimal absorption.[169-171] It is rapidly absorbed and reaches peak serum concentrations 1–2 hours after the dose, with a bioavailability of 76 percent.[172]

In infants and children, a dose of 5 mg/kg produces peak serum concentrations of 4.4 μg/ml (range: 0.3–8.8). The serum half-life varies from 1.6 hour (range: 1.0–2.4), when given in a suspension of 20 mg/ml on an empty stomach, to 2.3 hours (range: 0.9–11.7), when given as crushed tablets in applesauce.[173] The peak concentration occurs more rapidly and the mean peak values are 1.6 to 4 times higher in children receiving the suspension. For patients given the suspension, 67 percent had peak plasma concentrations $\geq 4\ \mu g/ml$.[173] The plasma half-life was longer after administration of crushed tablets. In another study doses of 3 and 10 mg/kg of the suspension produced mean peak serum concentrations of 0.5 and 2 $\mu g/ml$, respectively.[174]

Ketoconazole is almost entirely protein-bound (93–99 percent). The distribution of the drug is good in most tissues and fluids.[4,175,176] Penetration into the cerebrospinal fluid is poor, even in the presence of meningeal inflammation.[175–178] In children with coccidioidal meningitis receiving 200–400 mg/day of ketoconazole, cerebrospinal fluid concentrations ranged from 0.0 to 0.5 $\mu g/ml$.[178] Ketoconazole is metabolized by the liver and excreted in the bile as inactive metabolites. Only a small percentage of the active drug is excreted in the urine.[179] The pharmacokinetics of ketoconazole do not seem to be altered in patients with hepatic or renal impairment, but the drug should be used with caution in patients with hepatic disease.[175] The drug is not significantly removed by hemodialysis or peritoneal dialysis.

Clinical Studies

Patients with chronic mucocutaneous candidiasis respond very well to ketoconazole.[179–181] There are anecdotal reports demonstrating efficacy for systemic *Candida* infections.[182] Ketoconazole has demonstrated efficacy for treatment of disseminated and pulmonary histoplasmosis[75,76]; however, HIV-infected patients may have a higher failure rate.[74,183] Paracoccidioidomycosis responds well to ketoconazole, with cure or improvement in 88–95 percent of patients.[75,184] Cure rates of 81–100 percent have been achieved in patients with mild to moderate blastomycosis.[74,185]

Ketoconazole has shown some efficacy in coccidioidomycosis, but relapses occur frequently.[77,78] It is not efficacious for treatment of aspergillosis, cryptococcosis, chromomycosis, and sporotricosis.[186–189] In 160 patients who were given 400–2000 mg of ketoconazole once daily for various fungal infections, doses greater than 400 mg were more toxic without significantly increasing clinical efficacy.[178]

Clinical Indications and Posology

Ketoconazole is considered the drug of choice for prophylaxis and treatment of patients with chronic mucocutaneous candidiasis and for patients with paracoccidioidomycosis.[190] This drug represents a safe and effective alternative to amphotericin B for blastomycosis and histoplasmosis in immunocompetent hosts.[74] It is not recommended for disseminated fungal infections or for fungal meningitis. Ketoconazole should not be used as empiric antifungal therapy in neutropenic oncology

patients because of the lack of activity of this drug against *Aspergillus* sp. or *Candida tropicalis*.[191]

The manufacturer recommends the following doses in pediatrics: children <20 kg, 50 mg daily; children 20–40 kg, 100 mg daily; children >40 kg, 200 mg daily. Other recommendations are a dosage of 5–10 mg/kg/day.[173,174] The duration of therapy varies according to the type of infection and response to therapy. In cases with suboptimal response, serum concentrations of ketoconazole can be determined, and the physician should look for causes altering the absorption of ketoconazole, such as antacids, H_2 blockers, and anticholinergic agents, as well as possible drug interactions.

Side Effects

At the lower doses, ketoconazole is generally well tolerated. Anorexia, nausea, and vomiting are the most common side effects and are proportional to the ingested dose.[90] Three percent of patients report these symptoms at dosages lower than 400 mg/day, compared to 17 percent at 400 mg/day and 43 percent at 800 mg/day.[74,90] Skin rashes and pruritus occur in approximately 10 percent of patients.[74] Infrequent adverse effects are headaches, dizziness, somnolence, photophobia, and diarrhea. Gynecomastia, impotence, and menstrual irregularities have been reported.[192] Disulfiram-like reactions have also been reported.[193]

Asymptomatic elevation of liver enzymes occurs in 2–5 percent of patients. The hepatic injury is usually reversible if the drug is stopped.[194–198] Severe hepatotoxicity occurs in 1 case in 15,000 and is not dose-dependent.[197] The majority of cases appear in the first 3 months of therapy.[197] The medication should be discontinued if the hepatic enzymes are greater than three times the upper limit of normal.

Ketoconazole reversibly inhibits steroidogenesis in the adrenal gland,[199,200] blocks glucocorticoid receptors,[201,202] and inhibits testosterone synthesis.[203,204] In children ketoconazole impairs production of cortisol and aldosterone, but not sufficiently to require steroid replacement therapy at times of acute illness or surgery.[205]

Ketoconazole is embryotoxic and teratogenic in rats.[33] There are no data on its safety during pregnancy.[117] Ketoconazole is excreted in breast milk. Caution is advised for its use in pregnant or breast-feeding women.

Drug Interactions

Cimetidine and antacids decrease ketoconazole absorption.[135] Phenytoin delays the time to peak concentration of ketoconazole.[175] Rifampin reduces ketoconazole serum concentration by about 33 percent.[206,207] Ketoconazole prolongs the half-life of cyclosporine through interference with its hepatic metabolism.[208–211] There are contradictory reports on synergy or antagonism between ketoconazole and amphotericin B or flucytosine.[32–34] Interference with the laboratory assay for triglycerides has been reported in one study.[186]

MICONAZOLE

Miconazole (Monistat) belongs to the imidazole group. It is primarily used as a topical agent for superficial fungal infections and rarely as an intravenous or intrathecal drug.

Mechanism of Action

Miconazole blocks the synthesis of ergosterol, alters the permeability of fungal cell membranes, and interferes with intracellular enzymes, resulting in intracellular necrosis of the organism.[8,14]

Spectrum of Activity

Miconazole is active *in vitro* against *Coccidioides immitis, Histoplasma capsulatum, Paracoccidioides brasiliensis, Blastomyces dermatitidis, Cryptococcus neoformans,* and *Sporothrix schenckii.* It is less active against *Aspergillus* and *Candida* sp. (Table 27–1).

Formulation

Miconazole is available in 200-mg vials for I.V. injection. The dose should be diluted in either 0.9 percent sodium chloride or 5 percent dextrose to a final volume of 200 ml and infused over 1–2 hours. The optimal dilution for use in children is not known.

Pharmacology

Miconazole is only slightly soluble in water, and its oral absorption produces low serum levels with wide individual differences. There is no oral preparation, and only the intravenous formulation is available for use in systemic fungal infections.

Data are sparse on the pharmacokinetics and efficacy of miconazole in infants and children.[62,182,212–219] Peak serum concentrations of 0.53 and 1.26 μg/ml have been measured after doses of 4 and 7 mg/kg, respectively.[213,219] The pharmacokinetics in adult patients fit a three-compartment model with a terminal half-life of about 24 hours. The drug is highly protein-bound (90 percent) and diffuses into most tissues.[220] It penetrates the cerebrospinal fluid poorly, even in the presence of meningeal inflammation. Penetration into sputum is also poor. Miconazole is metabolized by the liver with only minimal urinary excretion. No dosage alteration is necessary in patients with renal impairment or undergoing hemodialysis.

Intrathecal or intraventricular (with an Ommaya reservoir) injection of 20 to 30 mg produces detectable cerebrospinal fluid levels for up to 3 days.[221]

Clinical Studies

Miconazole has been used for systemic infections and fungal meningitis,[221–223] especially in patients with coccidioidomycosis who failed to respond or could not tolerate amphotericin B therapy. The drug has been used in infants and older children with systemic candidiasis with some clinical response,[62,182,212–218] but treatment failures have been reported.[62,215,216] Intrathecal administration has been efficacious in some patients with cryptococcal and coccidioidal meningitis.[221]

Clinical Indications and Posology

Miconazole is considered the drug of choice for *Pseudoallescheria boydii* infections.[223] It has a potential role for other susceptible fungal infections when patients fail to respond to or cannot tolerate amphotericin B. Toxicity is a limiting factor in long-term therapy, and relapse often follows termination of the drug.

For children the total daily dose should be between 20 and 40 mg/kg/day in three divided doses, depending on the type and severity of infection.[224] The doses and duration of therapy vary according to the type of infection and response of the patient. The following guidelines have been suggested: candidiasis, 1–20 weeks; coccidioidomycosis, 3–20 weeks; cryptococcosis, 3–12 weeks; pseudoallescheriasis, 5–20 weeks. However, some patients may need a longer duration of therapy.

Intrathecal administration (20–30 mg of undiluted injectable miconazole) may be considered for some patients with cryptococcal or coccidioidal meningitis who fail to respond to standard therapy.

Side Effects

There are numerous side effects,[90] but they seem to be less important than those of amphotericin B. Phlebitis and pruritus are the most common side effects; nausea, vomiting, diarrhea, fever, chills, anaphylactic reactions, skin rashes, and drowsiness can occur. Hyponatremia develops in up to 45 percent of patients. Anemia, thrombocytopenia, leukopenia, and hyperlipidemia have been reported infrequently.[90,225] Cardiac arrhythmias and respiratory arrest may occur with rapid infusion.[214,226] Arachnoiditis has been reported after intrathecal administration.

Miconazole does not appear to be teratogenic in animals, but its safety in human pregnancy or in breast-feeding has not been established.[117,132,133]

Drug Interactions

There is a decreased anticandida effect when miconazole is used in combination with amphotericin B. Miconazole markedly increases the anticoagulant effect of coumarin drugs.[135]

FLUCONAZOLE

Fluconazole (Diflucan) is a newly marketed bis-triazole antifungal agent that can be administered either orally or intravenously.

Mechanism of Action

Fluconazole acts by inhibition of fungal ergosterol synthesis.[8,15-17]

Spectrum of Activity

Fluconazole offers a narrower spectrum of activity than ketoconazole or itraconazole. It is considerably less active *in vitro* than ketoconazole (Table 27-1) but seems to have a high efficacy *in vivo*.[227]

Formulation

Fluconazole is available in 100-mg and 200-mg tablets and in 200-mg and 400-mg vials (2 mg/ml) for I.V. injection. An oral suspension (10mg/ml and 40 mg/ml) is not commercially available but can be obtained from the company (Pfizer Laboratories).

Pharmacology

Fluconazole is a water-soluble, metabolically stable drug. Absorption is rapid and unaffected by the presence of food, with a bioavailability of >90 percent and a low protein binding (11 percent).[228] Peak serum concentrations are 1.4 μg/ml after a 1 mg/kg dose, 2.5-3.5 μg/ml after a 50-mg dose, and 4.5-8.0 μg/ml after a 100-mg dose.[229,230] After oral administration the plasma half-life is about 30 hours and the volume of distribution is 0.7 liter/kg, with a plasma clearance of 0.40 ml/min/kg and a renal clearance of 0.27 $\pm$ 0.07 ml/min/kg.

The distribution in the different tissues is good, including the central nervous system (cerebrospinal fluid/blood concentrations are 74-89 percent).[231] Its pharmacokinetics differ from those of ketoconazole, as fluconazole is 90 percent renally excreted (principally as unmetabolized drug), with urinary concentrations that are 10-fold higher than in plasma. Plasma clearance is decreased in the presence of impaired renal function.[230] Hemodialysis reduces plasma concentrations by about 50 percent.

Clinical Studies

For oropharyngeal candidiasis, fluconazole (50 mg daily) produced clinical and mycologic cure ranging from 69 to 100 percent.[232] For patients who could not tolerate conventional antifungal therapy, fluconazole was effective in 75 percent of those with either cryptococcal, coccidioidal, or candidal infections.[71] Fluconazole (50-400 mg/day) has been efficacious for coccidioidal meningitis as sole therapy; however, not every patient responds to therapy, and relapses occur.[233] Fluconazole may be the replacement drug for amphotericin B as maintenance therapy for cryptococcal meningitis.[70] There is a very limited experience with fluconazole in pediatric patients, and no pharmacokinetic data have yet been published. Children 3 to 13 years of age have been treated safely with 3-6 mg/kg of fluconazole once daily.

Clinical Indications and Posology

Fluconazole has been approved for oropharyngeal and esophageal candidiasis and for cryptococcal meningitis. It is also effective for other serious systemic candida infections, including urinary tract infections, pneumonia, and peritonitis. The exact posology has not been determined in children.

For oropharyngeal and esophageal candidiasis, a loading dose of 200 mg is recommended followed by 100 mg once daily for a minimum of 14-21 days. For systemic candidiasis and acute cryptococcal meningitis, a loading dose of 400 mg is recommended followed by 200 mg once daily for at least 4 weeks in systemic candidiasis, and for 10-12 weeks after cerebrospinal fluid cultures become sterile in cryptococcal meningitis. The maintenance dose for this disease is 200 mg daily. In renal insufficiency, patients with a creatinine clearance >40 ml/min may continue to receive the recommended doses every 24 hours, with a clearance of 21-40 ml/min every 48 hours and with a clearance of 10-20 ml/min every 72 hours.

Side Effects

Fluconazole appears less toxic than ketoconazole. From 16 to 29 percent of patients report one or more clinical adverse effects (more often in HIV-infected patients). Gastrointestinal side effects are the most frequent (14.2 percent), including nausea, vomiting, diarrhea, and abdominal pain. The next most frequent are central nervous system effects (9 percent), with dizziness, headaches, and seizures.[232] Rash occurs in approximately 4 percent of patients. Sixteen percent of patients develop laboratory abnormalities, principally anemia and increase in liver function tests. Severe hepatic injury is rare.

There are no data on toxicity or teratogenicity for the fetus during pregnancy. It is not known if fluconazole is excreted in breast milk.

Drug Interactions

Fluconazole potentiates the effects of warfarin and increases the plasma levels of phenytoin and oral hypoglycemic agents.[228] Cimetidine decreases the absorption of fluconazole, while rifampin decreases both the half-life and the area under the curve of fluconazole.[228] There are contradictory data on its interaction with cyclosporine A.[228,234] In contrast to ketoconazole, fluconazole has little effect on the biosynthesis of testosterone by mammalian cells.[235]

ITRACONAZOLE

Itraconazole is a new orally absorbed triazole derivative. It is licensed for use in several countries but is not commercially available in the United States.

Mechanism of Action

Itraconazole shares its basic principles of activity with ketoconazole and the other azoles.[236] It inhibits the synthesis of ergosterol and produces simultaneous accumulation of 14-α-methysterols. Its effect seems to be principally through inhibition of the cytochrome P-450 system.

Spectrum of Activity

The drug demonstrates a broad spectrum of activity against a number of fungal species (Table 27–1), including dermatophytes, *Malassezia furfur, Candida* sp., *Aspergillus* sp., *Sporothrix schenckii, Cryptococcus neoformans, Coccidioides immitis,* and *Histoplasma capsulatum.*[237]

Formulation

Itraconazole is available as 100-mg and 200-mg tablets.

Pharmacology

Itraconazole is a highly lipophilic drug that is better absorbed with food. The blood levels are low, but higher concentrations are obtained in the tissues after repeated dosing. There is wide interpatient variability. The absorption appears to be slow, with peak concentrations 3.0–6.0 hours after administration. At steady state the mean peak concentrations of itraconazole after doses of 100 mg daily, 200 mg daily, and 200 mg twice daily are 412, 1070, and 1980 ng/ml, respectively.[238] The half-life seems to be longer (20–30 hours) than that of ketoconazole.[239]

Itraconazole is metabolized by the liver into inactive metabolites that are excreted in the bile and urine.[240] The excretion in the feces is 3–18 percent. Tissue penetration of itraconazole is good except for the central nervous system.[241] Renal dysfunction, hemodialysis, or continuous peritoneal dialysis does not seem to alter itraconazole pharmacokinetics.[242] There are no published studies of the pharmacokinetics of itraconazole in infants and children.

Clinical Studies

Excellent results have been obtained with a 3-day regimen of 200 mg daily for a large number of women with vaginal candidiasis.[243] The drug has been used successfully for treatment of sporotrichosis, chromomycosis, and aspergillosis and has proven to be useful for therapy of some life-threatening infections when standard therapy has failed.[243–247] Itraconazole has been effective in therapy of children with chronic granulomatous disease and invasive *Aspergillus* infection.[248]

Clinical Indications and Posology

In some countries itraconazole has been licensed for the short-term treatment of vaginal candidiasis and dermatophytoses.[243,249] Current data suggest that itraconazole may have similar indications as ketoconazole, with possibly better efficacy and fewer side effects. For systemic infections the recommended daily dose is from 200 to 400 mg daily. Itraconazole is a promising agent, but further studies are needed to determine its precise role for prophylaxis and treatment of systemic mycoses in normal and immunocompromised hosts.

Adverse Effects

The tolerance to itraconazole is very good.[227,247] Side effects have been reported in 2–8 percent of patients and include mild elevations of liver enzymes, increase in creatinine levels, nausea, headache, pyrosis, and dysuria.[243] To date, there are no reports of serious hepatotoxicity. No impairment of cortisol synthesis has been demonstrated in patients receiving itraconazole.[239,250]

There are no data on toxicity or teratogenicity for the fetus during pregnancy. It is not known if itraconazole is excreted in breast milk.

Drug Interactions

Itraconazole does not alter the pharmacokinetics of warfarin, but serum concentrations of itraconazole are reduced with concomitant use of rifampin.[240] The pharmacokinetics of cyclosporine may be altered by concomitant administration of itraconazole.[240,251]

REFERENCES

1. Gallis HA, Drew RH, Pickard WW: Amphotericin B: 30 years of clinical experience. Rev Infect Dis 12:308–329, 1990
2. Norman AW, Demel RA, De Kruyff B, et al: Studies on the bio-

logic properties of polyene antibiotics: Comparison of other polyenes with filipin in their ability to interact specifically with sterol. Biochim Biophys Acta 290:1–14, 1972

3. Brajtburg J, Powderly WG, Kobayashi GS, et al: Amphotericin B: Current understanding of mechanisms of actions. Antimicrob Agents Chemother 34:183–188, 1990

4. Heel RC, Brogden RN, Carmine A, et al: Ketoconazole: A review of its therapeutic efficacy in superficial and systemic fungal infections. Drugs 23:1–36, 1982

5. Gold W, Stout HA, Pagano JF, et al: Amphotericin A and B, antifungal antibiotics produced by a streptomycete. Antibiot Annual 1955–56, p 579.

6. Seabury JH, Dascomb HE: Experience with amphotericin B. Ann NY Acad Sci 89:202, 1960

7. Brandsberg JW, French ME: In vitro susceptibility of isolates of *Aspergillus fumigatus* and *Sporothrix schenckii* to amphotericin B. Antimicrob Agents Chemother 2:402, 1972

8. McGinnis MR, Rinaldi MG: Antifungal drugs: Mechanisms of action, drug resistance, susceptibility testing, and assays of activity in biological fluids, in Lorian V (ed): Antibiotics in Laboratory Medicine, 2nd ed. Baltimore, Williams and Wilkins, 1986, pp 223–281

9. Rippon JW: Medical Mycology: The Pathogenic Fungi and the Pathogenic Actinomycetes. 3rd ed. Philadelphia, WB Saunders, 1988

10. Kucers A, Bennett NMK: The Use of Antibiotics: A Comprehensive Review with Clinical Emphasis, 4th ed. Philadelphia, JB Lippincott, 1987

11. Shadomy S: In vitro studies with 5-fluorocytosine. Appl Microbiol 17:871, 1969

12. Steer PL, Marks MI, Klite PD, et al: 5-Fluorocytosine: An oral antifungal compound. A report on clinical and laboratory experience. Ann Intern Med 75:6–15, 1972

13. Vandevelde AG, Mauceri AA, Johnson JE III: 5-Fluorocytosine in the treatment of mycotic infections. Ann Intern Med 77:43, 1972

14. Shadomy S, Paxton L, Espinel-Ingroff A, et al: In vitro studies with miconazole and miconazole nitrate. J Antimicrob Chemother 3:147, 1977

15. Espinel-Ingroff A, Shadomy S, Gebhart RJ: In vitro studies with R51,211 (itraconazole). Antimicrob Agents Chemother 26:5–9, 1984

16. Kobayashi GS, Travis S, Medoff G: Comparison of the in vitro and in vivo activity of the bis-triazole derivative UK 49,858 with that of amphotericin B against *Histoplasma capsulatum*. Antimicrob Agents Chemother 29:660–662, 1986

17. Rogers TE, Galgiani JN: Activity of fluconazole (UK 49,858) and ketoconazole against *Candida albicans* in vitro and in vivo. Antimicrob Agents Chemother 30:418–422, 1986

18. Van Cutsem J, Van Gerven F, Janssen PAJ: Activity of orally, topically, and parenterally administered itraconazole in the treatment of superficial and deep mycoses: Animal models. Rev Infect Dis 9(suppl 1):S15–S32, 1987

19. Galgiani JN: Susceptibility of *Candida albicans* and other yeasts to fluconazole: Relation between in vitro and in vivo studies. Rev Infect Dis 12(suppl 3):S272–S275, 1990

20. Fisher MA, Sten S-H, Haddad J, et al: Comparison of in vivo activity of fluconazole with that of amphotericin B against *Candida tropicalis, Candida glabrata,* and *Candida krusei.* Antimicrob Agents Chemother 33:1443–1446, 1989

21. Drutz DJ: In vitro antifungal susceptibilities testing and measurements of levels of antifungal in body fluids. Rev Infect Dis 9:392–397, 1987

22. Mertz W: *Candida lusitaniae:* Frequency of recovery, colonization and amphotericin B resistance. J Clin Microb 20:1194–1195, 1984

23. Mertz W, Sandford G: Isolation and characterization of a polyene resistant variant of C. tropicalis. J Clin Microb 9:677–680, 1979

24. Pappagianis D, Collins M, Hector R, et al: Development of resistance to amphotericin B in *Candida lusitaniae* infecting a human. Antimicrob Agents Chemother 16:123–126, 1979

25. Dick J, Mertz W, Saral R: Incidence of polyene-resistant yeasts recovered from clinical specimens. Antimicrob Agents Chemother 18:158–163, 1980

26. Guinet R, Chanas J, Goullier A, et al: Fatal septicemia due to amphotericin B-resistant C. *lusitaniae.* J Clin Microb 18:433–444, 1983

27. Lopez-Berstein G, Fainstein V, Hopfer R, et al: Liposomal amphotericin B for the treatment of systemic fungal infections in patients with cancer: A preliminary study. J Infect Dis 151:704–710, 1985

28. Bennett JE, Dismukes WE, Duma RJ, et al: A comparison of amphotericin B alone and combined with flucytosine in the treatment of cryptococcal meningitis. N Engl J Med 301:126–131, 1979

29. Smego RA, Perfect JR, Durack DT: Combined therapy with amphotericin B and 5-fluorocytosine for candida meningitis. Rev Infect Dis 6:791–801, 1986

30. Auwera PV, Ceuppens AM, Heymans C, et al: In vitro evaluation of various antifungal agents alone and in combination by using an automatic turbidimetric system combined with viable count determinations. Antimicrob Agents Chemother 29:997–1004, 1986

31. Medoff G: Controversial areas in antifungal chemotherapy: Short course and combination therapy with amphotericin B. Rev Infect Dis 9:403–407, 1987

32. Schaffner A, Frick PG: The effect of ketoconazole on amphotericin B in a model of disseminated aspergillosis. J Infect Dis 151:902–910, 1985

33. Van Tyle JH: Ketoconazole: Mechanism of action, spectrum of activity, drug interactions, adverse reactions, and therapeutic use. Pharmacotherapy 4:343–373, 1984

34. Eng RH: Susceptibility of zymocetes to amphotericin B, miconazole, and ketoconazole. Antimicrob Agents Chemother 20:688–690, 1981

35. Louria D: Some aspects of the absorption, distribution and excretion of amphotericin B in man. Antibiot Med Clin Ther 5:295–301, 1958

36. Kravetz H, Andriole V, Huber M, et al: Oral administration of solubilized amphotericin B. N Engl J Med 265:183–184, 1961

37. Ching M, Raymond K, Bury RW, et al: Absorption of orally administered amphotericin B lozenges. Br J Clin Pharm 16:106–108, 1983

38. Jagdis FA, Mongi N, Lawrence RM, et al: Distribution of radiolabelled amphotericin B methyl ester and amphotericin B in non-human primates, in Proceedings 16th Interscience Conference on Antimicrobial Agents and Chemotherapy, Abstract 305, Washington, DC, 1976

39. Block ER, Bennett JE, Livoti LG, et al: Flucytosine and amphotericin B: Hemodialysis effects on the plasma concentrations and clearance studies in man. Ann Intern Med 80:613–617, 1974

40. Bennett JE: Amphotericin B binding to serum beta lipoprotein, in Iwata K (ed) Recent Advances in Medical and Veterinary Mycology. Tokyo, University of Tokyo Press, 1977, pp 107–109

41. Atkinson AJ, Bennett JE: Amphotericin B pharmacokinetics in humans. Antimicrob Agents Chemother 13:271–276, 1978

42. Cherry JD, Lloyd CA, Quilty JF, et al: Amphotericin B therapy in children: A review of the literature and a case report. J Pediatr 75:1063–1069, 1969

43. Rao HKM, Myers GJ: Candida meningitis in the newborn. South Med J 72:1468, 1979

44. Ward RM, Sattler FR, Dalton AS: Assessment of antifungal therapy in an 800-gram infant with candidal arthritis and osteomyelitis. Pediatrics 72:234–238, 1983

45. Hall JE, Cox F, Karlson K, et al: Amphotericin B dosage for disseminated candidiasis in premature infants. J Perinatol 7:194–198, 1983

46. Benson JM, Nahata MC: Pharmacokinetics of amphotericin B in children. Antimicrob Agents Chemother 33:1989–1993, 1989

47. Starke JR, Mason EO Jr, Kramer WG, et al: Pharmacokinetics of amphotericin B in infants and children. J Infect Dis 155:766–774, 1987

48. Koren G, Lau A, Klein J, et al: Pharmacokinetics and adverse effects of amphotericin B in infants and children. J Pediatr 113:559–563, 1988

49. Drutz DJ, Spickard A, Rogers DE, et al: Treatment of dissemi-

nated mycotic infections. New approach to therapy with amphotericin B. Am J Med 45:405, 1968

50. Colette N, Van der Auwera P, Lopez AP, et al: Tissue concentrations and bioactivity of amphotericin B in cancer patients treated with amphotericin B-deoxycholate. Antimicrob Agents Chemother 33:362–368, 1989

51. Bindschadler DD, Bennett JE: A pharmacologic guide to the clinical use of amphotericin B. J Infect Dis 20:427–436, 1969

52. Craven PC, Ludden TM, Drutz DJ: Excretion pathways of amphotericin B. J Infect Dis 140:329–340, 1979

53. Felman HA, Hamilton JD, Gutman RA: Amphotericin B therapy in an anephric patient. Antimicrob Agents Chemother 4:402–405, 1973

54. Hill HR, Mitchell TG, Matsen JM, et al: Recovery from disseminated candidiasis in a premature infant. Pediatrics 53:48, 1974

55. Miller MJ: Fungal infections, in Remington JS, Klein JO (eds): Infectious Diseases of the Fetus and Newborn Infant. Philadelphia, WB Saunders, 1990, pp 475–515

56. Wilson R, Feldman S: Toxicity of amphotericin B in children with cancer. Am J Dis Child 133:731–734, 1979

57. Butler KM, Rench MA, Baker CJ: Amphotericin B as a single agent in the treatment of systemic candidiasis in neonates. Pediatr Infect Dis J 9:51–56, 1990

58. Johnson DE, Thompson TR, Green TB, et al: Systemic candidiasis in very low-birth-weight infants ($\leq$1500 gms). Pediatrics 73:138–143, 1984

59. Faix RG: Systemic Candida infections in infants in intensive care nurseries: High incidence of central nervous system involvement. J Pediatr 105:616–622, 1984

60. Bayer A, Blumenkrantz M, Montgomerie J, et al: Candida peritonitis: Report of 22 cases and review of the English literature. Am J Med 61:832–840, 1976

61. Klein JO, Yamauchi T, Horlick SP: Neonatal candidiasis, meningitis and arthritis: Observations and a review of the literature. J Pediatr 81:31, 1972

62. Duffty P, Lloyd DJ: Neonatal systemic candidiasis. Arch Dis Child 58:318, 1983

63. Baley JE, Kliegman RM, Fanaroff AA: Disseminated fungal infections in very low-birth-weight infants: Therapeutic toxicity. Pediatrics 73:153–157, 1984

64. Utz JP: Flucytosine. N Engl J Med 286:777–778, 1972

65. Robertson DM, Riley FC, Hermans PE: Endogenous Candida oculomycosis: Report of two patients treated with flucytosine. Arch Ophthalmol 91:33–38, 1974

66. Kohn DB, Uehling DT, Peters ME, et al: Short-course amphotericin B for isolated candiduria in children. J Pediatr 110:310–313, 1987

67. Wise G, Kozinn P, Goldberg P: Amphotericin B as a urologic irrigant in the management of noninvasive candiduria. J Urol 128:82–84, 1982

68. Stamm AM, Diasio RB, Dismukes WE, et al: Toxicity of amphotericin B plus flucytosine in 194 patients with cryptococcal meningitis. Am J Med 83:236–242, 1987

69. Meunier-Carpentier F: Cryptococcal meningitis: A case report and review of diagnostic procedures and therapy. Acta Clin Belg 36:300–302, 1981

70. Bennett JE: Overview of the symposium. Rev Infect Dis 12(suppl 3):S263–S266, 1990

71. Robinson PA, Knirsch AK, Joseph JA: Fluconazole for life-threatening fungal infections in patients who can not be treated with conventional antifungal drugs. Rev Infect Dis 12(suppl 3):S349–S363, 1990

72. Stamm AM, Dismukes WE: Current therapy of pulmonary and disseminated fungal diseases. Chest 83:911–917, 1983

73. Sarosi GA: Management of fungal diseases. Am Rev Resp Dis 127:250–253, 1983

74. National Institute of Allergy and Infectious Diseases Mycoses Study Group: Treatment of blastomycosis and histoplasmosis with ketoconazole. Results of a prospective randomized clinical trial. Ann Intern Med 103:861–872, 1985

75. Negroni R, Robles AM, Arechavala A, et al: Ketoconazole in the treatment of paracoccidioidomycosis and histoplasmosis. Rev Infect Dis 2:643–649, 1980

76. Hawkins SS, Gregory DW, Alford RH: Progressive disseminated

histoplasmosis: Favorable response to ketoconazole. Ann Intern Med 95:446–449, 1981

77. Stevens DA, Stiller RC, Williams PL, et al: Experience with ketoconazole in three major manifestations of progressive coccidioidomycosis. Am J Med 74(suppl 1B):58–63, 1983

78. Galgiani JN, Stevens DN, Graybill JR, et al: Ketoconazole therapy of progressive coccidioidomycosis. Comparison of 400 and 800 mg doses and observations at higher doses. Am J Med 84:603–610, 1988

79. Rahko P, Davey P, Wheat J, et al: Treatment of Torulopsis glabrata peritonitis with intraperitoneal amphotericin B. JAMA 249:1187–1188, 1983

80. Eisenberg ES, Leviton I, Saliro R: Fungal peritonitis in patients receiving peritoneal dialysis: Experience with 11 patients and review of the literature. Rev Infect Dis 8:309–321, 1987

81. Kennedy MS, Deeg HJ, Siegel M, et al: Acute renal toxicity with combined use of amphotericin B and cyclosporine after marrow transplantation. Transplantation 35:211–215, 1983

82. Lopez-Berestein G, Hopfer RL, Mehta R, et al: Liposome-encapsulated amphotericin B for the treatment of disseminated candidiasis in neutropenic mice. J Infect Dis 147:939–944, 1984

83. Lopez-Berestein G, Fainstein V, Hopfer RL, et al: Liposomal-amphotericin B for the treatment of systemic fungal infections in patients with cancer: A preliminary study. J Infect Dis 154:704–710, 1985

84. Lopez-Berestein G, Bodey GP, Fainstein V, et al: Treatment of systemic fungal infections with liposomal amphotericin B. Ann Intern Med 149:2533–2536, 1989

85. Brajtburg J, Powderly WG, Kobayashi GS, et al: Amphotericin B: Delivery systems. Antimicrob Agents Chemother 34:381–384, 1990

86. Schmitt HJ, Bernard EM, Häuser M, et al: Aerosol amphotericin B is effective for prophylaxis and therapy of pulmonary aspergillosis. Antimicrob Agents Chemother 32:1676–1679, 1988

87. Niki Y, Bernard EM, Schmitt HJ, et al: Pharmacokinetics of aerosol amphotericin B in rats. Antimicrob Agents Chemother 34:29–32, 1990

88. Posner J: Reservoirs for intraventricular chemotherapy. N Engl J Med 288:212–213, 1973

89. Block ER, Bennett JE: Stability of amphotericin B in the infusion bottle. Antimicrob Agents Chemother 4:648, 1973

90. Drutz D: Newer antifungal agents and their use, including an update on amphotericin B and flucytosine, in Remington J, Swartz M (eds): Current Clinical Topics in Infectious Diseases, vol 3. New York, McGraw-Hill, 1982, pp 97–135

91. Spitzer TR, Creger RJ, Fox RM, et al: Rapid infusion of amphotericin B: Effective and well-tolerated therapy for neutropenic fever. Pharmatherapeutica 5:305–311, 1989

92. Butler W, Bennett J, Hill G, et al: Electrocardiographic and electrolytes abnormalities caused by amphotericin B in dog and man. Proc Soc Exp Biol Med 116:857–863, 1964

93. Utz J: Amphotericin B toxicity: Combined clinical staff conference at the NIH. General side effects. Ann Intern Med 61:334–340, 1964

94. Craven PC, Gremillion DH: Risk factors of ventricular fibrillation during rapid amphotericin B infusion. Antimicrob Agents Chemother 27:868–871, 1985

95. Medoff G, Kobayashi G: Strategies in the treatment of systemic fungal infections. N Engl J Med 302:145–155, 1980

96. Durks L, Aisner J, Fortner C, et al: Meperidine for the treatment of shaking chills and fever. Arch Intern Med 140:483–484, 1980

97. Gigliotti F, Shenep JL, Lott L, et al: Induction of prostaglandin synthesis as the mechanism responsible for the chills and fever produced by infusing amphotericin B. J Infect Dis 156:784–789, 1987

98. Gelfand JA, Kimball K, Burke JF, et al: Amphotericin B treatment of mononuclear cells in vitro results in secretion of tumor necrosis factor and interleukin-1. Clin Res 36:456A, 1988

99. Googe JH, Walterspiel JN: Arrhythmia caused by amphotericin B in a neonate. Pediatr Infect Dis J 7:73, 1988

100. Wright D, Robichaud K, Pizzo P, et al: Lethal pulmonary reactions associated with the combined use of amphotericin B and leukocyte transfusions. N Engl J Med 304:1185–1189, 1981

101. Dana B, Durie B, White R, et al: Concomitant administration of granulocyte transfusions and amphotericin B in neutropenic patients: Absence of significant pulmonary toxicity. Blood 57:90–94, 1981
102. Bow E, Schroeder M, Louie T: Pulmonary complications in patients receiving granulocyte transfusions and amphotericin B. Can Med Assoc J 130:593–597, 1984
103. Dutcher JP, Kendall J, Norris D, et al: Granulocyte transfusion therapy and amphotericin B: Adverse reactions? Am J Hematol 31:102–108, 1989
104. Argov Z, Mastaglia FL: Disorders of neuromuscular transmission caused by drugs. N Engl J Med 301:409, 1979
105. Argov Z, Mastaglia FL: Drug induced peripheral neuropathies. Br Med J 1:664, 1979
106. Schiffman SS: Taste and smell in disease. Part 1. N Engl J Med 308:1277, 1983
107. Steinmetz PR, Lawson LR: Defect in urinary acidification induced in vitro by amphotericin. J Clin Invest 49:596–601, 1970
108. McCurdy DK, Frederic M, Elkington JR: Renal tubular acidosis due to amphotericin B. N Engl J Med 278:124, 1968
109. Butler WT, Bennett JE, Alling DW, et al: Nephrotoxicity of amphotericin B. Early and late effects in 81 patients. Ann Intern Med 61:175, 1964
110. Miller RP, Bates JH: Amphotericin B toxicity. Ann Intern Med 71:1089, 1969
111. Drutz DJ, Fan JH, Tai TY: Hypokalemic rhabdomyolysis and myoglobinuria following amphotericin B therapy. JAMA 211:824, 1970
112. Jacqze E, Branch RA, Heidermann H, et al: Prévention de la néphrotoxicité de l'amphotéricine B au cours du traitement des candidoses profondes. Ann Biol Clin 45:689–693, 1987
113. Smith SR, Galloway MJ, Reilly JT, et al: Amiloride prevents amphotericin B related hypokalaemia in neutropenic patients. J Clin Pathol 41:494–497, 1988
114. Lin AC, Goldwasser E, Bernard EM, et al: Amphotericin B blunts erythropoietin response to anemia. J Infect Dis 161:348–351, 1990
115. Chan CSP, Tuazon CU, Lessin LS: Amphotericin B-induced thrombocytopenia. Ann Intern Med 96:332–333, 1982
116. Neiberg AD, Mavromatis F, Dykes J, et al: *Blastomyces dermatitidis* treated during pregnancy: Report of one case. Am J Obstet Gynecol 128:911–912, 1977
117. Chow AW, Jenessan PJ: Pharmacokinetics and safety of antimicrobial agents during pregnancy. Rev Infect Dis 7:287–313, 1985
118. Ismail MA, Lerner SA: Disseminated blastomycosis in a pregnant woman. Am Rev Resp Dis 126:350–353, 1982
119. Cohen I: Absence of congenital infection and teratogenesis in three children born to mothers with blastomycosis and treated with amphotericin B during pregnancy. Pediatr Infect Dis J 6:76–77, 1987
120. Watts EA, Gard PD Jr, Tuthill SW: First reported cases of intrauterine transmission of blastomycosis. Pediatr Infect Dis 2:308–310, 1983
121. Catanzaro A: Pulmonary mycosis in pregnant women. Chest 86(suppl):14S–18S, 1984
122. Daniel L, Salit IE: Blastomycosis during pregnancy. Can Med Assoc J 131:759–761, 1984
123. McCoy MJ, Ellenberg JF, Killum AP: Coccidioidomycosis complicating pregnancy. Am J Obstet Gynecol 137:739, 1980
124. Feldman R: Cryptococcosis (torulosis) of the central nervous system treated with amphotericin B during pregnancy. South Med J 52:1415, 1959
125. Aitken GWE, Symonds EM: Cryptococcal meningitis in pregnancy treated with amphotericin B: A case report. J Obstet Gynaecol Br Commonw 69:677, 1962
126. Kuo D: A case of torulosis of the central nervous system during pregnancy. Med J Aust 49:558, 1962
127. Sanford WG, Rosch JR, Stonehill RB: A therapeutic dilemma: The treatment of disseminated coccidioidomycosis with amphotericin B. Ann Intern Med 56:553, 1962
128. Harris RE: Coccidioidomycosis complicating pregnancy. Report of 3 cases and review of the literature. Obstet Gynecol 28:401, 1966
129. Smale LE, Waechter KG: Dissemination of coccidioidomycosis in pregnancy. Am J Obstet Gynecol 107:356, 1970
130. Hadsall FJ, Acquarelli JJ: Disseminated coccidioidomycosis presenting as facial granulomas in pregnancy: A report of two cases and review of the literature. Laryngoscope 83:51, 1973
131. Curole DN: Cryptococcal meningitis in pregnancy. J Reprod Med 26:317–319, 1981
132. Antimicrobial agents in pregnancy. Med Lett 27:93–95, 1985
133. Briggs GG, Freeman RK, Yaffe SJ: Drugs in Pregnancy, 2nd ed. Baltimore, Williams and Wilkins, 1986, pp 21, 294
134. Ghannoum MA, Motwy MS, Abuhatab MA, et al: Interactive effects of antifungal and antineoplastic agents on yeasts commonly prevalent in cancer patients. Antimicrob Agents Chemother 33:726–730, 1989
135. Ellenhorn MJ, Barceloux DG: Medical Toxicology—Diagnosis and Treatment of Human Poisoning. New York, Elsevier, 1990, pp 117–129
136. Goren MP, Viar MJ, Shenep JL, et al: Monitoring serum aminoglycoside concentrations in children with amphotericin B nephrotoxicity. Pediatr Infect Dis J 7:698–703, 1988
137. Yee GC, Kennedy MS, Deeg HJ, et al: Cyclosporine-associated renal dysfunction in marrow transplant recipients. Transplant Proc 17(suppl 1):196–201, 1985
138. Tutschka PJ, Beschorner WE, Hess AD, et al: Cyclosporin-A to prevent graft-versus-host disease: A pilot study in 22 patients receiving allogeneic marrow transplantation. Blood 61:318–325, 1983
139. Antoniskis D, Larsen RA: Acute, rapidly progressive renal failure with simultaneous use of amphotericin B and pentamidine. Antimicrob Agents Chemother 34:470–472, 1990
140. Waldorf AR, Polak A: Mechanisms of action of 5-fluorocytosine. Antimicrob Agents Chemother 23:79–85, 1983
141. Medoff G, Comfort M, Kobnayashi GS: Synergistic action of amphotericin B and 5-fluorocytosine against yeast-like organisms. Proc Soc Exp Biol Med 138:571, 1971
142. Polak A: Synergism of polyene antibiotics with 5-fluorocytosine. Chemotherapy 24:2, 1978
143. Ashe WD Jr, Van Renken DE: 5-Fluorocytosine: A brief review. Clin Pediatr 16:365–366, 1977
144. Cutler RE, Blais AD, Kelly MR: Flucytosine pharmacokinetics in subjects with normal and impaired renal function. Clin Pharmacol Ther 24:333–342, 1978
145. Daneshend TK, Warnock DW: Clinical pharmacokinetics of systemic antifungal drugs. Clin Pharmacokinet 8:17–42, 1983
146. Holt RJ, Newman RC: The antimycotic activity of 5-fluorocytosine. J Clin Pathol 26:167–174, 1983
147. Drouhet E, Borderon JC, Borderon E, et al: Évolution des concentrations sériques de 5-fluorocytosine chez les prématurés. Bull Soc Fr Mycol Med 3:37–40, 1974
148. Block ER, Bennett JE: Pharmacological studies with 5-fluorocytosine. Antimicrob Agents Chemother 14:903–908, 1978
149. Diasio RB, Lakings DE, Bennett JE: Evidence for conversion of 5-fluorocytosine to 5-fluorouracil in humans: Possible factor in 5-fluorocytosine toxicity. Antimicrob Agents Chemother 14:903–908, 1978
150. Koechlin BA, Rubio F, Palmer S, et al: The metabolism of 5-fluorocytosine-2(^{14})C and of cytosine (^{14})C in the rat and the disposition of 5-fluorocytosine-2 (^{14})C in man. Biochem Pharmacol 15:435–446, 1966
151. Wise G, Weinstein S, Goldberg P, et al: Flucytosine in urinary candida infections. Urology 3:708–711, 1974
152. Wise G, Kozinn P, Goldberg P: Flucytosine in the management of genitourinary candidiasis: Five years of experience. J Urol 124:70–72, 1980
153. Mauceri AA, Cullen SI, Van de Velde AG, et al: Flucytosine. An effective oral treatment for chromomycosis. Arch Dermatol 109:873–879, 1974
154. Bennett J: Flucytosine. Ann Intern Med 86:319–322, 1977
155. Hawkins C, Armstrong D: Fungal infections in the immunocompromised host. Clin Haematol 13:599–630, 1984
156. Gold JWM: Opportunistic fungal infections in patients with neoplastic disease. Am J Med 76:458–463, 1984

157. Mina FA, Hopkins SJ, Richelo B: Parenteral 5-fluorocytosine in the therapy of systemic mycoses. Ann NY Acad Sci 544:571–574, 1989

158. Harris BE, Manning BW, Federle TW, et al: Conversion of 5-fluorocytosine to 5-fluorouracil by human intestinal microflora. Antimicrob Agents Chemother 29:44–48, 1986

159. Harder EJ, Hermans PF: Treatment of fungal infections with flucytosine. Arch Intern Med 135:231, 1975

160. White CA, Traube J: Ulcerating enteritis associated with flucytosine therapy. Gastroenterology 83:1127, 1982

161. Kauffman C, Frame P: Bone marrow toxicity associated with 5-FC therapy. Antimicrob Agents Chemother 11:244–247, 1977

162. Philpot CK, Lo D: Cryptococcal meningitis in pregnancy. Med J Aust 2:1005–1007, 1972

163. Schonebeck J, Segerbrand E: *Candida albicans* septicemia during first half of pregnancy successfully treated with 5-fluorocytosine. Br Med J 4:337–338, 1973

164. O'Neill MB, Hill JB, Arbus GS: False elevation of the serum creatinine level associated with the use of flucytosine. Can Med Assoc J 137:133–134, 1987

165. Mitchell RT, Marshall LH, Lefkowitz LB Jr, et al: Falsely elevated serum creatinine levels secondary to the presence of 5-fluorocytosine. Am J Clin Pathol 84:251–253, 1985

166. Graybill JR, Drutz DJ: Ketoconazole: A major innovation for treatment of fungal disease. Ann Intern Med 93:921–923.

167. Van den Bossche H, Willemsens G, Cools W, et al: In vitro and in vivo effects of the antimycotic drug ketoconazole on sterol synthesis. Antimicrob Agents Chemother 17:922–928, 1980

168. Dixon D, Shadomy S, Shadomy HJ, et al: Comparison of the in vitro antifungal activities of miconazole and a new imidazole R41,400. J Infect Dis 138:245–248, 1978

169. Van der Meer JWM, Kenning JJ, Scheijgrond HW, et al: The influence of gastric acidity on the bioavailability of ketoconazole. J Antimicrob Chemother 6:552–554, 1980

170. Mannisto PT, Mantyla R, Nykanen S, et al: Impairing effect of food on ketoconazole absorption. Antimicrob Agents Chemother 21:730, 1982

171. Daneshmend TK, Warnock DW, Ene MD: Influence of food on the pharmacokinetics of ketoconazole. Antimicrob Agents Chemother 25:1–3, 1984

172. Daneshmend TK, Warnock DW, Turner A, et al: Pharmacokinetics of ketoconazole in normal subjects. J Antimicrob Chemother 8:299–304, 1981

173. Ginsburg CM, McCracken GH Jr, Olsen KD: Pharmacology of ketoconazole suspension in infants and children. Antimicrob Agents Chemother 23:787–789, 1983

174. Bardare M, Tortorana AM, Pietrogrande MC, et al: Pharmacokinetics of ketoconazole and treatment evaluation in candidal infections. Arch Dis Child 59:1068–1071, 1984

175. Brass C, Galgiani JN, Blaschke TJ, et al: Disposition of ketoconazole, an oral antifungal, in humans. Antimicrob Agents Chemother 21:151–158, 1982

176. Graybill JR, Lundberg D, Donovan W, et al: Treatment of coccidioidomycosis with ketoconazole. Clinical and laboratory studies in 18 patients. Rev Infect Dis 2:661–673, 1980

177. Craven PC, Graybill JR, Jorgensen JH, et al: High dose ketoconazole for treatment of fungal infections in the central nervous system. Ann Intern Med 98:160, 1983

178. Sugar AM, Alsup SG, Galgiani JN, et al: Pharmacology and toxicity of high dose ketoconazole. Antimicrob Agents Chemother 31:1874–1878, 1987

179. Maksymiuk AW, Levine HB, Bodey GB: Pharmacokinetics of ketoconazole in patients with neoplastic diseases. Antimicrob Agents Chemother 22:43–46, 1982

180. Fanconi S, Seger R, Joller P, et al: Intermittent ketoconazole therapy for chronic mucocutaneous candidiasis in childhood. Eur J Pediatr 139:176–180, 1980

181. Rosenblatt HM, Byrne W, Ament ME, et al: Successful treatment of chronic mucocutaneous candidiasis with ketoconazole. J Pediatr 97:657–660, 1980

182. Tudehope DI, Rigby B: Neonatal systemic candidiasis treated with miconazole and hepaconazole. Med J Aust 1:480, 1983

183. Johnson PC, Khardori N, Najjar AF, et al: Progressive disseminated histoplasmosis in patients with acquired immunodeficiency syndrome. Am J Med 85:152–158, 1988

184. Restrepo A, Gómez I, Cano LE, et al: Treatment of paracoccidioidomycosis with ketoconazole: A three year experience. Am J Med 74(suppl 1B):48–52, 1983

185. Bradsher RW, Rice DC, Abernathy RS: Ketoconazole therapy for endemic blastomycosis. Ann Intern Med 103:872–879, 1985

186. Dismukes WE, Stamm AM, Graybill JR, et al: Treatment of systemic mycoses with ketoconazole: Emphasis on toxicity and clinical response in fifty-two patients. Ann Intern Med 98:13–20, 1983

187. Symoens J, Maens M, Dom J, et al: An evaluation of two years of clinical experience with ketoconazole. Rev Infect Dis 2:674–687, 1980

188. Perfect JR, Durack DT, Hamilton JD, et al: Failure of ketoconazole in cryptococcal meningitis. JAMA 247:3349–3351, 1982

189. Drouhet E, Dupont B: Laboratory and clinical assessment of ketoconazole in deep-seated mycoses. Am J Med 74(suppl 1B):30–47, 1983

190. Horsburgh C, Kirkpatrick CH: Long-term therapy of chronic mucocutaneous candidosis; experience with twenty-one patients. Am J Med 74(suppl 1B):23–29, 1983

191. Fainstein V, Bodey GP, Elting L, et al: Amphotericin B therapy of fungal infections in neutropenic cancer patients. Antimicrob Agents Chemother 31:11–15, 1987

192. Defelice R, Johnson DG, Galgiani JN: Gynecomastia with ketoconazole. Antimicrob Agents Chemother 19:1073–1074, 1981

193. Fazio RA, Wickremesinghe PC, Arsura EL: Ketoconazole therapy of candida oesophagitis—a prospective study of 12 cases. Am J Gastroenterol 79:261–264, 1983

194. Duarte P, Chow C, Simmons F, et al: Fatal hepatitis associated with ketoconazole therapy. Arch Intern Med 144:1069–1070, 1984

195. Heiberg J, Svejgaard E: Toxic hepatitis during ketoconazole treatment. Br Med J 283:825–826, 1981

196. Horsburgh C, Kirkpatrick C, Teusch C: Ketoconazole and the liver. Lancet 1:860, 1982

197. Lewis JH, Zimmerman HJ, Benson GD, et al: Hepatic injury associated with ketoconazole therapy—an analysis of 33 cases. Gastroenterology 86:503–513, 1984

198. Svejgaard E, Ramek L: Hepatic dysfunction and ketoconazole therapy. Ann Intern Med 96:788–789, 1982

199. Pont A, Williams PL, Loose DS, et al: Ketoconazole blocks adrenal steroid synthesis. Ann Intern Med 97:370–372, 1982

200. Loose DS, Kan PB, Hirst MA, et al: Ketoconazole blocks adrenal steroidogenesis by inhibiting cytochrome P450-dependent enzymes. J Clin Invest 71:1495–1499, 1983

201. Loose DS, Stover EP, Feldman D: Ketoconazole binds to glucocorticoid receptors and exhibits antagonist activity in culture cells. J Clin Invest 72:404, 1983

202. Tucker WS, Snell BB, Island DP, et al: Reversible adrenal insufficiency induced by ketoconazole. JAMA 253:2413–2414, 1985

203. Pont A, Williams S, Azhar S, et al: Ketoconazole blocks testosterone synthesis. Arch Intern Med 142:2137–2140, 1982

204. Grosso D, Boyden T, Parmentier R, et al: Ketoconazole inhibition of testicular secretion of testosterone and displacement of steroid hormones from serum transport proteins. Antimicrob Agents Chemother 23:207–212, 1983

205. Britton H, Shehab Z, Lightner E, et al: Adrenal response in children receiving high doses of ketoconazole for systemic coccidioidomycosis. J Pediatr 112:488–492, 1988

206. Engelhard D, Stutman HR, Marks MI: Interaction of ketoconazole with rifampin and isoniazide. N Engl J Med 311:1681–1683, 1984

207. Meunier F: Serum fungistatic and fungicidal activity in volunteers receiving antifungal agents. Eur J Clin Microb 5:103–109, 1986

208. Dieperink H, Møller J: Ketoconazole and cyclosporin. Lancet 2:1217, 1982

209. Daneshemend T: Ketoconazole–cyclosporine interaction. Lancet 2:1342–1343, 1982

210. Ferguson R, Sutherland D, Simmons R, et al: Ketoconazole, cyclosporin metabolism and renal transplantation. Lancet 2:882–883, 1982

211. Morgenstein G, Powles R, Robinson B, et al: Cyclosporin interaction with ketoconazole and melphalan. Lancet 2:1342, 1982
212. Clarke M, Davies DP, Odds F, et al: Neonatal systemic candidiasis treated with miconazole. Br Med J 281:354, 1980
213. Sung JP, Rajani K, Chopra DR, et al: Miconazole therapy for systemic candidiasis in a conjoined (Siamese) twin and a premature newborn. Am J Surg 138:688, 1979
214. Kanarek KS, Williams PR: Toxicity of intravenous miconazole overdosage in a preterm infant. Pediatr Infect Dis 5:486, 1986
215. McDougall PN, Fleming PJ, Speller DCE, et al: Neonatal systemic candidiasis: A failure of intravenous miconazole in two neonates. Arch Dis Child 57:884, 1983
216. Sutton A: Miconazole in systemic candidiasis. Arch Dis Child 58:319, 1983
217. Bennett JE, Remington JS: Miconazole in cryptococcosis and systemic candidiasis: A word of caution. Ann Intern Med 94:708, 1981
218. Tuck S: Neonatal systemic candidiasis treated with miconazole. Arch Dis Child 55:903, 1980
219. Fisher JF, Duma RJ, Markowitz SM, et al: Therapeutic failures with miconazole. Antimicrob Agents Chemother 13:965–968, 1978
220. Drouhet E, Dupont E: Evolution of antifungal agents: Past, present and future. Rev Infect Dis 9(suppl 1):S4–S14, 1987
221. Deresinski S, Lilly R, Levine H, et al: Treatment of fungal meningitis with miconazole. Arch Inter Med 137:1180–1185, 1977
222. Sung J, Grendahl J, Levine M: Intravenous and intrathecal miconazole therapy for systemic mycosis. West J Med 126:5–13, 1977
223. Lutwick LI, Rytel MW, Yanez JP, et al: Deep infections from Petriellidium boydii treated with miconazole. JAMA 241:272–273, 1979
224. Hell RC, Brogden RN, Pakes GE, et al: Miconazole: A preliminary review of its therapeutic efficacy in systemic fungal infections. Drugs 19:7–30, 1980
225. Bagnarello AG, Lewis LA, McHenry MC, et al: Unusual serum lipoprotein abnormality induced by the vehicle of miconazole. N Engl J Med 296:497, 1977
226. Fainstein V, Bodey G: Cardiorespiratory toxicity due to miconazole. Ann Intern Med 93:432–433, 1980
227. Phillips P, Fetchick R, Weisman I, et al: Tolerance and efficacy of itraconazole in treatment of systemic mycoses: Preliminary results. Rev Infect Dis 9(suppl 1):S87–S93, 1987
228. Lazar JD, Wilner KD: Drug interaction with fluconazole. Rev Infect Dis 12(suppl 3):S327–S333, 1990
229. Humphrey MJ, Jevans S, Tarbit MH: Pharmacokinetic evaluation of UK-49,858 a metabolically stable triazole antifungal drug, in animals and humans. Antimicrob Agents Chemother 28:648–653, 1985
230. Brammer KW, Farrow PR, Faulkner JK: Pharmacokinetics and tissue penetration of fluconazole in humans. Rev Infect Dis 12(suppl 3):S318–S326, 1990
231. Tucker RM, Williams PL, Arathoon EG, et al: Pharmacokinetics of fluconazole in cerebrospinal fluid and serum in human coccidioidal meningitis. Antimicrob Agents Chemother 32:369–373, 1988
232. Hay RJ: Overview of studies of fluconazole in oropharyngeal candidiasis. Rev Infect Dis 12(suppl 3):S334–S337, 1990
233. Tucker RM, Galgiani JN, Denning DW, et al: Treatment of coccidioidal meningitis with fluconazole. Rev Infect Dis 12(suppl 3):S380–S389, 1990
234. Krüger HU, Schuder U, Zimmerman R, et al: Absence of significant interaction of fluconazole with cyclosporin. J Antimicrob Chemother 24:781–786, 1989
235. Hanger DP, Jevans S, Shaw JTB: Fluconazole and testosterone: In vivo and in vitro studies. Antimicrob Agents Chemother 32:646–648, 1988
236. Van Cutsem J, Van Gerven F, Van de Ven M-A, et al: Itraconazole, a new triazole that is orally active in aspergillosis. Antimicrob Agents Chemother 26:527–534, 1984
237. Hay RJ, Dupont B, Graybill JR: First international symposium on itraconazole: A summary. Rev Infect Dis 9(suppl 1):S1–S3, 1987
238. Hardin TC, Graybill JR, Fetchick R, et al: Pharmacokinetics of itraconazole following oral administration to normal volunteers. Antimicrob Agents Chemother 32:1310–1313, 1988
239. Van Cauteren H, Heykants J, De Coster R, et al: Itraconazole: Pharmacologic studies in animals and humans. Rev Infect Dis 9(suppl 1):S43–S46, 1987
240. Heykants J, Michiels M, Meuldermans W, et al: The pharmacokinetics of itraconazole in animals and man: An overview, in Fromtling RA (ed) Recent Trends in the Discovery, Development and Evaluation of Antifungal Agents, Barcelona, JR Prous Science Publishers, 1987, pp 223–229
241. Perfect JR, Durack DT: Penetration of imidazoles and triazoles into cerebrospinal fluids in rabbits. J Antimicrob Chemother 27:579–583, 1986
242. Boelaert J, Schurgers M, Matthys E, et al: Itraconazole pharmacokinetics in patients with renal dysfunction. Antimicrob Agents Chemother 32:1595–1597, 1988
243. Cauwenbergh G, De Doncker P, Stoops K, et al: Itraconazole in the treatment of human mycoses: Review of three years of clinical experience. Rev Infect Dis 9(suppl 1):S146–S152, 1987
244. Borelli D: A clinical trial of itraconazole in the treatment of deep mycoses and leishmaniasis. Rev Infect Dis 9(suppl 1):S57–S63, 1987
245. Lavalle P, Suchii P, De Ovando F, et al: Itraconazole for deep mycoses: Preliminary experience in Mexico. Rev Infect Dis 9(suppl 1):S64–S70, 1987
246. Dupont B, Drouhet E: Early experience with itraconazole in vitro and in patients: Pharmacokinetic studies and clinical results. Rev Infect Dis 9(suppl 1):S71–S76, 1987
247. Ganer A, Arathoon E, Stevens DA: Initial experience in therapy for progressive mycoses with itraconazole, the first clinically studied triazole. Rev Infect Dis 9(suppl 1):S77–S86, 1987
248. Neijins HJ, Frankel J, de Muinck Keizer-Schoma SMPF, et al: Invasive *Aspergillus* infections in chronic granulomatous disease: Treatment with itraconazole. J Pediatr 115:1016–1019, 1989
249. Warnock DW: Itraconazole and fluconazole: New drugs for deep fungal infections. J Antimicrob Chemother 24:275–277, 1989
250. Phillips P, Graybill JR, Fetchick R, et al: Adrenal response during therapy with itraconazole. Antimicrob Agents Chemother 31:647–649, 1987
251. Shaw MA, Gumbleton M, Nicholls PJ: Interaction of cyclosporin and itraconazole. Lancet 2:637, 1987

28

CHLORAMPHENICOL

ARNOLD L. SMITH

Chloramphenicol was first isolated from *Streptomyces venezuela.* However, it is currently chemically synthesized from moderately simple starting products. This antibiotic has lipophilic as well as polar activities: it consits of an aromatic nitro moiety and an aliphatic side chain containing a dichloroacetamido group attached to 1′,3′-dipropanol (Figure 28–1). The resultant physical properties lead to a very poor solubility in water (approximately 2 mg/ml). Because of the poor solubility, more water-soluble derivatives are formulated for parenteral use and a palatable fatty acid ester is formulated for oral administration. Chloramphenicol is remarkably stable to the extremes of pH and temperature.[1]

MECHANISM OF ACTION

Bacterial protein synthesis is inhibited by the binding of chloramphenicol to the 50S subunit of the 70S ribosome.[2,3] At that site chloramphenicol inhibits peptidyl transferase activity, the step that adds an incoming amino acid to the growing polypeptide chain. In mammalian mitochondria—organelles thought to be genetically related to bacteria and containing 70S ribosomes—protein synthesis is inhibited by chloramphenicol[4]; however, serum concentrations >50 µg/ml are necessary to drive chloramphenicol into this organelle. For chloramphenicol to bind to the 70S ribosomal subunit, the 1′- and 3′-hydroxyl groups must be in synplanar position to one another. In addition, the group adjacent to the amide linkage in the side chain must be capable of removing electrons; the paranitro group can be replaced by any other. Recognizing the necessity of the synplanar relationship, Nagabushian and colleagues replaced the 3′-hydroxyl group with a fluorine—an atom whose Van der Walls radii are approximately the same as those of the hydroxyl group. We found that this compound, D(−)-threo-2-dichloroacetamido-1-paranitrophenyl-1′-hydroxyl, 3′-fluoropropane, had biologic activity equivalent to the parent compound.[5] The importance of the synthesis of this structural analog, designated SCH 29482, was that the 3′-hydroxyl group can no longer be a substrate for chloramphenicol acetyltransferase (CAT), the enzyme responsible for antibiotic inactivation. CAT is the major mechanism by which bacteria become resistant to this antibiotic.

SPECTRUM OF ACTIVITY

Chloramphenicol is active against a wide variety of bacteria. However, its exact potency is dependent upon the specific bacterium being tested. For example, virtually all *Haemophilus influenzae* and *Neisseria meningitidis* are killed by chloramphenicol at a concentration of 2 µg/ml.[6] Therefore, the drug is defined as bactericidal against these organisms (killing 99.9 percent of the inoculum). With Enterobacteriaceae, on the other hand, growth is inhibited but organisms are not killed at concentrations as high as 16 µg/ml.[6] Thus, most bacteria residing in the human gastrointestinal tract or causing infections in that focus are inhibited by chloramphenicol but not killed in the test conditions noted. Chloramphenicol is therefore defined as bacteriostatic for enteric organisms. A chloramphenicol-susceptible organism is defined by the National Committee for Clinical Laboratory Standards (NCCLS) as one whose growth is inhibited by concentrations of 16 µg/ml or less.[7] Susceptible organisms, however, are not routinely distinguished as to whether the antibiotic is bactericidal or bacteriostatic. In certain species a high proportion of the isolates are resistant to chloramphenicol by these criteria. These include most *Pseudomonas aeruginosa* and *Serratia marcescens* (see Table 28–1).

In certain genera, such as *Pseudomonas,* a variable proportion of this species is susceptible to chloramphenicol. Thus, if this antibiotic is to be used for an infection caused

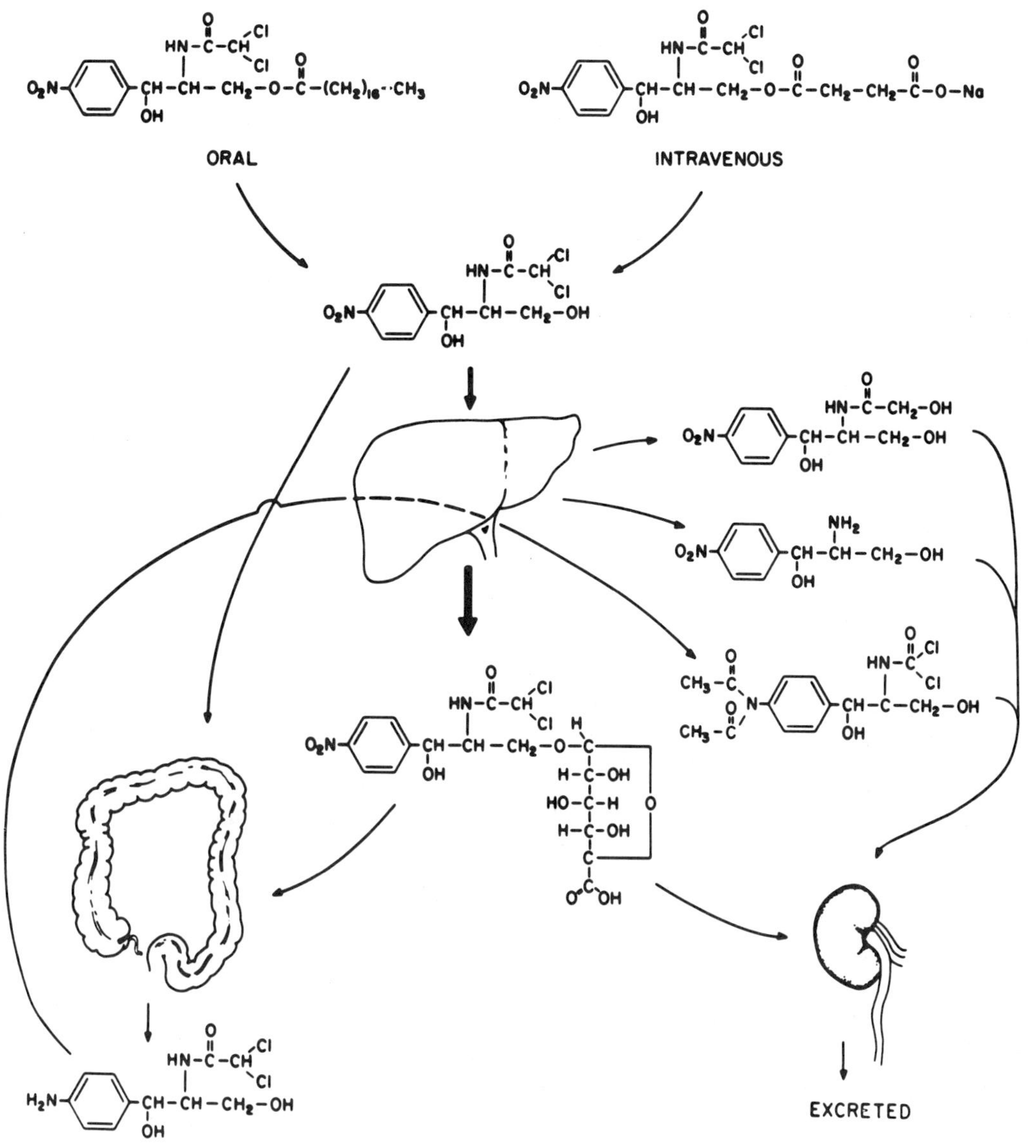

FIGURE 28–1. Chloramphenicol formulations and disposition. The 3′-palmitate ester (oral) or the 3′-succinate ester must be cleaved to yield a free 3′-hydroxyl, the group essential for biologic activity. Chloramphenicol glucuronide (bottom middle) is thought to be the major excretory product, and chloramphenicol alcohol, chloramphenicol base, and N-diacetylchloramphenicol the minor excretory products.

by these organisms, susceptibility testing should be performed.

RESISTANCE

Chloramphenicol-resistant bacteria occur "naturally." These bacteria are said to have intrinsic resistance. Bacteria can also acquire resistance. There are three basic ways in which a bacterium can become resistant to chloramphenicol: (1) modification of the target, i.e., the ribosome-binding site, so that the drug is no longer active; (2) failure of the drug to accumulate intracellularly (this may be due to decreased permeability; with other antibiotics,

e.g., tetracycline, it is due to the acquisition of a mechanism to pump drug extracellularly as it diffuses in); (3) modification of the drug so that it is no longer active (acetylation of the 3′-hydroxyl group). In cases where it has been examined, the overwhelmingly common mechanism of intrinsic resistance is failure of the drug to reach effective intracellular concentrations. In the strains examined to date, this mechanism, which is common in *P. aeruginosa* and *P. cepacia,* appears to be due to a modified porin. These water-filled permeability channels either are absent or are regulated, closing in the presence of chloramphenicol and preventing the antibiotic from entering the cell.

Acquired chloramphenicol resistance is invariably due to the acquisition of chloramphenicol acetyltransferase.[8] Chloramphenicol acetyltransferase is present in a wide

TABLE 28–1. ACTIVITY OF CHLORAMPHENICOL AGAINST BACTERIA INFECTING HUMANS

BACTERICIDAL
  Haemophilus influenzae
  Neisseria meningitidis

BACTERIOSTATIC
  Shigella sp.
  Salmonella sp.
  Escherichia coli
  Pasteurella multocida
  Streptococcus agalactiae
  Staphylococcus aureus
  Staphylococcus epidermidis
  Streptococcus pneumoniae
  Listeria monocytogenes
  *Pseudomonas cepacia**
  Bacteroides sp.

RESISTANT
  *Pseudomonas aeruginosa**
  Serratia marcescens

*Percentage susceptible or resistant varies; testing must be performed.

variety of gram-negative and gram-positive bacteria. The prototypic enzymes were first described and characterized in *Escherichia coli*. Subsequently, it was found that variants of these enzymes are present in streptococci, staphylococci, pneumococci, and *Haemophilus* sp. There is a wide diversity in the primary structure of these enzymes, suggesting divergent evolution. All the enzymes have one feature in common: the 3'-hydroxyl group of chloramphenicol is acetylated using acetyl-CoA as a donor. With the 3'-hydroxyl group acetylated, the antibiotic is no longer able to bind the ribosomes and it is biologically inactive. All the chloramphenicol acetyltransferases that have been described to date have been R-plasmid-mediated. In certain genera the variant enzymes appear to be very similar to the *E. coli* enzymes with nonessential portions of the gene deleted.[8] Bacteria producing chloramphenicol acetyltransferase are readily recognized by susceptibility testing[7] or by a direct test of the isolated colonies for enzyme activity.[9]

The spread of R-plasmids encoding chloramphenicol acetyltransferase throughout many genera depends on many factors, the most important of which is the frequency of administration of chloramphenicol. For example, in the United States invasive *H. influenzae* (type b strains) are very rarely resistant to chloramphenicol (<1 percent of all strains). In contrast, in Spain, where over-the-counter dispensing of chloramphenicol was not restricted until several years ago, the frequency of resistance in disease-causing isolates of the same genus and species (*H. influenzae* type b) is 75 percent. In those geographic areas with high prevalence of chloramphenicol resistance, the antibiotic cannot be used for treatment of common serious infections, for example, meningitis in Spain. Similarly, there have been "epidemics" of dissemination of a resistance plasmid in *Salmonella typhi* in Mexico. Thus, enteric infections in travelers, particularly those who have been to Spain, Mexico, or certain South American countries, cannot be assumed to have chloramphenicol-susceptible organisms. An alternative anti-

biotic should be administered until susceptibility testing has been completed.

PHARMACOKINETICS

Metabolism

Chloramphenicol is unique among widely used antibiotics in that there is an exceptionally large patient-to-patient variation in systemic clearance as well as volume of distribution. Thus, administration of "standard doses" must always be followed by measurement of the serum concentration at least twice during the dosing interval. Only in this way can one be assured that therapeutic yet nontoxic serum concentrations are the result of the dose selected.

Chloramphenicol is administered either orally or parenterally. As with any drug, the serum concentration seen at any point in time after administration depends on the rate of absorption from the administration site and the rate of clearance. Because of marked interpatient differences in both absorption and elimination, there is a highly variable peak concentration with a standard dose. It appears that metabolism is the primary mechanism responsible for a wide variability in serum chloramphenicol concentrations seen after administration by oral or parenteral routes. The major organ responsible for chloramphenicol metabolism is the liver. Chloramphenicol is disposed of by the liver by at least four active metabolic pathways: glucuronidation, dehydrodehalogenation, amidase activity, and a minor oxidation pathway (Figure 28–1). It is thought that the major metabolite (~80 percent) in children and adults is the glucuronide ether. This compound, in which there is a linkage between the 3'-hydroxyl group of chloramphenicol and glucuronic acid, is devoid of biologic activity, and as a weak organic acid it is rapidly excreted by the kidney. However, contemporary studies have not always documented that this route is as important as older studies indicated.[10,11] Each of the pathways producing chloramphenicol base and the chloramphenicol alcohol is thought to represent clearance of ~4 percent of the drug, the same amout excreted unchanged into the bile.[10,11] The paranitro constituent of chloramphenicol can also be reduced to an amine, either by the human liver[12] or by bacteria in the lumen of the gastrointestinal tract. Chloramphenicol reductase, which reduces the nitro to an amine, is present in many Enterobacteriaceae. Thus, the reabsorption of reduced chloramphenicol is another source of chloramphenicol amine. It appears that the chloramphenicol amine is excreted in the urine after diacetylation.[13] In addition, within the lumen of the gastrointestinal tract, chloramphenicol glucuronide can be hydrolyzed and the active parent drug reabsorbed.

The contribution of the minor metabolites (Figure 28–2) to chloramphenicol clearance is less certain. These compounds are suspected to be of importance in chloramphenicol toxicity. Many of the intermediates in the minor chloramphenicol oxidative pathway are reactive

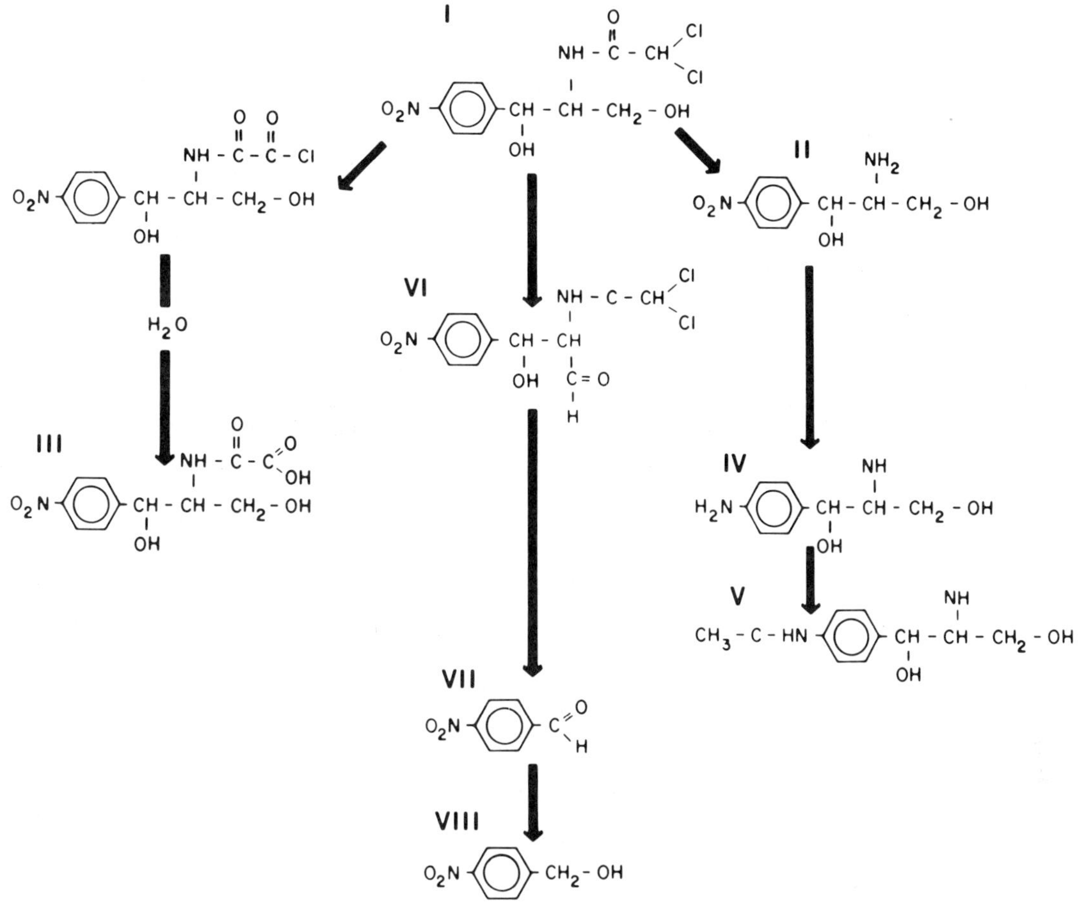

FIGURE 28-2. Oxidative metabolism of chloramphenicol (I). Hepatic cytochrome P-450 catalyzes oxidation of the dichloroacetamido group, which is unstable forming the oxamic derivative (III). Oxidation of the primary alcohol by the same enzyme system yields chloramphenicol aldehyde (VI). This β-hydroxybenzaldehyde undergoes retro-aldol decomposition yielding p-nitrobenzaldehyde (VII) and p-nitrobenzylalcohol (VIII). Amidase can cleave the dichloracetamido group to dichloroacetate and chloramphenicol base (II), which can be reduced (IV) and excreted as an acetylated derivative (V).

and/or nitroso derivatives. Such compounds, independently, have been felt to be important in the genesis of bone marrow aplasia. The identification of these metabolites has suggested that they may be the cause of the "idiosyncratic" aplasia following chloramphenicol administration. According to this hypothesis, the patients with a predominance of this pathway (because of environmental exposure or genetic predisposition) are at increased risk for aplasia.

Oral Administration

Chloramphenicol is administered by mouth in two formulations: the crystalline compound in capsules (the so-called base) or the palmitate ester in a suspension (Figure 28-1). The greatest bioavailability occurs with the crystalline compound. For example, in adults the mean area under the serum concentration–time curve (AUC) following administration of 1.5 gm by capsule was 143 μg h/ml, while in the same individuals the AUC after administration of the palmitate ester was 126 μg h/ml.[14] Since

palmitic acid is esterified to the 3'-hydroxyl group, hydrolysis of this bond must occur before biologically active chloramphenicol reaches the systemic circulation. It is not exactly clear where the hydrolysis occurs; animal studies suggested that there was intraluminal hydrolysis by pancreatic lipase.[15] These workers found that mixing rat duodenal contents with chloramphenicol palmitate yielded 96 percent hydrolysis of chloramphenicol palmitate in 2 hours at 38°C; other tissue such as spleen, kidney, or liver hydrolyzed less than 10 percent during the same interval. More recently, Dickinson et al.[16] studied the absorption of oral chloramphenicol in patients with cystic fibrosis. They found that in these patients with varying degrees of exocrine pancreatic insufficiency, 16,000 units of lipase (the amount administered to the patients to aid digestion) hydrolyzed only 50 percent of "small amounts" of chloramphenicol palmitate. This suggests that there may be some hydrolysis in the small bowel mucosa. Table 28-2 depicts the disposition of chloramphenicol after administration of chloramphenicol palmitate.

Since the total venous blood coming from the gastro-

TABLE 28–2. PHARMACOKINETICS OF CHLORAMPHENICOL AFTER ADMINISTRATION OF CHLORAMPHENICOL PALMITATE

REF.	SUBJECTS	N	AGE RANGE (yrs)	DOSE (mg/kg)*	C_{max} (μg/ml)	$t_{1/2}$ (h)	AUC (μg·h/ml)
16	Cystic fibrosis	10	13.6–23.8	19.5	3.2 ± 0.7	5.1 ± 1.9	32.5 ± 15
	Cystic fibrosis with lipase	10	13.6–23.8	19.5	5.4 ± 2.4	5.4 ± 2.0	49.7 ± 19
19	Infants with meningitis	15	0.17–7.0	18.75	25 ± 10	4.8 ± 1.6	131.7 ± 57
18	Infants with meningitis	18	0.17–18.0	25	27 ± 11	5.1 ± 1.8	110 ± 46

*Dose is expressed as milligrams of chloramphenicol equivalents per kilogram body weight.

intestinal tract enters the liver, one would predict that there might be presystemic chloramphenicol metabolism, i.e., the compound would be metabolized by the liver prior to reaching the systemic circulation. Evidence of this was obtained by Glazko et al.[17] They found that there was a dose-dependent increase in maximum serum chloramphenicol concentration after oral administration to adult human volunteers. When the oral dose of crystalline compound was increased from 0.5 to 1.5 gm, the amount of biologically active chloramphenicol in the serum increased from 55 percent of the total aromatic nitro compounds (the assay used at the time) to 90 percent of the total aromatic nitro compounds. This suggests that the increased dosing saturated those hepatic processes, converting chloramphenicol into inactive (or less active) biological compounds that still contained the paranitro moiety. For reasons to be described below, the oral route achieves greater serum AUC for a given dose than either intramuscular or intravenous administration.[18,19] In contrast to intravenous administration, the peak serum concentration is not as high, yet the apparent elimination half-life is always longer following oral administration.[18] This is probably due to the continued absorption during elimination along the large surface area of the small bowel.

Parenteral Administration

This route is used for patients whose gastrointestinal function is unknown or abnormal to ensure that the drug reaches the systemic circulation. Formulations for parenteral administration consist of chloramphenicol sodium succinate (Figure 28–1) or chloramphenicol in oil. As was the case with the palmitate ester, the 3'-succinate ester is devoid of biologic activity and was formulated to increase the solubility of chloramphenicol. Chloramphenicol in oil is a slow-release formulation prepared exclusively for intramuscular use; this formulation has been used almost exclusively in developing countries where a single dose is used for certain diseases. Data on the pharmacokinetics of this formulation are not available.

Intramuscular Administration

Glazko et al.[20] reported in an abstract the administration of chloramphenicol succinate intramuscularly and intravenously. There were five normal men in each group, and the authors reported that 2–4 hours later the plasma chloramphenicol concentration in the AUC was equivalent in each group. If anything, there was a bias with high or higher concentrations following intramuscular administration.[20] Ross and coworkers[21] studied four children without an intravenous comparison group, but from the dose administered (25 mg/kg) there appeared to be good absorption into the systemic circulation. However, DuPont et al.[22] administered chloramphenicol intramuscularly to 13 adult subjects; 4 comparison subjects received chloramphenicol by the oral route. They reported that the plasma chloramphenicol concentrations after oral administration were approximately twice as high as those after intramuscular administration. Because of this information, the intramuscular route was not recommended by the Food and Drug Administration (FDA) for chloramphenicol succinate administration. Because of the ease of intramuscular administration and its convenience in children, Shann et al.[23] compared serum concentrations after intramuscular administration to those obtained after intravenous administration in children between 1 month and 6 years of age. These workers found, both by chemical assay using high-performance liquid chromatography (HPLC) and by bioassay, that the serum concentrations after the first dose were only 5 percent higher after intramuscular than after intravenous injection. With subsequent doses, the intramuscular route gave higher concentrations according to the chemical assay. It is not clear why these data differ from those of DuPont et al.[22] It has been suggested that the adults may have had an intraadipose rather than an intramuscular injection, which would markedly affect the absorption of this partially polar compound. One striking feature of the Shann report[23] was the marked interpatient variation in peak serum concentration, which ranged from 15 to 75 μg/ml with a dose of 25 mg/kg body weight.

Another potential reason for the wide variability in the study of Shann et al. in comparison to that of DuPont et al. would be the magnitude of the illness in the subjects. Shann et al. studied children with a variety of infectious diseases in Papua New Guinea. The illnesses were unusually severe: 15 percent of 367 children with pneumonia studied by the same group died.[24] This is in contrast to the study of DuPont et al. in which experimental typhoid fever was induced in relatively healthy adults. It may well be that ill children have delayed renal clearance of the succinate prodrug but adequate hepatic esterase activity. In contrast, active renal tubular secretion of the prodrug in adults during slow absorption from muscle might lead to

TABLE 28–3. CHLORAMPHENICOL PHARMACOKINETICS FOLLOWING ADMINISTRATION OF THE SUCCINATE PRODRUG

REF.	SUBJECTS	N	AGE RANGE (YRS)	DOSE (mg/kg)	ROUTE	C_{max} (μg/ml)	MEAN $t_{1/2}$* (h)	AUC (μg·h/ml)
23	Infants with a variety of infections	11	0.08–6	25	I.M.	16.8 ± 7.4	12	101 ± 26
		8	0.08–6	25	I.V.	16.9 ± 6.4	12	108 ± 51
27	Infants with meningitis	13	0.3–6	25	I.V.	26 ± 14.5	4.6	NA
28	Infants with meningitis	17	0.3–6	18.75	I.V.	28.4 ± 16.8	3.98	66.7 ± 14
29	Infants with meningitis	14	0.4–2	25	I.V.	15.0 ± 8.3	4.0	195.9 ± 72

*Estimated from the author's data.
NA, not available.

the negligible serum concentrations. Table 28–3 depicts the serum chloramphenicol concentrations following intravenous administration of the succinate prodrug. Older data obtained from colorimetric assays or bioassays are not included.

Although the wide intrapatient variation in peak concentration and elimination half-life is lost when averages are viewed, the variability is remarkable. There is approximately an eightfold variation in peak serum concentration and a 10-fold patient-to-patient variation in plasma clearance with a standard dose (25 mg/kg) administered to an ill infant. With chloramphenicol succinate this variation is in part due to the effect of prodrug pharmacokinetics.

Chloramphenicol Succinate Pharmacokinetics

Chloramphenicol succinate is converted to chloramphenicol by the human liver. This process was studied by Yamakawa et al.[25] who characterized the hepatic hydrolytic activity against chloramphenicol succinate in autopsy specimens. They found an apparent K_m of 0.38 mM and a V_{max} of 6 μmol/gm/h shortly after birth; these kinetic constants did not change during the first year of life. From these data one would infer that the chloramphenicol succinate hydrolase could be saturated depending on either the rate of administration or the dose. Koup et al.[26] attempted to demonstrate dose dependence of chloramphenicol succinate kinetics in adolescent monkeys. These investigators found dose dependence: a dose of 25 mg/kg yielded a chloramphenicol succinate peak of 90 μg/ml, while increasing the dose to 100 mg/kg increased the serum chloramphenicol succinate concen-

tration to 650 μg/ml. In addition, the total body chloramphenicol succinate clearance decreased with increasing dose. However, the majority of the decrement in total body clearance was due to decreasing metabolic (nonrenal) clearance; this suggested saturation of certain enzymatic pathways, such as the hepatic hydrolase. However, because of the marked efficiency of the kidney in secreting chloramphenicol succinate, the resultant serum chloramphenicol concentration was relatively constant given the wide range of doses used. Renal chloramphenicol succinate clearance (Table 28–4) invariably equaled or exceeded the glomerular filtration rate. This observation suggests that there is active tubular secretion. We studied this question directly by seeking to determine if there was competition between ampicillin and chloramphenicol succinate in the kidney. In performing this study, we found that chloramphenicol serum concentrations were higher if chloramphenicol was coadministered with ampicillin immediately before the ampicillin dose. Renal secretion is extremely efficient: on the average, one-third of a dose of chloramphenicol succinate infused intravenously is excreted in the urine. More striking, however, is the wide intrapatient variation (Table 28–4). In some patients 82 percent of the amount infused intravenously was excreted by the kidney. This means that the actual dose of chloramphenicol was 18 percent of that sought by the prescribing physician. In contrast, other patients received 94 percent of the dose sought: i.e., only 6 percent of the prodrug was excreted unchanged in the urine. Also striking is the wide variation in the elimination half-life of the prodrug, which varies from 12 minutes to 4 hours. The majority of the variation in the apparent elimination half-life is due to variable renal excretion. In addition, nonrenal clearance (metabolic and presumably hydrolytic cleavage) also has some impact.

TABLE 28–4. PHARMACOKINETICS OF CHLORAMPHENICOL SUCCINATE

REF.	SUBJECTS	N	AGE RANGE (mos)	MEAN DOSE (mg/kg)	$t_{1/2}$ RANGE (h)	MEAN CLEARANCE (ml/min/M²) Plasma	MEAN CLEARANCE (ml/min/M²) Renal	% DOSE IN URINE (RANGE)
30	Infants with *H. influenzae* infection	26	0.1–192	25	0.35–1.25	356.4	150	6–80
20	Infants with meningitis	28	0.04–84	20.9	0.2–4.0	330.0	136.4	6–82
30	Infants with meningitis	16	2–168	25	NA	320.5	NA	6–73

NA, not available.

It is also known that chloramphenicol succinate, although a prodrug, distributes like other weak organic acids. Tuomanen et al.[18] found that 8 of 27 cerebrospinal fluid samples obtained during the treatment of meningitis had chloramphenicol succinate concentrations between 2.5 and 16 μg/ml. It is not clear whether chloramphenicol succinate is hydrolyzed to a significant extent by organs other than the liver or in fluid such as cerebrospinal fluid. Glazko and coworkers[10] studied the tissue distribution of chloramphenicol succinate in monkeys after dosing to steady state. Chloramphenicol was measured by a colorimetric method and expressed as equivalent to the amount of active drug. Liver, kidney, and lung concentrations exceeded serum concentrations, while muscle and fat concentrations were slightly less than serum concentrations. Additional information can be obtained from the original articles on chloramphenicol disposition.[27-30]

CLINICAL USE

Central Nervous System Infections

The primary use of chloramphenicol in the United States is for the treatment of meningitis and brain abscesses. Chloramphenicol penetrates the blood–brain barrier and the blood–cerebrospinal fluid barrier independently of the presence or absence of inflammation. Cerebrospinal fluid chloramphenicol concentrations range from 23 to 100 percent of the simultaneously obtained serum concentrations.[27,31,32] In the United States the most common indication for chloramphenicol administration to children appears to be H. influenzae type b meningitis. Nationwide approximately 25 percent of the strains causing this disease are resistant to ampicillin. To date less than 1 percent of the strains are resistant to chloramphenicol; thus, the recommended initial empiric therapy for an infant with meningitis until the organism is identified and susceptibility testing performed includes ampicillin and chloramphenicol. Chloramphenicol is active against H. influenzae type b whether or not the strain is ampicillin-resistant, and an in vitro antagonism cannot be demonstrated.[33] A disadvantage of the administration of chloramphenicol to children with this disease is the necessity of monitoring serum concentrations. Because of the aforementioned wide variation in peak serum concentration and elimination half-life, therapeutic monitoring is necessary to ensure safe, efficacious concentrations. When chloramphenicol was compared to cefotaxime or ceftriaxone for the treatment of H. influenzae meningitis,[33,34] there was no difference in the rate of resolution of the magnitude of inflammation in the cerebrospinal fluid or in the outcome as assessed on a short-term (acute) basis. When the cost of chloramphenicol administration is compared to that incurred by administration of third-generation cephalosporins for the treatment of meningitis, the net cost for a standard course of therapy comes out about the same. This is due to the high cost of monitoring chloramphenicol, a drug that costs one-tenth as much (or less) as the third-generation cephalosporins.

Brain abscesses are also treated with chloramphenicol. Chloramphenicol reaches concentrations in brain tissue that exceed the simultaneous serum concentrations by many orders of magnitude.[34] The penetration into brain and abscess tissue is thought to occur because of its high lipid solubility. There are no studies comparing chloramphenicol to other agents active against anaerobes (such as metronidazole) in children with brain abscesses.

Intraabdominal Abscesses

Chloramphenicol has been used in the treatment of intraabdominal abscesses in experimental systems and in adult patients. There are no data recorded on the comparative efficacy of the antibiotic for this infection. In the human studies that are available, there was no difference in the outcome measures used when chloramphenicol was combined with gentamicin and compared to clindamycin, a drug also active against anaerobes.[35] Other studies[36] using guinea pigs found chloramphenicol less active than metronidazole both therapeutically and in prevention of infections. However, the effect of species on drug distribution, elimination, and metabolism is not clear. The outcome may be a reflection of the differences in metabolism rather than in antimicrobial activity.

Rocky Mountain Spotted Fever

This infection is effectively treated with chloramphenicol. Therapeutic monitoring is absolutely essential because of the widespread metabolic changes accompanying the diffuse vasculitis that is the hallmark of the disease. The metabolic dysfunction and electrolyte imbalance common in Rocky Mountain spotted fever might be expected to perturb the pharmacokinetics of both chloramphenicol succinate and the biologically active compound.

Typhoid Fever

Chloramphenicol has been compared to ceftriaxone in the treatment of typhoid fever.[37] Chloramphenicol administration was associated with a greater probability of being afebrile after 7 days of treatment. However, 52 percent of the patients receiving chloramphenicol were bacteremic on day 3, while all in the ceftriaxone group had sterile blood cultures at that time. An advantage of chloramphenicol is that it may penetrate into fixed macrophages where S. typhi is sequestered. This would not be expected to occur to the same extent with ceftriaxone, a highly polar antibiotic.

Panophthalmitis

Chloramphenicol penetrates into both aqueous humor and vitreous humor. Because of these unique properties, it has been used for panophthalmitis due to a variety of organisms. There are no data, however, comparing this treatment of this rare infection to the more standard intravitreal injection. Chloramphenicol should not be used for bacterial conjunctivitis. There are many agents available that are efficacious for this benign, self-limited infection.

DRUG INTERACTIONS

Since chloramphenicol is metabolized by oxidative pathways, it is not surprising that there might be competition for cytochrome P-450s if this antibiotic is coadministered with other extensively metabolized drugs. Conversely, one might expect that prior administration of drugs that are known to induce hepatic cytochrome P-450 activity might increase the metabolic clearance of chloramphenicol, leading to lower steady-state plasma concentrations. Likewise, prior administration of a drug known to decrease P-450 activity is associated with delayed chloramphenicol clearance and increased serum concentrations. However, complicating the seemingly straightforward drug interactions is the ability of chloramphenicol per se to inhibit cytochrome P-450 activity.[38] Also complicating the interpretation of putative drug interaction (when other drugs are administered during a treatment course) is the observation that as the infectious disease abates, the total plasma clearance of chloramphenicol increases.[28,39] Thus, some of the effects of concomitant administration (such as that observed by Spika et al.[40] in which chloramphenicol clearance was apparently increased by acetaminophen) may be the normally occurring increase in clearance.[28,39] In virtually all these studies, the subjects were being treated for invasive *H. influenzae* type b infections.

Table 28–5 depicts the drugs affecting chloramphenicol disposition. In humans the concomitant administration of known inducers of hepatic cytochrome P-450 (rifampin and phenobarbital) increases plasma chloramphenicol clearance. This is reflected in both a lower C_{max} concentration and a shorter elimination half-life.

Phenytoin definitely prolongs the clearance of chloramphenicol (Table 28–5). Acetaminophen was purported to interfere with chloramphenicol metabolism[42]; however, in a subsequent well-controlled study in which the potential for interaction between acetaminophen and

chloramphenicol was thoroughly studied, i.e., controlled for dose and duration of administration, there was no interaction between these two drugs.[43]

Because of the wide intrinsic interpatient variability in chloramphenicol disposition and because of the potential for interaction, it is clear that in critically ill children receiving multiple drugs in addition to chloramphenicol, therapeutic monitoring of all drugs should be performed if possible.

TOXICITY

Two types of toxicity are seen with chloramphenicol: that due to drug accumulation and the so-called idiosyncratic reaction. The older literature suggested that most patients during a therapeutic course of chloramphenicol administration had depression in erythropoiesis, myelopoiesis, or both. These data were generated prior to the era of therapeutic drug monitoring. During this period (the 1950s), many reports indicated that chloramphenicol could cause aplastic anemia. The consensus from the literature at that time was that the suppression was "dose-related" (in reality plasma-concentration-related), while the aplasia was due to an individual reaction to drug administration. It is clear at this time that this distinction may not be absolute. Continued administration of a chloramphenicol dose that produces serum concentrations in excess of 59 μg/ml can suppress the marrow and, if the marrow is actively involved in erythropoiesis and myelopoiesis, can cause progression to aplasia.[44] In all the reported cases of chloramphenicol-associated aplasia, serum concentrations have not been measured. Thus, it is not clear whether the individual idiosyncratic reaction of patients demonstrating aplasia is not due to a lesion in drug elimination leading to drug accumulation with prolonged high blood concentrations. Genetic susceptibility is also a possibility (see later in text).

Toxicity Due to Decreased Elimination

The acute toxicity of chloramphenicol due to accumulation is age-dependent.[45,46] In the first 2 weeks of life, chloramphenicol clearance pathways do not have the

TABLE 28–5. DRUGS AFFECTING CHLORAMPHENICOL DISPOSITION

DRUG	SPECIES	PARAMETER MEASURED	MAGNITUDE OF EFFECT	REF.
Increased Clearance				
Phenobarbital	Dog	$t_{1/2}$	30% decrease	70
	Rat	$t_{1/2}$	16 → 3.5 min (fourfold decrease)	70
Phenobarbital	Human	Plasma clearance	286 → 483 ml/kg/h	71
Rifampin	Human	Plasma clearance	188 → 379 ml/kg/h	72
Phenobarbitone	Human	C_{max}	31 → 5 μg/ml	73
		$t_{1/2}$	438 → 246 min	
Decreased Clearance				
Phenytoin	Human	$t_{1/2}$	3.6 → 4.1 h	71
Acetaminophen	Human	$t_{1/2}$	3.3 → 15 h	42

activity seen in older infants and adults. It is commonly assumed that glucuronidation is the pathway that is rate-limiting for chloramphenicol elimination in a newborn.[45,46] These data were derived prior to the development of analytic methods distinguishing between chloramphenicol and its unconjugated metabolites. Accumulation of chloramphenicol in such infants is associated with the "gray syndrome." This illness is usually seen in a newborn who becomes lethargic and develops abdominal distention, hypotension, hypoxemia, and decreased peripheral perfusion; the hypoxemia and the decreased perfusion give rise to the gray appearance. The mechanism of this syndrome appears to be inhibition of mitochondrial function in the neonatal myocardium and liver. There is a severe unexplained systemic metabolic acidosis, and the cardiac ejection faction is markedly decreased. Often the first clue to the syndrome is the metabolic acidosis, which is due to lactate accumulation and is refractory to bicarbonate administration. On occasion there is concomitant hepatocellular dysfunction. At the time the syndrome is recognized, the serum chloramphenicol concentrations usually exceed 100 μg/ml; several cases have been reported with values as low as 75 μg/ml, but they are the exception. Six to 12 hours after the onset of the acidosis, the infant may lapse into shock. Most cases of gray syndrome in the past decade were the result of a medication error in which the desired dose was exceeded by many multiples. The treatment of choice for this syndrome appears to be exchange transfusion.[47] In theory, the chloramphenicol can be removed by charcoal hemoperfusion and dialysis.[48] However, because of the familiarity with exchange transfusion in most pediatric centers and its proven efficacy in removing chloramphenicol,[47] it is the procedure of choice in newborns. It is also important to remember that virtually any individual of any age who has markedly delayed clearance because of decreased intrinsic hepatic drug clearance or decreased hepatic perfusion can accumulate the drug and develop the gray syndrome. A report in a toddler[49] illustrates this point.

The reversible hematologic efforts of chloramphenicol also appear to be due to drug accumulation, but at a lower steady-state serum concentration. Examination of the bone marrow of patients with dose-related hematopoietic suppression showed vacuolization of early erythroblasts.[50] When these calls were examined with the electron microscope,[51] it was clear that the vacuoles were degenerating mitochondria. These changes are consistent with the inhibition of the synthesis of inner mitochondrial membrane enzymes; such inhibition can be seen *in vitro* at low concentrations (10 μg/ml).[4] In dogs the synthesis of one inner mitochondrial membrane enzyme, ferrochetalase (the enzyme inserting iron into protoporphyrin to synthesize heme), was also inhibited by chloramphenicol at concentrations usually considered therapeutic. This mechanism allows ready clinical prediction of chloramphenicol toxicity; i.e., without heme being synthesized, serum iron concentrations rise precipitously[51] and the reticulocyte count decreases. Several studies[50,53] have not been able to demonstrate an effect on hematopoiesis in normal adult volunteers administered standard chloramphenicol doses for 20 days. Indices of toxicity were seen only after 20 days

and consisted of reticulocytopenia and an increase in the serum iron concentration. These data are in contrast to those from patients with infection, in which reticulocytopenia can be seen as early as 5 days. The reason for the variation between these studies probably lies in the state of the bone marrow at the time of chloramphenicol administration. It is clear that if the marrow is recovering from an insult (such as vitamin B_{12} deficiency), chloramphenicol will suppress the response, i.e., the reticulocyte response with vitamin B_{12} administration. In general, chloramphenicol-associated hematopoietic suppression is more common in children between the ages of 6 and 15 years than in infants.[54,55]

We recently examined 74 children with *H. influenzae* meningitis who received chloramphenicol. All patients had their serum chloramphenicol concentrations adjusted on the basis of their peak serum and trough values every 3–5 days. In this study, even though anemia was associated with the underlying disease (*H. influenzae* meningitis), we could not show an effect of chloramphenicol on plasma heme, iron, iron-binding capacity, free erythrocyte protoporphyrin (FEP), or FEP/heme ratio. These data appear to substantiate the value of therapeutic monitoring.[56]

Idiosyncratic Aplasia

Idiosyncratic aplasia, in certain individuals, is due to a genetic metabolic defect in the bone marrow in which there is unusual susceptibility to chloramphenicol. This conclusion is derived from data in which there was concordance for chloramphenicol-induced aplasia in identical twins.[57] More important was the observation that DNA synthesis by bone marrow obtained from a father of a child with chloramphenicol-associated aplastic anemia was inhibited by concentrations commonly sought during the course of therapy: 25–30 μg/ml.[57] The incidence of aplasia is hard to estimate because the denominator, i.e., every patient receiving the drug, is not catalogued. From sales data and from assumptions about the amount of drug administered during standard therapy, the incidence of chloramphenicol-associated aplasia is estimated to be between 1 in 19,000 and 1 in 200,000 therapeutic courses.[58-63] In the usual case, pancytopenia is discovered 3–12 weeks after administration of chloramphenicol. In 75 percent of the cases, intermittent administration did not permit precise timing of the onset of aplasia after the first administration. The epidemiology of chloramphenicol-associated aplasia indicates that the complication is most common in females between 2 and 9 years of age who receive chloramphenicol by the oral route.[59,63]

Allergy

Allergy to chloramphenicol is extremely rare. There is one case in which topical administration was followed by urticaria and approximately 11 cases in which allergic responses occurred following oral administration.[64] Since chloramphenicol is administered to patients who are

TABLE 28–6. INHIBITORY EFFECT OF CHLORAMPHENICOL ON DRUG DISPOSITION

| | | VALUE | | |
DRUG	PARAMETER MEASURED	Alone	With Chloramphenicol	REF.
Phenytoin	Plasma $t_{1/2}$ (h)	13	26	74
Tolbutamide	Plasma $t_{1/2}$ (h)	5	14	74
Dicoumarol	Plasma $t_{1/2}$ (h)	10	27	74
Phenytoin	Plasma clearance (ml/min)	38.2	18.9	75
Phenobarbital	Plasma clearance (ml/min)	8.7	4.3	75

acutely ill with a variety of infections, it is not always certain that the drug was the etiologic agent. It is of interest, however, that most of the reported cases of "anaphylaxis due to chloramphenicol" occurred following oral administration.[64] This is in contrast to anaphylaxis following β-lactam administration, which is almost exclusively associated with parenteral administration. The message seems to be that allergic reactions can occur but are extremely infrequent.

THERAPEUTIC MONITORING

Several methods exist for the quantitation of chloramphenicol in serum specimens. One widely used is an enzyme-linked immunoassay (EMIT, SYVA Corporation, Palo Alto, CA). In this method, antibody reacts specifically with chloramphenicol and not with the succinate prodrug or with known metabolites. The other commonly used method is HPLC. The value of the latter method is that in addition to estimating chloramphenicol concentration, the technique allows for simultaneous quantitation of chloramphenicol succinate. This additional information aids in identifying specimens collected during or shortly after intravenous infusion of the succinate.

It is very clear that because of the wide interpatient variation in drug disposition, the effects of a resolving infection on clearance, and a potential for drug interaction, serum concentrations should be monitored in virtually all patients receiving the drug, if at all possible. This point has been made repeatedly in the English language.[65-68] When therapeutic monitoring is undertaken, it is not surprising to find that the parenteral dose of chloramphenicol succinate that maintains therapeutic concentrations in infants and children ranges from 20 to 400 mg/kg/day. Monitoring must be prospective, with a turnaround time within a dosing interval. In one study in which drug assays were performed some time later,[69] 10 of 70 infants (including 58 newborns) developed toxic reactions, including the gray baby syndrome, and one died.

REFERENCES

1. Malik VS: Chloramphenicol. Adv Appl Microbiol 15:297, 1972
2. Pestka S: Inhibitors of ribosome function. Annu Rev Microbiol 25:487, 1971
3. Nierhaus D, Hieihaus KH: Identification of the chloramphenicol binding protein in E. coli ribosomes by partial reconstitution. Proc Natl Acad Sci USA 70:22, 1973
4. Martelo OJ, Manyan DR, Smith US, et al: Chloramphenicol and bone marrow mitochondria. J Lab Clin Med 74:927, 1969
5. Wong K, Roberts MC, Smith AL: The activity of Sch 29482 against type b Haemophilus influenzae lacking or possessing detectable beta-lactamase activity. J Antimicrob Chemother 9:163, 1982
6. Turck D: A comparison of chloramphenicol and ampicillin as bactericidal agents for H. influenzae type b. J Med Microbiol 10:127, 1977
7. National Committee on Clinical Laboratory Standards: Performance Standards for Disc Susceptibility. ASM, Villanova, PA, 1985
8. Shaw WV: Comparative enzymology of chloramphenicol resistance. Ann NY Acad Sci 182:234, 1971
9. Azemun P, Stull T, Roberts M, et al: Rapid detection of chloramphenicol resistance in Haemophilus influenzae. Antimicrob Agents Chemother 20:168, 1981
10. Glazko AJ, Wolf LM, Dill WA, et al: Biochemical studies on chloramphenicol (chloromycetin). J Pharm Exp Ther 96:445, 1949
11. Glazko AJ, Dill WA, Rebstock MC: Biochemical studies on chloramphenicol (chloromycetin). J Biol Chem 183:679, 1950
12. Salem Z, Murray T, Yunis AA: The nitroreduction of chloramphenicol by human liver tissue. J Lab Clin Med 97:881, 1981
13. Henry NK, Anhalt JP: Detection of the N-Acetyl aryl amine of chloramphenicol in serum from patients receiving chloramphenicol. Abstracts of the Annual Meeting of the American Society of Microbiology, 1982
14. Glazko AJ, Dill WA, Kazenko A, et al: Physical factors affecting the rate of absorption of chloramphenicol esters. Antibiot Chemother 8:516, 1958
15. Glazko AJ, Edgerton WH, Dill WA, et al: Chloromycetin palmitate—A synthetic ester of chloromycetin. Antibiot Chemother 2:234, 1952
16. Dickinson CJ, Reed MD, Stern RC, Aronoff SC, Yamashita TS, Blumer JL: The effect of exocrine pancreatic function on chloramphenicol pharmacokinetics in patients with cystic fibrosis. Pediatr Res 23:388, 1988
17. Glazko AJ, Kinkel AW, Alegnani WC, et al: An evaluation of the absorption characteristics of different chloramphenicol preparations in normal human subjects. Clin Pharm 4:472, 1968
18. Tuomanen EI, Powell KR, Marks MI, et al: Oral chloramphenicol in the treatment of Haemophilus influenzae meningitis. J Pediatr 99:968, 1981
19. Kauffman RE, Thirumoorthi MC, Buckley JA, et al: Relative bioavailability of intravenous chloramphenicol succinate and oral chloramphenicol palmitate in infants and children. J Pediatr 99:963, 1981
20. Glazko AJ, DIll WA, Kinkel AW, Goulet JR, Holloway WJ, Buchanan RA: Absorption and excretion of parenteral doses of chloramphenicol sodium succinate in comparison with peroral doses of chloramphenicol. Clin Pharmacol Ther 21:104, 1977
21. Ross S, Puig JR, Zaremba EA: Chloramphenicol acid succinate (sodium salt). Antibiot Annu 1957-1958:803, 1958
22. DuPont HL, Hornick RB, Weiss CF, Snyder MJ, Woodward TE: Evaluation of chloramphenicol acid succinate therapy of induced typhoid fever and Rocky Mountain spotted fever. N Engl J Med 282:53, 1970
23. Shann F, Linnemann V, Mackenzie A, Barker J, Gratten M, Crinis N: Absorption of chloramphenicol sodium succinate after intramuscular administration in children. N Engl J Med 313:410–414, 1985

24. Shann F, Barker J, Poore P: Chloramphenicol alone versus chloramphenicol plus penicillin for severe pneumonia in children. Lancet 1:684, 1985

25. Yamakawa T, Itoh S, Onishi S, Isobe K, Hosoe A, Nishimura Y: Developmental changes in hepatic esterase activity towards chloramphenicol succinate and its Michaelis–Menten constant of liver, kidney and lung in human. Dev Pharmacol Ther 7:205, 1984

26. Koup JR, Weber A, Smith AL: Chloramphenicol succinate pharmacokinetics in Macaca nemestrina: Dose dependency study. J Pharm Exp Ther 219:316, 1981

27. Friedman CA, Lovejoy FC, Smith AL: Chloramphenicol disposition in infants and children. J Pediatr 95:1071, 1979

28. Sack CM, Koup JR, Smith AL: Chloramphenicol pharmacokinetics in infants and young children. Pediatrics 66:579, 1980

29. Yogev R, Kolling WM, Williams T: Pharmacokinetic comparison of intravenous and oral chloramphenicol in patients with Haemophilus influenzae meningitis. Pediatrics 67:656, 1981

30. Kauffman RE, Miceli JN, Strebel L, et al: Pharmacokinetics of chloramphenicol and chloramphenicol succinate in infants and children. J Pediatr 98:315, 1981

31. Windorfer A, Pringsheim W: Studies on the concentration of chloramphenicol in the serum and CSF of neonates, infants and small children. Eur J Pediatr 124:129, 1977

32. Dunkle LM: Central nervous system chloramphenicol concentration in premature infants. Antimicrob Agents Chemother 13:317, 1978

33. Cole FS, Daum RS, Teller L, et al: Effect of ampicillin and chloramphenicol alone and in combination on ampicillin-susceptible and resistant Haemophilus influenzae type b. Antimicrob Agents Chemother 15:415, 1979

34. Kramer PW, Griffith RS, Campbell RL: Antibiotic penetration of the brain. J Neurosurg 31:295, 1969

35. Harding GKM, Buckwold F, Ronald AR, et al: Prospective, randomized comparative study of clindamycin, chloramphenicol and ticarcillin, each in combination with gentamicin in therapy for intra-abdominal and female genital tract sepsis. J Infect Dis 142:384, 1980

36. Onderdonk AB, Kasper DL, Mansheim BJ, et al: Experimental animal models for anaerobic infections. Rev Infect Dis 1:291, 1979

37. Islam A, Butler T, Nath SK, Alam NH, Stoeckel K, Houser HB, Smith AL: Randomized treatment of patients with typhoid fever by using ceftriaxone or chloramphenicol. J Infect Dis 158:742–747, 1988

38. Halpert J, Balfour C, Miller NE, Morgan ET, Dunbar D, Kaminsky LS: Isozyme selectivity of the inhibition of rat liver cytochromes P-450 by chloramphenicol in vivo. Molec Pharmacol 28:290–296, 1985

39. Nahata MC, Powell DA: Chloramphenicol serum concentration falls during chloramphenicol succinate dosing. Clin Pharmacol Ther 33:308, 1983

40. Spika JS, Davis DJ, Martin SR, Beharry K, Rex J, Aranda JV: Interaction between chloramphenicol and acetaminophen. Arch Dis Child 61:1121, 1986

41. Sack CM, Koup JR, Smith AL: Chloramphenicol pharmacokinetics in infants and young children. Pediatrics 66:579, 1980

42. Buchanan N, Moodley GP: Interaction between chloramphenicol and paracetamol. Br Med J 2:307, 1979

43. Kearns GL, Bocchini JA Jr, Brown RD, Cotter DL, Wilson JT: Absence of a pharmacokinetic interaction between chloramphenicol and acetaminophen in children. J Pediatr 107:134, 1985

44. Daum RS, Cohen DL, Smith AL: Fatal aplastic anemia following apparent dose-related chloramphenicol toxicity. J Pediatr 94:403, 1979

45. Sutherland JM: Fatal cardiovascular collapse of infants receiving large amounts of chloramphenicol. Am J Dis Child 97:761, 1959

46. Burns LE, Hodgman JE, Cass A: Fatal circulatory collapse in infants receiving chloramphenicol. N Engl J Med 621:1318, 1959

47. Kessler DL, Smith AL, Woodrum DE: Chloramphenicol toxicity in a neonate treated with exchange transfusion. J Pediatr 96:140, 1980

48. Mauer SM, Chavers BM, Kjellstrand CM: Treatment of an infant with severe chloramphenicol intoxication using charcoal column hemoperfusion. J Pediatr 96:136, 1980

49. Graft AW, Brocklebank JT, Hey EN: The grey toddler. Arch Dis Child 49:235, 1974

50. Saidi P, Wallerstein RO, Aggeler PM: Effect of chloramphenicol on erythropoiesis. J Lab Clin Med 57:247, 1961

51. Schober R, Kosek JC, Wolf PL: Chloramphenicol-induced vacuoles: Their ultrastructure in bone marrow pronormoblasts and immature myeloid cells. Arch Pathol 94:298, 1972

52. Rubin D, Weisberger AS, Botti RE, et al: Changes in iron metabolism in early chloramphenicol toxicity. J Clin Invest 37:1286, 1958

53. Jiji RM, Gangarosa EJ, de la Macorra F: Chloramphenicol and its sulfamayl analogue. Arch Intern Med 111:70, 1968

54. Hughes DNO: Possible determinants and progress of hemopoietic toxicity during chloramphenicol therapy. Med J Aust 2:1142, 1973

55. Suhrland LG, Weisberger AS: Delayed clearance of chloramphenicol from serum in patients with hematologic toxicity. Blood 34:466, 1969

56. Sherry B, Smith AL, Kronmal RA: Anemia during Haemophilus influenzae type b meningitis: Lack of an effect of chloramphenicol. Dev Pharmacol Ther 12:188, 1989

57. Nagao T, Mauer AM: Concordance for drug-induced aplastic anemia in identical twins. N Engl J Med 281:7, 1969

58. Yunis AA: Drug-induced bone marrow injury. Adv Intern Med 15:357, 1969

59. Best WR: Chloramphenicol-associated blood dyscrasis. JAMA 201:99, 1967

60. Smick KM, Condit PK, Proctor RL, et al: Fatal aplastic anemia. J Chron Dis 17:899, 1964

61. Clarke WTW: Fatal aplastic anemia and chloramphenicol. Can Med Assoc J 97:815, 1967

62. Yunis AA, Bloomberg GR: Chloramphenicol toxicity: Clinical features and pathogenesis. Progr Hematol 4:138, 1964

63. Wallerstein RO, Condit PK, Kasper GK, et al: Statewide study of chloramphenicol therapy and fatal aplastic anemia. JAMA 208:2045, 1969

64. Palchick BA, Funk EA, McEntire JE, Hamory BH: Anaphylaxis due to chloramphenicol. Am J Med Sci 288:43, 1984

65. Black SB, Levine P, Shinefield HR: The necessity for monitoring chloramphenicol levels when treating neonatal meningitis. J Pediatr 92:235, 1978

66. Ekblad H, Ruuskanen O, Lindberg R, Iisalo E: The monitoring of serum chloramphenicol levels in children with severe infections. J Antimicrob Chemother 15:489, 1985

67. Rosin H, Crea A, Forster J: The benefits of drug monitoring in patients with bacterial meningitis, e.g., chloramphenicol monitoring. Pediatr Pharmacol 3:175, 1983

68. Rajchgot P, Pruber CG: Soldin SJ, Good F, Harding E, Golas C, MacLeod S: Toward optimization of therapy in the neonate. Clin Pharmacol Therapeut 33:551, 1983

69. Mulhall A, De Louvois J, Hurley R: Efficacy of chloramphenicol in the treatment of neonatal and infantile meningitis: A study of 70 cases. Lancet 1:284, 1983

70. Palmer DL, Despopoulos A, Rael ED: Induction of chloramphenicol metabolism by phenobarbital. Antimicrob Agents Chemother 1:112, 1972

71. Krasinski K, Kusmiesz H, Nelson JD: Pharmacologic interactions among chloramphenicol, phenytoin and phenobarbital. Pediatr Infect Dis 1:232, 1982

72. Kelly HW, Couch RC, Cushing AH, Knott R: Interaction of chloramphenicol and rifampin. J Pediatr 112:817, 1988

73. Bloxham RA, Durbin GM, Johnson T, Winterborn MH: Chloramphenicol and phenobarbitone—A drug interaction. Arch Dis Child 54:76, 1979

74. Christensen LK, Skovsted L: Inhibition of drug metabolism by chloramphenicol. Lancet 2:1397, 1969

75. Koup JR, Gibaldi M, McNamara P, Hilligoss DM, Colburn WA, Bruck E: Interaction of chloramphenicol with phenytoin and phenobarbital. Clin Pharmacol Ther 24:571, 1978

29
ANTICONVULSANTS

TAKASHI MIMAKI, PHILIP D. WALSON, *and* YASUHIRO SUZUKI

Until recently the drug treatment of seizures has been largely static and empirical. This has begun to change because of improved understanding of seizure mechanisms and anticonvulsant pharmacokinetics and pharmacodynamics, as well as the development of new, more effective, and potentially less toxic regimens. There is also growing awareness and understanding of the medical and social problems faced by patients with seizures, fostered by various epilepsy interest groups. The development of new diagnostic methods [such as computed tomography (CT), positron emission tomography (PET), magnetic resonance imaging (MRI), and electroencephalographic (EEG) mapping], improved hospital and ambulatory seizure monitoring techniques, increased receptor knowledge, and neurotransmitter and neuropsychological research has also helped to make the clinical pharmacology of anticonvulsant drugs a dynamic field. The changing nature of the subject requires an overview of this field to provide a framework for understanding both current and future therapeutic developments rather than an encyclopedic review of the voluminous data available on anticonvulsant drugs, which is already available in many excellent texts.[1-7]

Specific treatment (such as glucose for hypoglycemic seizures) should be given whenever possible; however, for most seizures the cause is not identifiable. Until research clarifies the pathophysiology of seizures, most treatment will involve the empirical use of anticonvulsant drugs. Therefore, only nonspecific seizure treatment will be considered. Also, discussion of the timing and relative importance of various diagnostic tests, including skull films, lumbar punctures, CT scans, MRI, EEGs, or various biochemical tests, is beyond the scope of the chapter.[8,9]

Rather than attempt to review all available literature, only those pharmacologic principles necessary to incorporate new data, evaluate new drugs, and objectively individualize therapy will be covered. Much of this information is available elsewhere in a number of basic textbooks and reviews.

NATURAL HISTORY

The natural history of any disease must be known before the effects of any therapeutic intervention can be assessed. This is especially true for seizure disorders, where patients may have large variations in seizure frequency or severity (including total remission) with or without changes in therapy. This is why it is important to document, whenever possible, seizure frequency both prior to and during treatment and to be familiar with the natural history of the specific seizure type treated. A seizure log, especially when combined with medication history and results of therapeutic drug monitoring, can be very useful for monitoring the response to drug therapy if the limitations of the data are appreciated.

Seizure frequency and severity can be difficult to document, even in a health care facility. Documentation in the home environment is limited by observer bias and training as well as diagnostic uncertainty and time spent unobserved. For example, seizure frequency may artificially appear to increase immediately after the initial diagnosis because previously unrecognized seizures begin to be more accurately detected by the patient or family. This can lead to false interpretations of the response to therapy, as can incomplete or inaccurate medication histories as well as suboptimal collection, measurement, or interpretation of drug concentrations.[10]

RISK/BENEFIT RATIO

Seizures are such dramatic, emotionally charged events that insufficient consideration may be given to the risk/benefit analysis of treatment. When therapy totally prevents seizures without toxicity, the benefits of therapy clearly outweigh the risks. However, this is not always clear, especially at the extremes of seizure frequency. The patient treated to prevent very infrequent seizures obtains little benefit (i.e., small reduction in seizure frequency) and yet is exposed to definite risks from chronic anticonvulsant use. A recent report[11] indicates that the risk of a second seizure is less than half in children even if no treatment is given. Similarly, some patients with very frequent seizures have little or no decrease in seizure frequency despite multiple drug toxicities. Finally, some patients even experience increased seizures as an adverse effect of drug use.[12,13] However, there is very low morbidity or mortality associated with the empirical, aggressive management of status epilepticus.[14] Many feel that early treatment of any type of childhood epilepsy is beneficial,[15,16] but not all agree. Although it is a difficult decision, the clinician must always weigh the risk, cost, inconvenience, and toxicity of anticonvulsant therapy against a given decrease in seizure frequency for each patient.[1,7,17–19] The risk/benefit ratio must be repeatedly reassessed, where possible in collaboration with the patient or parents, whenever drug dosages are changed or drugs added to a regimen. Risk/benefit analysis must also be considered in the choice of the initial drug.

TREATMENT

Initial Drug Choice by Seizure Type

A lack of studies adequately comparing treatments, and the inexact classification of seizures or patients in the studies that do exist, make anticonvulsant selection imprecise. Also, many patients have ill-defined, changing, or multiple seizure types. Nevertheless, initial therapy chosen empirically on the basis of seizure types is fairly effective.[17,20] Treatment is initiated with a single drug with efficacy for as many of the seizure types present as possible. A list of drug classes useful for each major clinical seizure type is presented in Figure 29–1. Recommendations for a given seizure type change frequently as more comparative studies become available, as new drugs and formulations progress through preclinical and clinical trials, and as patient classification is refined.[4,21]

The "Therapeutic Drug Concentration" Concept

The concept of a "therapeutic range" is useful when initiating therapy.[2,22,23] These ranges are drug concentrations that are found to be associated with a high probability of seizure control and a low probability of toxicity. The ranges are not absolute. Optimal control may be achieved at levels above or below these ranges for any given patient.[22] The optimal concentration for a given patient is determined by many factors, including age (Figures 29–2 and 29–3), sex, disease state, the presence of other drugs (Figure 29–4), duration of treatment, altered protein binding, time of sampling, physiologic variables (e.g., pH, pO_2, glucose, etc.), and intrinsic variability in disease activity or end-organ responsiveness.[2] Most therapeutic

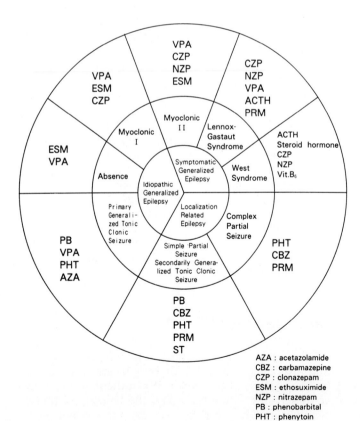

AZA : acetazolamide
CBZ : carbamazepine
CZP : clonazepam
ESM : ethosuximide
NZP : nitrazepam
PB : phenobarbital
PHT : phenytoin
PRM : primidone
VPA : valproate sodium
ST : sulthiame

FIGURE 29–1. Current drugs of choice by class for various seizure types. *Not available in many countries. (From Ohtahara,[77] with permission.)

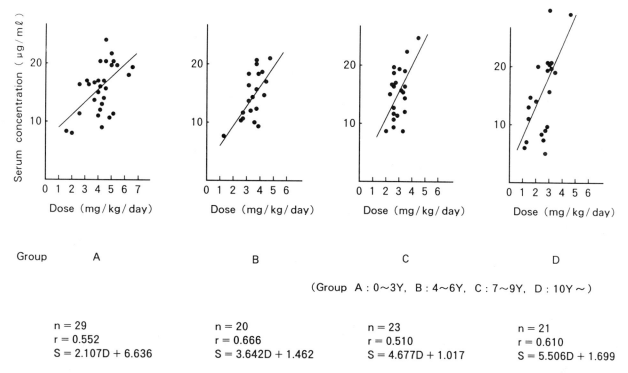

(Group A : 0~3Y, B : 4~6Y, C : 7~9Y, D : 10Y ~)

n = 29	n = 20	n = 23	n = 21
r = 0.552	r = 0.666	r = 0.510	r = 0.610
S = 2.107D + 6.636	S = 3.642D + 1.462	S = 4.677D + 1.017	S = 5.506D + 1.699

FIGURE 29–2. Phenobarbital dose and serum concentration in each age group. (Modified from Takizawa et al.,[78] with permission.)

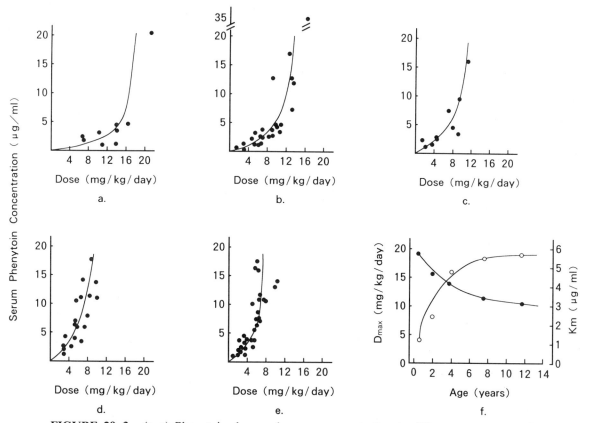

FIGURE 29–3. (a–e) Phenytoin dose and serum concentration in different age groups. (f) Change of V_{max} (●) and K'_m (○) with advancing age. (Modified from Nishihara et al.,[79] with permission.)

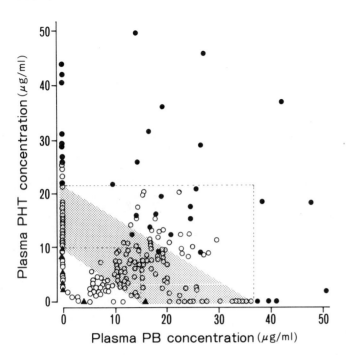

Proposed therapeutic zone
Patients with toxic manifestation
Patients with clinical seizures

FIGURE 29–4. Proposed therapeutic range of plasma phenobarbital and phenytoin concentrations in patients treated with both phenobarbital and phenytoin. (From Honda et al.,[80] with permission.)

ranges used for children are in fact based on adult studies or relatively few pediatric patients. Despite these limitations, the therapeutic range can be used in a practical approach to initial individualization of therapy.

Initial Dosing

Once a drug is chosen, the initial dosage and dosing frequency are chosen empirically (see Table 29–1) and continued either until toxicity occurs or until the drug concentration is expected, on the basis of drug and patient characteristics, to have reached steady state and drug concentration is measured. If seizure control is not adequate but toxicity is present, an alternative drug should be considered. If neither toxicity nor control of seizures is present, even if the concentration is "therapeutic," the dosage is increased until either seizure control is achieved or toxicity occurs and the process is repeated. Drug concentrations ("levels") should be measured (a) at each new steady state, (b) whenever toxicity or poor compliance is suspected, (c) once seizure control is first achieved, or (d) whenever seizure control is lost. Concentration changes on the same regimen indicate either improper sampling or measurement, altered compliance or absorption, or changes in distribution, binding, or clearance. Loss of sei-

zure control at previously effective concentrations may indicate disease progression, decreased end-organ responsiveness (i.e., tolerance), decreased unbound drug concentrations, altered physiology, or changes in sample collection or analysis.

When toxicity occurs before seizure control, despite proper choice of drug and appropriate drug concentrations, the clinician and patient must decide to either decrease the dose, switch drugs, add another drug, or accept incomplete seizure control. Decreasing the dose despite seizures and "therapeutic levels" is also a pharmacologically sound but often neglected possibility. The decision to do so involves accepting some risk of increased seizures in order to decrease toxicity. Switching to another drug involves adding a drug prior to withdrawal of the first drug. When this is done, there is a tendency to continue both drugs (even if the second drug alone might work) because of the risk of withdrawal seizures during the transition period or even poorer control on the new drug.

Accepting incomplete seizure control is also a logical if seldom chosen alternative. This is especially true for patients with infrequent or non-life-threatening seizures. Accepting incomplete control should be discussed with patients and parents as an alternative to increasing dosages, switching to a different drug, or adding medication. The occurrence of breakthrough seizures despite "adequate" single-drug therapy does *not* necessarily require adding or switching to a second drug. Adding a drug can decrease compliance and increase the chances of drug reactions and interactions (e.g., altered clearance, binding, or absorption). Adding drugs can also result in artifactual changes in seizure frequency due to observer bias or altered surveillance rather than actual changes in seizure frequency. Despite the fact that there is little or no evidence that multiple drug therapy is superior to monotherapy,[22] the decision is commonly made to add a drug.[24] Certainly a second drug should not be added until dosage increases result in unacceptable toxicity from a single drug, regardless of the dosage used or the concentration reached. "Maximal" dosages are determined by individual response rather than textbook recommendations or even the attainment of "supra" therapeutic concentration. Published maximal dosages are often inadequate to achieve effective, nontoxic concentrations, especially in young children. And some patients do not experience toxicity or even require concentrations above those generally accepted as therapeutic or toxic.

When an additional drug is needed, it is selected on the basis of previous therapy, response, seizure type(s), and individual clinical variables. Polypharmacy may occasionally be necessary, but only in patients with multiple seizure types that do not respond to a single drug, such as myoclonic epilepsies of infants and children (e.g., Lennox-Gastaut syndrome).[25]

There has been a move away from multidrug treatment of "drug-resistant" (intractable) seizures because of the problems of such therapy, and because it has been shown that multiple drugs seldom produce better seizure control than individualized, single-drug therapy combined with proper therapeutic drug monitoring.[22,26,27]

TABLE 29–1. PHARMACOKINETIC CHARACTERISTICS OF ANTIEPILEPTIC DRUGS

DRUG	MAINTENANCE DOSE (mg/kg/day)	USUAL ADULT DOSE (mg/day)	THERAPEUTIC RANGE (mg/liter) MONOTHERAPY	$t_{1/2}$ (h)	PEAK TIME (h)	V_d (liters/kg)	PROTEIN BINDING (%)	ELIMINATION ROUTE L: LIVER K: KIDNEY	ACTIVE METABOLITES KNOWN
Phenobarbital	2–5	120	10–40	36–144	6–18	0.5–0.7	40–60	L + K	
Mephobarbital	1–10	400–600	*	30–70	2.5–7	0.8–4.1	58–68	L	+
Metharbital	5–15	100–800	*	—	—	—		L	
Primidone	5–15	500–1,500	5–15	3–13	3.2 ± 10	0.7–1.0	0–50	L	+
Phenytoin	2–12	300	5–25	Dose-dependent	4–8	0.6–0.7	87–93	L	
Mephenytoin	3–15	200–600	—	—	—	—	—	L	
Ethotoin	50	2000–3000	15–50	3–6	1–2	—	—	L	
Trimethadione	40	300–1,500	—	—	0.5–2	—	0	L	+
Paramethadione	A	300–900	—	B	—	—	—	L	
Ethosuximide	15–40	250–1,500	40–120	16–60	2–3	0.7	0	L + K	
Methsuximide	5–20	300–1,200	8–12	2–3	<3	—	<10	L	+
Phensuximide	C	1000–3000	—	4	1–4	—	<10	D	
Diazepam	0.1–1.0	20–40	>0.6	10–40	Diazepam:1–2 Desmethyl:24–48	2.2–2.6	94–98	L	+
Clonazepam	0.02–0.2	Maximum<20	0.01–0.10	20–60	1.2	1.5–5.5	82	L	
Carbamazepine	5–20	400–1200	4–12	4–20	2–6	0.7–1.4	60–80	L	+
Valproic acid	10–50	500–1500	40–150	6–15	1–4	0.1–0.4	85–95	L	

*See phenobarbital.

A: | Age | Initial dose (mg) |
0–2 yr 300
2–6 yr 600   Dosage may be gradually increased at weekly intervals until seizures are controlled or toxic symptoms appear.
> 6 yr 900

B: Paramethadione has been reported to have biphasic half-life of 1.2 h for the first phase and 24 h for the second phase.

C: 1–3 gm, regardless of age.

D: Very little is known about the metabolism of phensuximide.

PHARMACOKINETICS

Therapeutic Drug Level Monitoring (TDM)

TDM, the measurement and proper interpretation of drug concentrations in biologic samples (plasma, blood, serum, cerebrospinal fluid, brain, saliva, or urine), has improved the efficacy and decreased the toxicity of anticonvulsant drugs. A full discussion of the rationale, techniques, mathematical and pharmacologic basis, applications, and limitations of TDM is beyond the scope of this chapter, and several reviews are available to the interested reader.[1,10,22,28,29] Only some commonly unappreciated principles are emphasized.

Appropriate sampling is a minimum requirement for proper TDM. For example, the exact sampling time must be known in relation to the dosing regimen, the drug, the patient's clinical response, and the expected approach to steady state. Concentrations can seldom be usefully interpreted without a complete medical and medication history including the clinical response, the time on the regimen, the formulation, other drugs taken, and the time between the last dose and sample collection. Knowledge of the drug's pharmacology and kinetics is also required.

In general, steady-state, predose concentrations are monitored as a measure of efficacy in preventing seizures. Concentrations should also be measured at the time of unexpected seizure occurrences or when toxicity occurs. Concentrations and clinical data should be used to establish individual concentration–response relationships. Many patients do well only with drug concentrations outside published therapeutic ranges.[22,30] Measurements of drug concentrations, if properly interpreted and continued for at least a year, allow as many as 85–95 percent of seizure patients to be controlled with a single drug.[16,31] However, randomly collected samples that are reported merely as being below, within, or above a published range have not been shown to improve seizure control. Unfortunately, few physicians are adequately trained in all aspects of TDM. Many measured drug concentrations are ignored or responded to improperly.[10] Both the physicians who order drug assays and the laboratory services that analyze samples and interpret results should be aware of the many factors that affect drug level interpretation.

ABSORPTION AND "PEAK" LEVELS

A discussion of drug absorption is beyond the scope of this chapter, but an appreciation of the variables that may affect the rate or extent of absorption is required to properly interpret drug concentrations and to select appropriate sampling times.

It may be useful to use peak concentrations as a measure of maximal pharmacologic effect, especially if toxicity is suspected. In practice, however, variability in both the rate of absorption and individual rates of elimination makes it difficult to measure peak levels, even with multiple samples. This is because the time of the peak level is a function of both absorption and elimination rates. Drug concentration rises until the rate of absorption equals the *rate* of elimination. Absorption is usually first-order, that is, proportional to the amount of drug in the intestine. The rate of absorption is maximal initially, decreases with time, and is usually faster than the rate of elimination. Peak levels are reached when the rate of absorption decreases enough to equal the rate of drug clearance. Contrary to popular impression, absorption continues long beyond the peak. The time of the peak is not predictable from knowledge of only the rate or the completeness of absorption. Anticonvulsant peaks are often both delayed and unpredictable because both drug clearance and absorption rates are slow and vary widely among patients, drugs, and products.

Peak concentrations may occur earlier in children due to more rapid clearance rather than to any increase in rate (or extent) of absorption in children. This principle also explains the discrepancies between serum "half-lives" determined after oral and intravenous administration. When absorption is much slower than clearance, the fall in drug concentration reflects absorption rate rather than elimination. For these reasons it is very difficult to use peak concentrations to monitor therapy, especially for drugs such as phenytoin that have variable (e.g., dose-dependent) elimination or absorption characteristics.[32] This is why predose, steady-state levels are usually used to monitor prophylactic therapy and why toxicity can occur at any time in a dosing regimen, not merely at the time of "expected" peaks.

VARIABLES AFFECTING STEADY-STATE LEVELS

Most drugs obey linear kinetics. The average drug concentration at steady state (C_{ss}) for these drugs can be determined by the equation

$$C_{ss} = (F/Cl) (D/\lambda)$$

where F is the fraction absorbed (or taken), D is the dose given, λ is the dosing interval, and Cl is the total body clearance. Note that the dose absorbed per unit time ($F \cdot D/\lambda$) is determined by compliance, bioavailability, and the dosage regimen prescribed.

Poor compliance is a frequent cause of variations in drug concentrations and seizure control. Altered compliance should always be suspected when levels unexpectedly change. However, changes in sampling time, assay technology, drug regimen or preparation used, use of additional drugs, or altered clearance due to changes in renal or hepatic function all can cause variations in drug concentrations on the same regimen. An appreciation of how these factors alter drug concentrations is required to correctly interpret measured drug concentrations. For phenytoin, interpretation also requires an appreciation of nonlinear or saturation kinetics.

Most anticonvulsants are metabolized by enzyme systems that are saturable at some drug concentration.

Once saturation occurs, metabolism is determined by Michaelis–Menten (nonlinear or saturation) kinetics:

$$\text{Rate of metabolism} = \frac{V_{max} \times C}{K_m + C}$$

where C is the plasma concentration of the drug at the enzyme site, V_{max} is the maximum velocity of the enzyme reaction (determined by the total amount of enzyme present), K_m is the drug concentration at which metabolism is one-half maximum, and $1/K_m$ is a measure of the affinity between the drug and the enzyme. Once the enzyme becomes saturated, the rate of metabolism approaches a maximal rate (V_{max}) that remains constant no matter how high the drug concentration rises. Among the consequences of this saturation is that there is no "half-life."

For most drugs saturation kinetics are only observed at the concentrations seen after massive overdoses. However, for most patients given phenytoin, saturation occurs well within the therapeutic range. The concentration at which this occurs is not easily predicted, because there is considerable interpatient, and perhaps even intrapatient, variation in K_m and V_{max}. In practical terms, this means that even a small increase or decrease in dose (Figure 30-3), clearance, or fraction absorbed can result in a disproportionately large increase or decrease, respectively, in concentration. Failure to fully understand nonlinear kinetics can significantly decrease the clinician's ability to use phenytoin effectively (see discussion of phenytoin in the section on hydantoins).

CLEARANCE AS A FUNCTION OF AGE

The change in concentration over a dosing interval is determined by drug clearance, absorption, and distribution, all of which change with age.[3]

As a general rule, clearance is very low in the neonate (especially the premature) but increases rapidly within the first year of life, then changes more slowly with adolescence.[3] Although variable, clearance usually reaches or exceeds adult values in young children.

Drug absorption may also vary with age. In general, significant differences in absorption are usually related more to use of different formulations than to altered physiologic processes. However, differences in both the rate and extent of absorption are seen in children, especially for slowly absorbed preparations, because of rapid intestinal transit times, dosage measurement errors, or high first-pass effects that alter the fraction absorbed.

Clinically significant differences in absorption characteristics have been well documented for anticonvulsants. Both the amount absorbed and the rate of absorption (bioavailability) may be clinically important. Whenever possible, patients should be maintained on the same formulation. The use of brand-name drugs minimizes, but does not eliminate, bioavailability problems. Even brand-name drugs may be manufactured by different suppliers or manufacturing processes.[33] Changes in dosage regimen can alter concentration, since the route of administration, type of preparation (suspension, tablet, capsule, suppository, etc.), measurement errors, and compliance may each alter rate or extent of absorption.

Differences in clearance or absorption are most critical for drugs with nonlinear kinetic behavior. For such drugs, even small changes produce disproportionate changes in drug concentrations,[22,34] effects, or the time necessary to reach a new steady state.[35] Phenytoin is the best example of this type of drug, but data exist which indicate that other anticonvulsants, including phenobarbital and ethosuximide,[36] may also exhibit dose-dependent kinetics (especially at concentrations above the therapeutic range.[2,37]

Alterations in drug distribution also occur with age, clinical condition, and other drug treatment. Distribution affects both the rate of clearance and the relationship between the drug concentration in blood and brain. Clinically important distribution considerations exist for many anticonvulsant drugs.

ASSAY VARIABILITY

Assay variability is an important factor in the interpretation of drug concentrations. The clinician must be aware of the type, accuracy, linearity, specificity, and sensitivity, as well as the reproducibility, of assays used. Neither the use of sophisticated instrumentation nor the theoretical reproducibility of results guarantees the reliability of a clinical measurement. Only laboratories that have been shown to consistently produce reliable results by an external, national (or international) interlaboratory quality control system[38,39] should be used.

Recently developed reagent strip methods that are accurate when tested under controlled conditions may not always produce equally accurate results when performed in the office setting. Finally, not even all hospital laboratories produce reliable results, even with identified test samples.[10]

It must also be appreciated that published therapeutic ranges are often based on studies that used older, less specific analytic methods than those currently in use. It is known that intermethod variability occurs, but it is unclear how significant these variations are.[37]

UNBOUND VERSUS TOTAL DRUG

Most clinical laboratories measure and report only total drug concentrations. This is the sum of the protein-bound and unbound (free) drug concentrations. Yet the unbound concentration is more directly related to the pharmacologic effect. For highly bound drugs (e.g., phenytoin), even a small change in protein binding may result in a large change in drug effect.

Variation in unbound concentrations accounts for at least some of the intrapatient variability in response to a given concentration (Figure 29–5).

Routine measurement of unbound rather than total

drug concentrations should theoretically improve anticonvulsant use, but except in unusual patients (e.g., renal failure patients) this impression has not been substantiated. Such monitoring is both expensive and not routinely available.

ANTICONVULSANTS—GENERAL

This chapter addresses only the major anticonvulsant classes. Many less useful agents (e.g., bromides, acetazolamide, paraldehyde, or phenacemide), numerous rarely used agents (e.g., ACTH, steroids, amphetamines, lidocaine, imipramine, quinacrine, sulthiane, etc.), and non-drug treatments (including surgery, biofeedback, or behavior modification) will not be covered.

Barbiturates (Phenobarbital, Metharbital, Mephobarbital, and Primidone)

Since the introduction of phenobarbital, literally thousands of related compounds have been synthesized. Only a few are useful anticonvulsants at subanesthetic doses. The four clinically useful drugs are structurally similar. Some are metabolically interconverted. Phenobarbital, for example, is a metabolite of both mephobarbital and primidone. The barbiturates are effective for generalized tonic clonic seizures and status epilepticus. They are less useful for complex partial, myoclonic, and akinetic seizures. However, despite years of use, relatively few rigorous or comparative studies of efficacy or toxicity exist.

Generally accepted therapeutic ranges for the barbiturates are presented in Table 29–1. These ranges are poorly defined because of many factors, including the presence of active metabolites, pH-dependent ionization and distribution, and the occurrence of metabolic and pharmacodynamic tolerance. The ionization characteristics of these drugs, especially phenobarbital, are such that physiologic changes in pH alter both drug distribution and elimination. Other drugs, or disease states that alter plasma, tissue, or urinary pH, may alter barbiturate kinetics or effects.

Absorption is rapid and complete for all members of the class. Significant bioavailability problems have not been identified. Renal elimination is relatively unimportant, at least for unchanged parent drugs, since clearance is principally by hepatic metabolism. However, when metabolism is slow, renal clearance does become important (e.g., during overdose and in newborns). Metabolic clearance is age-dependent, being slowest in prematures but as fast in young children as in adults, if not faster. Autoinduction as well as induction by other drugs occurs. Metabolic saturation does not occur at therapeutic concentrations but may occur at high concentrations of phenobarbital and primidone. Empirical dosage regimens are given in Table 29–1. Larger doses are required in young children (<30 kg) than in newborns, older children, or adults (Figure 29–2). However, even in young children, phenobarbital is eliminated so slowly that single daily dosing is usually adequate except in the rare child in whom unwanted peak pharmacologic responses (sedation or hyperactivity) are observed.[40] Since phenobarbital is a metabolite of both primidone and mephobarbital, it is possible that less frequent dosing of these drugs is possible as well, but except for phenobarbital, studies are lacking comparing the efficacy or toxicity of various barbiturate dosage regimens.

Phenobarbital is the most useful drug of the class. It is a safe, inexpensive, and effective drug. Its use in children is limited by the relatively common occurrence of altered behavior or cognitive function and "paradoxical" central nervous system (CNS) excitement.[41] Depression may also occur.[42] Its long half-life both makes once-daily administration reasonable and necessitates using loading doses (of about 10–20 mg/kg) to rapidly achieve steady-state concentrations followed by much lower (2–6 mg/kg/day) maintenance doses. Without loading doses it can take 2 weeks to achieve steady state.

The anecdotal claims that mephobarbital is less toxic, less potent, better tolerated, or more useful for absence seizures than phenobarbital are difficult to reconcile with the fact that the drug is readily metabolized to phenobarbital.

Metharbital is the oldest (and longest-acting) barbiturate, but it is rarely used. Except for anecdotal claims of superiority in myoclonic epilepsy, it has no apparent advantage over phenobarbital, especially since metharbital has more anesthetic and sedative properties. Once-daily administration appears to be possible but may be limited by the excessive sedation that occurs with initial large doses.

Although structurally slightly different, primidone may be considered a barbiturate. It is metabolized by a saturable process to phenobarbital.[1] It is still unclear how much anticonvulsant activity primidone has in humans above that of its two active metabolites (phenylethylmalonamide, PEMA and phenobarbital). Initial doses should be small with gradual increases depending on efficacy, toxicity, and the appreciation that the metabolites (especially phenobarbital) will continue to accumulate for weeks before steady state is achieved.[2,34] Primidone concentrations are difficult to interpret without measurement of its active metabolites, especially phenobarbital.

The most common toxic effect of the barbiturates is excitement and hyperactive behavior.[43] The reported adverse effect of phenobarbital on intelligence after long-term use, although of small magnitude, is important if confirmed.[44] The incidence of excitement and hyperactivity is difficult to establish, but they occur frequently in young children. Withdrawal, tolerance and hypersensitivity reactions (especially rashes), and hemorrhage also occur in infants born to phenobarbital-treated women. Less common or less well-documented effects include gastrointestinal upset, jaundice, and megaloblastic anemia.

Another important side effect of the barbiturates is their ability to stimulate drug metabolism, including their own. This effect must be considered when adjusting the dosage of coadministered drugs, especially when starting or stopping barbiturates in an already stabilized patient.

These drugs have been used for many years, but because they were introduced before legislation required more data, few rigorous studies of drug efficacy or toxicity exist.[44] Some recent studies have compared the various barbiturates to more recently introduced agents, but most of the available literature is anecdotal. Studies documenting the occurrence of behavior disorders in children[41] or adverse effects on intelligence[44] make the need for studies on relative efficacy even more acute.

Hydantoins (Ethotoin, Mephenytoin, and Phenytoin)

Of the hydantoins, only three have had appreciable use. Phenytoin was the first introduced and is still the only one routinely used. Most of the therapeutic literature on the hydantoins is anecdotal. However, a large body of older and an expanding number of more recent comparative studies indicate that phenytoin, by an unknown mechanism, suppresses simple partial, complex partial, and secondarily generalized tonic clonic seizures. Phenytoin is also of some use in status epilepticus, but its relative efficacy when compared to newer, less toxic alternative agents has not been defined. The amount of discussion of phenytoin is less an indication of the relative use of phenytoin than a reflection of the fact that more data may exist on phenytoin than any other anticonvulsant.

The therapeutic range for phenytoin (Table 29–1) was first established by a prospective study of a small group of hospitalized patients.[45] Although most studies support this range, some recent retrospective studies have found conflicting associations between drug concentrations and seizure control.[21,46] Both a lack of correlation[47] and even a negative correlation[48] between phenytoin concentrations and seizure control have been reported. It is unclear whether these discrepancies are the result of poor design, inadequate sample collections or analyses, or a biphasic level response relationship for phenytoin.

One of the most convincing studies of the therapeutic range for phenytoin was a 3-year prospective (but unblinded) study of 32 adult and child epileptic outpatients.[49] In these patients the mean phenytoin plasma concentrations were increased from 6.1 to 11.7 to 15.0 μg/ml during the first, second, and third study year, respectively. This was accompanied by a decrease in the annual mean generalized tonic clonic seizure frequency per patient from 5.8 to 4.1 to 1.6, respectively.

The accepted therapeutic range for phenytoin (5–25 μg/ml) is based on many studies, but for a given patient the optimal concentration may vary greatly.[22] To some degree the optimal concentration is determined by the severity and duration of the seizure disorder. Patients with mild or infrequent seizures may be best titrated to a lower concentration. Although there are few objective data, patients with more severe disorders may have increasing benefit at concentrations even higher than 25 mg/liter.[50,51] However, some studies have documented increasing seizure frequency at higher phenytoin concentrations.[1,12] Such a negative correlation between concentration and effect may be an artifact of patient selection. Patients without seizures don't take their medication, and difficult-to-control patients take more drug. However, in some patients seizure frequency does increase with increasing anticonvulsant concentrations (i.e., a biphasic level response or so-called paradoxical seizures). When this occurs, it usually is associated with phenytoin concentrations above 35 $\mu g/ml$. This may cause increased absence or generalized tonic clonic seizures. It is important to consider this phenomenon whenever seizure frequency increases along with (or in spite of) concentrations at the top of or above the therapeutic range, especially since this may occur without other signs of toxicity (e.g., nystagmus).

The absorption characteristics of phenytoin are complicated by its chemical characteristics, the various preparations available, and its kinetic behavior. Numerous problems with phenytoin bioavailability have been documented.[3] The intramuscular route of administration produces particularly unpredictable absorption and should be avoided.[2] Although there are many generic products that are as well absorbed as the standard (Parke-Davis) preparation,[52] it is best to avoid switching products since the dose-dependent clearance of phenytoin makes even small changes in availability potentially dangerous.

As with phenobarbital, larger[53] and more frequent daily phenytoin doses are required to maintain therapeutic levels in some children (Figure 29–3). Differences in body composition, absorption, relative organ sizes, distribution, and more rapid drug metabolism are probably all responsible.[2,40] Few studies of effective concentrations in children exist, but it appears that the therapeutic range in children is similar to, if somewhat wider than, that in adults.[22,54,55] This range is difficult to define because the concentration–response relationship may be altered by many factors, including liver or kidney disease, the presence of other drugs (Figure 29–4) or metabolites, folic acid balance, pregnancy, or the amount of protein binding.[2] Protein binding is especially important for phenytoin because both effects and clearance are determined by the amount of unbound drug.

Phenytoin is almost totally metabolized (hydroxylated) in the liver to inactive metabolites by a process that is saturable (capacity-limited) at concentrations within the therapeutic range. Saturation results in nonlinear kinetic behavior, where small changes in dose result in inordinately large changes in blood concentration, clearance, and effect (see the preceding discussion). Also, drug accumulation continues for progressively longer periods for each increase in dose after saturation occurs. Small changes in the dose or the amount absorbed may result in large changes in both the eventual concentration and the time it takes to reach maximal concentrations.

A number of methods have been devised to dose phenytoin.[56] Phenytoin is a classic example of a drug for which drug concentration monitoring can be useful. There is a narrow therapeutic margin; large interpatient variability in clearance occurs; there is a relatively good concentration–response relationship; and some toxic effects (e.g., cognitive dysfunction) are only suspected clinically when concentrations are very elevated. Drug concentrations should be measured after initiating therapy and after any change in clinical condition, dosage regimen, formulation used, or concomitant drug therapy.

Drug monitoring is especially important in children,[56] since children appear to require higher maintenance dosages than adults (up to even 12–16 mg/kg/day), compliance is often a problem, dosage measurement errors often occur, intestinal transit time is variable, and erratically absorbed preparations are often used. Also, many toxic neuropsychologic effects are more difficult to recognize in children, and other toxic effects, including gum hypertrophy, hypertrichosis, altered vitamin metabolism, neonatal bleeding, and possible teratogenic or immunologic effects, are either of special importance to or have greater impact on children.[1,2]

The most common toxic side effects are neurologic and are correlated with blood concentrations. The actual incidence of toxicity at various blood concentrations is unknown. Generally, however, neurologic signs are uncommon below 15 $\mu g/ml$,[2] nystagmus appears above 20 $\mu g/ml$, ataxia above 30 $\mu g/ml$, paradoxical seizures above 35 $\mu g/ml$, and mental changes above 40 $\mu g/ml$.[57]

Less common adverse neurologic effects that occur only rarely in children include peripheral neuropathy, dizziness, insomnia, nervousness, irritability, muscle twitching, diplopia, fatigue, depression, tremor, headache, and psychotic disturbances. Children, especially those who have abnormal neurologic function before treatment, may be unable or unwilling to report many of these effects. In addition, children often are treated long-term. Toxicity appears to be related to both blood, plasma, or serum concentrations, and duration of therapy. It is possible that prolonged, excessive levels may produce permanent CNS lesions, including Purkinje cell degeneration.[58] This possibility is of particular importance in the developing child. However, even if all CNS toxicity is reversible, the effect of even temporary cognitive or psychomotor impairment during the rapid learning period needs special consideration. Since alternative treatments are usually available, special caution should be taken before phenytoin is used in any child in whom the early signs of CNS toxicity would be difficult or impossible to recognize.

Numerous nonspecific gastrointestinal symptoms and a variety of both minor and serious dermatologic conditions are also reported. Cross hypersensitivity reactions between the barbiturates and the structurally similar hydantoins also occur.

A wide range of both serious and relatively benign hematologic disorders occur rarely, including thrombocytopenia, leukopenia or leukocytosis, granulocytopenia, agranulocytosis, pancytopenia, eosinophilia, monocytosis, and anemias, as well as a malignant or premalignant lymphoproliferative disorder.

Numerous other uncommon reactions have also been reported, including altered vitamin D metabolism in children who receive multiple drugs and have limited sun exposure.[1,2] The two most common and distressing side effects (hirsutism and gum hypertrophy) are cosmetic, but both can be particularly distressing to children. Drug monitoring and good oral hygiene may decrease but not eliminate the chances of these adverse effects.

Phenytoin appears to be safer than the barbiturates in acute overdoses. It does cause an acute cerebellar delirium syndrome, but rarely coma. Oral overdose rarely causes the cardiac toxicity seen with rapid intravenous administration. This is at least in part because much of the toxicity of intravenous phenytoin is secondary to the diluent used for the parenteral preparation (pH > 12 and 40 percent propylene glycol). A less toxic intravenous prodrug formulation under development may decrease the toxicity associated with intravenous administration.

Use in pregnancy may be associated with neonatal bleeding[59] or teratogenesis. Although the teratogenic risk is increased two- to threefold in phenytoin-treated epileptic mothers, it is difficult to separate drug- from disease-related risks.[60] Decisions on treatment during pregnancy are based on the relative risks of alternative or no drug treatment and seizures versus the increased risk of malformations (especially cleft lip and congenital heart lesions). Both the doses required and the effective drug concentrations may be lower in pregnant women.

Phenytoin and the other hydantoins are very effective drugs. The use of any hydantoin is limited more by toxicity than by lack of efficacy, and only some of this toxicity can be avoided by careful clinical and laboratory monitoring.

Mephenytoin is chemically and pharmacologically very similar to phenytoin. Its metabolism appears to be more rapid than that of phenytoin but has been less well studied. Mephenytoin is claimed to be therapeutically superior to phenytoin, but serious toxicity (especially rashes and fatal blood dyscrasias) limits its use. Its N-demethylated metabolite is active and is responsible for some therapeutic as well as toxic effects. Mephenytoin is similar to many other hydantoins that are effective but seldom used because of toxicity. Ethotoin, on the other hand, appears to be both less toxic and less efficacious than phenytoin. Few useful data exist on the pharmacokinetic behavior of either of these other hydantoins in children. Since less-toxic alternatives to phenytoin usually can be found, these drugs have little use.

Numerous drugs have been reported to increase phenytoin concentrations or effects due to altered metabolism or protein binding (Table 29–2). Isoniazid, coumarin anticoagulants, disulfiram, chloramphenicol, chloridiazepoxide, methylphenidate, chlorpromazine, estrogens, ethosuximide, and phenylbutazone all have been reported to cause interactions. Decreased total phenytoin

TABLE 29–2. DRUG INTERACTIONS OF ANTIEPILEPTIC DRUGS

PRIMARY DRUG	MAY INTERACT WITH	POTENTIAL EFFECT ON PRIMARY DRUG	MANAGEMENT AND HOW TO AVOID
Phenobarbital or primidone	Sulthiame	Marked increase	Monitor serum phenobarbital levels
			Reduce dose of phenobarbital or primidone if necessary
	Sodium valproate	Marked sedation	Reduce dose of phenobarbital or primidone
	Phenytoin	Increase Decrease	Monitor serum phenobarbital levels
	Pheneturide	Increase	Monitor serum phenobarbital levels
	Dicoumarol	Decrease	Avoid this combination
	Phenylbutazone	Decrease	Avoid this combination
	Aminopyrine	Decrease	Avoid this combination
Primidone	Isoniazid	Reduced conversion to phenobarbitone and PEMA	Avoid this combination
Phenytoin	Sulthiame	Increase	Monitor serum phenytoin levels
	Pheneturide	Increase	Reduce dose if necessary
	Phenobarbital	Variable	Monitor serum levels of both drugs
	Carbamazepine	Decrease	Usually not of clinical importance because of added effect of interfering drug
	Diazepam	Decrease	
	Sodium valproate	Rise in free (not total) phenytoin, producing transient increase in drug effects	Monitor serum free phenytoin
Phenytoin	Imipramine Isoniazid Chloramphenicol Dicoumarol Phenyramidol Disulfiram	Increase drug effects, producing risk of drug intoxication	Avoid this combination
	Phenylbutazone Sulphafurazole Salicylic acid Diazoxide	Rise in free levels, producing transient increase in drug effects	Monitor free phenytoin Avoid this combination
	Ethanol	Decrease	Avoid this combination
Carbamazepine	Primidone	Decrease	Monitor serum carbamazepine levels
	Phenytoin	Decrease	
	Warfarin	Decrease	
	Triacetyloleandomycin	Increase	Avoid this combination
	Erythromycin	Increase	Avoid this combination
	Valproic acid	Altered disposition	

levels have been reported with phenobarbital, primidone, carbamazepine, and valproic acid, but the latter is associated with increased unbound levels.[2]

Oxazolidinediones (Trimethadione and Paramethadione)

The era of selective anticonvulsants began with the introduction of trimethadione. Although chemically similar to both the barbiturates and hydantoins, the oxazolidinediones (trimethadione and paramethadione) appear to be effective only for absence seizures. Although most older literature is anecdotal, newer controlled studies support the claims of efficacy of these drugs for classical absence epilepsy. Other seizure types, including atypical absence seizures (Lennox-Gastaut syndrome), do not respond.

The therapeutic ranges have not been well described. For paramethadione this is partly due to the presence of its slowly cleared, active metabolite (dimethadione) and the fact that steady-state ratios of metabolite to parent drug (up to 20:1) are reached only after weeks of therapy.[1] Few data exist for paramethadione.

Both trimethadione and paramethadione are well absorbed, freely distributed into body water, and cleared mainly by hepatic demethylation to active metabolites (especially dimethadione), which are then cleared by the kidney. Increased toxicity occurs with either hepatic or renal dysfunction. There is evidence that dimethadione inhibits hepatic demethylation and causes progressive increases in duration of action.[61] There is no objective evidence for the therapeutic superiority of either drug. Dosage recommendations are given in Table 29-1. Once-daily trimethadione dosing is possible since it is slowly (and almost totally) demethylated to dimethadione, which in turn is very slowly cleared.

Toxic side effects, especially visual ones, are commonly seen. Visual toxicity is said to be less common in children, but children are often less willing or able to complain about such effects. Renal glomerular changes, proteinuria, and a nephrotic syndrome have been reported, especially with paramethadione. Less common but more serious reactions involve the skin, bone marrow, and liver. Any rash should be viewed with concern because a lupus-like syndrome, erythema multiforme, alopecia, pruritus, or severe exfoliative dermatitis can occur. Fatalities have been reported secondary to these dermatologic diseases as well as to hepatitis, nephrosis, and blood dyscrasias. Nonspecific gastrointestinal symptoms such as hiccups, nausea, vomiting, abdominal pain, or anorexia occur both alone and as a prelude to more serious toxicity.

Personality changes, headaches, fatigue, and paresthesia as well as a myasthenic syndrome occur and are difficult to recognize in children. Prophylactic combination treatment with a drug for generalized tonic clonic seizures is often recommended because it is known that absence seizures may increase briefly, and because other seizure types (especially generalized tonic clonic seizures) may begin or increase when these drugs are first given. The decision to begin with combination therapy in a child must be individualized on the basis of the clinical presen-

tation, the risk of generalized tonic clonic seizures, and the toxicity of the drugs in question. Such prophylactic therapy may be justified if the history is suggestive of generalized tonic clonic seizures or if the electroencephalogram (EEG) contains more than classic absence discharges (i.e., 3 or 4 cps generalized spike-and-wave complex discharges).

Although these drugs are teratogenic,[1] this should rarely be a problem because absence seizures are uncommon in women of reproductive age and because alternative drugs are available. These drugs are already rarely used. Future use of these drugs will depend on the results of comparative studies and clinical perceptions of the effectiveness of other less toxic agents.

Succinimides (Ethosuximide, Phensuximide, and Methsuximide)

The succinimides are less-toxic alternatives to the oxazolidinediones for the treatment of absence seizures. Both anecdotal and well-controlled studies indicate that ethosuximide is the drug of choice (over phensuximide) for absence seizures. Methsuximide is also occasionally useful for complex partial seizures that cannot be controlled with other drugs.[62]

Because absence seizures rarely occur outside the pediatric age group, the therapeutic range for ethosuximide has been described in children. Significant interpatient variability occurs, but most patients are controlled at ethosuximide concentrations of 40–120 µg/ml. The therapeutic range for methsuximide is more difficult to define because of its active metabolite (N-desmethylsuximide), which may be present in concentrations many times higher than the parent drug.[62] It has been claimed that efficacy begins at a methsuximide concentration of 8–12 µg/ml, and toxicity usually occurs at 20–25 µg/ml.[63] Toxicity may be seen with N-desmethylsuximide concentrations of more than 40–50 µg/ml.[62] Plasma protein binding is low and unlikely to cause changes in effects.

Ethosuximide clearance is largely by hepatic metabolism, which appears to be more rapid in children ($t_{1/2}$ = 39 hours) than in adults ($t_{1/2}$ = 60 hours).[1,2] Methsuximide is cleared more rapidly ($t_{1/2}$ = 2–3 hours), but its metabolite (N-desmethylsuximide) is cleared much more slowly.[36]

Little is known about the effects of disease state on drug efficacy or toxicity. Initial doses should be small, and dosage increases should be gradual and guided by monitoring of drug concentrations, which has been shown to significantly increase both compliance and control.[1,3] Seizure frequency may dramatically decrease with low doses or concentrations, even before steady state is achieved. The most common side effects are eosinophilia (10 percent), nausea, vomiting, ataxia, and drowsiness. Serious bone marrow disorders, liver disorders, renal disorders, neurologic dyskinesias, and psychiatric disorders may occur. Repeated blood counts and liver and renal function tests are recommended. Less common side effects include many dermatologic, neuropsychiatric, and urinary conditions that are either difficult to diagnose in children or of particular importance in the growing child. Some of the behavioral effects are virtually impossible to distinguish from presenting symptoms, especially in emotionally disturbed children. It is in these children that careful examinations and drug monitoring are most useful. Renal and hepatic toxicity appears to be more common with methsuximide. Because some patients develop generalized tonic clonic seizures after starting a suximide,[1,2,64] some authors recommend combining a drug for generalized tonic clonic seizures with a suximide. There are not enough objective data on the risks or benefits of such combination therapy to recommend its routine use, especially when compared to monotherapy with a single drug that is effective for both seizure types.

Benzodiazepines (Diazepam and Clonazepam)

Of the hundreds of benzodiazepines introduced, only two (diazepam and clonazepam) are labeled for anticonvulsant use in the United States, but other agents (e.g., nitrazepam, lorazepam, midazolam, and oxazepam) are effective as well.

Intravenous diazepam is the drug of choice for status epilepticus, but clonazepam may be equally or more effective. Both also have at least short-term efficacy for myoclonic, akinetic, and absence seizures.

All benzodiazepines are chemically similar heterocyclic compounds, many of which can be metabolically interconverted. All have pharmacokinetic properties similar to diazepam. Many metabolites are active. The chemical configuration of the benzodiazepines is similar to phenytoin. These drugs all interfere with the kinetics of several neurotransmitters, especially γ-aminobutyric acid (GABA). Specific endogenous benzodiazepine receptors exist, especially in the limbic system, thalamus, and hypothalamus, in association with GABA and adenosine receptors and the chloride channel. However, the exact relationship among any or all of these facts and the mechanism(s) of action is still unclear.

Therapeutic ranges for the benzodiazepines (Table 29–1) are poorly described because of many factors, including tissue distribution, active metabolites, and pharmacologic tolerance. The concentration–response relationship is influenced by the amount of time on the medication, body composition, age, and the presence of metabolites or other drugs.

Diazepam is a lipid-soluble, but water-insoluble, compound that is rapidly and completely absorbed after oral or rectal, but not intramuscular, administration. It is rapidly distributed into fatty tissues. It is slowly metabolized in the liver to an active metabolite (desmethyldiazepam), which is subsequently hydroxylated ($t_{1/2}$ = 25–50 hours) to another active metabolite (oxazepam). Oxazepam is glucuronidated and then renally excreted. Some metabolites undergo hepatic recirculation.

Plasma half-life is prolonged at both extremes of age and by the presence of liver disease. The daily oral dose of diazepam (0.1–1.0 mg/kg) is usually given in divided doses, but once-daily administration should be possible. Only oxazepam has been reported to have a short enough half-life to require multiple daily dosing to avoid wide variations in drug concentrations. However, prolonged distribution may be associated with wide swings in post-dosing concentration for all benzodiazepines, especially clonazepam (personal observation). When chronic oral clonazepam is used, a low starting dose (0.02 mg/kg) is suggested to minimize drowsiness, but chronic doses of up to 0.2 mg/kg are sometimes required. However, dosage regimens need to be individualized on the basis of adverse peak drug effects rather than drug concentrations. Diazepam is the drug of choice in status epilepticus, where 0.2–0.5 mg/kg should be given (undiluted) directly into as large a vein as possible. Rectal, but not intramuscular, administration of the intravenous preparation is also effective and should be considered for nonhospital use. Clonazepam appears to be as effective as diazepam for the treatment of status epilepticus at very low intravenous doses (0.005–0.02 mg/kg).

Compared to the anticonvulsant classes already discussed, the benzodiazepines are very safe drugs. The most common side effects in children are sedation and hypersalivation. Numerous other neurologic and psychiatric symptoms can occur, many of which may be difficult to recognize in children, especially children with abnormal neurologic function or emotional problems. Paradoxical excitement, giddiness, aggression, or irritability can occur at any age but are more common in children and the elderly. Respiratory symptoms occur and are related to respiratory depression and hypersecretion. Hirsutism, hair loss, skin rashes, peripheral edema, and a variety of nonspecific gastrointestinal, urinary, musculoskeletal, hepatic, and hematopoietic effects have been reported rarely. Habituation, dependence, and withdrawal can all occur, but pharmacologic tolerance is perhaps the most limiting property.

Despite the fact that the quality of the therapeutic literature for the benzodiazepines is better than for many older drugs, there is a definite need for long-term controlled studies comparing the various benzodiazepines to agents in the same and other drug classes. There has been a recent resurgence of interest in these drugs. However, long-term studies are particularly needed because of the pharmacologic tolerance that has been described with use of these agents. Their use to prevent or treat febrile convulsions (especially by the rectal route) would be especially interesting in view of recent concerns about both the safety and efficacy of phenobarbital.[44]

Carbamazepine

Carbamazepine is a unique anticonvulsant that is chemically related to the tricyclic antidepressants. Approval for anticonvulsant use was delayed in the United States by early reports of significant hematologic and hepatic toxicity and deaths. Fortunately, the incidence of serious toxicity appears to be low, especially in children.[65]

Even though carbamazepine is a relatively new agent, there is a large amount of uncontrolled and anecdotal data as well as very good controlled and comparative data on efficacy and toxicity. Not all patients or seizure types respond, but efficacy appears at least comparable to that of phenytoin or phenobarbital for generalized tonic clonic seizures and both simple and complex partial seizures. There is little effect on absence, and there are variable effects on combined or other seizure types. Carbamazepine appears to be especially useful for complex partial seizures, in children who experience excessive sedation with other agents, or in patients with depressive symptoms. Carbamazepine has replaced both phenytoin and phenobarbital as the first-choice anticonvulsant for a number of pediatric seizure disorders.

Despite the presence of an active metabolite (carbamazepine epoxide), there is a narrow therapeutic range when carbamazepine is used as monotherapy (see Table 29–1). The therapeutic range is lower (4–8 mg/liter) when combined with other drugs. Drug monitoring is especially important because of the wide range (at least fourfold) in dosages required to achieve effective concentrations. Measurement of epoxide concentrations can be useful but is not required. The concentration–response relationship for carbamazepine is altered by other drugs, by active metabolite, and perhaps by alterations in protein binding. Anecdotal reports of lower efficacy in young children despite high dosages are probably related to increased clearance in children.

Carbamazepine is well absorbed, has an apparent distribution volume equal to that of body water, and is moderately (60–80 percent) bound to plasma proteins. It is metabolized in the liver to at least one active metabolite (epoxide) at a variable rate.[1] Plasma half-lives have a wide range (8–60 hours) and may be both shorter and more variable in newborns and young children.[1-3] Its metabolic clearance may be genetically controlled (polygenic), as has been described for other tricyclics. Metabolism may be induced by other drugs as well as by carbamazepine itself. In some patients autoinduction may shorten the half-life enough to justify two or even three daily doses. Changes in the EEG do not correlate with efficacy, but drug monitoring is useful to guide dosage adjustments and has been shown to increase efficacy.

Knowledge of the toxicity of carbamazepine is evolving.[63] Transient leukopenia is common, but significant bone marrow depression (including fatal agranulocytosis) appears to be rare in children. The long-term efficacy and toxicity of carbamazepine are still being clarified. Many adverse effects have been reported, including nystagmus, ataxia, diplopia, blurred vision, lens opacities, gastrointestinal disturbances, bone marrow suppression, serious skin reactions, hepatic damage, altered cardiovascular function, hyponatremia from inappropriate ADH secretion, bladder dysfunction, and worsening of seizures at high concentrations. Cognitive dysfunction is much less common than with phenytoin or phenobarbital but can occur even within the therapeutic range,[66] especially if carbamazepine is used in polytherapy.[67]

Testicular atrophy as well as hepatic and genital tumors have been found in rats after chronic dosing. Bladder discoloration is seen in dogs after high doses. The importance of these findings for humans is unclear, but the possibility of long-term gonadal toxicity is of special importance in children. Baseline and periodic followup of blood and platelet counts, liver and renal function, and periodic ophthalmologic examinations are recommended in addition to drug concentration monitoring. The occurrence of even minor skin rashes, if not otherwise explained, should probably result in discontinuation, since serious dermatologic conditions such as Stevens-Johnson syndrome, exfoliative dermatitis, erythema multiforme, erythema nodosa, and lupus erythematosus have all been reported.

Other problems with carbamazepine include its ability to alter valproate disposition,[2] the lack of an intravenous carbamazepine preparation, which limits its usefulness, and the possibility of teratogenic effects, which has raised concern about use in pregnant women.

The role of carbamazepine in seizure treatment, while changing, continues to be very promising because of its efficacy for multiple seizure types, limited toxicity, and apparent ability to improve mood, motor function, and behavior. The latter is especially useful for institutionalized or retarded patients. Of note are reports of anticonvulsant activity of another tricyclic antidepressant (imipramine).[68]

Valproic Acid (Valproate)

Although valproic acid has been known chemically since 1881, it was not introduced in Europe as an anticonvulsant until 1963 and was not approved for anticonvulsant use in the United States until 1978. Valproic acid (2-propylvaleric dipropyl acetic acid) is a simple saturated aliphatic carboxylic acid whose mechanism of action is unknown. Many salts of the acid have been made. The sodium salt (sodium valproate) is currently marketed in the United States, but the free acid as well as the magnesium and calcium salts are also used. The preparations differ slightly in their rate and completeness of absorption and the incidence of gastrointestinal upset, but it is not clear whether or not they differ significantly in their clinical effects. A divalent sodium form, depakote, which appears to decrease intestinal upset, is also available.

A number of studies have documented the efficacy of valproic acid in most seizure types. It appears to be especially useful for absence seizures, but it is also useful for generalized tonic clonic, simple partial and complex partial, sensory, minor myoclonic, and akinetic seizures.

There is a poor relationship between drug concentration and therapeutic effect, but effective predose concentrations are said to range between 40 and 150 mg/ml. The relationship between concentration and toxicity is even less well defined, but there is some evidence that the production of hepatotoxic metabolites is dose- or concentration-dependent.

Little is known about factors that alter the concentration–response relationship. Absorption is rapid but is delayed by food. The drug is distributed in body water and is 85–95 percent bound to plasma proteins.[1,2] It is conjugated to the glucuronide in the liver and then excreted in the urine. Very little unchanged drug can be recovered. Metabolites that have been described include the di-acid (2-propy gluturic acid) and a ketone metabolite that causes a false positive urine ketone reaction.

Little is known about the effects of disease states on valproic acid kinetics or effects. Liver disease, as well as disease-related or genetically determined alterations in glucuronidation or short-chain fatty acid metabolism, might be of importance. Overdosage is associated with prolonged half-lives.[2] Wide variations in serum concentration and clearance occur with therapeutic use. Reported plasma half-lives in patients vary from 6 to 15 hours, with shorter half-lives (and more toxicity) in patients receiving multiple drugs. A prolonged half-life has been reported in a newborn.[1] Unexplained wide swings in plasma concentration occur even when the drug is given in multiple daily doses (humans) or by infusion (animals). Despite the poorly defined therapeutic ranges, drug monitoring may be useful because of the unpredictability of compliance or concentration changes with dosage adjustment, the wide range of dosages used, and the ability of other anticonvulsants to alter valproic acid clearance.

Doses must be individualized on the basis of response. It may take weeks for full effects to be seen. Doses higher than 60 mg/kg may be required, but the recommended initial dose is between 10 and 15 mg/kg, with gradual increases up to 30–45 mg/kg. It may be necessary to give multiple doses per day with food to decrease gastrointestinal side effects (nausea and vomiting).[1]

Sedation, hypersalivation, hair loss, changes in weight, pancreatitis,[69] alterations in platelet function, and fatal liver damage have been reported. Long-term experience with toxicity is lacking.[1] Dose-related teratogenic effects and testicular toxicity occur in animals.[38] Teratogenicity in humans (neural tube defects) has been documented.[1,70]

Numerous drug–drug interactions involving valproic acid have been described.[1,2,71,72] Phenytoin, phenobarbital, primidone, and carbamazepine have all been reported to shorten valproic acid half-lives.[2,3] Valproic acid also increases total phenobarbital[72] and carbamazepine concentrations. When combined with clonazepam, valproate may induce absence status.[3,73]

Future Drugs

The Food and Drug Administration (FDA) cooperated with the medical community and the pharmaceutical industry in the introduction of valproic acid. The introduction of valproic acid is only one example of the response to the growing need for sponsorship of drugs with limited markets, including new, less toxic anticonvulsants. The Epilepsy Branch of the National Institutes of Neurological Diseases and Stroke has supported the investigation of a number of promising compounds with anticonvulsant activity.[74] These efforts have produced a number of well-designed laboratory and clinical investigations. It is paradoxical that there are often more good comparative therapeutic studies on the newest agents than there are on much older compounds. There are also some good data on relative toxicity, although (as for all new drugs) long-term or delayed toxicity data will not be available for some time. Although initial studies often demonstrate efficacy for newer agents, it must be remembered that the initial enthusiasm for many drugs can fade with time, as has been seen with a number of drugs (e.g., gamma vinyl GABA, oxycarbazepine, progabide, cin-

romide). Many of these and others (e.g., flunarazine zonisamide, gabapentin, lamotrigine, Org 6370) are still being investigated or used in some countries.[74] Literally dozens of other drugs are being investigated in animal models.[75] Vigabatrin, an inhibitor of GABA transaminase recently introduced in the United Kingdom, has been hailed as the "first successful rational approach to the treatment of chronic epilepsy."[76]

DOSAGES AND REGIMENS

Most dosage regimens are empirical. The need for individualized dosing based on clinical response, toxicity, serum concentrations, and patient characteristics cannot be overemphasized. The doses, dosage frequencies, and therapeutic ranges given (see text and Table 29–1) are meant only as general guidelines. Contrary to many published guidelines, there are no absolute minimum or maximum dosages, especially where reliable therapeutic drug monitoring services (not just concentration measurements) are available. The more unusual the response or concentration on a standard regimen, the more likely it is that unusual pharmacokinetic behavior, disease processes, or patient characteristics exist. At all times, the lowest dose and dosage frquency compatible with adequate control and minimal toxicity is the ideal, if difficult, goal in therapy.

CONCLUSION

Anticonvulsant therapy is changing. Trials of old, new, and potential agents are increasingly reported. Long-neglected areas of research are becoming active. A variety of chemically unique as well as related compounds are progressing through preclinical and clinical investigation. The federal government has become increasingly active in the marketing and testing of less toxic, alternative anticonvulsants in an attempt to decrease "the drug lag" and to sponsor nonprofitable therapies. The role of the government continues to become more active at every stage of drug development, including the postmarketing phases.

The future holds promise for more rational, more effective, and less toxic anticonvulsant therapy and the possibility of more objective data on the clinical pharmacology of anticonvulsants in children.

REFERENCES

1. Levy RH, Dreifuss FE, Mattson RH, Meldrum BS, Penry JK (eds): Antiepileptic Drugs, 3rd ed. New York, Raven Press, 1989
2. Taylor WJ, Caviness MD (eds): A Textbook for the Clinical Application of Therapeutic Drug Monitoring. Abbott Laboratories, Texas, 1986
3. Morselli PL, Pippenger CE, Penry JK (eds): Antiepileptic Drug Therapy in Pediatrics. New York, Raven Press, 1983

4. Roger J, Dravet C, Bureau M, Dreifuss FE, Wolf P (eds): Epileptic Syndromes in Infancy, Childhood and Adolescence. London, John Libber, 1985

5. Behrman RE, Vaugham VC III (eds): Nelson Textbook of Pediatrics, 13th ed. Philadelphia, W. B. Saunders, 1987

6. Browne TR, Feldman RG (eds): Epilepsy Diagnosis and Management. Boston, Little, Brown and Company, 1983

7. Aicardi J (ed): The International Review of Child Neurology. Epilepsy in Children. New York, Raven Press, 1986

8. Erenberg G: Initial evaluation and management of the child with seizures. Cleveland Clinic J Med 56:S202–S205, 1989

9. Rothner AD: Not everything that shakes is epilepsy. Cleveland Clinic J Med 56:S206–S213, 1989

10. Cox S, Walson PD: Providing effective TDM services. Therapeut Drug Monitoring 11:310–322, 1989

11. Shinnar S, Berg AT, Moshe SL, Petix M, Maytal J, Kang H, Goldensohn ES, Hauser WA: Risk of seizure recurrence following a first unprovoked seizure in childhood: A prospective study. Pediatrics 85:1076–1085, 1990

12. Troupin AS, Ojelmann LM: Paradoxical intoxication: A complication of anticonvulsant administration. Epilepsia 16:753–758, 1975

13. Snead OC III, Hosey LC: Exacerbation of seizures in children by carbamazepine. N Engl J Med 313:916–921, 1985

14. Maytal J, Shinnar S, Moshe SL, Alvarez LA: Low morbidity and mortality of status epilepticus in children. Pediatrics 83:323–331, 1989

15. Verity CM: When to start anticonvulsant treatment in childhood epilepsy: The case for early treatment. Br Med J 297:1528–1530, 1988

16. Freeman JM: Status epilepticus: It is not what we thought or taught. Pediatrics 83:444–445, 1989

17. Menkes JH (ed): Textbook of Child Neurology, 3rd ed. Philadelphia, Lea & Febiger, 1985

18. Hauser WA: Should people be treated after a first seizure? Arch Neurol 43:1287–1288, 1986.

19. Hart RG, Easton JD: Seizure recurrence after a first unprovoked seizure. Arch Neurol 43:1289–1290, 1986

20. Drugs for epilepsy: Medical Letter on Drugs and Therapeutics 31(783):1–4, 1989

21. Commission on Classification and Terminology of the International League Against Epilepsy: Proposal for classification of epilepsies and epileptic syndromes. Epilepsia 26:268–278, 1985

22. Choonara IA, Rane A: Therapeutic drug monitoring of anticonvulsants state of the art. Clin Pharmacokinet 18:318–328, 1990

23. Feldman RG, Pippenger CE: The relation of anticonvulsant drug level to complete seizure control. J Clin Pharmacol 3:51–59, 1976

24. Bourgeois BFD: Problems of combination drug therapy in children. Epilepsia 29:S20–S24, 1988

25. Bourgeois BFD: The rational use of antiepileptic drugs in children. Cleveland Clinic J Med 56:S248–S253, 1989

26. Schmidt D: Reduction of two drug therapy in intractable epilepsy. Epilepsia 24:368–376, 1983

27. Theodore WH, Porter RJ: Removal of sedative-hypnotic antiepileptic drugs from the regimen of patients with intractable epilepsy. Ann Neurol 13:320–324, 1983

28. Hvidberg EF, Dam M: Clinical pharmacokinetics of anticonvulsants. Clin Pharmacokinet 1:161–188, 1976

29. Scheiner LB, Tozer TN: Clinical pharmacokinetics: The use of plasma concentrations of drugs, in Melmon KL, Morelli HF (eds): Clinical Pharmacology—Basic Principles in Therapeutics. New York, MacMillan, 1978

30. Vajda FJE, Aicardi J: Reassessment of the concept of a therapeutic range of anticonvulsant plasma levels. Dev Med Child Neurol 25:660–671, 1983

31. Reynolds EH, Shorvon SD: Monotherapy or polytherapy for epilepsy? Epilepsia 22:1–10, 1981

32. Jung D, Powell JR, Walson PD, Perrier D: Effect of dose on phenytoin absorption. Clin Pharmacol Ther 28:479–485, 1980

33. Walson PD: Bioavailability: A clinician's viewpoint, in Blanchard J, Sawchuch RJ, Brodie BB (eds): Principles and Perspectives in Drug Bioavailability. New York, S. Karger, 1979, pp 274–289

34. Richens A, Robins A (eds): Drug Treatment of Epilepsy. London, Henry Kimptom Publishers, 1976

35. Allen JP, Ludden TM, Burrow SR, Clementi WA, Stavchansky SA: Phenytoin cumulation kinetics. Clin Pharmacol Ther 26:445–448, 1979

36. Smith GA, McKauge L, Dubetz D, Tyrer JH, Eadie MJ: Factors influencing plasma concentrations of ethosuximide. Clin Pharmacokinet 4:38–52, 1979

37. Janz D, Meinardi H, Sherwin: Clinical Pharmacology of Anti-Epileptic Drugs. New York, Springer-Verlag, 1975

38. Pippenger CE, Penry JK, White BG, et al: Interlaboratory variability in determination of plasma antiepileptic drug concentrations. Arch Neurol 33:351–355, 1976

39. Pippenger CE, Paris-Kutt H, Penry JK, Daly DD: Antiepileptic drug level quality control program: Interlaboratory variability, in Pippenger CE, Penry JK, Kutt H (eds): Antiepileptic Drugs: Qualitative Analysis and Interpretation. New York, Raven Press, 1978, pp 187–197

40. Walson PD, Mimaki T, Curless R, Mayersohn M, Perrier D: Once daily doses of phenobarbital in children. J Pediatr 97:303–305, 1980

41. Trimble MR, Cull C: Children of school age: The influence of antiepileptic drugs on behavior and intellect. Epilepsia 29:S15–S19, 1988

42. Brent DA, Crumrine PK, Varma R, Brown RV, Allan MJ: Phenobarbital treatment and major depressive disorder in children with epilepsy: A naturalistic follow-up. Pediatrics 85:1086–1091, 1990

43. Herranz JL, Armijo JA, Artega R: Clinical side effects of phenobarbital, primidone, phenytoin, carbamazepine, and valproate during monotherapy in children. Epilepsia 29:794–804, 1988

44. Farwell JR, Lee YJ, Hirtz DG, Sulzbacher SI, Ellenberg JH, Nelson KB: Phenobarbital for febrile seizures—effects on intelligence and on seizure recurrence. N Engl J Med 322:364–369, 1990

45. Buchthal F, Svensmark O, Schiller PJ: Clinical and electroencephalographic correlations with serum levels of diphenylhydantoin. Arch Neurol 2:624–630, 1960

46. Kutt H, McDowell F: Management of epilepsy with diphenylhydantoin sodium. JAMA 203:969–972, 1968

47. Haerer AF, Grace JB: Studies of anticonvulsant levels in epileptics. Acta Neurol Scand 45:18–31, 1969

48. Travers RD, Reynolds EH, Gallagher BB: Variation in response to anticonvulsants in a group of epileptic patients. Arch Neurol 27:29, 1972

49. Lund L: Anticonvulsant effects of diphenylhydantoin relative to plasma levels. A prospective 3 year study in ambulant patients with generalized epileptic seizures. Arch Neurol 31:289–294, 1974

50. Schmidt D, Einicke I, Haenel F: The influence of seizure type on the efficacy of plasma concentrations of phenytoin, phenobarbital and carbamazepine. Arch Neurol 43:263–265, 1986

51. Cobos JE: High-dose phenytoin in the treatment of refractory epilepsy. Epilepsia 28:111–114, 1987

52. Melikian AP, Straughn AB, Slywka GWA, Whyatt PL, Meyer MC: Bioavailability of 11 phenytoin products. J Pharmacokinet Biopharm 5:133–146, 1977

53. Curless RG, Walson PD, Carter DE: Phenytoin kinetics in children. Neurology 26:715–725, 1976

54. Borofsky LG, Louis S, Kutt H, Roginsky M: Diphenylhydantoin: Efficacy, toxicity and dose-serum level relationships in children. J Pediatr 81:995–1002, 1972

55. Norell E, Lilienberg G, Gamstorp I: Systematic determination of the serum phenytoin level as an aid in the management of children with epilepsy. Eur Neurol 13:232–244, 1975

56. Yuen G, Patimer PT, Littlefield LC, Mackey RW: Phenytoin dosage predictions in paediatric patients. Clin Pharmacokinet 16:254–260, 1989

57. Kutt H, Winters W, Kohenge R, McDowell F: Diphenylhydantoin metabolism, blood levels, and toxicity. Arch Neurol 11:642–648, 1964

58. Reynolds EH: Chronic antiepileptic toxicity: A review. Epilepsia 16:319–352, 1975

59. Solomon GE, Hilgartner MW, Kutt H: Coagulation defects caused by diphenylhydantoin. Neurology 22:1165–1171, 1972

60. Janz D: The teratogenic risk of antiepileptic drugs. Epilepsia 16:159–169, 1975

61. Frey HH, Schulz R: Time course of the demethylation of trimethadione. Acta Pharmacol Toxicol 28:477–483, 1970
62. Miles MV, Tennison MB, Greenwood RS: Pharmacokinetics of N-desmethylmethsuximide in pediatric patients. J Pediatr 144:647–650, 1989
63. Porter RJ, Penry JK, Lacy JR, Newmark ME, Kupferberg HJ: Plasma concentrations of phensuximide, methsuximide and their metabolites in relation to clinical efficacy. Neurology 29:1509–1513, 1979
64. Lorentz de Haas AM, Kuilman M: Ethosuximide and grand mal. Epilepsia 5:90–96, 1964
65. Durelli L, Massazza U, Cavallo R: Carbamazepine toxicity and poisoning: Incidence, clinical features and management. Med Toxicol Adverse Drug Exp 4:95–107, 1989
66. O'Dougherty M, Wright FS, Cox, S, Walson PD: Carbamazepine plasma concentration. Relationship to cognitive impairment. Arch Neurol 44:863–867, 1987
67. Gillham RA, Williams N, Wiedmann K, Butler E, Larkin JG, Brodie MJ: Concentration–effect relationships with carbamazepine and its epoxide on psychomotor and cognitive function in epileptic patients. J Neurol Neurosurg Psychiatr 51:929–933, 1988
68. Fromm GH, Wessel HB, Glass JD, et al: Imipramine in absence and myoclonic seizure. Neurology 28:953–967, 1978
69. Wyllie E, Wyllie R, Cruse RP, Erenberg G, Rothner AD: Pancreatitis associated with valproic acid therapy. Am J Dis Child 138:912–914, 1984
70. Lindhout D, Meinardi H: Spina bifida and in-utero exposure to valproate. Lancet 2:396, 1984
71. Levy RH, Koch KM: Drug interaction with VPA. Drugs 24:543–556, 1982
72. Wilder BJ, Willmore LJ, Bruni J, Villarreal HJ: Valproic acid: Interaction with other anticonvulsant drugs. Neurology 28:892–896, 1978
73. Jeavons PM, Clark JE, Maheshwari M: Treatment of generalized epilepsies of childhood and adolescence with sodium valproate (Epilim). Dev Med Child Neurol 19:9–25, 1977
74. Porter RJ: New antiepileptic drugs. Cleveland Clinic J Med 56:S260–265, 1989
75. Loscher W, Schmidt D: Which animal models should be used in the search for new antiepileptic drugs? A proposal based on experimental and clinical considerations. Epilepsy Res 2:145–181, 1988
76. Reynolds EH: Vigabatrin: Rational treatment for chronic epilepsy. Br Med J 300:277–278, 1990
77. Ohtahara S: The classification of epilepsy and antiepileptic drug therapy. Adv Pediatr Neurol 15:77–93, 1986
78. Takizawa K, Mimaki T, Yabuuchi H, Yamatodani A: Relationship between serum levels and daily dose of phenobarbital in children. Jpn Pediatr Practice 48:459–464, 1985
79. Nishihara K, Kohda Y, Saitoh Y, Nakagawa F, Tamura Z, Hosaka A, Ishikawa N: Dose-dependence of plasma phenytoin concentration in children. Igaku-No-Ayumi 107:512–515, 1978
80. Honda H, Nishihara K, Saitoh H, Kohda Y: Combined use of phenytoin and phenobarbital. Proposal of a therapeutic concentration zone. Brain & Develop (Domestic Ed) 12:140–147, 1980

30
ANTIHISTAMINES

C. WARREN BIERMAN, F. ESTELLE R. SIMONS, *and* KEITH J. SIMONS

A knowledge of the role of histamine in health and disease is essential for the understanding of agents that compete with histamine for receptors. In this chapter the initial focus will be on various aspects of histamine, including synthesis, metabolism, function as a regulator of homeostasis in health, role in inflammation and immediate hypersensitivity, mechanisms that control histamine secretion, and ways that this control can be modified *in vitro*. Next, histamine receptors and their various functions in humans will be discussed. H_1-receptor antagonists will be discussed in greater depth than H_2-receptor antagonists. Recently described H_3 receptors, agonists, and antagonists will be discussed only briefly, as their potential clinical importance is unknown at present.

HISTORY

Histamine was the first of a series of amines released during inflammation to be identified, synthesized, and studied. In 1907 Vogt synthesized histamine chemically. Barger and Dale[1] in 1910 found that it caused isolated guinea pig ileum to constrict. In the same year, it was identified as a uterine stimulant in extracts of ergot. Bacteria were found to be capable of synthesizing it by decarboxylation of an α-histadine. From 1911 to 1919 in a series of experiments, Dale and Laidlaw[2] found that histamine induced a shock-like syndrome when injected into frogs and mammals. Histamine also caused bronchoconstriction, especially in the guinea pig, cardiac and pulmonary artery constriction, and stimulation of cardiac contraction. It caused generalized capillary dilation that resulted in a pooling of blood in the capillary bed, a fall in systemic blood pressure, and a substantial loss of plasma through capillary endothelium, with the result that the animal developed hemoconcentration, increased blood viscosity, and a fall in body temperature.

Lewis[3] in 1927 described the triple response of the skin

consisting of erythema followed by a wheal-and-flare formation in response to trauma. The cutaneous vascular changes of redness and wheal were caused by histamine released from endogenous stores by pressure, while the flare was the result of a local histamine-induced axon reflex.

In 1937 Bonet and Straub[4] discovered a group of phenolic ethers that could block the effects of histamine. 929F, the first compound studied, could protect guinea pigs from histamine-induced anaphylaxis, but its toxicity precluded its use. A second compound, 1571F (1939), had greater antihistamine properties, but it also was toxic. In 1942 Halpern[5] developed Antergan in France, the first antihistamine to undergo clinical trials in humans (1944). Bonet[6] introduced Neo-Antergan, a drug even more potent and less toxic.

Meanwhile, because of World War II, American studies proceeded independently of the European work. In 1945 Loew[7] developed diphenhydramine, while Yonkman and coworkers[8] developed tripelennamine, both of which are still in clinical use. Thereafter, scores of additional drugs were developed.

Riley[9] discovered in 1952 that the mast cell was a major source of histamine. In 1953 Riley described two distinct cell types: elongated, densely staining ovoid cells embedded in adventitia close to small blood vessels (type I) and larger, regularly shaped cells scattered around capillaries and in interstices away from blood vessels (type II). Certain organic bases—stilbamidine, propamidine, and compound 48/80—produced histamine-like changes when injected subcutaneously in humans. When injected intravenously in the cat or dog, they induced liberation of large quantities of histamine into the circulation and induced specific changes in these cell types. The type II cells showed degranulation and vacuolation, though the type I cells had fewer changes. Riley and West[10] showed a correlation between the number of mast cells and the histamine content in a variety of tissues, including mast cell tumors in animals and solitary urticaria pigmentosa lesions in humans. In blood they found histamine exclu-

303

sively in basophils, except in the rabbit where they identified it in platelets.

In 1953 Mongar and Schild[11] published the first of a series of studies concerning the mechanism of histamine secretion from mast cells. Subsequent studies, such as those of Foreman,[12] focused on the role of calcium and on histamine release by antigen and other ligands.

In 1966 Ash and Schild[13] proposed the name H_1 for receptors blocked by known antihistamines. Actions of histamine such as stimulation of gastric secretion, inhibition of rat uterine contraction, and stimulation of isolated atria not blocked by these drugs are mediated through a second group of receptors now known as H_2 receptors.

In 1972 Black and coworkers[14] confirmed the existence of the H_2 receptor by synthesizing a group of drugs that specifically blocked them. This has led to the development of H_2-antagonist drugs now in widespread use in the treatment of gastric acid hypersecretory states in adults. These will be discussed later.

Histamine H_3 receptors and their specific agonists and antagonists were identified by Arrang and coworkers[31] in 1987. By using ^{3}H-labeled probes, they showed reversible binding of these agents to sites in the cerebral cortex of both animal and human brain as well as in membranes of guinea pig lung. They speculate that the H_3 receptors may control mast cell histamine formation and, possibly, release. Whether H_3-receptor antagonists will have clinical relevance must await further studies.

Synthesis and Metabolism of Histamine

Figure 30-1 shows the pathways for synthesis and metabolism of histamine worked out largely by Schayer.[15] Histamine is formed by decarboxylation of L-histidine by a highly specific enzyme, L-histamine decarboxylase. Though specific inhibitors of this enzyme have been found, they are not in clinical use. Histamine is stored in mast cell granules, where turnover is slow, as well as in gastric tissues, where turnover is more rapid. Histamine is metabolized by two routes: by methylation to methylhistamine and by deamination.

Most, if not all, tissues have the capacity to degrade histamine. In humans only a small percentage of labeled histamine appears unchanged in the urine. Blockade of one pathway shifts the metabolism to the alternate pathway.

FUNCTION OF HISTAMINE IN HEALTH AND DISEASE

Histamine appears to be important in homeostasis. Its actions range from local and systemic cardiovascular effects[2] to regulating the microcirculation,[15] mediating gastric secretion, and acting as a neurotransmitter in the central nervous system. In disease, histamine release is associated with tissue injury, inflammation, and immediate and late-phase hypersensitivity reactions.[16]

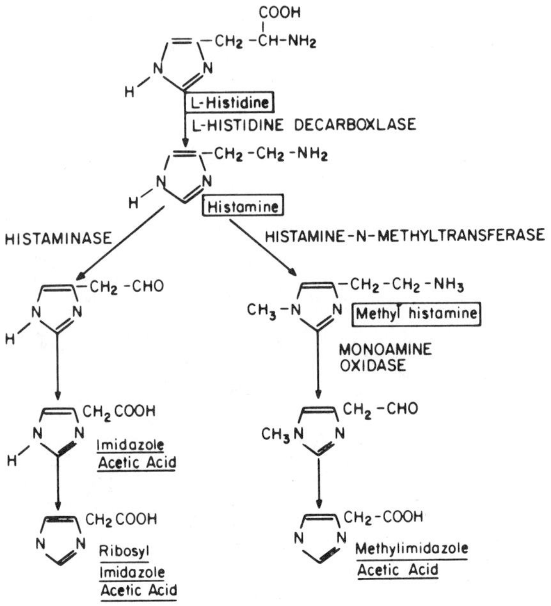

FIGURE 30-1. Pathways of synthesis and metabolism of histamine.

Cardiovascular Effects

Histamine has been reported to have a variety of different actions in the cardiovascular system.[17] Some of these actions appear to be contradictory, depending on the experimental conditions and the mammalian species. In humans intravenous histamine has been reported both to raise and to lower blood pressure. Small doses increase coronary blood flow, while larger doses may decrease it.

In general, histamine appears to dilate postcapillary venules, while it contracts larger microvessels and large blood vessels. Histamine can induce changes in the permeability of the microvascular wall in all areas of the mammalian circulation, acting selectively on the venular side of the microcirculatory bed. It is possible that histamine increases molecular transport both by increasing the number of available pores or endothelial gaps and by enhancing the rate of vesicular transport.[18]

Regulation of the Microcirculation

The regulation of the microcirculation within tissues appears to be mediated by interaction of blood-borne substances and nervous stimuli. Schayer[19] has proposed that histamine is synthesized continually in the small blood vessels, so-called nascent histamine, where its accumulation and washout could then account for spontaneous opening and closing of these vessels in the vascular bed. There is no direct evidence for this hypothesis. Whether histamine has any physiologic role in the regulation of the microcirculation[20] is still controversial.

Increased synthesis also occurs in rapidly growing fetal tissue and in tissues undergoing repairs, such as granulation tissue, regenerating liver tissue, and some tumor tissue.[21]

Regulation of Gastric Secretion

MacIntosh[22] in 1938 showed that histamine was released from the stomach during vagal stimulation. Only with the development of H_2 antagonists was the importance of histamine for gastric secretion proven. Histamine itself acts directly on the parietal cells through H_2 receptors that are apparently linked to adenylate cyclase to activate a proton pump. Gastrin and acetylcholine also stimulate these parietal cells directly through separate receptors, though histamine may play a role in this process.

Histamine in the Central Nervous System

Histamine, histidine decarboxylase, and histamine N-methyltransferase have been found in relatively high concentration in the hypothalmus and are present in the midbrain, cortex, and cerebellum of the rat, mouse, and monkey.[23] Here histamine is not associated with mast cells and has a relatively high turnover rate that is increased by stress and decreased by anesthesia. It increases adenylate cyclase activity selectively in the hypothalmus. The exact function of histamine in the brain and its role in neurotransmission is not clear. With the identification of an H_3-receptor agonist and antagonists, rapid advances in this area can be anticipated.

Role in Inflammation and Allergy

Histamine is released from mast cells or basophils in humans by conditions such as trauma, burns, infections, and allergy. Symptoms in patients with atopic diseases such as anaphylaxis, urticaria, allergic rhinitis, asthma, and atopic dermatitis are partially mediated by histamine.

The plasma membrane of both mast cells and basophils possesses unique high-affinity receptors[24] for the Fc portion of immunoglobulin E (IgE). In the presence of specific antigen, bridging of IgE molecules occurs with resulting cell activation. Upon activation, mast cells and basophils release preformed mediators from their secretory granules into the extracellular environment and generate *de novo* lipid metabolites from the cell membranes.[25] Mast cells are the chief source of histamine in tissues, and basophils are the chief source of histamine among circulating cells. Histamine in the granule is ionically bound to acidic groups in a heparin–protease matrix. Upon release of the granule contents, the histamine becomes freely soluble. Elevated plasma histamine levels are present in patients experiencing anaphylaxis, in patients with mastocytosis, and in patients with antigen-induced bronchial asthma.[26] Though histamine was the first mediator of inflammation identified, numerous other mediators have now been found either preformed in the granules or newly formed from the cell membrane, as noted in Table 30–1.

These substances are all involved actively in allergic inflammatory reactions. Mast-cell degranulation results in the influx of inflammatory cells such as eosinophils,

TABLE 30–1. INFLAMMATORY MAST-CELL-DERIVED MEDIATORS

SUBSTANCE	BIOLOGIC ACTIVITY
Preformed in granule	
Histamine	Vasodilation, vasopermeability, pruritus, bronchoconstriction
Proteases	Degradation of blood vessel basement membrane, generation of vasoactive complement and angiotensin metabolites
Heparin	Formation of complexes with proteases
Eosinophil chemotactic factor	Eosinophil chemotaxis
Neutrophil chemotactic factor	Neutrophil chemotaxis
Newly formed from membrane	
Prostaglandin D_2	Vasopermeability, bronchoconstriction
Leukotrienes C_4, D_4, E_4	Vasopermeability, bronchoconstriction
Platelet-activating factor	Aggregation of platelets, vasopermeability, bronchoconstriction, chemotaxis

Modified from Serafin and Austin,[26] with permission.

neutrophils, and lymphocytes through the action of a variety of chemotactic factors derived from membrane. The activated human lung mast cell makes both prostaglandin D_2 and sulfidopeptide leukotrienes, whereas basophils synthesize only leukotrienes.[27] Prostaglandin D_2 when injected into the skin induces a wheal-and-flare reaction similar to histamine and when inhaled produces bronchoconstriction 10 times greater than histamine.[28] Leukotrienes C_4, D_4, and E_4 induce wheal-and-flare reactions when injected in a dosage of 1 nmol and induce bronchospasm when inhaled. Platelet-activating factor causes a wheal-and-flare response in a dosage of 0.2 nmol and severe bronchospasm when administered by aerosol to baboons, an activity 1000 times greater than histamine.[29] Thus it would appear that the release of histamine sets the stage for formation and release of a cascade of progressively more potent chemical mediators leading to tissue inflammation.

Other Factors Affecting Histamine Secretion

Drugs can induce histamine release either by an immunologic mechanism, as with penicillin allergy (anaphylactic reaction), or directly, by such drugs as curare or opiates, by an unknown mechanism (anaphylactoid reaction).

Other factors affecting histamine release include extracellular calcium ions, pH, and cyclic AMP. If calcium-binding sites are occupied by lanthanum, then histamine release is inhibited; if calcium is carried into the mast cell by treatment with ionophore A 23187, histamine release is enhanced. The interaction between hydrogen and calcium ions in histamine secretion may be related to transmembrane H^+ movement or may reflect ionization of molecules involved in calcium transport. Cyclic AMP appears to have a physiologic role in controlling histamine release by limiting calcium entry into the cell.[30]

HISTAMINE RECEPTORS

The name H_1 *receptor* was proposed by Ash and Schild[13] for receptors blocked by known antihistamines. They presented evidence that the actions of histamine not blocked by these drugs were mediated through a second type of receptor. Black[14] proposed the term H_2 *receptor* to describe those receptors blocked by a new series of antagonists. These two types of receptors could be distinguished by 2-methylhistamine, which was an exclusive agonist for H_1 receptors, and 4-methylhistamine, which was an agonist mainly for H_2 receptors. To date H_3 receptors have been identified only in the brain and lung.[31] Their function has yet to be identified. Table 30–2 shows the effects of H_1-, H_2-, and H_3-receptor stimulation. In many tissues only H_1 or H_2 receptors are present; in some both are present and act synergistically.

Histamine Receptors in the Cardiovascular System

In the vascular tree both H_1- and H_2-receptor stimulation elicits vasodilation. H_1 receptors, however, have a high affinity for histamine and mediate only a short-lived response. H_2 receptors, by contrast, induce dilation that develops more slowly but is sustained. In capillaries H_1 receptors promote permeability, while the role of H_2 receptors, if any, is slight. In the heart histamine increases the force of contraction and speeds heart rate. Virtually all of these effects appear to be due to H_2 receptors. The net effect of these actions is to induce a fall in blood pressure in which both H_1 and H_2 receptors participate.[32]

Histamine Receptors in the Lung

Histamine is important in asthma. H_1-receptor stimulation decreases airway caliber by contracting bronchial smooth muscle, augmenting intraluminal serous fluid, and increasing capillary permeability resulting in mucosal edema. H_2-receptor stimulation might decrease airway caliber by augmenting intraluminal mucus but might increase airway caliber by relaxing smooth muscle. Thus H_2-receptor stimulation might have a variable effect on airway obstruction, whereas H_1-receptor stimulation clearly contributes to airway constriction.[33] H_3-receptor stimulation inhibits acetylcholine release from vagal nerves in human airways, inhibits neurogenic microvascular leakage in the airways, and may play some defense role against excess bronchoconstriction.

H_1-RECEPTOR ANTAGONISTS

Preclinical Pharmacology and Classification

Most compounds that, at low concentrations, are pharmacologic antagonists of histamine at H_1-receptor sites may be described by the general structure (I) where Ar is aryl (including phenyl) and Ar^1 is arylmethyl (Ar CH_2) or a second aryl group.

$$Ar \diagdown$$
$$x—C—C—N$$
$$Ar^1 \diagup$$

-aminoethyl

(I)

$$Ar \diagup$$
$$x—C—C—N$$
$$Ar \diagdown$$

(II)

Tricyclic derivatives (II) in which the two aromatic rings are bridged have essentially the same general structure. Most H_1 antagonists have structures that comprise a double-aromatic unit linked by a two- or three-atom chain to a tertiary amino basic group. Histamine itself is a molecule of similar structure but differs from its antagonists in possessing only a single aromatic (imidazole) feature and in being levorotatory whereas antagonists are dextrorotatory. Most antihistamines are chemically stable, water-soluble salts.

H_1-receptor antagonists have been traditionally classified according to their chemical structures into groups: ethanolamines, ethylene diamines, aklylamines, piperazines, piperidines, and phenothiazines.[34] Although this classification has some usefulness, drugs within each group vary considerably in their antihistaminic potency and adverse effects, and many of the second-generation nonsedating H_1-receptor antagonists do not fit readily into the traditional classification system.

H_1-receptor antagonists, at low concentrations, are reversible competitive inhibitors of the actions of hista-

TABLE 30–2. ACTIVITY OF THE HISTAMINE RECEPTORS IN VARIOUS TISSUES

	H_1	H_2	H_3
Hypotension	+ + +	+	—
Skin			
Erythema	+ + +	—	—
Edema	—	+ + +	—
Gastric secretion	—	+ + +	—
Bronchoconstriction	+ + +	±	?
Contraction of GI smooth muscle	+ + +	—	—
Dilation of microblood vessels < 80μm in diameter	+ + + +	+ +	—
Nasal mucosal edema	+ + +	—	—
CNS effects	—	—	+ + + +

+ + + + = strong effect; + + + = moderate effect; + + = mild effect; + = slight effect; — = no effect.

mine. They block histamine from entering into a relationship with H_1 receptors in the mucous glands of the nasal mucosa, the itch receptors of the nasal mucosa and skin, and the smooth muscle of the gastrointestinal and respiratory tracts. They antagonize the action of histamine on the capillaries, resulting in reduced capillary permeability and reduced edema and wheal formation. In larger blood vessels, they partially inhibit the vasodilator effect of histamine; residual vasodilation reflects the involvement of H_2-receptor antagonists. Unlike H_2 antagonists, H_1-receptor antagonists do not inhibit gastric secretion, however.

In addition to being pharmacologic antagonists of histamine, many H_1-receptor antagonists also prevent release of inflammatory mediators from sensitized mast cells and basophils[35]; some, such as cetirizine, also have an anti-inflammatory effect. First-generation H_1-receptor antagonists may possess weak anticholinergic effects and suppress salivary and lacrimal secretions. Other first-generation H_1-receptor antagonists, such as promethazine, possess α-adrenergic blocking ability. In concentrations higher than required to antagonize histamine, some H_1-receptor antagonists possess local anesthetic effects. Some, such as cyproheptadine, are effective inhibitors of both histamine and 5-hydroxytryptamine activity.

First-generation H_1-receptor antagonists cross the blood–brain barrier and cause a variety of unwanted central nervous system effects. Some useful central nervous system effects are also found, for example, the ability of dimenhydrinate and diphenhydramine to combat motion sickness and the usefulness of diphenhydramine in decreasing rigidity and improving voluntary movement in patients with drug-induced extrapyramidal symptoms and other neurologic disorders. The second-generation H_1-receptor antagonists, such as terfenadine, astemizole, loratadine, and cetirizine, are relatively lipophobic and do not cross the blood–brain barrier.

Pharmacokinetics and Pharmacodynamics of H_1-Receptor Antagonists

H_1-receptor antagonists are reasonably well absorbed when administered by mouth, with peak serum concentrations being reached approximately 2 hours after dosing. All the first-generation H_1-receptor antagonists and most of the the second-generation H_1-receptor antagonists are metabolized by the hepatic cytochrome P-450 system. Clearance rates and serum elimination half-life values are extremely variable (Table 30–3), with half-life values in adults ranging from 24 hours or less for chlorpheniramine, diphenhydramine, hydroxyzine, terfenadine, and loratadine to 9.5 days for astemizole and its active metabolites.[36-58] Volumes of distribution tend to be large and are usually not corrected for bioavailability because intravenous formulations are generally unavailable for comparison with oral formulations.

Children have shorter elimination half-life values for H_1-receptor antagonists than do adults (Figure 30–2) (Table 30–3).[38,40,44,47,50] The elimination half-life of an H_1-receptor antagonist increases with increasing age of the patients (Figure 30–3).[36-38,40-48,50-55,57,58] The serum elim-

TABLE 30–3. PHARMACOKINETICS AND PHARMACODYNAMICS OF H_1-RECEPTOR ANTAGONISTS

H_1-RECEPTOR ANTAGONIST	B-PHASE SERUM ELIMINATION HALF-LIFE (h)	SIGNIFICANT WHEAL SUPPRESSION (h)*
Chlorpheniramine	24.4 (11.0)†	24
Brompheniramine	24.9	3–9
Triprolidine	2.0	—
Hydroxyzine	20.0 (7.1)†	2–36
Cetirizine	8.0–9.0 (7.0)†	24
Loratadine	11.0	24
Terfenadine‡	17.0	12–24
Astemizole	9.5 days§	0 (single dose); weeks (short course)

†Serum elimination half-life value in children.
‡Terfenadine metabolite I.
*Dose-dependent; see specific references on page 308 for doses used.
§Includes $t_{1/2}$ of hydroxylated metabolites.

ination half-life of H_1-receptor antagonists is prolonged in patients with hepatic dysfunction.[56]

Cetirizine, the relatively nonsedating carboxylic acid metabolite of hydroxyzine, has unique pharmacokinetic properties. Unlike other H_1-receptor antagonists, it is not metabolized by the hepatic cytochrome system; rather, 70 percent of a dose of cetirizine appears as unchanged drug in the urine within 72 hours.[47,57] In adults, it has a serum elimination half-life value of 8–9 hours, except in patients with renal failure, in whom the half-life value may be 18 hours.[58]

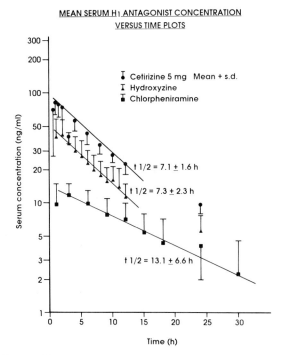

FIGURE 30–2. Mean serum elimination half-life values for H_1-receptor antagonists are shorter in children than they are in adults; for example, for cetirizine 7.1 h (8.0–9.0 h in adults) hydroxyzine 7.3 h (14.1–20.0 h in adults) and chlorpheniramine 13.1 h (21.0–24.4 h in adults). (From Simmons et al.)[40,44,47]

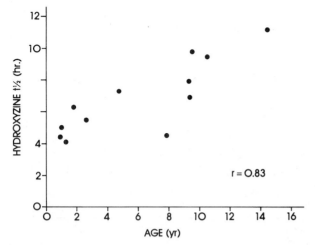

FIGURE 30–3. Hydroxyzine serum elimination half-life versus age in 12 patients aged 1–14 years, $r = .83$. (From Simons et al.,[44] with permission.)

Breast milk concentration versus time curves parallel serum concentration versus time curves in single-dose studies of H_1-receptor antagonists.[59]

Maximum antihistaminic effects of the H_1-receptor antagonists occur several hours after peak serum concentrations have passed (Figures 30–4 and 30–5) and persist even when serum concentrations of the parent compound have declined to the lowest limits of analytic detection, probably because of the presence of active metabolites. H_1-receptor antagonists should therefore be given *before* an anticipated allergic reaction, if possible, in order to achieve maximum efficacy. The duration of action of these drugs, as assessed by suppression of the histamine-

induced wheal and flare in the skin or by suppression of symptoms, is much more prolonged than might be expected from consideration of the serum elimination half-life values (Figure 30–4 and 30–5; Table 30–3).[39,40,43–45,47,49–51,54–56,60] H_1-receptor antagonists reduce the wheal-and-flare response to histamine and to allergens and must therefore be discontinued days or, in the case of astemizole, weeks before diagnostic skin testing.

Traditionally, first-generation H_1-receptor antagonists were usually administered three or four times daily, but this type of dosage regimen, or use of sustained-action formulations, may be unnecessary for many of these medications, at least in adults.[36,37,39,42,45,51,61] Terfenadine is generally administered in a dose of 60 mg every 12 hours, but 120 mg every 24 hours is just as effective.[62] Astemizole is generally administered in a dose of 10 mg daily; a short course of astemizole may suppress the histamine-induced wheal and flare for weeks.[63] Loratadine 10 mg daily significantly suppresses the histamine-induced wheal and flare for 12–24 hours. Cetirizine 10 mg once daily suppresses the histamine-induced wheal and flare for 24 hours.

Subsensitivity

Chronic administration of first-generation H_1-receptor antagonists may be associated with an *apparent* decrease in efficacy over weeks or months.[64–68] This has been attributed to autoinduction of hepatic metabolism and shortening of half-life values, based on limited data obtained in dogs administered diphenhydramine or chlorcyclizine by mouth for several weeks.[69] In a more recent study, however, dogs administered hydroxyzine daily for 150 days, intramuscularly to ensure compliance, have had somewhat higher mean serum hydroxyzine concentrations at the end of the treatment course than on the first day of treatment, and significantly longer mean

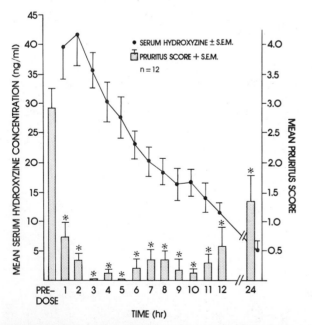

FIGURE 30–4. Serum hydroxyzine concentration versus time curve and suppressive effect of hydroxyzine on pruritus in children with severe atopic dermatitis. (From Simons et al.,[44] with permission.)

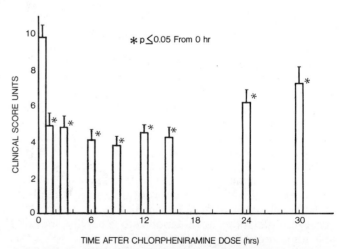

FIGURE 30–5. Suppression of the clinical score for rhinitis symptoms in children following a single dose of chlorpheniramine. Significant suppression of symptoms occurred for 30 hours. (From Simons et al.,[40] with permission.)

serum half-life values on days 30, 60, and 120 than on day 1.[70]

Furthermore, humans do not eliminate chlorpheniramine or terfenadine more rapidly during long-term chronic dosing than during short-term dosing. The efficacy of chlorpheniramine, loratadine, terfenadine, or cetirizine in suppressing the histamine-induced wheal and flare does not diminish over 4–8 weeks in studies in which compliance has been monitored rigorously (Figure 30–6a and b).[47,55,68,71] Additional studies of the "subsensitivity" phenomenon in humans are necessary in view of the long-term treatment often required with H_1-receptor antagonists.

Interactions with Other Medications

The first-generation H_1-receptor antagonists interact adversely with ethanol and diazepam and enhance the adverse psychomotor effects of these compounds.[72] The second-generation H_1-receptor antagonists terfenadine, astemizole, loratadine, and cetirizine do not interact with or potentiate the effects of ethanol.[72-75] Terfenadine does not interact with theophylline.[76]

Adverse Effects

Considering the enormous amounts of H_1-receptor antagonists used, with and without physician supervision, singly and in combination with a variety of other drugs, severe toxic reactions are uncommon, attesting to the relative safety of this class of drugs. First-generation H_1-receptor antagonists may cause sedation, impairment of cognitive function, diminished alertness, slowed reaction times, confusion, dizziness, tinnitus, and anticholinergic effects such as dry mouth, blurred vision, and urinary retention. Others, such as tripelennamine, are prone to cause adverse effects in the gastrointestinal tract, including anorexia, nausea, vomiting, epigastric distress, diarrhea, and constipation. Some of these symptoms, particularly central nervous system suppression, correlate with peak serum concentrations. Elderly patients[54] and patients with hepatic dysfunction[56] are particularly prone to these adverse effects. Ingestion of large doses of the second-generation H_1-receptor antagonists terfenadine, astemizole, loratadine, and cetirizine has not been reported to cause sedation.

Less common adverse effects have been recognized,[43] such as facial dyskinesia or the excitation experienced by young children and infants after ordinary therapeutic doses of first-generation H_1-receptor antagonists. A neonatal withdrawal syndrome has been described in infants born to mothers receiving large therapeutic doses of hydroxyzine before parturition. Some H_1 blockers, such as cyproheptadine and astemizole, cause appetite stimulation and inappropriate weight gain. A few patients on terfenadine or astemizole, most of whom admitted to taking a massive overdose, have had torsade de pointes, syncope, and cardiac arrest.[77,78] Although teratogenic effects

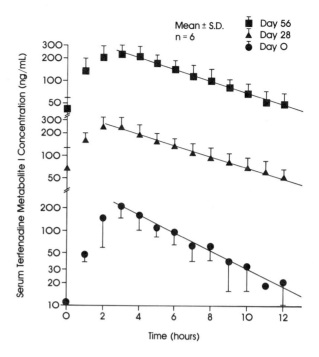

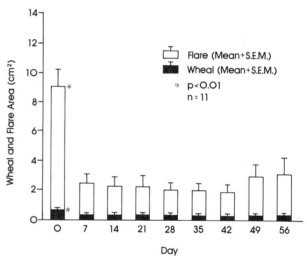

FIGURE 30–6(a). Lack of change in pharmacokinetics of terfenadine metabolite I before and during the 6 days of treatment with terfenadine 60 mg b.i.d. in adults. **(b).** Lack of subsensitivity to terfenadine as evidenced by continued suppression of the histamine-induced wheal and flare. Tests were performed every 7 days for 56 days. (From Simons et al.,[55] with permission.)

of piperazine compounds have been noted in animals,[79] fetal anomalies in humans have not been proven to be due to any H_1-receptor antagonist.

Allergic Disorders in Which H_1-Receptor Antagonists May be Useful

H_1-receptor antagonists provide relief of symptoms in patients with allergic rhinitis and/or allergic conjunctivitis; allergic skin disorders such as atopic dermatitis, urticaria, and dermographism; asthma; and anaphylaxis. Their use in otitis media with effusion or in upper respiratory infections is controversial, although widespread. Formulations and recommended dosages of representative H_1-receptor antagonists are listed in Table 30–4.

Allergic Rhinitis

H_1-receptor antagonists are effective in the management of seasonal and perennial allergic rhinitis symptoms such as rhinorrhea, nasal itching, and sneezing. None of the H_1-receptor antagonists, including the new, relatively nonsedating medications, prevent nasal blockage in antigen challenge tests, and none relieve nasal blockage as well as they prevent and relieve rhinorrhea, itching, and sneezing. Addition of an α-adrenergic agent such as pseudoephedrine to an H_1-receptor antagonist significantly improves relief of nasal congestion compared to the relief of congestion achieved by the H_1-receptor antagonist alone.[80,81]

In prospective, double-blind studies of the efficacy of the new H_1-receptor antagonists, most of which have been performed in adults, the medications have been found to be superior to placebo and comparable to chlorpheniramine in relieving the symptoms of nasal discharge, itching, and sneezing. In children weighing greater than 35 kg, terfenadine 60 mg twice daily is superior in efficacy to placebo (Figure 30–7).[82] In adults, in most but not all studies, terfenadine 60 mg twice daily is equal in efficacy to chlorpheniramine 8 mg twice daily, loratadine 10 or 40 mg daily, and mequitazine 5 mg twice daily.[83–90] Astemizole 10 mg daily is more potent than placebo or than pheniramine or chlorpheniramine, and as potent or more potent than terfenadine 60 mg twice daily.[87,91–94] Astemizole has a longer lag time to peak onset of action than any other H_1-receptor antagonist and is not suited for sporadic use. For optimal effectiveness of astemizole, either a loading dose of 30 mg daily should be given in the first week of treatment,[95] or astemizole treatment should be started well in advance of the peak pollen season in patients with chronic allergic rhinitis.[87,92] Loratadine 10 mg once daily is superior to placebo and equal in efficacy to chlorpheniramine twice daily and terfenadine 60 mg twice daily. Loratadine 10 mg once daily is also equal in efficacy to clemastine 1 mg twice daily and mequitazine 5

TABLE 30–4. FIRST GENERATION H₁ ANTIHISTAMINES

GENERIC NAME	PROPRIETARY NAME	FORMULATION	CHILDREN'S DOSE	ADULT DOSE
First Generation				
Azatadine maleate	Optimine	Tablet 1 mg	0.5–1 mg b.i.d.	1 mg b.i.d.
Brompheniramine maleate	Dimetane	Syrup 2 mg/5 ml Tablets 4 mg Time-release 8, 12 mg	0.35 mg/kg/24h	8–12 mg b.i.d.
Chlorpheniramine maleate	Chlortrimeton	Syrup 2.5 mg/5 ml Tablets 4 mg Time-release 8, 12 mg Parenteral solution 10 mg/ml	0.35 mg/kg/24h	8–12 mg b.i.d.
Cyproheptadine hydrochloride	Periactin	Syrup 2 mg/5 ml Tablets 4 mg	0.25 mg/kg/24h	4–20 mg daily in divided doses. Do not exceed 0.5 mg/kg q24h
Diphenhydramine hydrochloride	Benadryl	Elixir 12.5 mg/5 ml capsules 25, 50 mg solution for injection 50 mg/mL	2.5–5 mg/kg/24h	25–50 mg q4–6h
Hydroxyzine hydrochloride	Atarax	Syrup 10 mg/5 ml Capsules 10, 25, 50 mg	2 mg/kg/24th	25–50 mg o.d. (hs)-t.i.d.
Promethazine hydrochloride	Phenergan	Syrup 10 mg/5 ml Tablets 10, 25, 50 mg solution for injection 25 mg/ml	0.5 mg/kg at bedtime	25 mg at bedtime
Second Generation				
Terfenadine	Seldane; Marion Merrell Dow	Suspension 30mg/5 ml*; Tablets 60 mg, 120 mg*	3–6 yr, 15 mg b.i.d. 7–12 yr, 30 mg b.i.d.	60 mg b.i.d. or 120 mg
Astemizole	Hismanal; Janssen	Suspension 10mg/5 ml*; Tablets 10 mg	<6 yr, 0.2 mg/kg/24 hr 6–12, 5 mg o.d.	10 mg o.d.
Loratadine	Claritin; Schering-Plough	Tablets 10 mg*		10 mg o.d.
Certirizine	Reactine; Pfizer	Tablets 10 mg*		10 mg o.d.

*not available in the United States at the time of publication

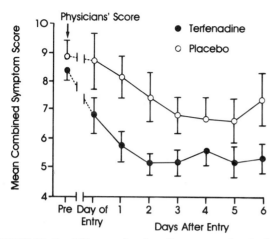

FIGURE 30-7. Efficacy of terfenadine versus placebo in children with allergic rhinitis. (From Guill et al.,[82] with permission.)

mg twice daily.[81,84,96–98] Cetirizine 5–20 mg daily is superior to placebo and in a 10 mg daily dose is as effective as terfenadine 60 mg twice daily in controlling the symptoms of seasonal and perennial allergic rhinitis.[99]

There is renewed interest in topical application of H_1-receptor antagonists to the nasal mucosa. Azatadine inhibits the early release of histamine and concomitant symptoms after antigen and histamine challenge intranasally,[100] although not after cold dry air challenge. Topically applied levocabastine, which has the highest potency of any H_1-receptor antagonist described so far (1500 times that of chlorpheniramine), provides highly significant protection against allergen-triggered allergic rhinitis symptoms.[101,102]

H_1- and H_2-receptor antagonists administered together topically or by mouth are significantly more effective in blocking nasal congestion than either the H_1- or the H_2-receptor antagonists alone. The synergistic effects are not large and have not been found universally in all studies; while of theoretical interest, they are probably not clinically important.[103–104]

Allergic Conjunctivitis

In patients with allergic conjunctivitis, H_1-receptor antagonists administered by mouth are useful for the relief of ocular symptoms such as itching, tearing, and erythema.[80–99,105–106] Applied topically to the conjunctivae, potent H_1-receptor antagonists such as levocabastine also provide relief of allergic conjunctivitis symptoms.[101,102,107]

Allergic Skin Disorders (Atopic Dermatitis, Urticaria, and Dermographism)

H_1-receptor antagonists are commonly prescribed for symptomatic relief of itching in these disorders. Itching is difficult to quantify in allergic skin disorders, as the chemical mediator for it has not been identified and no animal models exist. Nevertheless, it is known that H_1-receptor antagonists have a greater antipruritic effect in allergic skin disorders than in other types of pruritic skin disorders. The mechanism of the antipruritic effect is unknown, but it is not entirely central.

Assessment of the antipruritic effect of H_1-receptor antagonists has been subjective, depending on the patient's perception of the amount of itch and observed healing of lesions. In children with atopic dermatitis, hydroxyzine has a significantly greater antipruritic effect than cyproheptadine; a single dose of hydroxyzine will significantly suppress the itching of widespread atopic dermatitis for at least 24 hours (Figure 30–4).[44] Second-generation H_1-receptor antagonists such as astemizole are not as effective as hydroxyzine in relieving pruritus in atopic dermatitis, suggesting that the sedative effect provided by the first-generation H_1-receptor antagonists contributes to the relief of pruritus.[108]

In suppression of histamine-induced wheals and flares and of dermographism, hydroxyzine is more effective than other first-generation H_1-receptor antagonists such as diphenhydramine, chlorpheniramine, promethazine, and cyproheptadine. In double-blind studies in patients with urticaria, hydroxyzine has also generally proven superior to other first-generation H_1-receptor antagonists. In prospective, double-blind, long-term studies in adults with urticaria, the second-generation H_1-receptor antagonists such as terfenadine, astemizole, and cetirizine are well tolerated and result in significant remission of symptoms.[109–111]

Asthma

In numerous well-designed double-blind studies, it has been shown that H_1-receptor antagonists such as chlorpheniramine, hydroxyzine, clemastine, terfenadine, azelastine, and cetirizine have a modest, dose-related bronchodilator effect. In bronchial challenge studies, pretreatment with an H_1-receptor antagonist given by mouth, intravenously, or by inhalation prevents histamine-, antigen-, and exercise-induced asthma but not methacholine-induced asthma.[112–117] The long-term bronchodilator effects of H_1-receptor antagonists such as chlorpheniramine or astemizole administered for several months to patients with chronic asthma have been confirmed.[117,118]

H_1-receptor antagonists are not drugs of first choice for chronic asthma; however, previous concerns about the potential adverse effects of H_1-receptor antagonists in asthma have been exaggerated. If required for chronic rhinitis treatment or for treatment of pruritus in patients with allergic skin disorders, H_1-receptor antagonists should not be withheld from patients with concurrent asthma.

Anaphylaxis

The initial treatment of choice for anaphylaxis consists of administration of a potent physiologic antagonist of the immediate hypersensitivity response, which will prevent further mediator release and "turn off" the adverse reaction. Epinephrine is the drug of first choice. H_1-receptor antagonists such as hydroxyzine and diphenhydramine may be useful adjuncts to epinephrine, particularly for control of symptoms such as rhinorrhea and pruritus. However, H_1-antagonists should never replace epinephrine in the treatment of anaphylaxis.

Otitis Media

H_1-receptor antagonists, often in combination with α-adrenergic agonists, are frequently prescribed for children with acute otitis media or otitis media with effusion. Few well-designed, placebo-controlled, double-blind clinical studies in which there is repeated objective assessment of tympanic membrane compliance can be cited to support any beneficial effect of these medications on Eustachian tube function.[119]

Otitis media with effusion has a high spontaneous remission rate. In a large, well-controlled, double-blind, randomized trial of a chlorpheniramine–pseudoephedrine combination versus placebo in nonallergic infants and children with otitis media with effusion, there was no difference in outcome between the two treatment regimens.[120] In another large, double-blind randomized study by the same investigators in children with otitis media with effusion, treated with a 2-week course of amopicillin, the addition of a 4-week course of a chlorpheniramine–pseudoephedrine preparation did not hasten resolution.[121] In a third study by different authors, triprolidine, either alone or in combination with pseudoephedrine, did not shorten the course of chronic serous otitis media significantly compared with placebo, although in patients treated with the combination of medications, the mean pressure gradient across the tympanic membrane was significantly improved.[122]

Studies of the efficacy of H_1-receptor antagonists such as chlorpheniramine and brompheniramine in combination with decongestants in acute otitis media have generally not shown statistically significant effects on symptom resolution or prevention of persistent middle ear effusion.[123,124] In one double-blind study, however, chlorpheniramine in combination with phenylpropanolamine and phenyltoloxamine was more effective than placebo in acute otitis media.[125]

There is conflicting evidence as to whether H_1-receptor antagonists in combination with decongestants prevent acute otitis media from developing in children with upper respiratory infections.[126] In one double-blind study, the incidence of acute otitis media was almost identical in the group of children receiving brompheniramine and in children who received placebo.

Upper Respiratory Infections

Antihistamines used alone and in combination with other drugs have been promoted for treatment of viral upper respiratory infections since the late 1940s. Many of the reports suggesting their usefulness were conducted decades ago and were not randomized, double-blind, placebo-controlled clinical trials. Although studies can be

found in which H_1-receptor antagonists such as chlorpheniramine or terfenadine were apparently superior to placebo in ameliorating the symptoms of the common cold,[127,128] most recent, well-designed, placebo-controlled studies do not support the use of oral or topical H_1-receptor antagonists in prevention or relief of upper respiratory infections.[129]

Preparations and Dosage

Table 30–4 lists representative antihistamines by generic and proprietary names, types of formulation, and suggested dosages for children and adults. It also includes second-generation antihistamines, which are not yet available in the United States, although some are available in Canada at the time of writing of this chapter.

Overdosage

Fatal or near-fatal intoxication of children has been reported rarely following ingestion of large doses of H_1-receptor antagonists such as diphenhydramine, hydroxyzine, chlorpheniramine, tripelennamine, and dimenhydrinate. Symptoms develop rapidly after ingestion, often within 15 to 30 minutes, and death can occur within 2 hours. Older children, like adults, usually manifest lethargy, extreme drowsiness, or coma after overdose, but young children may suffer from excitation, irritability, hyperactivity, insomnia, visual hallucinations, and seizures. Patients generally exhibit evidence of autonomic imbalance, such as dryness of the mucous membranes, fever, flushed facies, pupillary dilation, urinary retention, decreased gastrointestinal motility, hypotension, and tachycardia. Cardiorespiratory arrest and death may occur.[130,131]

Treatment consists of general supportive measures, such as evacuation of stomach contents. If the child is seen shortly after ingestion of H_1-receptor antagonists with strong antiemetic effects, gastric lavage may be more effective than centrally acting emetics such as ipecac. Short-acting anticonvulsants such as thiopental or diazepam should be used for seizures; mechanical ventilation may be required for respiratory arrest.

H_2 ANTIHISTAMINES

The inability of conventional antihistaminic drugs to inhibit histamine-stimulated gastric acid secretion led to the search for specific antagonists of this action. The first such useful drug, developed as a result of the systematic modification of the histamine molecule, was burimamide, a specific competitive antagonist of histamine for H_2 receptors, with no specific interaction with H_1 receptors, catecholamine β-receptors, or acetylcholine receptors. Burimamide, like histamine, is an imidazole derivative substituted by a simple polymethylene chain terminating in a polar nitrogen atom, but the side chain is larger and the nitrogen atom is uncharged. Burimamide was shown to inhibit histamine- and pentagastrin-stimulated gastric acid secretion, but not vagally stimulated gastric acid secretion, in animals and humans.

Burimamide was relatively inactive orally, and further chemical substitution produced cimetidine, which won rapid acceptance for the treatment of duodenal ulcer and gastric hypersecretory conditions. Subsequently ranitidine, which possesses a substituted furan ring, and is 4–10 times more potent than cimetidine, was introduced.[132]

The H₂ blockers are reversible, competitive antagonists of the action of histamine on H₂ receptors. They inhibit both fasting and nocturnal gastric acid secretion as well as that stimulated by food, fundic distention, insulin, or caffeine. They reduce both the volume of gastric juice secreted and its hydrogen ion concentration.

H₂-blockers are sometimes administered concurrently with H₁-blockers to adult patients with chronic urticaria in order to reduce itching and whealing. H₂-blockers are being investigated for their ability to enhance cell-mediated immunity in patients with primary and secondary immunodeficiency disorders.

Pharmacokinetics

Both cimetidine and ranitidine are rapidly and completely absorbed orally, with peak plasma concentrations appearing in 1–2 hours. Absorption is not affected by food or antacids; however, first-pass hepatic metabolism results in bioavailability of approximately 50 percent. Their elimination half-life is about 2–3 hours. Elimination occurs primarily via the kidneys; at least 60 percent of these drugs appear in the urine unchanged, while most of the remainder is metabolized.

Adverse Reactions and Side Effects

The incidence of side effects is low and adverse reactions are generally minor. Many side effects are drug-specific. Cimetidine, for example, binds to the androgen receptor and may induce impotence and gynecomastia which disappear if ranitidine is substituted. Cimetidine also binds to cytochrome P-450 and diminishes the activity of hepatic microsomal drug-metabolizing enzymes, hence patients receiving theophylline must have a dosage adjustment to avoid toxicity. Cimetidine may cause central nervous system confusion, and may rarely cause bone marrow depression. These side effects are not seen with ranitidine.

These drugs are not fully approved for use in children but may be useful in treating such conditions as gastroesophageal reflux and gastric hypersecretory states in the pediatric age group.

Addendum: For updated information about H₁-receptor antagonists please see:

Simons, F.E.R.: H₁-receptor antagonists: Clinical pharmacology and therapeutics. J Allergy Clin Immunol, 84:845–863, 1990.

Simons, F.E.R. and Simons, K.J.: Second-generation H₁-receptor antagonists. Annals of Allergy, 66:5–21, 1991.

REFERENCES

1. Barger G, Dale HH: The presence in ergot and physiological activity of beta-imidazolylethylene. J Physiol 40:38–40, 1910
2. Dale HH, Laidlaw PP: The physiological action of β-iminozolylethylamine. J Physiol 41:318–344, 1910
3. Lewis T, Grant RT: Vascular reactions of the skin to injury. Heart 11:209–265, 1924
4. Bonet D, Straub AM: Action protectrice des éthers phénoliques au cours de l'intoxication histaminique. Soc Biol 124:547–549, 1937
5. Halpern BN: Les antihistaminiques de synthèse: Essais de chimiothérapie des états allergiques. Arch Int Pharmacodyn 68:339–408, 1942
6. Bovet D, Horclois R, Walthert F: Propriétés antihistaminiques de la N-p-methoxybenzyl-N-dimethylaminoéthyl à aminopyridine. Compt Rend Soc Biol 138:99–100, 1944
7. Loew ER, Kaiser ME, Moore V: Synthetic benzhydryl alkamine ethers effective in preventing fatal experimental asthma in guinea-pigs exposed to atomized histamine. J Pharmacol Exp Ther 83:120–129, 1945
8. Yonkman FF, Chess D, Mathieson D, Hansen N: Pharmacodynamic studies of a new antihistamine agent. N'-pyridyl-N' benzyl-N-dimethyl-ethylene diamine HCl, pyribenzamine HCl. J Pharm Exp Ther 87:256–264, 1946
9. Riley JF, West GB: Histamine in tissue mast cells. J Physiol 117:72P–73P, 1952
10. Riley JF, West GB: The occurrence of histamine in mast cells, in Rocha e Silva (ed): Handbook of Experimental Pharmacology, vol XVIII. Histamine and Antihistamines, Part I. New York, Springer-Verlag, 1966, pp 116–135
11. Mongar JL, Schild HO: Quantitative measurement of the histamine-releasing activity of a series of monoalkylamines using minced guinea-pig lung. Br J Pharmacol 8:103–109, 1953
12. Foreman J, Mongar JL: The control of secretion from mast cells, in Pepys J, Edwards AM (eds): The Mast Cell in Health and Disease. Tunbridge Wells (England), Pitman Medical, 1980, pp 30–37
13. Ash ASF, Schild HO: Receptors mediating some actions of histamine. Br J Pharmacol 27:427–439, 1966
14. Black JW, Duncan WAM, Durant CJ, Ganellin CR, Parsons EM: Definition and antagonism of histamine H₂-receptors. Nature 236:385–390, 1972
15. Schayer RW: The metabolism of histamine in various species. Br J Pharmacol 11:472–3, 1956
16. Warner JA, Pienkowskui SM, Plaut M, Normal PS, Lichtenstein LM: Identification of histamine releasing factor(s) in the late phase of cutaneous IgE-mediated reactions. J Immunol 136:2583–2587, 1986
17. Altura BM, Halevy S: Cardiovascular actions of histamine, in Rocha e Silva (ed): Handbook of Experimental Pharmacology, vol. XVII/2. Histamine II and Antihistamines. New York, Springer-Verlag, 1978, pp 1–21
18. McNamee JE, Grodins FS: Effect of histamine on microvasculature of isolated dog gracilis muscle. Am J Physiol 229:119–125, 1975
19. Schayer RW: Histamine and microcirculation. Life Sci 15:391–401, 1974
20. Altura BM: Retiendo-endothelium system function and histamine release in shock and trauma: relationship to micro-circulation. Klin Wochenschr 60:882–890, 1982
21. Kahlson G, Rosengren E: New approaches to the physiology of histamine. Physiol Rev 48:155–196, 1968
22. Douglas WW: Histamine and 5-hydroxytryptamine (serotonin) and their antagonists, in Gilman AG, Goodman LS, Rall TW, Murad F (eds): Goodman and Gilman's The Pharmacological Basis of Therapeutics, 7th ed. New York, Macmillan, 1985, p 614
23. Snyder SH, Taylor KM: Histamine in brain: A neurotransmitter, in Snyder SH (ed): Perspectives in Neuropharmacology. New York, Oxford University Press, 1972, pp 43–73
24. Coleman JW, Godfrey RC. The number and affinity of IgE receptors on dispersed human lung mast cells. Immunology 44:859–863, 1981
25. Lewis RA, Austen KF. Mediation of local homeostasis and

inflammation by leukotrienes and other mast cell-dependent compounds. Nature 293:103–108, 1981

26. Serafin WE, Austin KF: Mediators of immediate hypersensitivity reactions. N Engl J Med 317:30–34, 1987
27. Lewis RA, Austen KF: The biologically active leukotrienes: Biosynthesis, metabolism, receptors, functions, and pharmacology. J Clin Invest 73:889–897, 1984
28. Hardy CC, Robinson C, Tattersfield AE, Holgate ST. The bronchoconstrictor effect of inhaled prostaglandin D_2 in normal and asthmatic men. N Engl J Med 311:209–213, 1984
29. Henocq E, Vargaftig BB: Accumulation of eosinophils in response to intracutaneous PAF-acether and allergens in man. Lancet 1:1378–1379, 1986
30. Foreman JC, Hallett MB, Mongar JL: The relationship between histamine secretion and ^{45}calcium uptake by mast cells. J Physiol 271:193–214, 1977
31. Arrang JM, Garbarg M, Lancelot JC, Lecomte JM, Pollard H et al: Highly potent and selective ligands for histamine H_3 receptors. Nature 327:117–123, 1987
32. Douglas WW: Histamine and 5-hydroxytryptamine (serotonin) and their antagonists, in Gilman AG, Goodman LS, Rall TW, Murad F (eds): Goodman and Gilman's The Pharmacological Basis of Therapeutics, 7th ed. New York, Macmillan, 1985, pp 607–612
33. Joad J, Casale TB. Histamine and airway caliber. Ann Allergy 61:1–7, 1988
34. Douglas WW: Histamine and 5-hydroxytryptamine (serotonin) and their antagonists, in Gilman AG, Goodman LS, Rall TW, Murad F (eds): Goodman and Gilman's The Pharmacological Basis of Therapeutics, 7th ed. New York, Macmillan, 1985, pp 605–638
35. Church MK, Gradidge CF: Inhibition of histamine release from human lung in vitro by antihistamines and related drugs. Br J Pharmac. 69:663–667, 1980
36. Vallner JJ, Needham TE, Chan W, Viswanathan CT: Intravenous administration of chlorpheniramine to seven subjects. Curr Ther Res 26:449–453, 1979
37. Yacobi A, Stoll RG, Chao GC, Carter JE, Baaske DM, et al: Evaluation of sustained-action chlorpheniramine-pseudoephedrine dosage forms in humans. J Pharm Sci 69:1077–1081, 1980
38. Thompson JA, Bloedow DC, Leffert FH: Pharmacokinetics of intravenous chlorpheniramine in children. J Pharm Sci 70:1284–1286, 1981
39. Simons FER, Frith EM, Simons KJ: The pharmacokinetics and antihistaminic effects of brompheniramine. J Allergy Clin Immunol 70:458–464, 1982
40. Simons FER, Luciuk GH, Simons KJ: Pharmacokinetics and efficacy of chlorpheniramine in children. J Allergy Clin Immunol 69:376–381, 1982
41. Garteiz DA, Hook RH, Walker BJ, Okerholm RA: Pharmacokinetics and biotransformation studies of terfenadine in man. Arzheim.-Forsch./Drug Res. Huang SM 32:1185–1190, 1982
42. Huang SM, Athanikar NK, Sridhar K, Huang YC, Chiou WL: Pharmacokinetics of chlorpheniramine after intravenous and oral administration in normal adults. Eur J Clin Pharmacol 22:359–365, 1982
43. Simons FER, Simons KJ: H_1-receptor antagonists: Clinical pharmacology and use in allergic disease. Pediatr Clin North Am 30:899–914, 1983
44. Simons FER, Simons KJ, Becker AB, Haydey RP: Pharmacokinetics and antipruritic effects of hydroxyzine in children with atopic dermatitis. J Pediatr 104:123–127, 1984
45. Simons FER, Simons KJ, Frith EM: The pharmacokinetics and antihistaminic effects of the H_1-receptor antagonist hydroxyzine. J Allergy Clin Immunol 73:69–75, 1984
46. Heykants J: Pharmacokinetics and metabolism of astemizole in man, in Astemizole: A New, Non-Sedative, Long-Acting H_1-Antagonist. Oxford, Medical Education Services, 1984, pp 25–34
47. Watson WTA, Simons KJ, Chen XY, Simons FER: Cetirizine: a pharmacokinetic and pharmacodynamic evaluation in children with seasonal allergic rhinitis. J Allergy Clin Immunol 84:457–464, 1989
48. Sorkin EM, Heel RC: Terfenadine: A review of its pharmacodynamic properties and therapeutic efficacy. Drugs 29:34–56, 1985
49. Simons KJ, Singh M, Gillespie CA, Simons FER: An investigation of the H_1-receptor antagonist triprolidine: Pharmacokinetics and antihistaminic effects. J Allergy Clin Immunol 77:326–330, 1986
50. Simons FER, Watson WTA, Simons KJ: The pharmacokinetics and pharmacodynamics of terfenadine in children. J Allergy Clin Immunol 80:884–890, 1987
51. Gengo FM, Dabronzo J, Yurchak A, Love S, Miller JK: The relative antihistaminic and psychomotor effects of hydroxyzine and cetirizine. Clin Pharm Ther 42:265–272, 1987
52. Hilbert J, Radwanski E, Weglein R, Perentesis G, Symchowicz S, et al: Pharmacokinetics and dose proportionality of loratadine. J Clin Pharmacol 27:694–698, 1987
53. Hilbert J, Moritzen V, Parks A, Radwanski E, Perentesis G, Symchowicz S, Zampaglione N: The pharmacokinetics of loratadine in normal geriatric volunteers. J Int Med Res 16:50–60, 1988
54. Simons KJ, Watson WTA, Chen XY, Simons FER: Pharmacokinetic and pharmacodynamic studies of the H_1-receptor antagonist hydroxyzine in the elderly. Clin Pharmcol Ther 45:9–11, 1989
55. Simons FER, Watson WTA, Simons KJ: Lack of subsensitivity to terfenadine during long-term terfenadine treatment. J Allergy Clin Immunol 82:1068–1075, 1988
56. Simons FER, Watson WTA, Chen XY, Minuk GY, Simons KJ: The pharmacokinetics and pharmacodynamics of hydroxyzine in patients with primary biliary cirrhosis. J Clin Pharmacol 29:809–815, 1989
57. Wood SG, John BA, Chasseaud LF, Yeh J, Chung M: The metabolism and pharmacokinetics of ^{14}C-cetirizine in humans. Ann Allergy 59:31–34, 1987
58. Matzke GR, Yeh J, Awni WM, Halstenson CE, Chung M: Pharmacokinetics of cetirizine in the elderly and patients with renal insufficiency. Ann Allergy 59:25–30, 1987
59. Hilbert J, Radwanski E, Affrime MB, Perentesis G, Symchowicz S, et al: Excretion of loratadine in human breast milk. J Clin Pharmacol 28:234–239, 1988
60. Huther KJ, Renftle G, Barraud N, Burke JT, Koch-Weser J: Inhibitory activity of terfenadine on histamine-induced skin wheals in man. Eur J Clin Pharmacol 12:195–199, 1977
61. Georgitis JW, Shen D: Nasal pharmacodynamics of brompheniramine in perennial rhinitis. Arch Otolaryngol Head Neck Surg 114:63–67, 1988
62. Murphy-O'Connor JC, Renton RL, Westlake DM: Comparative trial of two dose regimens of terfenadine in patients with hay fever. J Int Med Res 12:333–337, 1984
63. Lantin JP, Huguenot C, Pecoud AR: Effect of astemizole on skin tests with histamine, codeine and allergens. J Allergy Clin Immunol 81:213, 1988
64. Monash S: Development of refractory condition of skin towards antihistaminic drugs after antihistaminic therapy as determined by histamine iontophoresis. J Invest Dermatol 15:1–2, 1950
65. Dannenberg TB, Feinberg SM: The development of tolerance to antihistamines: A study of the quantitative inhibiting capacity of antihistamines on the skin and mucous membrane reaction to histamine and antigens. J Allergy 22:330–339, 1951
66. Long WF, Taylor RJ, Wagner CJ, Leavengood DC, Nelson HS: Skin test suppression by antihistamines and the development of subsensitivity. J Allergy Clin Immunol 76:113–117, 1985
67. Taylor RJ, Long WF, Nelson HS: The development of subsensitivity to chlorpheniramine. J Allergy Clin Immunol 76:103–107, 1985
68. Bantz EW, Dolen WK, Chadwick EW, Nelson HS: Chronic chlorpheniramine therapy: subsensitivity, drug metabolism, and compliance. Ann Allergy 59:341–346, 1987
69. Burns JJ, Conney AH, Koster R: Stimulatory effect of chronic drug administration on drug-metabolizing enzymes in liver microsomes. Ann NY Acad Sci 104:881–893, 1963
70. Simons KJ, Simons FER: The effect of chronic administration of hydroxyzine on hydroxyzine pharmacokinetics in dogs. J Allergy Clin Immunol 79:928–932, 1987

71. Roman IJ, Kassem N, Gural RP, Herron J: Suppression of histamine-induced wheal response by loratadine (SCH 29851) over 28 days in man. Ann Allergy 57:253–256, 1986
72. Moser L, Huther KJ, Koch-Weser J, Lundt PV: Effects of terfenadine and diphenhydramine alone or in combination with diazepam or alcohol on psychomotor performance and subjective feelings. Eur J Clin Pharmac 14:417–423, 1978
73. Rombaut N, Heykants J, Vanden Bussche G: Potential of interaction between the H₁-antagonist astemizole and other drugs. Ann Allergy 57:321–324, 1986
74. Doms M, Vanhulle G, Baelde Y, Coulie P, Dupont P, Rihoux J-P: Lack of potentiation by cetirizine of alcohol-induced psychomotor disturbances. Eur J Clin Pharmacol 34:619–623, 1988
75. Hindmarch I, Bhatti JZ: Psychomotor effects of astemizole and chlorpheniramine, alone and in combination with alcohol. Int Clin Psychopharmacol 2:117–119, 1987
76. Luskin AT, Luskin SS, Fitzsimmons WF, Macleod CM: Pharmacokinetic evaluation of the terfenadine-theophylline interaction. J Allergy Clin Immunol 81:320, 1988
77. Craft TM: Torsade de pointes after astemizole overdose. Br Med J 292:660, 1986
78. Simons FER, Kesselman MS, Giddins NG, Pelech AN, Simons KJ: Astemizole-induced torsade de pointes. Lancet 78 volume no. is 2.:624, 1988
79. King CTG, Howell J: Teratogenic effect of buclizine and hydroxyzine in the rat and chlorcyclizine in the mouse. Am J Obstet Gynecol 95:109–111, 1966
80. Diamond L, Gerson K, Cato A, Peace K, Perkins JG: An evaluation of triprolidine and pseudoephedrine in the treatment of allergic rhinitis. Ann Allergy 47:87–91, 1981
81. Dockhorn RJ, Shellenberger MK, Hassanien R, Trachelman L: Efficacy of SCH434 (loratadine plus pseudoephedrine) versus components and placebo in seasonal allergic rhinitis. J Allergy Clin Immunol 81:178, 1988
82. Guill MF, Buckley RH, Rocha W, Kemp JP, Segal AT, et al: Multicenter, double-blind, placebo-controlled trial of terfenadine suspension in the treatment of fall-allergic rhinitis in children. J Allergy Clin Immunol 78:4–9, 1986
83. Brostoff J, Lockhart JDF: Controlled trial of terfenadine and chlorpheniramine maleate in perennial rhinitis. Postgrad Med J 58:422–423, 1982
84. Bruttmann G, Pedrali P: Loratadine (SCH 29851) 40 mg once daily versus terfenadine 60 mg twice daily in the treatment of seasonal allergic rhinitis. J Int Med Res 15:63–70, 1987
85. Gutkowski A, Del Carpio J, Gelinas B, Schulz J, Turenne Y: Comparative study of the efficacy, tolerance, and side-effects of dexchlorpheniramine maleate 6 mg bid with terfenadine 60 mg bid. J Int Med Res 13:284–288, 1985
86. Horak F, Bruttmann G, Pedrali P, Weeke B, Frolund L, et al: A multicentric study of loratadine, terfenadine and placebo in patients with seasonal allergic rhinitis. Arzneim-Forsch/Drug Res 38:124–128, 1988
87. Howarth PH, Holgate ST: Comparative trial of two non-sedative H₁ antihistamines, terfenadine and astemizole, for hay fever. Thorax 39:668–672, 1984
88. Hugonot L, Hugonot R, Beaumont D: A double-blind comparison of terfenadine and mequitazine in the symptomatic treatment of acute pollinosis. J Int Med Res 14:124–130, 1986
89. Kemp JP, Buckley CE, Gershwin ME, Buchman E, Cascio FL, et al: Multicenter, double-blind, placebo-controlled trial of terfenadine in seasonal allergic rhinitis and conjunctivitis. Ann Allergy 54:502–509, 1985
90. Rokenes HK, Andersson B, Rundcrantz H: Effect of terfenadine and placebo on symptoms after nasal allergen provocation. Clin Allergy 18:63–69, 1988
91. Wihl J-A, Petersen BN, Petersen LN, Gundersen G, Bresson K, et al: Effect of the non-sedative H₁-receptor antagonist astemizole in perennial allergic and non-allergic rhinitis. J Allergy Clin Immunol 75:720–727, 1985
92. Grillage MG, Harcup JW, Mayhew SR, Huddlestone L: Astemizole suspension in the maintenance treatment of paediatric hay fever: a comparison with terfenadine suspension. Pharmatherapeutica 4:642–647, 1986
93. Howarth PH, Emanuel MB, Holgate ST: Astemizole, a potent histamine H₁-receptor antagonist: effect in allergic rhinoconjunctivitis, on antigen- and histamine-induced skin weal responses and relationship to serum levels. Br J Clin Pharm 18:1–8, 1984
94. Richards DM, Brogden RN, Heel RC, Speight TM, Avery GS: Astemizole: A review of its pharmacodynamic properties and therapeutic efficacy. Drugs 28:38–61, 1984
95. Gendreau-Reid L, Simons KJ, Simons FER: Comparison of the suppressive effect of astemizole, terfenadine, and hydroxyzine on histamine-induced wheals and flares in humans. J Allergy Clin Immunol 77:335–340, 1986
96. Meltzer EO, Ellis EF, Rosen JP, Shapiro GG, Siegel SC, et al: A comparison of loratadine, chlorpheniramine, and placebo suspensions in children with seasonal allergic rhinitis. J Allergy Clin Immunol 81:177, 1988
97. Skassa-Brociek W, Bousquet J, Montes F, Verdier M, Schwab D. et al: Double-blind placebo-controlled study of loratadine, mequitazine, and placebo in the symptomatic treatment of seasonal allergic rhinitis. J Allergy Clin Immunol 81:725–730, 1988
98. Dockhorn RJ, Bergner A, Connell JT, Falliers CJ, Grabiec SV, et al: Safety and efficacy of loratadine (Sch-29851): A new nonsedating antihistamine in seasonal allergic rhinitis. Ann Allergy 58:407–411, 1987
99. Berman B, Buchman E, Dockhorn R, Leese P, Mansmann H, et al: Cetirizine therapy of perennial allergic rhinitis. J Allergy Clin Immunol 81:177, 1988
100. Togias A, Proud D, Kagey-Sobotka A, Norman P, Lichtenstein L, et al: The effect of a topical tricyclic antihistamine on the response of the nasal mucosa to challenge with cold, dry air and histamine. J Allergy Clin Immunol 79:599–604, 1987
101. Bende M, Pipkorn U: Topical levocabastine, a selective H1 antagonist, in seasonal allergic rhinoconjunctivitis. Allergy 42:512–515, 1987
102. Pecoud A, Zuber P, Kolly M: Effect of a new selective H₁-receptor antagonist (levocabastine) in a nasal and conjunctival provocation test. Int Arch All Appl Immunol 82:541–543, 1987
103. Havas TE, Cole P, Parker L, Oprysk D, Ayiomamitis A: The effects of combined H₁ and H₂ histamine antagonists on alterations in nasal airflow resistance induced by topical histamine provocation. J Allergy Clin Immunol 78:856–860, 1986
104. Secher C, Kirkegaard J, Borum P, Maansson A, Osterhammel P, et al: Significance of H₁ and H₂ receptors in the human nose: rationale for topical use of combined antihistamine preparations. J Allergy Clin Immunol 70:211–218, 1982
105. Beswick KBJ, Kenyon GS, Cherry JR: A comparative study of beclomethasone dipropionate aqueous nasal spray with terfenadine tablets in seasonal allergic rhinitis. Curr Med Res Opin 9:560–567, 1985
106. Wood SF: Oral antihistamine or nasal steroid in hay fever: A double-blind double-dummy comparative study of once daily oral astemizole vs twice daily nasal beclomethasone dipropionate. Clin Allergy 16:195–201, 1986
107. Pipkorn U, Bende M, Hedner J, Hedner T: A double-blind evaluation of topical levocabastine, a new specific H₁-receptor antagonist in patients with allergic conjunctivitis. Allergy 40:491–496, 1985.
108. Roberts JE, Simons FER, Simons KJ, Gillespie CA: The antipruritic effect of placebo versus hydroxyzine versus hydroxyzine versus astemizole in children with severe atopic dermatitis. J Allergy Clin Immunol 81:210, 1988
109. Juhlin L, de Vos C, Rihoux J-P: Inhibiting effect of cetirizine on histamine-induced and 48/80-induced wheals and flares, experimental dermographism, and cold-induced urticaria. J Allergy Clin Immunol 80:599–602, 1987
110. Krause LB, Shuster S: A comparison of astemizole and chlorpheniramine in dermographic urticaria. Br J Dermatol 112:447–453, 1985
111. Salisbury J, Bor S, Blair C: A double-blind placebo controlled study of terfenadine in the treatment of chronic idiopathic urticaria. Br J Clin Pract 41:859–861, 1987
112. Chan TB, Shelton DM, Eiser NM: Effect of an oral H₁-receptor

antagonist, terfenadine, on antigen-induced asthma. Br J Dis Chest 80:375–384, 1986

113. Clee MD, Ingram CG, Reid PC, Robertson AS: The effect of astemizole on exercise-induced asthma. Br J Dis Chest 78:180–183, 1984

114. Patel KR: Terfenadine in exercise-induced asthma. Br Med J 288:1496–1497, 1984

115. Patel KR: Effect of terfenadine on methacholine-induced bronchoconstriction in asthma. J Allergy Clin Immunol 79:355–358, 1987

116. Rafferty P, Holgate ST: Terfenadine (Seldane) is a potent and selective histamine H_1-receptor antagonist in asthmatic airways. Am Rev Respir Dis 135:181–184, 1987

117. Lewiston NJ, Johnson S, Sloan E: Effect of antihistamine on pulmonary function of children with asthma. J Pediatr 101:458–460, 1982

118. Holgate ST, Emanuel MB, Howarth PH: Astemizole and other H_1 antihistaminic drug treatment of asthma. J Allergy Clin Immunol 76:375–380, 1985

119. Stillwagon PK, Doyle WJ, Fireman P: Effect of an antihistamine/decongestant on nasal and eustachian tube function following intranasal pollen challenge. Ann Allergy 58:442–446, 1987

120. Cantekin EI, Mandel EM, Bluestone CD, Rockette HE, Paradise JL et al: Lack of efficacy of a decongestant antihistamine combination for otitis media with effusion ("secretory" otitis media) in children. N Engl J Med 308:297–301, 1983

121. Mandel EM, Rockette HE, Bluestone CD, Paradise JL, Nozza RJ: Efficacy of amoxicillin with and without decongestant-antihistamine for otitis media with effusion in children. N Engl J Med 316:432–437, 1987

122. Pierson WE, Kraemer MJ, Perkins GJ & Bierman CW: Antihistamine and decongestant therapy for eustachian tube dysfunction in allergic children. J Allergy Clin Immunol 69:143, 1982

123. Bhambhani K, Foulds DM, Swamy KN, Eldis FE, Fischel JE: Acute otitis media in children: Are decongestants or antihistamines necessary? Ann Emerg Med 12:13–16, 1983

124. Schnore SK, Sangster JF, Gerace TM, Bass MJ: Are antihistamine-decongestants of value in the treatment of acute otitis media in children? J Family Pract 22:39–43, 1986

125. Moran DM, Mutchie KD, Higbee MD, Paul LD: The use of an antihistamine-decongestant in conjunction with an anti-infective drug in the treatment of acute otitis media. J Pediatr 101:132–136, 1982

126. Randall JE, Hendley JO: A decongestant-antihistamine mixture in the prevention of otitis media in children with colds. Pediatrics 63:483–485, 1979

127. Henauer SA, Glück U: Efficacy of terfenadine in the treatment of common cold. A double-blind comparison with placebo. Eur J Clin Pharmacol 34:35–40, 1988

128. Howard Jr JC, Kantner TR, Lilienfield LS, Princiotto JV, Krum RE et al: Effectiveness of antihistamines in the symptomatic management of the common cold. JAMA 242:2414–17, 1979

129. Gaffey MJ, Gwaltney JM, Sastre A, Dressler WE, Sorrentino JV, Hayden FG: Intranasally and orally administered antihistamine treatment of experimental rhinovirus colds. Am Rev Respir Dis 136:556–560, 1987

130. Hestand HE, Teske DW: Diphenhydramine hydrochloride intoxication. J Pediatr 90:1017–1018, 1977

131. Wyngaarden JB, Seevers MH: The toxic effects of antihistaminic drugs. JAMA 145:277–282, 1951

132. Douglas WW: Histamine and 5-hydroxytryptamine (sevotonin) and their antagonists, in Gilman AG, Goodman LS, Rall TW, Murad F (eds): Goodman and Gilman's The Pharmacological Basis of Therapeutics, 7th ed. New York, Macmillan, 1985, pp 624–627

31

ADVANCES IN THE PHARMACOLOGIC MANAGEMENT OF ASTHMA

MALCOLM R. HILL *and* STANLEY J. SZEFLER

Recently there has been a dramatic increase in understanding of the pathophysiology of asthma. This information has led to a reevaluation of the therapeutic approaches to the treatment of asthma. This review will first highlight current concepts regarding the pathophysiology of asthma as a foundation for a discussion on the clinical pharmacology of antiasthma medications.

CHARACTERIZATIONS OF ASTHMA

Success in the treatment of any disease is achieved when drug therapy is directed toward specific pathophysiologic mechanisms. Despite recent gains in understanding the pathophysiology of asthma, a clearly defined mechanism cannot be elucidated. Multiple pathways are likely involved in the initiation and continuation of the disease.

Asthma is "characterized by increased responsiveness of the trachea and bronchi to various stimuli and manifested by widespread narrowing of the airways that changes in severity, either spontaneously or as a result of therapy."[1] Indeed, it is increased responsiveness or hyperreactivity of the airways to a variety of stimuli which is the most consistent finding in asthmatic patients.[2]

Increased airway reactivity follows exposure of the asthmatic to a variety of environmental factors, including allergens, exercise, cold air, viral upper respiratory tract infections, and other environmental factors such as chemicals, smoke, air pollution, medications, etc.[3] The course and severity of asthma are quite variable, with some patients having subclinical disease, some with mild intermittent exacerbations, and others experiencing persistent signs and symptoms of asthma. Asthma can remit spontaneously, while other patients may improve with the removal of an essential precipitant or as the result of therapeutic intervention. Some patients only rarely require therapy, while others need continuous intensive medical regimens, including chronic systemic corticosteroids (Figure 31–1).

There remains little doubt that there is a hereditary component in determining which children are at risk for development of asthma. Young males tend to be affected approximately twice as often as females; however, this ratio evens out as adulthood is reached. Although there is a tendency for asthma to improve from mid-childhood to adolescence, denial of symptoms in adolescence may mask impairment of pulmonary function. One of the most important goals for treatment of asthma in children is to achieve a near normal life-style. Normal exercise tolerance, good school attendance, quality and quantity of sleep, and appropriate social interactions need to be considered as therapeutic endpoints for pharmacologic management of asthma.

CELLULAR AND BIOCHEMICAL FEATURES OF ASTHMA

The enhanced bronchial responsiveness and airway obstruction observed in asthma is theoretically the result of an abnormal inflammatory response within the lung. Histologic studies show bronchial smooth muscle hypertrophy, mucosal edema, hypersecretion, and airway inflammation. Marked inflammatory changes with extensive damage to the epithelial lining of the airway are also observed in patients with mild intermittent to moderately severe chronic asthma.[4] Similar alterations are seen in patients who have died from acute attacks.[5] The relationship of underlying airway reactivity and inflammation will be addressed through a discussion of the inflammatory cells, mediators of inflammation, and the neural mechanisms involved (Figure 31–2).

Inflammatory Cells

Asthma is associated with desquamation of bronchial epithelium and infiltration of the airway lining with mast cells, eosinophils, and lymphocytes.[5] The role and func-

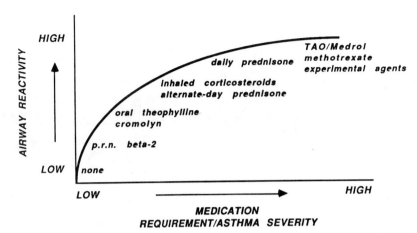

FIGURE 31–1. Schematic representation of the relationship between asthma severity and medication requirement.

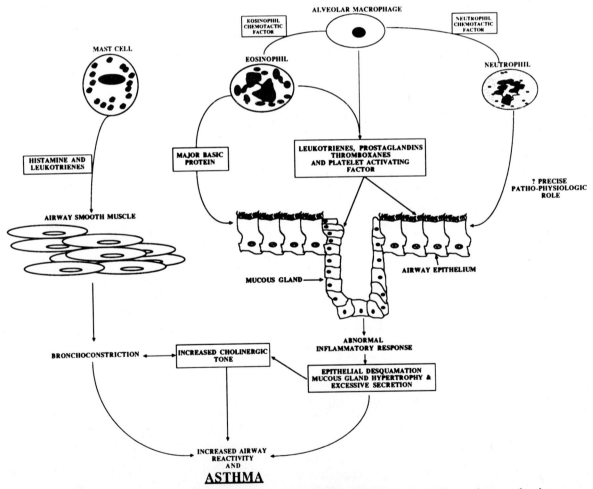

FIGURE 31–2. Schematic diagram of inflammatory cells and mediators and the resultant pathophysiologic effects that result in asthma. See text for details.

tion of eosinophils,[6] mast cells,[7-9] macrophages,[10] neutrophils,[11] and basophils[12] in the pathogenesis of asthma have been investigated extensively.

The mast cell initiates an immediate response to allergen in sensitive individuals. Once binding of allergen to cell-bound immunoglobulin E (IgE) occurs, there is release of mediators including histamine, eosinophil and neutrophil chemotactic factors, leukotrienes C_4, D_4, and E_4, prostaglandins, platelet-activating factor (PAF), and many others.[7] When allergic asthmatics receive airway challenge with antigen, a significant rise in histamine concentration recovered from bronchoalveolar lavage fluid is observed, most likely a result of lung mast cell degranulation.[8] Histamine release from mast cells is inhibited by both β-agonists and, to a lesser extent, cromolyn sodium.[13] Conversely, there is no evidence that corticosteroids inhibit the degranulation of human lung mast cells.[14]

The eosinophil is also a major contributor to the pathogenesis of asthma.[6] Granules present in the eosinophil contain major basic protein (MBP), which is responsible for damage to airway epithelium.[15] Since MBP is present in very high quantities in the sputum of patients with asthma,[16] the damage to airway epithelium caused by eosinophil degranulation may contribute to the development of airway hyperreactivity. Despite the probable importance of eosinophils in asthma, surprisingly little is known regarding the pharmacology of this cell type. Corticosteroids have a marked eosinopenic effect and also reduce eosinophil adherence and inhibit chemotaxis, resulting in diminished recruitment of these cells to inflammatory sites.[17] However, the effects of other antiasthma medications such as theophylline or β-agonists on the eosinophil are not known.

The potential role of alveolar macrophages and neutrophils in the pathogenesis of asthma is evolving. These cells ordinarily serve as "scavengers" to engulf and digest bacteria and other foreign materials.[18] They may play a role in the initiation and amplification of inflammation in allergic asthma.[19] A partial list of mediators produced by alveolar macrophages includes PAF, LTB_4, LTC_4, and LTD_4. Additionally, alveolar macrophages attract inflammatory cells including neutrophils and eosinophils.[19]

Inflammatory Mediators in Asthma

There has been an explosion of information regarding the role of mediators in asthma, summarized recently by Smith and Henson[20] and by Abraham and Wanner.[21] Although many substances are implicated, further investigation is needed to clarify their significance in the pathogenesis of asthma. We will highlight those mediators considered as major contributors.

HISTAMINE

Histamine, a mediator released from mast cells, induces smooth muscle contraction, mucosal edema, and mucus secretion that contributes to bronchospasm.[7] Lung mast cells are an important source of histamine, and its release can be induced by a physical stimulus, such as exercise, or by allergen exposure. Although histamine may elicit an asthmatic response, antihistamines are relatively ineffective in the treatment of asthma. This may be related to an insufficient dose or short duration of action of currently available antihistamines, or to the failure to block the actions of other mediators that produce similar effects in the airway.

Membrane-Derived Lipid Mediators

Phospholipids are present in the membranes of most inflammatory cells, and mediators derived from membrane phospholipids include the prostaglandins (PGs), leukotrienes (LTs), and PAF.

Certain prostaglandins, such as PGD_2, are potent bronchoconstricting agents.[22] PGD_2, however, has a short duration of effect, due to rapid metabolism, and thus its role in clinical asthma remains to be determined. Similarly, $PGF_{2\alpha}$ is a potent bronchoconstrictor in asthmatic patients and enhances the effect of histamine.[23] The origin of this compound in the lung is currently unknown, and it is not clear whether this substance has any other pathophysiologic effects. Another cyclooxygenase product that is produced in the lung, prostacyclin (PGI_2),[24] contributes to inflammation and edema due to its vasodilator properties. Finally, other cyclooxygenase products, such as thromboxane A_2 (TXA_2), which is produced within the lung by alveolar macrophages, fibroblasts, epithelial cells, neutrophils, and platelets,[21] may have bronchoconstricting properties and be involved in the late response to antigen exposure. These substances have also been implicated in the development of airway inflammation and hyperreactivity in some animal models. The thromboxane synthetase inhibitors that have recently become available will be crucial tools in understanding the role of thromboxanes in clinical asthma.

The lipoxygenase pathway of arachidonic acid metabolism results in synthesis of leukotrienes,[21] including leukotrienes C_4, D_4, and E_4 (sulfidopeptideleukotrienes) that were formerly referred to as slow-reacting substance of anaphylaxis (SRS-A). Leukotrienes have potent effects on airway smooth muscle, mucociliary function, and microvascular permeability.[25] However, the available potent leukotriene antagonists have not had significant antiasthmatic effect in humans.

Another phospholipid-derived mediator, PAF, is released upon stimulation of alveolar macrophages, neutrophils, and platelets. PAF, when administered directly to the lung, results in sustained bronchoconstriction, edema formation, and cellular changes associated with a generalized inflammatory response.[26] Moreover, PAF produces airway hyperresponsiveness in humans that peaks in 3 days and continues for 1–4 weeks after PAF inhalation.[27] The relevance of PAF in asthma and allergic diseases will be clarified once clinical trials are conducted with specific PAF antagonists.

THE NERVOUS SYSTEM IN ASTHMA

The parasympathetic and sympathetic nervous systems play an integral role in the regulation of airway tone. A brief description of airway smooth muscle innervation will provide background information for discussion of the mechanism of action of bronchodilator medications.

Parasympathetic Nervous System

Virtually all asthmatics have profound bronchoconstriction in response to cholinergic agonists, such as methacholine or carbachol, suggesting an abnormality in the parasympathetic nervous system. Sensory nerve endings within the airway interact with the central nervous system through the afferent vagus nerve. Nerve impulses return to the lung via the efferent vagus. Postganglionic nerves located in airway smooth muscle release acetylcholine which produces bronchoconstriction. Anticholinergic bronchodilators, such as atropine and its derivative ipratropium bromide, are cholinergic receptor antagonists. The parasympathetic nervous system also regulates mucus secretion,[28] and airway inflammation can result in increased exposure of sensory nerve endings contributing to bronchial hyperreactivity.[29]

Sympathetic Nervous System

In contrast to the extensive distribution of the parasympathetic system, the airway is poorly innervated by sympathetic nervous system. Although there is minimal direct innervation of airway smooth muscle,[30] there is a rich supply of β-adrenergic receptors in airway smooth muscle.[31] Furthermore, clinical observation verifies the importance of the sympathetic nervous system. For example, β-adrenergic antagonists have little or no effect on airway tone in nonasthmatics but can produce profound bronchoconstriction in asthmatics.[32] Moreover, β-adrenergic agonists have little effect in normals yet are potent bronchodilators in asthmatics. Therefore, the sympathetic nervous system may not be important as a homeostatic mechanism in healthy humans but is very important in reversing bronchoconstriction in response to adverse stimuli in asthmatics. β_2-Receptors are involved in bronchodilatory effects, as stimulation of pulmonary β_1-receptors does not produce bronchodilator effects in asthmatic humans.[33] Other functional aspects of β-receptor stimulation include increased mucociliary clearance, inhibition of antigen-induced release of mediators from mast cells, and prevention of microvascular leakage induced by histamine.[34] Although β_2-receptors are located throughout the lung,[35] radioligand studies have demonstrated β_2-receptors located in cardiac tissue as well.[36] The function of the cardiac receptors is not clear, but stimulation appears to produce inotropic rather than chronotropic effects.

DRUGS USED IN THE TREATMENT OF ASTHMA

Bronchodilator Antiasthma Drugs

β-Adrenergic Agonists

Clinical Pharmacology

β-Adrenergic agonists (β-agonists) are the most potent bronchodilators. These agents produce maximal smooth muscle relaxation *in vitro* against a wide variety of constrictor agents, including leukotrienes, prostaglandins, carbachol, and histamine.[37] Activity results from β-adrenergic receptor stimulation, which activates adenylate cyclase, conversion of ATP, increased intracellular cyclic AMP, and consequent relaxation of smooth muscle. Stimulation of these receptors in other tissues results in enhanced mucociliary transport, increased mucus and water secretion into the airways, and inhibition of antigen-induced release of mast cell mediators.[34]

PHARMACOKINETICS. Recently developed β-agonists, specifically terbutaline and albuterol, have a greater β_2-selectivity, longer duration of action, and improved oral bioavailability, since they are not metabolized by catechol-O-methyltransferase or monoamine oxidase enzymes. Terbutaline is incompletely absorbed as a result of gut wall sulfation and has an average bioavailability of 15 percent.[38] Absorption of albuterol is slightly greater, with overall bioavailability of approximately 50 percent.[39] An extended-release formulation of albuterol is available (Proventil Repetabs, Schering, Kenilworth, NJ), which is designed to release half of the dose immediately and the remaining half 2–4 hours later. A true sustained-release formulation of albuterol is in clinical trials (Volmax, Glaxo, Research Triangle Park, NC) and will likely be introduced for twice-daily dosing.

After parenteral administration, terbutaline and albuterol display multicompartment disposition. The terminal phase half-life for terbutaline is 17 hours,[40] while that for albuterol is 3–4 hours.[39] There is a good relationship between single parenteral doses of terbutaline and effect on pulmonary function.[41] The pharmacokinetics of the inhaled route are not as well characterized, for several reasons. First, the dose of drug that arrives within the lung for absorption varies depending on the administration technique. Second, systemic absorption of any drug that may be swallowed will falsely elevate estimates of bioavailability. Finally, the doses of drug administered via metered-dose inhaler are relatively low, and suitable assay methodologies have not been developed to detect the concentrations of drug that are present.

The relatively slow elimination of these compounds contrasts with their short duration of action. Single-dose studies indicate that bronchodilation may persist for up to 6 hours.[42] Bitolterol, the prodrug of the active moeity colterol, is slightly longer-acting than albuterol, but these differences may not be clinically relevant.[43]

Perhaps more important than the duration of the bronchodilatory effect is the duration of the functional antagonism to bronchoconstriction, or the antireactivity effect, provided by various β-agonists. With appropriate study design, serial bronchoprovocation with nonspecific challenges such as histamine, methacholine, or exercise may be more clinically relevant. The duration of the bronchodilator effect of inhaled metaproterenol outlasted the ability to protect from exercise-induced bronchospasm by several hours.[44] The antireactivity effect of metered-dose aerosols of metaproterenol and albuterol was investigated using serial bronchoprovocational challenges with histamine.[45] Two puffs of albuterol had a greater initial effect than two puffs of metaproterenol, but neither treatment was different from placebo by 4 hours postdose. Similar information is now available for bitolterol, terbutaline, and fenoterol, as summarized in Table 31–1.

ROUTE OF ADMINISTRATION. The optimal method for administration of β-agonists is via the inhaled route. The onset of effect occurs within minutes, and peak intensity occurs soon thereafter. Moreover, the inhaled route offers the potential to maximize the inherent β_2-selectivity by applying the drug to the desired intrapulmonary site and bypassing systemic delivery, thereby lowering the potential for adverse effects. Finally, inhaled β-agonists effectively block exercise-induced bronchospasm, whereas oral β-agonists do not.[46]

The theoretical advantage of parenteral β-agonists in the treatment of acute severe asthma is that the drug reaches peripheral airways blocked by intense bronchoconstriction and mucosal edema. Although this seems intuitively correct, aerosolized terbutaline has been shown to be as effective as intravenous terbutaline.[47] If the clinical response to nebulized doses of β-agonists is inadequate, a subcutaneous dose of epinephrine may be effective while other treatments, such as intravenous corticosteroids and aminophylline, are instituted.

Intravenous isoproterenol is occasionally used in the treatment of acute severe asthma associated with a rising pCO$_2$ and impending respiratory failure. It can be effective despite maximal use of subcutaneous epinephrine, intravenous corticosteroids and aminophylline, and appropriate oxygen and hydration.[48] As this therapy is only indicated in critically ill patients and is associated with significant toxicity,[49,50] its use should be limited to the pediatric intensive care unit with experienced physicians.

TOLERANCE. Tolerance, subsensitivity, or tachyphylaxis refers to diminished responsiveness in receptor-mediated systems following prolonged exposure of the receptor to an agonist. For the β-agonists, tolerance that develops after several weeks of chronic therapy is mostly manifested as decreased intensity and duration of bronchodilator action. At least 10 clinical investigations have demonstrated some degree of tolerance.[51] Overall, the peak intensity declined by a range of 14–58 percent, and the time that pulmonary function remained 15 percent above baseline was reduced by 50 percent. Therefore, the degree of bronchodilator activity during chronic therapy is reduced as compared to single doses. Furthermore, when assessing clinical trials, the use of β-agonists prior to initiation of the study period should be carefully reviewed.

Present Status

Inhaled β-agonists are effective in all stages of asthma therapy. They are the first to be prescribed for control of mild intermittent asthma, the most effective agents in preventing exercise-induced bronchospasm, and extremely useful for chronic asthma therapy in combination with theophylline, cromolyn, and inhaled or systemic corticosteroids. Oral β-agonists may be useful adjunctive therapy in the treatment of nocturnal asthma, and the new long-acting formulations are currently in clinical trials. Dosing guidelines for children and adults are provided in Table 31–2.

Future Considerations

In providing reversal and protection from symptoms of asthma with potent, long-acting β-agonists, are we masking a smoldering inflammatory process in the lung? Historically, β-agonists have been used for years in patients, including young children, with mild asthma without progression of the underlying disease. It therefore appears that this form of therapy is safe and efficacious. Continuing research in patients with chronic asthma will alleviate these concerns.

Theophylline

Clinical Pharmacology

There is a tremendous volume of literature devoted to the clinical pharmacology of theophylline, and several excellent, detailed reviews are available.[52] This discussion will therefore be limited to major and recent information,

TABLE 31–1. DURATION OF ANTIREACTIVITY EFFECT FOR VARIOUS β-AGONISTS*

AGENT (DOSAGE)	RELATIVE AEROSOL POTENCY†	DURATION OF EFFECT (h)	REF.
Albuterol (180 μg/2 puffs)	1.0	4–5	45
Metaproterenol (1300 μg/2 puffs)	0.37	3–4	45
Terbutaline (400 μg/2 puffs)	0.43	4–5	171
Bitolterol (1050 μg/3 puffs)	Not determined	4–5	172
Fenoterol (400 μg/2 puffs)	1.88‡	5–6	173

*Adapted with permission from Jenne JW, Ahrens RC: Pharmacokinetics of beta-adrenergic compounds, in Jenne JW, Murphy S (eds): Drug Therapy for Asthma: Research and Clinical Practice. New York, Marcel Dekker, 1987, pp 213–258.
†Equivalent number of puffs of albuterol required to produce initial effects equal to 1 puff of medication tested.
‡Based on a study of bronchodilation.

TABLE 31–2. RECOMMENDED DOSAGES OF ADRENERGIC BRONCHODILATORS

DRUG (TRADE NAME)	RECEPTOR SPECIFICITY	ROUTE	ADULT DOSE	PEDIATRIC DOSE	COMMENTS
Epinephrine (Adrenalin)	α, β_1, β_2	Subcutaneous	0.3 ml (0.3 mg) of 1:1000 dilution every 20 min (3 doses maximum)	0.01 ml/kg of 1:1000 dilution (up to 0.3 ml max) every 20 min (3 doses max)	Duration <1 h injection solution contains sodium bisulfite
Epinephrine suspension (Sus-Phrine)	α, β_1, β_2	Subcutaneous	0.15–0.3 ml (0.75–1.5 mg) of 1:200 dilution every 6 h	0.005 ml/kg of 1:200 dilution (up to 0.15 ml) every 6 h	Doses should be repeated only when necessary
Isoetharine (Bronkosol) Beta-2 (Bronkometer)	β_1, β_2	Nebulization Metered-dose inhaler	0.25–1.0 ml (2.5–10 mg) every 2–4 h 1–2 actuations (340 μg/act) every 2–4 h	0.02 ml/kg up to 0.5 ml* every 2–4 h No specific pediatric guidelines	Solutions contain sodium bisulfite
Metaproterenol	β_1, β_2	Nebulization	0.3 ml (15 mg) every 2–6 h	Acute: 0.01 ml/kg up to 0.3 ml[a] every 2–6 h	See footnote for use with intermittent nebulizers†
		Metered-dose inhaler Tablet or syrup	1–2 activations (650 μg/act) every 2–6 h 20 mg every 6 h	Not recommended in patients <12 yrs‡ 6–9 yrs (<60 lb): 10 mg every 6 h 9–12 years (>60 lb): 20 mg every 6 h	Safety and efficacy have been demonstrated in patients <6 yrs receiving 1.3–2.6 mg/kg/day
Terbutaline (Brethine, Bricanyl)	β_2	Oral (tablet) Subcutaneous	5 mg every 8 h 0.3 ml (0.3 mg) every 20 min (3 doses max)	Not recommended in patients <12 yrs 0.01 ml/kg (up to 0.3 ml) every two min (3 doses max)	Significant bronchodilation has been documented in children (>5 yrs) in doses of 50–100 μg/kg/dose every 8 h§
		Nebulization	Acute: 2 ml (2 mg) every 2–4 h	Acute: 0.03 ml/kg (up to 2 ml max) every 2–4 h*	Benefit from use on a chronic prophylactic basis can be outweighed by cost factors (see discussion)
(Brethaire)		Metered-dose inhaler	2 actuations (200 μg/act) every 4–6 h	Safety and efficacy in patients <12 yrs not established‡	
Bitolterol (Tornalate)	β_2	Metered-dose inhaler	2–3 actuations (370 μg/act) every 6–8 h, not to exceed 2 actuations every 4 h	Safety and efficacy in patients <12 yrs not established‡	Theoretical advantage in longer duration of action; however, more evluation indicated (bitolterol is the esterified prodrug of active colterol)

with special emphasis on the use of theophylline in children.

The mechanism of action of theophylline is probably not related to a single effect, but likely includes several pathways. One potential mechanism is related to inhibition of phosphodiesterase activity. Inhibition of this enzyme would lead to intracellular accumulation of cyclic AMP, resulting in smooth muscle relaxation. At therapeutic concentrations, however, theophylline is a poor inhibitor of phosphodiesterase.[53] Furthermore, other phosphodiesterase inhibitors do not have antiasthma properties. Recent reports suggest that theophylline potentiates β-adrenergic receptor activity and thereby relaxes airway smooth muscle.[54]

Adenosine, an endogenous neurotransmitter, produces bronchoconstriction in asthmatic humans[55] and has other effects that may lead to the development of asthma.[37] However, the methylxanthine bronchodilator enprofylline lacks adenosine antagonistic effect, suggesting that adenosine antagonism may not be a significant contributor to the bronchodilator effect of theophylline.[56]

Recently, Pauwells and coworkers[57] demonstrated that theophylline and enprofylline attenuate the immediate and late asthmatic response to allergen exposure. Although theophylline and enprofylline do not completely block the allergic response, theophylline may be a potent functional antagonist for certain mediators.

Finally, there is indirect evidence that theophylline has a membrane-stabilizing effect on pulmonary capillary endothelium, preventing release of plasma-borne mediators into the interstitial and alveolar space and preventing interaction of these mediators with inflammatory cells.[58] Further investigation is needed to understand the mechanism of action of theophylline.

BRONCHODILATOR EFFECT. The bronchodilator effect of theophylline correlates directly with its serum concentration, and bronchodilator effects are observed in both chronic and acute asthmatics.[59,60] The beneficial effects

TABLE 31–2. RECOMMENDED DOSAGES OF ADRENERGIC BRONCHODILATORS *Continued*

DRUG (TRADE NAME)	RECEPTOR SPECIFICITY	ROUTE	ADULT DOSE	PEDIATRIC DOSE	COMMENTS
Pirbuterol (Max Air)	β_2	Metered-dose inhaler	2 actuations (200 μg/act) every 4–6 h	Safety and efficacy in patients <12 yrs not established‡	May have slightly lower incidence of side effects than albuterol, but more data are needed
Albuterol	β_2	Oral (tablet or syrup)	2–4 mg every 8 h initally. Max dose 8 mg every 8 h	2–6 yrs: 0.1 mg/kg (2 mg max) every 8 h 6–14 yrs: 2 mg every 8 h	
		Repetab	4–8 mg every 12 h	Safety and efficacy in patients <12 yrs not established‡	Repetab formulation releases 50% of dose immediately and 50% within 2–4 h postdose for a longer duration of action
		Metered-dose inhaler	2 actuations (90 μg/act) every 4–6 h	Safety and efficacy in patients <12 yrs not established‡ Experience suggests 1–2 puffs every 4–6 h and prior to exercise is safe in children‡	
		Nebulization	0.5–1.0 ml (2.5–5.0 mg) every 4–6 h. Experience suggests doses of albuterol can be administered repeatedly at 20-min intervals. In these situations heart rate should be monitored carefully	Safety and efficacy in patients <12 yrs not established‡ Safe dose appears to be 0.05–0.15 mg/kg every 2–6 h as needed¶	

*Rachelefsky G, Siegel S: J Allergy Clin Immunol 76:409–425, 1985.
†Investigations at National Jewish Center for Immunology and Respiratory Medicine have shown that when used with intermittent nebulizers, which operate only on inspiration, a much smaller dose is required to produce equal bronchodilator effect vs the dose recommended by the manufacturer, when administered by continuous nebulization. For intermittent nebulization of metaproterenol, 0.08 ml (4 mg) in 1.2 cc total volume every 4–6 h for adults and 0.0025 ml/kg in 1.2 cc total volume every 2–6 h for children are appropriate doses.
‡These metered-dose inhalers are not aproved for use in children by the FDA. However, they are commonly prescribed for children as young as 5 years of age using doses similar to adults. They are useful in prevention and treatment of bronchospasm with similar side effects to those seen in adults. Clinicians prescribing these drugs should document that other forms of treatment are not optimal and inform patient and parent that the drug is being used in a nonapproved manner.
§Ardel B, et al: J Pediatr 93:305–307, 1978.
¶Kelly HW, Murphy S, Jenne JW, in Drug Therapy for Asthma, Appendix II, Marcel Dekker, pp 1025–1031.
Physicians Desk Reference—source of information.

are observed over the concentration range of 5–20 μg/ml.[61]

BRONCHOPROTECTIVE EFFECT. Theophylline attenuates the immediate[61] and late[57] asthmatic response to allergen exposure. Theophylline can also reduce nonspecific airway reactivity to histamine or methacholine when serum theophylline concentrations are between 10 and 20 μg/ml.[62] In addition, exercise-induced bronchospasm in asthmatics is markedly reduced in the presence of theophylline when serum concentrations are at least 10 μg/ml[63] and perhaps more effective at 15 μg/ml.[64]

CHRONIC ASTHMA. Theophylline therapy has been associated with a significant decrease in symptomatology associated with chronic asthma,[65] even in patients who require oral and inhaled corticosteroids,[66] by improving exercise tolerance and by reducing nocturnal symptoms and supplemental β-agonist requirements. As compared to inhaled albuterol four times daily, theophylline is superior, especially in controlling nighttime awakening from asthma and morning wheeze.[67] Brenner and coworkers[68] recently demonstrated the importance of maintenance theophylline in severe, steroid-requiring asthmatics. In this double-blind, controlled study, stabilized patients were randomized to receive placebo or individualized doses of sustained-release theophylline in addition to concomitant antiasthmatic agents, including inhaled cromolyn and β-agonists and inhaled and oral corticosteroids. Following transfer to palcebo treatment, severe exacerbations of asthma developed, necessitating acute hospitalization or additional corticosteroid therapy. Theophylline is therefore an important medication in the management of severe chronic asthma.

ACUTE ASTHMA. Beneficial effects of theophylline (as aminophylline) for acute severe asthma were first reported in the late 1930s,[69] and its use increased until it became standard therapy for the treatment of acute severe asthma. Recent reports suggest that intravenous aminophylline has no benefit over aggressive nebulized β-

agonist therapy alone in acute severe asthma.[70] In contrast, Vozeh and coworkers[71] demonstrated a more rapid therapeutic effect in patients with asthma or chronic obstructive pulmonary disease with dosage schemes designed to achieve serum theophylline concentrations of 19 μg/ml, as compared to a similar group treated with dosage regimens providing average concentrations of 10 μg/ml. In the treatment of acute asthma, it is reasonable to optimize β-agonist therapy and consider earlier use of corticosteroids to compensate for the limited bronchodilator properties of theophylline.

TOXICITY. Adverse effects can be directly related to serum theophylline concentration. Jenne et al.[72] observed that most toxicity, including nausea, vomiting, and anorexia, occurred in patients with serum theophylline concentrations greater than 13 μg/ml and was most common in patients with concentrations greater than 20 μg/ml. More serious toxicity can occur at concentrations greater than 20 μg/ml, including irritability and insomnia. At concentrations greater than 35 μg/ml, cardiac arrhythmias, hypotension, seizures, and death have been observed.[73] Oral doses of activated charcoal increase theophylline elimination[74] and are useful in the treatment of acute or chronic toxicity.

Certain adverse effects appear unrelated to serum theophylline concentrations. Since theophylline decreases gastroesophageal sphincter tone,[75] it is postulated that this could worsen asthma via aspiration or neurally mediated reflex bronchoconstriction. However, a recent investigation failed to associate the use of sustained-release theophylline formulations with gastroesophageal reflux in patients with asthma.[76] The possibility of gastroesophageal reflux as a precipitant of asthma should be evaluated in patients with severe asthma, especially those with a nocturnal component.

The possible association between the use of theophylline and abnormalities in learning and behavior in children is also a concern.[77] Rachelefsky and coworkers[78] studied 20 mildly asthmatic children in a double-blind, randomized parallel trial of theophylline versus placebo. Extensive neuropsychological testing as well as parental evaluations did not detect differences between treatments. However, composite scores from schoolteachers recognized deficits in attention and classroom behavior in children receiving theophylline. Unfortunately, the only available studies to date on theophylline and behavior are limited in both sample size and study duration (see Table 31–3) and must be considered preliminary until larger, well-controlled investigations of sufficient duration are available. There is no doubt that theophylline has the potential to affect learning and behavior in some patients. Until these effects are understood more clearly, it may be advisable to seek alternative antiasthma medications such as cromolyn if a clearly identifiable adverse effect is observed by a parent or teacher.

CLINICAL PHARMACOKINETICS. The pharmacokinetics of theophylline have been studied extensively and were recently reviewed in great detail by Hendeles et al.[79] Since the absorption and elimination of theophylline have unique features, this area will be highlighted.

Dosage Requirements in Children. There is a significant positive correlation between patient age and theophylline clearance such that age becomes the major determinant in estimation of the proper theophylline dosage for a specific child. Age-dependent dosage guidelines are widely published. Milavetz and coworkers[80] recently demonstrated the relationship between dosage and age in a large population of asthmatics (Figure 31–3).

Alterations in the dietary protein content are known to affect theophylline elimination. Increased protein content can substantially increase elimination, while decreasing protein can result in decreased elimination of theophylline.[81] The growing and developing child may occasionally experience relevant changes in dietary protein con-

TABLE 31–3. PROSPECTIVE, RANDOMIZED, DOUBLE-BLIND, PLACEBO-CONTROLLED STUDIES EVALUATING THE NEUROPSYCHOLOGIC EFFECTS OF THEOPHYLLINE IN ASTHMATICS

REF.	ASTHMA SEVERITY CLASSIFIED	PRESENCE OF A NONASTHMA CONTROL GROUP	SAMPLE SIZE (AGE–RANGE)	CROSSOVER	DURATION*
174	Yes	No	13 (8–13)	Yes	4 weeks
175	Yes	No	20 (6–12)	No	4 weeks
176	Yes	No	18 (13–70)	Yes	3 months
177	No	No	29 (7–12)	No	2 weeks

PARAMETERS ASSESSED/DETRIMENTAL EFFECT†

REF.	ATTENTION	LEARNING & MEMORY	VISUAL-SPATIAL‡ PLANNING	MOTOR CONTROL ASSESSMENT	PARENTAL ASSESSMENT OF CHILD BEHAVIOR	SCHOOL TEACHER ASSESSMENT OF CHILD BEHAVIOR	DEPRESSION	OBSESSIVE-COMPULSIVE BEHAVIOR
174	Yes/−	Yes/−	Yes/+	No	No	No	No	No
175	Yes/−	Yes/−	Yes/−	No	Yes/−	Yes/+	No	No
176	Yes/−	Yes/−	Yes/−	Yes/+	No	No	No	No
177	No	Yes/−	Yes/−	No	Yes/+	No	Yes/+	Yes/+

*Minimum duration of study to allow for evaluation of normal fluctuation in testing may be 3 months or longer.
†Parameters assessed are indicated with a yes or no. If a given parameter was assessed and was found to be associated with a detrimental effect, it is indicated as positive (+) or, if no effect, a negative (−) indicator.
‡Ability to comprehend imaginary movements in three-dimensional space or ability to manipulate objects in the imagination.

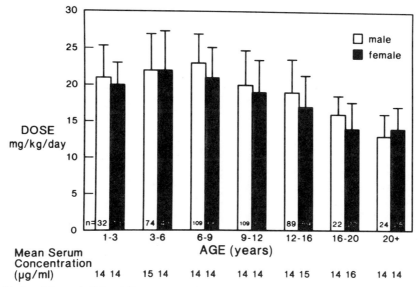

FIGURE 31–3. Mean ± S.D. daily dosages of theophylline (mg/kg/day) required to produce serum theophylline concentrations between 10 and 20 μg/ml. A greater than three-fold variation in dosage requirement is seen in each age group. Therapy was initiated with doses unlikely to produce adverse effects, followed by two incremental increases of 25 to 50 percent at 3-day intervals, if tolerated. Adjustment of the final dosage was by measurement of serum theophylline concentration. (From Milavetz et al.[80] with permission.)

tent when feeding patterns are altered. This may need to be considered when changes in theophylline dosage requirements are observed.

Sustained-Release Oral Formulations. Although the absorption of liquids and plain tablets of theophylline is rapid and complete, the relatively rapid elimination in children necessitates frequent dosing at 6-hour intervals. Sustained-release formulations facilitate convenient dosage intervals. Of the more than 25 formulations available in the United States, only a few are absorbed slowly enough to permit twice-daily administration with acceptable fluctuations in serum theophylline concentration. Theo-Dur tablets are completely absorbed and have less than 100 percent fluctuation (peak − trough/trough serum theophylline concentration) in most children.[82] Similarly, Slo-Bid Gyrocaps have acceptable fluctuation in serum theophylline concentration; an additional advantage is the possibility of emptying the capsules on soft food for administration to young children.[83] An investigational formulation by Riker Labs (Noctelin) appears to have slow enough absorption for once-daily administration in many children[84] but has not been completely evaluated in children less than 8 years of age. Finally, a sustained-release liquid theophylline is currently being evaluated for twice-daily administration in children, but it may not be suitable for those who are rapid metabolizers.[85]

Another consideration is the effect of food on the rate and extent of absorption with certain sustained-release formulations. Significant alterations in theophylline absorption occur with Uniphyl (Purdue-Frederick) and Theo-24 (Searle). With these formulations, absorption is incomplete in the fasting state, and both the rate and extent of absorption increase in the presence of a high-fat-content meal.[86,87] Food also affects Theo-Dur Sprinkle, a

formulation intended for pediatric dosing, in the opposite fashion. When administered with a meal, the extent of absorption is decreased to approximately 50 percent of the dose.[88] This food–drug interaction is often misinterpreted as representing unusually rapid metabolism, necessitating high theophylline dose requirements.

Absorption Variability. In most patients theophylline absorption from sustained-release dosage forms is relatively consistent. In younger children and adolescents, a diurnal pattern in theophylline absorption occurs such that serum theophylline concentrations are lower following the evening dose.[89] This is related to a decreased rate of absorption at night, possibly correlated with postural changes.[90] Dose-to-dose and day-to-day variation in the rate and extent of theophylline absorption may also present as a problem in certain patients[91] and may require careful evaluation. When faced with erratic serum theophylline concentrations, it is important to consider poor patient compliance as a confounding variable, but equally important to consider the possibility of variable absorption in patients who appear to be compliant.

Present Concerns/Future Considerations

Theophylline is a useful adjunct in the treatment of chronic asthma. Concerns regarding the effects of theophylline on learning and behavior in children have raised questions regarding the appropriate application of theophylline. Unfortunately, there is insufficient information to relieve these concerns. At the same time, efforts are being made to develop more convenient dosage forms, specifically once-daily products, suitable for use in young children. Finally, more information is needed on the potential anti-inflammatory mechanisms of action for theophylline.

Anticholinergics

Clinical Pharmacology

Historically, anticholinergic drugs were used as bronchodilators long before the advent of sympathomimetics. They fell into disfavor as the sympathomimetics appeared to be more effective. With increased understanding of the role of the cholinergic nervous system in regulation of airway tone, there was a resurgence of interest in anticholinergic bronchodilators.

Anticholinergics induce bronchodilation by preventing acetylcholine binding at postganglionic muscarinic receptors located along airway smooth muscle. This receptor-mediated antagonism decreases the activity of guanylate cyclase, resulting in deceased formation of cyclic 3′,5′-guanosine monophosphate and thereby inducing airway relaxation.[92]

Atropine sulfate is a tertiary ammonium compound administered as a 1–2 mg/ml solution in water or saline via nebulizer. A quaternary ammonium compound derived from atropine, ipratopium bromide (Atrovent, Boehringer-Ingelheim), formerly known as SCH1000, has been available commercially in Europe since the mid-1970s and in the United States since late 1987. Atropine methylnitrate is a quaternary ammonium derivative that is only available experimentally. The advantage of the quaternary ammonium derivatives is their poor absorption from the lung and other sites of deposition. Atropine sulfate, although variably absorbed, does yield systemic concentrations of drug[93] that have been associated with toxicity.[94] Conversely, when quaternary ammonium compounds such as ipratropium are administered via inhalation, the drug is virtually nonabsorbable.[95] In addition to minimal systemic side effects, ipratropium is not associated with increasing sputum viscosity, despite diminished total sputum volume in patients with chronic bronchitis.[96]

BRONCHODILATOR EFFECTS. There is an extensive body of literature describing the bronchodilator effects of anticholinergics in patients with chronic obstructive pulmonary disease as well as asthma, and these have been summarized recently.[97] Ipratropium generally provides a significant bronchodilator effect but is not as potent as albuterol.[98,99] The onset of action is delayed in comparison to β-agonists, with maximal effect being reached within 60–120 minutes postdose.[98] There is some additive effect when ipratropium is combined with albuterol in the treatment of acute severe asthma in children.[100] The duration of action of ipratropium may be as long as 6–8 hours. Since anticholinergics are receptor antagonists, they do not induce tolerance or tachyphylaxis. Tolerance has not been observed in long-term studies in adult patients with chronic obstructive lung disease.[101] Rebound airway hyperresponsiveness to methacholine may occur following discontinuation of inhaled ipratropium.[102] It is not clear whether this hyperresponsiveness is present if measured by a nonspecific challenge agent such as histamine, and it is not considered a significant clinical problem in asthmatics discontinuing inhaled ipratropium therapy.

BRONCHOPROTECTIVE EFFECTS. Inhaled anticholinergics are generally ineffective as bronchoprotective agents.

Ipratropium does not block exercise-induced bronchospasm,[103] nor does it have any effect on the immediate or late asthmatic response to allergen,[104] despite significant bronchodilation prior to the challenge. Ipratropium completely blocks methacholine-induced bronchoconstriction, while having no effect on histamine-induced bronchoconstriction.[105] In summary, anticholinergics are ineffective agents for prevention of bronchospasm as a result of exposure to a variety of adverse stimuli, with the exception of the muscarinic agent methacholine.

Present Status

The use of inhaled anticholinergics is currently limited in the treatment of asthma. β-Agonists are more potent bronchodilators, have more rapid onset of action, and are effective in a broader spectrum of patients. Although ipratropium may have a longer duration of effect, this may not be clinically significant. Occasionally, inhaled anticholinergics may be useful in the treatment of acute severe asthma in patients who do not respond adequately to aggressive β-agonist therapy. Inhaled ipratropium may be beneficial in older patients with emphysema or chronic bronchitis who do not respond to β-agonists. Patients should be informed that the onset of action is slow and beneficial effects may not be observed immediately. Maximal bronchodilation may take as long as 2 hours after the dose.

Future Considerations

One reason that anticholinergics have not received much attention in asthma is their relative lack of potency as compared with agents such as albuterol. A possible explanation for their low potency is that the recommended dose may be too low. The use of ipratropium with its relative absence of adverse effects may lend itself to more aggressive dosing regimens and better bronchodilation.

Nonbronchodilator Antiasthma Drugs

Cromolyn

Clinical Pharmacology

Cromolyn sodium (disodium cromoglycate) is a synthetic derivative of a natural furanochrome from the Mediterranean plant *Ammi visnaga*.[106] Although the precise biologic and functional activity of cromolyn in asthma is unknown, there are three proposed areas of activity.

First, cromolyn acts as a mast cell–stabilizing agent. Flint and coworkers[107] demonstrated that cromolyn inhibits mediator release from human lung mast cells obtained via bronchoalveolar lavage. This mast cell–stabilizing effect likely explains its efficacy in blocking antigen-induced mast cell histamine release following antigen challenge,[8] and development of the subsequent immediate asthmatic response.[104] Second, cromolyn has inhibitory effects on neutrophil activation following bronchial provocation with allergen.[108] Third, cromolyn and its congener nedocromil inhibit activation of eosinophils[109] and subsequent secretion of eosinophil granules.[110] If cromolyn inhibits secretion of MPB from eosinophils, then perhaps it prevents desquamation of airway epithelium and consequent airway hyperreactivity.

In addition to its effects on inhibition of the early and late asthmatic response to allergen challenge, a number of clinical studies show that cromolyn inhibits bronchoconstriction in response to a variety of nonspecific stimuli such as exercise,[111] cold air,[112] and sulfur dioxide.[113] These observations suggest an effect of cromolyn on afferent vagal tone, which modulates irritant receptor–mediated bronchoconstriction.

Present Status

In long-term treatment cromolyn decreases airway reactivity in allergic subjects, especially during the pollen season,[114] reduces signs and symptoms of chronic asthma,[115] and may be comparable in overall effect to theophylline.[116] It is recommended that cromolyn be administered for a minimum of 4 weeks before being considered ineffective. Since there are no clinical criteria to predict responders to cromolyn, it is important to ensure adequate duration of therapy, proper inhalation technique, and compliance. Additionally, adjunctive therapy with inhaled β-agonists and perhaps a short course of oral prednisone to establish optimal pulmonary function and symptom control prior to beginning cromolyn may be necessary.

Future Considerations

The use of cromolyn as a first-line drug in the treatment of chronic asthma in the United States is likely to increase. The reasons for this are multifactorial.[117]

A convenient, metered-dose inhaler delivering 1 mg cromolyn per actuation is now available in addition to the Spinhaler (20 mg/capsule) and the nebulizer solution (20 mg/vial). Despite the absence of well-controlled studies demonstrating the metered-dose inhaler to be as effective as the Spinhaler, there is some information demonstrating that this dosage form is better than placebo.[118,119]

Another advantage of cromolyn is that it is virtually devoid of significant side effects,[120] placing cromolyn in a favorable position as first-line therapy, especially in children. This is not due to the superior clinical effects of cromolyn as compared to theophylline, but more to recent concern regarding the potential effects of theophylline on learning and behavior in children (see theophylline discussion).

Finally, with insight into the pathophysiology of asthma and its association with inflammatory processes, attention is turning toward drugs with potential anti-inflammatory effects, such as cromolyn and corticosteroids.[121] However, this increased attention must be carefully evaluated. When cromolyn was introduced as a steroid-sparing agent in the treatment of asthma,[122] it soon fell into disfavor, as the beneficial effects in this patient population were minimal. With the resurgence in use, primarily as a first-line agent, it is once again being used for patients requiring inhaled or oral corticosteroids where clinical benefit was not previously apparent.[123,124] Therefore, one must be cautious in utilizing cromolyn in more severe asthmatics or in milder asthmatics already receiving inhaled corticosteroids.

Corticosteroids

Clinical Pharmacology

The beneficial effect of corticosteroids in asthma is related to prevention or suppression and resolution of airway inflammation. Pharmacologic effects include reduction of mediator production and release, reduction of inflammatory cell recruitment and infiltration, and decreased vascular permeability. Important clinical effects are prevention or inhibition of mucus secretion and airway edema.

The corticosteroids useful in the treatment of asthma and other inflammatory diseases are those that selectively bind to intracellular glucocorticoid receptors.[125] After binding occurs, the receptor complex is transferred from the cytoplasm to the nucleus. Once the receptor complex is bound to DNA, gene expression occurs, resulting in formation of messenger RNA and consequent protein synthesis. One of these proteins, lipocortin, is believed to exert its anti-inflammatory effects via inhibition of phospholipase A_2 and diminished formation of arachidonic acid and subsequent mediators.[126] Corticosteroids also increase the density and binding affinity of β-adrenergic receptors on peripheral leukocytes as well as smooth muscle cells cultured from human lung.[127,128] Moreover, administration of methylprednisolone restores the bronchoprotective effect of isoproterenol after induced tachyphylaxis.[129] This mechanism of action may be important in the treatment of acute severe asthma.

SYSTEMIC CORTICOSTEROIDS. The magnitude of effect of any medication is dependent on the dose administered and may be modified by conditions that affect absorption, distribution, and elimination. The time course of the effect is also dependent on the pharmacodynamic activity or the so-called biologic half-life of the corticosteroids.

Corticosteroids such as cortisol, prednisolone, and methylprednisolone are hydrophobic, lipophilic compounds. Structural modifications, including esterification to form methylprednisolone sodium succinate and hydrocortisone sodium succinate, increase solubility for parenteral administration. The most frequently used corticosteroid for oral administration is prednisone, which is itself inactive and requires reduction of the C-11 ketone to generate the active form prednisolone. This conversion step is rapid and complete after oral administration of prednisone; maximal plasma prednisolone concentrations are measured at 1–2 hours and are generally five times greater than plasma prednisone concentrations. Although there is interpatient variability in prednisolone elimination, patients with corticosteroid-requiring asthma do not differ from the normal population.[130] Moreover, asthmatics who require daily prednisone do not metabolize prednisolone more rapidly than those maintained on alternate-day prednisone.[131] More importantly, however, may be the evaluation of corticosteroid absorption and elimination in patients with poorly controlled asthma despite aggressive therapy, and especially in those patients who do not develop systemic side effects. Important abnormalities such as decreased absorption or unusually rapid metabolism have been observed.[132]

INHALED CORTICOSTEROIDS. The proposed advantages of inhaled corticosteroids are the potent topical anti-inflammatory effect in the airway and the minimal systemic effects. The ideal inhaled corticosteroid would have the following properties: (1) high degree of topical potency, (2) minimal systemic absorption from the lung, (3) rapid deactivation of any corticosteroid that is absorbed, and (4) absence of local or systemic side effects. According to these criteria, the ideal corticosteroid for inhaled use is not currently available. Inhaled corticosteroids available in the United States include beclomethasone dipropionate, triamcinolone acetonide, and flunisolide. Budesonide, which is not available in the United States, has many favorable features,[133] but some questions regarding adverse effects observed in animal studies remain unanswered.

Beclomethasone dipropionate aerosol is completely absorbed from the lung but is rapidly deactivated via reduction pathways and subsequently eliminated.[134] When administered in doses of 800 μg/day for 1 month to asthmatic adolescents, there is a significant decrease in urinary free cortisol, suggesting some systemic effect.[135] However, response to adrenocorticotropic hormone (ACTH) stimulation was unaffected. Triamcinolone acetonide is effective in contolling asthma symptoms and improving pulmonary function tests, without a significant decrease in morning plasma cortisol concentration.[136]

Dysphonia and candidiasis are local adverse effects associated with inhaled corticosteroid administration.[137] Dysphonia is a dyskinesia of the muscles that control phonation, while candidiasis is caused by overgrowth of candidal organisms in the immunosuppressed oropharynx. Fortunately, both are dose-related and generally resolve after discontinuation of the inhaled corticosteroid. Use of a spacer device is effective in maximizing intrapulmonary deposition and also in minimizing these local effects. Oropharyngeal candidiasis may be treated locally with nystatin, and recurrences may be reduced or prevented by rinsing the mouth with water after corticosteroid inhalation.

TIME COURSE OF EFFECTS. Although the cellular effects of corticosteroids are immediate, the intricate processes necessary to attain the desired pharmacologic effect result in a lag time between corticosteroid administration and clinical effect. The plasma half-lives for cortisol and prednisolone are 0.5–1.0 and 2–3 hours, respectively. The biologic half-lives, based on the duration of ACTH suppression following single doses, for cortisol and prednisolone are 8–12 and 12–36 hours, respectively.[138] To successfully prevent an immediate asthmatic response to antigen challenge in an animal model, intravenous corticosteroid must be administered at least 3 hours prior to allergen exposure.[139] The late asthmatic response can be blocked by corticosteroid administration just prior to allergen challenge.[140] Inhaled corticosteroids can block both the immediate and the late asthmatic response after several weeks of therapy.[141]

Present Status

ACUTE ASTHMA. Although corticosteroids are used in the treatment of acute severe asthma, their beneficial effect is occasionally questioned.[142,143] Multiple trials have been conducted with variable and usually negative results. This confusion is often due to poor study design, questionable dosage strategies, and poor selection of outcome variables. As recently as 1983, a series of randomized, double-blind, placebo-controlled clinical investigations using high-dose and early corticosteroid administration demonstrated their efficacy.[144,145] The specific corticosteroid effect in this clinical situation is not clearly understood but likely includes most effects described previously. The onset of clinical effect may, however, be as long as 6 hours.

CHRONIC ASTHMA. Chronic systemic corticosteroid therapy, especially daily dosing, must be avoided.[138] Although alternate-day therapy is less harmful, it is still not without adverse effects. Inhaled corticosteroids are useful in reducing systemic corticosteroid requirements. In the United States inhaled corticosteroids are selected as first-line therapy (as a supplement to β-agonists) in only 22 percent of adults and 8 percent of children, whereas oral theophylline is preferred in over 70 percent of adults and children.[146] Certainly, the efficacy of inhaled corticosteroids is substantial, but large, detailed, multicenter clinical trials comparing oral theophylline and inhaled corticosteroids are not available. Triamcinolone acetonide may be more convenient for use, as it is available with a built-in spacer device. The incidence of cough is less with triamcinolone acetonide than with beclomethasone.[147] Flunisolide is likely to produce similar beneficial clinical effects as compared to beclomethasone dripropionate.[148] The systemic potencies and effects after inhalation of triamcinolone acetonide or flunisolide are not well characterized.

FUTURE CONSIDERATIONS. With increased emphasis on the inflammatory component of asthma and the inherent anti-inflammatory effect of corticosteroids, the use of inhaled corticosteroids in the United States will likely increase as it has in the United Kingdom.[149] The role of inhaled corticosteroids in the reduction of underlying airway reactivity is important. In a recent study comparing oral prednisolone and inhaled beclomethasone dipropionate in doses that produced similar improvement in pulmonary function, beclomethasone dipropionate resulted in a signficant decrease in underlying airway hyperreactivity.[150]

CONCEPTS OF TREATMENT

The principles of pathophysiology and various characteristics of asthma are important in designing a treatment regimen for individual patients. Optimal care of the asthmatic patient will reduce the degree to which individual features of asthma evolve. Unique pharmacologic approaches to therapy may be required for adequate treatment.

Exercise-Induced Asthma

The cough and wheeze associated with exercise are a manifestation of bronchial hyperreactivity.[151] The temporary bronchoconstriction following a short period of intense exercise is termed exercise-induced asthma or bronchoconstriction. The degree of bronchoconstriction observed is related to the amount of heat and/or water loss from the airways during the exercise period.[152] Exercise-induced asthma may be the only clinical feature in a patient with mild asthma and is a relatively consistent finding in patients with moderate to severe disease. Fortunately, it can be attenuated in the majority of patients by prophylactic treatment with inhaled β-agonists and, to a lesser degree, by cromolyn and theophylline. Occasionally, combination therapy may be required to sufficiently inhibit exercise-induced asthma.

Asthmatic Response to Allergen Exposure

When sensitive individuals are exposed to inhaled allergen, two general patterns of airway obstruction may be observed. The immediate asthmatic response (IAR) occurs shortly after exposure and may last from 30 minutes to 2 hours.[153] Subsequently, the late asthmatic response (LAR) occurs in many subjects within several hours after allergen exposure (Figure 31–4), and the airway obstruction may last up to 12 hours.[154] This biphasic pattern in airway obstruction is further differentiated by the classes of medications that are active in reversing or preventing bronchoconstriction.[155] The IAR occurs alone or in conjunction with an LAR, whereas the LAR rarely occurs as an isolated event. The optimal therapy is obviously avoidance. Certain patients with specific allergen sensitivity may respond to immunotherapy. β-Agonists are only effective in preventing the IAR.[104] Whereas cromolyn prevents the IAR and LAR, multiple doses of corti-

costeroids only prevent development of the LAR.[104,156,157] However, in some studies regular use of inhaled corticosteroids also reduces the IAR. Theophylline and enprofylline attenuate the LAR.[57] Ipratropium, in contrast, has no effect on the IAR or LAR.[104] Pharmacotherapy therefore consists of cromolyn use prior to a single or seasonal allergen exposure. Similarly, inhaled corticosteroids may serve as prophylaxis in reducing airway reactivity and seasonal exacerbations of asthma.

Nocturnal Asthma

Worsening of asthma that occurs during sleep is termed nocturnal asthma. Asthmatics with this component are also called "morning dippers," since there is a signficant decrease in pulmonary function between bedtime and awakening. The pathophysiologic mechanisms responsible for this symptom complex are not clear, but it is associated with diurnal patterns in endogenous secretion of cortisol and circulating epinephrine[158] and an accumulation of inflammatory cells in the bronchoalveolar space.[159] Medical factors such as sinusitis and gastroesophageal reflux should be considered in the evaluation and management of these patients.[160] Bedtime dosing of theophylline may be effective in the treatment of nocturnal worsening of asthma.[161] The introduction of sustained-release oral β-agonists and longer-acting inhaled β-agonists may also prove helpful in the management of these patients.

Moderate and Severe Chronic Asthma

Patients with chronic asthma have frequent episodic or persistent bronchconstriction and a compromised life-style. They have exercise-induced bronchospasm, nocturnal symptoms, and may experience seasonal exacerbations. Since they require continuous aggressive pharmacotherapy, they are at significant risk for adverse effects from medications, particularly corticosteroids.

In order to minimize the dose of oral corticosteroids, these patients receive optimal courses of β-agonists and theophylline to relieve episodic bronchoconstriction and nocturnal exacerbations. Although cromolyn and aerosol

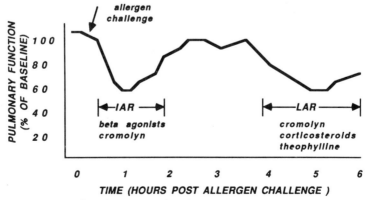

FIGURE 31–4. Pulmonary function versus time in a typical sensitized patient who demonstrates an immediate asthmatic response (IAR) and a late asthmatic response (LAR) following inhalation of a specific allergen. Drugs that inhibit or antagonize the IAR or LAR are shown.

corticosteroids are used to reduce inflammation and airway reactivity, arguments can be made that cromolyn may add little to concomitant corticosteroid therapy[123,124]; however, its unique effect on both the IAR and the LAR and its rare incidence of adverse effects result in its continued application.

Oral corticosteroids are usually required either in periodic bursts or as chronic maintenance therapy for severe chronic asthma. Attempts are made to define the minimum maintenance dose by careful titration and observation. Monitoring daily peak flow is extremely useful in defining this maintenance dose. Occasional patients fail to respond adequately despite aggressive corticosteroid therapy. Several therapeutic options are now available and should be considered in those patients at risk for adverse corticosteroid effects.

Troleandomycin, a macrolide antibiotic, may be beneficial in up to 75 percent of severe steroid-requiring asthmatic patients. It is most effective when combined with methylprednisolone.[162] Of interest is the fact that methylprednisolone, but not prednisolone, elimination is impaired in the presence of troleandomycin.[163] The primary mechanism of action is related to inhibition of corticosteroid metabolism; however, independent effects of troleandomycin have not been adequately studied. The use of combination troleandomycin–methylprednisolone therapy requires careful dosage titration, as described by Wald et al.[164] Patients who cannot reach alternate-day steroid therapy within 6 weeks, or those who cannot be maintained on a dose of methylprednisolone less than 12 mg every other day, should be considered nonresponders and troleandomycin should be discontinued.

Methotrexate has received recent interest as adjunctive therapy that facilitates significant steroid dose reduction. A double-blind, crossover trial in 14 patients reported by Mullarkey et al.[165] resulted in a 35 percent steroid dose reduction in the methotrexate treatment period, with significant subjective improvement and maintenance of pulmonary function. The low-dose methotrexate protocol resulted in a limited incidence of adverse effects, specifically nausea and an evanescent rash. More extensive clinical experience is needed to substantiate the use of methotrexate in the treatment of severe asthma.

Similarly, limited experience with gold therapy[166] and perhaps intravenous gamma globulin[167] indicates potential beneficial effects in the treatment of severe asthma. Ongoing research is directed at defining the safest and most effective therapy from those previously described and, most important, the appropriate time to begin treatment.

FUTURE DIRECTIONS

While the recent emphasis on inflammation and airway reactivity has revolutionized the treatment of asthma, it has also prompted questions regarding alternative forms of therapy. Potent effects of prostaglandins, leukotrienes, PAF, and thromboxane A_2 have stimulated investigations with drugs that inhibit synthesis or directly antagonize these mediators. Trials with medications that antagonize the effects of prostaglandins and leukotrienes have been disappointing. With the availability of specific antagonists for PAF and thromboxane A_2 synthetase inhibitors, the clinical significance of these mediators in asthma will be examined.

Perhaps we will find that blocking a specific mediator is a futile effort because of the release of multiple mediators. In that case, a generalized, broad-spectrum approach, similar to that identified for corticosteroids, would be much more successful. An attempt has been made to introduce nonbronchodilator antiasthma medications, particularly in oral form, similar in properties to inhaled cromolyn. These attempts have met with limited success, since their beneficial effect is not readily apparent in all patients. A recent Task Force on Nonbronchodilator Antiasthma Drugs provided guidelines for future investigation of this category of medications.[168]

Given the mechanisms of cell activation in the course of inflammation, calcium channel blockers would appear to offer unique effects. However, clinical trials suggest that this mode of therapy provides no antiasthma effect.[169] Perhaps a cell-specific calcium channel blocker or an inhibitor of cellular mechanisms at a more proximal or generalized site (such as an inhibitior of protein kinase C activity) would prove more effective.

There is no doubt that we already have potent medications to relieve bronchospasm and reduce inflammation. Unfortunately, they have not signficantly reduced the morbidity and mortality associated with asthma.[170] Directions for the future must include not only the development of new medications, but also careful scrutiny of the methods used to deliver health care, including patient education, access to treatment centers, and more effective use of available medications.

A comprehensive overview of the diagnosis and management of asthma has recently been published.[178] Continuing analysis of these interventions is required to determine the impact on asthma morbidity and mortality.

REFERENCES

1. American Thoracic Society Committee on Diagnostic Standards for Nontuberculous Respiratory Diseases: Definitions and classification of chronic bronchitis, asthma and pulmonary emphysema. Am Rev Respir Dis 85:762–768, 1962
2. Boushey HA, Holtzman MJ, Sheller JR, Nadel JA: Bronchial hyperreactivity. Am Rev Respir Dis 121:389–413, 1980
3. Bleecker ER: Airways reactivity and asthma: Significance and treatment. J Allergy Clin Immunol 75:21–24, 1985
4. Laitinen LA, Heino M, Laitinen A, Kava T, Haahtela T: Damage of airway epithelium and bronchial reactivity in patients with asthma. Am Rev Respir Dis 131:599–606, 1985
5. Dunhill MS, Massarella GR, Anderson JA: A comparison of the quantitative anatomy of the bronchi in normal subjects, in status asthmaticus, in chronic bronchitis and emphysema. Thorax 24:176–179, 1969
6. Frigas E, Gleich GJ: The eosinophil and the pathology of asthma. J Allergy Clin Immunol 77:527–537, 1986
7. Kaliner M: Mast cell mediators and asthma. Chest 87:2S–4S, 1985 (suppl)
8. Casale TB, Wood D, Richerson HB, Zehr B, Zavala D, Hunninghake GW: Direct evidence of a role for mast cells in the pathogenesis of antigen-induced bronchospasm. J Clin Invest 80:1507–1511, 1987
9. Holgate ST, Hardy C, Robinson C, Agius RM, Howarth PH: The

mast cell as a primary effector cell in the pathogenesis of asthma. J Allergy Clin Immunol 77:274–282, 1986

10. Lee TH: Interactions between alveolar macrophages, monocytes, and granulocytes: Implications for airway inflammation. Am Rev Respir Dis 135:514–517, 1987

11. Murphy KR, Wilson MC, Irvin CG, Glezen L, Marsh WR, Haslett C, Henson PM, Larsen GL: The requirement for polymorphonuclear leucocytes in the late asthmatic response and heightened airways reactivity in an animal model. Am Rev Respir Dis 134:62–68, 1986

12. Schleimer R, Fox C, Naclerio R: Role of human basophils in the pathogenesis of allergic diseases. J Allergy Clin Immunol 76:369–374, 1985

13. Holgate ST, Church MK: Mediator release from human lung mast cells. Respiration 46 (suppl 1):22–23, 1984

14. Schleimer RP, Schulman ES, MacGashan DW, Peters SP, Hayes EC, Adams K, Lichtenstein LM, Adkinson NF: Effects of dexamethasone on mediator release from human lung fragments and purified lung mast cells. J Clin Invest 71:1830–1835, 1983

15. Gleich GJ, Frigas E, Loegering DA, Wassom DL, Steinmuller D: Cytotoxic properties of eosinophil major basic protein. J Immunol 123:2925–2927, 1975

16. Frigas E, Loegering DA, Solley GO, Farrow GM, Gleich GJ: Elevated levels of eosinophil granule major basic protein in the sputum of patients with bronchial asthma. Mayo Clin Proc 56:345–353, 1981

17. Altman LC, Hill JS, Hairfield WM, Mullarkey MF: Effects of corticosteroids on eosinophil chemotaxis and adherence. J Clin Invest 67:28–36, 1981

18. Brain JD: Lung macrophages: How many are there? What do they do? Am Rev Respir Dis 137:507–509, 1987

19. Rankin JA, Askenase PW: The potential role of alveolar macrophages as a source of pathogenic mediators in allergic asthma, in Lichenstein LM, Austen KF (eds): Asthma: Physiology, Immunopharmacology, and Treatment. London, Academic Press, 1984

20. Smith HR, Henson PM: Mediators of asthma. Semin Respir Med 8:287–301, 1987

21. Abraham WM, Wanner A: Inflammatory mediators of asthma. Pediatr Pulmonol 4:237–247, 1988

22. Hardy CC, Robinson C, Tattersfield AE, Holgate ST: The bronchoconstrictor effect of inhaled prostaglandin D-2 in normal and asthmatic men. N Engl J Med 311:209–213, 1984

23. Fish JE, Jameson LS, Albright A, Norman PS: Modulation of the bronchomotor effects of chemical mediators by prostaglandin F2-alpha in asthmatic subjects. Am Rev Respir Dis 130:571–574, 1984

24. Patterson R, Harris KE, Greenberger RA: Effect of prostaglandin D-2 and I-2 on the airways of rhesus monkeys. J Allergy Clin Immunol 65:269–273, 1980

25. Goetzl EJ: Leukocyte recognition and metabolism of leukotrienes. Fed Proc 42:3128–3131, 1983

26. Barnes PJ, Chung KF, Page CP: Platelet activating factor as a mediator of allergic disease. J Allergy Clin Immunol 81:919–934, 1988

27. Cuss FM, Dixon CMS, Barnes PJ: Effects of inhaled platelet activating factor on pulmonary function and bronchial responsiveness in man. Lancet 2:189–192, 1986

28. Boushey HA, Holtzman MJ: Autonomic regulation of airways: Parasympathetic nervous system, in Weiss EB, Segal MS, Stein M (eds): Bronchial Asthma: Mechanisms and Therapeutics. Boston, Little, Brown and Co, 1985

29. Holtzman MJ, Fabbri LM, O'Byrne PM, Gold BD, Aizawa H, Walters EH, Alpert SE, Nadel JA: Importance of airway inflammation for hyperresponsiveness induced by ozone. Am Rev Respir Dis 127:686–690, 1983

30. Richardson JB: Nerve supply to the lungs. Am Rev Respir Dis 119:758–803, 1979

31. Zaagsma J, van der Heijden PJCM, van der Schaar MWG, Bank CMC: Comparison of functional beta-adrenoceptor heterogeneity in central and peripheral airways smooth muscle of guinea-pig and man. J Receptor Res 3:89–106, 1983

32. Singh BN, Whitlock RML, Comber RH, Williams FH, Harris EA: Effects of cardioselective beta adrenoceptor blockade on specific airways resistance in normal subjects and in patients

with bronchial asthma. Clin Pharmacol Ther 19:493–501, 1976

33. Lofdahl C-G, Svedmyr N: Effects of prenalterol in asthmatic patients. Eur J Clin Pharmacol 23:297–303, 1982

34. Barnes PJ: Airway receptors, in Jenne JW, Murphy S (eds): Drug Therapy for Asthma: Research and Clinical Practice. New York, Marcel Dekker, 1987, pp 67–95

35. Barnes PJ, Basbaum CB, Nadel JA, Roberts JM: Localization of beta-adrenoceptors in mammalian lung by light microscopic autoradiography. Nature 299:444–447, 1982

36. Hedberg A, Kempf F, Josephson ME, Molinoff PB: Coexistence of beta-1 and beta-2 adrenergic receptors in the human heart: Effects of treatment with receptor antagonists or calcium entry blockers. J Pharmacol Exp Ther 234:561–568, 1985

37. Persson CGA, Karlsson J-A: In Vitro responses to bronchodilator drugs, in Jenne JW, Murphy S (eds): Drug Therapy for Asthma: Research and Clinical Practice. New York, Marcel Dekker, 1987, pp 129–159

38. Davies DS: Pharmacokinetics of terbutaline after oral absorption. Eur J Respir Dis 65 (suppl 134):111–117, 1984

39. Morgan DJ, Paull JD, Richmond BH, Wilson-Evered E, Ziccone SP: Pharmacokinetics of intravenous and oral salbutamol and its sulphate conjugate. Br J Clin Pharmacol 22:587–593, 1986

40. Nyberg L: Pharmacokinetic parameters of terbutaline in healthy men. An overview. Eur J Respir Dis 65 (suppl 134):149–160, 1984

41. Oosterhuis B, Braat MCP, Roos CM, Werner J, Boxtel CJ: Pharmacokinetic pharmacodynamic modeling of terbutaline bronchodilation in asthma. Clin Pharmacol Ther 40:469–475, 1986

42. Dulfano MJ, Glass P: The bronchodilator effects of terbutaline: Route of administration and patterns of response. Ann Allergy 37:357–366, 1976

43. Orgel HA, Kemp JP, Tinkelman DG, Webb DR: Bitolterol and albuterol metered-dose aerosols: Comparison of two long acting beta2-adrenergic bronchodilators for the treatment of asthma. J Allergy Clin Immunol 75:55–62, 1985

44. Sly M, Heimlich EM, Ginsburg J, Busser RJ, Strick L: Exercise-induced bronchospasm: Evalution of metaproterenol. Ann Allergy 26:253–258, 1968

45. Ahrens RC, Harris JB, Milavetz G, Annis L, Ries R: Use of bronchial provocation with histamine to compare the pharmacodynamics of inhaled albuterol and metaproterenol in patients with asthma. J Allergy Clin Immunol 79:876–882, 1987

46. Anderson SD, Seale JP, Rozea P, Bandler L, Theobald G, Lindsay DA: Inhaled and oral salbutamol in exercise-induced asthma. Am Rev Respir Dis 114:493–500, 1976

47. Williams SJ, Winner SJ, Clark TJH: Comparison of inhaled and intravenous terbutaline in acute severe asthma. Thorax 36:629–631, 1981

48. Herman JJ, Noah ZL, Moody RR: Use of intravenous isoproterenol for status asthmaticus in children. Crit Care Med 11:716–720, 1983

49. Matson JR, Loughlin GM, Strunk RC: Myocardial ischemia complicating the use of isoproterenol in asthmatic children. J Pediatr 92:776–778, 1978

50. Kurland G, Williams J, Lewiston NJ: Fatal myocardial toxicity during continuous infusion intravenous isoproterenol therapy of asthma. J Allergy Clin Immunol 63:407–411, 1979

51. Nelson HS: Beta adrenergic agonists. Chest 82 (suppl):33–38, 1982

52. Hendeles L, Weinberger M: Theophylline: A state of the art review. Pharmacotherapy 3:2–44, 1983

53. Bersgrand H: Phosphodiesterase inhibition and theophylline. Eur J Respir Dis 61(suppl 109):37–44, 1980

54. MacKay AD, Baldwin CJ, Tattersfield AE: Action of intravenously administered aminophylline in normal airways. Am Rev Respir Dis 127:609–613, 1983

55. Cushley MJ, Tattersfield AE, Holgate ST: Inhaled adenosine and guanosine on airway resistance in normal and asthmatic subjects. Br J Clin Pharmacol 15:161–165, 1983

56. Persson CGA, Erjfat I, Karlsson J-A: Adenosine antagonism: A less desirable characteristic of xanthine drugs? Acta Pharmacol Toxicol 49:317–320, 1981

57. Pauwels R, Van Renterghem D, Van Der Straeten M, Johannesson N, Persson CGA: The effect of theophylline and enprofyl-

line on allergen-induced bronchoconstriction. J Allergy Clin Immunol 76:583–590, 1985

58. Persson CGA: Xanthines as airway anti-inflammatory drugs. J Allergy Clin Immunol 81:615–617, 1985

59. Jackson RH, McHenry JI, Moreland FB, Raymer WJ, Etter RL: Clinical evaluation of Elixophyllin with correlation of pulmonary function studies and theophylline serum levels in acute and chronic asthmatic patients. Dis Chest 45:75–85, 1964

60. Jenne JW, Wyze E, Rood FS, MacDonald FM: Pharmacokinetics of theophylline: Application to adjustment of the clinical dose of aminophylline. Clin Pharmacol Ther 13:349–360, 1972

61. Martin GL, Atkins PC, Dunsky EH, Zweiman B: Effects of theophylline, terbutaline, and prednisone on antigen-induced bronchospasm and mediator release. J Allergy Clin Immunol 66:204–212, 1980

62. McWilliams BC, Menendez R, Kelley HW, Howick J: Effects of theophylline on inhaled methacholine and histamine in asthmatic children. Am Rev Respir Dis 130:193–197, 1984

63. Bierman CW, Shapiro GG, Pierson WE, Dorsett CS: Acute and chronic theophylline therapy in exercise-induced bronchospasm. Pediatrics 60:845–849, 1977

64. Pollock J, Kiechel F, Cooper D, Weinberger M: Relationship of serum theophylline concentration to inhibition of exercise-induced bronchospasm and comparison with cromolyn. Pediatrics 60:840–844, 1977

65. Weinberger MM, Bronsky EA: Evaluation of oral bronchodilator therapy in asthmatic children. J Pediatr 84:421–427, 1974

66. Nassif EG, Weinberger MM, Thompson R, Huntley V: The value of maintenance theophylline in steroid dependent asthma. N Engl J Med 304:71–75, 1981

67. Joad JP, Ahrens RC, Lindgren SD, Weinberger M: Relative efficacy of maintenance therapy with theophylline, inhaled albuterol, and the combination for chronic asthma. J Allergy Clin Immunol 79:78–85, 1987

68. Brenner AM, Berkowitz R, Marshall N, Strunk RC: Need for theophylline in severe steroid-requiring asthmatics. Clin Allergy 18:143–150, 1988

69. Herrmann G, Aynesworth MB, Martin J: Successful treatment of persistent dyspnea "status asthmaticus." J Lab Clin Med 23:135–148, 1937

70. Fanta CH, Rossing TH, McFadden ER: Treatment of acute asthma. Is combination therapy with sympathomimetics and methylxanthines indicated? Am J Med 80:5–10, 1986

71. Vozeh S, Kewitz G, Perruchoud A, Taschan M, Kopp C, Heitz M, Follath F: Theophylline serum concentrations and therapeutic effect in severe acute bronchial obstruction: The optimal use of intravenously administered aminophylline. Am Rev Respir Dis 125:181–184, 1982

72. Jenne JW, Wyze E, Rood FS, MacDonald FM: Pharmacokinetics of theophylline: Application to adjustment of the clinical dose of aminophylline. Clin Pharmacol Ther 13:349–360, 1972

73. Hendeles L, Bighley L, Richardson RH, Hepler CD, Carmichael J: Frequent toxicity from IV aminophylline infusions in critically ill patients. Drug Intell Clin Pharm 11:12–18, 1977

74. Berlinger WG, Spector R, Goldberg MJ, Johnson GF, Quee CK, Berg MJ: Enhancement of theophylline clearance by oral activated charcoal. Clin Pharmacol Ther. 33:351–354, 1983

75. Stein MR, Towner TG, Weber RW, Mansfield LE, Jacobson KW, McDonnell JT, Nelson HS: The effect of theophylline on lower esophageal sphincter pressure. Ann Allergy 45:238–241, 1980

76. Hubert D, Gaudric M, Guerre J, Lockhart A, Marsac J: Effect of theophylline on gastroesophageal reflux in patients with asthma. J Allergy Clin Immunol 81:1168–1174, 1988

77. Weinberger M, Lindgren S, Bender B, Lerner JA, Szefler SJ: Effects of theophylline on learning and behavior: Reason for concern or concern without reason? J Pediatr 111:472–473, 1987

78. Rachelefsky GS, Wo J, Adelson J, Mickey MR, Spector SL, Katz RM, Siegel S, Rohr AS: Behavior abnormalities and poor school performance due to oral theophylline use. Pediatrics 78:1133–1138, 1986

79. Hendeles L, Massanari M, Weinberger M: Theophylline, in Evans WE, Schentag JJ, Jusko WJ (eds): Applied Pharmaco-

kinetics: Principles of Therapeutic Drug Monitoring, 2nd ed. Spokane, Applied Therapeutics, 1986, pp 1105–1188

80. Milavetz G, Vaughn LM, Weinberger MM, Hendeles L: Evaluation of a scheme for establishing and maintaining dosage of theophylline in ambulatory patients with chronic asthma. J Pediatr 109:351–354, 1986

81. Juan D, Worwag EM, Schoeller DA, Kotake AN, Hughes RL, Fredriksen NC: Effects of dietary protein on theophylline pharmacokinetics and caffeine and aminopyrine breath tests. Clin Pharmacol Ther 40:187–194, 1987

82. Hendeles L, Iafrate RP, Weinberger M: A clinical and pharmacokinetic basis for the selection and use of slow release theophylline products. Clin Pharmacokinet 9:95–135, 1984

83. Sallent J, Hill M, Stecenko A, MacKenzie M, Hendeles L: Bioavailability of a slow release theophylline capsule given twice daily to preschool children with asthma: Comparison with liquid theophylline. Pediatrics 88:116–120, 1988

84. Pedersen S, Steffensen G: Absorption characteristics of once-a-day slow-release theophylline preparation in children with asthma. J Pediatr 110:953–959, 1987

85. Guill MF, Pruitt AW, Altmana RE, Lawless TE, Brown DA, DuRant RH, Bottini PB: Clinical and pharmacokinetic evaluation of a sustained-release liquid theophylline preparation. J Allergy Clin Immunol 82:281–286, 1988

86. Karim A, Burns T, Wearley L, Streicher J, Palmer M: Food-induced changes in theophylline absorption from controlled-release formulations. Part I. Substantial increased and decreased absorption with Uniphyl tablets and Theo-Dur Sprinkle. Clin Pharmacol Ther 38:77–83, 1985

87. Hendeles L, Weinberger M, Milavetz G, Hill M, Vaughn L: Food-induced "dose-dumping" from a once-a-day theophylline product as a cause of theophylline toxicity. Chest 87:758–765, 1985

88. Pedersen S, Moller-Peterson J: Erratic absorption of a slow-release theophylline sprinkle product. Pediatrics 74:534–538, 1984

89. Scott PII, Tabachnick E, MacLeod S, Correia J, Newth C, Levison H: Sustained-release theophylline for childhood asthma: Evidence for circadian variation of theophylline pharmacokinetics. J Pediatr 99:476–479, 1981

90. Warren JB, Cuss F, Barnes PJ: Posture and theophylline kinetics. Br J Clin Pharmacol 19:707–709, 1985

91. Szefler SJ: Theophylline and its fickle unpredictability of absorption. Ann Allergy 55:580–583, 1985

92. Gross N, Skorodin M: State of the Art. Anticholinergic, antimuscarinic bronchodilators. Am Rev Respir Dis 129:856–870, 1984

93. Kradjan WA, Smallridge RC, Davis R, Verma P: Atropine serum concentrations after multiple inhaled doses of atropine sulfate. Clin Pharmacol Ther 38:12–15, 1985

94. Karpel JP, Appel D, Breidbart D, Fusco MJ: A comparison of atropine sulfate and metaproterenol sulfate in the emergency room treatment of asthma. Am Rev Respir Dis 133:727–729, 1986

95. Deckers W: The chemistry of new derivatives of tropane alkaloids and the pharmacokinetics of a new quaternary compound. Postgrad Med J 51(suppl 7):76–81, 1975

96. Ghafouri MA, Patil KD, Kass I: Sputum changes associated with the use of ipratropium bromide. Chest 86:387–393, 1984

97. Gross NJ: Ipratropium bromide. N Engl J Med 319:486–494, 1988

98. Ruffin RE, Fitzgerald JD, Rebuck AS: A comparison of the bronchodilator activity of Sch 1000 and salbutamol. J Allergy Clin Immunol 59:136–141, 1977

99. Bell R, Sahay JN, Barber PV, Chatterjee SS, Cox G: A therapeutic comparison of ipratropium bromide and salbutamol in asthmatic patients. Curr Med Res Opinion 8:242–246, 1982

100. Beck R, Robertson C, Galdes-Sebaldt M, Levison H: Combined salbutamol and ipratropium bromide by inhalation in the treatment of severe acute asthma. J Pediatr 107:605–608, 1985

101. Ashutosh K, Lang H: Comparison between long-term treatment of chronic bronchitic airway obstruction with ipratropium bromide and metaproterenol. Ann Allergy 53:401–406, 1984

102. Newcomb R, Tashkin DP, Hui KK, Conolly ME, Lee E, Dau-

phine B: Rebound hyperresponsiveness to muscarinic stimulation after chronic therapy with an inhaled muscarinic antagonist. Am Rev Respir Dis 132:12–15, 1985

103. Borut TC, Tashkin DP, Fisher TJ, Katz R, Rachelefsky G, Siegel SC, Lee E, Harper C: Comparison of aerosolized atropine sulfate and SCH 1000 on exercise-induced bronchospasm in children. J Allergy Clin Immunol 60:127–133, 1977

104. Howarth PH, Durham SR, Lee TH, Kay AB, Church MK, Holgate ST: Influence of albuterol, cromolyn sodium and ipratropium bromide on the airway and circulating mediator responses to allergen bronchial provocation in asthma. Am Rev Respir Dis 132:986–992, 1985

105. Woenne R, Kattan M, Orange RP, Levison H: Bronchial hyperreactivity to histamine and metacholine in asthmatic children after inhalation of SCH 1000 and chlorpheniramine. J Allergy Clin Immunol 62:119–124, 1978

106. Cox JSG: Review of chemistry, pharmacology, toxicity, metabolism, specific side-effects, anti-allergic properties in-vitro and in-vivo of disodium cromoglycate, in Pepys J, Frankland AW (eds): Disodium Cromoglycate in Allergic Airway Disease. London, Butterworth, 1970

107. Flint KC, Leung KBP, Pearce FL, Hudspith BN, Brostoff J, Johnson NM: Human lung mast cells recovered by bronchoalveolar lavage: Their morphology, histamine release, and the effects of sodium cromoglycate. Clin Sci 68:427–432, 1985

108. Kay AB, Wardlaw AJ, Moqbel R, Buchanan DR, Cromwell O, Fitzharris P: Leukocytes in the asthma process, in Kay AB (ed): Allergy and Inflammation. London, Academic Press, 1987, pp 203–223

109. Moqbel R, Walsh GM, MacDonald AJ, Kay AB: Effect of disodium cromoglycate on activation of human eosinophils and neutrophils following reversed (anti-IgE) anaphylaxis. Clin Allergy 16:78–83, 1986

110. Spry CJF, Kumardswami V, Tai PC: The effect of nedocromil sodium on secretion from human eosinophils. Eur J Respir Dis 69(suppl 147):241–243, 1986

111. Godfrey S, Konig P: Suppression of exercise-induced asthma by salbutamol, theophylline, atropine, cromolyn, and placebo in a group of asthmatic children. Pediatrics 56:930–934, 1975

112. Latimer KM, Roberts R, Morris MM, Hargreave FE: Inhibition by sodium cromoglycate of bronchoconstriction stimulated by respiratory heat loss: Comparison of pressurized aerosol and powder. Thorax 39:277–281, 1984

113. Sheppard D, Nadel JA, Boushey HA: Inhibition of sulfur dioxide-induced bronchoconstriction by disodium cromoglycate in asthmatic subjects. Am Rev Respir Dis 124:257–259, 1981

114. Lowhagen O, Rak S: Modification of bronchial hyperreactivity after treatment with sodium cromoglycate during pollen season. J Allergy Clin Immunol 75:460–467, 1985

115. Bernstein IL, Siegel SC, Brandon ML, Brown EG, Evans RR, Feinberg AR, Freidlander S, Krumholtz RA, Hadley RA, Handelman NI, Thurston D, Yamate M: A controlled study of cromolyn sodium sponsored by the Drug Committee of the American Academy of Allergy. J Allergy Clin Immunol 50:235–245, 1972

116. Furukawa CT, Shapiro GG, Kraemer MJ, Pierson WE, Bierman CW: A double-blind study comparing the effectiveness of cromolyn sodium and sustained-release theophylline in childhood asthma. Pediatrics 74:453–489

117. Bernstein IL: Cromolyn sodium in the treatment of asthma: Coming of age in the United States. J Allergy Clin Immunol 76:381–388, 1985

118. Geller-Bernstein C, Levin S: Sodium cromoglycate pressurized aerosol in childhood asthma. Curr Ther Res 34:345–349, 1983

119. Cordier R: Sodium cromoglycate delivered by pressurized aerosol in the treatment of adult asthma. Clin Trials J 21:483–491, 1984

120. Settipane GA, Klein DE, Boyd GK, Struam JH, Freye HB, Weltman JK: Adverse reactions to cromolyn. JAMA 23:811–813, 1979

121. McFadden ER: Corticosteroids and cromolyn sodium as modulators of airway inflammation. Chest 94:181–183, 1988

122. Chai H, Molk L, Falliers CJ, Miklich D: Steroid sparing effects of

123. disodium cromoglycate (DSC) in children with severe clinical asthma, in Serafini (ed): New Concepts in Allergy and Clinical Immunology. Amsterdam, Excerpta Medica, 1971, pp 385–391

123. Toogood JH, Jennings B, Lefcoe NM: A clinial trial of combined cromolyn/beclomethasone treatment for chronic asthma. J Allergy Clin Immunol 67:317–324, 1981

124. Mitchell I, Paterson IC, Cameron SJ, Grant IWB: Treatment of childhood asthma with sodium cromoglycate and beclomethasone dipropionate aerosol singly and in combination. Br Med J 4:457–458, 1976

125. Rao GS: Mode of entry of steroid and thyroid hormones into cells. Mol Cell Endocrinol 21:97–108, 1981

126. Hirata F, Schiffmann E, Venkatasubramanian K, Salomon D, Axelrod J: A phospholipase A2 inhibitory protein in rabbit neutrophils induced by glucocorticoids. Proc Natl Acad Sci USA 77:2533–2536, 1980

127. Fraser CM, Venter JC: The synthesis of beta-adrenergic receptors in cultured human lung cells: Induction by glucocorticoids. Biochem Biophys Res Commun 94:390–397, 1980

128. Davies AO, Lefkowitz RJ: In-vitro desensitization of beta-adrenergic receptors in human neutrophils: Attenuation by corticosteroids. J Clin Invest 71:565–571, 1983

129. Stephan WC, Chick TW, Avner BP, Jenne JW: Tachyphylaxis to inhaled isoproterenol and the effect of methylprednisolone in dogs. J Allergy Clin Immunol 65:105–109, 1980

130. Rose JQ, Nickelsen JA, Middleton E, Yurchak AM, Park BH, Jusko JW: Prednisolone disposition in steroid dependent asthmatics. J Allergy Clin Immunol 66:366–373, 1980

131. Greenberger PA, Choe MJ, Atkinson AJ, Ambre JJ, Patterson R: Comparison of prednisolone kinetics in patients receiving daily or alternate-day prednisone for asthma. Clin Pharmacol Ther 39:163–168, 1986

132. Hill MR, Szefler SJ, Ball BD, Bartoszek M, Brennner AW: Monitoring glucocorticoid therapy: A pharmacokinetic approach. Clin Pharmacol Ther 48:390–398, 1990

133. Toogood JH, Baskerville JC, Jennings B, Lefcoe NM, Johansson SA: Influence of dosing frequency and schedule on the response of chronic asthmatics to the aerosol steroid, budesonide. J Allergy Clin Immunol 70:288–298, 1982

134. Martin LE, Harrison C, Tanner RJN: Metabolism of beclomethasone by animals and man. Postgrad Med J 51(suppl 4):11–20,1975

135. Bisgaard H, Nielsen MD, Andersen B, Andersen P, Foged N, Fuglsang G, Host A, Leth C, Pedersen M, Pelck I, Stafanger G, Osterballe O: Adrenal function in children with bronchial asthma treated with beclomethasone dipropionate or budesonide. J Allergy Clin Immunol 81:1088–1095, 1988

136. Bernstein IL, Chervinsky P, Falliers CJ: Efficacy and safety of triamcinolone acetonide aerosol in chronic asthma. Chest 81:20–26, 1981

137. Toogood JH, Jennings B, Greenway RW, Chuang L: Candidiasis and dysphonia complicating beclomethasone treatment of asthma. J Allergy Clin Immunol 65:145–153, 1980

138. Harter JG: Corticosteroids: Their physiologic use in allergic diseases. NY State J Med 66:827–849, 1966

139. Delehunt JC, Yerger L, Ahmen T, Abraham WM: Inhibition of antigen-induced bronchoconstriction by methylprednisolone succinate. J Allergy Clin Immunol 73:479–483, 1984

140. Booij-Noord H, de Vries K, Sluiter HJ, Orie NGM: Late bronchial obstructive reaction to experimental inhalation of house-dust extract. Clin Allergy 2:43–61, 1972

141. Burge PS, Efthimiou J, Turner-Warwick M, Nelmes PTJ: Double-blind trials of inhaled beclomethasone dipropionate and fluocortin butyl ester in allergen-induced immediate and late asthmatic reactions. Clin Allergy 12:523–531, 1982

142. Fiel SB: Should corticosteroids be used in the treatment of acute, severe asthma? I. A case for the use of corticosteroids in acute severe asthma. Pharmacotherapy 5:327–331, 1985

143. Mok J, Kattan M, Levison H: Should corticosteroids be used in the treatment of acute severe asthma? II. A case against the use of corticosteroids in acute, severe asthma. Pharmacotherapy 5:331–335, 1985

144. Fanta CH, Rossing TH, McFadden ER: Glucocorticoids in acute

asthma: A controlled clinical trial. Am J Med 74:845–851, 1983

145. Haskell RJ, Wong BM, Hansen JE: A double-blind, randomized clinical trial of methylprednisolone in status asthmaticus. Arch Intern Med 143:1324–1327, 1983

146. Hodkin JE: United States audit of asthma therapy. Chest 90(suppl):62–69, 1986

147. Shim CS, Williams MH: Cough and wheezing from beclomethasone dipropionate aerosol are absent after triamcinolone acetonide. Ann Intern Med 106:700–703, 1987

148. Dry J, Sors C, Gervais P, van Straaten L, Perrin-Fayolle M, Paramelle B: A comparison of flunisolide inhaler and beclomethasone dipropionate inhaler in asthma. J Int Med Res 13:289–292, 1985

149. Clark TJH: Asthma therapy in the United Kingdom. Chest 90(suppl):67–70, 1986

150. Jenkins CR, Woolcock AJ: Effect of prednisone and beclomethasone dipropionate on airway responsiveness in asthma: A comparative study. Thorax 43:378–384, 1988

151. McFadden ER: Exercise induced asthma. Am J Med 68:471–472, 1980

152. Anderson SD: Is there a unifying hypothesis of exercise-induced asthma? J Allergy Clin Immunol 73:660–665, 1984

153. Larsen GL: Late phase reactions: Observations on pathogenesis and prevention. J Allergy Clin Immunol 76:665–669, 1985

154. Pelikan Z, Pelikan M, Kruis M, Berger MPF: The immediate asthmatic response to allergen challenge. Ann Allergy 56:252–260, 1986

155. Cartier AC, Thompson NC, Frith PA, Roberts R, Hargreave FE: Allergen-induced increase in bronchial responsiveness to histamine: Relationship to the late asthmatic response and change in airways caliber. J Allergy Clin Immunol 70:170–177, 1982

156. Pelikan Z, Pelikan-Filipek M, Shoemaker MC, Berger MPF: Effects of beclomethasone dipropionate on the asthmatic response to allergen challenge. I. Immediate response. Ann Allergy 60:211–216, 1988

157. Pelikan Z, Pelikan-Filipek M, Remejer L: Effects of disodium cromoglycate and beclomethasone dipropionate on the asthmatic response to allergen challenge. II. Late response. Ann Allergy 60:217–225, 1988

158. Barnes P, Fitzgerald G, Brown M, Dollery C: Nocturnal asthma and changes in circulating epinephrine, histamine and cortisol. N Engl J Med 303:263–267, 1980

159. Martin RJ, Cicutto LC, Ballard RD, Szefler SJ: Airway inflammation in nocturnal asthma. Am Rev Respir Dis 137:284, 1988

160. Ballard RD, Martin RJ: Nocturnal asthma. Semin Resp Med 8:302–307, 1987

161. Barnes PJ, Greening AP, Neville L, Timmers J, Poole GW: Single-dose slow release aminophylline at night prevents nocturnal asthma. Lancet 1:299–301, 1982

162. Spector SL, Katz FH, Farr RS: Troleandomycin: Effectiveness in steroid-dependent asthma. J Allergy Clin Immunol 54:367–379, 1974

163. Szefler SJ, Ellis EF, Brenner M, Rose JQ, Spector SL, Yurchak A, Andrews F, Jusko WJ: Steroid-specific and anticonvulsant interaction aspects of troleandomycin-steroid therapy. J Allergy Clin Immunol 69:455–462, 1982

164. Wald JA, Friedman BF, Farr RS: An improved protocol for using troleandomycin (TAO) in the treatment of steroid-requiring asthma. J Allergy Clin Immunol 78:36–44, 1986

165. Mullarkey MF, Blumenstein BA, Andrade WP, Bailey GA, Olason I, Wetzel LE: Methotrexate in the treatment of corticosteroid-dependent asthma: A double-blind crossover study. N Engl J Med 318:603–607, 1988

166. Bernstein DI, Bernstein IL, Bodenheimer SS, Pietrusko RG: An open study of Auranofin in the treatment of steroid dependent asthma. J Allergy Clin Immunol 81:6–16, 1988

167. Pay R, Friday G, Stillwagon P, Skoner D, Caliguiri L, Fireman P: Asthma and selective immunoglobulin subclass deficiency: Improvement of asthma after immunoglobulin replacement therapy. J Pediatr 112:12–130, 1988

168. Bernstein IL (ed): Report of the American Academy of Allergy and Immunology Task Force on guidelines for clinical investigation of nonbronchodilator antiasthmatic drugs. J Allergy Clin Immunol 78(part 2):489–546, 1986

169. Massey KL, Hill M, Harman E, Rutledge DR, Ahrens R, Hendeles L: Dose response of inhaled gallopamil (D600), a calcium channel blocker in attenuating airway reactivity to methacholine and exercise. J Allergy Clin Immunol 81:912–918, 1988

170. Sheffer AL, Buist AS: Proceedings of the Asthma Mortality Task Force. J Allergy Clin Immunol 80:361–516, 1987

171. Harris JB, Ahrens RC, Milavetz G, Ries RA, Annis L, Eddy MA: Relative potencies and rates of decline in effect of inhaled albuterol and terbutaline (Abstr.). J Allergy Clin Immunol 77:147, 1986

172. Harris JB, Ahrens RC, Annis L, Ries RA, Milavetz G, Hendricker C: Comparison of peak effects and rates of decline of albuterol and bitolterol via metered-dose inhaler (Abstr.). Ann Allergy 56:520, 1986

173. Salome CV, Schoeffel RE, Woolcock HJ: Effect of aerosol fenoterol on the severity of bronchial hyperreactivity in patients with asthma. Thorax 38:854–858, 1983

174. Springer C, Goldenberg B, BenDov I, Godfrey S: Clinical, physiologic, and psychologic comparison of treatment by cromolyn or theophylline in childhood asthma. J Allergy Clin Immunol 76:64–69, 1985

175. Rachelefsky GS, Wo J, Adelson J, Mickey MR, Spector SL, Katz RM, Siegel SC, Rohr AS: Behavior abnormalities and poor school performance due to oral theophylline use. Pediatrics 78:1133–1138, 1986

176. Joad JP, Ahrens RC, Lindgren SD, Weinberger MM: Extrapulmonary effects of maintenance therapy with theophylline and inhaled albuterol in patients with chronic asthma. J Allergy Clin Immunol 78:1147–1153, 1986

177. Furukawa CT, Duhamel TR, Weimer L, Shapiro G, Pierson WE, Bierman CW: Cognitive and behavioral findings in children taking theophylline. J Allergy Clin Immunol 81:83–88, 1988

178. Guidelines for the diagnosis and management of asthma. National Heart, Lung, and Blood Institute Asthma Education Program Expert Panel Report. Pediatr Asthma Allergy Immunol 5:57–186, 1991

32

ANTIPYRETICS

JAMES G. LINAKIS *and* FREDERICK H. LOVEJOY, JR.

The treatment of fever is one of the most common therapeutic interventions carried out by the pediatrician.[1] In fact, fever is one of the leading reasons that children are brought for medical attention.[2] In one study some 20 percent of children presenting to emergency departments had fever,[3] and in one group of private practitioners, 10.5 percent of children seen between the ages of 1 and 24 months of age had a temperature $\geq 38.3°C.$[4] Yet, despite the prevalence of fever in the pediatric age group, the number of agents used for their antipyretic effect is small.

ANTIPYRETIC AGENTS

Medications commonly considered for use as antipyretics are listed in Table 32–1. They include salicylates (aspirin; sodium, calcium, choline, and other salts or esters of salicylic acid; and salicylamide); aminophenols (including acetaminophen, acetanilid, and phenacetin); propionic acid–derived nonsteroidal anti-inflammatory agents (including ibuprofen and naproxen, hereafter referred to as nonsteroidals); and phenylpyrazoles (including antipyrine, aminopyrine, dipyrone, and phenylbutazone). Phenacetin and acetanilid have been used as alternatives to aspirin, but methemoglobinemia, hemolysis, and nephritis have restricted their general use.[5] The various salicylates and related compounds are effective antipyretic, analgesic, and anti-inflammatory agents, except for salicylamide, which was found to be relatively ineffective clinically for these purposes after a considerable period of initial popularity.[1] Acetaminophen, which is an active metabolite of both acetanilid and phenacetin, is relatively free of renal and hematologic toxicity. Phenylpyrazoles, such as dipyrone, have antipyretic activity, but their clinical usage is limited because of a prohibitive incidence of aplastic anemia.[1] Propionic acid–derived nonsteroidal anti-inflammatory agents have considerable analgesic, anti-inflammatory, and antipyretic activity. Concern over toxic side effects has limited their use in

children,[6] but two of the nonsteroidals, naproxen and ibuprofen, are currently used in children for their anti-inflammatory effects and antipyretic properties.[7,8] Other nonsteroidals have also been demonstrated to have antipyretic effects in clinical studies performed in Europe.[9] However, none of these drugs is approved in the United States for simple antipyresis. In fact, in spite of the relatively large number of antipyretic agents theoretically available, toxicity and limited experience have, in effect, limited the choices in children to aspirin and acetaminophen (although certain of the nonsteroidal anti-inflammatory drugs are gaining increasing favor as antipyretic agents. While aspirin offers analgesic, anti-inflammatory, and antipyretic activity, acetaminophen's pharmacologic effects are limited to antipyresis and analgesia. Unfortunately, because of its association with Reye's syndrome, the clinical indications for use of aspirin in pediatrics have been reduced substantially.[10,11]

MECHANISM OF FEVER AND ITS REDUCTION

Fever is an elevation of body temperature above normal as a result of altered temperature regulation.[12] Temperature is regulated by the hypothalamus through a complex feedback system, and fever results from the activation by the hypothalamus of thermoregulatory effectors so as to maintain body temperature at a level higher than normal. The postulated mechanism suggests that various substances produce or act as exogenous pyrogens.[13] These substances include many bacteria, viruses, fungi, and polynucleotides, and the exogenous pyrogen is thought to act on monocytes and fixed-tissue macrophages causing the production and release of endogenous pyrogen (also called interleukin-1). This endogenous pyrogen enters the central nervous system and, in ways that are poorly understood, acts to raise the temperature "set point," perhaps by local release of prostaglandins

335

**TABLE 32–1. CLASSIFICATION, CHARACTERISTICS, AND
PEDIATRIC DOSES OF ANTIPYRETIC DRUGS***

	ADDITIONAL EFFICACIES		Suggested Oral Antipyretic Dose†
	Analgesia	Anti-inflammatory	
Salicylates Aspirin Sodium salicylate Calcium salicylate Choline salicylate	+	+	10–15 mg/kg q4–6h
Aminophenols Acetaminophen Acetanilid Phenacetin	+	−	10–15 mg/kg q4–6h 5–10 mg/kg q6h
Propionic acids Ibuprofen Naproxen‡	+	+	5–10 mg/kg q4–6h 7.5 mg/kg q12h
Phenylpyrazoles Antipyrine Aminopyrine Dipyrone Phenylbutazone Oxyphenbutazone	+	+	Toxic§
Mefenamic acid‡	+	+	6.5 mg/kg q6h
Indomethacin	+	+	Toxic§

*Adapted from Lovejoy FJ Jr, Done AK: The use of antipyretics, in Yaffe SJ (ed): Pediatric Pharmacology: Therapeutic Principles in Practice, 1st ed. New York, Grune & Stratton, 1980
†Doses are recommended by the authors only for drugs whose antipyretic usefulness in children has been well established or at least evaluated in controlled trials, though not necessarily approved for pediatric use.
‡Not presently approved for pediatric use as antipyretic.
§Toxic indicates that a drug's potential for adverse reactions precludes recommendations for simple antipyresis.

within the hypothalamus.[12] Interleukin-1 also acts on lymphocytes to activate an immune response, primarily through its mitogenic activity.

Both aspirin and acetaminophen, and apparently the nonsteroidals as well, reduce fever through an alteration in response of the hypothalamus to pyrogens. Presumably this occurs by returning the temperature set point toward normal through an inhibition of prostaglandin synthesis.[14] The lowering of the set point brings into action physiologic mechanisms for heat loss, including vasodilation and sweating.

A distinction should be made between fever and heat illness, since treatment of the two entities is quite different.[15] *Fever* refers to an elevation in body temperature that results from a thermoregulatory response to an elevated set point. In *heat illness,* on the other hand, body temperature is elevated without a concomitant rise in the temperature set point. Within this context, there are three different pathophysiologic mechanisms responsible for temperature elevation, and the appropriate therapeutic response is different in each instance.[16] In the first situation, in which a high set point is the mechanism for fever (for example, in infection, malignancy, and collagen vascular disease), the appropriate therapy is the administration of antipyretic drugs to lower the hypothalamic set point. Removal of heat by ice-water sponging, without a pharmacologic change in the set point, will lower body temperature only briefly and will lead to an increased metabolic rate with increased discomfort. In the second situation, in which heat production is excessive and the

hypothalamic set point is normal (for example, in hyperthyroidism and aspirin overdose), attempts to lower the set point by drug administration will be without benefit. In the third situation, in which heat loss is impaired and the hypothalamic set point is normal (for example, in ectodermal dysplasia and heat stroke), pharmacologic lowering of the set point will again be without benefit.

THE TREATMENT DECISION

The decision to lower temperature and some of the risk–benefit issues to be evaluated are important considerations in the therapy of fever. Several arguments exist to suggest that temperature should not be lowered[17]:

1. Fever may be protective to the host by providing an unfavorable environment for the infecting organism.[1] Temperature elevations seen clinically are detrimental to the growth of certain organisms, such as gonococci and some treponemes. In addition, fever may also inhibit the growth of pneumococci and some viruses,[18,19] although the clinical relevance of these experimental findings is presently unclear. Evidence now exists that fever plays an important role in enhancing the immune response.[20] Numerous host defense mechanisms appear to be augmented in the presence of an increase in body temperature, including leukocyte

migration,[21] bactericidal activity of leukocytes,[22] lymphocyte transformation,[22] and interferon activity.[23] Whether these *in vitro* findings will ultimately be shown to be qualitatively important *in vivo* remains to be seen.

2. The treatment of fever may be inadvisable if it obscures clinical findings of diagnostic or prognostic value or diverts attention away from the establishment of an etiology for the fever.[24] Fever may cause sufficient symptomatic morbidity to lead to earlier medical evaluation. Furthermore, although reduction of fever may improve the clinical appearance of the child, the absence of bacteremia is not predicted by either reduction in fever or improvement in clinical appearance after antipyresis.[25,26] Home treatment with antipyretics might therefore delay appropriate medical treatment.

3. The risk of treatment may outweigh the morbidity of the symptoms. The adverse reactions seen in overdose or at pharmacologic doses for both aspirin and acetaminophen may outweigh the benefits derived from antipyretic therapy in certain age groups and in certain groups of patients who are at risk when treated with these drugs. In addition, the relationship between aspirin and Reye's syndrome[10,11] has dramatically shifted the perceived risks associated with that drug.

4. Fever in the child is generally self-limited, rarely of serious consequence, and usually well tolerated.

On the other hand, arguments in support of lowering temperature include the following[17]:

1. In children with a history of febrile seizures, prompt temperature lowering is a logical therapeutic approach, although to date no study has conclusively demonstrated that aggressive treatment of fever decreases the incidence of febrile seizures.[2]

2. Although fever rarely poses a serious threat, it clearly creates discomfort, and its reduction will often settle an apprehensive home environment.[1]

3. Excessive temperature in certain uncommon clinical situations (such as familial dysautonomia) may cause direct damage to the central nervous system.

4. *In vitro* and animal studies have suggested that certain aspects of the immunologic response (e.g., phagocytosis by polymorphonuclear leukocytes) may be impaired by high fever.[27,28]

CLINICAL EFFICACY

When aspirin, acetaminophen, and certain nonsteroidal agents have been compared to placebo, a statistically significant antipyretic effect has been demonstrated.[29–31] Controlled and uncontrolled studies comparing the antipyretic activity of aspirin and acetaminophen have not, however, demonstrated a significant difference in the rate or the degree of lowering of temperature when the drugs have been used in equal doses.[32–36] Two nonsteroidal anti-inflammatory agents, ibuprofen and naproxen, have been studied with regard to their antipyretic activity in chil-

dren. Both medications appear to be at least as effective as aspirin and acetaminophen in their antipyretic effect,[7,8,36–41] although the use of naproxen as an antipyretic has not been approved by the Food and Drug Administration (FDA) in the United States. A third nonsteroidal, suprofen, has also been shown to have significant antipyretic activity in children.[9,42,43] Suprofen is not marketed in the United States. With aspirin and acetaminophen, as well as the nonsteroidal anti-inflammatory drugs, reduction in temperature generally begins within 30 minutes of administration of the drug, and a reduction of 1–2 degrees celsius can be expected within 1 hour. With all of the antipyretics mentioned, the degree of the antipyretic effect appears to increase until at least 2 hours after administration. With acetaminophen this effect is maintained for 3–3.5 hours, while with aspirin it may persist for 4–4.5 hours.[36] The antipyretic activity of ibuprofen and naproxen appears to have an even longer duration, with the effect lasting 6–8 hours with ibuprofen,[39a] and 8–12 hours with naproxen.[7,40] In the individual patient, factors such as the quantity of the stomach contents, the severity of the clinical illness, and the concomitant use of other drugs may cause small alterations in this pattern of response.

An interest in using the two most accepted drugs, either simultaneously or alternately, to augment fever control is understandable. A combination of aspirin and acetaminophen has been demonstrated to be more effective in reducing fever in children than when either drug is used alone.[36] The rate and degree of temperature reduction are generally greater with the combination of aspirin and acetaminophen, and the duration of the effect is significantly more sustained (average 6 hours). While this study disclosed no signs of toxicity with the combined therapy, there has been some suggestion that undesirable effects may be increased with the combination.[44] Further, salicylate may have deleterious effects on the absorption and metabolism of acetaminophen.[45,46] Finally, the apparent association of aspirin with Reye's syndrome, particularly within the context of chickenpox or influenza, suggests that combined therapy that involves aspirin use should be reserved for special circumstances (e.g., difficult-to-control fevers associated with malignancy). A similar combination of acetaminophen and ibuprofen has not been studied to date.

The use of sponging along with antipyretic medication should also be considered. Investigation comparing the effectiveness of sponging with tepid water, ice water, and equal parts of 70 percent isopropyl alcohol and water in combination with acetaminophen has shown the combination of the antipyretic agent and sponging to be superior in lowering temperature to sponging or the antipyretic agent alone.[47] In the same study, sponging with ice water or with alcohol in water was equally effective and significantly superior to sponging with tepid water. Sponging with tepid water, however, offered greater comfort during the sponging procedure, and is presumably safer than sponging with alcohol.

Selection of a specific antipyretic will be dictated by the complex of symptoms to be treated. In most children with fever and mild noninflammatory pain, acetaminophen will generally be the drug of choice. Nevertheless, because acetaminophen is a relatively poor anti-inflammatory agent in comparison to aspirin and ibuprofen or naproxen, it is not the optimal antipyretic agent to be used when fever is accompanied by inflammation. When this is the case, aspirin (assuming no contraindication) or one of the nonsteroidal anti-inflammatory drugs should be more efficacious.

PHARMACOLOGY OF ASPIRIN

Absorption

Rapid absorption of aspirin tablets occurs in the acid environment of the stomach as well as through the large absorptive surface of the duodenum and jejunum.[48,49] The rate-limiting step to absorption is the dissolution of the aspirin tablet. Factors slowing absorption include exercise, a recent meal, and cold solids or liquids, while an empty stomach and hot liquids augment absorption.[48] Salicylates may be found in serum as early as 15–30 minutes following oral administration, and peak levels occur by 1–1.5 hours. Both rectally administered and enteric-coated aspirin result in delayed absorption and variable peaks and levels.[49]

Distribution

Aspirin is hydrolyzed to salicylic acid in the intestinal wall and during the first pass through the liver.[49] A significant percentage (50–80 percent) is bound to albumin and is pharmacologically and toxicologically inactive. This bound fraction is in equilibrium with an unbound portion of the drug which is highly pH-dependent and pharmacologically active.[49] In the blood at pH 7.4, it exists predominantly in its ionized form, with a smaller nonionized portion being in equilibrium with tissues. With a lowering of serum pH, the ratio of ionized to nonionized drug will shift in the direction of greater nonionization and increased lipid solubility, with increased permeability through membranes and increased transfer of drug to tissue sites. Conversely, with increasing serum pH, greater ionization, decreased lipid solubility, and decreased permeability through membranes will occur.

A number of drugs compete with salicylate for plasma protein binding sites. Examples of medications where this interaction may occur are phenytoin, oral hypoglycemic agents, and phenylbutazone.[50] In addition, a decrease in the plasma albumin concentration will result in a decrease in the number of protein binding sites for salicylic acid. As a result, there has been concern that while decreased protein binding will not be reflected in changes in serum salicylate concentrations, it may result in greater pharmacologic and toxicologic effect due to an increase in the amount of free salicylate.[51] Nevertheless, such an increase in toxicity secondary to decreased protein binding has not been well documented in the clinical literature. Finally, the volume of distribution of salicylates increases with increasing amounts of drug ingested.[52] This

finding has important implications for increased effects of aspirin at toxic serum levels.

The effect of pH on the ratio of ionized to nonionized drug has important pharmacokinetic significance. Aspirin has a pKa of 3. Thus, in the acid medium of the stomach, 50 percent of an aspirin dose is in its nonionized form, resulting in prompt absorption. In the alkaline environment of the small bowel, the drug is mainly ionized. In this form absorption would be expected to be slow, yet because of the large absorptive surface area of the duodenum and jejunum, rapid absorption occurs.[48] In the blood at pH 7.4, the majority of the unbound drug is in its ionized form, resulting in a considerable proportion of salicylic acid remaining in the vascular compartment, with a resultant low volume of distribution (0.15–0.2 liter/kg). Clinical conditions that result in either a metabolic or a respiratory acidosis, however, will increase the nonionized fraction of the drug, with increased transfer of unbound drug into tissues leading to augmented pharmacologic activity.[53,54] Furthermore, in overdose, when high levels of salicylic acid exist, either medications or clinical states that create a respiratory or a metabolic acidosis will increase toxicity through enhanced entrance of salicylate into the central nervous system.[55,56]

Elimination

Salicylate elimination occurs through both hepatic metabolism and renal excretion. At therapeutic doses, hepatic metabolism accounts for the majority of salicylate elimination; hepatic metabolism consists primarily of conjugation with glycine and glucuronic acid. Nevertheless, at doses above therapeutic levels, the conjugation pathways become saturated, and the elimination kinetics switch from first-order to zero-order, thus decreasing the rate of elimination.

The plasma half-life of aspirin at therapeutic doses is about 15 minutes, although the half-life of its active metabolite, salicylic acid, is approximately 2.5 hours. This half-life may be prolonged to 12 hours at higher doses.

The contribution of renal excretion to the overall elimination of salicylates increases in overdose. Initial urinary excretion of aspirin occurs as early as 30 minutes following ingestion and can be confirmed by a positive Phenistix or ferric chloride test in the urine (burgundy-colored urine following boiling and addition of 5–10 drops of 10 percent ferric chloride solution).[57] Renal excretion of hepatically formed metabolites is highly efficient, preventing accumulation of metabolites in the serum or tissues.[58]

Urinary salicylate excretion may be augmented by increasing glomerular filtration through enhanced intravenous fluids, diuretics, or osmotic agents. Additionally, renal excretion of salicylate is increased by an alkaline urine (pH 7.0–8.0). At this pH, the unbound drug passing through the renal tubules is trapped in the urine and is maintained in an ionized state with poor membrane permeability, decreased tubular reabsorption, and increased urinary excretion.[59] This forms the basis for treatment of aspirin overdose with alkalinization of the urine.

PHARMACOLOGY OF ACETAMINOPHEN

Absorption

Acetaminophen is dispensed in liquid form and as chewable tablets. These preparations help circumvent the time necessary for dissolution of the nonchewable tablets. Absorption from the stomach and upper small intestine thus occurs rapidly, and initial serum levels may be expected as early as 30 minutes following ingestion.[60] Peak levels generally occur by 1 hour, even in the nonchewable tablet preparation.

Acetaminophen is also available as rectal suppositories. The potency of the suppository formulation is reportedly substantially less than that of the oral preparations. In addition, the bioavailability of acetaminophen in suppositories is highly variable, resulting in variable serum concentrations.

Distribution

Binding of acetaminophen to plasma protein is variable but small (about 20–30 percent), with the majority of drug remaining in the free state. Distribution is to most body tissues, with a volume of distribution of 0.8–1.0 liter/kg.

Elimination

Removal of acetaminophen occurs through hepatic metabolism and subsequent renal excretion of hepatic metabolites. Only about 3 percent is excreted in the urine as the parent compound. The plasma half-life is about 2 hours. At therapeutic doses, acetaminophen is eliminated mainly via conjugation to sulfate or glucuronic acid; a small amount (5–15 percent) appears in the form of mercapturic acid. The formation of mercapturic acid proceeds through a reaction in which acetaminophen is metabolized by the hepatic cytochrome P-450 system to a reactive intermediary and then conjugated with the sulfhydryl group of glutathione. Evidence now suggests that the unconjugated intermediary of the cytochrome P-450 system metabolism of acetaminophen is responsible for its toxicity in overdose.[61,62] With overdose the pathways of conjugation to sulfate and glucuronic acid become saturated, and an increasing fraction of the drug is metabolized by the cytochrome P-450 system. Ordinarily the reactive intermediates formed as the result of the action of the cytochrome P-450 system are made innocuous by reacting with hepatic glutathione. Liver glutathione becomes depleted, however, when the acetaminophen burden is great, and thus the reactive intermediates are permitted to bind covalently to hepatocytes and cause centrilobular hepatic necrosis.[63] The kidneys also metabolize small amounts of acetaminophen to a toxic intermediary, and rare cases of acetaminophen-associated acute renal failure have been reported.[64]

Overall, the findings suggest that with hepatic compromise, where drug might accumulate, acetaminophen may not be advisable. In these situations an alternative antipyretic should be considered.

PHARMACOLOGY OF NONSTEROIDAL ANTI-INFLAMMATORY DRUGS

Absorption

Naproxen and ibuprofen are available in both liquid and tablet forms. Ibuprofen and naproxen are both well absorbed from the gastrointestinal tract, although ibuprofen is absorbed more rapidly. Absorption is delayed by the presence of food in the stomach. Peak plasma concentrations of ibuprofen occur in 1–2 hours from the time of ingestion, whereas naproxen concentrations peak within 2–4 hours.

Distribution

Ibuprofen and naproxen are both nearly completely (99 percent) bound to plasma protein at therapeutic doses. As a result, the volume of distribution of both drugs is small (0.10–0.17 liter/kg).[65] Because of the high degree of protein binding, the nonsteroidals may compete with other drugs for protein binding sites.

Elimination

Ibuprofen is excreted in the urine as inactive metabolites or their conjugates. The major metabolites are a carboxylated compound and a hydroxylated compound. Less than 3 percent of the parent drug is excreted unchanged by the kidney. The plasma half-life of ibuprofen at therapeutic doses is approximately 2 hours.

Naproxen and its metabolites are also almost entirely excreted in the urine. Approximately 30 percent of the drug undergoes 6-demethylation, and this metabolite and naproxen itself are excreted as the glucuronide or other conjugates. The elimination half-life of naproxen is about 14 hours.

ADVERSE REACTIONS

Aspirin

Wide usage of aspirin has resulted over the years in the recording of a sizeable number of adverse reactions. Perhaps the most serious toxicity associated with the therapeutic use of aspirin has come to light only recently. Epidemiologic data have demonstrated a significant association between aspirin use in some children and Reye's syndrome.[10] Although reports of these data have been the subject of much criticism regarding methodology,[66] a recent study designed specifically to circumvent these methodologic problems also suggested a significant biologic relationship between aspirin use and Reye's syndrome.[11] In light of these findings, it would appear most judicious to avoid aspirin use at least in children with chickenpox and influenza-like illnesses.

A growing body of literature has also addressed the issue of the risk of gastric bleeding in association with the use of aspirin. Aspirin in a dose of 1–3 gm/day in adults will result in occult gastrointestinal blood loss of approximately 3–5 ml/day (normal loss is less than 1 ml).[67–69] Two factors may be responsible for these findings. First, aspirin causes an increased rate of epithelial desquamation and exfoliation, leading to a loss of integrity of the gastric mucosal barrier.[70,71] Gastroscopy has shown the presence of hemorrhagic erosions adjacent to undissolved aspirin tablets. Second, blood loss may be worsened by a prolonged bleeding time induced by aspirin's effect on platelets.[72] With chronic use of aspirin, occult gastrointestinal bleeding may lead to iron deficiency anemia.[73] The incidence of massive gastrointestinal bleeding in association with the use of aspirin is less clear. Patients taking aspirin at least 4 days a week for a 12-week period have greater likelihood of gastrointestinal blood loss, but the rate of major bleeding is extremely low (15 per 100,000 per year).[74] These findings would suggest an increased risk with aspirin usage in patients (1) on medications that have an inherent toxicity for the gastric mucosa (such as potassium salts and steroids); (2) with illnesses predisposing to gastric ulceration, such as central nervous system disease, burns, or sepsis; and (3) with a history of prior gastric ulceration or esophageal varices.[75]

Aspirin in overdose or when chronically administered at high doses may produce prolongation of the prothrombin time. This defect is corrected by the administration of vitamin K. In addition, the bleeding time is prolonged through aspirin-induced increased fibrinolytic activity,[76] as well as through the inhibition of formation of platelet aggregates, with resultant diminished platelet adhesiveness.[77–79] This effect is seen with a single dose of 0.3–0.6 grams of aspirin and is accentuated in patients with hemophilia.[80] Since the platelet life span is 8 days, hemostasis may be impaired for 4–7 days following the cessation of aspirin therapy.[78] This qualitative platelet defect is rapidly corrected by transfusion of fresh platelets. Sodium or choline salicylate and acetaminophen[81] in normal subjects and in patients with hemophilia[82] do not prolong bleeding time. These findings suggest an increased risk with aspirin in the following clinical situations: (1) the patient with clotting or platelet disorders,[80] (2) the patient undergoing a surgical procedure,[35] and (3) the patient receiving drugs that decrease hemostasis (reduce available vitamin K, depress circulating platelets, inhibit platelet aggregation, or increase fibrinolysis).[83] In these situations, where mild analgesia or antipyresis is desired acetaminophen would offer an advantage.[84]

The infant born to a mother who has taken aspirin during the last week of pregnancy may be at risk for bleeding and premature closure of the ductus arteriosus. Petechiae, purpura, cephalohematoma, melena, and massive gastrointestinal bleeding have all been described.[85–88] Qualitative platelet abnormalities present at birth have persisted for 3 weeks following delivery.[85,86] The use of aspirin in the week prior to delivery is inadvisable and is associated with particular risk during difficult or traumatic deliveries and in the presence of known hemostatic defects in the mother or the newborn.

Aspirin in overdose or when used in patients with certain clinical diseases may be hepatotoxic.[89,90] Liver biopsy reveals hepatocellular necrosis with periportal inflammation and fatty changes. These changes may simulate the changes seen in Reye's syndrome, although the absence of mitochondrial changes in salicylate toxicity aids in the differentiation. Increased serum enzyme activity (aspartate aminotransferase, alanine aminotransferase), elevated alkaline phosphatase, and hyperbilirubinemia may occur when aspirin is used in high therapeutic doses for the treatment of rheumatic fever,[91] rheumatoid arthritis,[89,92] and lupus erythematosus.[90,94] The reaction is dose-related, is rarely serious, and is reversible on lowering or discontinuing the medication. Rarely, a fulminant reaction has been reported in children receiving aspirin for rheumatoid arthritis, characterized by an acute alteration in sensorium in association with increased serum enzyme activity, hyperammonemia, and hyperbilirubinemia.[95] These abnormalities abate with discontinuation of the medication and have recurred when the drug was reinstituted.

Cutaneous allergic reactions, asthma, and anaphylaxis may all occur as hypersensitivity reactions to aspirin.[94,96] An additional serious reaction occurring with aspirin use, labeled aspirin intolerance, manifests with rhinorrhea, nasal polyps, a prolonged bleeding time, asthma, and shock.[97] The prevalence of this reaction is probably less than 0.2 percent in the general population. It is frequent in adults with asthma and infrequent in adolescents. As no *in vitro* test will presently identify patients at risk, a positive history for aspirin intolerance should exclude further use of aspirin.

When aspirin is administered at higher than recommended doses or at too frequent intervals, relatively minor increases in dosage will result in large increases in serum concentrations with resultant clinical toxicity.[29] A number of studies have offered an explanation for these characteristics of accumulation based on the kinetics of elimination.[98,99] As with any drug, aspirin administered repetitively at therapeutic doses accumulates in the body until the amount entering equals the amount removed by excretion and biotransformation ("steady state," by definition). At sufficiently high doses, however, hepatic mechanisms for the removal of aspirin become saturated, resulting in a shift from first-order to mixed first- and zero-order kinetics and a pronounced increase in serum concentration. The child receiving recommended antipyretic doses of aspirin at recommended intervals acquires a steady-state serum level of 15–20 mg/dl.[29] Signs of toxicity generally appear at levels of greater than 30–35 mg/dl. Vomiting, diarrhea, inadequate fluid intake, and the excretion of an acid urine (common with relative starvation) will narrow this margin of safety by decreasing renal clearance of the dug and increasing the serum concentration. Metabolic acidosis will also increase the diffusion of salicylates across membranes to tissue sites, resulting in increased toxicity.[29,53] The margin of safety with aspirin may thus be narrowed and exceeded with relative ease.

The most commonly recognized adverse effect of aspirin is acute overdose. Due to the frequent use of aspirin and its easy accessibility, acute aspirin poisoning still remains quite common. Nevertheless, growing awareness of the drug's potential risk in overdose, the relative increase in frequency of other types of poisonings, and the institution of safety caps may be factors accounting for the drop in aspirin overdoses since 1965.[59,100] Numerous excellent reviews exist detailing the clinical manifestations and treatment for this overdose.[59,101]

Acetaminophen

The frequency of adverse effects from therapeutic doses of acetaminophen appears to be less than with aspirin. This may, however, only be a reflection of the shorter period of time that acetaminophen has been in use. To date, manifestations of acetaminophen toxicity at therapeutic levels have been very infrequent and largely non-dose-related. These have included neutropenia, leukopenia, thrombocytopenia, hypersensitivity reactions (maculopapular rash, laryngeal edema, urticaria, angioedema, and anaphylactic reactions), drug fever, and hypoglycemia.[102] Moderate doses of acetaminophen also appear to increase the incidence of hepatotoxicity in chronic alcohol abusers.[103] There have also been rare case reports of nephrotoxicity associated with therapeutic use of acetaminophen.[104] Unlike aspirin, therapeutic doses of acetaminophen do not cause gastric irritation, and gastric ulceration and bleeding do not occur with its use.[105] In addition, while large doses have been reported to potentiate the effect of oral anticoagulants, small doses have no effect on prothrombin time.

In the 1960s and early 1970s, acute overdose from acetaminophen was limited to Europe, where the drug was in common use. In the past several years, with increased availability and usage in the United States, acetaminophen has become one of the substances most frequently involved in poison exposures.[106] Initial toxicity, irrespective of the size of the overdose, is limited to nausea, vomiting, and diaphoresis.[107,108] The acid–base abnormalities seen with aspirin are not part of the picture of acetaminophen overdose. In large overdose, elevated hepatic enzyme activity occurs 24–36 hours following ingestion.[108] Patients who recover undergo improvement in their clinical condition and liver function parameters by the end of the first week. The phenomenon is dose-related[109]: it occurs in 2- to 3-year-olds at doses of 2–3 grams and in adolescents at doses of greater than 8 grams.[108]

Whether hepatotoxicity is produced by lesser doses of acetaminophen in patients with reduced hepatic glutathione stores (e.g., from relative starvation in a sick child) remains unclear. This explanation may account for the hepatotoxicity seen with moderate doses of acetaminophen in alcoholics.[103] It is known that agents which induce the enzymes responsible for the formation of the hepato-

toxic metabolite (e.g., phenobarbital, phenytoin) do predispose to hepatotoxicity.[110] Overdose of acetaminophen has also been associated with acute renal failure,[64,111] apparently secondary to toxic intermediate metabolites formed in the kidney.

Oral N-acetylcysteine is the only antidote currently approved for treatment of acetaminophen poisoning in the United States. Oral methionine and intravenous N-acetylcysteine are used in the United Kingdom and Canada. N-Acetylcysteine provides effective protection from hepatotoxicity in 93 percent of high-risk patients when given within 10 hours of the overdose and in 70 percent of patients when given between 10 and 16 hours postingestion.[62] N-Acetylcysteine is thought to act by replenishing hepatic glutathione reserves, thus providing additional stores for detoxification of the reactive intermediate.

Nonsteroidal Anti-Inflammatory Agents

By far the most common adverse effect associated with use of the nonsteroidal anti-inflammatory drugs is gastritis. Nevertheless, in contrast to most nonsteroidals, ibuprofen causes comparatively little gastrointestinal irritation,[112] and the incidence of severe reactions to ibuprofen appears to be less than that of the salicylates. Allergic reactions are rare but may include pruritus, nonspecific dermatitis, and urticaria. Other less frequent side effects have included headache, dizziness, tinnitus, and thrombocytopenia, and in rare cases, toxic amblyopia, renal failure, and hepatic damage. The latter may be more common in children than in adults.[112]

With naproxen, the most commonly reported side effects are gastrointestinal, such as heartburn, nausea, and dyspepsia. Again, these occur less frequently than when therapeutically equivalent doses of aspirin are administered.[113] Serious gastrointestinal bleeding has been rare with naproxen, but a few fatalities have been reported. Central nervous system side effects include dizziness, headache, drowsiness, and depression. Other less common side effects include pruritus and other dermatologic problems, angioneurotic edema, thrombocytopenia, agranulocytosis, and jaundice.[113] Rare cases of naproxen-associated elevations in liver function tests and renal failure have been reported, and again, there is some concern that these may occur more frequently in the pediatric population.[114] Since, to date, the nonsteroidal anti-inflammatory drugs have not been used extensively in the pediatric population, it seems likely that the full range of adverse reactions is still unknown.

THE USE OF ANTIPYRETICS IN THE CLINICAL SETTING

Because aspirin, acetaminophen, and the nonsteroidals all have excellent antipyretic activity, specific clinical contraindications will often dictate the selection of one drug over the other. Strong contraindications to the use of aspirin include:

1. Any child with varicella or an influenza-like illness, because of the risk of developing Reye's syndrome. Some feel that aspirin is contraindicated in any child with fever of infectious etiology.
2. The presence of or the past history of esophageal varices or gastric or duodenal ulcer.
3. Clinical situations where an increased risk of gastric ulceration is recognized, including fulminant disease in the neonate, serious illness involving the central nervous system (meningitis, encephalitis, etc.), and extensive burns.
4. Seven to ten days prior to and following major surgery because of the potential for clotting dysfunction.
5. Clinical situations with clotting or platelet abnormalities or in association with drugs with a capacity to impair hemostasis.
6. For a week prior to childbirth.
7. In well-documented instances of allergic manifestations to aspirin.

Clinical situations also exist where strong contraindications to the use of aspirin do not exist, yet the risk of aspirin may exceed the benefit. In these situations a simple adjustment in the dose or alertness to potential side effects may be all that is required. These situations include:

1. Renal failure.
2. High-dose aspirin in association with vomiting, decreased oral intake, dehydration, or metabolic or respiratory acidosis.
3. Hypoalbuminemia.
4. Concomitant use of drugs with high protein binding.

Contraindications to the use of acetaminophen are less frequent, but in the following situations aspirin or a nonsteroidal would be the favored antipyretic agent (assuming no contraindications exist):

1. Clinical disease where an anti-inflammatory effect is needed (rheumatoid arthritis, rheumatic fever, etc.).
2. Acute inflammatory liver disease and/or liver failure.

The relatively brief clinical experience with nonsteroidal anti-inflammatory drugs in children would suggest that their use for that purpose should be reserved for special circumstances. These might include instances where:

1. Combined antipyretic and anti-inflammatory properties are needed and aspirin is contraindicated.
2. The prolonged antipyretic effect is more desirable.

In summary, in most instances of fever in children the current antipyretic of choice will be acetaminophen. In some cases, however, the special properties of aspirin or the nonsteroidal anti-inflammatory agents may make them the preferable treatment.

REFERENCES

1. Done AK: Antipyretics. Pediatr Clin North Am 19:167–177, 1972
2. Schmitt BD: Fever in childhood. Pediatrics 74(suppl):929–936, 1984
3. McCarthy PL: Controversies in pediatrics: What tests are indicated for the child under 2 with fever. Pediatr Rev 1:51–56, 1979
4. Hoekelman R, Lewin EB, Shapira MB, et al: Potential bacteremia in pediatric practice. Am J Dis Child 133:1017–1019, 1979
5. Beaver WT: Mild analgesics, a review of their clinical pharmacology. Am J Med Sci 250:577–604, 1965
6. Mills JA: Nonsteroidal anti-inflammatory drugs. N Engl J Med 290:1002–1005, 1974
7. Cashman TM, Starns RJ, Johnson J, et al: Comparative effects of naproxen and aspirin on fever in children. J Pediatr 95:626–629, 1979
8. Amdekar YK, Desai RZ: Antipyretic activity of ibuprofen and paracetamol in children with pyrexia. Br J Clin Pract 39:140–143, 1985
9. Burgio GR, Nespoli L, Michos N, et al: Open study of clinical effect of suprofen syrup in children. Arzneim-Forsch/Drug Res 36:968–971, 1986
10. Hurwitz ES, Barrett MJ, Bregman D, et al: Public Health Service Study of Reye's syndrome and medications: Report of the main study. JAMA 257:1905–1911, 1987
11. Forsyth BW, Horwitz RI, Acampora D, et al: Aspirin and Reye's syndrome: Biologic fact or methodologic error? (Abstr.) Pediatr Res 23(4, part 2):291A, 1988
12. Dascombe MJ: The pharmacology of fever. Prog Neurobiol 25:327–373, 1985
13. Atkins E: Fever: The old and the new. J Infect Dis 149:339–348, 1984
14. Done AK: Treatment of fever in 1982: A review. Am J Med 74:27–35, 1983
15. Lorin MI: Fever: Pathogenesis and treatment, in Feigin RD, Cherry JD (eds): Textbook of Pediatric Infectious Diseases. Philadelphia, W.B. Saunders Company, 1987
16. Stern RC: Pathophysiologic basis for symptomatic treatment of fever. Pediatrics 59:92–98, 1977
17. Lovejoy FH Jr: Aspirin and acetaminophen: A comparative view of their antipyretic and analgesic activity. Pediatrics 62:904–909, 1978
18. Carmichael LE, Barnes FD, Percy DH: Temperature as a factor in resistance of young puppies to canine herpesvirus. J Infect Dis 120:669–678, 1969
19. Enders JF, Shaffer MF: Studies on natural immunity to pneumococcus type III: The capacity of pneumococcus type III to grow at 41°C and their virulence for rabbits. J Exp Med 64:7–18, 1936
20. Jampel HD, Duff GW, Gershon RK, et al: Fever and immunoregulation III. Hyperthermia augments the primary in vitro humoral immune response. J Exp Med 157:1229–1238, 1983
21. Bernheim HA, Bodel PT, Askenase PW, et al: Effects of fever on host defense mechanisms after infection in the lizard Dipsosaurus dorsalis. Br J Pathol 59:76–84, 1978
22. Roberts NJ, Steigbigel RT: Hyperthermia and human leukocyte function: Effects on response of lymphocytes to mitogen and antigen and bactericidal capacity of monocytes and neutrophils. Infect Immun 18:673–679, 1977
23. Heron I, Berg K: The actions of interferon are potentiated at elevated temperature. Nature 274:508–510, 1978
24. Pizzo PA, Lovejoy FH Jr, Smith DH: Prolonged fever in children: Review of 100 cases. Pediatrics 55:468–473, 1975
25. Torrey SB, Henretig F, Fleisher G, et al: Temperature response to antipyretic therapy in children: Relationship to occult bacteremia. Am J Emerg Med 3:190–192, 1985
26. Tiller T, Baker RC: Changes in clinical toxicity following fever reduction in febrile children: Correlation with diagnosis (Abstr.). Am J Dis Child 142:394–395, 1988
27. Austin TW, Truant G: Hyperthermia, antipyretics and function of polymorphonuclear leukocytes. Can Med Assoc J 118:493–495, 1978

28. Vaughn LK, Kluger MJ: Fever and survival in rabbits infected with Pasteurella multocida. J Physiol 282:243–251, 1978
29. Done AK, Yaffe SJ, Clayton JM: Aspirin dosage for infants and children. J Pediatr 95:617–625, 1979
30. Hunter J: Study of antipyretic therapy in current use. Arch Dis Child 48:313–315, 1973
31. Simila S, Kouvalainen K, Keinanen S: Oral antipyretic therapy: Evaluation of ibuprofen. Scand J Rheumatol 5:81–83, 1976
32. Tarlin L, Landrigan P, Babineau R, et al: A comparison of the antipyretic effect of acetaminophen and aspirin. Am J Dis Child 124:880–882, 1972
33. Eden AN, Kaufman A: Clinical comparison of three antipyretic agents. Am J Dis Child 114:284–287, 1967
34. Colgan MT, Mintz AA: The comparative antipyretic effect of N-acetyl-p-aminophenol and acetylsalicylic acid. J Pediatr 50:552–555, 1957
35. Reuter SH, Montgomery WW: Aspirin vs acetaminophen after tonsillectomy. Arch Otolaryngol 80:214–217, 1964
36. Steele RW, Young FSH, Bass JW, et al: Oral antipyretic therapy, evaluation of aspirin-acetaminophen combination. Am J Dis Child 123:204–206, 1972
37. Kandoth PW, Joshi MK, Joshi VR, et al: Comparative evaluation of antipyretic activity of ibuprofen and aspirin in children with pyrexia of varied aetiology. J Int Med Res 12:292–297, 1984
38. Wilson G, Guerra AJMS, Santos NT: Comparative study of the antipyretic effect of ibuprofen (oral suspension) and paracetamol (suppositories) in paediatrics. J Int Med Res 12:250–254, 1984
39. Katob A: A comparative study of two dosage levels of ibuprofen syrup in children with pyrexia. J Int Med Res 13:122–126, 1985
39a. Walson PD, Galletta G, Braden NJ, et al: Ibuprofen, acetaminophen, and placebo treatment of febrile children. Clin Pharmacol Ther 46:9–17, 1989
40. Szorady I, Martonyi E, Santa A: Antipyretic effect of naprosyn syrup in childhood. Ther Hung 33:201–206, 1985
41. Ayeemuddin SK, Vega RA, Kim TH, et al: The effect of naproxen on fever in children with malignancies. Cancer 59:1966–1968, 1987
42. Giovannini M, Longhi R, Besana R, et al: Clinical experience and results of treatment with suprofen in pediatrics. 5th communication: A single-blind study on antipyretic effect and tolerability of suprofen syrup versus metamizole drops in pediatric patients. Arzneim-Forsch/Drug Res 36:959–964, 1986
43. Weippl G, Baerlocher K, Michos N: Open study of the clinical effects of suprofen drops in children. Arzneim-Forsch/Drug Res 36:965–967, 1986
44. Cotty VF, Sterbenz FJ, Mueller F, et al: Augmentation of human blood acetylsalicylate concentrations by the simultaneous administration of acetaminophen with aspirin. Toxicol Appl Pharm 41:7–13, 1977
45. Whitehouse LW, Paul CJ, Wong LT, et al: Effect of aspirin on a subtoxic dose of ^{14}C-acetaminophen in mice. J Pharm Sci 66:1399–1403, 1977
46. Whitehouse LW, Paul CJ, Thomas BH: Effect of acetylsalicylic acid on a toxic dose of acetaminophen in the mouse. Toxicol Appl Pharm 38:571–582, 1976
47. Steele RW, Tanaka PT, Lara RP, et al: Evaluation of sponging and of oral antipyretic therapy to reduce fever. J Pediatr 77:824–829, 1970
48. Smith MJH, Smith PK: The Salicylates: A Critical Bibliographic Review. New York, Interscience Publishers, 1966
49. Levy G: Clinical pharmacokinetics of aspirin. Pediatrics 62:867–872, 1978
50. Mills JA: Nonsteroidal anti-inflammatory drugs. N Engl J Med 290:781–784, 1974
51. Yacobi A, Levy G: Intraindividual relationships between serum protein binding of drugs in normal human subjects, patients with impaired renal function and rats. J Pharm Sci 66:1285–1289, 1977
52. Levy G, Yaffe SJ: Relationship between dose and apparent volume of distribution of salicylate in children. Pediatrics 54:713–717, 1974
53. Hill JB: Experimental salicylate poisoning: Observations on the effects of altering blood pH on tissue and plasma salicylate concentrations. Pediatrics 47:658–665, 1971
54. Hill JB: Salicylate intoxication. N Engl J Med 288:1110–1113, 1973
55. Buchanan N, Rabinowitz L: Infantile salicylism—A reappraisal. J Pediatr 84:391–395, 1974
56. Proudfoot AT, Brown SS: Acidaemia and salicylate poisoning in adults. Br Med J 2:547–550, 1969
57. Johnson PK, Free HM, Free AH: A simplified urine and serum screening test for salicylate intoxication. J Pediatr 63:949–953, 1963
58. Levy G, Tsuchiya T, Amsel LP: Limited capacity for salicyl phenolic glucuronide formation and its effect on the kinetics of salicylate elimination in man. Clin Pharmacol Ther 13:258–268, 1972
59. Snodgrass WR: Salicylate toxicity. Pediatr Clin North Am 33:381–391, 1986
60. Peterson RG, Rumack BH: Pharmacokinetics in children. Pediatrics 62:877–879, 1978
61. Black M: Acetaminophen hepatotoxicity. Gastroenterology 78:382–392, 1980
62. Rumack BH: Acetaminophen overdose in children and adolescents. Pediatr Clin North Am 33:691–701, 1986
63. Clark R, Thompson RPH, Borirakchanyavat V, et al: Hepatic damage and death from overdose of paracetamol. Lancet 1:66–69, 1973
64. Cobden I, Record CO, Wark MK, et al: Paracetamol-induced acute renal failure in the absence of fulminant liver damage. Br Med J 284:21–22, 1982
65. Verbeeck RK, Blackburn JL, Loewen GR: Clinical pharmacokinetics of non-steroidal anti-inflammatory drugs. Clin Pharmacokinet 8:297–331, 1983
66. Daniels SR, Greenberg RS, Ibrahim MA: Scientific uncertainties in the studies of salicylate use and Reye's syndrome. JAMA 249:1311–1316, 1983
67. Leonards JR, Levy G, Niemczura R: Gastrointestinal blood loss during prolonged aspirin administration. N Engl J Med 289:1020–1022, 1973
68. Leonards JR, Levy G: Gastrointestinal blood loss from aspirin and sodium salicylate tablets in man. Clin Pharmacol Ther 14:62–66, 1973
69. Leonards JR, Levy G: Reduction or prevention of aspirin-induced occult gastrointestinal blood loss in man. Clin Pharmacol Ther 10:571–575, 1969
70. Fromm D: Salicylate and gastric mucosal damage. Pediatrics 62:938–942, 1978
71. Croft DN: Exfoliative cytology of the stomach after administration of salicylates, in Dixon AJ, Martin BK, Smith MJH, et al (eds): Salicylates: An International Symposium. London, Churchill, 1963
72. Mills DG, Borda IT, Philip RB, et al: Effects of in vitro aspirin on blood platelets of gastrointestinal bleeders. Clin Pharmacol Ther 15:187–192, 1973
73. Heggarty H: Aspirin and anemia in childhood. Br Med J 1:491–492, 1974
74. Levy M: Aspirin use in patients with major upper gastrointestinal bleeding and peptic ulcer disease. N Engl J Med 290:1158–1162, 1974
75. Hussey HH: Aspirin can be dangerous. JAMA 228:609, 1974
76. Memon IS: Aspirin and blood fibrinolysis. Lancet 1:364, 1970
77. Quick AJ: Salicylates and bleeding: The Aspirin Tolerance Test. Am J Med Sci 252:265–269, 1966
78. Weiss HJ: The pharmacology of platelet inhibition, in Spaet TH (ed): Progress in Hematology and Thrombosis. New York, Grune and Stratton, 1972
79. Willis AL: An enzymatic mechanism for the anti-thrombotic and anti-hemostatic action of aspirin. Science 183:325–327, 1974
80. Kaneshiro MM, Mielke CH, Kasper CK, et al: Bleeding time after aspirin in disorders of intrinsic clotting. N Engl J Med 281:1039–1042, 1969
81. Sutor AH, Bowie EJW, Owen CA: Effect of aspirin, sodium salicylate and acetaminophen. Mayo Clin Proc 46:178–181, 1971
82. Binder RA, Durocher J, Mielke H: Treatment of pain in hemophilia. Am J Dis Child 127:371–373, 1974
83. Soloway HB: Drug induced bleeding. Am J Clin Pathol 61:622–627, 1974

84. Weiss HJ: Aspirin—A dangerous drug? JAMA 229:1221–1222, 1974

85. Bleyer WA, Breckenridge RT: Studies on the detection of adverse drug reactions in the newborn. JAMA 213:2049–2053, 1970

86. Haslam RR, Ekert H, Gillam MB: Hemorrhage in a neonate possibly due to maternal ingestion of salicylate. J Pediatr 84:556–557, 1974

87. Corby DG, Schulman I: The effects of antenatal drug administration on aggregation of platelets of newborn infants. J Pediatr 79:307–313, 1971

88. Levy G, Garrettson LK: Kinetics of salicylate elimination by newborn infants of mothers who ingested aspirin before delivery. Pediatrics 53:201–210, 1974

89. Ritch RR, Johnson JS: Salicylate hepatotoxicity in patients with juvenile rheumatoid arthritis. Arthritis Rheum 16:1–9, 1973

90. Wolfe JD, Metzger AL, Goldstein RC: Aspirin hepatitis. Ann Intern Med 80:74–76, 1974

91. Manso C, Taranta A, Nydick I: Effect of aspirin administration on serum glutamic oxalo acetic and glutamic pyruvic transaminases in children. Proc Soc Exp Biol Med 93:84–88, 1956

92. Koppes GM, Arnett FC: Salicylate hepatotoxicity. Postgrad Med 56:193–195, 1974

93. Seaman WE, Ishak KG, Plotz PH: Aspirin induced hepatotoxicity in patients with systemic lupus erythematosus. Ann Intern Med 80:1–8, 1974

94. Weinberger M: Analgesic sensitivity in children with asthma. Pediatrics 62:910–915, 1978

95. Schaller JG: Chronic salicylate administration in juvenile rheumatoid arthritis: Aspirin "hepatitis" and its clinical significance. Pediatrics 62:916–925, 1978

96. Asad SI, Kemeny DM, Youlten LJF, et al: Effect of aspirin in "aspirin sensitive" patients. Br Med J 288:745–748, 1984

97. Samter M, Beers RF Jr: Intolerance to aspirin: Clinical studies and consideration of its pathogenesis. Ann Intern Med 68:975–983, 1968

98. Levy G, Tsuchiya T: Salicylate accumulation kinetics in man. N Engl J Med 287:430–432, 1972

99. Levy G: Pharmacokinetics in salicylate elimination in man. J Pharm Sci 54:959–967, 1965

100. McIntire MS, Angle CR: Aspirin fatalities: The new taxonomy. Pediatrics 69:249–250, 1982

101. Brenner BE, Simon RR: Management of salicylate intoxication. Drugs 24:335–340, 1982

102. Sutton E, Soyka LF: How safe is acetaminophen? Clin Pediatrics 12:692–694, 1973

103. Seeff LB, Cuccherini BA, Zimmerman HJ, et al: Acetaminophen hepatotoxicity in alcoholics: A therapeutic misadventure. Ann Intern Med 104:399–404, 1986

104. Gabriel R, et al: Acute tubular necrosis, caused by therapeutic doses of paracetamol? Clin Nephrol 18:269–271, 1982

105. Pearson HA: Comparative effects of aspirin and acetaminophen on hemostasis. Pediatrics 62:926–929, 1978

106. Litovitz TL, Martin TG, Schmitz B: 1986 Annual Report of the American Association of Poison Control Centers National Data Collection System. Am J Emerg Med 5:405–445, 1987

107. Rumack BH, Matthew H: Acetaminophen poisoning and toxicity. Pediatrics 55:871–876, 1975

108. Lovejoy FH Jr, Goldman P: Acetaminophen toxicity. Pediatr Rev 1:117–121, 1979

109. Prescott LF, Roscoe P, Wright N, et al: Plasma paracetamol half-life and hepatic necrosis in patients with paracetamol overdosage. Lancet 1:519–522, 1971

110. Mitchell JR, Jollow DJ, Potter WZ, et al: Acetaminophen-induced hepatic necrosis. I. Role of drug metabolism. J Pharm Exp Therap 187:185–194, 1973

111. Curry RW, Robinson JD, Sughrue MJ: Acute renal failure after acetaminophen ingestion. JAMA 247:1012–1014, 1982

112. Royer GL, Seckman CE, Welshman IR: Safety profile: Fifteen years of clinical experience with ibuprofen. Am J Med 77(suppl.):25–34, 1984

113. Segre EJ: Naproxen, in Huskisson EC (ed): Anti-Rheumatic Drugs. New York, Praeger, 1983

114. Laxer RM, Silverman ED, Balfe JW, et al: Naproxen-associated renal failure in a child with arthritis and inflammatory bowel disease. Pediatrics 80:904–908, 1987

33

CARDIAC DRUGS

RAFAEL GORODISCHER *and* GIDEON KOREN

DRUGS USED IN THE MANAGEMENT OF CONGESTIVE HEART FAILURE

General Considerations

Clinical and experimental studies have documented that the heart of the young infant responds in a more limited fashion to inotropic agents than that of the older child or adult.[1-5] This is due to the biologic immaturity and restricted functional reserve of the young heart, as well as to the different pathogenesis of cardiac decompensation in infants with left-to-right shunts.[6,7] A lower ratio of active myofilaments to noncontractile elements,[8] greater stiffness of the ventricle,[9,10] underdeveloped cardiac sympathetic nerves,[11,12] and higher cardiac output per unit surface area[13] are characteristic features of the immature compared to the fully developed heart. Differences in electrolyte concentrations and in a number of metabolic reactions have also been described in the newborn myocardium.[14,15]

Over the years, digitalis glycosides and diuretics have become key drugs in the management of congestive heart failure. Concern with the low therapeutic/toxic ratio of digitalis has led to increased use of natural and synthetic catecholamines in acute situations and introduction of novel inotropic agents.

On the other hand, it has been recently recognized that little is achieved in many infants with congenital heart defects by attempting to increase myocardial contractility. Their myocardium may already be working at the peak of its contractile force but be unable to sustain adequate blood flow because of volume overload (due to left-to-right shunting in patent ductus arteriosus and ventricular septal defect) or pressure overload (in obstructive lesions).[1,6,7] Awareness of the dissociation between the function of the heart as a pump (pump function) and the contractile performance of the myocardium (myocardial function) has resulted in novel strategies in the management of cardiac failure. Growing experience is being gained with the use of systemic vasodilators that reduce cardiac workload in infants and children in heart failure.

Inotropic Agents in Acute Situations

Catecholamines

A variety of adrenergic compounds exert a positive inotropic effect by acting directly on β_1-adrenergic receptors of the myocardium. They may be used temporarily in the management of congestive heart failure (except in congestive failure due to obstructive lesions) until a more permanent therapy is established; clinical use of these agents is limited by their positive chronotropic action and tendency to exacerbate cardiac arrhythmias. Their actions in the heart include stimulation of adenyl cyclase, increased intracellular concentration of cyclic AMP, and Ca^{2+} delivery to cardiac contractile proteins. These effects seem to be mediated by cyclic AMP–dependent protein kinases.[16] Clinical use of these agents is summarized in Table 33–1.

Epinephrine (adrenaline), the major hormone secreted by the adrenal medulla, it a potent stimulator of both α- and β- adrenergic receptors and thus exerts complex effects on various organs. Following subcutaneous or slow intravenous administration, it increases the force of myocardial contraction and the heart rate, with a resultant increase in cardiac output and systolic pressure; diastolic pressure usually falls because of its effect on β_2-adrenergic receptors of skeletal muscle vasculature. The increased work of the heart is achieved at the expense of greater oxygen consumption and decreased cardiac efficiency. In the kidneys epinephrine increases vascular resistance and decreases plasma flow. Epinephrine also induces automaticity of the myocardium, and its intravenous administration may cause cardiac arrhythmias.

Whereas noncatecholamine sympathomimetic amines act indirectly on the heart (through release of norepineph-

TABLE 33–1. USE OF SELECTED INOTROPIC AGENTS

DRUG	INDICATIONS	ROUTE AND DOSE	REF.
Epinephrine (adrenaline)	Cardiac resuscitation	I.V. or intratracheal 0.01 mg/kg/dose	3,25,26
	Cardiac decompensation following cardiac surgery	I.V. 0.1–1.0 μg/kg/min	
	Anaphylactic shock	S.C. 0.01 mg/kg/dose	
Isoproterenol (Isuprel)	Failure of other inotropic agents; bradycardia	I.V. Initially: 0.05–0.1 μg/kg/min; increase if necessary (heart rate, peripheral perfusion) up to 1 μg/kg/min	3,25
Dopamine	Heart failure (asphyxiated neonates, following cardiac surgery), shock (cardiogenic, septic), renal failure	I.V. 2–30 μg/kg/min	3,21,25,27,28
Dobutamine	Acute cardiac decompensation	I.V. 5–20 μg/kg/min	3,25,29

rine), epinephrine directly stimulates β_1-adrenergic receptors of cardiac muscle, pacemaker, and conductive tissue.

Epinephrine is administered only parenterally; after oral administration it is readily metabolized in the gut and liver. Due to its constrictive effect on subcutaneous blood vessels, absorption is more rapid following intramuscular than subcutaneous injection. It is readily absorbed by the mucosa of the tracheobronchial tree, a route employed in cardiac resuscitation. Epinephrine is rapidly inactivated by catecholamine-0-methyl transferase (COMT) and monoaminooxidase (MAO) of the liver and other tissues, and its metabolites are excreted in the urine.

Toxic effects include restlessness, anxiety, fear, headache, tremor, pallor, dizziness, and palpitations. Fatal ventricular arrhythmias may develop following intravenous injection. Interaction between epinephrine and halogenated hydrocarbon anesthetics may result in ventricular fibrillation.

Epinephrine for injection is a sterile solution of epinephrine hydrochloride in water. When administered intracardially or intratracheally, the 1:1000 solution should never be used undiluted.

Norepinephrine (levarterenol, l-noradrenaline), the neurotransmitter of sympathetic postganglionic fibers and of certain tracts in the central nervous system, constitutes 1/10 to 1/5 of the catecholamines in the adrenal medulla. It stimulates mainly β_1-adrenergic receptors and has little action of β_2-receptors.

Intravenous infusion of norepinephrine causes an increase in peripheral resistance and a rise in systolic and diastolic blood pressure, with no change (or a decrease) in cardiac output; therefore, its use is limited to the management of hypotension and has no indication in situations that require increased myocardial contraction force. The mechanisms and extent of absorption, metabolism, and excretion are similar to those of epinephrine.

It is administered by intravenous infusion at an initial dose of 0.1 μg/kg/min and increased until the desired effect is obtained or up to 1 μg/kg/min.

Isoproterenol (isoprenaline) acts on β_1- and β_2-adrenergic receptors, with minimal effect on α-receptors. Intravenous infusion of isoproterenol causes positive inotropic and chronotropic effects, decreased peripheral resistance and diastolic pressure, and increased renal blood flow. The resulting greater cardiac output may raise systolic pressure.

Isoproterenol is rapidly absorbed when administered as aerosol, and it is metabolized primarily by COMT. Although less pronounced, its side effects are similar to those of epinephrine.

Dopamine. This sympathomimetic amine is a metabolic precursor of norepinephrine and epinephrine and acts as a central neurotransmitter. It has a positive inotropic effect on the myocardium resulting from direct stimulation of β_1-adrenergic receptors and also from the effect of norepinephrine released by cardiac sympathetic nerve terminals. It has a less marked chronotropic effect than isoproterenol. At low therapeutic doses (2–5 μg/kg/min), it has a predominant β_1-adrenergic action, and the increase in cardiac output parallels the increase in heart rate; at higher doses dopamine has increasing α-adrenergic action. Also, at low doses it causes renal vasodilation and promotes diuresis by stimulating renal dopaminergic receptors, and increases systolic pressure with little or no effect on diastolic pressure. Because it increases pulmonary artery pressure, it should be used with caution, if at all, in patients with elevated pulmonary vascular resistance. At high doses (>10 μg/kg/min), it stimulates arteriolar α-adrenergic receptors, causing vasoconstriction (including renal vasoconstriction) and hypertension. In contrast to the response to isoproterenol, which is equal at all ages, the inotropic response to dopamine in the young animal increases with advancing age[2]; this may be due to the decreased levels of releasable norepinephrine of the immature myocardium. Dopamine therapy is free from central nervous system effects because it does not cross the blood–brain barrier. It is metabolized by MAO and COMT and therefore is effective only when given parenterally.

No adverse effects have been recorded in infants, children, and adolescents with a dose of 0.3–25 μg/kg/min.[17] However, excessive dosage can cause side effects that represent enhanced sympathomimetic activity. Extravasation may cause ischemic necrosis. Phentolamine may be used when gangrene of the fingers or toes is feared following prolonged administration of the drug.

Dobutamine is a synthetic β-sympathomimetic amine that has a potent inotropic action but little effect on heart rate. It is a mixture of L- and D-isomers, and its pharmacologic effects are explained by their different action on α_1- (L-isomer) and β_1- and β_2-adrenergic (D-isomer) receptors. It does not stimulate renal dopamine receptors and has no effect on renal vasculature; low-dose dopamine may be added to the dobutamine infusion if increased renal cortical flow is desired. High dosages of dobutamine may cause elevation of systemic arterial pressure. Increasing plasma concentrations between 40 and 190 μg/ml correlate with progressive improvement in cardiac function in adults with low output failure.[18] It seems less effective in infants under 1 year of age than in older children.[5] Few pharmacokinetic data on this agent are available.

Newer Inotropic Agents

Some patients in cardiac failure remain symptomatic despite conventional therapy, including diuretics, vasodilators, and digoxin. New cardiotonics recently studied may be used in these patients. These new inotropic agents not only increase the contractility of the myocardium but also have vasodilating properties and the potential of a greater therapeutic index as compared to digoxin. Their inotropic effect is obtained by a mechanism different than inhibition of Na^+,K^+-ATPase or β-adrenergic receptor stimulation. Some of them have been released for general use, while others are still under investigation. Few data are available at present on these agents in the developing organism, and their routine use in pediatrics should await reports of carefully performed clinical trials.[19,20]

Amrinone and *milrinone* are potent bipyridine derivatives that inhibit the cyclic AMP—specific cardiac phosphodiesterase. Their positive inotropic action is additive to that of digitalis. In addition, they increase heart rate and decrease systemic vascular resistance.

Both of them are well absorbed following oral administration, rapidly distributed in the body, and excreted in the urine; amrinone undergoes biotransformation in the liver to an N-acetyl derivative and other metabolites. The plasma elimination half-lives of amrinone and milrinone in adults are around 4 and 1.5 hours, respectively. The body clearance of both drugs is reduced in cardiac failure.

Amrinone acts rapidly following intravenous administration, whereas after oral dosage its effect peaks within 3 hours and lasts for 4–6 hours. The inotropic action of amrinone is age-dependent; it has no effect in the neonatal period.[4,21]

Toxicity is related to dose and route of administration and includes gastrointestinal intolerance, hepatotoxicity, fever, and thrombocytopenia. Milrinone is better tolerated than amrinone.

Enoximone is an imidazole derivative available in intravenous and oral form that has a wide margin of safety. In addition to its positive inotropic effect, it causes vasodilation. Its terminal plasma half-life is 6 hours in the adult, and it is excreted in the urine as a sulfoxide metabolite.[22] No relationship has been established between the plasma concentration of the parent drug or its sulfoxide metabolite and the pharmacologic effect. Adverse effects (nausea, diarrhea, headache, abnormal liver function tests) occur in as many as one-fourth of the patients.[23]

Other newer inotropic agents presently under investigation include *piroximone* and *ibopamine* (an ester derivative of deoxyepinephrine); they also exhibit vasodilating properties and may be used orally.[19,20]

Preload- and Afterload-Reducing Drugs

Experience with drugs that modify the workload of the heart in children has increased in the past years. The aim of preload-reducing therapy is to decrease the elevated pressure and congestion in the venous bed (systemic or pulmonary), the ventricular filling, and the ventricular dilation of the patient in heart failure. On the other hand, arteriolar vasodilators (afterload-reducing agents) tend to lower the elevated resistance to left ventricular ejection (afterload) and to improve stroke volume. The increased systemic vascular resistance in heart failure is caused by compensatory homeostatic mechanisms that aim to maintain systemic arterial pressure, i.e., elevated sympathetic tone and circulating catecholamines, and stimulation of the renin–angiotensin system.

It has been shown that systemic vasodilators are particularly useful in severe mitral or aortic regurgitation, systemic hypertension, cardiomyopathy, myocardial ischemia, and in postoperative cardiac surgical patients. Because volume or pressure loading may decrease myocardial contractility, systemic vasodilators used in severe cardiac failure are usually administered in combination with inotropic drugs. The effect of systemic vasodilators, as opposed to inotropic agents and diuretics, on the Frank–Starling curve of the failing ventricle is illustrated in Figure 33–1. For a detailed analysis of the theoretical rationale of vasodilator therapy in cardiac failure, the reader is referred to other reviews.[6,24]

Preload- and afterload-reducing drugs cause variable regional vasodilation. As opposed to the rather uniform arteriolar and/or venous vasodilation caused by direct-acting agents (hydralazine, nitroprusside, nitrates), the effect of α-adrenergic blocking agents and angiotensin-converting enzyme inhibitors is limited to specific beds. Table 33–2 summarizes the main systemic vasodilators

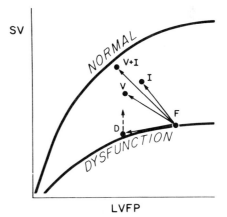

FIGURE 33–1. Frank–Starling left ventricular function curve relating left ventricular filling pressure (LVFP) to stroke volume (SV). Depressed curve of heart failure can be shifted toward normal by inotropic drugs (I) or vasodilator drugs (V), and these effects are complementary when the drugs are infused together (V + I). Note that diuretics (D) usually reduce filling pressure (F) without augmenting output. The dashed line suggests that stroke volume may later rise, perhaps by virtue of a gradual improvement in ventricular function. (From Cohn and Franciosa: Vasodilator therapy of cardiac failure. N Engl J Med 297:27, 1977, with permission.)

TABLE 33–2. SELECTED VASODILATORS USED IN CONGESTIVE HEART FAILURE

DRUG	MECHANISM OF ACTION	ROUTE AND DOSE	REF.
Venous muscle relaxants			
Nitroglycerine	Direct vasodilation (increase in cyclic GMP)	I.V. 0.5–20 μg/kg/min (max 60 μg/kg/min)	6,29
Arteriolar vasodilators			
Hydralazine	Direct vasodilation (increase in cyclic GMP?)	I.V. 1.5 μg/kg/min or 0.1–0.5 mg/kg q6h P.O. 0.5–7 mg/kg/day q6–8h (max 200 mg/day)	6,29,31,32
Nifedipine	Ca channel blocker	P.O. or sublingual 0.1–0.5 mg/kg/dose q6–8h (caution in neonates)	29
Mixed vasodilators			
Nitroprusside	Direct vasodilatation (increase in cyclic GMP)	I.V. 0.5–8 μg/kg/min	6,29,33–35
Phentolamine	Competitive α_1- and α_2-adrenergic blocker	I.V. 2.5–15 μg/kg/min	29
Prazosine	Competitive α_1-adrenergic blocker	P.O. first dose 5 μg/kg; increase as needed up to 100 μg/kg/day (q6h)	6,29,30
Captopril	Angiotensin-converting enzyme inhibitor	P.O. Neonates: 0.1–0.4 mg/kg/dose q6–24h Infants: 0.5–6 mg/kg/day (q6–24h) Older children: 12 mg/dose q12–24 h	6,29,30,36,37
Enalapril	Angiotension-converting enzyme inhibitor	P.O. 0.08 mg/kg/dose q12–24 h (older children)	29

used in the treatment of cardiac failure in infants and children and their presently recommended doses. This simplified classification reflects their main site of action; however, the physiologic response to vasodilation is often more complex in the patient in heart failure. The pharmacology of specific systemic vasodilators is reviewed in Chapter 39, Antihypertensive Agents.

ANTIARRHYTHMIC AGENTS

A great number of antiarrhythmic drugs are available today. None of them is universally effective. Most produce frequent or severe side effects, and extensive pediatric use has been limited to only a few. Insufficient pharmacokinetic data are available concerning the majority of both "classical" and "newer" antiarrhythmic agents in infants and children, and dosage is derived from clinical experience. As many arrhythmias are rare or occur as emergencies, the use of antiarrhythmic agents in children is not based on classical randomized, controlled trials. Although historical controls could be used, limited experience does not allow rigorous analysis of the relative efficacy and safety of the host of new antiarrhythmic agents available today. The risk/benefit ratio and the personal experience of the clinician with the various drugs, the specific type of arrhythmia present, and the overall conditions of the child should be considered in the selection of the particular agent. Final recommendations of rational dosages should await reports on the relationship of phar-

macokinetic processes to their therapeutic and toxic effects.

Classification of antiarrhythmic agents is complex; they exert multiple actions that vary in different tissues, and they generate active metabolites that produce different effects than the parent drug. For these reasons a system that classifies antiarrhythmic actions rather than drugs (the Vaughan Williams classification) is preferred today (Table 33–3).[38]

The therapeutic indications and dosages of antiarrhythmic agents are summarized in Tables 33–4 and 33–5, and the untoward effects in Table 33–6. Drug interactions, both pharmacokinetic and pharmacodynamic, are common in combination therapy for cardiac arrhythmias and between antiarrhythmic agents and other drugs (Tables 33–7 and 33–8). For a more extensive review of the use of antiarrhythmic agents in pediatrics and the pharmacologic profile of these drugs in adults (few pharmacokinetic data are available in children), the reader is referred to other sources.[39–42]

β-Adrenergic Blocking Agents

Propranolol is a nonselective β_1- and β_2-adrenergic blocking agent used in diseases of the cardiovascular system such as hypertension, tetralogy of Fallot, hypertrophic obstructive cardiomyopathy, and arrhythmias, as well as in neonatal thyrotoxicosis[43] and other conditions.

Propranolol exerts negative inotropic and chronotropic actions on the heart that result in decreased cardiac out-

TABLE 33–3. CLASSIFICATION OF ANTIARRHYTHMIC AGENTS BY THEIR MECHANISM OF ACTION

CLASS	MECHANISM OF ACTION	DRUGS	EFFECT ON ECG
I	Fast sodium channel blockade: depress phase 0 depolarization and prolong conduction		
IA	Prolong repolarization and refractory period	Quinidine Procainamide Disopyramide	Prolong QRS and QTc
IB	Shorten repolarization	Lidocaine Tocainide Mexiletine Phenytoin	Minimal effect on PR, QRS, and QTc
IC	Slow conduction; little effect on repolarization	Encainide Flecainide Lorcainide Propafenone	Prolong PR, QRS, and QTc
Uncl	Combined effects of IA, IB, and/or IC	Ethmozine	May prolong PR and QRS
II	β-adrenergic blockade	Propranolol Timolol Metoprolol	Prolong PR
III	Prolong repolarization and refractory period	Amiodarone Bretylium	Prolong PR and QTc
IV	Slow calcium channel blockade	Verapamil Diltiazem Nifedipine	Prolong PR

Abbreviations: Uncl: unclassified; QTc: QT interval corrected for heart rate.

TABLE 33–4. THERAPEUTIC INDICATIONS OF ANTIARRHYTHMIC DRUGS

DRUG	THERAPEUTIC INDICATIONS	COMMENTS
Quinidine	PVD, VT	Contraindicated in long QT syndrome
Procainamide	PVD, VT	Contraindicated in myasthenia gravis and complete heart block
Disopyramide	PVD, VT (non-life-threatening)	
Lidocaine	VT	
Phenytoin	Digoxin-induced tachyarrhythmias	Infuse slowly
Mexiletine	VA in CHD	May replace phenytoin in patients with phenytoin side effects
Encainide	PJRT, SVT refractory to digoxin, propranolol, verapamil	Greater efficacy when combined with verapamil or propranolol
Flecainide	Refractory and life-threatening arrhythmias	
Propafenone	Life-threatening postoperative JET	Infuse colloid during loading to maintain BP
Ethmozine	AET originating in right atrium	
Propranolol	SVA, VA, digitalis-induced arrhythmias	Contraindicated in asthma and heart block
Amiodarone	Refractory and life-threatening arrhythmias in CHD, myocarditis, cardiomyopathies	Screen thyroid function, monitor HR in sick sinus syndrome, use with caution with other antiarrhythmics. Decrease digoxin dose to ½ (kinetic and dynamic interaction)
Verapamil	Reentrant SVT	Contraindicated in severe low cardiac output, intracardiac right to left shunt, patients receiving beta blockers. Use with extreme caution in infants

Abbreviations: SVT = supraventricular tachycardia; SVA = supraventricular arrhythmia; PAF = paroxysmal atrial flutter/fibrillation; PJRT = permanent junctional reciprocating tachycardia (atypical atrioventricular node reentry); VA = ventricular arrhythmia; PVD = premature ventricular depolarization; VT = ventricular tachycardia; VF = ventricular fibrillation; JET = junctional ectopic tachycardia; CHD = congenital heart disease; HR = heart rate; BP = blood pressure.

TABLE 33–5. DOSES OF ANTIARRHYTHMIC AGENTS

DRUG	ROUTE	DOSE	REF.
Quinidine	P.O.	15–60 mg/kg/day (q6h) (Test dose 2 mg/kg)	65
Procainamide (Pronestyl)	I.V. P.O.	Initial: 3–6 mg/kg over 5 min (max dose 500 mg); maintenance: 0.02–0.08 mg/kg/min (max 60 mg/kg/day) 15–50 mg/kg/day (q4–6h) (max 4 gm/day)	65
Disopyramide	P.O.	3–6 mg/kg/day (q6h) adjusted for plasma conc >2 μg/ml	68
Lidocaine (Xylocaine)	I.V.	Initial: 1–5 mg/kg; maintenance: 0.01–0.05 mg/kg/min	65
Phenytoin	I.V. P.O.	2–4 mg/kg over 5 min 2–5 mg/kg/day (q12h)	65
Mexiletine		4–15 mg/kg/day (q8h)	40
Encainide	P.O.	60–120 mg/m^2/day (q6–8h)	40
Flecainide	I.V. P.O.	0.4–2 mg/kg over 5–10 min 3–6 mg/kg/day (q8–12h) increase if necessary to max 20 mg/kg	66,67
Propafenone	I.V.	Loading: boluses of 0.2 mg/kg q10min until ventricular rate < 150/min or max 2 mg/kg Maintenance: 0.004–0.0077 mg/kg/min	40
Ethmozine	P.O.	200 mg/m^2/day (q8h)	40
Propranolol (Inderal)	I.V. P.O.	0.01–0.02 mg/kg over 10 min (may repeat q6–8h) 0.2–4 mg/kg/day (q6–8h)	65
Amiodarone	I.V. P.O.	5–7 mg/kg over 30 min, followed by 1–2 mg/kg/h for 24–48 h Loading: 10 mg/kg/day (q12h) for 7–10 days maintenance: 5 mg/kg/day for 1–2 mos; then decrease (to 2.5 mg/kg/day) or increase (to 10–15 mg/kg/day) according to response	61 40
Verapamil	I.V. P.O.	0.1 mg/kg over 30 s; may repeat $\times$2 after 15-min intervals 0.01–0.3 mg/kg/day (q6–8h)	58

put. The effective refractory period of the AV node is increased by propranolol, and thus this agent slows the ventricular response to rapid atrial arrhythmias and abolishes supraventricular arrhythmias which require reentry in the AV node.[43a] This electrophysiologic effect explains most of the antiarrhythmic actions of propranolol. At high concentrations (rarely needed for arrhythmia control), it has nonspecific "quinidine-like" actions, such as a decrease in membrane responsiveness of Purkinje cells.[44] Important noncardiac effects of propranolol include decreased blood glucose concentration and plasma renin activity, and bronchoconstriction.

Propranolol has complex pharmacokinetics.[44] Following oral dosage it is effectively absorbed in the intestine; however, the liver extracts large amounts of the drug from the venous portal blood before it reaches the systemic circulation.[44a] This first-pass effect results in a low bioavailability (30–60 percent of the dose) and marked interindividual differences in plasma concentrations after oral doses. Elimination of propranolol decreases when hepatic blood flow decreases (such as in conditions associated with low cardiac output). For those reasons the use of propranolol based on unit of body weight or surface area is only an approximation for initial treatment.

Following maternal dosage, the infant receives propranolol by placental transfer and by breast milk. Reported plasma concentrations of propranolol following birth have been up to 24 and 36 ng/ml in neonates and their mothers, respectively.[45,46] As compared to propranolol, newer β-adrenergic blocking agents (atenolol, acebutolol) appear to cross more effectively into breast milk,

probably due to substantially lower protein binding, and cases of neonatal toxicity with these agents have been described. The use of propanolol in pregnancy has been associated with several fetal, obstetric, and neonatal complications: decreased placental size and intrauterine growth retardation, fetal depression at birth, and postnatal hypoglycemia, bradycardia, and hyperbilirubinemia.[46] The increased muscular tone of the uterus and decreased uterine flow induced by propranolol and/or effects of this drug on maternal heart rate or blood pressure could explain the decreased placental size and retardation of fetal growth.

Clinical improvement has been reported with the use of propranolol in infants and children with tetralogy of Fallot and with hypertrophic obstructive cardiomyopathy[47,48]; treatment failures correlate with low doses (and low serum concentrations) in infants.[47] A dose of 2–6 mg/kg/day is recommended for the management of hypoxemic spells in infants with tetralogy of Fallot.[47] Although it is not a drug of choice today, much higher doses were recommended in the long-term management of supraventricular tachycardia and hypertension in children; these doses (up to 16 mg/kg) resulted in plasma concentrations in the range of 100–700 ng/ml with no side effects. However, caution should be exercised with the use of high doses; due to its β-adrenergic blocking properties, propranolol may decrease cardiac contractility and produce AV conduction disturbances, bradycardia, hypo- or hyperglycemia, gastrointestinal alterations, and bronchospasm.

In patients scheduled for cardiac surgery, it has been

TABLE 33–6. UNTOWARD EFFECTS OF ANTIARRHYTHMIC DRUGS

DRUG	UNTOWARD EFFECT
Quinidine	Cardiotoxicity (SA and AV blocks, VT, asystole), hypotension, cinchonism, nausea, vomiting, diarrhea, hypersensitivity reactions
Procainamide	Cardiotoxicity, hypotension, nausea, vomiting, psychosis, systemic lupus syndrome, hypersensitivity reactions
Disopyramide	Atropine-like symptoms (dry mouth, constipation, blurred vision, urinary retention), nausea, vomiting, cardiac depression
Lidocaine	Paresthesias, behavior changes, hypocusia, convulsions, respiratory arrest
Phenytoin	Nystagmus, ataxia, vertigo, nausea
Mexiletine	Headache, tremor, paresthesias, mood changes, nausea, rash
Encainide	Headache, fatigue, dizziness, proarrhythmic effects, heart failure, blurred vision, tremor
Flecainide	Proarrhythmic events, nausea
Propafenone	Hypotension, nausea, vomiting, congestive heart failure, proarrhythmic events, personality changes, sleep disturbances
Ethmozine	Headache, allergic reactions, neurologic, gastrointestinal, and proarrhythmic effects
Propranolol	Hypotension, heart failure, AV block, asystole
Amiodarone	Corneal microdeposits, gritty eyes, rash, headache, peripheral neuropathy, abnormal thyroid function, sleep disturbances, personality changes, photosensitivity, gray pigmentation of skin, abnormal liver function, liver failure, encephalopathy, cardiotoxicity (sinus bradycardia, AV block, deterioration of sinus or AV node function, VT, VF, Torsade de pointes with QTc prolongation. Pulmonary fibrosis (in adults)
Verapamil	Cardiotoxicity (sinus node depression, bradycardia, AV block, asystole, heart failure), hypotension, shock, nausea, vomiting, constipation, hepatotoxicity

Abbreviations: see Table 34–4.

recommended that propranolol therapy be discontinued several days prior to the operative procedures.[49]

Calcium Channel Blockers

These drugs are a heterogeneous group of highly lipid-soluble compounds that inhibit the entry of calcium ions into the cell or their mobilization from intracellular stores. Their pharmacologic effects are most prominent and have been best characterized in the cardiovascular system, but they also affect other tissues (central nervous, respiratory, endocrine, and gastrointestinal systems; uterus; and platelets).

Verapamil has more potent cardiac effects than nifedipine at doses sufficient to produce vasodilation. It was originally used as an antianginal drug; later it was found useful in the management of cardiac arrhythmias[50,51] and

of hypertrophic cardiomyopathy in adults and children.[52] Of the three main calcium channel blockers in clinical use (verapamil, nifedipine, and diltiazem), only verapamil has been extensively used in cardiac arrhythmias, and today it is a drug of choice in the treatment of reentrant supraventricular tachycardia. Verapamil prolongs atrioventricular junctional conduction time (antero- and retrograde) and the refractory period of the AV node, and depresses sinus node automaticity. It also causes direct negative chronotropic and inotropic effects, resulting in worsening of the ventricular function in patients with congestive heart failure. The potentially more advantageous diltiazem has similar electrophysiologic effects as verapamil and minimal negative inotropic effects; however, experience with this agent in cardiac arrhythmias is limited.

Verapamil improves left ventricular diastolic relaxation and filling, and symptomatology in adults and children with hypertrophic cardiomyopathy[52]; it is unclear, however, whether the long-term prognosis of this condition is also improved.

Verapamil is well absorbed following oral administration but only about 20 percent reaches the systemic circulation, due to a marked first-pass effect. It undergoes N-demethylation to the biologically active norverapamil. Its bioavailability increases and the degree of its biotransformation decreases during chronic therapy, which results in prolongation of its plasma half-life and in higher plasma concentrations.[53] Pharmacokinetic data for verapamil are similar in adults and infants,[54] but older children have a longer plasma half-life and a smaller body clearance than adults.[55]

In children with supraventricular tachycardia, verapamil is used mainly intravenously. Adverse effects of verapamil are dose-related and an extension of its pharmacology. Severe sinus bradycardia may occur following initiation of verapamil therapy in patients with sick sinus syndrome. Serious side effects may occur in infants after

TABLE 33–7. ELECTROPHYSIOLOGIC AND HEMODYNAMIC INTERACTIONS IN COMBINATION ANTIARRHYTHMIC THERAPY[40,69]

DRUG I	DRUG II	RESULTING INTERACTION
Verapamil	Propranolol	Hypotension, sinus arrest, congestive heart failure
Amiodarone	Propranolol	Potential of increased toxicity due to effects on sinus automaticity and AV conduction
Amiodarone	Class IA agents	Marked QT prolongation, Torsade de pointes
Amiodarone	Class I agents	Symptomatic bradycardia in latent sinus node dysfunction
Amiodarone	Verapamil	Potential increased toxicity
Amiodarone	Diltiazem	Potential increased toxicity
Amiodarone	Mexiletene	Synergism
Propranolol	Mexiletene	Synergism
Beta blockers	Class I agents	Symptomatic bradycardia in latent sinus node dysfunction

TABLE 33–8. PHARMACOKINETIC INTERACTIONS WITH ANTIARRHYTHMIC AGENTS[41,45,69]

ANTIARRHYTHMIC AGENT	INTERACTING DRUG	RESULTANT INTERACTION
Quinidine	Cimetidine	Inhibition of quinidine metabolism
	Phenytoin Phenobarbital	Induction of quinidine and reduced serum quinidine concentrations
	Warfarin	Increased prothrombin time
	Digoxin	Digoxin toxicity
	Debrisoquine	Inhibits specific liver cytochrome P-450
	Nitroglycerin	Postural hypotension
	Amiodarone	Increased serum quinidine
Disopyramide	Phenytoin Phenobarbital	Induction of disopyramide metabolism
Mexiletine	Phenobarbital Phenytoin Rifampin	Increased clearance of mexiletine
Mexiletine	Cimetidine	Slows mexiletine absorption
Encainide	Cimetidine	Increased serum concentration of encainide and metabolites
Amiodarone	Various drugs	Amiodarone blocks cytochrome P-450 metabolism
Amiodarone	Warfarin	Potentiation of warfarin effect
Amiodarone	Digoxin	Increased serum digoxin
Amiodarone	Procainamide	Increased serum procainamide
Amiodarone	Flecainide	Increased serum flecainide
Lidocaine	Beta blockers Cimetidine	Increased serum lidocaine

even a single standard intravenous dose; therefore, it should be used with great caution in this age group.[56,57] Intravenous calcium chloride (10 mg/kg) followed by normal saline (10 ml/kg, rapidly) and/or sympathomimetic amines and atropine (0.01 mg/kg) are recommended if hypotension, sinus bradycardia, and/or advanced AV block occurs as a result of verapamil therapy.[58] The use of verapamil with β-adrenergic blockers is contraindicated; both agents prolong the refractory period of the AV node, and combination therapy may result in hypotension, bradycardia, asystole, and death. Coadministration of verapamil and disopyramide may also be lethal.[58] Simultaneous administration of verapamil (but not nifedipine or diltiazem) with digoxin increases serum digoxin concentrations; this seems to be due to inhibition of the renal tubular secretion of digoxin.[59] Administration of verapamil to patients on warfarin therapy may cause prolongation of prothrombin time, perhaps as a result of warfarin displacement from protein binding sites.[58]

Amiodarone is a new and highly effective agent used in a variety of severely symptomatic and uncontrolled life-threatening arrhythmias. Chemically, it is an iodinated benzofuran with a structure similar to thyroxine. Initially studied for its antianginal properties, it was found also to have important electrophysiologic effects. It prolongs the action potential of all cardiac cell types and lengthens AV nodal conduction. In addition, it has α- and β-blocker effects.[60]

Amiodarone has unique and complex pharmacokinetic properties[39] that have not been well characterized in children. Its absorption following oral administration is slow and erratic, its bioavailability is low (22–50 percent), and its onset of action is delayed for days (4–10) in children and several weeks in adults. Due to its long terminal life (between 10 and 55 days), its effects may persist for a considerable period after discontinuation of the drug. A major metabolite, desethylamiodarone, accumulates in the plasma during long-term oral treatment; its antiarrhythmic potency is unclear. At effective doses, lower serum concentrations of amiodarone and desethylamiodarone are reached in children than in adults; at similar plasma concentrations of amiodarone, lower concentrations of desethylamiodarone are reached in infants than in children.[61] While serum concentrations of amiodarone correlate with dosage in adults, such a correlation has not been found in children. Serum concentrations of amiodarone and desethylamiodarone do not distinguish between responders and nonresponders. On the other hand, severe toxicity seems to correlate with amiodarone serum concentrations >2.5 μg/ml and desethylamiodarone >3.0 μg/ml.[62] Transplacental passage of amiodarone and desethylamiodarone has been estimated as 10 and 25 percent, respectively. Maternal milk contains higher concentrations of amiodarone and desethylamiodarone than plasma; in one study daily ingestion by a breast-fed infant was estimated as 1.5 and 0.5 mg/kg body weight, respectively, with no untoward effects.[63] When used in children, a loading dose is given for 10 to 14 days and then the dose is reduced to that minimally effective. Higher dosages may be required in ventricular than in supraventricular tachycardia in children.[64]

Although it is often stated that serious side effects as seen in adults do not occur in children, an 8-year-old girl with fatal hepatic failure and encephalopathy associated with amiodarone therapy has been described.[70] Other side effects have been reported in older children, but not in young children or infants (Table 33–6).[71]

REFERENCES

1. White RD, Lietman, PS: A reappraisal of digitalis for infants with left-to-right shunts and "heart failure." J Pediatr 92:867–870, 1978
2. Driscoll DJ, Gillete PC, Ezrailson EG, et al: Inotropic response of the neonatal canine myocardium to dopamine. Pediatr Res 12:42, 1978
3. Friedman WF, George BL: New concepts and drugs in the treatment of congestive heart failure. Pediatr Clin N Am 31:1197–1227, 1984
4. Binah O, Legato MJ, Danilo P Jr, et al: Developmental changes in the cardiac effects of amrinone in the dog. Circ Res 52:747–752, 1983
5. Perkin RM, Levin DL, Webb R, et al: Dobutamine: A hemodynamic evaluation in children with shock. J Pediatr 100:977–983, 1982
6. Friedman WF, George BL: Treatment of congestive heart failure by altering loading conditions of the heart. J Pediatr 106:697–706, 1985
7. Rudolph AM: Developmental considerations in neonatal failure. Hosp Pract 20:53–70, 1985
8. Sheldon CA, Friedman WF, Sybers HD: Scanning electron microscopy of fetal and neonatal lamb cardiac cells. J Molec Cell Cardiol 8:853–862, 1976
9. McPherson RA, Kramer MF, Covell JW, et al: A comparison of the active stiffness of fetal and adult cardiac muscle. Pediatr Res 10:660–664, 1976
10. Romero TE, Friedman WF: Limited left ventricular response to volume overload in the neonatal period: A comparative study with the adult animal. Pediatr Res 13:910–915, 1979
11. Geis WP, Tatooles CJ, Priola DV, et al: Factors influencing neurohormonal control of the heart in the newborn. Am J Physiol 228:1685–1689, 1975
12. Pappano AJ: Ontogenic development of autonomic neuroeffector transmission and transmitter reactivity in embryonic and fetal hearts. Pharmacol Rev 29:3, 1977
13. Klopfenstein HS, Rudolph AM: Postnatal changes in the circulation and responses to volume loading in sheep. Circ Res 42:839–845, 1978
14. Goldberg BP, Baskin SI: The effect of age on sodium and potassium concentrations and fluxes in cardiac muscle. Fed Proc 33:476, 1974
15. Battaglia FC, Meschia G: Principal substrates of fetal metabolism. Physiol Rev 58:449, 1978
16. Tsien RW: Cyclic AMP and contractile activity in the heart. Adv Cyclic Nucleotide Res 8:363, 1977
17. Driscoll DJ, Gillette PC, McNamara DC: The use of dopamine in children. J Pediatr 92:309–314, 1978
18. Leier CV, Unverferth DV: Dobutamine. Ann Int Med 99:490–496, 1983
19. Colucci WS, Wright RF, Braunwald E: New positive inotropic agents in the treatment of congestive heart failure. N Engl J Med 314:290–299, 349–358, 1986
20. Rocci ML, Wilson H: The pharmacokinetics and pharmacodynamics of newer inotropic agents. Clin Pharmacokinet 13:91–109, 1977
21. Bina O, Rosen MR: Developmental changes in the interactions of amrinone and ouabaine in canine ventricular muscle. Dev Pharmacol Ther 6:333–346, 1983
22. Okerholm RO, Chan KY, Lang JF, et al: Biotransformation and pharmacokinetic overview of enoximone and its sulfoxide metabolite. Am J Cardiol 60:21C–26C, 1987
23. Jessup M, Ulrich S, Samaha J, Helfer D: Effects of low dose enoximone for chronic congestive heart failure. Am J Cardiol 60:80C–84C, 1987
24. Cohn JN, Franciosa JA: Vasodilator therapy in cardiac failure. N Engl J Med 297:27–31, 254–258, 1977
25. American Academy of Pediatrics. Committee on Drugs: Emergency drug doses for infants and children. Pediatrics 81:462–465, 1988
26. Orlowski, JP: Cardiopulmonary resuscitation in children. Pediat Clin N Am 27:495–512, 1980
27. DiSessa TG, Leitner M, Ti CC, et al: The cardiovascular effects of dopamine in the severely asphyxiated neonate. J Pediatr 99:772–776, 1981
28. Lang P, Williams RG, Norwood WI, Castaneda A: The hemodynamic effects of dopamine in infants after corrective cardiac surgery. J Pediatr 96:630–634, 1980
29. Artman M, Graham TP: Guidelines for vasodilator therapy of congestive heart failure in infants and children. Am Heart J 113:994–1005, 1987
30. Beekman RH, Rocchini AP, Dick M, et al: Vasodilator therapy in children: Acute and chronic effects in children with left ventricular dysfunction or mitral regurgitation. Pediatrics 73:43–51, 1984
31. Artman M, Parrish MD, Appleton S, et al: Hemodynamic effects of hydralazine in infants with idiopathic dilated cardiomyopathy and congestive heart failure. Am Heart J 113:144–150, 1987
32. Artman M, Parrish MD, Boerth RC, et al: Short term hemodynamic effects of hydralazine in infants with complete atrioventricular canal defects. Circulation 69:949–954, 1984
33. Appelbaum A, Blackstone EH, Kouchoukos NT, Kirklin JW: Afterload reduction and cardiac output in infants early after intracardiac surgery. Am J Cardiol 39:445–451, 1977
34. Dillon TR, Janos GG, Meyer RA, et al: Vasodilator therapy for congestive heart failure. J Pediatr 96:623–629, 1980
35. Beekman RH, Rocchini AP, Rosenthal A: Hemodynamic effects of nitroprusside in infants with a large ventricular septal defect. Circulation 64:553–558, 1981
36. Shaw NJ, Wilson N, Dickinson DF: Captopril in heart failure secondary to a left to right shunt. Arch Dis Child 63:360–363, 1988
37. Shaddy RE, Teitel DF, Brett C: Short term hemodynamic effects of captopril in infants with congestive heart failure. Am J Dis Child 142:100–105, 1988
38. Harrison DC: Antiarrhythmic drug classification: New science and practical applications. Am J Cardiol 50:185–187, 1985
39. Nestico PF, Morganroth J, Horowitz LN: New antiarrhythmic drugs. Drugs 35:286–319, 1988
40. Moak JP, Smith RT, Garson A: Newer antiarrhythmic drugs in children. Am Heart J 113:179–185, 1987
41. Woosley RL, Funck-Brentano C: Overview of the clinical pharmacology of antiarrhythmic drugs. Am J Cardiol 61:61A-69A, 1988
42. Benet LZ, Sheiner LB: Design and optimization of dosage regimens: Pharmacokinetic data, in Gilman AG, Goodman LS,

Rall TW, Murad F (eds): Goodman and Gilman's The Pharmacological Basis of Therapeutics, 7th ed. New York, Macmillan, Company, 1985, pp 1663–1733

43. Pemberton PJ, McConell B, Shanks RG: Neonatal thyrotoxicosis treated with propranolol. Arch Dis Child 49:813–815, 1974

43a. Wu D, Denes P, Dhingra R, Khan A, and Rosen KM: The effects of propranolol in induction of AV nodal resistant paroxsymal tachycardia. Circulation 50:665–677, 1974

44. Nies AS, Shand DG: Clinical pharmacology of propranolol. Circulation 52:6–15, 1975

44a. Nies AS, Shand DG, Wilkinson GR: Metered hepatic blood flow and drug disposition. Clin Pharmacokinet 1:135–155, 1976

45. Langer A, Hung GT, McA'Nulty JA, et al: Adrenergic blockade: A new approach to hyperthyroidism during pregnancy. Obstet Gynecol 44:181, 1974

46. Habib A, McCarthy JS: Effects on the neonate of propranolol administered during pregnancy. J Pediatr 91:808, 1977

47. Garson A Jr, Gillette PC, McNamara DG: Propranolol: The preferred palliation for tetralogy of Fallot. Am J Cardiol 47:1098–1104, 1981

48. Shand DG, Sell CG, Oates JA: Hypertrophic obstructive cardiomyopathy in an infant. Propranolol therapy for three years. N Engl J Med 285:843, 1971

49. Viljoen JF, Estafanous FG, Kellner GA: Propranolol and cardiac surgery. J Thorac Cardiovasc Surg 64:826, 1972

50. Shahar E, Barzilay Z, Frand M: Verapamil in the treatment of paroxysmal supraventricular tachycardia in infants and children. J Pediatr 98:323–326, 1981

51. Porter CJ, Gilette PC, Garson A, et al: Effects of verapamil on supraventricular tachycardia in children. Am J Cardiol 48:487, 1981

52. Shaffer EM, Rocchini AP, Spicer RL, et al: Effects of verapamil on left ventricular diastolic filling in children with hypertrophic cardiomyopathy. Am J Cardiol 61:413–417, 1988

53. Hamman SR, Blouin RA, McAllister RG Jr: Clinical pharmacokinetics of verapamil. Clin Pharmacokinet 9:26–41, 1984

54. De Vonderweid U, Benettoni A, Piovan D, Padrini R: Use of oral verapamil in long term treatment of neonatal paroxysmal supraventricular tachycardia. A pharmacokinetic study. Int J Cardiol 5:581, 1984

55. Wagner JG, Rocchini AP, Vasiliades J: Prediction of steady-state verapamil plasma concentrations in children and adults. Clin Pharmacol Ther 32:172–181, 1982

56. Cho C, Pruitt AW: Therapeutic uses of calcium-channel blocking drugs in the young. Am J Dis Child 140:360–366, 1986

57. Epstein ML, Kiel EA, Victorica BE: Cardiac decompensation following verapamil therapy in infants with supraventricular tachycardia. Pediatrics 75:737–740, 1985

58. Porter CJ, Garson A, Gilette PC: Verapamil: An effective calcium blocking agent for pediatric patients. Pediatrics 71:748–755, 1983

59. Koren G, Soldin S, MacLeod SM: Digoxin-verapamil interaction: in vitro studies in rat tissue. J Cardiovasc Pharmacol 5:443, 1983

60. Singh BN: Amiodarone: Historical development and pharmacologic profile. Am Heart J 106:788–797, 1983

61. Bucknall CA, Keeton BR, Curry PVL, et al: Intravenous and oral amiodarone for arrhythmias in children. Br Heart J 56:278–284, 1986

62. Kannan R, Yabek SM, Garson A, et al: Amiodarone efficacy in a young population: Relationship to serum amiodarone and desethylamiodarone levels. Am Heart J 114:283–287, 1987

63. Latini T, Tognoni G, Kates RE: Clinical pharmacokinetics of amiodarone. Clin Pharmacokinet 9:136, 1984

64. Dick M, Campbell RM: Advances in the management of cardiac arrhythmias in children. Pediat Clin N Am 31:1175–1195, 1984

65. Gelband H, Rosen MR: Pharmacologic basis for the treatment of cardiac arrhythmias. Pediatrics 55:59–67, 1975

66. Till WA, Rowland E, Shinebourne EA, Ward DE: Treatment of refractory supraventricular arrhythmias with flecainide acetate. Arch Dis Child 62:247–252, 1987

67. Wren C, Campbell RWF: The response of paediatric arrhythmias to intravenous and oral flecainide. Br Heart J 57:171–175, 1987

68. Baker AU, Hayler AM, Curry PV, et al: Measurement of plasma disopyramide as a guide to paediatric use. Int J Cardiol 10:65–69, 1984

69. Levy S: Combination therapy for cardiac arrhythmias. Am J Cardiol 61:95A–101A, 1988

70. Yagupsky P, Gazala E, Sofer S, et al: Fatal hepatic failure and encephalopathy associated with amiodarone therapy. J Pediatr 107:967–979, 1985

71. Costigan DC, Holland FJ, Daneman D, et al: Amiodarone therapy effects on childhood thyroid function. Pediatrics 77:703–708, 1986

34

DIGOXIN

GIDEON KOREN *and* RAFAEL GORODISCHER

Despite being one of the most widely prescribed group of drugs for over two centuries, the role of digitalis glycosides in pediatric therapy is far from being consensual. In fact, after many years of research, serious questions are currently emerging concerning its clinical efficacy in infants and children and the role of therapeutic drug monitoring in optimizing patient care.

For practical purposes this chapter will deal mainly with digoxin, which is by far the most common digitalis glycoside in pediatric use. An attempt will be made to put currently available experience and controversies in a clinical perspective and to suggest an approach for individualization of digoxin therapy.

CHEMISTRY

The term "digitalis" describes the entire group of cardiac glycoside inotropic and chronotropic drugs. Cardiac glycosides of medicinal importance are extracted from *Digitalis purpurea* Linné (Fam. Scrophulariacaeae) (digitoxin, digitalis, gitalin), *D. lanata* Ehrhart (Fam. Scrophulariaceae) (digoxin, digitoxin, lanatoside C, deslanoside, acetyldigitoxin), *Strophanthus gratus* (ouabain), and *Acocanthera schimperi* (ouabain).[1-4]

Digitalis glycosides have a characteristic ring structure (aglycone or genin) to which one or more sugars are attached. The aglycone consists of a steroid nucleus and an α,β-unsaturated five- or six-membered lactone ring at the C-17 position of the steroid nucleus. The hydroxyl groups at C-3 and C-14 are in the β-configuration. The sugars are attached usually through the C-3 hydroxyl (Figure 34–1).

Mechanism of Action

The cardiac glycosides specifically inhibit membrane $Na^+–K^+$ exchange, and it is generally accepted that the positive inotropic effects of digitalis result from specific binding to Na^+,K^+-ATPase.[5-6] Inhibition of the sodium pump causes an increase in intracellular Na^+ concentration, leading to an enhanced intracellular CA^{2+} concentration through the $Na^+–Ca^{2+}$ exchange system.[5] The augmented intracellular Ca^{2+} is associated with improved cardiotonicity. When measured simultaneously, a good correlation exists between the specific binding of [^{3}H]ouabain to an isolated, electrically stimulated heart muscle and its force of contraction. However, this view is not universally accepted. It was shown that the cardiotonic effect of the cardiac glycosides is sustained long after inhibition of the NA^+,K^+-ATPase has resolved. Moreover, a positive inotropic effect can be measured at concentrations that do not cause changes in cation fluxes.[5-6] In addition, there is a serious discrepancy between the *in vivo* situation, where digoxin exerts its effect at a concentration of 10^{-9} M, and the *in vitro* setting, where 10^{-7} M is needed to elicit an effect in isolated cardiac muscle.[6] A possible explanation for this discrepancy is the multiplicity of cardiac glycoside receptors in the heart. Both high- and low-affinity binding sites have been demonstrated, suggesting that different receptors produce the pharmacologic effects *in vivo* and *in vitro*.[6]

Recently, several studies have documented both in animals and in humans apparent differences between neonatal and adult Na^+,K^+-ATPase.[7-10] In animals a higher density of receptor sites in neonatal heart and erythrocytes correlates with an apparently lower effect at a similar serum concentration of digoxin. In humans the notion of a "lower sensitivity" of the neonatal myocardium to the clinical and toxic effects of the glycoside has been proposed but has never been proven. Gorodischer et al.[11] found that myocardial uptake of digoxin is nearly twice as great in infants as in adults at the same serum concentrations, as would be expected from the larger distribution volume of digoxin in infants.

It has been suggested that infants and young children may need a higher daily dose of digoxin relative to their body size than older children and adults to achieve equiv-

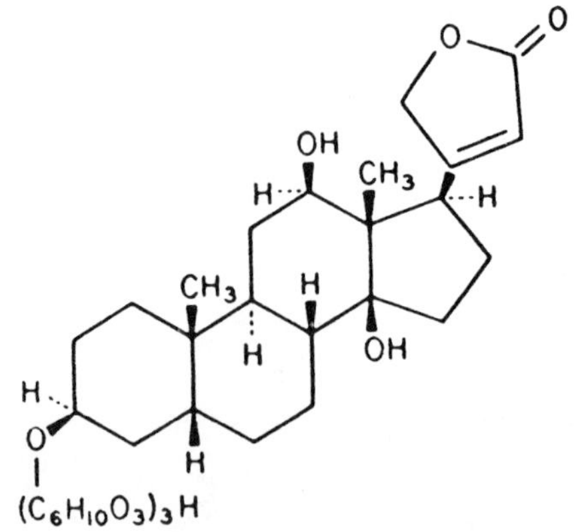

FIGURE 34–1. Structure of digoxin and digitalis compounds.

alent serum concentrations, due to a faster clearance rate of the drug[12]; however, analysis of available studies does not support this possibility (Table 34–1).

Effects of Digitalis on the Kidney

After their introduction to clinical use, it was assumed that the main effect of digitalis glycosides in the treatment of dropsy (edema) was diuretic. In the early twentieth century, it became apparent that the primary effect of the digitalis glycosides is on the heart. However, it was impossible to explain the relief of edema only by the chronotropic and inotropic cardiac effects. A recent controlled study in infants showed that clinical benefit from digoxin was not always associated with echocardiographic evidence of inotropic effect.[13] Other studies have demonstrated that the administration of digoxin to normal, hypertensive patients or patients with chronic congestive heart failure results in reduction in plasma renin activity, thus presumably ameliorating the angiotensin-mediated vasoconstriction and aldosterone-mediated sodium retention in many patients.[14-16] This may be due to a decrease in tubular sodium reabsorption induced by digoxin.

CLINICAL PHARMACOKINETICS

Table 34–1 summarizes pharmacokinetic values of digoxin in a variety of pediatric age groups and compares them to adults.

Absorption

The systemic bioavailability of digoxin tablets administered orally varies (55–85 percent) from one preparation to the next, and instances of toxic digoxin concentrations could be attributed to transferring a patient from one digoxin formulation to another.[25-27] The rate and extent of gastrointestinal absorption are generally greater for digoxin in an elixir form than for tablets. Intestinal motility may affect the absorption of digoxin tablets. For example, malabsorption syndromes that are characterized by intestinal hypermotility, as well as motility-stimulating

drugs such as metoclopramide, decrease absorption. Drugs that retard gastrointestinal motility, such as the anticholinergics, tend to increase bioavailability.[28,29] It has been shown that some intestinal bacteria are capable of metabolizing digoxin to dihydro derivatives.[30] Consequently, the route of administration and concomitant use of antibiotics may affect the amount of the parent compound in the systemic circulation. Recent studies have shown the existence of significant enterohepatic circulation of digoxin. Digoxin was administered intravenously to healthy volunteers who received activated charcoal concomitantly by the oral route. Activated charcoal has the capacity to bind digoxin present in the gastrointestinal lumen. Digoxin half-life was significantly shorter when activated charcoal was given than when the glycoside was infused alone.[31] This indicates that digoxin given systemically reaches the gastrointestinal lumen and can be trapped there by the charcoal. Important implications for the treatment of digoxin toxicity may be derived from these observations. The bioavailability of digoxin administered orally to the neonate is not appreciably different from that in older infants or adults.

Distribution

Digoxin is characterized by a large distribution volume (3–10 liters/kg). At steady state only about 1 percent of the body load of digoxin is circulating in the bloodstream. The remainder is found in various tissues, with high concentrations recorded in the skeletal and cardiac muscles, kidneys, liver, and skin.[32-34] This large volume of distribution has several important clinical pharmacokinetic implications:

1. In cases of toxicity, it is clinically useless to try to remove the drug from the blood using hemodialysis, hemoperfusion, exchange transfusion, or peritoneal dialysis, because the vast majority of the body load resides in the peripheral tissue and compartments and is not accessible to these modalities.

2. Small changes in the distribution of the drug may cause dramatic alterations in serum concentrations. For example, a decrease in tissue binding from 99 to 98 percent of the body load will result in doubling the circulating levels of digoxin (from 1 to 2 percent). This mechanism has been shown to be operative in some drug interactions with digoxin (see subsequent discussion).

3. Because of the extreme discrepancy between blood and tissue concentrations of digoxin, it is conceivable that the blood/tissue concentration ratio will be variable. Indeed, a variety of studies have shown large variability in the correlation between serum and cardiac muscle concentrations of digitalis compounds.[35-37] This creates problems in interpreting serum concentrations of digoxin, because one of the important conditions necessary for the rational application of therapeutic drug monitoring is the existence of a good correlation between blood and target organ concentrations.

4. The distribution phase of digoxin from the blood is relatively slow, with a half-life of about 30 minutes follow-

TABLE 34–1. AGE-DEPENDENT PHARMACOKINETICS OF DIGOXIN IN HUMANS*

| | CLEARANCE RATE (ml/min/m²) | | | |
	Lisalo[18]	Halkin[19]	$t_{1/2}$(h)	V_d(liters/kg)[39]
Preterm	53		57 (38–88)	3.3 ± 1
< 1 mo	69	33	69 ± 25	
1–3 mos	87	60	45.5 ± 7.3	
4–6 mos	106			9.8 ± 2.6
7–12 mos		88	12–42	
> 2 yrs		144		
Adults		82–223	15–70	5.1–7.3

*Data from refs. 17–24, 39.
 Comparison of values between different studies is difficult due to variability in patient populations, methodology of drug administration, and pharmacokinetic calculation. Therefore we have preferred to bring two studies (References 18 and 19) which compare clearance values over a large range of ages.

ing intravenous or oral administration of the drug.[38] This means that, initially, very high concentrations of digoxin can be measured in the serum. The practical implication of this slow distributive phase is that initial levels measured close to the time of administration may be erroneously interpreted as potentially toxic.[39]

Elimination and Metabolism

For many years it was believed that most of the body load of digoxin is eliminated through the kidney by glomerular filtration. This assumption was supported by the fact that the elimination of digoxin is proportional to renal function and is prolonged in renal insufficiency. Similar to adults, in children there is a good correlation between serum creatinine and elimination half-life of digoxin.

In 1974 Steiness[40] revealed that in humans the renal clearance of digoxin by far exceeds the inulin clearance, suggesting net tubular secretion of the glycoside. Koren et al.[41] recently documented the tubular secretion of digoxin using the *in vivo* multiple indicator dilution technique. Although the exact mechanism of tubular secretion of digoxin is not yet clear, it appears to be modulated by renal blood flow and age, with children having a more predominant tubular secretion.[41] Coadministration of quinidine, verapamil, amiodarone, and spironolactone has been shown to inhibit the net tubular secretion of digoxin without affecting the glomerular filtration rate.[42] In the case of quinidine, this effect is caused by a decrease in renal blood flow.[43] Digoxin tubular secretion does not appear to participate in the organic acid or organic base transport mechanisms.[44] Currently, it is apparent that the contribution of net tubular secretion of digoxin to the renal clearance of the drug may exceed that of filtration.

The extrarenal elimination of digoxin varies in different studies in adults and may be as high as 50 percent in some cases, with both digoxin and its metabolites found in the bile. Some years ago it was believed that relatively polar glycosides such as digoxin, deslanoside, and ouabain were not metabolized appreciably.[45–47] Today, it is appreciated that digoxin metabolism can be extensive and can involve reduction of the lactone ring to form dihydrodigoxin and the stepwise removal of sugar molecules, followed by epi-

merization of the 3β-hydroxy to the 3α-(epi) position and conjugation to give the polar metabolites 3-epi-glucuronide and 3-epi-sulfate.[48–51]

Gault et al.[50] showed that in some patients extensive biotransformation of digoxin takes place, with polar metabolites predominating. Six hours after the dose, only 58 and 64 percent of the radioactivity present in the serum samples was associated (cochromatographed) with digoxin in those individuals with impaired and normal renal function, respectively.

Clark and Kalman[51] reported urinary dihydrodigoxin to account for 7–47 percent of the labeled digoxin products present. It is assumed that the dihydro derivatives are formed by the intestinal bacterial flora; consequently, the route of administration will govern the extent of conversion to these compounds. No studies are available to date on the degree of biotransformation of digoxin in the pediatric age group.

The different metabolites of digoxin have various degrees of cardioactivity (Table 34–2). Stepwise removal of the sugar residues leads to a stepwise loss of cardioactivity, whereas reduction of the lactone ring results in almost total loss of pharmacologic activity.[52–54] Most important for the therapeutic drug monitoring of digoxin is the fact that its metabolites cross-react with the available immunoassays (Table 34–3).

Unlike digoxin, most of the body load of digitoxin is metabolized by the liver.[1] However, elimination is not prolonged in patients with hepatic insufficiency, probably owing to the high capacity of the metabolizing system. Unlike digoxin, the elimination of digitoxin is not affected by renal insufficiency, and therefore it has been

TABLE 34–2. PERCENTAGE OF CARDIOACTIVITY OF DIGOXIN METABOLITES*

METABOLITE	% ACTIVITY RELATIVE TO DIGOXIN
Dihydrodigoxin	2–6
Dihydrodigoxigenin	2
Digoxigenin	4–21
Digoxigenin monodigitoxiside	66
Digoxigenin bisdigitoxiside	77

*Data from refs. 52–54.

TABLE 34–3. CROSS-REACTIVITY OF DIGOXIN AND ITS METABOLITES WITH THE FPIA METHOD FOR DIGOXIN MEASUREMENT*

METABOLITE	METABOLITE CONCENTRATION (nmol/liter)	DIGOXIN CONCENTRATION (nmol/liter)	APPARENT VALUE OF DIGOXIN MEASURED BY FPIA
Digoxigenin	10.2	0	13.8
Monodigitoxiside	7.7	0	10.0
Bisdigitoxiside	6.1	0	6.05
Digitoxin	10.5	0	9.6
Digoxigenin monodigitoxiside bisdigitoxiside dihydrodigoxin	0.64 of each	2.56	5.2

*Source: From Reference 73.
FPIA: Fluorescent polarization immunoassay (TDx, Abbott).

suggested as the cardiac glycoside of choice in patients with various degrees of renal insufficiency.[1] The elimination half-life of digoxin in healthy individuals is 24–50 hours, whereas that of digitoxin is 7 days.[1] Digitoxin metabolites are excreted appreciably by the kidney. Ouabain is eliminated by the kidney, mainly through glomerular filtration with no evidence of tubular secretion or reabsorption.

Measurement of Digoxin in Body Fluids

Table 34–3 documents the apparent measurements of digoxin caused by the various metabolites, as assessed by the commonly used fluorescent polarization immunoassay (FPIA) method. It has been argued that the serum half-life of these polar metabolites is short and therefore their potential contribution to digoxin immunoreactivity is marginal; however, the new studies by Gault[50] indicate that this assumption may not be true in all patients, and accumulation of metabolites may contribute to the apparent reading of digoxin.

During the past two decades, digoxin has been routinely measured in body fluids by various immunoassay procedures.[2,55–60] Although liquid chromatographic and gas chromatographic–mass spectrometric procedures have been described,[35,61–64] they have not been widely applied in the routine clinical chemistry laboratory, owing to their lack of sensitivity, which would necessitate lengthy sample preparation and large sample size. The lack of specificity of the present immunoassays for digoxin is a serious shortcoming in therapeutic drug monitoring.

Endogenous Digoxin-Like Substances (EDLS)

The discovery that digoxin immunoreactivity can be measured in animals and humans known never to have received the drug has changed our understanding of digoxin pharmacokinetics. These measurements have been made in newborn infants, pregnant women, and patients with renal and hepatic insufficiency and with hypertension.[65–67]

In a group of newborn infants not treated with digoxin and not exposed to it *in utero,* measured levels of the glycosides were within the therapeutic range in most instances. Levels tended to decrease with increasing gestational age.[68] When digoxin was added to samples containing EDLS, apparent levels were additive; consequently, upon dosing an infant with the recommended schedule, digoxin readings may reach the "toxic" range due to substantial concentrations of EDLS. Consequently, pharmacokinetic parameters of clearance, distribution volume, and elimination half-life determined in infants and children with significant EDLS levels may be erroneous. We have found that in newborn infants with EDLS levels between 0.6 and 1.5 ng/ml, the calculated $t_{1/2}$ will appear to be falsely prolonged and the V_d and cl falsely smaller. Consequently, doses based on these miscalculations may be smaller than really needed.[68]

Considerable interest has been generated by the finding of EDLS, with many investigators believing that they are on the brink of discovering a natriuretic hormone.

The postulated natriuretic hormone has been isolated from plasma, placenta, and brain[66,69–71]; it cross-reacts with digoxin antisera, inhibits Na^+,K^+-ATPase, and also causes a natriuresis and diuresis. Studies by Gault et al.,[65] Hamblyn et al.,[72] and Devynck et al.[69] lend credence to the concept previously postulated by LaBella and others.[73] Gault's group showed in a preliminary study that the concentration of digitalis-like factors in plasma more than doubled in patients with mild hypertension in response to both an intravenous salt load and a high-salt diet.[65] Hamblyn et al.,[72] using a kinetic Na^+,K^+-ATPase assay, demonstrated a significant correlation between concentrations of an inhibitor of Na^+,K^+-ATPase activity in plasma and the mean arterial blood pressure of normotensive and hypertensive individuals. Devynck et al.[69] found that in two-thirds of untreated hypertensives and several of the normotensive subjects with a family history of hypertension, the potency of the digitalis-like compound, as measured by its interference with ouabain binding to the erythrocyte, was significantly greater than in the controls.

Recent fast-atom bombardment mass spectrometric and nuclear magnetic resonance data on EDLS purified from placenta indicated the possible presence of unsaturated fatty acids and monoglycerides. Similar compounds are known to cross-react in digoxin immunoassays.[74] Moreover, unsaturated fatty acids and unsaturated monoglycerides possess considerable ability, in micromolar concentrations, to inhibit ^{86}Rb uptake and/or interfere with the binding of [^{3}H]ouabain to Na^+,K^+-ATPase.[75] Data recently published by Tamura et al.[76] indicate that linoleic and oleic acids act as endogenous Na^+,K^+-ATPase inhibitors; these compounds were isolated and identified from porcine plasma after the pigs had undergone volume-expansion experiments. It can be speculated that EDLS are a family of unsaturated fatty acids and unsaturated monoglycerides that play some role as endogenous regulators of the enzyme Na^+,K^+-ATPase.

Clinical Efficacy of Digoxin in Fetuses, Infants, and Children

Whereas the efficacy of cardiac glycosides in supraventricular arrhythmias is well established,[1] similar evidence for efficacy in congestive heart failure is controversial. In infants recent studies suggest inotropic agents may not improve hemodynamics substantially.[12,39,77–82] Because the cardiac failure stems from a congenital malformation in most of these cases (for example, ventricular septal defect or persistent ductus arteriosus), it has been argued that the already hyperactive and presumably healthy myocardium may not benefit from digitalis. Most infants and children with congestive heart failure are treated with both digoxin and diuretics, which makes it difficult to assess the net effect of the glycoside.

A study by Berman et al.,[13] in which infants with ventricular septal defect were treated with digoxin alone, has addressed this question. The dose of digoxin was adjusted to achieve a mean steady-state concentration of 1.6 ng/ml. Only 6 of the 21 infants had an inotropic response as reflected by echocardiographic measurements, but the drug was judged to be of clinical benefit to an additional 6 infants. Although the authors concluded that "not all infants with a congested circulatory status due to a ventricular septal defect benefit from digoxin therapy," the drug was efficacious in more than 50 percent of the cases.

Although Sahn and colleagues[79] described echocardiographic improvement in infants and children 6–12 hours after digitalization with 35–45 μg/kg, Pinsky et al.[80] could not observe changes in the ratio of preejection period to left ventricular ejection time (PEP/LVET) in preterm infants with persistent ductus arteriosus (PDA) loaded with 20–30 μg/kg digoxin. Lundell and Boreus[81] could not detect a favorable clinical effect when digoxin was administered to preterm infants with PDA, evidenced by heart rate, LVET, or preejection intervals. Conversely, Sandor and colleagues[82] could show digoxin to be beneficial in neonates with heart failure whether serum concentration was high (mean 3.4 μg/ml) or low (2 ng/ml). Warburton and colleagues[39] could not detect echocardiographic differences in preterm infants receiving either 20 or 40 μg/kg digoxin.

The preceding studies document the controversy about the role of digoxin in the treatment of pediatric heart failure.

In adults Mulrow and coworkers[83] have critically appraised the published clinical evidence of digitalis efficacy using standardized methodologic criteria. Between 1960 and 1982, 16 studies published in English tried to address this question. Only two double-blind, placebo-controlled trials provided clinically useful information. In one study digoxin could be successfully withdrawn in elderly patients with stable congestive heart failure, while the other showed objective benefit in patients with severe congestive heart failure following digoxin treatments.

This survey suggests that more controlled studies are needed in order to define specific groups of cardiac patients who would benefit from digoxin. This is especially important in view of the low therapeutic index of digoxin and therefore its high rate of toxicity, even when used in recommended doses. It well may be that many pediatric patients with left-to-right shunt do not benefit from digoxin, whereas many others do. More accurate end point measurements and large controlled studies are needed in order to rationalize digoxin therapy in the pediatric age group during the third century of its clinical use.

In the treatment of arrhythmias, and especially supraventricular tachycardia, digoxin is efficacious beyond doubt due to both direct and indirect (autonomic) effects. It slows the rate of the sinus node through the vagal nerve and increases the refractory period, thus abolishing reentry supraventricular tachycardia.

Because protracted periods of fetal tachyarrhythmias (supraventricular tachycardia, atrial flutter, and atrial fibrillation) may cause congestive heart failure and fetal death, transplacental therapy with digoxin as well as other antiarrhythmics (e.g., quinidine, verapamil, amiodarone) has been successfully tried in a variety of cases. Maternal digitalization appears to be the treatment of choice in such cases, relying on the excellent transplacental distribution of the glycoside. In a few cases where the fetus suffered from severe cardiac failure due to Rh incompatibility, digoxin was injected into the fetal peritoneum at the time of blood transfusion.

Toxicity

It has been estimated that a substantial proportion (up to 25 percent) of hospitalized adults receiving digoxin experience some degree of adverse effects related to the drug.[84] Although similar figures are lacking in pediatric patients, there is a clinical impression that toxicity is not as common in children. As discussed above, these differences have been attributed to age-related changes in quality and quantity of the digitalis receptor, the membrane Na^+,K^+-ATPase receptor. It should be noted, however, that large controlled studies are needed in infants and children to prove their relative responsiveness or unresponsiveness to digitalis.

Table 34–4 summarizes the most common adverse effects of digitalis. The arrhythmias induced by digitalis are more likely to occur and are more severe in patients with cardiac disease. Hypokalemia, hypocalcemia, hypomagnesemia, and hypoxia are likely to increase the risk of toxicity; consequently, kaliuretic diuretics, which are

TABLE 34–4. COMMON ADVERSE EFFECTS OF DIGITALIS

Cardiac
  Sinus bradycardia
  Disturbances in A-V conduction
  A-V block
  Complete S-A block
  Ventricular premature depolarization (bigemini, trigemini)
  Ventricular tachycardia
  Ventricular fibrillation

Gastrointestinal
  Nausea
  Vomiting
  Anorexia
  Diarrhea
  Abdominal discomfort

Central Nervous System
  Dizziness
  Headache
  Fatigue
  Malaise
  Neurologic pain of lower face, extremities or lumbar area
  Blurred vision
  Yellow, green, or white vision
  Aphasia
  Confusion
  Delirium
  Hallucinations

Other
  Gynecomastia

often coadministered with digoxin, are a common reason for its toxicity.

Therapeutic Monitoring of Digoxin Therapy

The rationale for the therapeutic monitoring of concentrations of a particular drug stems from the following criteria:

- a specific and reliable method must be available for its measurement;

- a well-defined association between serum concentrations and therapeutic and toxic effects of the drug should exist;

- the drug should have a low therapeutic index, with a danger of causing toxicity when administering therapeutic doses;

- a poor correlation should exist between dose and serum concentration;

- the effect of the drug should not be easily measurable under routine clinical practice.

Digoxin does not meet the first two criteria. There are major problems in accurately measuring concentrations of digoxin with currently available immunoassays, as discussed previously. This is especially important in newborn infants and in pregnancy, where the existence of EDLS may lead to falsely elevated measurements of the glycoside.

Recently Gault et al.[84] proposed a simple methanol extraction method for digoxin-like factors, digoxin, and metabolites of digoxin prior to measurement of immunoassay. They proposed to use this technique in patient populations known to have EDLS.

There is no accurate definition of a "therapeutic window" for digoxin. As noted previously, few blinded, controlled studies have tried to prove digitalis efficacy in congestive heart failure. More importantly, sparse information exists on the correlation of serum concentrations of cardiac glycosides with inotropic effects. More information exists on the putative correlation between serum concentrations of digoxin and its antiarrhythmic effects.

Some investigators have observed a good correlation whereas others have not.[35–37,85,86]

Most authorities regard the therapeutic range of digoxin to be 0.5–2.0 ng/ml. With digoxin concentrations above 2 ng/ml, there is an increased risk of digitalis toxicity, including nausea, vomiting, anorexia, yellow vision, malaise, and cardiac arrhythmias. However, there is a wide "gray zone" of levels that may be toxic in one individual and nontoxic in another. In a recent study, Koren et al.[87] demonstrated that even at serum concentrations above 5 ng/ml, about one-third of pediatric patients would not show symptoms or signs of toxicity.[87] A variety of clinical conditions, including hypokalemia, hypocalcemia, hypomagnesemia, and chronic heart disease, may increase the risk of toxicity of digitalis glycosides.

Despite the limitations outlined, the therapeutic monitoring of digoxin concentrations is indicated in routine therapy for several reasons:

1. *To assess patient compliance.* Here, therapeutic drug monitoring may be an important guideline for the assessment of therapeutic failures.

2. *To tailor an optimal dosing schedule.* If an infant receives a given dose of digitalis in the hospital, does not respond clinically, and is found to have a steady-state serum concentration of 0.8 ng/ml, the pediatrician can gradually and safely increase the dose without achieving potentially toxic concentrations.

3. *To confirm a clinical impression of toxicity.* Many of the symptoms and signs of digitalis toxicity (anorexia, cachexia, nausea, vomiting, arrhythmias) may be caused by the underlying cardiac condition. The only available way to differentiate between these two diagnostic possibilities is by measuring the serum concentration of the glycoside. If the measured level is, for example, 0.7 ng/ml, it is very unlikely that drug toxicity caused the symptoms; if, however, the measured concentration is 3.8 ng/ml, it is conceivable that drug-related toxicity has occurred.

During the last decade, several drugs that are commonly coadministered with digoxin have been shown to interfere with the disposition of cardiac glycosides and to cause potentially toxic serum concentrations.[42] Quinidine, verapamil, and amiodarone may cause significant elevation in the serum concentration of digoxin, which is often associated with signs of digoxin toxicity. Spironolactone has been shown to decrease digoxin clearance, but no cases of toxicity have been reported. Pharmacokinetic studies have shown that all these drugs decrease the renal clearance of digoxin without affecting the glomerular filtration rate (GFR), suggesting an inhibition of the tubular secretion of the glycoside as the putative mechanism. In addition, they significantly decrease the extrarenal clearance of digoxin and diminish the volume of distribution of the glycoside. Preliminary studies with quinidine in both humans and animals show that, similar to the inhibition of the renal tubular secretion of digoxin, it can inhibit the transport of the glycoside into bile.[43,88]

In children the significant increase in serum concentration of digoxin associated with amiodarone therapy has been shown to correlate with a decrease in the renal clearance of digoxin without changing creatinine clearance. Similarly, concomitant therapy with quinidine resulted in a significant increase in digoxin serum concentrations, whereas spironolactone did not appear to do so.[42] Whenever these drugs are coadministered with digoxin, the dose of the cardiac glycoside should be decreased, with careful monitoring of its steady-state serum concentrations.

Several drugs that are known to decrease the GFR may cause potentially toxic accumulation of digoxin. These include indomethacin, often used to facilitate closure of the patent ductus arteriosus in preterm infants,[89] and cyclosporine A, used in patients undergoing cardiac transplantation.[90]

Several pharmacokinetic principles have to be considered for the rational interpretation of digitalis concentrations:

1. It takes four to five elimination half-lives of the drug to achieve a steady state with an unchanged dose. Any determination of concentration before steady state is achieved will yield a lower concentration and could result in an erroneous increase in dose. The half-life of digoxin may be prolonged in infants with very low birth weights and in infants and children with renal insufficiency. Thus, it may take several weeks to achieve a steady-state concentration. To shorten this time lag, a loading dose is often administered.

2. The distribution of digoxin from the blood into various tissue compartments is relatively slow. Therefore, very high concentrations can be measured in the blood after a dose. Eventually, in the postdistributive phase, less than 1 percent of digoxin will remain in the circulation and the resultant concentrations will be low. Levels obtained from sampling soon after the administration of a dose may be erroneously interpreted as excessive, and the following drug dose may, as a result, be withheld. In a recent analysis of the reasons for digoxin levels above 5 ng/ml in children, we found that 40 percent of the cases in the Hospital for Sick Children in Toronto stemmed from an inappropriate sampling time. In many of these cases, administration of the drug was stopped even when it appeared to be clinically needed. Some reasons for excessive serum concentrations of cardiac glycosides are shown in Table 34–5.

Figure 34–2 is an algorithm currently used at the Hospital for Sick Children in Toronto for digoxin dose schedule in pediatric patients.

The pediatrician or clinical pharmacologist may be asked to assist in a forensic investigation of digoxin toxicity. Several important issues need to be considered:

1. After death, digoxin is redistributed from various tissues back into the blood.[91,92] Therefore an excessive postmortem level cannot be interpreted as an excessive level before death. Conversely, if the postmortem concen-

TABLE 34–5. INTERPRETATION OF EXCESSIVE SERUM CONCENTRATIONS OF DIGITALIS GLYCOSIDES

1. A dose too large for age group
2. Improved bioavailability of a new product
3. Renal insufficiency
4. Interaction with other drugs: quinidine, verapamil, amiodarone, indomethacin, cyclosporine
5. Presence of endogenous digoxin-like factors
6. Poisoning: accidental in children, old people; suicide attempt; intentional (homicidal); or iatrogenic (medication error)
7. Inappropriate sampling time

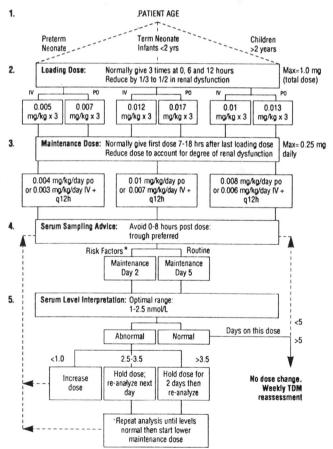

FIGURE 34–2. Algorithm for digoxin dose schedule in pediatric patients. (From Lee DuPuis (Ed.) Formulary of the Hospital for Sick Children. The Hospital for Sick Children, 1991. Reprinted with permission.)

tration is not excessive, it is suggestive that the antemortem level was not in the toxic range.[93]

2. In very severe agonal states in the intensive care unit, antemortem levels may increase long after cessation of digoxin therapy.[94] This is presumably due to EDLS, redistribution of the glycoside, and the development of acute renal failure.

3. Significant digoxin concentrations measured by immunoassay are frequently recorded after death in patients not receiving digoxin.

In summary, it appears that only through definitive methods such as mass spectrometry of HPLC can one positively identify and possibly implicate digoxin as a cause of death.

New Approaches to Life-Threatening Digoxin Toxicity

Two recent advances may change the therapeutic approach to life-threatening digoxin toxicity:

1. *Treatment of digoxin toxicity with Fab antibody fragments.* The concept of using hapten-specific antibodies to reverse the toxic effects of a drug has been previously advanced.[95-98] More recently, digoxin-specific Fab antibody fragments have been purified and used to treat patients with advanced, life-threatening digoxin toxicity.[99] In such circumstances, an immunologic approach is feasible, can be life-saving, and has been used experimentally for over 10 years. Recently the Fab antibody fragments became commercially available. The fascinating side of this new approach is that it can neutralize the pharmacologic effects of a drug with a very large distribution volume that cannot be effectively removed by hemodialysis or hemoperfusion.

2. *Treatment with oral activated charcoal.* In the last few years, several studies have documented that treatment with oral activated charcoal significantly reduces the elimination half-life of digoxin given intravenously.[31] This means that a clinically significant portion of digoxin undergoes enterohepatic circulation and can be trapped by the charcoal in the gastrointestinal tract. This "intestinal dialysis" method may prove helpful as an additional means to treat life-threatening poisoning by one of the digitalis glycosides.

SUMMARY

Despite continuous controversy associated with a variety of aspects of the pharmacology of the cardiac glycosides, it appears that these agents will continue to be widely used in the future.

Current methods for measurement of digoxin are unreliable and allow measurement of both cardioinactive metabolites of digoxin and EDLS. As a result, the therapeutic monitoring of digoxin concentrations should, for the most part, be limited to an assessment of patient compliance and confirmation of a clinical impression of drug toxicity.

REFERENCES

1. Gilman AG, Goodman LS, Rall TW, Murad F (eds): Goodman and Gilman's The Pharmacological Basis of Therapeutics, 7th ed. New York, Macmillan, 1985, pp 716–743
2. Smith TW: Digitalis glycosides, Part I. N Engl J Med 288:719–722, 1973
3. Wade A: Martindale—The Extra Pharmacopoeia, 27th ed. London, Pharmaceutical Press, 1977, pp 485–598
4. Wilson CO, Gisvold O, Doerge RF: Textbook of Organic, Medicinal and Pharmaceutical Chemistry, 7th ed. Philadelphia, Lippincott, 1977, pp 797–809
5. Akera T, Brody TM: Sodium ion and the cardiac actions of digitalis. Trends Pharmacol Sci 6:296–298, 1985
6. Erdmann E, Werdan K, Brown L: Multiplicity of cardiac glycoside receptors in the heart. Trends Pharmacol Sci 6:293–295, 1985
7. Koren G, Long D, Klein J, Beatie D, Bologa-Campeanu M, Livne A, Kirpalani H: Comparison of the digitalis receptor in erythrocytes from preterm infants and adults. Pediatr Res 23:414–417, 1988
8. Berman WJ, Musselman J, Shortencarrier R: The physiological effects of digoxin under steady state drug conditions in newborn and adult sheep. Circulation 62:1165–1171, 1980
9. Rosen KG, Sigstrom L: The influence of age on Na$^+$, K$^+$ ATPase activity in erythrocytes in fetal and newborn guinea pigs. J Perinatal Med 6:154–159, 1978
10. Kelliter GJ, Roberts J: Effects of age on the cardiotoxic action of digitalis. J Pharmacol Exp Ther 197:18–29, 1976
11. Gorodischer R, Jusko WJ, Yaffe SJ: Tissue and erythrocyte distribution of digoxin in infants. Clin Pharmacol Ther 19:256–263, 1976
12. Wettrell G, Andersson KE: Clinical pharmacokinetics of digoxin in infants. Clin Pharmacokinet 2:17–31, 1977
13. Berman W Jr, Yabek SM, Dillan T, Christensen D, et al: Effects of digoxin in infants with a congested circulatory state due to a ventricular septal defect. N Engl J Med 308:363–366, 1983
14. Antonello A, Cargnielli G, Ferrari M, et al: Effect of digoxin on plasma renin activity in man. Lancet 2:850, 1976
15. Covit AB, Schaer GL, Sealey JE, et al: Suppression of the renin angiotensin by intravenous digoxin in chronic congestive heart failure. Am J Med 75:445–447, 1983
16. Montanaro D, Antonello-Baggio B, Finotti P, et al: Effect of digoxin on plasma renin activity in hypertensive patients. Int J Clin Pharmacol Ther Toxicol 18:322–823, 1980
17. Morselli PL, Franco-Marselli R, Bossi L: Clinical pharmacokinetics in newborns and infants, in Gibaldi M, Prescott L, (eds): Handbook of Clinical Pharmacokinetics, vol 2. New York: ADIS Health Sciences Press, 1983, pp 98–141
18. Lisalo E, Dahl E: Serum levels and renal excretion of digoxin during maintenance therapy in children. Acta Paediatr Scan 63:699–702, 1974
19. Halkin H, Radomsky M, Millman P, et al: Steady state serum concentrations and renal clearance of digoxin in neonates, infants and children. Eur J Clin Pharmacol 13:113–117, 1978
20. Morselli PL, Assael BM, Gomeni R, et al: Digoxin pharmacokinetics during human development, in Morselli PL, Garattini S, Sereni F (eds): Basic and Therapeutic Aspects of Perinatal Pharmacology New York, Raven Press, 1975
21. Wettrel G: Distribution and elimination of digoxin in infants. Eur J Clin Pharmacol 11:329, 1977
22. Roberts RJ: Drug therapy in infants. Philadelphia, W.B. Saunders Co., 1984
23. Hastreiter AR, Somonton RL, van der Harst RL, et al: Digoxin pharmacokinetics in premature infants. Pediatr Pharmacol 2:23–27, 1982
24. Gorodischer R, Jusko WJ, Yaffe SJ: Renal clearance of digoxin in young infants. Res Commun Chem Pathol Pharmacol 16:363, 1977
25. Greenball DJ, Duhme DW, Koch-Wesen J, et al: Evaluation of digoxin bioavailability in single dose studies. N Engl J Med 289:651–654, 1975
26. Huffman DH, Azarnoff DL: Absorption of orally given digoxin preparations. JAMA 222:957–960, 1972
27. Lindenbaum J, Mellow MH, Blockstone MO, et al: Variation in biologic availability of digoxin from four preparations. N Engl J Med 285:1344–1347, 1981

28. Heizer WD, Smith TW, Goldfinger SE: Absorption of digoxin in patients with malabsorption syndromes. N Engl J Med 285:257–259, 1971

29. Manninen V, Melin J, Apajalahti A, et al: Altered absorption of digoxin in patients given propantheline and metoclopramide. Lancet 1:398–400, 1973

30. Lindenbaum J, Rund D, Butler VP, et al: Inactivation of digoxin by the gut flora: Reversal by antibiotic therapy. N Engl J Med 305:789–794, 1981

31. Lalonde RL, Deshpande R, Hamilton PP, et al: Acceleration of digoxin clearance by activated charcoal. Clin Pharmacol Ther 37:367–371, 1985

32. Andersson K-E, Bertler A, Wettrell G: Post-mortem distribution and tissue concentrations of digoxin in infants and adults. Acta Paediatr Scand 64:497–504, 1975

33. Doherty JE, Perkins WH, Flanigan WJ: The distribution and concentration of tritiated digoxin in human tissues. Ann Intern Med 66:116–124, 1967

34. Lichey J, Havestatt CH, Weinmann J, et al: Human myocardium and plasma digoxin concentration in patients on long-term digoxin therapy. Int J Clin Pharmacol 16:460–462, 1978

35. Kim YI, Noble RJ, Zipes DP: Dissociation of inotropic effect of digitalis from its effect on atrioventricular conduction. Am J Cardiol 36:459–467, 1975

36. Shapin W, Narahara K, Taubert K: Relationship of plasma digitoxin and digoxin to cardiac response following intravenous digitalization in man. Circulation 42:1065–1072, 1970

37. Steiness E, Waldorf S, Hansen P, et al: Reduction of digoxin-induced inotropism during quinidine administration. Clin Pharmacol Ther 27:791–795, 1980

38. Koup JR, Greenblatt DJ, Jusko WJ, et al: Pharmacokinetics of digoxin in normal subjects after intravenous bolus and infusion doses. J Pharmacokinet Biopharm 3:181–192, 1975

39. Warburton D, Bell EF, Oh W: Pharmacokinetics and echocardiographic effects of digoxin in low birth weight infants with left-to-right shunting due to patent ductus arteriosus. Dev Pharmacol Ther 1:189–000, 1980

40. Steiness E: Renal tubular secretion of digoxin. Circulation 50:103–107, 1974

41. Koren G. Clinical pharmacokinetic significance of the renal tubular secretion of digoxin. Clin Pharmacokinetics 13:334–343, 1987

42. Koren G: Interaction between digoxin and commonly coadministered drugs in children. Pediatrics 75:1032–1037, 1985

43. Koren G, Klein J, Giesbrecht E, BenDayan R, Soldin S, Sellers E, MacLeod SM, Silverman M: The effect of quinidine on the renal tubular and biliary transport of digoxin; In vivo and in vitro studies in the dog. J Pharmacol Exp Ther 247:1193–1198, 1988

44. Koren G, Klein J, MacLeod SM, et al: Cellular mechanisms of digoxin transport and toxic interactions in the kidney. Vet Hum Toxicol 1986 (in press)

45. Doherty JE: Digitalis glycosides: Pharmacokinetics and their clinical implications. Ann Intern Med 79:229–238, 1973

46. Marks BH, Dutta S, Gautheir J, et al: Distribution in plasma, uptake by the heart and excretion of ouabain-H₃ in human subjects. J Pharmacol Exp Ther 145:351–356, 1964

47. Seldon R, Margolies MN, Smith TW: Renal and gastrointestinal excretion of ouabain in dog and man. J Pharmacol Exp Ther 188:615–623, 1974

48. Doherty JE: Metabolism of digitalis in man, in Marks BH, Weissler, AM (eds): Basic and Clinical Pharmocology of Digitalis, Springfield, Il. Charles C. Thomas, pp 11–20, 1972

49. Gault MH, Kalra J, Longerich L, et al: Digoxigenin biotransformation. Clin Pharmacol Ther 31:695–704, 1982

50. Gault MH, Longerich L, Loo JCK, et al: Digoxin biotransformation. Clin Pharmacol Ther 35:74–82, 1984

51. Clark DB, Kalman SM: Dihydrodigoxin: A common metabolite of digoxin in man. Drug Metab Dispos 2:148–150, 1974

52. Bach EJ, Reiter M: The differences in velocity between the lethal and inotropic action of dihydrodigoxin. Arch Exp Pathol Pharmakol 248:437–449, 1964

53. Brown BT, Stafford A, Wright SE: Chemical structure and pharmacologic activity of some derivatives of digitoxigenin and digoxigenin. Br J Pharmacol 18:311–324, 1962

54. Lage GL, Spratt JL: Structure-activity correlation of the lethality

55. Cerceo E, Elloso CA: Factors affecting the radioimmunoassay of digoxin. Clin Chem 18:539–543, 1972

56. Glassman A, Tilden R, Bruno F: Radioimmunoassay of digoxin. South Med J 63:1367, 1970

57. Rawal N, Leung FY, Henderson AR: Fluorescence polarization immunoassay of serum digoxin: Comparison of the Abbott immunoassay with the Amerlex radioimmunoassay. Clin Chem 29:586, 1983

58. Rumley AG, Trope A, Rowe DJF, et al: Comparison of digoxin analysis by EMIT with Immunophase and Dac-Cel radioimmunoassay. Ann Clin Biochem 17:315–318, 1980

59. Schermann JM, Bourdon R: Effect of deproteinization on determination of serum digoxin by fluorescence polarization immunoassay. Clin Chem 30:337–338, 1984

60. Smith TW, Butler VP, Haber E: Characterization of antibodies of high affinity and specificity for the digitalis glycoside digoxin. Biochemistry 9:331, 1970

61. Castle MC: Isolation and quantitation of picomole quantities of digoxin, digitoxin and their metabolites by high-pressure liquid chromatography. J Chromatogr 115:437–445, 1975

62. Fujii Y, Fujii H, Yamazaki M: Separation and determinations of cardiac glycosides in Digitalis purpurea leaves by micro high performance liquid chromatography. J Chromatogr 258:147–153, 1983

63. Jogestrand T, Ericsson R, Sundquist K: Skeletal muscle digoxin concentration during digitalization and during withdrawal of digoxin treatment. Eur J Clin Pharmacol 19:97–105, 1981

64. Watson E, Clark DR, Kalman SM: Identification by gas chromatography-mass spectroscopy of dihydrodigoxin, a metabolite of digoxin in man. J Pharmacol Exp Ther 184:424–431, 1973

65. Koren G, Farine D, Grundmann H, Heyes J, MacLeod SM, Soldin S, Taylor J: Endogenous digoxin like substance in uneventful and high risk pregnancies. Dev Pharmacol Ther 11:82–87, 1988

66. Gault MH, Vasedv SC, Longerich LL, et al: Plasma digitalis-like factors(s) increase with salt loading. N Engl J Med 309:1459, 1984

67. Graves SW, Brown B, Valdes R: An endogenous digoxin like substance in patients with renal impairment. Ann Intern Med 99:604–608, 1983

68. Koren G, Farine D, Marlsky D, Taylor J, Heyes J, Soldin S, MacLeod SM: Significance of the endogenous digoxin-like substance in infants and mothers. Clin Pharmacol Ther 36:759–764, 1984

69. Devynck M-A, Pernollet MG, Rosenfeld JB, Meyer P: Measurements of digitalis-like compound in plasma: Application in studies of essential hypertension. Br Med J 287:631–634, 1983

70. Gruber KA, Whitaker JM, Buckalew VM Jr: Endogenous digitalis-like substance in plasma of volume-expanded dogs. Nature 287:743–745, 1980

71. Fishman MC: Endogenous digitalis-like activity in mammalian brain. Proc Natl Acad Sci USA 75:4661–4663, 1979

72. Hamblyn JM, Ringel R, Schaeffer J, et al: A circulating inhibitor of Na⁺/K⁺ ATPase associated with essential hypertension. Nature 300:650–652, 1982

73. LaBella FA: Is there an endogenous digitalis? Trends Pharmacol Sci 3:334–335, 1982

74. Soldin SJ, Papanastasiou-Diamandi A, Heyes J, et al: Are immunoassays for digoxin reliable? Clin Biochem 17:317–320, 1984

75. Young A, Giesbredt E, Soldin SJ: A study of lipid effects on the digoxin immunoassay and on the binding to and activity of Na⁺/K⁺-ATPase. Clin Biochem 19:195–200, 1986

76. Tamura M, Kuwano H, Kinoshita T, Inagami T: Identification of linoleic acid and oleic acids as endogenous Na⁺/K⁺ ATPase inhibitors from acute volume-expanded hog plasma. J Biol Chem 260:9672–9677, 1985

77. Baylen B, Meyer RA, Korfhagen J, Benzing G III, Bubb ME, Kaplan S: Left ventricular performance in the critically ill premature infant with patent ductus arteriosus and pulmonary disease. Circulation 55:182–188, 1977

78. Park SC, Steinfeld L, Dimich I: Systolic time intervals in infants with congestive heart failure. Circulation 47:1281–1288, 1973

79. Sahn DJ, Vaucher Y, Williams DE, et al: Echocardiographic detection of large left to right shunts and cardiomyopathies in infants and children. Am J Cardiol 73:73–76, 1976

and central effects of selected glycosides. J Pharmacol Exp Ther 152:501–508, 1966

80. Pinsky WW, Jacobsen JR, Gillette PC, et al: Dosage of digoxin in premature infants. J Pediatr 96:639–643, 1979

81. Lundell BPW, Boreus LO: Digoxin therapy and left ventricular performance in premature infants with patent ductus arteriosus. Acta Pediatr Scand 72:339–344, 1983

82. Sandor GGS, Bloom KR, Izukawa T, et al: Noninvasive assessment of left ventricular function related to serum digoxin levels in neonates. Pediatrics 65: 541–000, 1980

83. Mulrow CD, Feussner JR, Velez R: Reevaluation of digitalis efficacy. Ann Int Med, 101:113–117, 1984

84. Longerich L, Dowe M, Vasdev S, Gault H: A simple method to assay digoxin in sera with metabolites and/or digitalis like factor. Clin Invest Med 9:A18, 1986

85. Belz GG, Aust PE, Munkes R: Digoxin plasma concentrations and nifedipine. Lancet 1:844-845, 1981

86. Ford AR, Aronson JK, Grahame-Smith DG, et al: Changes in cardiac receptor sites, 86-rubidium uptake and intracellular sodium concentrations in the erythrocytes of patients receiving digoxin during the early phases of treatment of cardiac failure in regular rhythm and of atrial fibrillation. Br J Clin Pharmacol 8:125–134, 1979

87. Koren G, Parker R: Interpretation of excessive serum concentrations of digoxin in children. Am J Cardiol 55:1210–1214, 1985

88. Ben-Itzhak J, Bassan HM, Shor R, Laniz A: Digoxin quinidine interaction: A pharmacokinetic study in the isolated perfused rat liver. Life Sci 37:411–415, 1985

89. Koren G, Zarfin Y, Perlman M, MacLeod SM: Effects of indomethacin on digoxin pharmacokinetics in preterm infants. Pediatr Pharmacol 4:25–30, 1984

90. Strauss MH, Dorian P, Cardella C, David T, Ogilvie RI: Digoxin cyclosporine interaction: A new phenomenon. Clin Invest Med 9:A16, 1986

91. Koren G, MacLeod SM: Postmortem redistribution of digoxin in rats. J Forens Med 30:92–96, 1985

92. Spiehler VR, Fischer WR: Digoxin like immunoreactive substance in postmortem blood of infants and children. J Forens Med 30:86–91, 1985

93. Koren G, Beatie D, Soldin SJ, Einarson T: Interpretation of excessive postmortem concentration of digoxin. Arch Path Lab Med 113:758–761, 1989

94. Koren G, Beatie K, Soldin S: Agonal elevation in digoxin serum concentrations in critically ill patients. Crit Care Med 16:793–795, 1988

95. Butler VP Jr, Chen JP: Digoxin-specific antibodies. Proc Natl Acad Sci USA 57:71–78, 1967

96. Curd J, Smith TW, Jaton J-C, et al: The isolation of digoxin-specific antibody and its use in reversing the effects of digoxin. Proc Natl Acad Sci USA 68:2401–2406, 1971

97. Schmidt DH, Butler VP Jr: Reversal of digoxin toxicity with specific antibodies. J Clin Invest 50:1738–1744, 1971

98. Smith TW, Butler VP Jr, Haber E: Cardiac glycoside-specific antibodies in the treatment of digitalis intoxication, in Haber E, Krause R (eds): Antibodies in Human Diagnosis and Therapy. New York, Raven Press, 1977, pp 365–389

99. Smith TW, Butler VP Jr, Haber E, et al: Treatment of life-threatening digitalis-specific Fab antibody fragments. N Engl J Med 307:1357–1362, 1982

35

ANTIVIRAL CHEMOTHERAPY

JANAK A. PATEL *and* PEARAY L. OGRA

In the past 30 years, with improved hygiene, the availability of better health care, and the practice of large-scale immunization, many viral diseases such as smallpox, poliomyelitis, measles, mumps, and rubella have been brought under control in many parts of the world. However, infections caused by viruses in the upper and lower respiratory tracts, herpesviruses, and human immunodeficiency virus (HIV), among other agents, continue to cause significant morbidity and mortality.

With the advent of newer, more specific, safer, and easier-to-administer antiviral agents and the development of rapid diagnostic methods such as immunofluorescent microscopy, radio immunoassays, enzyme immunoassays, and DNA hybridization, the field of antiviral therapy has been thrust into the forefront and offers exciting opportunities for treatment of several viral infections. Currently, effective treatment is available for infections with herpes simplex viruses (HSV), respiratory syncytial virus (RSV), varicella–zoster virus (VZV), and influenza viruses.

Important milestones in the evolution of antiviral chemotherapy to date include the development of thiosemicarbazone in the early 1950s, the recognition of interferons as natural antiviral substances in the late 1950s, and the availability of idoxyuridine in the early 1960s, amantadine in the mid-1960s, vidarabine (Ara-A) in the mid-1970s, and, finally, acyclovir and ribavirin in the late 1970s.

This chapter will review major aspects of the development and usage of antiviral drugs in mammalian systems. The clinical application of these drugs in the management of illnesses caused by various viruses will be discussed. Many antiviral drugs have not been properly evaluated in the pediatric population. In such situations, relevant studies carried out in adults and in animal models will also be discussed.

HOST REQUIREMENTS FOR VIRAL GROWTH

Viruses depend on the cellular machinery of the host for their replication and utilize the host cell substrates, enzymes, and nucleotides. Only a few steps of viral replication are regulated by virus-specific enzymes that are independent of the host cell substrates. These steps have been used as potential targets for selective inhibition of viral multiplication by antiviral agents. Since viruses are metabolically active only inside the cell, antivirals should be able to penetrate the cell membrane and achieve adequate intracellular levels. The fact that viruses depend on host cell machinery for their multiplication and that the steps of host cell and virus replication are often similar may account for the high *in vivo* toxicity and low therapeutic index of many antiviral agents. The development of clinical symptoms frequently follows viral multiplication and dissemination to systemic sites. Therefore, in order for the antiviral agents to be effective against clinical infections, they must be introduced into the host very early, preferably prior to dissemination and establishment of infection in the susceptible cells. Such prompt intervention requires rapid and accurate diagnosis. Antiviral agents may also need to be effective in the latent intracellular stage of diminished viral protein synthesis, in order to prevent relapses.

REPLICATION PATTERNS OF HUMAN VIRUSES

The basic steps in the replication of DNA and RNA viruses are represented in Figure 35–1.

365

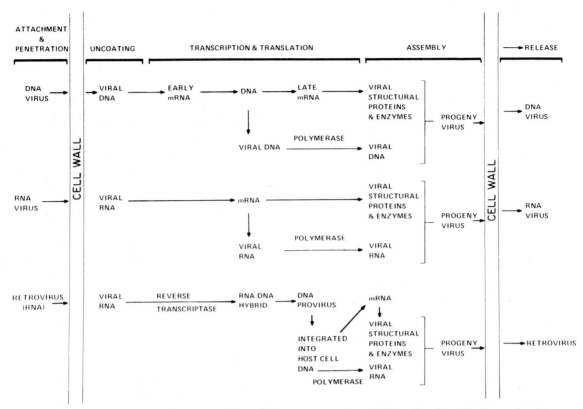

FIGURE 35–1. Schematic representation of the events associated with replication of DNA and RNA viruses.

Attachment, Penetration, and Uncoating

Attachment of a virus to the host cell is accomplished either by electrostatic forces that bind the virus to the cell surface receptors or by steric compatibility. The viral penetration occurs either through fusion of the viral envelope with the cytoplasmic membrane or by engulfment of the virus by the cell. Uncoating of the nucleocapsid protective outer coat of the virus follows, thereby exposing viral nucleic acid to cell cytoplasm. Host cell enzymes appear to participate in this process.

Transcription and Translation

Following uncoating, the viral nucleic acids are transported to the site of replication either in the cytoplasm (DNA viruses with large genome) or in the nucleus (DNA viruses with small genome and most RNA viruses except influenza). The nucleic acids serve two purposes: (1) to act as a template for transcription of messenger RNA (mRNA) and (2) to act directly as a messenger. The mRNA, in turn, is translated into viral proteins. In the case of retrovirus, the nucleic acids are transcribed with the help of reverse transcriptase into a minus-strand DNA. Synthesis of a complementary DNA is then initiated, which migrates to the nucleus and becomes integrated as proviral DNA in host chromosomes.

Synthesis of Viral Proteins

The synthesis of component viral proteins is an essential step in the eventual viral genome replication. The synthesis of most structural proteins of RNA viruses is associated with the synthesis of RNA-dependent RNA polymerase. However, the synthesis of early mRNA in DNA viruses corresponds only to the translation of early viral proteins, which include uncoating enzymes and other proteins that alter host cell metabolism to facilitate viral nucleic acid and protein synthesis, and enzymes involved in DNA replication. The progeny DNA serves as a template for the transcription of late mRNA and is associated with synthesis of viral structural proteins for DNA viral genome replication. In the case of retrovirus, the integrated proviral DNA template is transcribed by host DNA polymerase into viral RNA. The latter acts either as genomic RNA or as mRNA for protein synthesis.

Steps in Assembly, Maturation, and Release

Following synthesis, the viral structural proteins and viral genome are reorganized in a precise conformational order to form a viral nucleocapsid. This activity does not seem to require any specific enzyme action. For enveloped viruses, the nucleocapsid acquires its envelope by budding through the host cell membrane.

APPROACHES TO CHEMOTHERAPY OF VIRAL INFECTIONS

The mechanisms of action of antiviral agents are summarized in Table 35-1.

Inhibition of Attachment and Penetration

Specific antibodies, with or without the cooperation of complement, bind to the virus and thereby inhibit the attachment of virus to the host cell. Amantadine and rimantadine inhibit uncoating of the envelope of influenza A virus prior to host cell penetration.[1,2] HIV attachment to the CD_4 lymphocyte receptor can be inhibited by AL721, a lipid compound that alters viral cell lipid content.[3] Similarly, peptide T, an oligopeptide chain that corresponds to a small conserved region on the HIV envelope gp120, blocks HIV attachment to the CD_4 receptor of lymphocytes.[4]

Inhibition of Reverse Transcriptase

Retroviral reverse transcriptase can be inhibited by enzyme-binding compounds such as suramin (nonselective)[5] and zidovudine (selective).[6] It can also be inhibited

TABLE 35-1. IMPORTANT ANTIVIRAL AGENTS AND THEIR MECHANISMS OF ACTION

AGENT	SUSCEPTIBLE VIRUS	MECHANISM(S) OF ACTION
Acyclovir (ACV)	Herpes simplex 1 & 2 Varicella-zoster Epstein-Barr	1. Selectively activated by HSV- and VZV-specified TK to ACV-MP 2. Further activation by host enzymes to ACV-TP which acts as chain terminator of viral DNA and inactivates DNA polymerase
Vidarabin (Ara-A)	Herpes simplex 1 & 2 Varicella zoster	1. Phosphorylation by cellular adenosine kinase and deoxycytidine kinase to active form of Ara-ATP 2. Ara-ATP inhibits viral DNA polymerase
Ribavirin	Respiratory syncytial virus Parainfluenza virus type 3 Influenza virus A and B Arenavirus (Lassa fever) Adenoviruses Measles Hepatitis A Human immunodeficiency virus	1. Resembles guanosine; active through metabolite: ribavirin-5-monophosphate (RMP) 2. RMP competitively inhibits GMP 3. Inhibits DNA and RNA viruses by altering virus nucleoside pool and messenger RNA formation
Zidovudine	Human immunodeficiency virus	1. Thymidine analog that is phosphorylated *in vivo* by cellular enzymes to the 5'-triphosphate form, which in turn inhibits viral reverse transcriptase and terminates viral DNA chain elongation
Ganciclovir (DHPG)	Cytomegalovirus Herpes simplex 1 and 2 Varicella zoster Epstein-Barr	1. Phosphorylated by virus-induced cellular thymidine kinase to DHPG-MP. It is further activated by host enzymes to DHPG-TP which inactivates viral DNA polymerase
Amantadine	Influenza A	1. Inhibits uncoating of envelope prior to host cell penetration 2. Inhibits M_2 protein in assembly of progeny virions
Rimantadine	Influenza A	Similar to Amantadine
Phosphonoformate	Herpes simplex 1 & 2 cytomegalovirus Epstein-Barr Human immunodeficiency virus	1. Selectively inhibits herpesvirus DNA polymerase 2. Noncompetitive inhibitor as a substrate and template for reverse transcriptase activity
Disoxaril	Rhinoviruses Enteroviruses	1. Incorporation of drug by replacement into peptide chains of the virus coat proteins. This resists viral uncoating after penetration into the cell
Interferons	Rhinoviruses Papillomavirus Chronic hepatitis B, non-A non-B, or delta virus infection Cytomegalovirus Herpes simplex 1 and 2 Varicella zoster	1. Alters metabolism of the mammalian cell so that the synthesis and assembly of viral components are impeded
Immune serum globulin	Enteroviruses Respiratory syncytial virus Cytomegalovirus	1. Extracellular virus coating by specific antibody with or without complement, thereby preventing virus attachment to host cell
Interleukin-2	Herpes simplex	1. Stimulates B cells to proliferate and differentiate into immunoglobulin-producing cells 2. Stimulates NKCs that mediate antibody-dependent cellular cytotoxicity (ADCC)

by reverse transcriptase substrate and template analogs such as phosphoroformate (PFA) and zidovudine (AZT).

Inhibition of Transcription and Translation

Nucleoside analogs can interfere with nucleic acid synthesis by depletion of enzyme substrates. For example, ribavirin, which resembles guanosine, acts by the formation of ribavirin-5'-monophosphate (RMP), thereby reducing the pool of native guanosine triphosphate (GTP).[7] Nucleoside analogs can also utilize virus-specific enzymes to form compounds that inhibit viral DNA polymerase. Acyclovir achieves such activity by utilizing virus-specific thymidine kinase (TK) for phosphorylation to acycloguanosine triphosphate, which, in turn, inhibits viral DNA polymerase.[8] On the other hand, adenine arabinoside (Ara-A) is converted entirely by cellular enzymes to triphosphate, which inhibits viral DNA polymerase at a lower concentration than cellular DNA polymerase.[9] Similarly, ganciclovir (DHPG) utilizes virus-specific TK, leading to DHPG triphosphate formation that results in DNA polymerase inhibition of human cytomegalovirus.[10] Idoxyuridine resembles thymidine and is phosphorylated in HSV-infected cells and incorporated into viral DNA, resulting in breaks in the nucleic acid.[11]

Inhibition of Assembly and Release

Agents such as thiosemicarbazones lead to inhibition of the production of structural proteins for assembly by defective processing of late structural proteins of vaccinia virus.[12] The interferons lead to the production of other cellular proteins that have antiviral activity which ultimately leads to the inhibition of assembly and release of mature virions.[13]

ANTIVIRAL AGENTS

Like any ideal antimicrobial therapeutic agent, an antiviral should have selective specificity against viral replication without any significant toxicity to the host cell, i.e., a high therapeutic index. It should be available in both orally and systemically administered formulations. It should also attain high levels in body fluids and intracellularly, with the ability to concentrate effectively in the susceptible tissues during a specific viral infection. It should be excreted favorably.

Nucleoside Analogs

The purine or pyrimidine analogs act by their incorporation into the nucleic acids of viral DNA or RNA, which leads to abnormal transcription and translation resulting in the loss of antiviral infectivity. They also act by phosphorylation to triphosphates that are inhibitors of DNA and RNA polymerases.

Purine Nucleosides

Acyclovir [ACV; Zovirax; 9-(2-Hydroxyethoxymethyl)guanine]

The structure of acyclovir resembles that of deoxyguanosine (Figure 35–2). It is phosphorylated by virally specified TK of infected cells and does not require cellular kinase. This activity leads to the formation of acyclovir monophosphate (ACV-MP), which is further converted to di- and triphosphates (ACV-TP) by cellular enzymes.[8] The amount of ACV-TP formed is, therefore, 40–100 times greater in HSV- or VZV-infected cells than in uninfected cells,[14] thus accounting for the high therapeutic index and few side effects. ACV-TP is a potent antiviral substance because it inhibits DNA polymerase, leading to chain termination.[15] These mechanisms are very effective in suppressing replication of HSV types 1 and 2 (HSV-1 and HSV-2) and VZV. However, acyclovir is 10 to 50 times more effective *in vitro* against HSV than VZV.[16,17]

Epstein-Barr virus (EBV) does not specify its own TK and the amount of ACV-TP formed by cellular enzymes is very small, but its viral DNA polymerase is exquisitely sensitive to small amounts of ACV-TP.[18,19] This stops replication of EBV *in vitro* but has no effect on virus latency in treated patients.[20]

Human cytomegalovirus (CMV) neither specifies its own TK nor is susceptible to small amounts of ACV-TP formed by cellular enzymes.[21] This may explain the lack of effect of acyclovir on replication of CMV.

PHARMACOKINETICS AND CLINICAL APPLICATIONS. Acyclovir is available in three forms: intravenous, oral, and topical. When it is given intravenously, peak plasma levels are reached at 1 hour that are much higher than concentrations required to inhibit susceptible herpesviruses. Its half-life is under 4 hours in neonates (0–3 months),[22,23] 2–3 hours in older infants (3 months–1 year),[23] and about 3 hours in adults.[23] It is well distributed in the body, with the steady-state distribution approximately equal to the volume of body fluid, and it achieves therapeutic concentrations in many organs, including the brain and vesicle fluids.[23] Acyclovir is primarily excreted unchanged by glomerular filteration, accounting for 70 percent of total dose. The remainder is excreted by tubular secretion.[24] When given orally in liquid, capsule, or tablet forms, its absorption is slow and variable, with about 15–20 percent entering the circulation[25] and reaching a peak level 2–3 hours after a dose. These peak levels are well within the concentrations required for inhibition of HSV-1 and HSV-2. In infants and children, the peak serum concentration of acyclovir after an oral dose with liquid suspension may be about 40 percent of the expected peak level in adults with identical dosage regimens,[26] whereas in neonates it produces a higher peak concentration and a longer half-life, which reflects immature renal function in this age group. Limited data are currently available on the pharmacokinetics and efficacy of oral acyclovir in children and infants, but it has been used with some success in the treatment of mild VZV or HSV infections in those at risk of disseminated disease.[27,28] The use of acyclovir in clinical conditions is discussed in detail in Therapeutic Uses of Antiviral Agents.

Guanosine Analogs

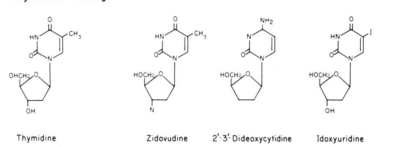

Guanosine   Ribavirin   Acyclovir   Ganciclovir

Thymidine Analogs

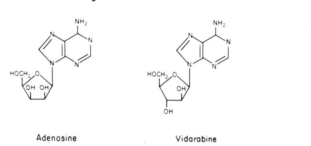

Thymidine   Zidovudine   2'-3'-Dideoxycytidine   Idoxyuridine

Adenosine Analog

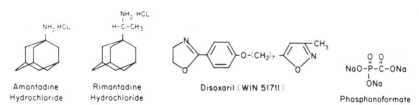

Adenosine   Vidarabine

Other Antivirals

Amantadine Hydrochloride   Rimantadine Hydrochloride   Disoxaril (WIN 51711)   Phosphonoformate

FIGURE 35–2. Structural formulas of antiviral agents.

In renal insufficiency, dosage adjustments are required.[23] For creatinine clearance of 50 ml/min/1.73 m² or above, adjustments are not necessary (given every 8 hours). For creatinine clearance of 25–50 ml/min/1.73 m², the dosage interval is lengthened to every 12 hours; for creatinine clearance of 10–25 ml/min/1.73 m², the dosage interval is lengthened to every 24 hours; and for creatinine clearance of less than 16 ml/min/1.73 m², each dose is reduced by 50 percent and the interval lengthened to every 24 hours. Hemodialysis performed over 6 hours reduces plasma acyclovir levels by 50–60 percent.[29]

TOXICITY. Toxicity of acyclovir is relatively mild. When intravenously administered in less than 1 hour, plasma creatinine elevations have been noted.[30] This may be due to microcrystallization of acyclovir in the renal collecting systems.[31] It can be avoided by infusing acyclovir over 1 hour and maintaining adequate hydration. Other possible types of toxicity are rare but are reported to be more frequent among bone marrow transplant patients.[32] These include bone marrow suppression, and neurotoxicity as manifested by lethargy, agitation, tremor, disorientation, or transient hemiparesis. Serum transaminase elevation, allergic reactions, and phlebitis at the intravenous site have also been observed.[33]

Vidarabine (Adenine Arabinoside; Ara-A; 9-β-D-Arabinofuranosyl-adenine)

Vidarabine is identical to adenosine except that the sugar moiety is arabinose rather than ribose (Figure 35–

2). It is phosphorylated to the active form Ara-ATP by cellular adenosine kinase and deoxycytidine kinase. Ara-ATP then blocks viral DNA synthesis by inhibiting viral DNA polymerase.[9] Vidarabine is incorporated into the viral DNA molecule, but to a lesser extent than into cellular DNA[34]; hence, this mechanism does not seem to be important for viral inhibition.

PHARMACOKINETICS AND CLINICAL APPLICATION. The plasma half-life of vidarabine is about 4 hours. After 12 hours of constant infusion of 10 mg/kg, the unchanged form is detectable at levels of 0.2–0.4 µg/ml.[35] These levels are below the *in vitro* inhibitory concentration required for herpesviruses. However, *in vivo,* a relatively low level seems sufficient for intracellular activation and viral inhibition. The established clinical efficacy is only against infections with HSV-1, HSV-2,[35–37] and VZV.[38,39] The main degradative pathway to the less active form, Ara-hypoxanthine (Ara-HX), probably occurs in the erythrocytes.[35,40]

A major drawback of vidarabine is its relatively low solubility, approximately 0.7 mg/ml. The extra fluid load may prove detrimental in a patient with preexisting brain edema. The large volumes of fluid needed for dilution also prevent intramuscular use. Oral administration cannot be used because of deamination following intestinal absorption. Topical preparations are available for ophthalmic use and are associated with lesser irritation than idoxuridine.[37] The use of vidarabine in clinical conditions is discussed in detail in Therapeutic Uses of Antiviral Agents.

Vidarabine is most highly concentrated in the kidneys, liver, and spleen. Lower levels are found in the skeletal muscles and brain. Vidarabine and its metabolites can be found in the cerebrospinal fluid (CSF) at a level approximately 50 percent of that in the serum and persist for up to 10 days after therapy.[35] It is cleared from the body by the kidney with about 60 percent of a single dose excreted as Ara-HX within 24 hours.[40] In severe renal insufficiency, the plasma half-life of vidarabine can be as long as 4–7 hours,[41] which necessitates a reduction in dose. Ara-HX is cleared by hemodialysis in a linear fashion.[41]

Vidarabine monophosphate (Ara-AMP), a more soluble product than vidarabine, has been developed.[42] It can be given intravenously or intramuscularly in small volumes. However, it has no established clinical role in antiviral therapy at present.

TOXICITY. In general, vidarabine has a fairly high therapeutic index. Common adverse effects are nausea, with or without vomiting, and diarrhea.[43] Less common adverse effects are mainly due to neurotoxicity.[43] These include faintness, dizziness, fatigue, and tremors.

Ganciclovir [GCV; DHPG; BW B759U; B10LF-62; 9-[2'-Hydroxy-1-(hydroxymethyl)ethoxymethyl] guanine]

Ganciclovir (DHPG) is a derivative of acyclovir (Figure 35–2) which contains an additional hydroxymethyl group on the side chain. Similar to acyclovir, it is phosphorylated by the HSV- and VZV-specified TKs. The monophosphate (DHPG-MP) is further phosphorylated by guanylate kinase to the triphosphate (DHPG-TP). DHPG-MP is a better substrate than acyclovir monophosphate (ACV-MP)[10] and results in an approximately 10-fold higher level of DHPG-TP in HSV-infected cells and a 20-fold higher level in VZV-infected cells.[8] However, DNA polymerases of HSV-1 and VZV are more sensitive to ACV-TP, resulting in similar inhibitory values of acyclovir and ganciclovir for HSV-1, HSV-2, and VZV.[8] Another difference between the two compounds is that ganciclovir incorporation into viral DNA does not lead to termination of the nucleoside chain, which probably explains its increased toxicity.[10] But the most important difference between acyclovir and ganciclovir is in their activities against CMV. Phosphorylation of ganciclovir is much higher than that of acyclovir in CMV-infected cells.[44] Although TK and deoxycytidine kinase levels in CMV-infected cells are at their peak 3 days after infection, the peak phosphorylation of ganciclovir and acyclovir occurs considerably later.[45] The nature of the intracellular enzyme responsible for ganciclovir phosphorylation is not yet known. The inhibition of EBV replication by ganciclover is not as great as for CMV, but DHPG is about six times more sensitive than acyclovir.[46] However, the clinical efficacy of DHPG against EBV is not yet known. The use of DHPG in clinical conditions is discussed in detail in Therapeutic Uses of Antiviral Agents.

PHARMACOKINETICS. The pharmacokinetics of ganciclovir are similar to those of acyclovir. Its peak serum levels after an intravenous infusion are similar to those of acyclovir, and the mean serum half-life is 3.6 hours,[47] which is slightly longer than that of acyclovir. Its volume of distribution is about 1.6 liters/kg.[47] Ganciclovir is not metabolized in the body and 99 percent is excreted unchanged through the kidneys, which necessitates dosage adjustments in renal insufficiency.[47] Hemodialysis reduces the plasma level of DHPG to about 53–60 percent of its previous level.[47] When given orally, its absorption is very poor and bioavailability varies from 3 to 6 percent. In a pharmacokinetic study of oral ganciclovir administered to adult volunteers at a dose of 20 mg/kg given every 6 hours, therapeutic peak plasma levels were achieved.[48]

TOXICITY. Neutropenia is the most common adverse reaction to ganciclovir and occurs in about 40 percent of patients; its occurrence appears to be related to the duration of treatment and the size of dose.[49] Other less common reactions are thrombocytopenia, nausea, vomiting, hepatitis, and central nervous system dysfunction with disorientation and psychosis.[49] Allergic reactions with skin rash and eosinophilia also have been reported. Phlebitis and local pain with severe tissue reaction have been observed after extravasation of intravenously administered drug, which is attributed to its alkalinity (pH 10). Azoospermia has been observed in all animal species tested.

Ribavirin (Virazole; 1-β-D-Ribofuranosyl-1,2,4-triazole-3-carboxamide)

Ribavirin is a nucleoside-like compound that is similar to guanosine and inosine (Figure 35–2). It has a wide spectrum of antiviral activity *in vitro* and *in vivo* against RNA and DNA viruses. It is phosphorylated by cellular adenosine kinase to ribavirin monophosphate and further phosphorylated by other cellular enzymes to a triphosphate (RV-TP).[7] These steps are nonspecific and probably result in antiviral levels of RV-TP in all tissues. RV-TP is a potent inhibitor of RNA polymerase and also inhibits formation of the 5' "cap" of viral messenger RNA, which is essential in viral replication.[7] It also acts as a chain terminator of viral RNA. Some antiviral effect may be due to reduction in guanosine triphosphate pools by competitive inhibition of cellular inosine monophosphate dehydrogenase.[50] A combination of these mechanisms of action gives ribavirin a broad antiviral activity against agents such as Lassa fever virus, adenoviruses, human herpesviruses, HIV, influenza A and B viruses, CMV, parainfluenza virus types 1 and 2, RSV, vaccinia virus, rhinovirus, bunyaviruses, and togaviruses.[51] Its use in clinical conditions is discussed in Therapeutic Uses of Antiviral Agents (Table 35–2).

PHARMACOKINETICS. Ribavirin is available in oral, intravenous, and aerosol forms. Aerosolized ribavirin is given by a small-particle aerosol generator that uses a solution concentration of 20 mg/ml. The method of delivery can be by face mask, intranasal tube, "tent," or endotracheal tube. However, the endotracheal route is fraught with technical problems related to crystallization of the drug in the ventilator air circuits. Nonetheless, this problem can be surmounted by rigorous attention to cleansing and by modification of the mechanical ventilating apparatus.[52]

About 70 percent of the aerosolized drug is deposited in the respiratory tree. The mean concentration of ribavirin in tracheal secretions after an 8-hour aerosol therapy is 7700 μM, which is more than 1000-fold higher than in plasma.[53] The respiratory secretion concentrations far exceed the minimum inhibitory concentrations required for common respiratory viruses. *In vitro* inhibitory concentrations of ribavirin are 4–100 μM for influenza A and B viruses, 16–64 μM for RSV, and 12–130 μM for parainfluenza virus types 1 and 3.[53] Ribavirin is cleared rapidly from the airway, probably by diffusion across the membrane and elimination upwards through the airway. The mean half-life in respiratory secretions is 1.4–2.5 hours.[53] After administration of ribavirin by face mask for 20 hours for 5 days, pediatric patients have plasma concentrations of 1.5–14.3 μM (mean = 6.8 μM).[54]

The plasma half-life of ribavirin given as an aerosol is long. This is partly due to a prolonged terminal excretion phase and partly due to continued diffusion from the respiratory epithelium into the plasma. For example, when it is given by aerosol for 8 hours for 3 consecutive days, the mean peak plasma level rises from 3.3 μM on the first day to 6.1 μM on the third day. Under these circumstances, the plasma half-life is over 9 hours.[53]

After an oral dose, 50 percent of the drug is absorbed from the intestinal tract.[55] Serum peak levels are reached in 1–1.5 hours, and the plasma half-life is about 10–12 hours.[56] Because of accumulation of RV-TP in erythrocytes due to inefficient dephosphorylation, the half-life of ribavirin in erythrocytes is 40 days.[56]

Ribavirin is degraded in plasma and tissues to an inactive form. In experimental animals the major metabolite is triazole-3-carboxamide. However, in humans a majority of the drug is excreted unchanged in the urine. After an oral dose of ribavirin is given to adults, approximately 54 percent is excreted in the urine over a 72- to 80-hour period.[56]

TOXICITY. Adverse effects of ribavirin have been reported infrequently. Bronchospasm and worsening of respiratory function have occurred. In some patients other adverse effects such as apnea, cardiac arrest, hypotension, digitalis toxicity, jaundice, rash, and conjuctivitis have been reported, although very rarely, and it is not clear whether there is a causal relationship. Development of anemia has been observed when ribavirin is given orally or by intravenous route in high doses over 10–14 days.[57] This may occur becuase ribavirin is concentrated 100-fold in red blood cells, with a slow excretory rate.[56] This has not been observed with aerosol administration.

Zidovudine (Azidothymidine; AZT; Retrovir; 3' - Azido-3'-deoxythymidine)

Zidovudine is a thymidine analog (Figure 35–2) that was initially developed as an anticancer drug in the 1960s. In 1974 it was found to inhibit *in vitro* replication of C-type murine retrovirus. In 1985 Mitsuya et al.[58] demonstrated *in vitro* activity of zidovudine against HIV. It is converted by cellular kinases to the 5'-triphosphate form (AZT-TP), which inhibits HIV reverse transcriptase approximately 100 times more effectively than it does cellular DNA polymerase alpha.[59] In addition, AZT monophosphate (AZT-MP) is incorporated into the growing DNA strand by HIV reverse transcriptase.[59] This leads to 3' modification and prevents further 5'→3' phosphodiester links, resulting in termination of viral DNA chain synthesis.[59] HIV replication is inhibited *in vitro* at a concentration of 0.5 μM under conditions of high viral excess and by concentrations as low as 10 nM at low viral doses. Inhibition of multiplication of uninfected lymphocytes requires concentrations of more than 1mM.[59]

PHARMACOKINETICS. Zidovudine is available in both parenteral and oral forms. After an oral dose of 5 mg/kg or an intravenous dose of 2.5 mg/kg over 1 hour, plasma concentrations of 5 μM have been shown to be achieved in adult studies.[60] Bioavailability after an oral dose is approximately 60 percent. Zidovudine has a short plasma half-life of only 1 hour and therefore must be given as frequently as every 4 hours.[60] Blood–brain barrier penetration is adequate for HIV inhibition in the central nervous system.[61] Zidovudine is metabolized by glucoronidation in the liver[62] and excreted by the kidney.

TOXICITY. Toxic effects of zidovudine in acquired immunodeficiency syndrone (AIDS) or AIDS-related complex (ARC) patients include megaloblastic anemia requiring blood transfusions in approximately 21 percent of patients and neutropenia in about 16 percent.[63] Headaches, nausea, myalgia, and insomnia are more common. All the side effects are apparently reversible but may necessitate either reduction of dosage or temporary withdrawal of zidovudine.[64] Concurrent administration of drugs such as acetaminophen that are glucoronidated by

TABLE 35–2. SUMMARY OF USES OF ANTIVIRAL AGENTS

VIRUS AND CLINICAL CONDITION	TREATMENT REGIMEN	COMMENTS
HSV		
Neonatal	Acyclovir 10 mg/kg/dose, I.V. over 1 h, every 8 h for 10–14 days	Treatment of choice
	Vidarabine 30 mg/kg/day, I.V. over 12–24 h for 10–14 days	Problem of excessive fluid administration
Encephalitis	Acyclovir Children & adults: 10 mg/kg/dose, I.V. over 1 h every 8 h for 10–14 days	Relapse may occur
	Vidarabine Children & adults: 15–30 mg/kg/day, I.V. over 12–24 h for 10–14 days	
Primary genital	Topical acyclovir 5% ointment every 3–4 hours for 7 days	Oral acyclovir preferable to topical form
	Systemic acyclovir Children: 600 mg/m^2/dose, P.O. four times a day for 10 days or 250 mg/kg/m^2/dose, I.V. over 1 h every 8 h for 5 days Adults: 200 mg, P.O. five times a day for 10 days or 5 mg/kg/dose, I.V. over 1 h, every 8 h for 5 days	Not tested in children for genital infection
Recurrent genital	Intermittent oral acyclovir Children: 600 mg/m^2/dose, P.O. four times a day for 5 days Adults: 200 mg, P.O. five times a day for 5 days	Initiate at the earliest sign of symptoms
	Chronic suppressive oral acyclovir Children: untested Adults: 200 mg, P.O. three times a day for up to 6 months	Effectiveness of treatment duration longer than 6 months not known
Immunocompromised host Mild mucocutaneous	Acyclovir Children: 600 mg/m^2/dose, P.O. four times a day until resolution of symptoms Adults: 200 mg, P.O. five times a day until resolution of symptoms	Oral therapy efficacious
Severe mucocutaneous, e.g., esophagitis	Acyclovir Children: 250 mg/m^2/dose, I.V. over 1 h, every 8 h for 7 days Adults: 5 mg/kg/dose, I.V. over 1 h, every 8 h for 7 days	
Seropositive transplant patients	Acyclovir Children and adults: I.V. dose as above, start 3–7 days prior to transplant and continue for 3–5 weeks afterwards	Efficacious to prevent reactivation during therapy
Keratitis	Trifluridine 1% ophthalmic sol., one drop per eye, every 2 h while awake for 14–21 days Vidarabine 3% ophthalmic ointment, apply to lower lid, five times a day for 21 days	Must have ophthalmologic evaluation. Trifluridine is the treatment of choice in the U.S.
	Acyclovir 3% ophthalmic ointment, apply to lower lid five times a day for 14 days	Not available in the U.S. but may be better than trifluridine and vidarabine
VZV		
Immunocompromised host	Acyclovir Neonates and children: 500 mg/m^2, I.V. over 1 h every 8 h for 7 days Or children: 600 mg/m^2, P.O. five times a day for 10 days Adults: 10–15 mg/kg, I.V. over 1 h every 8 h for 7 days	Efficacious
Herpes zoster	Acyclovir Children: untested Adults: I.V. as above or 800 mg P.O. five times a day for 7–10 days	Efficacious

372

Virus / Condition	Drug / Dosage	Comments
CMV Disseminated in immunocompromised host	Ganciclovir (DHPG) Neonate: untested Children and adults: 2.5 mg/kg, I.V. over 1 h, every 8 h, or 5 mg/kg, I.V. every 12 h for 14 days	Investigational
Transplant patients prevention of primary CMV infection	Chronic suppressive therapy: 2.5–7.5 mg/kg/day, I.V. over 1 h once daily	Investigational
	Ganciclovir Children and adults: 2–5 mg/kg, I.V. over 1 h, every 8 h for 3–5 weeks	Investigational
	CMV immunoglobulin 150 mg/kg, I.V. within 72 h of transplant, then 100 mg/kg at 2 and 4 weeks, then 50 mg/kg at 6, 8, 12, and 16 weeks	Investigational
	IVIG 500 mg/kg, I.V. at transplant, then at 2 and 4 weeks, then 250 mg/kg at 6 and 8 weeks	Investigational
EBV Infectious mononucleosis	Acyclovir Children: untested Adults: 10 mg/kg/dose, I.V. over 1 h every 8 h for 7 days or 800 mg, P.O. five times a day for 7 days	Investigational
RSV	Ribavirin as aerosol, 20 mg/ml Infants: 1.42 mg/kg/h over 8–20 h for 3–7 days Older children: aerosol at 0.82 mg/kg/h over 8–20 h for 3–7 days IVIG: I.V., one dose at 2 gm/kg over 12–24 hours	Use with mechanical ventilators requires special skills Investigational
Influenza A virus Pneumonia	Amantadine Children: 5–8 mg/kg/day, P.O. once or in two divided doses for 7–10 days (maximum daily dose 200 mg/day) Adults: 200 mg, P.O. once or in two divided doses for 5 days Rimantadine: 5 mg/kg/day once or in two divided doses for 7–10 days Ribavirin aerosol: used as in RSV infection Ribavirin (oral) Adults: loading dose of 1200 mg, P.O. at 0.1 and 2 h, then 1200 mg every 12 h for four doses	Investigational but efficacious Investigational Investigational
High risk group prophylaxis	Amantadine or rimantadine as above for 4–8 weeks during epidemic season	
Influenza B Pneumonia	Ribavirin aerosol and oral therapy as above	Investigational
Rhinovirus Prophylaxis in upper respiratory infection	IFN-α Adults: intranasal spray at 3–10 mu/day for 1 week throughout the season of rhinoviral activity	Investigational
	Eviroxime Adults: nasal spray at 568–2720 μg four to six times per day in the season of activity	Investigational
HIV	Zidovudine Children: Therapy undetermined (Phase 1 study completed) Adults: 250 mg, P.O. or I.V. every 4 h	Investigational Needs to be given indefinitely. Combination therapy with other agents under study
Enteroviruses Chronic enteroviral meningoencephalitis	IVIG Children and adults: adjust dose and frequency to maintain adequate serum IgG concentrations. Intraventricular: (pH 7.4) give commercial IVIG via ventricular access: 1–2 ml/day and may increase up to 10 ml/day, once daily or b.i.d. until CSF is normal	Probable benefit, necessary to determine specific antiviral antibody titer (≥ 1:16)
	Disoxaril (WIN51711) No clinical study	Investigational

Table continued on following page

TABLE 35-2. SUMMARY OF USES OF ANTIVIRAL AGENTS *Continued*

VIRUS AND CLINICAL CONDITION	TREATMENT REGIMEN	COMMENTS
Papilloma virus Laryngeal papillomatosis	IFN-α Children: 5 mu/m^2 daily for 28 days and then three times weekly for 5 months	Investigational
Anogenital warts	IFN-α Adults: intralesional at 1 × 10^6 IU three times a week for 3 weeks	Investigational
Chronic Hepatitis B	IFN-α Adults: steroid withdrawal, followed by interferon 5 × 10^{6}U daily, S.C. for 90 days	Investigational
Chronic non-A, non-B hepatitis	IFN-α Adults: 0.5–5 mu, S.C. daily or three times weekly for 12 months	Investigational
Lassa fever	Ribavirin Adults: 2 gm I.V. loading dose and then 1 gm I.V. every 6 h for 4 days, then 0.5 gm every 8 h for another 6 days *or* 2 gm P.O. loading dose, then 1 gm P.O. every 8 h for 10 days	Used in West Africa Oral therapy is investigational
Measles	Ribavirin Children: 10 mg/kg/day, P.O. for 5–7 days	Investigational
Hepatitis A	Ribavirin Adults: 13 mg/kg/day, P.O. for 14 days	Investigational

the liver seems to prolong the half-life of zidovudine and may be associated with increased toxicity.[63]

Pyrimidine Nucleosides

Idoxyuridine (Iododeoxyuridine, IUdR); Trifluridine (Trifluorothymidine, TFT)

IUdR and TFT are halogenated pyrimidine analogs (Figure 35–2). They are both first-generation antivirals. They are phosphorylated by virus-specific TK and thymidylate kinase to the mono-, di-, and triphosphates. The triphosphates competitively inhibit viral DNA polymerase.[8] However, the principal antiviral activity is due to their incorporation into viral DNA, leading to abnormal transcription and translation.[8]

These agents are available only in topical forms. IUdR is available as a 0.1 percent ophthalmic solution or a 0.5 percent ointment. TFT is available as a 1 percent ophthalmic solution. Their primary use is in the treatment of HSV keratitis. TFT and IUdR are effective in 95 and 76 percent of treated patients, respectively. However, they produce conjunctival irritation and do not affect the rate of recurrence. At the moment, TFT is the drug of choice for treatment of herpetic keratitis (ophthalmic acyclovir preparation, a more tolerable product, is not available in the United States). Intravenous preparations have been shown to be too toxic for clinical use.

Other Antiviral Agents

Amantadine (1-Adamantanamine hydrochloride)

Amatadine is the 1-amino derivative of a complex acyclic compound, amantine (Figure 35–2). Most viruses susceptible to amantadine are enveloped RNA viruses. *In vitro* amatadine has been shown to inhibit uncoating of the viral genome at the early stage.[2] It is also known to elevate the pH of polyendosomes containing the virus,[65] thereby inducing a conformational change in the glycoproteins. However, the peak levels obtained after an oral dose are too low to provide antiviral effect *in vivo* by these means. It has been suggested that amantadine activity against influenza A virus at low concentrations is due to inhibition of a protein that has been termed M_2.[65] This protein is unique to influenza A virus, and it is incorporated into the plasma membrane of infected cells.[65] The present data suggest that the M_2 protein may have a role in the assembly of progeny virions and that amantadine can inhibit this function.

PHARMACOKINETICS. Amantadine is available only as an oral compound, and it is well absorbed after oral administration. After a recommended dose, plasma peak levels are reached in 2–4 hours. The serum half-life is 12–18 hours.[66] It penetrates well into pulmonary tissues with concentrations that are two-thirds of those in serum.[67] Concentrations in salivary and nasal secretions are equal to those in serum.[66] The volume of distribution is about 4–10 liters/kg. This is much larger than the plasma compartment. Amantadine is not metabolized by the body, and more than 90 percent is excreted unchanged in the

urine by renal tubular secretion and glomerular filtration.[68] Urinary alkalinization slows excretion, whereas acidification enhances elimination. Because clearance of amantadine is mainly dependent on renal function, dosage adjustments are necessary with reduced creatinine clearance rates.[69] Because of the extremely large volume of distribution of amantadine and its large total body store, hemodialysis is ineffective, removing less than 5 percent of an oral dose.[69]

TOXICITY. Amantadine is generally well tolerated. However, the major side effects, which occur in 10–33 percent of recipients, involve the central nervous system.[67,70] These side effects are dopaminergic and are primarily those of jitteriness, insomnia, fatigue, difficulty in concentrating, anxiety, depression, and, rarely, hallucinations. They are dose-related and are usually mild and reversible upon cessation of the drug. However, they can be increased with concomitant administration of antihistamines, which are anticholinergics, and reversed by physostigmine administration. Other, less common, side effects, for which causal relationship to amantadine is not established, include deterioration of congestive heart failure, livedo reticularis, and arrhythmias.

Rimantadine (α-Methyl-1-adamatanemethylamine Hydrochloride)

Rimantadine is a closely related derivative of amantadine (Figure 35–2). It is similar to amantadine in its mechanism of action and antiviral spectrum, although rimantadine is reported to be more active against certain strains of influenza A virus.[71]

PHARMACOKINETICS. Rimantadine and amantadine differ markedly in their pharmacokinetic profiles. Rimantadine is well absorbed orally (>90 percent) but has delayed bioavailability, with peak levels achieved at 4.0–4.5 hours after oral administration.[67] The peak plasma concentrations in adults after oral doses of 100 and 200 mg are about 0.2 and 0.3 μg/ml, respectively. The peak plasma concentrations in children given a single dose of 6.6 mg/kg average 0.7 μg/ml.[72] These concentrations are approximately half of those achieved with amantadine.[66] However, the plasma rimantadine concentrations required for *in vitro* inhibition of influenza A viruses are lower than those of amantadine.

Approximately 40 percent of rimantadine is bound to plasma proteins. Its volume of distribution is very large (about 10–15 liters/kg). Unlike amantadine, rimantadine is extensively metabolized, presumably by the liver, to ortho-, para-, and meta-hydroxylated metabolites. Only 25–40 percent of an orally ingested dose is excreted in the urine, of which 90 percent is in the form of metabolites.[66] The half-life of rimantadine is 25–36 hours.[66,67] Because of the large volume of distribution, hemodialysis is ineffective in removing rimantadine. Therefore, in renal insufficiency dosage changes are necessary.

Rimantadine appears to be well concentrated in respiratory secretions, with levels that approach or exceed those found in plasma and are greater than those achieved with amantadine.[66]

TOXICITY. Adverse side effects of rimantadine are rare and significantly less than those of amantadine. The central nervous system side effects observed have been similar to those for placebo groups (4–6 percent).[67] This is thought to be due to low blood levels of rimantadine. When the levels approach those of amantadine, central nervous system side effects are similar. Other adverse effects are related to minor gastrointestinal complaints, including loss of appetite and nausea, which occur in about 16 percent of patients receiving rimantadine and are similar to those for amantadine.

Phosphonoformate (Foscarnet Sodium; PFA)

Phosphonoformate is a pyrophosphate analog (Figure 35–2). It interacts with the pyrophosphate-binding site, inhibiting herpesvirus DNA polymerase without prior phosphorylation.[73] It has been known to be an effective inhibitor of HSV-1 and HSV-2, VZV, CMV, and EBV *in vitro*[74] and also to inhibit reverse transcriptase activity of a variety of animal retroviruses.[75] Phosphonoformate acts as a noncompetitive inhibitor of reverse transcriptase with respect to the substrate and template. Recently, HIV replication *in vitro* has been shown to be inhibited at doses ranging from 0.1 to 0.5 μM.[76]

PHARMACOKINETICS AND CLINICAL APPLICATION. Phosphonoformate is available in topical (3 percent cream) and intravenous forms. The topical preparation has been shown to be effective in shortening the vesicular period of early herpes labialis and genital infections.[77] It also inhibits the development of new lesions. However, comparative clinical trials with acyclovir are needed, and therefore the potential clinical utility of phosphonoformate in the treatment of HSV infections remains unclear.

Intravenous administration requires continuous infusion because of a short half-life and instability at low pH.[78] Most of the drug is eliminated from soft tissues, and about 60–80 percent is excreted intact into the urine. Some of the drug is deposited in the bone matrix without any adverse effect. Preliminary studies of phosphonoformate have shown efficacy in HIV infection[79] and severe disseminated CMV infections in AIDS patients and transplant patients.[78]

TOXICITY. In humans toxicity related to intravenously administered phosphonoformate is low. It may induce anemia and rise in serum creatinine,[78,80] which are reversible. It may be inadvisable to use phosphonoformate concurrently with other nephrotoxic agents. Other minor side effects are nausea, tremor, and phlebitis. Relapses are high (90 percent) after a course of treatment, usually within 1 month of therapy.[80] Therapy requires continuous intravenous infusion, which is a problem in terms of patient compliance.

Further studies are required to evaluate intermittent maintenance therapy and comparative efficacy of phosphonoformate with other anti-CMV agents such as ganciclovir.

Disoxaril (WIN 51711)

Disoxaril is representative of a new structural class of compounds (Figure 35–2). It has antipicornaviral activity.[81] Picornaviruses are RNA-containing viruses that include rhinoviruses and enteroviruses.

Disoxaril inhibits picornavirus replication through viral uncoating (disassembly) following penetration of the cell membrane.[82] It has been shown to achieve antiviral effect in rhinoviruses by binding of the drug by displacement in the peptide chains in the virus coat proteins (VP$_1$).[83]

In vitro studies have shown that rhinovirus serotypes are generally less sensitive than enteroviruses. Among the various classes of enteroviruses, the echovirus group is the most sensitive.[84] *In vivo* studies of orally administered disoxaril in mice have shown efficacy against poliovirus and echovirus infections.[84] Presently, it is not approved for clinical use. Early clinical trials in humans are underway.

Immunomodulators

Interferons

Interferons (IFNs) are naturally occurring host-coded proteins that were first described by Issacs and Lindeman in 1957. They were identified as antiviral factors that appeared in the supernatants of chick chorioallantoic membrane cultures after incubation with ultraviolet-inactivated influenza virus.

Interferon synthesis is induced after an appropriate stimulus of the cell and seems to require both RNA and protein synthesis.[85] Liberated interferons bind and aggregate at the specific receptors on the plasma cell membrane.[86] They are internalized by endocytosis. This triggers events that lead to the production of enzymes and proteins, with eventual establishment of the antiviral state. There are at least three different types of human interferon[87]: IFN-α (leukocyte), produced by lymphocytes and macrophages; IFN-β (fibroblast), produced by fibroblasts and epithelial cells; and IFN-γ (immune), produced by T lymphocytes. IFN-α usually appears after natural infection with viruses or after immunization with double-stranded RNA-containing agents. In general, RNA viruses are more effective interferon inducers than DNA viruses. IFN-β is produced by similar stimuli as IFN-α but has shown a lesser range of effect in viral diseases. IFN-γ is produced after stimulation by mitogens and specific foreign antigens and may be clinically less important as an antiviral substance. All three classes of interferon can now be produced by recombinant techniques, resulting in improved supply and specific activity.

PHARMACOKINETICS. Interferons can be applied locally (intralesionally or topically) or parenterally. When given orally, they are probably inactivated by the proteolytic enzymes in the gastric juices. Interferons behave similarly to plasma proteins in that they pass interchangeably between intravascular and extravascular fluid compartments.[88] Therefore, lower levels are detected in the CSF, aqueous and vitreous humor of the eye, and fetal blood and amniotic fluids. After an intravenous infusion over 24 hours, there is a rapid clearance with plasma half-life of 2–4 hours.[89] After an intramuscular injection, peak levels range from 6 to 8 hours[90] and may be at undetectable levels by 18–36 hours. The half-lives of subcutaneously and intranasally administered interferon are 8–10 hours and 20 minutes, respectively. Even though the plasma half-life of interferon seems short, the antiviral effect persists much longer. Interferon metabolism is less well defined and probably occurs in the liver, skeletal muscles, and lung.[87] It is catabolized mainly by the kidney.[91] Filtered interferons are taken up by the renal tubules and degraded; hence, interferons are rarely recovered from urine.

TOXICITY. The toxicity of intranasally applied interferons is dose-dependent and reversible and includes nasal stuffiness, bloody mucus, and mucosal erosions that have been found in up to 12–25 percent of treated individuals.[87,92,93] Intradermal (intralesional) interferons may produce local inflammation 2–4 hours after administration. This may partly be related to prostaglandin synthesis *in vivo*.[87] With parenteral administration, the most common side effects are fever, chills, and myalgias.[94–96] Less common adverse effects include headaches, fatigue, nausea, anorexia, bone marrow suppression, weight loss, hypotension, confusion, coma, and electroencephalographic changes.[94]

CLINICAL APPLICATIONS. Topical interferons have been used in prophylaxis and treatment of certain respiratory viral infections such as influenza A, rhinoviruses, and coronavirus.[87,92,97] They have also been used in ocular virus infections such as herpes keratitis, adenovirus conjunctivitis, and enterovirus-70 conjunctivitis, and in the treatment of papilloma virus lesions such as condyloma acuminatum,[98] verruca vulgaris, and laryngeal papillomatosis.[99–102] Parenterally administered interferons have been used in viral hepatitis due to hepatitis B[95,103,104] and non-A, non-B viruses.[105] They have also been utilized in the treatment of localized and disseminated HSV-1 and HSV-2 infections; disseminated VZV infections; and CMV infections that occur in renal transplant recipients or other immunosuppressed patients or that are acquired congenitally.[87] Lately, high-dose parenteral interferons have also been used in patients with AIDS and associated Kaposi's sarcoma.[106] Other applications have included intrathecal administration in treatment of subacute sclerosing panencephalitis[107] due to measles virus and in rabies encephalitis.[108]

Clinical applications, however, are limited, and significant clinical responses have been noted only in rhinovirus common colds, herpetic keratitis, condyloma acuminatum, and laryngeal papillomatosis. Moreover, less than 50 percent of published studies reporting improvement have been performed with appropriate controls. The use of interferons may be limited by their high costs and toxicity and the availability of other antiviral agents. Future uses may include combination therapy with steroids and with other antiviral agents. At the moment, interferons are unlicensed for general use in the United States. Therefore, better studies that focus on increasing understanding of the mechanisms of toxicity in addition to devising controlled clinical trials alone or in combination with other forms of therapy are necessary.

Immune Serum Globulin (ISG)

Immunoglobulins (gamma globulins) are proteins that function as the effector molecules (antibody) of B-cell-mediated immunity. There are at least five major classes of immunoglobulin: IgG, IgM, IgA, IgD, and IgE. Apart from IgD, all classes of immunoglobulin have antiviral activity. IgG is the major class of antibody that is present in immunoglobulin preparations available for immunotherapy. These products also contain adequate amounts of the various subclasses of IgG (IgG$_1$, IgG$_2$, IgG$_3$, and IgG$_4$). The specific antiviral activity has been associated with the subclasses IgG$_1$ and IgG$_3$, and less frequently with other subclasses.

PHARMACOKINETICS. The commercially available preparations are licensed for intramuscular and intravenous use. The intramuscular route of administration has several disadvantages, such as pain and discomfort, limitation of volume of administration due to muscle mass size, limitation of frequency of administration, slow and only modest elevation of IgG (maximum levels at 2 days to 2 weeks), and antibody degradation at the site of injection. Intravenous administration, therefore, is the preferred method. It can be given rapidly and repeatedly and in high doses with little discomfort. Intravenous immunoglobulin (IVIG) preparations are prepared by pooling plasma from several hundred to several thousand donors. Therefore there may be a lot-to-lot variation in antibody to viral pathogens. There are also differences in antibody levels between different pharmaceutical preparations. Many of these lots may have high titers by enzyme-linked immunosorbent assay (ELISA) but variable functional activity as determined by viral neutralization, which may be critical for prevention or treatment of viral diseases.

CLINICAL APPLICATIONS. IVIG has been used with variable degrees of success as an antiviral therapeutic and prophylactic agent against a variety of viral diseases. It may improve oxygenation and reduce viral shedding in RSV pneumonia.[109] It can ameliorate the severity of disease expression in primary CMV infection in bone marrow transplant patients.[110,111] It has also been used in the treatment of chronic enteroviral meningoencephalitis in agammaglobulinemic patients, in whom it has been given either intravenously[112,113] or intraventricularly. IVIG therapy may also modify other viral diseases, such as adenovirus pneumonia in immunocompromised patients, in whom uncontrolled treatment trials have shown some efficacy. Virus-specific immunoglobulin has been employed for prophylaxis against measles, hepatitis A, hepatitis B, varicella, rubella, and rabies exposure in susceptible individuals. Administration of immunoglobulin for established viral diseases has not produced beneficial results for these infections.

TOXICITY. Adverse effects of IVIG administration are usually acute and mild. These include flushing of the face, nausea, vomiting, sweating, muscle cramps, headaches, shortness of breath, and fever. These reactions do not warrant discontinuation of therapy. Slowing or stopping the infusion for 15–30 minutes will usually stop the reactions, and IVIG administration can then be resumed. Hypotension and anaphylaxis are much less common and may be more frequent in children with IgA immunodeficiency who have been sensitized to certian immunoglobulin components, such as IgA, as a result of multiple immunoglobulin infusions.[114] Although most currently available products are low in IgA, the minute amounts present can potentially cause production of anti-IgA antibodies.

The risk of transmission of viral infections by IVIG is exceedingly small. The Cohn ethanol method of fractionating human plasma has been shown to eliminate the infectivity of viruses including hepatitis B and HIV. However, transmission of non-A, non-B hepatitis has been reported in a few cases.[115] Since 1985 all commercial products are tested for HIV antibody and the positive preparations are not utilized. However, physicians cannot consider the use of IVIG to be totally without risks.

Interleukin-2 (IL-2)

Interleukin-2 is a lymphokine that is secreted by helper T cells. It participates in expansion and maturity of T-cell and B-cell function. It is important for the stimulation of B cells to proliferate and differentiate into immunoglobulin-secreting cells. IL-2 is also known to stimulate natural killer cells (NKC),[116] which can function as effector cells that mediate antibody-dependent cellular cytotoxicity (ADCC). This can result in the lysis of virus-infected cells. This activity can be augmented by interferon.

Human IL-2 is now available from recombinant technology. Its clinical use, however, is not yet established in treatment of viral diseases. *In vivo* studies of IL-2 have shown enhanced virus killing in HSV-infected animals.[117,118] *In vitro* it also enhances natural killing of VZV-infected cells.[119] Hosts such as neonates with diminished NKC activity are susceptible to severe viral infections, such as those caused by HSV and VZV. However, *in vitro* data suggest that in human neonates, the use of IL-2 alone without concomitant administration of adult leukocytes fails to protect against HSV infection.[120] At the moment, the best potential seems to be in therapy of patients with HIV infection. It has been reported that administration of IL-2 to patients with defective NKC can enhance lysis of HIV-infected cells.[121] Initial clinical studies in patients with AIDS have shown some benefit.[122] IL-2 must be given intravenously. Its half-life is less than 1 hour; hence, constant infusions seem to be indicated.[123] Its metabolism in humans is unknown. Animal studies suggest renal tubular catabolism of filtered IL-2.[123]

TOXICITY. The toxic effects of IL-2 are frequent and can be very severe. In a study involving cancer patients, all patients developed fever, fatigue, hypoalbunemia, eosinophilia, erythematous rash with pruritus and scaling, and anemia that required blood transfusions.[124] Other frequent side effects were nausea, diarrhea, stomatitis, and oliguria with fluid retention. Further studies regarding the dosage, mode, and duration of administration are necessary to achieve less toxic side effects before large-scale clinical trials of efficacy in viral diseases can be attempted.

Ampligen

Ampligen is a mismatched double-stranded RNA (dsRNA) containing Poly(1):Poly($C_{12}U$) ribonucleotide chains. dsRNAs promote production of various lymphokines such as tumor necrosis factor (TNF) and interferons. Ampligen, as a mismatched dsRNA, retains this activity without having the known dsRNA toxicities. It is known to augment NKC and monocyte activities and aid in B-cell maturation through the interferon effect.[125] *In vitro* studies have shown anti-HIV activity when used singly or in synergistic combination with zidovudine.[126] A recent small clinical study has shown some benefit in patients with ARC/LAC, with improvement in symptoms and immune augmentation for both T- and B-cell function.[127] Ampligen was not toxic when given intravenously. It may, therefore, be useful in combination therapy with zidovudine and interferon, and may allow dosage reductions of other agents to reduce toxicity. An added benefit is the ability of ampligen to cross the blood–brain barrier. Appropriately controlled, long-term studies are needed to establish its use in clinical practice.

THERAPEUTIC USES OF ANTIVIRAL AGENTS

Respiratory Infections

Viral respiratory tract infections account for about 30–40 percent of illnesses warranting a pediatrician's attention. Most of these are self-limited and do not require specific antiviral chemotherapy. The following viruses may require therapy when indicated. Treatment regimen is summarized in Table 35–2.

Respiratory Syncytial Virus (RSV)

Lower respiratory tract infections such as bronchiolitis and pneumonia due to RSV are of concern in infants younger than 2 months of age and those with cardiopulmonary disease or immunodeficiency. Patients in these high-risk groups and those hospitalized with moderate-to-severe infection have been shown to benefit from aerosolized ribavirin.[128,129] This is given via a small-particle generator, SPAG-2. The standard concentration of ribavirin in the reservoir of the aerosol generator is 20 mg/ml. The estimated dose for infants less than 1 year of age is 1.42 mg/kg/h, and for older children it is 0.82 mg/kg/h.[130] It can be administered over 8–20 hours via a face mask, oxygen hood, or nasal tube. Delivery via a ventilator is difficult because of crystallization of the drug in the apparatus. This should be attempted only in tertiary care units experienced in the use of the drug and capable of constant patient observation.[52] The duration of therapy varies from 3 to 7 days. The best results are obtained if therapy is instituted within the first 3 days of the onset of lower respiratory disease. Improvement in oxygenation is usually seen within the first 24 hours after the initiation of therapy. However, the duration of hospitalization and the mortality rate remain unaffected. There is presently a debate on selection criteria for the high-risk patient and on the cost and benefit of the therapy.[131]

Recently, IVIG has been tried in a study of children with pneumonia or bronchiolitis.[109] IVIG was given at a dose of 2 gm/kg over 12–24 hours. This resulted in significant reductions in nasal RSV shedding and in improvements in transcutaneous oximetry readings. However, the mean duration of hospitalization was not reduced. Theoretically, IVIG may be more effective when given in combination with ribavirin. The use of IVIG needs to be considered with caution, because of a lot-to-lot variation in titers of neutralizing antibody to RSV. Further studies are necessary before general recommendations can be made.

Influenza Viruses

Prophylaxis and treatment of influenza A infection can be achieved with oral amantadine and rimantadine. Both drugs have been tested in children and found to be safe and efficacious.[132–136] Rimantadine has fewer adverse effects; however, it is not yet licensed for general use in the United States.

The dosage of amantadine in prophylaxis of children is 5–8 mg/kg/day divided every 12 hours (maximum 200 mg/day). The dosage for treatment of uncomplicated influenza A infection is the same continued for 7 days. It should be started within 48 hours of onset of clinical symptoms. The dosage of rimantadine for prophylaxis is 5 mg/kg/day.

Ribavirin aerosol used in a manner similar to the treatment of RSV has been shown to be effective against influenza A and B infections.[137] However, a recent study has failed to show efficacy against influenza B infection.[138] Ribavirin has also been used orally. When high-dose therapy was given in a double-blind, placebo-controlled study,[139] it produced better efficacy results than in earlier studies using lower doses.[140] The high-dose regimen was given as an initial loading dose of 1200 mg repeated 1 and 2 hours later and maintained at 1200 mg every 12 hours for 2 days. It was tolerated well.

Rhinoviruses

These agents account for 30–50 pecent of common colds. Because of the frequency and associated morbidity of common colds, various methods of therapeutic interventions have been attempted. Rhinoviruses also frequently cause lower respiratory infections in children.

Natural and recombinant human interferons have received the most comprehensive clinical testing involving adult subjects. Prophylactic efficacy trials have shown high-level efficacy. Intranasal spray of IFN-α_2 (rIFN-a$_2$) has been used most extensively in research trials. Doses for IFN-α_2 vary from 3 to 10 million units (MU)[87,92] per day during peak periods for rhinoviral activity in the community. It has also been used at 5 MU per day administered for 1 week after exposure to illness in the family setting.[93] Other forms of interferons, such as rIFN-a$_2$, rIFN-a(Ly), and HuIFN-b, have been used with similar results. However, the 12–15 percent rate of nasal irritation and mucous membrane destruction is sufficient to discourage use for prevention of mild illnesses like common colds. Therapeutic trials for established rhinoviral infection have met with little success.

Enviroxime, a benzimidazole derivative, has *in vitro* inhibitory activity against many serotypes of rhinoviruses and has been tested in oral and topical forms in rhinoviral infections.[97] Prophylactic trials using a nasal spray at doses ranging from 568 to 2720 μg four to six times per day have shown efficacy that ranges from modest to none. Similarly, oral therapy has shown poor absorption and efficacy. Therapeutic trials of enviroxime have shown no significant benefit in naturally occurring rhinovirus colds.[141]

Coronaviruses

These agents are responsible for 7–20 percent of common colds. Prophylactic trials of interferon rIFN-a in experimentally induced colds using adult volunteers have shown modest efficacy when high doses (9.0 MU/day) were employed.[87] As in rhinoviral infections, no practical therapy is available for children.

Herpesvirus Infections

Herpes Simplex Virus (HSV) Infections

Mucocutaneous Infections

Examples of this form of HSV infection are gingivostomatitis, genital herpes, keratitis, herpetic whitlow, and eczema herpeticum. Oral herpes in the form of gingivostomatitis has not been studied regarding specific antiviral therapy. In severe cases requiring hospitalization, intravenous acyclovir may be expected to be as effective as in primary genital infection. Topical therapy with 5 percent acyclovir ointment has produced disappointing results for recurrent oral lesions. No controlled clinical trials of acyclovir therapy for primary oral lesions have been undertaken.

Genital Herpes

Acyclovir is the drug of choice. Topical, oral, and intravenous forms are all beneficial (see Table 35–2 for dosage guide). However, oral and intravenous forms are superior in the treatment of primary genital herpes.[142] Oral administration is more practical for outpatient use and cheaper than intravenous treatment, although both are equally efficacious. It is given for 10 days. Intravenous treatment should be reserved for the acutely ill requiring hospitalization or for those who cannot take oral medication. Therapy should be initiated as soon as possible in primary herpes. Treatment with acyclovir has no effect on future recurrences unless it is used as a chronic suppressive therapy.[143,144] This is recommended for those with six or more recurrences per year. Prophylactic acyclovir in children for recurrent herpes lesions has been untested. In adults, studies extending up to 1 year have shown good efficacy and safety.[143] Presently, acyclovir is approved in the United States for use up to 6 months.

HSV Keratitis

Topical preparations such as idoxyuridine, vidarabine, trifluridine, acyclovir, and interferon have been tested. Idoxyuridine is less efficacious and more toxic than other available agents.[145] At the moment, trifluridine in a 1 percent ophthalmic solution is the drug of choice for primary or recurrent HSV keratitis or lid infection. It is used as one drop per eye every 2 hours while awake until healing occurs. Vidarabine ophthalmic ointment is less effective than trifluridine.[37] A topical ophthalmic preparation of acyclovir has been shown to be useful[146,147] but is unavailable in the United States for clinical use.

Neonatal HSV

Babies with neonatal HSV can have localized disease in the skin, eye, mouth, or central nervous system, or it can be disseminated with manifestations of hepatitis, disseminated intravascular coagulation, and pneumonitis, with or without evidence of encephalitis. The morbidity and mortality of this disease is significant.

Neonatal HSV treatment trials have included therapy with intravenous idoxyuridine, cytosine arabinoside, vidarabine,[148] and acyclovir. Vidarabine and acyclovir have been shown to have comparable efficacy in a placebo-controlled trial in the newborn.[149,150] At the moment acyclovir seems preferable to vidarabine because acyclovir avoids the problems associated with vidarabine, such as excessive fluid administration during the 12-hour or longer infusion period and the need for another intravenous access for other medications. However, acyclovir is yet to be approved by the Food and Drug Administration (FDA) in the United States for use in the newborn. The recommended dose of acyclovir is 10 mg/kg/dose given intravenously every 8 hours for 10–14 days. Vidarabine is recommended to be used at doses of 30 mg/kg/day given as a 12- to 24-hour infusion for 10–14 days. Therapy should be instituted at the earliest suspicion of the disease. Although untested in clinical trials, prophylactic therapy seems warranted in high-risk babies such as those born to mothers with primary herpes at the time of delivery. In this situation all appropriate cultures must be obtained prior to initiating therapy. Babies with ocular involvement should receive topical antiviral medication such as trifluridine, idoxyuridine, or vidarabine in addition to parenteral therapy.

Herpes Simplex Encephalitis (HSE)

HSE occurs at all ages (25–30 percent of cases in children), in all races, and throughout the year. It primarily involves the inferior and medial portion of the temporal lobe and the orbitofrontal region of the frontal lobe. Well-controlled trials have shown that acyclovir has therapeutic superiority over vidarabine.[151,152] Mortality 6 months after starting acyclovir treatment has dropped to 20 percent as compared to 40 percent for those treated with vidarabine.

The recommended dose of intravenous acyclovir is 10 mg/kg/dose every 8 hours for 10–14 days. At this point, though, the optimal dosage and duration are not yet known. There is about a 5 percent rate of relapse after therapy.[151–153] Future recommendations may involve longer therapy of at least 14–21 days. In cases of relapse, a second 14-day course of acyclovir should be given.

HSV in the Immunocompromised Host

HSV in the immunocompromised host can cause acute and severe mucocutaneous disease, which may become persistent. The risk of dissemination and death is low. Topical, oral, and intravenous administrations of acyclovir have shown benefit in several studies. Oral and intravenous therapy used prophylactically in seropositive transplant patients[28,32,154,155] and in leukemic patients undergoing induction chemotherapy has shown efficacy in preventing infection. However, the appropriate dosage and duration of therapy are yet to be determined.

Pharmacokinetic studies in children indicate that an oral dose of 600 mg/m² given four times a day is needed to achieve therapeutic levels.[26,156] Lower plasma levels, though, have shown efficacy in prophylaxis trials.[155] In adolescents and adults, an oral dose of 200–400 mg is given five times daily. If patients cannot tolerate oral medications, intravenous acyclovir should be given at 250 mg/m² or 5 mg/kg every 8 hours. Prophylactic therapy has been instituted 3–7 days prior to transplantation and continued for 3–5 weeks in some of the studies. Patients with recurrent disease may be placed on chronic suppressive therapy. In established mucocutaneous infections in children, milder manifestations can be treated orally at 600 mg/m² given four times a day, and severe manifestations such as herpes esophagitis should be treated intravenously at 15 mg/kg (10 mg/kg in neonates) per dose given every 8 hours. Vidarabine has also been shown to be effective, but substantially less than acyclovir, in the treatment of mucocutaneous HSV infection in the immunocompromised host.

Varicella-Zoster Virus (VZV) Infections

Treatment of VZV in otherwise healthy children does not seem warranted. In immunocompromised children, VZV infections can be severe, with cutaneous and visceral dissemination and a high rate of mortality. This can occur from both primary varicella (chickenpox) and varicella zoster (shingles). Both vidarabine[39] and acyclovir have been shown to be efficacious. However, acyclovir is shown to be much better in reducing the clinical disease and halting the dissemination[157] and therefore seems to be the drug of choice. It is given intravenously at 500 mg/m² every 8 hours for 7 days. It must be started within 72 hours of onset of infection. VZV requires higher inhibitory concentrations of acyclovir than that necessary to inhibit HSV-1 and HSV-2. Oral dosage for children may have to exceed 600 mg/m²/dose. No clinical trials have been conducted in children regarding oral therapy. A small and uncontrolled study of 10 children receiving oral doses of 250–650 mg/m²/dose given five times a day for 10 days showed good efficacy.[28] A study conducted in adults showed that 800 mg of acyclovir given five times a day for 7 days is effective in modifying acute herpes zoster.[158]

Future efforts may focus on 6-deoxyacyclovir,[159] the prodrug of acyclovir, which when given orally is converted to acyclovir and produces fourfold higher plasma concentrations.

Cytomegalovirus (CMV) Infections

Infection due to CMV is usually asymptomatic in previously well hosts. However, in the congenital form and the acquired form in an immunocompromised host, it can affect the central nervous system resulting in mental retardation, hearing impairment, encephalitis, and retinitis, and involve other organs producing pneumonia, colitis, hepatitis, hemolytic anemia, thrombocytopenia, and graft rejection. In the normal host, it may also produce CMV mononucleosis.

Treatment in the immunocompromised host has been largely unsuccessful with agents such as idoxyuridine, vidarabine, acyclovir, and Ara-C. Ganciclovir seems to be the most effective anti-CMV agent yet developed. It has been shown to produce clinical and virologic improvement,[6,49,160,161] but efficacy in patients with advanced CMV pneumonia has been less encouraging.[6,162] It has not yet been studied in congenital CMV infections. In bone marrow transplant patients and organ recipients, a short course of ganciclovir for 2 weeks may be adequate to reduce various manifestations of CMV infection in the high-risk period after transplantation.[161] In contrast, patients with longer-lasting immunosuppression associated with AIDS and neoplasms may require chronic suppressive therapy to prevent relapses. Ganciclovir is used at a dose of 2.5 mg/kg given intravenously over 1 hour at 8-hour intervals or 5 mg/kg at 12-hour intervals.[49,160,162] Maintenance therapy has been attempted at 2.5–7.5 mg/kg/day[49,160] given as a single intravenous dose for 5–7 days/week; however, appropriate dose and duration are yet undetermined. Although pediatric patients of various ages have been included in larger studies of treatment with intravenous ganciclovir that involved patients of all age groups, there have been no controlled clinical trials exclusively in children. Therefore, efficacy and toxicity in children are undetermined. At present, ganciclovir is an investigational drug.

CMV immune globulin[110,163] and high-titer intravenous immunoglobulin[111,164,165] have been shown to be beneficial for prophylaxis in renal transplant patients who are at high risk for primary CMV disease. These agents may decrease the incidence of clinically evident disease but may not affect the rates of viral isolation or seroconversion.[110] No standard therapeutic regimen exists. In one study, CMV immune globulin was given intravenously at a dose of 150 mg/kg within 72 hours after transplantation, then 100 mg/kg 2 and 4 weeks after transplantation, then 50 mg/kg 6, 8, 12, and 16 weeks after transplantation.[110] Commercially available unselected lots of IVIG have been used at a regimen of 500 mg/kg at the time of transplant and at 2 and 4 weeks, followed by 250 mg/kg at 6 and 8 weeks.[164] The use of immunoglobulin is considered investigational, and careful virologic and immunologic monitoring is required.

Prophylaxis with human and recombinant IFN-α has been shown to suppress viremia and clinical signs of CMV infection,[87] although this is disputed by other studies. In one trial, human IFN-α given intramuscularly at 3 MU/day three times a week for 6 weeks and then twice a week for 8 weeks provided clinical benefit.[166]

It is possible that combination therapy with the above agents may be more effective.

Epstein-Barr Virus (EBV) Infections

EBV infection can be asymptomatic or cause infectious mononucleosis with occasional fatality, or it may follow a chronic or recurrent course. In the immunocompromised host, it has been associated with the development of lymphoproliferative disorders, hemophagocytic syndrome, lymphocytic interstitial pneumonia, and possibly oral hairy leukoplakia. It is also thought to be related to malignancies such as African Burkitt's lymphoma, nasopharyngeal carcinoma, and thymic carcinoma.

Clinical symptoms in infectious mononucleosis are thought to be due to cellular cytotoxic reactions against infected B cells. This reaction may also be responsible for other manifestations of EBV. Recent therapeutic trials have concentrated mostly on acyclovir because of its *in vitro* inhibition of EBV within achievable plasma levels and relative safety.[18] Thus far, its effects on the clinical course of infectious mononucleosis and chronic infections, including chronic fatigue syndrome, have been found to be discouraging. In infectious mononucleosis, it is shown to inhibit oropharyngeal secretion of EBV, which resumes after discontinuation of acyclovir.[20,167] This may be because it does not eliminate latent infection from infected B cells. In one study it was shown to reduce the oropharyngeal symptoms but had no effect on systemic clinical manifestations such as lymphadenopathy, spleen and liver enlargement, or elevated levels of liver enzymes. Intravenous acyclovir at a dose of 10 mg/kg given every 8 hours for 7 days[20] and oral acyclovir at a dose of 800 mg five times a day for 7 days[167] have produced similar results in two different studies. It is postulated that acyclovir given early in the course of the disease and for longer duration may be more efficient.[167] In chronic fatigue syndrome, a well-controlled study demonstrated no efficacy when acyclovir was given intravenously at 500 mg/m^2 every 8 hours for 7 days, followed by 800 mg by mouth four times a day for 30 days.[168] At present, the role of acyclovir in the management of EBV infections is not clear, although sporadic reports exist of its benefit in a few severely ill patients.

Other agents of potential benefit include ganciclovir, which has *in vitro* activity against EBV but has not been tried in clinical settings. Interferon prophylaxis in renal transplant recipients has not been shown to significantly reduce reactivation of EBV.[169]

Enteroviral Infections

The human enteroviruses include the polioviruses, coxsackieviruses A and B, echoviruses, and other serotypes of enteroviruses that are labeled only by numbers.

Although enteroviruses may cause poliomyelitis and myocarditis, most enteroviral illnesses are asymptomatic or very mild in the immunologically normal individual. There are two groups of individuals who are at risk for severe infection due to enteroviruses: (1) Infants in the perinatal period are at high risk for succumbing to meningitis, encephalitis, myocarditis, and/or hepatitis. (2) Persons with antibody deficiencies, in particular X-linked agammaglobulinemic patients, are prone to vaccine-associated paralytic poliomyelitis and to chronic enteroviral meningoencephalitis (CEMA).

Presently, the treatment of enterovirus infections is supportive. Patients with CEMA have been given gamma globulin preparations in an uncontrolled manner. Intramuscular gamma globulins have been unsatisfactory as maintenance prophylaxis. IVIG seems to offer hope in preventing infection, but in infected individuals it does not prevent the slow loss of cognitive function and periodic relapses.[112] It is suggested that the virus isolated from these patients be serotyped and specific neutralizing antibody titers tested. The effective neutralizing titer is not known, but titers of 1:16 or more may be adequate. Antibodies to most common enteroviral serotypes are usually well represented in commercial IVIG preparations. It is recommended that these patients be given IVIG at a dose and frequency adequate to maintain trough IgG concentrations of 900–1000 mg/dl and peak concentrations of > 1500 mg/dl, with periodic testing of virus-specific antibody titers in the patient's serum. Some patients whose condition did not improve have then been given immunoglobulin via intraventricular catheters or reservoirs.[113] This treatment involves giving immunoglobulin preparations with a neutralizing antibody titer of ≥1:16 against the patient's isolate and a pH as close to 7.4 as possible. One to two milliliters is given daily and may be increased up to 10 ml/day, given once or divided in twice-daily doses. The duration of therapy has not been established, but therapy has been recommended to be given until all viral cultures of both ventricular and lumbar fluid have been negative on at least two occasions. The results of this therapy have been mixed.

One promising therapeutic modality of the future is an agent called disoxaril (WIN51711) that has been shown to have antienteroviral activity *in vitro* and *in vivo* in animal models.[84,170] There have been no clinical trials of this drug.

Interferon in synergism with antibody has been shown to neutralize some enteroviruses *in vitro*.[171] However, there are no published reports of its use in CEMA patients.

Human Immunodeficiency Virus (HIV) Infection

HIV-infected children can be asymptomatic or symptomatic with AIDS characterized by opportunistic infections such as *Pneumocystis carinii* pneumonia, neurologic abnormalities, interstitial pneumonitis, and recurrent bacterial infections.

In vitro reverse transcriptase inhibitory activity has been demonstrated with suramin, phosphonoformate, zidovudine, 2′, 3′-dideoxycytidine (ddC), ribavirin, rifamycin derivatives, ampligen, IFN-α, and HPA-23. Of these, only zidovudine is undergoing clinical testing in children. A phase 1 study of pediatric AIDS patients has evaluated the safety and efficacy of zidovudine at 80, 120, or 160 mg/m^2/dose given intravenously every 6 hours, followed by chronic oral zidovudine at one to five times the intravenous dose.[172] It was tolerated well, but some patients developed anemia, neutropenia, and transient elevation of liver enzymes. Studies in adult patients with AIDS and ARC have reached a more advanced stage.[60,63,173] A recently completed double-blind, placebo-controlled trial of zidovudine[173] in these patients demonstrated that zidovudine recipients (250 mg every 4 hours by mouth) had improved survival, weight gain, skin test reactivity, number of opportunistic infections, and CD4 lymphocyte numbers in peripheral blood. This has led to approval of zidovudine for adults who have symptomatic HIV infection and have a history of cytologically confirmed *P. carinii* pneumonia or an absolute CD4 lymphocyte count of less than 200/mm^3 in peripheral blood. At present, zidovudine is unapproved for use in children. Further controlled studies are necessary to determine the appropriate dose, frequency, duration, and efficacy in children.

Another agent of promise is ddC, a dideoxynucleoside (Figure 35–2) that is 10 times more potent *in vitro* than zidovudine. Recently, a phase 1 clinical trial of ddC in adult AIDS/ARC patients was completed.[174] ddC was given intravenously for 14 days at different doses: 0.03 mg/kg every 8 hours, 0.03 mg/kg every 4 hours, or 0.25 mg/kg every 8 hours. This was followed by oral ddC at the same dose for an additional 4 weeks. This study showed that ddC can be tolerated in the short term with *in vitro* virostatic drug levels and that it is well absorbed. Immunologic and virologic improvement was seen. Some patients were also given combination therapy of zidovudine alternating with ddC.[174] Patients received 200 mg zidovudine orally every 4 hours for 7-day periods, alternating with 0.03 mg/kg ddc orally every 4 hours for 7-day periods for a total of 9 or more weeks. This regimen also was well tolerated with immunologic and virologic benefits. It was also noted that this combination therapy reduced the incidence of anemia associated with the use of zidovudine alone; however, the use of ddC over a prolonged period was associated with painful peripheral neuropathy. Larger controlled studies of these regimens need to be done.

Phosphonoformate has been shown in preliminary studies to achieve adequate virostatic levels in serum and CSF. A pilot study using continuous phosphonoformate[79] at a dose of 20 mg/kg/h for 3 weeks was associated with inhibition of reverse transcriptases but no increase in CD4$^+$ cells. Orally bioavailable analogs of phosphonoformate have been developed. Phase 1 trials utilizing intravenous and oral phosphonoformate are currently underway.

Ribavirin, a well-known antiviral agent, also has *in vitro* HIV inhibitory activity. A phase 1 study involving oral ribavirin has been conducted in HIV-infected adults.[175] It was given at varying doses. Long-term therapy involved a loading dose of 1200 mg twice daily for 3 days, followed by 300 mg twice daily for 1 year. It was tolerated well. However, review of data from ribavirin trials by the FDA has indicated no substantial evidence of efficacy. Further clinical trials are currently underway to evaluate its role in the treatment of AIDS. Combination therapy of ribavirin with zidovudine needs caution because of the antagonism shown *in vitro*.[176]

AL721, which is thought to interfere with attachment of HIV to CD4 receptors on cells, has *in vitro* inhibitory activity against HIV.[3] In preliminary trials in human elderly subjects given 10–15 gm of AL721 per day by mouth, it was well tolerated without adverse effects.[3] Preliminary studies in AIDS patients have shown promising results.[177,178] Recently, phase 1 clinical trials in patients with ARC and HIV-related persistent generalized lymphadenopathy have begun.

Acyclovir has weak activity against HIV; however, it potentiates *in vitro* activity of zidovudine due to unknown mechanisms. Equivalent anti-HIV activity can be obtained *in vitro* with lower concentrations of zidovudine. A phase 1 study has been done that involved administration of 100 mg of zidovudine orally every 4 hours for 7 days, followed by 100 mg of zidovudine and 800 mg of acyclovir orally every 4 hours for an additional 9 weeks.[179] This was conducted in patients with AIDS and ARC who received zidovudine at half the recommended dose. This regimen was well tolerated with improved immunologic and virologic parameters. It was also associated with lesser bone marrow toxicity than seen with zidovudine therapy alone. Further large-scale controlled studies are required before this therapy can be recommended.

Other reverse transcriptase inhibitors, such as HPA-23 (a mineral-condensed polyanion containing tungsten and antimony)[180] and suramin,[181] have been tested in AIDS patients with limited clinical improvement. Peptide T, an octapeptide that blocks the binding of the viral envelope to the CD4 receptor,[4] has been tested in a small number of patients with encouraging results.[182] Further clinical testing is now underway.

Immunomodulators such as IL-2, IFN-α, and ampligen have also received therapeutic trials. Small clinical studies of intravenously given natural product or recombinant human IL-2 have been conducted in cancer[124] and AIDS[122,183] patients. These studies have shown improved immunologic response. In patients with AIDS, it was given at doses ranging from 250 to 10^7 U/day by continuous intravenous infusion. Serious nonopportunistic bacterial infections developed in a significant number of patients. The explanation for this is unknown, but the use of IL-2 needs very careful study. Recombinant IFN-α has also been given to patients with AIDS at a concentration of 1×10^7 U/mg protein and a dose of 0.001–1.0 mg/m²/day.[122] The virologic and immunologic parameters with this therapy have not been discussed, but it was tolerated well with no serious side effects. Ampligen has also undergone phase 1 clinical trials, with good tolerance and probable efficacy.[127]

In summary, anti-HIV chemotherapy in children with HIV infection is not yet available. Zidovudine is the only agent tested so far in children and needs further study. It seems that combination therapy may be more effective, with lesser toxicity of individual agents. Treatment of asymptomatic children needs to be defined, which theoretically should be more helpful in suppressing the progression of HIV infection.

Human Papillomavirus (HPV) Infections

HPV infection in adults is a sexually transmitted disease that involves mucus membranes and skin. It is manifested by formation of warts (condylomata acuminata) on the penis, anus, vulva, vagina, and cervix. HPV may be acquired from the maternal genital tract during delivery and is known to cause laryngeal papillomatosis, a progressive intractable condition that presents primarily in preschool children. This may produce life-threatening obstruction. HPV also has oncogenic potential. Effective anti-HPV therapy is therefore necessary.

For the treatment of laryngeal papillomatosis in children, a double-blind, placebo-controlled study using IFN-α_{N1} given intramuscularly at a dose of 5 MU/m² daily for 28 days and three times weekly for 5 months has shown significant improvement when it was used as an adjuvant to surgery.[99] However, another clinical trial has found diminished efficacy during the posttreatment followup period.[102] A recent review of toxicity of this therapy[94] has shown controllable and reversible side effects, such as fever, headache, chills, myalgia, nausea, fatigue, neurologic manifestations, and growth retardation. However, in view of the serious nature of this disease, these effects may be considered tolerable. At the moment, the optimum dosage, frequency, and duration are undetermined and its use is to be considered experimental.

Anogenital warts have long been treated with weekly topical application of 25 percent podophyllin ointment, with cure rates of less than 30 percent. The practical use of podophyllin is also limited by systemic toxic effects, potential teratogenicity, and unsuitability for application on the cervix, anus, and urethra. It is contraindicated in children because they may digitally transfer some of the ointment to other body areas. Cryotherapy, electrical cautery, and CO_2 laser application are effective and are the treatments of choice. Intralesional IFN-α therapy has been tried in the treatment of anogenital warts.[96,98] It may be useful adjunct therapy for older and intractable warts. However, response is generally better for younger warts. IFN-α_{2b} was found to be effective and tolerable in a large, multicenter, randomized, double-blind study.[96] Patients received intralesional interferon at a dose of 1×10^6 IU given three times weekly for 3 weeks and observed for 13 weeks. Warts decreased in size in 62.4 percent of patients and disappeared completely in 35 percent. However, in the latter group, there was a relapse rate of 21 percent. Because of the large doses and multiple frequency of injections required, interferon may be less useful in the treatment of multiple warts. Also, interferon therapy for warts in HIV-infected patients seems less effective.[96]

At present, interferon therapy for anogenital warts seems a promising modality, but it is unlicensed for use in the United States and its use must be considered experimental.

Hepatitis B Virus (HBV) Infection

HBV disease can be acute or chronic. Infants who are infected within the first year of life have a more than 90 percent chance of developing chronic HBV infection, as compared to 5–10 percent among adults. Chronic HBV infection seems to be associated with an increased rate of cirrhosis and hepatoma.

Treatment of acute HBV infection is supportive. For chronic HBV infection, various therapeutic modalities have been studied. Among these, therapy with corticosteroids, vidarabine, Ara-AMP, and acyclovir has generally been unsuccessful. The interferons seem to be the most promising agent yet studied. IFN-α given intramuscularly at 5–10 MU/day for 2–4 months has produced a response in 30–40 percent of patients.[103] However, termination of HBV infection is rare. When IFN-α was used with Ara-AMP as a combination therapy, it was found to be ineffective.[184] A recent study of adult patients, using a combination of steroid withdrawal followed by recombinant human IFN-α_{2b} given subcutaneously at a dose of 5 MU daily for 90 days, has shown the best results thus far.[95] However, these patients have not been followed far enough, and large well-controlled studies are necessary before conclusions can be drawn. In view of the extremely high rate of chronicity after HBV infection in infants, studies are also warranted in this age group. Treatment is likely to be most effective if initiated in the first year of chronic HBV infection before HBV can become integrated into the host cell genome.

Non-A, Non-B Hepatitis Infection

An agent associated with this disease is yet unidentified, and reliable serologic markers have not been developed. Nonetheless, it is an important cause of chronic liver disease, and in 15–25 percent of infected individuals it leads to cirrhosis, portal hypertension, and hepatic failure.

There is currently no effective therapy for chronic non-A, non-B hepatitis infection. Therapy with corticosteroids has been unsuccessful. Recently, subcutaneously administered recombinant human IFN-α given at varying doses of 0.5–5 MU daily, every other day, or three times a week for up to 12 months showed efficacy in controlling the disease activity.[105] Further controlled studies are needed to assess the role of interferon therapy in the treatment of this disease.

Lassa Fever, Hepatitis A, and Measles

Lassa fever is a disease caused by Lassa virus that is endemic in parts of West Africa and has a mortality rate of 15–20 percent from irreversible hypovolemic shock. It has been successfully treated in adults with intravenous ribavirin given as a 2-gm loading dose and then 1 gm every 6 hours (55 mg/kg) for another 6 days.[57] The best results were obtained when ribavirin was used during the first 6 days of illness. Oral ribavirin is also effective, but the proper dosage regimen has not yet been established.[57]

Oral ribavirin has been tested against measles outside the United States. Reports of efficacy have been published from Mexico, Brazil, and the Phillipines.[185] Three double-blind, placebo-controlled studies have shown ribavirin to be effective in reducing the severity, duration of illness, and complications of measles. The dose used is 10 mg/kg for 5–7 days.

Favorable results have been reported for oral ribavirin treatment of hepatitis A virus infection.[186] It is used at 13 mg/kg/day for 14 days. Treatment was associated with rapid recovery from illness and return to normal liver function parameters. However, ribavirin is not approved for use in the United States in the treatment of measles or hepatitis A virus infections.

POTENTIAL PROBLEMS OF ANTIVIRAL THERAPY

Resistance to Antiviral Agents

As more antiviral agents become available, their use is also expected to increase, sometimes in an inappropriate manner. With the selective pressure of antiviral agents, mutant viruses are likely to emerge. As of now, the most evident example is that of the emergence of HSV mutants against nucleoside analogs. Three basic mechanisms of resistance have been described. First, HSV and VZV mutants deficient in TK may be selected.[187] This results in lack of phosphorylation of nucleoside analogs that depend on viral TK. It is also the most important mechanism of resistance of HSV against acyclovir. Second, HSV mutants that possess altered TK may be selected.[188] These mutants phosphorylate thymidine but not acyclovir (altered substrate specificity). Third, HSV mutants with an altered DNA polymerase activity may be selected.[187] Because nucleoside analogs also exhibit antiviral activity by inhibition of DNA polymerase, these mutants can be resistant to all nucleoside analogs and also to phosphonoacetic acid.

The development of resistance to nucleoside analogs is important to recognize because it may lead to therapeutic failure and potential spread through the susceptible human reservoir. In clinical practice, resistance to acyclovir in HSV infection has been noted almost exclusively in immunocompromised patients receiving systemic and chronic therapy. In most cases, the occurrence of these isolates has been associated with prolonged viral shedding and low-grade infection.[189] However, progressive and destructive lesions have been described in a few cases.[190,191] Almost all of the mutant isolates from patients have exhibited diminished TK activity. Overall, resistant strains emerge much less readily, probably because TK-defective strains have reduced virulence.

Other resistant viruses have also been reported. A CMV

mutant that phosphorylates ganciclovir poorly has been described.[192] Influenza A virus resistant to amantadine[193] and rimantadine has been demonstrated experimentally. Heider et al.[194] have reported two virus isolates from an H3N2 influenza A epidemic that were relatively resistant to amantadine and rimantadine.[194] Similarly, Hall et al.[134] have reported isolation of rimantadine-resistant influenza A virus from infected children who were treated with rimantadine. This was associated with rebound in viral shedding. Its occurrence, however, is not widespread and the exact mechanism of resistance is unknown.

The need for prevention of the development of resistant viruses must be appreciated. It should be approached with concern while new antiviral agents are being developed. Unnecessary and excessive use of antiviral agents must be avoided. The full importance of this problem can be understood only if the emergence of resistance is carefully monitored.

Teratogenicity and Oncogenicity of Antiviral Agents

The long-term complication arising from brief or prolonged therapy with antiviral agents is unknown. Because many antiviral agents are incorporated into nucleic acids, they have potential for oncogenicity and mutagenicity. This has been demonstrated in cell culture systems with vidarabine and acyclovir.[195,196] Vidarabine has also been demonstrated to have teratogenicity in animals.[196] It is only prudent, therefore, to avoid antiviral agents during pregnancy and inadvisable to conceive children while on therapy except under exceptional circumstances.

FUTURE PROSPECTS

Antiviral therapy is making rapid advances. As our knowledge of molecular events of viral replication expands, more effective antiviral compounds will inevitably be developed, especially for chronic and latent infections. The final goal should be to develop drugs that are biologically active only in virus-infected cells, can be given orally, have a prolonged half-life, can be delivered to proper sites, and have a high therapeutic index with little or no potential for development of resistance.

The use of combination therapy now seems to be gaining a wider acceptance. Additive or synergistic combination may have the true advantages of improving selective inhibition of viral replication, increasing killing of the virus, suppression of resistant strains, and diminution in drug toxicity. Whether or not long-term intermittent combination therapy will eradicate latent viral infection is presently not known.

Finally, it is hoped that proper pharmacokinetic studies and well-controlled clinical trials for evaluation of efficacy and safety of new antiviral agents will be performed in pediatric patients on which sound recommendations for future use can be based.

REFERENCES

1. Steel R: Antiviral agents for respiratory infections. Pediatr Infect Dis J 7:457–461, 1988
2. Richmann DD, et al: Fate of influenza A virion proteins after entry into subcellular fractions of LLC cells and the effect of amantadine. Virology 151:200, 1986
3. Sarin P, et al: Effects of a novel compound (AL721) on HTLV-III infectivity in vitro. N Engl J Med 313:313–314, 1985
4. Pert CB, et al: Octapeptides deduced from the neuropeptide receptor like pattern of antigen T4 in brain potently inhibit human immunodeficiency virus receptor binding and T-cell infectivity. Proc Natl Acad Sci USA 83:9254, 1986
5. De Clercq E: Suramin in the treatment of AIDS: Mechanism of action. Antiviral Res 7:1, 1987
6. Koretz S, et al: Treatment of serious cytomegalovirus infections with 9-(1,3-dihydroxy-2-propoxymethl) guanine in patients with AIDS and other immunodeficiences. N Engl J Med 314:801–805, 1986
7. Gilbert B, et al: Biochemistry and clinical applications of ribavirin. Antimicrob Agents Chemother 30:201–205, 1986
8. Elion GB: History, mechanism of action, spectrum, and selectivity of nucleoside analogues, in Mills J, Corey L (eds): Antiviral Chemotherapy. New York, Elsevier, 1986, p 118
9. Shipman C, et al: Antiviral activity of arabinosyladenine (Ara-A) and arabinosylhypoxanthine in herpes simplex virus-infected KB cell. I. Selective inhibition of viral DNA synthesis in synchronized suspension cultures. Antimicrob Agents Chemother 9:120–127, 1976
10. Cheng YC, et al: Unique spectrum of activity of 9-[(1,3-dihydroxy-2-propoxy)methyl]guanine against herpesviruses in vitro and its mode of action against herpes simplex virus type 1. Proc Natl Acad Sci USA 80:2667–2670, 1983
11. Eidinoff ML, et al: Incorporation of unnatural pyrimidine bases into deoxyribonucleic acid of mammalian cells. Science 129:1550–1551, 1959
12. Woodson B, Joklik WK: The inhibition of vaccine virus multiplication by Isatin-B-thiosemicarbazone. Proc Natl Acad Sci USA 54:946–953, 1965
13. Floyd-Smith G, et al: Interferon action: RNA cleavage pattern of a (2′-5′)oligoadenylate-dependent endonuclease. Science 212:1030, 1981
14. Elion GB: Mechanism of action and selectivity of acyclovir. Am J Med 73(1A):7–13, 1982
15. McGuirt PV, Furman PA: Acyclovir inhibition of viral DNA chain elongation in Herpes simplex virus-infected cells. Am J Med 73(1A):67–71, 1982
16. Biron KK, Ellion GB: Sensitivity of varicella-zoster virus in vitro to acyclovir. 19th Interscience Conference on Antimicrobial Agents and Chemotherapy, Boston, 1979
17. Bryson YJ, Hebblewaite D: The in vitro sensitivity of clinical isolates of varicella-zoster to virostatic and virocidal concentrations of acyclovir. International Conference on Human Herpesviruses, Atlanta, Georgia, March, 1980
18. Pagano JS, Datta AK: Perspectives on interaction of acyclovir with Epstein-Barr and other herpes viruses. Am J Med 73(1A):18–26, 1982
19. Colby B, et al: Effect of acyclovir on Epstein-Barr virus DNA replication. J Virol 34:560–568, 1980
20. Anderson J, et al: Effect of acyclovir on infectious mononucleosis: A double-blind, placebo-controlled study. J Infect Dis 153:283–290, 1986
21. St. Clair MH, et al: Inhibition of cellular alpha and virally induced deoxyribonucleic acid by the triphosphate of acyclovir. Antimicrob Agents Chemother 18:741–745, 1980
22. Hintz M, et al: Neonatal acyclovir pharmacokinetics in patients with herpes virus infections. Am J Med 73(1A):210–214, 1982
23. Blum MR, et al: Overview of acyclovir pharmacokinetic disposition in adults and children. Am J Med 73(1A):186–192, 1982
24. Laskin LO, et al: Pharmacokinetics and tolerance of acyclovir; a new anti-herpesvirus agent in humans. Antimicrob Agents Chemother 21:393–398, 1982
25. de Miranda P, Blum MR: Pharmacokinetics of acyclovir after intravenous and oral administration. J Antimicrob Chemother 12:29–37, 1983

26. Sullender W, et al: Pharmacokinetics of acyclovir suspension in infants and children. Antimicrob Agents Chemother 31:1722–1726, 1987
27. Novelli V, et al: Acyclovir administered perorally in immuno-compromised children with varicella-zoster infections. J Infect Dis 149:478, 1984
28. Novelli V, et al: High dose oral acyclovir for children at risk of disseminated herpesvirus infections. J Infect Dis 151:372, 1985
29. Laskin LO, et al: Effect of renal failure on the pharmacokinetics of acyclovir. Am J Med 73(1A):197–201, 1982
30. Brigden D, et al: Renal function after acyclovir intravenous injection. Am J Med 73(1A):182–185, 1982.
31. Tucker WE, et al: Preclinical safety evaluation of Zovirax (BW248U). Abstract 64, 18th Interscience Conference on Antimicrobial Agents and Chemotherapy, American Society for Microbiology, 1978, Washington, DC
32. Saral R, et al: Acyclovir prophylaxis of herpes simplex virus infections: A randomized, double-blind, controlled trial in bone marrow transplant recipients. N Engl J Med 305:63–67, 1981
33. Keeney RE, et al: Acyclovir tolerance in humans. AM J Med 73(1A):197–201, 1982
34. Pelling JC, et al: Internucleotide incorporation of arabinosyladenine into herpes simplex virus and mammalian cell. Virology 109:323–335, 1981
35. Whitley RJ, et al: Vidarabine: A preliminary review of its pharmacological properties and therapeutic use. Drugs 20:267–282, 1980
36. Whitley RJ, et al: Adenine arabinoside therapy of biopsy-proved herpes simplex encephalitis: National Institute of Allergy and Infectious Diseases Collaborative Antiviral Study. N Engl J Med 297:289–294, 1977
37. Hyndink RA, et al: Herpetic keratitis–Clinical evaluation of adenine arabinoside and idoxuridine, in Pavan-Landston D, Buchanan RA, Alford CA Jr. (eds): Adenine Arabinoside: An Antiviral Agent. New York, Raven Press, 1975, pp 331–335.
38. Whitley RJ, et al: Early vidarabine therapy to control the complications of herpes zoster in immunosuppressed patients. N Engl J Med 304:313–318, 1981
39. Whitley RJ, et al: Vidarabine therapy of varicella in immunosuppressed patients. J Pediatr 101:125–131, 1982
40. LePage GA, et al: Studies of 9-β-arabinofuranosyladenine in man. Drug Metab Dispos 1:756–759, 1973
41. Arnoff GR, et al: Hypoxanthine-arabinoside pharmacokinetics after adenine arabinoside administration to a patient with renal failure. Antimicrob Agents Chemother 18:212–214, 1980
42. Whitley RJ, et al: Pharmacology, tolerance and antiviral activity of vidarabine monophosphate in humans. Antimicrob Agents Chemother 18:709–715, 1980
43. Ross AH, et al: Toxicity of adenine arabinoside in humans. J Infect Dis 133(suppl):192–198, 1976
44. Mar EC, et al: Inhibition of cellular DNA polymerase alpha and human Cytomegalovirus-induced DNA polymerase by the triphosphates of 9-(2-hydroxyethoxymethyl)guanine and 9-(1,3-dihydroxy-2-propoxymethyl)guanine. J Virol 53:776–780, 1985
45. Biron KK, et al: Metabolic activation of the nucleoside analog 9-([2-hydroxy-1(hydroxymethyl)ethoxy]methyl)guanine in human diploid fibroblasts infected with human cytomegalovirus. Proc Natl Acad Sci USA 82:2473–2477, 1985
46. Lin JC, et al: Herpes viruses and virus chemotherapy, in Kano R (ed): Amsterdam, Elsevier Publishers, pp 225–227
47. Sommadossi JP, et al: Clinical pharmacokinetics of ganciclovir in patients with normal and impaired renal function. Rev Infect Dis 10(suppl 3):S507–514, 1988
48. Jacobson M, et al: Human pharmacokinetics and tolerance of oral ganciclovir. Antimicrob Agents Chemother 31:1251–1254, 1987
49. Buhles NC, et al: Ganciclovir treatment of life or sight threatening cytomegalovirus infection: Experience in 314 immunocompromised patients. Rev Infect Dis 10(suppl 3):S495–S504, 1988
50. Wray SK, et al: Mode of action of ribavirin: Effect of nucleotide pool alterations on influenza virus ribonucleoprotein synthesis. Antiviral Res 5:29–37, 1985
51. Sidwell RW: In vitro and in vivo inhibition of DNA viruses by ribavirin, in Smith RA, Knight V, Smith JA (eds): Clinical Applications of Ribavirin. New York, Academic Press, 1984, pp 19–31
52. Outwater KM: Ribavirin administration to infants receiving mechanical ventilation. Am J Dis Child 142:512–515, 1988
53. Connor JD: Comparative pharmacology of nucleoside analogs with antiviral activity, in Mills J, and Corey L (eds): Antiviral Chemotherapy. New York, Elsevier Press, 1986, pp 138–154
54. Connor JD, et al: Ribavirin pharmacokinetics in children and adults during therapeutic trials, in Smith RA, Knight V, Smith JA (eds): Clinical Applications of Ribavirin. New York, Academic Press, 1984, pp 107–123
55. Smith RA, Wade MJ: Studies with a broad spectrum antiviral agent. Royal Society of Medicine, International Congress and Symposia Session 108:31, 1986
56. Catlin DM, et al: ¹⁴C-Ribavirin: Distribution and pharmacokinetic studies in rats, baboons and man, in Smith RA, Kirkpatric W (eds): Ribavirin: A broad spectrum antiviral agent. New York, Academic Press, 1980, pp 83–98
57. McCormick J, et al: Lassa fever: Effective therapy with ribavirin. N Engl J Med 314:20–26, 1986
58. Mitsuya H, et al: 3'-Azido-3'-deoxythymidine (BWA509U): An antiviral agent that inhibits the infectivity and cytopathic effect of human T-lymphotropic virus type III/lymphadenopathy-associated virus in vitro. Proc Natl Acad Sci USA 82:7096–7100, 1985
59. Furman PA, et al: Phosphorylation of 3'-azido-3'-deoxythymidine and selective interaction of the 5'-triphosphate with human immunodeficiency virus reverse transcriptase. Proc Natl Acad Sci USA 83:8333, 1986
60. Yarchoan R, et al: Administration of 3'-azido-3'-deoxythymidine, an inhibitor of HTLV-III replication, to patients with AIDS and AIDS-related complex. Lancet 1:575, 1986
61. Yarchoan R, et al: Response of human-immunodeficiency virus associated neurological disease to 3'-azido-3'-deoxythymidine. Lancet 1:132, 1987
62. Yarchoan R, et al: Development of antiretroviral therapy for the acquired immunodeficiency syndrome and related disorders. N Engl J Med 316:557–564, 1987
63. Richman D, et al: The toxicity of azidothymidine (AZT) in the treatment of patients with AIDS and AIDS-related complex. N Engl J Med 317:192–197, 1987
64. Bach MC: Zidovudine for lymphocytic interstitial pneumonia associated with AIDS. Lancet 2:796, 1987
65. Hay AJ, et al: The molecular basis of the specific antiinfluenza action of amantadine. EMBO J 4:3021, 1985
66. Hayden FG, et al: Comparative single dose pharmacokinetics of amantadine hydrochloride and rimantadine hydrochloride in young and elderly adults. Antimicrob Agents Chemother 28:216, 1985
67. Dolin R: Clinical efficacy, pharmacology, and toxicity of amantadine and derivatives, in Mills J, Corey L (eds): Antiviral Chemotherapy. New York, Elsevier, 1986, pp 58–62
68. Bleidner WE, et al: Absorption, distribution and excretion of amantadine hydrochloride. J Pharmacol Exp Ther 150:484–490, 1965
69. Horadam VW, et al: Pharmacokinetics of amantadine hydrochloride in subjects with normal and impaired renal function. Ann Intern Med 94:454, 1981
70. Bryson YJ, et al: A prospective double-blind study of side effects associated with the administration of amantadine for influenza A virus prophylaxis. J Infect Dis 141:543–547, 1980
71. Tsunoda A, et al: Antiviral activity of alpha-methyl-1-adamantine-methylamine hydrochloride. Antimicrob Agents Chemother XX:1965, 553
72. Anderson EL, et al: Single dose pharmacokinetics of rimantadine in children, in Ishigami I (ed): Recent Advances in Chemotherapy: Antimicrobial Section 3. Tokyo, Tokyo University Press, 1985, pp 1955–1956
73. Mao JCH, et al: Inhibition of DNA polymerase from herpes simplex virus-infected WI-38 cells by phosphonoacetic acid. J Virol 15:1281–1283, 1975
74. Oberg B: Antiviral effects of Phosphonoformate (PFA, Foscarnet sodium). Pharmacol Ther 19:387–415, 1983
75. Eriksson B, et al: Inhibition of reverse transcriptase activity of

avian myeloblastosis virus by pyrophosphate analogues. Antiviral Res 2:81, 1982

76. Sandstrom EG, et al: Inhibition of human T-cell lymphotropic virus type III in vitro by phosphonoformate. Lancet 1:1480–1482, 1985

77. Wallin J, et al: Treatment of recurrent herpes labialis with trisodium phosphonoformate in Nelson JD, Gracci C (eds): Current Chemotherapy and Infectious Diseases. Washington, DC, American Society for Microbiology, 1980, pp 1361–1362

78. Ringden C, et al: Pharmacokinetics, safety, and preliminary clinical experiences using Foscarnet in the treatment of cytomegalovirus infections in bone marrow and renal transplant recipients. J Antimicrob Agents Chemother 17:373–387, 1986

79. Farthing CF, et al: Pilot study on the treatment of AIDS and ARC patients with intravenous Foscarnet (Abstr.). Proc Int Confer AIDS, Paris, June 23–25, 1986, p 35

80. Walmsley S, et al: Treatment of cytomegalovirus retinitis with trisodium phosphonoformate hexahydrate (Foscarnet). J Infect Dis 157:569–572, 1988

81. Otto MJ, et al: In vitro activity of WIN 51711: A new broad spectrum antipicornavirus drug. Antimicrob Agents Chemother 27:883–886, 1985

82. Fox MP, et al: The prevention of rhinovirus and poliovirus uncoating by WIN 51711: A new antiviral drug. Antimicrob Agents Chemother 30:110–116, 1986

83. Smith TJ, et al: The site of attachment in human rhinovirus 14 for antiviral agents that inhibit uncoating. Science 233:1286–1293, 1986

84. McKinley MA, Frank JA: WIN 51711–A novel drug for the treatment of enterovirus infections, in Mills J, Cory L (eds): Antiviral Chemotherapy. New York, Elsevier, 1986, pp 90–96.

85. Preble OT, Friedman RM: Biology of disease. Interferon induced alterations in cells. Relevance to viral and nonviral disease. Lab Invest 49:4, 1983

86. Blalock JE, Stanton JD: Common pathways of interferon and hormonal action. Nature 283:406, 1980

87. Greenberg S: Human interferon in viral disease. Infect Dis Clin North Am 1:383–423, 1987

88. Wills RJ, et al: Interferon kinetics and adverse reactions after intravenous, intramuscular and subcutaneous injection. Clin Pharmacol Ther 35:722, 1984

89. Jordan GU, et al: Administration of human leukocyte interferon in herpes zoster. J Infect Dis 130:56–62, 1974

90. Jordan GU, et al: Recombinant leukocyte A interferon: Pharmacokinetics, single-dose tolerance, and biologic effects in cancer patients. Ann Intern Med 96:549–556, 1982

91. Bocci V, et al: The kidney is the main site of interferon catabolism. J Interferon Res 2:309, 1982

92. Hayden F, et al: Prevention of natural colds by contact prophylaxis with intranasal alpha$_2$-interferon. N Engl J Med 314:71–75, 1986

93. Douglas R, et al: Prophylactic efficacy of intranasal alpha$_2$-interferon against rhinovirus infections in the family setting. N Engl J Med 314:65–70, 1986

94. Crockett D, et al: Side effects and toxicity of interferon in the treatment of recurrent respiratory papillomatosis. Ann Otol Rhinol Laryngol 96:601–607, 1987

95. Perrilo R, et al: Prednisone withdrawal followed by recombinant alpha interferon in the treatment of chronic type B hepatitis: A randomized, controlled trial. Ann Intern Med 109:95–100, 1988

96. Eron L, et al: Interferon therapy for condylomata acuminata. N Engl J Med 315:1059–1064, 1986

97. Sperber S, et al: Chemotherapy of rhinovirus colds. Antimicrob Agents Chemother 32:409–419, 1988

98. Geffen J, et al: Intralesional administration of large doses of human leukocyte interferon for the treatment of condylomata acuminata. J Infect Dis 150:612–615, 1984

99. Kashima H, et al: Interferon alpha-N1 (Wellferon) in juvenile onset of recurrent respiratory papillomatosis: Results of a randomized study in twelve collaborative institutions. Laryngoscope 98:334–340, 1988

100. Bomholt, A: Interferon therapy for laryngeal papillomatosis in adults. Arch Otolaryngol 109:550–552, 1983

101. Haglund S, et al: Interferon therapy for juvenile laryngeal papillomatosis. Arch Otolaryngol 107:327–332, 1981

102. Healey GB, et al: Treatment of recurrent respiratory papillomatosis with human leukocyte interferon. N Engl J Med 319:401–407, 1988

103. Davis G, et al: Interferon in viral hepatitis: Role in pathogenesis and treatment. Hepatology 6:1038–1041, 1986

104. Alexander G, et al: Loss of HBsAg with interferon therapy in chronic hepatitis B virus infection. Lancet 1:66–69, 1987

105. Hoofangle J, et al: Treatment of chronic non-A, non-B hepatitis with recombinant human alpha interferon. N Engl J Med 315:1575–1578, 1986

106. Rios A, et al: Treatment of acquired immunodeficiency syndrome-related Kaposi's sarcoma with lymphoblastoid interferon. J Clin Oncol 3:506, 1985

107. Behan PO: Interferon in the treatment of subacute sclerosing panencephalitis. Lancet 1:1059, 1981

108. Merigan TC, et al: Human leukocyte interferon administration to patients with symptomatic and suspected rabies. Ann Neurol 16:82, 1984

109. Hemming V, et al: Intravenous immunoglobulin treatment of respiratory syncytial virus infections in adults and young children. Antimicrob Agents Chemother 31:1882–1886, 1987

110. Snydman D, et al: Use of cytomegalovirus immune globulin to prevent cytomegalovirus disease in renal transplant recipients. N Engl J Med 317:1049–1054, 1987

111. Chehimi J, et al: Selection of an intravenous immune globulin for the immunoprophylaxis of cytomegalovirus infections: An in vitro comparison of currently available and previously effective immune globulins. Bone Marrow Transplant 2:395–402, 1987

112. McKinney R, et al: Chronic enteroviral meningoencephalitis in agammaglobulinemic patients. Rev Infect Dis 9:334–356, 1987

113. Erlendsson K, et al: Successful reversal of echovirus encephalitis in x-linked hypogammaglobulinemia by intraventricular administration of immunoglobulin. N Engl J Med 312:351–353, 1985

114. Bjorkander J, et al: Immunoglobulin prophylaxis in patients with antibody deficiency syndromes and anti-IgA. J Clin Immunol 7:8–15, 1987

115. Williams PE, et al: Non-A, non-b hepatitis transmission by intravenous immunoglobulin. Lancet, August 27, 1988

116. Henney CS, et al: Interleukin-2 augments natural killer activity. Nature 291:335–338, 1981

117. Kohl S, et al: Use of interleukin-2 and macrophages to treat herpes simplex virus infection in neonatal mice. J Infect Dis 157:1187–1192, 1988

118. Weinberg A, et al: Acute genital infection in guinea pigs: Effect of recombinant interleukin-2 on herpes simplex virus type 2. J Infect Dis 154:134–140, 1986

119. Ito M, et al: Interleukin-2 enhances natural killing of varicella-zoster virus-infected targets. Clin Exp Immunol 65:182–189, 1986

120. Kohl S, et al: Defects in interleukin-2 stimulation of neonatal natural killer cytotoxicity to herpes simplex virus-infected cells. J Pediatr 112:976–981, 1988

121. Bonavida B, et al: Mechanism of defective NK cell activity in patients with acquired immunodeficiency syndrome (AIDS) and AIDS-related complex. J Immunol 137:1157–1163, 1986

122. Murphy P, et al: Marked disparity in incidence of bacterial infections in patients with the acquired immunodeficiency syndrome receiving interleukin-2 or interferon-gamma. Ann Intern Med 108:36–41, 1988

123. Donohue JH, Rosenberg SA: The fate of interleukin-2 after in vivo administration. J Immunol 130:2203–2208, 1983

124. West W, et al: Constant infusion of recombinant interleukin-2 in adoptive immunotherapy of advanced cancer. N Engl J Med 316:898–905, 1987

125. Carter WA, et al: Preclinical studies with ampligen (mismatched double-stranded RNA). J Biol Res Mod 4:495–502, 1985

126. Mitchell WM, et al: Mismatched double-stranded RNA (ampligen) reduces concentration of zidovudine (azidothymidine) required for in vitro inhibition of human immunodeficiency virus. Lancet 1:892, 1987

127. Carter W, et al: Clinical, immunological and virological effects of

ampligen, a mismatched double-stranded RNA, in patients with AIDS or AIDS-related complex. Lancet 1:1286–1292, 1987

128. Hall CB, et al: Aerosolized ribavirin treatment of infants with respiratory syncytial viral infection. N Engl J Med 308:1443–1447, 1983

129. Taber LH: Ribavirin aerosol treatment of bronchiolitis associated with respiratory syncytial virus infection in infants. Pediatrics 72:613–618, 1983

130. Rodriguez WJ, et al: Ribavirin aerosol treatment of serious respiratory syncytial virus infection in infants. Infect Dis Clin North Am 1:425–457, 1987

131. Wald ER, et al: Ribavirin for RSV infections: Editorial correspondence–Reply. J Pediatr 113:418, 1988

132. Steven S, et al: Rimantadine prophylaxis in children: A follow-up study. Pediatr Infect Dis J 7:379–383, 1988

133. Clover RD, et al: Effectiveness of rimantadine prophylaxis of children within families. Am J Dis Child 140:706–709, 1986

134. Hall CB, et al: Children with influenza A infections: Treatment with rimantadine. Pediatrics 80:275–282, 1987

135. Quilligan JJ, et al: The suppression of A2 influenza in children by the prophylactic use of amantadine. J Pediatr 69:572–575, 1966

136. Bryson YJ: The use of amantadine in children for prophylaxis and treatment of influenza A infections. Pediatr Infect Dis 1:44–46, 1982

137. Knight V, Gilbert BE: Ribavirin aerosol treatment of influenza. Infect Dis Clin North Am 1:441–457, 1987

138. Bernstein D, et al: Ribavirin small-particle aerosol treatment of influenza B virus infection. Antimicrob Agents Chemother 32:761–764, 1988

139. Stein D, et al: Oral ribavirin treatment of influenza A and B. Antimicrob Agents Chemother 31:1285–1287, 1987

140. Smith C, et al: Lack of effect of oral ribavirin in naturally occurring influenza A virus (H1N1) infection. J Infect Dis 141:548–554, 1980

141. Miller F, et al: Controlled trial of enviroxime against natural rhinovirus infections in a community. Antimicrob Agents Chemother 27:102–106, 1985

142. Corey J, et al: Treatment of primary first episode genital HSV infection with acyclovir: Results of topical, intravenous and oral therapy. J Antimicrob Chemother 12(B):79, 1983

143. Mertz GJ, et al: Suppression of frequently recurring genital herpes with oral acyclovir (ACV): Long term efficacy and toxicity Abstract 1183, 26th Interscience Conference on Antimicrobial Agents and Chemotherapy, New Orleans, Sept 29–Oct 1, 1986, p 312

144. Douglas JM, et al: Prevention of recurrent genital herpes simplex virus infection with daily oral acyclovir: A double-blind trial. N Engl J Med 310:1551, 1984

145. Pavan-Langston D, Foster CS: Trifluorothymidine and idoxuridine therapy of ocular herpes. Am J Ophthalmol 84:818–825, 1977

146. Laibson P, et al: Acyclovir and vidarabine for the treatment of herpes simplex keratitis. Am J Med 73(1A):281–285, 1982

147. La Lau C, et al: Multicenter trial of acyclovir and trifluorothymidine in herpetic keratitis. Am J Med 73(1A):305–306, 1982

148. Whitley, RJ: Therapeutic approaches to herpes simplex encephalitis and neonatal herpes simplex virus infections in Mills J, Corey L (eds): Antiviral Chemotherapy. New York, Elsevier, 1986, pp 155–166

149. Whitley R, et al: Vidarabine versus acyclovir therapy of neonatal herpes simplex virus, HSV, infection. Pediatr Res 20:323A, 1986

150. Whitley RJ, et al: Interim summary of mortality in herpes simplex encephalitis and neonatal herpes simplex virus infections: Vidarabine versus acyclovir. J Antimicrob Chemother 12(suppl):B105–B112, 1984

151. Skoldenberg B, et al: Acyclovir versus vidarabine in herpes simplex encephalitis. Randomized multicentre study in consecutive Swedish patients. Lancet 2:707–711, 1984

152. Whitley R, et al: Vidarabine versus acyclovir therapy in herpes simplex encephalitis. N Engl J Med 314:144–149, 1986

153. VanLandigham K, et al: Relapse of herpes simplex encephalitis

after conventional acyclovir therapy. JAMA 259:1051–1053, 1988

154. Prentice HG: Use of acyclovir for prophylaxis of herpes infections in severely immunocompromised patients. J Antimicrob Chemother 12(suppl):B153–B159, 1983

155. Gluckman E, et al: Oral acyclovir prophylactic treatment of herpes simplex infection after bone marrow transplantation. J Antimicrob Chemother 12(suppl):B161–B167, 1983

156. Arvin A: Oral therapy with acyclovir in infants and children. Pediatr Infect Dis J 6:56–58, 1987

157. Shepp D, et al: Treatment of varicella-zoster infection in severely immunocompromised patients. N Engl J Med 314:208–212, 1986

158. McKendrick MW, et al: Oral acyclovir in acute herpes zoster. Br Med J 293:1529–1532, 1986

159. Bridgen D, Whitman P: The clinical pharmacology of acyclovir and its prodrugs. Scand J Infect Dis 47:33–39, 1985

160. Erice A, et al: Ganciclovir treatment of cytomegalovirus disease in transplant recipients and other immunocompromised hosts. JAMA 257:3082–3087, 1987

161. Snydman DR: Ganciclovir therapy for cytomegalovirus disease associated with renal transplants. Rev Infect Dis 10(suppl 3):S554–S562, 1988

162. Shepp DM, et al: Activity of 9-[2-hydroxy-1-(hydroxymethyl)ethoxymethyl]guanine in the treatment of cytomegalovirus pneumonia. Ann Intern Med 103:368–373, 1985

163. Bowden R, et al: Cytomegalovirus immune globulin and seronegative blood products to prevent primary cytomegalovirus infection after marrow transplantation. N Engl J Med 314:1006–1010, 1986

164. Steinmuller D, et al: The use of immunoglobulin infusions as prophylaxis for cytomegalovirus infection for living related donor renal transplantation. Am J Kidney Dis 1:A21, 1988

165. Winston DJ, et al: Intravenous immune globulin for prevention of cytomegalovirus infection and interstitial pneumonia after bone marrow transplantation. Ann Intern Med 106:12–18, 1987

166. Hirsch MS, et al: Effects of interferon-alpha on cytomegalovirus reactivation syndromes in renal transplant patients. N Engl J Med 308:1489, 1983

167. Andersson J, et al: Acyclovir treatment in infectious mononucleosis: A clinical and virologic study. Infection 15(suppl 1):S14–S20, 1987

168. Strauss S, et al: Acyclovir (ACV) treatment of a chronic fatigue syndrome with unusual EBV serologic profiles: Lack of efficacy in a controlled trial. Clin Res 35(3):618A, 1987

169. Cheesman S et al: Epstein-Barr virus infection in renal transplant recipients: Effects of antithymocyte globulin and interferon. Ann Intern Med 93:39–42, 1980

170. McKinley M, et al: Recent developments in antiviral chemotherapy. Infect Dis Clin North Am 1:479–493, 1987

171. Langford MP, et al: Antibody and interferon act synergistically to inhibit enterovirus, adenovirus and herpes simplex virus infection. Infect Immun 41:214–218, 1983

172. Wilfert C: Safety and tolerance of zidovudine (ZDV, Retrovir) during a phase 1 study in children. Pediatr Res 379A:1066, 1988

173. Fischl M, et al: The efficacy of azidothymidine (AZT) in the treatment of patients with AIDS and AIDS-related complex. N Engl J Med 317:185–191, 1987

174. Yarchoan R, et al: Phase I studies of 2′,3′-dideoxycytidine in severe human immunodeficiency virus infection as a single agent and alternating with zidovudine (AZT). Lancet 1:76–81, 1988

175. Crumpacker C, et al: Ribavirin treatment of the acquired immunodeficiency syndrome (AIDS) and AIDS-related complex (ARC). Ann Intern Med 107:664–674, 1987

176. Baba M, et al: Ribavirin antagonizes inhibitory effects of pyrimidine 2′, 3′-dideoxynucleosides but enhances inhibitory effects of purine 2′,3′-dideoxynucleosides on replication of human immunodeficiency virus in vitro. Antimicrob Agents Chemother 31:1613–1617, 1987

177. Yust I, et al: Reduction of circulating HIV antigen in seropositive patients after treatment with AL-721 (Abstr.). IV Intl Conf AIDS, Stockholm, 1988

178. Grieco M, et al: Open study of AL-721 in HIV-infected subjects with generalized lymphadenopathy syndrome (LAS). Abstract TP223, III Intl Conf AIDS, Washington, DC, 1987

179. Surbone A, et al: Treatment of the AIDS and AIDS-related complex with a regimen of 3'-azido-2',3'-dideoxythymidine (azidothymidine or zidovudine) and acyclovir. Ann Intern Med 108:534–540, 1988

180. Vittecoq D, et al: Evaluation of antiviral activity and tolerance of HPA23 in 38 patients with HIV related disorders. Abstract WP216, III Intl Conf AIDS, Washington, DC, 1987

181. Levine AM, et al: Suramin antiviral therapy in the acquired immunodeficiency syndrome. Ann Inter Med 105:32, 1986

182. Wetterberg L, et al: Peptide T treatment of AIDS. Lancet 1:159, 1987

183. Ernst M, et al: Effects of systemic in vivo interleukin-2 in reconstitution in patients with acquired immunodeficiency syndrome (AIDS) and AIDS-related complex (ARC) on phenotypes and functions of peripheral blood mononuclear cells (PBMC). J Clin Immunol 6:170–181, 1986

184. Garcia G, et al: Adenine arabinoside monophosphate (vidarabine phosphate) in combination with human leukocyte interferon in the treatment of chronic hepatitis B. Ann Intern Med 107:278–285, 1987

185. Bank G, Fernandez H: Clinical use of ribavirin in measles: A summarized review, in Smith RA, Smith JA, Knight V (eds): Clinical Applications of Ribavirin. New York, Academic Press, 1984, pp 203–209

186. Sanchez FA, et al: Treatment of type A hepatitis with ribavirin, in Smith RA, Smith JA, Knight V (eds): Clinical Applications of Ribavirin. New York, Academic Press, 1984, pp 193–201

187. Schnipper LE, Crumpacker CS: Resistance of herpes simplex virus to acycloguanosine: Role of viral thymidine kinase and DNA polymerase loci. Proc Natl Acad Sci USA 77:2265–2269, 1980

188. Darby G, et al: Altered substrate specificity of herpes simplex virus thymidine kinase confers acyclovir resistance. Nature 289:81–83, 1981

189. Wade JC, et al: Frequency and significance of acyclovir-resistant herpes simplex virus isolated from bone marrow transplant patients receiving multiple courses of treatment with acyclovir. J Infect Dis 148:1077–1082, 1983

190. Norris S, et al: Severe, progressive herpetic whitlow caused by an acyclovir-resistant virus in a patient with AIDS. J Infect Dis 157:209–210, 1987

191. Sibrack CD, et al: Pathogenicity of acyclovir-resistant herpes simplex virus type 1 from an immunodeficient child. J Infect Dis 146:673–682, 1982

192. Biron KK, et al: A human cytomegalovirus mutant resistant to the nucleoside analog 9-[(2-hydroxy-1-(hydromethyl) ethoxy)methyl]guanine (BWB759U) induces reduced levels of BWB759U triphosphate. Proc Natl Acad Sci USA 83:8769–8773, 1986

193. Oxford J, et al: In vivo selection of an influenza A2 strain resistant to amantadine. Nature 226:82–83, 1970

194. Heider H, et al: Occurrence of amantadine- and rimantadine-resistant influenza A virus strains during the 1980 epidemic. Acta Virol 25:395, 1981

195. Tucker WE: Preclinical toxicology profile of acyclovir: An overview. Am J Med 73(1A):27–30, 1982

196. Kurtz SM: Toxicology of adenine arabinoside, in Pavan-Langston D, Buchanan RA, Alford CA (eds): Adenine Arabinoside: An Antiviral Agent. New York, Raven Press, 1975, pp 145–157

36

ANTINEOPLASTIC AGENTS

WILLIAM P. PETROS *and* WILLIAM E. EVANS

Approximately 6600 American children are diagnosed with malignancies every year.[1] Over one-half of these individuals will be cured of their disease. However, cancer is still the second leading cause of death in the pediatric population. A summary of the distribution of the major types of pediatric cancers is provided in Figure 36–1.[2] Response rates to treatment vary considerably according to type and extent of disease, with some malignancies demonstrating a dismal prognosis despite aggressive treatment, while others show excellent cure rates with current therapy. The potential role of clinical pharmacology in oncologic therapy is tremendous, considering that most antineoplastics have a low therapeutic index, wide interpatient variability in drug disposition, and potentially severe toxicities. There is accumulating evidence that application of clinical pharmacologic principles can lead to improvements in survival and/or minimization of adverse events associated with chemotherapy of selected childhood malignancies. Unfortunately, the clinical pharmacodynamics of many anticancer drugs have not been rigorously defined for many pediatric cancers, precluding the widespread application of pharmacologic principles to individualized therapy in all children with cancer. However, much is known about the clinical pharmacology of many anticancer drugs, and this knowledge can serve as a useful guideline for development of optimal therapeutic regimens.

This chapter summarizes selected clinical pharmacologic principles that are important in current anticancer therapy. For a more comprehensive review of general therapeutic strategies for childhood cancers, the reader is referred to texts in pediatric oncology[3,4] or oncolytic pharmacology.[5]

OVERVIEW OF TREATMENT MODALITIES

Major treatment modalities currently being utilized in cancer therapy include surgery, irradiation, chemother-

apy, and immunotherapy. Modern treatment strategies against malignancies often include combinations of these approaches, with the aim of achieving synergistic or additive oncolytic effects without excessive toxicity.

Surgery may be performed prior to other interventions for purposes of staging or debulking a tumor, as depicted in Figure 36–2. In very rare situations, surgery may be the only therapy necessary for cure. Because at least 10^9 tumor cells (translating into a volume of approximately 1 cc) are required for detection in common clinical practice, substantial tumor burden may be present prior to diagnosis or after surgical removal of primary tumor. One role of surgery is to reduce tumor cell volume to a point where intensive chemotherapy can produce enough cytotoxicity for a potential cure. In some situations, such as stage C neuroblastoma, chemotherapy may be used as the initial intervention to reduce tumor margins prior to surgery. Most often, surgery is followed by additional therapy for gross or microscopic residual disease or for adjuvant therapy when no detectable disease is present.

Many chemotherapy regimens are divided into several sections according to the planned timing and/or intensity of treatment. For example, early therapy of leukemia by combining different agents that are likely to be active has frequently been termed *induction therapy*. In theory, drug combinations with different mechanisms of oncolytic action, given in "adequate" doses, may circumvent preferential selection of initially resistant clones or acquisition of clones resistant to only one agent.[6] Examples of pediatric cancers currently being treated with regimens designed around this hypothesis include acute lymphocytic leukemia, Hodgkin's and non-Hodgkin's lymphoma, and brain tumors.[7–9] The goal of induction therapy is to rapidly eradicate as many tumor cells as possible, usually resulting in a tumor burden that is not clinically detectable. After induction, some type of additional intensive therapy (sometimes referred to as *consolidation therapy*) may be utilized to further enhance the initial cell kill and eradicate residual tumor cells in sites not commonly reached with the usual systemic doses. This may include local therapy, such as intrathecal injections, or

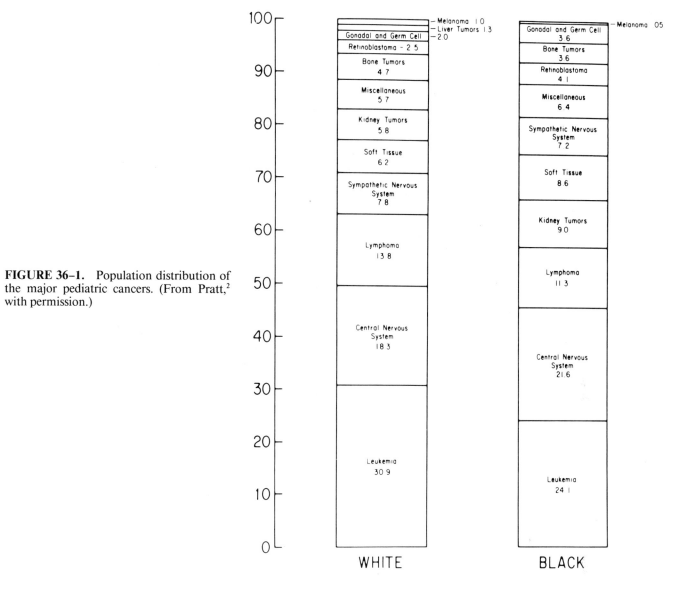

FIGURE 36–1. Population distribution of the major pediatric cancers. (From Pratt,[2] with permission.)

intensified systemic therapy (e.g., high-dose methotrexate). *Maintenance therapy (continuation therapy)* often consists of multiple drugs given in lower doses over a longer duration; however, some recent treatment regimens include intermittent administration (e.g., every 4–6 weeks) of higher doses of several drugs on an alternating basis (referred to as intensive *pulses* of therapy). Although these various terms are often useful to describe different components of the entire treatment, their definitions are somewhat arbitrary. Moreover, for potentially curable

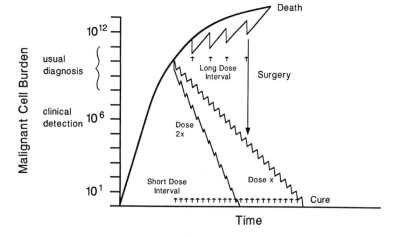

FIGURE 36–2. Potential influence of treatment regimens on a theoretical tumor growth curve. (Adapted from Dorr and Fritz,[66] with permission.)

diseases, it is essential to consider the individual components of therapy within the context of the total therapeutic strategy. That is, one cannot design a "phase" of therapy that is so intensive (i.e., toxic) that it significantly compromises the delivery of other components of therapy and thereby reduces the number of patients cured. The actual schedule of therapy for an entire protocol is dictated by the balance between the malignant cell kill and growth rate, and the time required by normal cells to recover from toxicity. Figure 36–2 demonstrates the potential effect of treatment schedule and dose on tumor cell kill and cure for three hypothetical treatment regimens, one with a long interval between courses, the second with a short course interval, and the third with two times the dose on a given course.

Recombinant DNA technology has recently enabled specific manipulation of the body's hematopoietic and immune systems with exogenously administered agents generically termed biologic response modifiers (BRMs). Adult trials exclusively using a BRM have shown favorable responses against some refractory tumors.[10,11] These agents will probably be of most benefit when combined with chemotherapy, particularly because their toxicities do not overlap with that of many traditional agents. A group of BRMs known as colony-stimulating factors are being used in conjunction with antineoplastics to improve their therapeutic index by reducing the degree and/or duration of myelosuppression.

PHARMACOLOGIC MECHANISMS OF CHEMOTHERAPY

Pharmacologic characteristics of many antineoplastic drugs used to treat childhood cancers are displayed in Figure 36–3. Traditional antineoplastic agents exert their therapeutic effects predominantly by alteration of DNA and/or RNA at various steps in the cell cycle, depending on the specific mechanism of action. In general, mechanisms can be classified into several groups: inhibition of active enzyme sites necessary for cell growth, presentation of a false substrate for an essential cellular enzyme, and direct binding to DNA or cellular proteins. Further classification segregates agents based on their dependency on target cell growth. Drugs whose action is predominantly dependent on the fraction of cells in a specific phase of the cell cycle (e.g., bleomycin) may exhibit a theoretical ceiling to their oncolytic dose–response curve, depending on the number of cells in the specific cell cycle phase at the time of drug exposure. In contrast, drugs working by cell cycle–independent mechanisms (e.g., alkylating agents) may show dose-related cytotoxicity that is unrelated to the fraction of cells in a particular cycle phase.

Combining drugs of different pharmacologic actions may potentiate the effects of both agents. Cells may be selectively recruited into a phase of the growth cycle by one drug, making them relatively more sensitive to a second agent that is cycle-dependent. Alternatively, drugs

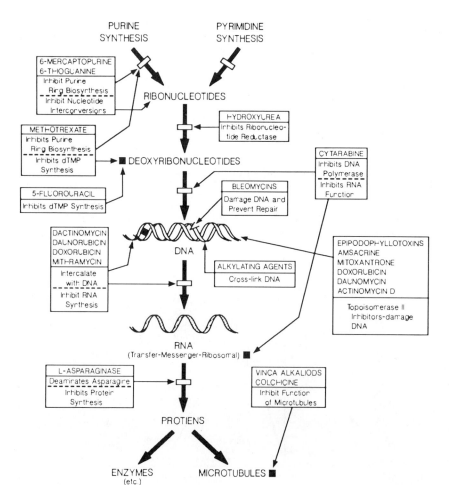

FIGURE 36–3. Pharmacologic mechanisms of action for important anticancer drugs. (Adapted from Gilman et al.,[67] with permission.)

TABLE 36-1. CLINICAL ACTIVITY OF ANTICANCER DRUGS USED IN PEDIATRIC PATIENTS

AGENT	LEUKEMIAS			LYMPHOMAS					Brain Tumors	Neuro blastoma	Wilms' Tumor	SARCOMAS			CARCINOMAS				
	ALL	AML	CML	Hodgkin's Disease	Lympho-cytic	Burkitt's	Large cell	Histio-cytosis				Osteogenic	Ewing's	Rhabdomyo	Small Cell	Retino-blastoma	Testic-ular	Terato	Ovarian
Antimetabolites																			
Methotrexate	*	+	−	+	*	*	*	*	+	−	−	+	+	+	−	−	+	−	−
Ara-C	+	*	*	−	*	*	−	−	−	−	−	−	−	−	−	−	−	−	−
6-TG	+	*	±	−	*	−	−	−	−	−	−	−	−	−	−	−	−	−	−
6-MP	*	+	+	−	*	−	−	−	−	−	−	−	−	−	−	−	−	−	−
5-Azacytidine	−	+	+	−	−	+	+	+	−	−	−	−	−	−	−	−	−	−	+
5-FU	−	−	−	−	−	−	−	−	±	±	−	±	±	−	+	+	+	+	+
Alkylating agents																			
Cyclophosphamide	+	±	+	*	*	*	*	*	±	*	+	+	+	+	+	*	*	+	*
Nitrogen mustard	−	−	−	*	±	−	±	±	+	+	−	−	−	−	±	±	+	−	−
Chlorambucil	−	−	−	*	−	−	−	−	−	−	−	−	−	−	−	−	+	+	+
Melphalan	−	−	±	−	±	±	−	−	−	−	−	±	−	−	−	−	+	−	−
Busulfan	−	−	*	−	−	−	−	−	−	−	−	−	−	−	−	−	−	−	*
Antibiotics																			
Doxorubicin	+	*	−	*	*	−	*	−	−	*	*	*	*	*	*	*	+	+	+
Daunorubicin	*	*	±	+	*	+	+	+	±	±	*	±	+	+	+	+	+	+	+
Actinomycin D	±	±	−	−	−	−	−	−	+	*	*	+	*	+	−	−	*	±	±
Bleomycin	−	−	−	*	−	−	−	−	+	−	−	−	−	−	−	*	*	−	−
Vinca alkaloids																			
Vincristine	*	+	+	*	*	*	*	*	*	*	*	*	*	*	*	*	+	+	+
Vinblastine	−	−	−	*	+	−	+	*	*	±	−	−	−	−	−	−	*	−	−
Miscellaneous Agents																			
Prednisone	*	±	−	*	*	±	*	*	+	±	−	−	−	−	−	−	−	−	−
CCNU-BCNU	±	−	−	*	*	−	−	−	*	−	−	±	−	−	−	−	−	±	−
DTIC	−	−	−	*	*	−	−	−	*	−	−	±	+	+	−	−	−	−	−
Procarbazine	−	−	−	*	±	−	−	−	*	*	−	−	−	−	−	−	−	−	−
L-Asparaginase	*	−	−	−	*	−	±	±	−	*	−	−	−	−	−	−	−	−	−
Cis-platinum	−	±	−	−	*	−	−	−	±	*	+	+	+	−	+	+	*	±	+
Hydroxyurea	±	+	+	+	*	−	−	−	+	*	±	±	−	−	+	−	−	±	−
Teniposide (VM-26)	+	−	−	+	*	−	−	−	+	*	±	±	±	−	+	+	+	+	+
Etoposide (VP-16)	+	+	−	+	+	+	+	±	+	+	+	+	+	−	+	*	+	+	+
Mitoxantrone	+	+	±	+	−	−	+	±	+	−	−	−	−	−	*	−	−	−	−
Amsacrine	+	±	−	+	−	−	−	±	−	−	−	−	−	−	−	−	−	−	−
Ifosfamide	+	−	−	+	+	−	−	−	+	+	+	+	+	+	+	+	+	+	+

*Used in primary therapy.
+Active.
−Effectiveness not demonstrated or determined.
Abbreviations: ALL, acute lymphocytic leukemia; AML, acute myelogenous leukemia; CML, chronic myelogenous leukemia.

that act on interrrelated cellular biochemical pathways may disrupt a pathway sequentially or complementarily to one another, enhance tumor cell kill, and/or decrease the likelihood of resistance.

Table 36–1 summarizes the clinical activity of drugs important in the treatment of childhood malignancies. Most therapeutic regimens in use combine active drugs from several classifications.

DETERMINANTS OF PEDIATRIC DOSAGES FOR CANCER CHEMOTHERAPY

Strategies for selecting the pediatric dose of chemotherapy have traditionally evolved from standard phase 1 toxicity studies. In these initial dose-finding studies, the objective is to determine the maximum tolerated dosage (MTD), defined as the dosage (in mg/kg or mg/m^2) that produces an "acceptable" level of toxicity. In most studies, the MTD is based on toxicities observed at various doses that have been empirically escalated and administered to groups of three to six patients at each dosage level. Although phase 1 and 2 studies in children have traditionally been delayed until after these studies have been completed in adults, surveys have indicated that MTDs in adults are not always informative for children[12] (see Table 36–2). Moreover, phase 1 and 2 studies in children and adults typically ignore the fact that interpatient pharmacokinetic variability is usually so great that it results in extensive overlap in systemic drug exposure at various dose levels evaluated in these initial clinical trials.[13] These recognized shortcomings in initial pediatric trials have led to suggestions on how the drug development process might be modified to yield more meaningful data.[14,15]

Several types of pediatric cancers are potentially curable with established treatment regimens; however, there remains a percentage of children who are not cured despite apparently similar prognostic characteristics and treatment regimens. Further investigation into this area has demonstrated that *dose intensity* can be a major determinant of outcome for drug-sensitive cancers such as acute lymphocytic leukemia[16] and Hodgkin's disease.[17] This term can be defined in a number of different ways, as described in the following sections; however, dose intensity generally refers to the amount of drug given to a patient per unit of time (e.g., mg/m^2/week). This is then used as a measure of the amount of anticancer therapy that has potential to act against malignant cells in a given patient. As described in the following sections, there are a variety of options for measuring dose intensity.

Protocol Dose Intensity

As response rates for some childhood cancers improved, additional attention was focused on biologic and pharmacologic basis for interpatient variability in response to therapy. Pinkel and coworkers[18] were among the first to investigate the possible relationship of dose to outcome. In their study, children with acute lymphocytic leukemia were randomized to receive either half or full dosages of 6-mercaptopurine, cyclophosphamide, and methotrexate during maintenance therapy. Those treated with the half-dosage regimen experienced significantly shorter durations of complete remission compared to the full-dose group. Subsequently, many studies in adults and children have shown that the dose and the dose intensity of cancer chemotherapy can have a significant effect on response in several drug-sensitive cancers.[14,19]

Although these studies have demonstrated a dose–response relationship for many anticancer drugs, we now know that there are many variables that can confound this relationship. Fortunately, several of these confounding variables (e.g., pharmacokinetic variability) can either be controlled or measured to evaluate the extent to which they affect the dose–response relationship for cancer chemotherapy (Figure 36–4).

TABLE 36–2. MAXIMUM TOLERATED DOSE (MTD) OF SOME ANTICANCER DRUGS IN CHILDREN AND ADULTS

DRUG	SCHEDULE	MTD (mg/m^2) Children	MTD (mg/m^2) Adults	RATIO MTD CHILDREN/ MTD ADULTS
Dianhydrogalactitiol	q.d. × 5	25	30	0.83
5-Azacytidine	q.d. × 5	200	225	0.89
TIC mustard	q.d. × 5	900	1000	0.90
Piperazinedione	q.d. × 5	3	3	1.0
VP16-213	Biweekly	150	125	1.20
Diglycoaldehyde	q.d. × 5	7500+	6000	1.25
m-AMSA	q.d. × 5	50	40	1.25
Daunomycin (mg/kg)	q.d. × 4	1.0	0.8	1.25
Adriamycin (mg/kg)	q.d. × 4	0.8	0.6	1.33
VM-26 (mg/kg)	Biweekly	4.0	3.0	1.33
3-Deazauridine (leukemia patients)	q.d. × 5	8.2	6.0	1.40
Azaserine (mg/kg) (total dose)	q.d.	156	108	1.44
Anhydro-5-fluoro-cyclocytidine	q.d.	300+	200+	1.50
Dihydroxyanthracenedione	Every 3 weeks	18	12	1.5
3-Deazauridine (solid tumors)	q.d. × 5	2.8	1.5	1.85
Cyclocytidine	q.d. × 10	600	300	2.00
ICRF-187	q.d. × 3	>2750	1250	>2.20

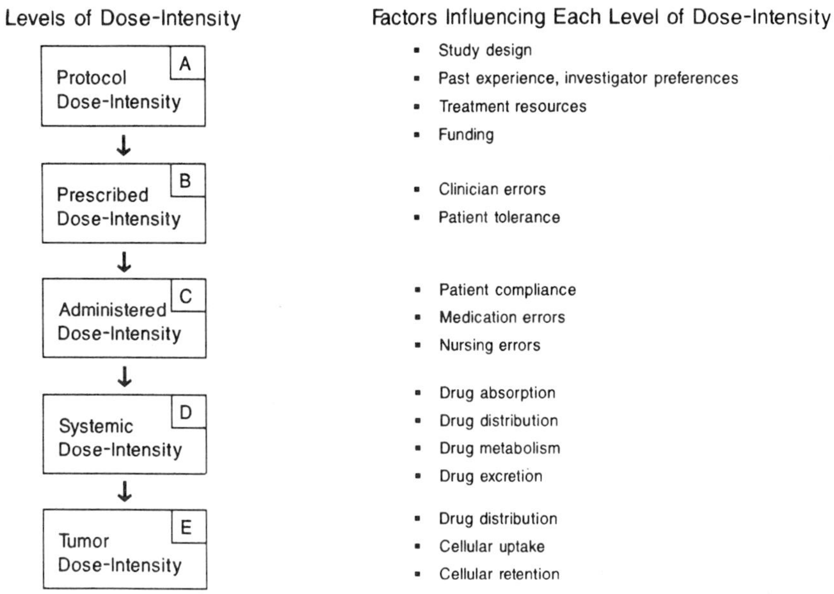

Levels of Dose-Intensity

Factors Influencing Each Level of Dose-Intensity

FIGURE 36–4. Scheme of various levels at which dose intensity (DI) can be defined and the corresponding factors that may influence DI at each level. Level A represents the DI written in any given treatment protocol; level B represents the DI actually prescribed for the patient; level C represents the DI actually taken by the patient; level D represents the extent and duration of systemic exposure achieved in the patient (e.g., area under the concentration–time curve in the patient's plasma); level E represents the actual exposure in the tumor cell. If the intracellular drug target is known (e.g., dihydrofolate reductase for MTX), level F (not depicted) might be the "drug target" DI. (From Evans,[14] with permission.)

Protocol Dose-Intensity — A
- Study design
- Past experience, investigator preferences
- Treatment resources
- Funding

Prescribed Dose-Intensity — B
- Clinician errors
- Patient tolerance

Administered Dose-Intensity — C
- Patient compliance
- Medication errors
- Nursing errors

Systemic Dose-Intensity — D
- Drug absorption
- Drug distribution
- Drug metabolism
- Drug excretion

Tumor Dose-Intensity — E
- Drug distribution
- Cellular uptake
- Cellular retention

Prescribed Dose Intensity

If one could design a protocol with optimal drug doses and schedules, there would be no certainty that this therapy would actually be given to all patients. Prescribed dose intensity is a factor usually thought to be easily controlled; however, a recent study has shown that physician adherence to a treatment protocol was a significant factor in the outcome of a group of children treated for acute lymphocytic leukemia.[20] Those children who relapsed were prescribed significantly less methotrexate than those in complete remission. This type of treatment variability may be of the greatest detriment to patients not enrolled in stringent protocols, when subjectively initiated alterations are made in the planned treatment schedule.

Traditionally, chemotherapy protocols have included provisions for dose reduction in patients experiencing excessive toxicity. A good example of such is the use of 6-mercaptopurine and methotrexate during maintenance therapy of acute lymphocytic leukemia. Clinicians are often given guidelines for dose reductions when myelosuppression secondary to these agents reaches unacceptable limits (e.g., WBC $<2000/mm^3$). Conversely, some patients may not demonstrate significant myelosuppression with standard protocol dosing (see the following for potential reasons). Yet escalation of dosages in patients failing to demonstrate a measurable pharmacologic effect (e.g., WBC $>4000/mm^3$), as suggested by some,[21] is not common practice.

Administered Dose Intensity

Patient compliance with the prescribed therapy is often a major determinant of the amount of scheduled therapy actually received (i.e., administered dose intensity). With today's complex cancer treatment regimens, many factors can influence the amount of planned therapy that is actually given. Such variables include patient tolerance to adverse effects, nutritional status, medication errors,

access to investigational drugs, availability of supportive care, and financial issues such as the extent of third-party coverage. Although the impact of many of these issues has not been systematically evaluated, surveys of patient/parent compliance with medication administration and clinic appointments have demonstrated an obvious need for continuous counseling in these areas.[22]

Many current treatment regimens require elaborate, labor-intensive therapy from laboratory, pharmacy, and nursing staffs. Examples include on-site manufacture of liposomal infusions, *in vitro* manipulation of an individual's lymphocytes, and administration of therapeutic agents via a variety of ambulatory infusion devices and by multiple routes. Tremendous advances in venous access techniques have enabled children to receive parenteral chemotherapy and supportive care for the duration of their therapy. Thus, careful documentation of administration variables is essential to adequately interpret response to therapy in an individual subject. In some situations this quality control measure can be easily accomplished by documenting on a protocol treatment calendar the time and amount of drug administered by the caregiver. For some drugs, long-term compliance can be objectively assessed by pharmacologic monitoring. One example is the use of erythrocyte methotrexate polyglutamate concentrations to assess the extent to which chronic compliance has occurred,[23] although the precision of this method and its relation to therapeutic outcome have not been established.

Systemic Dose Intensity

Careful diligence on the part of physicians, pharmacists, nurses, parents, and other clinicians can help to ensure that protocol therapy is given as planned. However, additional variables, such as patient-to-patient differences in drug disposition, can influence response to therapy, even if the administered dose is rigorously controlled.

In pediatric patients plasma concentrations of anticancer drugs can vary over a 2- to 10-fold range, even when uniform dosages are administered based on body weight or body surface area.[24] The pharmacokinetics of many anticancer drugs have been evaluated in children; these drugs include methotrexate, cyclophosphamide, bleomycin, etoposide, teniposide, and doxorubicin.[24] In most cases the pharmacokinetic variability cannot be predicted by routine clinical laboratory tests (serum creatinine, total bilirubin, etc.). The metabolism and elimination of a drug may also change over time within a patient due to the effects of concurrent drug therapy, changes in organ function, nutritional status, maturational changes, or possibly as a result of successful initial treatment of the primary disease process.[25]

Intuitively, one would expect this variability to be a potentially important determinant of response to a single drug. More importantly, evaluation of pharmacokinetic characteristics may help distinguish whether one drug in a multiagent regimen is being under- or overdosed, especially if these agents have overlapping therapeutic and/or toxic effects, precluding dosage adjustments based solely on a biologic measure of drug effects (e.g., WBC). While the pharmacokinetic characteristics of antineoplastic agents are often evaluated in phase I and II studies, relatively few data are available that evaluate the relationship of pharmacokinetics and response (i.e., pharmacodynamics). The following sections focus on some potentially important clinical pharmacodynamic data for anticancer drugs.

Absorption

Most cytotoxic agents used in pediatric oncology are administered parenterally; exceptions include the use of oral 6-mercaptopurine and methotrexate during maintenance therapy of acute lymphocytic leukemia. Considerable variability in the bioavailability of each of these drugs has been demonstrated. For example, approximately 5–37 percent of a 6-mercaptopurine dose reaches the systemic circulation.[26] The extent of systemic exposure following oral administration may be influenced by drugs such as allopurinol, which inhibits metabolism of 6-mercaptopurine by xanthine oxidase, and possibly by the time of day it is administered.[27] Given the effectiveness of 6-mercaptopurine for childhood acute lymphocytic leukemia, despite its poor and variable oral bioavailability, one might anticipate the potential value of using intravenous 6-mercaptopurine. Several clinical trials are under way to test this possibility.

Both interpatient and intrapatient variability in the systemic bioavailability of oral methotrexate have also been demonstrated. The fraction of methotrexate absorbed is dose-related, with approximately 40 percent bioavailability in doses less than 40 mg/m^2 and less than 25 percent at higher doses.[28] A study of children with acute lymphocytic leukemia receiving oral methotrexate retrospectively segregated patients into two groups depending on the methotrexate absorption rate.[29] The children not achieving a selected plasma concentration (slow absorbers) were more likely to experience a relapse in their disease. This provocative finding remains to be validated in a larger, prospective study. We currently utilize parenteral methotrexate for weekly maintenance therapy in our acute lymphocytic leukemia protocols because of wide interpatient variability in oral absorption.

Leucovorin is another drug with saturable oral absorption that is given either orally or parenterally. Rescue of normal cells from methotrexate cytotoxicity with leucovorin is a common and essential practice with high-dose methotrexate regimens. Although leucovorin doses are usually 15–30 mg, doses exceeding 50 mg may be required in some cases. Oral bioavailability studies have demonstrated that 90 percent of a 15-mg dose is bioavailable, compared to 75 percent of a 50-mg dose, and that saturation of absorption occurs with oral doses greater than 50 mg.[30,31] For this reason, high doses of leucovorin (although only rarely required) are given as parenteral injections to ensure complete bioavailability.

Distribution

The extent of drug penetration into various compartments of the body, as well as into tumors, is determined by several factors, including the drug's chemical composition, pharmacokinetics, protein binding, route of administration, and tumor hemodynamics. Methotrexate distribution characteristics have been well studied and provide a good model for determination of clinically important characteristics. Methotrexate sequestration can occur in pleural effusions and in ascitic fluid, and this can be clinically important when methotrexate is administered in high doses (over 250 mg/m^2).[30] These reservoirs may produce prolonged systemic exposure to cytotoxic concentrations of methotrexate, rendering the patient at increased risk for toxicity if adequate rescue measures (leucovorin) are not continued. One reason for the use of high-dose methotrexate regimens is to provide potentially cytotoxic concentrations to areas where the drug does not normally distribute well, such as the cerebrospinal fluid (CSF) or the testes. Intrathecal methotrexate is also utilized in the treatment of sensitive malignancies with high potential for central nervous system (CNS) involvement, such as acute lymphocytic leukemia.[32] Bleyer et al.[33] noted much lower CSF concentrations of methotrexate in pediatric patients compared to adults when intrathecal doses were based on the patient's body surface area (BSA) (Figure 36–5). A good relationship was found when the CSF concentration was related to patient age. This corresponds to the age-adjusted volume of CSF, with adult volumes being reached at approximately 3 years of age. In at least one study, dosing intrathecal methotrexate based on patient age has resulted in more consistent methotrexate concentrations in the CSF and a reduced incidence of CNS leukemia relapsing in the CNS.[32]

Metabolism/Excretion

Substantial variability in metabolism and/or excretion is often the most important factor determining the wide range of systemic exposure when uniform dosages (mg/

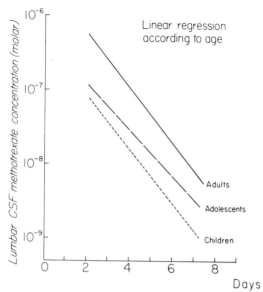

FIGURE 36–5. Regression of methotrexate CSF concentrations after intrathecal injection of 12 mg/m² in adults, adolescents, and children. (From Bleyer,[33] with permission.)

m²) are administered to children. Drug metabolism may be important not only for detoxification, but also for conversion of a parent drug to an active metabolite. Cyclophosphamide and ifosfamide are examples of drugs that require extracellular metabolic activation for efficacy. There are also inactive parent drugs that undergo intracellular activation (e.g., 6-mercaptopurine, Ara-C) as well as active parent drugs that have active metabolites (e.g., etoposide, doxorubicin, and methotrexate). Regulation of the enzymes involved in these activation pathways may be under monogenic control and/or influenced by developmental and pathologic processes. Unfortunately, a child who does not respond to a specific anticancer therapy is often wrongly believed to have a disease that is resistant to that therapy. One could also postulate that lack of response in an individual may be secondary to inadequate metabolic function necessary for drug activation and/or enhanced rates of drug inactivation and elimination. Investigations are currently under way to evaluate these premises.

Phase I and II studies in clinical oncology are conducted to assess a potential oncolytic agent against various tumors that are considered refractory to standard therapy. Traditionally, drug dosages based on BSA are escalated in every three to six patients until an MTD is achieved.[34] An alternative strategy for evaluating new drugs and establishing the optimal (i.e., maximum) dosage in children was recently implemented at St. Jude Children's Research Hospital.[13] Using teniposide as a prototype, 23 children with refractory acute lymphocytic leukemia or solid tumors were given 72-hour continuous infusions at escalating doses. Pharmacokinetic/pharmacodynamic relationships were investigated in these subjects at dosage levels of 450, 600, and 750 mg/m²/72 h. A 10-fold range in systemic clearance of teniposide was found, producing variability such that some subjects in the lowest dosage group had higher systemic exposure (area under the concentration × time curve) to the parent

drug than those receiving the highest dosage, and vice versa. The relationships between systemic exposure and response or toxicity were both highly significant. Predictably, there was a poor correlation between dose administered and response. These results indicate that interpatient variability in drug disposition may be so great that there are no differences in systemic drug exposure at the different dosage levels of a typical phase I or II trial. Results of the St. Jude trial and those of Egorin and others[35] support evaluation of selected new oncolytic phase I and II studies based on maximal tolerated systemic exposure as an end point, rather than maximal tolerated dosage.

Patients who rapidly eliminate antineoplastics may achieve less benefit from their prescribed dose than patients with slow elimination. This premise was tested in a group of 154 children with acute lymphocytic leukemia at St. Jude Children's Research Hospital receiving high-dose methotrexate for remission therapy.[16] Methotrexate systemic clearances during 24-hour continuous infusion were found to vary over a three-fold range. After a median followup of 3.5 years, multivariate analysis demonstrated that patients with methotrexate systemic clearance greater than 76 ml/min/m² were three times more likely to have a relapse during therapy ($p = .01$). When this population was compared to 254 historical controls who received the same backbone of maintenance therapy, but no high-dose methotrexate, only children with systemic clearances less than 76 ml/min/m² had significantly better disease-free survival compared to the control group. While this pharmacodynamic relationship has been supported by others,[36] it does not establish a therapeutic range for methotrexate. One can state that, given this group of patients and therapy regimen, 1000 mg/m² of methotrexate was not optimal for patients with relatively fast high-dose methotrexate systemic clearance.[16]

The pharmacodynamic data described above for methotrexate and teniposide have been utilized to design a prospective study to assess the therapeutic value of individualizing therapy based on each patient's pharmacokinetic characteristics, thus ensuring that patients with rapid clearance do not have relatively low systemic exposure to these drugs.[37] The clinical feasibility of this strategy was initially assessed in a pilot study of 18 children with relapsed acute lymphocytic leukemia given 24- and 36-hour continuous infusions of methotrexate and teniposide, respectively. Plasma samples were obtained during the infusions to determine individual pharmacokinetic parameters, and doses were adjusted to achieve steady-state concentrations of 10 μm for methotrexate and 10 mg/liter for teniposide. The actual mean steady-state concentrations produced after dose adjustment were 12.4 mg/liter for teniposide and 9.7 μm for methotrexate, demonstrating feasibility and accuracy in the clinical setting.

Tumor Dose Intensity

Ultimately one would like to know how much drug is available at the site of action inside both malignant cells (efficacy) and normal cells (toxicity). For some drugs and malignancies, the extracellular drug disposition will reflect what is occurring in the intracellular environment. However, in many cases, the relationship between extracellular and intracellular events may be complex and difficult to determine.

Variables such as tumor blood flow may play a role in determining the amount of drug presented to a malignant cell for intracellular transport. Tumor microcirculation is thought to be heterogeneous, with significant flow differences demonstrating time- and location-dependent characteristics. A number of factors have been shown to account for altered blood flow through a tumor cell bed. These include differences in perfusion pressures, blood viscosity, and vessel geometry.[38] Before a xenobiotic can reach the malignant cell, it usually has to pass from the microcirculation through the tumor interstitium. The latter compartment may also have substantially different structural and functional characteristics compared to normal tissue, potentially affecting drug transport. Briefly, some features of neoplastic tissue that distinguish it from normal interstitial tissue are a larger interstitial space, lower proteoglycan and hyaluronate concentrations, higher collagen content, and altered lymphatic function.[39]

Membrane transport of anticancer drugs can contribute to the development of drug resistance for some malignancies. Such work has recently focused on overexpression of a membrane glycoprotein responsible for augmentation of drug efflux in resistant cells.[40] These cells seem to exhibit cross-resistance between anthracyclines, vinca alkaloids, and epipodophyllotoxins. Some drugs have been shown to competitively inhibit this efflux mechanism *in vitro*, with the prototype agent being verapamil.[41] Clinical studies of efflux inhibitors, such as verapamil, in combination with oncolytics are currently being conducted for drug-resistant cancers.[42]

Intracellular metabolism is important in the activation or detoxification of several oncolytics. Both Ara-C and 6-mercaptopurine are metabolically converted within the cell to their active metabolites, Ara-CTP and 6-thioguanine nucleotide, respectively. Clinical evaluations of intracellular Ara-C disposition in patients with acute myelocytic leukemia have shown a correlation between intracellular metabolite retention and response to therapy or duration of remission.[43,44] Prospective studies have demonstrated the feasibility of individualizing Ara-C therapy based on measured intracellular active metabolite concentrations,[45] although clear relationships of these to efficacy or toxicity have not yet been completely evaluated.

Detoxification of the parent compound or its active metabolic products may also occur within the cellular environment. Glutathione-S-transferase enzymes catalyze such activity by accelerating conjugation of glutathione to electrophilic compounds. Increased activity of these enzymes has been demonstrated in some cells with acquired resistance to oncolytic agents and thus represents another pathway of developing resistant tumor cells.[46]

In summary, more complete knowledge of the cellular pharmacokinetics and biochemical pharmacology of anticancer drugs has provided guidelines for more rational therapy and should lead to more effective treatment.

BONE MARROW TRANSPLANT

Although aklylating agents and other anticancer drugs may exhibit steep dose-response characteristics, the dose one can safely administer is often limited by bone marrow toxicity in the host. Bone marrow support or transplantation procedures have enabled delivery of high-dose systemic therapy without permanent damage to hematopoietic function.

There are three basic types of bone marrow transplants: autologous, syngeneic, and allogeneic. Autologous transplants, now commonly termed *bone marrow support,* use the patient's own marrow, usually obtained while the disease is in remission. *In vitro* purging regimens may be used to rid the marrow of residual malignant cells. Infusion of marrow from an identical twin is termed syngeneic transplantation. Use of marrow from siblings or others who possess similar tissue antigens (e.g., human lymphocyte antigens, HLA) to the marrow recipient is termed allogeneic transplantation.

Bone marrow transplants have been utilized with some success in a number of pediatric malignancies, including acute lymphocytic leukemia (in second remission), acute nonlymphocytic leukemia (in first remission), neuroblastoma, preleukemia, and non-Hodgkin's lymphoma.[47-50]

The use of marrow transplants or marrow support procedures has permitted the administration of much higher dosages of several anticancer drugs, and there are examples where this higher dose intensity has yielded improved results in refractory cancers. However, syngeneic and allogeneic transplants are not without risk. Adverse events from this treatment can generally be divided into four categories: acute graft failure, infections, graft-versus-host disease, and delayed effects.[51] Graft failure is the least common of the four; however, it may result in significant mortality. The gastrointestinal tract, liver, and skin are frequently affected by graft-versus-host disease, which can be subdivided into acute (usually occurring < 100 days posttransplant) and chronic (occurring > 100 days posttransplant). Pharmacologic manipulation of the immune system is required for treatment of graft-versus-host disease. Agents used include corticosteroids, azathioprine, cyclosporine, antithymocyte globulin, methotrexate, cyclophosphamide, and monoclonal antibodies.[51] Combinations of these drugs are sometimes utilized. Infectious complications following bone marrow transplant include bacterial and fungal disease occurring most frequently during the initial hypoplasia. Subsequent interstitial processes involve organisms such as *Pneumocystis carinii,* cytomegalovirus, herpes simplex virus, and varicella–zoster virus. Delayed effects of transplants are usually attributed to side effects of the preparative regimen. Those reported include second malignancies, cataract formation, sterility, and pulmonary disease.

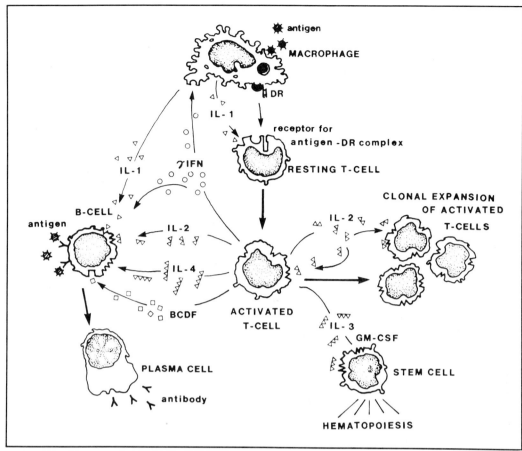

FIGURE 36–6. Effects of antigenic challenge on cytokine dynamics. Antigen first is processed by macrophage with subsequent activation of the resting T cell in the presence of the histocompatibility molecule (DR) and interleukin-1. The cell then produces various cytokines, which result in clonal expansion, differentiation, and activation of B cells. (From Dinarello and Mier,[69] with permission.)

IMMUNOTHERAPY

Relatively nonspecific immune modulators such as bacillus Calmette-Guérin (BCG) have been studied for a number of years. Only recently have more specific agents been available for widespread clinical trials. Most BRMs under current clinical evaluation alter either lymphocyte function or cytokine production. Figure 36–6 shows the interrelationship and actions of various cytokines. One of the most extensively evaluated cytokines is interleukin-2, which is produced *in vivo* by activated lymphocytes. Its potential mechanisms of antitumor activity include the proliferation of antigen-primed T cells, the induction of interferon-γ secretion, increased activity of natural killer cytotoxic T cells, and the production of lymphokine-activated killer (LAK) cells.[52] The latter population of cells is defined as those which can kill tumor cells resistant to natural killer cells. Clinical trials in adults have used both *in vivo* and *in vitro* interleukin-2 to generate LAK cell activity against cancers for which traditional chemotherapy alone would probably not be efficacious.[10,11]

Interferons have been classified into three principal subtypes: α, β, and γ. In general, these agents help to induce antigen expression and augment natural killer cell activity. However, each possesses pharmacologic characteristics differentiating it from the others. The exact mechanism responsible for antitumor effects of interferons is unclear.[53] Nonetheless, numerous clinical trials of these cytokines are under way to assess their activity in the treatment of pediatric malignancies.

Monoclonal antibodies are anticipated to have future clinical use in the diagnosis, monitoring, and treatment of malignancies. Diagnostically, they are already being utilized in situations such as the determination of acute lymphocytic leukemia lineages. Therapeutic use will most likely be in the form of conjugates to a cytotoxic agent or radionuclide, thus targeting the therapeutic agent to the antigenic area recognized by the antibody. The obstacles that must be overcome for these conjugates to be used clinically include specificity to tumor cells, affinity to the antigenic site, and stability of the cytotoxin–antibody conjugate.[54]

ADVERSE EFFECTS OF THERAPY

Drugs utilized to treat malignancies are derived from many different pharmacologic classifications, and thus their adverse effect profiles encompass a wide range of

TABLE 36–3. ROUTES OF ADMINISTRATION AND TOXICITIES OF SOME ANTICANCER DRUGS USED IN PEDIATRIC PATIENTS

AGENT	ROUTE OF ADMINISTRATION*	COMMON TOXICITIES	UNCOMMON TOXICITIES
Antimetabolites			
Methotrexate	P.O., I.M., I.V., I.T.	Myelosuppression, mucositis, hepatitis, dermatitis	Nephrotoxicity, neurotoxicity, osteoporosis, pneumonitis, cirrhosis
Ara-C	S.C., I.M., I.V., I.T.	Myelosuppression, nausea and vomiting, diarrhea, conjunctivitis, mucositis	Hepatitis, neurotoxicity, encephalopathy with I.T. administration
6-TG	P.O., (I.V.)	Myelosuppression	Nausea and vomiting
6-MP	P.O., (I.V.)	Myelosuppression; nausea, vomiting, and abdominal pain; hepatitis	Mucositis
5-Azacytidine	I.V.	Nausea and vomiting, myelosuppression	Hepatitis
5-FU	I.V., P.O. unreliable	Myelosuppression, anorexia, nausea and vomiting, mucositis, diarrhea	Dermatitis, alopecia, hyperpigmentation, cerebellar ataxia, hypersensitivity reactions, cardiotoxicity
Alkylating Agents			
Cyclophosphamide	P.O., I.V.	Myelosuppression, hemorrhagic cystitis, nausea and vomiting, alopecia	Mucositis, hyperpigmentation, hypo-osmolarity, infertility
Mechlorethamine	I.V., I.C., avoid extravasation	Nausea and vomiting, myelosuppression, diarrhea	Mucositis, alopecia
Chlorambucil	P.O.	Myelosuppression	Nausea and vomiting, hepatitis, seizures
Mephalan	P.O. (I.V.), avoid extravasation	Myelosuppression	Anorexia, nausea and vomiting
Busulfan	P.O.	Myelosuppression	Nausea and vomiting, alopecia, hyperpigmentation, diarrhea, pneumonitis
Ifosfamide	I.V.	Myelosuppression, hemorrhagic cystitis, nausea and vomiting	Confusion
Antibiotics			
Doxorubicin/ daunorubicin	I.V., avoid extravasation	Myelosuppression, nausea and vomiting, alopecia, mucositis	Cardiomyopathy
Actinomycin D	I.V., avoid extravasation	Myelosuppression, nausea and vomiting, mucositis, alopecia	Dermatitis, hyperpigmentation, radiation recall
Bleomycin	S.C., I.M., I.V., I.C.	Nausea and vomiting, dermatitis, hyperpigmentation, alopecia, fever	Pulmonary fibrosis, mucositis, hypersensitivity reactions
Vinca alkaloids			
Vincristine	I.V., avoid extravasation	Peripheral neuropathy, jaw pain, constipation, alopecia	Cranial nerve palsies, seizures, myelosuppression, hemolysis, inappropriate ADH secretion
Vinblastine	I.V. (P.O.), avoid extravasation	Myelosuppression, nausea and vomiting, mucositis	Peripheral neuropathy, alopecia
Miscellaneous agents			
Steroids	P.O., I.V.	Cushing's syndrome, diabetes, hypertension, growth delay	Hypokalemia, myopathy, osteoporosis, psychosis, adrenal insufficiency
CCNU/BCNU	P.O./I.V., avoid extravasation	Nausea and vomiting, delayed immunosuppression, myelosuppression	Hepatitis, stomatitis, pulmonary fibrosis
DTIC	I.V., avoid extravasation	Myelosuppression, nausea and vomiting, stomatitis, diarrhea	Hepatitis, alopecia, photosensitivity

TABLE 36–3. ROUTES OF ADMINISTRATION AND TOXICITIES OF SOME ANTICANCER DRUGS USED IN PEDIATRIC PATIENTS *Continued*

AGENT	ROUTE OF ADMINISTRATION*	COMMON TOXICITIES	UNCOMMON TOXICITIES
Procarbazine	P.O.	Nausea and vomiting, myelosuppression, lethargy, dermatitis, disulfiram-like reaction with alcohol	Stomatitis, peripheral neuropathy, seizures, myopathy/myalgias
L-Asparaginase	I.M., I.V.	Hypersensitivity reactions, coagulopathy, hyperglycemia, hepatic dysfunction	Encephalopathy, pancreatitis, abdominal pain
Cis-platinum	I.V.	Nausea and vomiting, nephrotoxicity, ototoxicity	Myelosuppression, seizures, peripheral and autonomic neuropathy, hypomagnesemia, hypocalcemia
Hydroxyurea	P.O. (I.V.)	Myelosuppression	Nausea and vomiting, mucositis, dermatitis, alopecia
Teniposide (VM-26)	I.V., avoid extravasation	Myelosuppression	Nausea and vomiting, alopecia, hypersensitivity reactions
Etoposide (VP-16)	P.O., I.V.	Myelosuppression, nausea and vomiting, alopecia	Hypersensitivity reactions, hypotension
Amsacrine	I.V., avoid extravasation	Nausea and vomiting, myelosuppression, alopecia	Anaphylaxis, stomatitis, ventricular arrhythmias, hepatic toxicity
Mitoxantrone	I.V., avoid extravasation	Nausea and vomiting, myelosuppression, blue-green sclera and urine	Cardiotoxicity, stomatitis, alopecia
Interferon	I.M., S.C.	Fever, chills, fatigue, headache, arthralgias	Hypotension, myelosuppression, anorexia
Interleukin-2	I.V.	Fluid retention, hypotension, nausea and vomiting, diarrhea	Anemia, thrombocytopenia, nephrotoxicity

*P.O. = oral, I.M. = intramuscular, S.C. = subcutaneous, I.V. = intravenous, I.T. = intrathecal, I.C. = intracavitary, ( ) = investigational.

toxicities. Toxicologic profiles of many antineoplastic agents used in pediatric oncology are listed in Table 36–3. Many of these effects are reversible or treatable, such as nausea and vomiting, alopecia, stomatitis, diarrhea, hyperuricemia, and bone marrow suppression. Unfortunately, some reactions, such as those affecting the heart, lungs, kidneys, or neurologic system, are irreversible and may be dose-limiting. (Reviews of specific end-organ toxicities may be found in reference 55.)

Bone marrow suppression occurs with many antineoplastics; notable exceptions include standard doses of vincristine, corticosteroids, bleomycin, and some BRMs. When cytotoxic drugs do produce bone marrow suppression, the typical nadir of affected cells occurs between 7 and 14 days, with recovery in 21–28 days. A delayed pattern of myelosuppression can be manifested after therapy with carmustine BCNU/lomustine CCNU or procarbazine. Cytokines known as colony-stimulating factors (CSFs) demonstrate an ability to stimulate bone marrow production and/or differentiation of progenitor cells. These substances vary in their specificity for cell lines. Interleukin-3, also known as multi-CSF, stimulates the production of neutrophilic, monocytic, erythrocytic, and megakaryocytic cell precursors, whereas G-CSF predominantly stimulates the production of granulocytes.[56,57] Figure 36–7 outlines CSF subclasses and their functional capacity. CSFs have produced a more rapid recovery from chemotherapy-induced bone marrow suppression in preliminary clinical studies.[58–60] It is hoped that this will enable the safe administration of higher doses of some anticancer drugs and potentially shorten the period of hypoplasia after bone marrow transplantation procedures. Evaluations must prove that malignant cell growth is not concomitantly potentiated by selected CSFs, prior to their widespread clinical use.

Other treatment strategies that alter the course of oncolytic toxicity are shown in Table 36–4. Probably the most impressive of these has involved measures taken to prevent host toxicity from high-dose methotrexate infusions. Lethal gastrointestinal, hepatic, and bone marrow toxicities associated with these regimens have been virtually eliminated by aggressive hydration, early identification of patients at increased risk for toxicity, and pharmacokinetically adjusted leucovorin rescue. Criteria for patients at high risk for toxicity may include delayed methotrexate excretion in the first 24 hours of exposure, gastrointestinal obstruction, or patients with "third spaces" (e.g., ascites or pleural effusions).[30] A history of renal dysfunction or previous methotrexate toxicity necessitates pharmacokinetic monitoring, even with low-dose regimens. Interac-

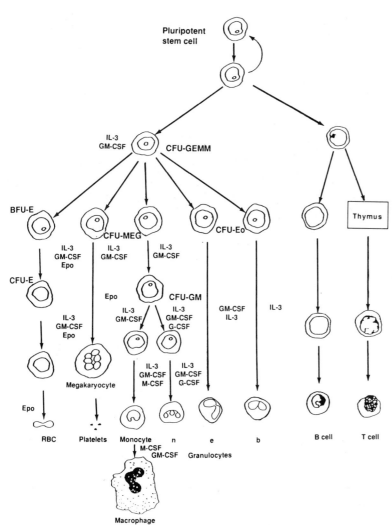

FIGURE 36–7. Subclassifications of colony-stimulating factors relating to their function. Abbreviations: CFU, colony-forming unit; b, basophil; BFU, burst-forming unit; e, eosinophil; E, erythrocyte; Epo, erythropoietin; m, monocyte; M, megakaryocyte. (From Clark and Kamen,[70] with permission.)

tions with drugs that alter renal function (e.g., nonsteroidal anti-inflammatory drugs) may also predispose to high-dose methotrexate toxicity, especially in patients with preexisting renal dysfunction.

The toxicity profile of an antineoplastic agent in children may differ from that encountered in adults. Anthracycline-induced cardiotoxicity can usually be related to total dose given over the patient's lifetime in both the adult and pediatric populations. Interestingly, at least one study has demonstrated that pediatric patients experience this effect at lower normalized doses (mg/m²) than do adults, as shown in Figure 36–8.[60]

Irreversible hearing loss can occur with cisplatin therapy, potentially affecting a child's speech and language development skills. The proportion of pediatric solid tumor patients experiencing significant hearing loss with cisplatin therapy has been shown to increase as the cumulative dosage increases (Figure 36–9). Younger children experience this effect at lower cumulative doses[61]; however, toxicity is not well studied in very young children

TABLE 36–4. TREATMENT/PREVENTION OF CHEMOTHERAPY-INDUCED TOXICITIES

CHEMOTHERAPY	ADVERSE EFFECT	TREATMENT
Cyclophosphamide	Hemorrhagic cystitis	Mesna (2-mercaptoethane sulfonate Na)
Methotrexate	GI toxicity Myelosuppression	Leucovorin Hydration Alkalinization Thymidine
Cis-platinum	Nephrotoxicity	NaCl Hydration Mannitol
Alkylating agents, epipodophyllotoxins	Myelosuppression	Colony-stimulating factors

due to methodologic problems of audiologic testing in this population.

The planned dose of an antineoplastic agent for the treatment of a pediatric malignancy is frequently based on the patient's BSA. A child with BSA < 1 m² may have a substantially greater BSA in relation to body weight than an older child or an adult. This relationship was thought to be responsible for a high incidence of severe neuropathies reported when vincristine was prescribed to a group of infants based on their BSA. Normalized to weight, the infants received over 1.5 times the dose given to older children.[62] Based on these data, calculation of vincristine dosage by body weight has been recommended for younger children, although the pharmacologic and physiologic basis has not been established.

In general, younger children have a relatively larger BSA per body weight and thus are prescribed larger doses in mg/kg if dosages are based on BSA. However, this may be appropriate for many drugs, since the clearance of many drugs is comparable in children and adults when normalized to BSA, but greater in children when normalized to body weight.[24,63] These relationships may not hold for infants, in whom greater toxicity has been observed when standard mg/m² doses were given. For example, infants with Wilms' tumor treated with vincristine and dactinomycin dosed on BSA had much higher death rates secondary to toxicity than did older children.[64]

The cure rates and survival of many childhood cancers are generally greater than those of most adult cancers. As these cure rates have escalated, late effects thought to be related to past disease or its therapy have been noted. The onset of symptoms may vary from months to years after therapy. Commonly reported toxicities include sterility,

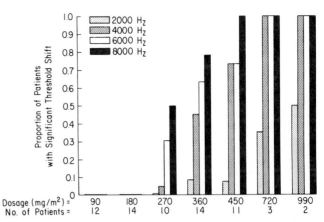

FIGURE 36–9. Proportion of pediatric solid tumor patients experiencing significant hearing loss in relation to their cumulative dose of cisplatin. (The important speech frequency range is 500–2000 Hz.) (From McHaney et al.,[61] with permission.)

hypogonadism, developmental delays, growth retardation, and second malignancies. Attempts to correlate these effects to risk factors are obviously difficult, due to the small numbers of patients evaluated and heterogeneous control groups. However, some initial cancer types and treatment modalities (as well as prescribed doses) have demonstrated elevated risk. The timing of therapy in relation to pubertal status has been shown to be important for gonadal toxicity, with gonadal quiescence conferring a protective effect in some.[65] In summary, one cannot truly know the overall risk of adverse events attributable to a drug or treatment regimen until its extensive use has resulted in durable cures that can be followed for prolonged periods.

SUMMARY AND CONCLUSIONS

Clinical pharmacology has played an extensive role in the design and evaluation of pediatric oncology studies. These data have proven useful in developing guidelines for the rational use of anticancer drugs in children. More recently, clinical pharmacologic principles have provided insights into why some children may fail to respond to therapy that is known to be curative in a majority of children with the same diagnosis. Prospective clinical trials are needed to clarify the importance of many clinical pharmacologic principles and to define their role in the design of curative therapy for childhood cancers.

ACKNOWLEDGMENTS: Supported in part by NIH MERIT award R37 CA36401, Leukemia Program Project CA20180, Solid Tumor Program Project CA23066, and Cancer Center CORE grant CA21765; a Centers of Excellence grant from the State of Tennessee; and ALSAC.

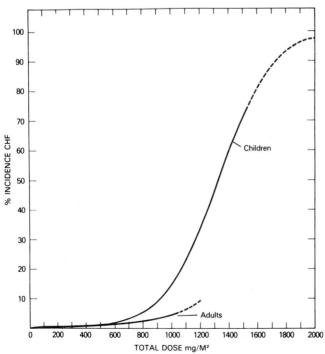

FIGURE 36–8. Percent incidence of daunomycin-induced congestive heart failure in adult and pediatric patients. (From von Hoff et al.,[60] with permission.)

REFERENCES

1. Cancer Facts and Figures–1988. New York, American Cancer Society, 1988

2. Pratt CB: Some aspects of childhood cancer epidemiology. Pediatr Clin N Am 32:541–556, 1985

3. Sutow WW, Fernbach DJ, Vietti TJ (eds): Clinical Pediatric Oncology. St. Louis, C.V. Mosby, 1983

4. Levine AS (ed): Cancer in the Young. New York, Masson, 1982

5. Chabner B, Collins JM (eds): Cancer chemotherapy: Principle and practice. Philadelphia, Lippincott. 1990

6. Goldie JH, Coldman AJ: A mathematical model for relating the drug sensitivity of tumors to their spontaneous mutation rate. Cancer Treat Rep 63:1727–1733, 1979

7. Coleman M: Chemotherapy for large-cell lymphoma: Optimism and caution. Ann Intern Med 103:140–142, 1985

8. Pendergrass TW, Milstein JM, Geyer JR, et al: Eight drugs in one day chemotherapy for brain tumors: Experience in 107 children and rationale for preradiation chemotherapy. J Clin Oncol 5:1221–1231, 1987

9. Bonadonna G, Valagussa P, Santoro A: Alternating non-cross-resistant combination chemotherapy or MOPP in stage IV Hodgkin's disease. Ann Intern Med 104:739–746, 1986

10. Rosenberg SA, Lotze MT, Muul LM, et al: A progress report on the treatment of 157 patients with advanced cancer using lymphokine-activated killer cells and interleukin-2 or high-dose interleukin-2 alone. N Engl J Med 316:889–897, 1987

11. West WH, Tauer KW, Yannelli JR, et al: Constant-infusion recombinant interleukin-2 in adoptive immunotherapy of advanced cancer. N Engl J Med 316:898–905, 1987

12. Glaubiger DL, von Hoff DD, Holcenberg JS, et al: The relative tolerance of children and adults to anticancer drugs. Front Radiat Ther Oncol 16:42–49, 1982

13. Rodman JH, Abromowitch M, Sinkule JA, et al: Clinical pharmacodynamics of continuous infusion teniposide: Systemic exposure as a determinant of response in a phase I trial. J Clin Oncol 5:1007–1014, 1987

14. Evans WE: Clinical pharmacodynamics of anticancer drugs: A basis for extending the concept of dose-intensity. Blut 56:241–248, 1988

15. Sulkes A, Collins JM: Reappraisal of some dosage adjustment guidelines. Cancer Treat Rep 71:229–233, 1987

16. Evans WE, Crom WR, Abromowitch M, et al: Clinical pharmacodynamics of high-dose methotrexate in acute lymphocytic leukemia. Identification of a relation between concentration and effect. N Engl J Med 314:471–477, 1986

17. Carde P, MacKintosh FR, Rosenberg SA: A dose and time response analysis of the treatment of Hodgkin's disease with MOPP chemotherapy. J Clin Oncol 1:146–153, 1983

18. Pinkel D, Hernandez K, Borella L, et al: Drug dosage and remission duration in childhood lymphocytic leukemia. Cancer 27:247–254, 1971

19. Frei E, Canellos GP: Dose: A critical factor in cancer chemotherapy. Am J Med 69:585–594, 1980

20. Peeters M, Koren G, Jakubovicz D, et al: Physician compliance and relapse rates of acute lymphoblastic leukemia in children. Clin Pharmacol Ther 43:228–232, 1988

21. Pieters R, Huismans DR, Veerman AJP: Are children with lymphoblastic leukaemia resistant to 6-mercaptopurine because of 5'-nucleotidase? Lancet 2:1471, 1987

22. Snodgrass W, Smith S, Trueworthy R, et al: Pediatric clinical pharmacology of 6-mercaptopurine: Lack of compliance as a factor in leukemia relapse. Proc Am Soc Clin Oncol 3:204, 1984

23. Schroder H, Clausen N, Ostergaard E, et al: Pharmacokinetics of erythrocyte methotrexate in children with acute lymphocytic leukemia during maintenance treatment. Cancer Chemother Pharmacol 20:248–252, 1987

24. Crom WR, Glynn-Barnhart AM, Rodman JH, et al: Pharmacokinetics of anticancer drugs in children. Clin Pharmacokinet 12:168–213, 1987

25. Relling MV, Crom WR, Pieper JA, et al: Hepatic drug clearance in children with leukemia: Changes in clearance of model substrates during remission-induction therapy. Clin Pharmacol Ther 41:651–660, 1987

26. Zimm S, Collins JM, Riccardi R, et al: Variable bioavailability of oral mercaptopurine—Is maintenance chemotherapy in acute lymphoblastic leukemia being optimally delivered? N Engl J Med 308:1005–1009, 1983

27. Langevin AM, Koren G, Soldin SJ, et al: Pharmacokinetic case for giving 6-mercaptopurine maintenance doses at night. Lancet 2:505–506, 1987

28. Teresi ME, Crom WR, Choi KE, et al: Methotrexate bioavailability after oral and intramuscular administration in children. J Pediatr 110:788–792, 1987

29. Craft AW, Rankin A, Aherne W: Methotrexate absorption in children with acute lymphocytic leukemia. Cancer Treat Rep 65(suppl 1):77–81, 1981

30. Evans WE, Crom WR, Yalowich JC: Methotrexate, in Evans WE, Schentag JJ, Jusko WJ (eds): Applied Pharmacokinetics: Principles of Therapeutic Drug Monitoring. Spokane, Applied Therapeutics, 1986, pp 1009–1056

31. Straw JA, Szapary D, Wynn WT: Pharmacokinetics of the diastereoisomers of leucovorin after intravenous and oral administration to normal subjects. Cancer Res 44:3114–3119, 1984

32. Bleyer WA, Coccia PF, Sather HN, et al: Reduction in central nervous system leukemia with a pharmacokinetically derived intrathecal methotrexate dosage regimen. J Clin Oncol 1:317–323, 1983

33. Bleyer WA: Clinical pharmacology of intrathecal methotrexate. II. An improved dosage regimen derived from age-related pharmacokinetics. Can Treat Rep 61:1419–1425, 1977

34. Collins JM, Zaharko DS, Dedrick RL, Chabner BA: Potential for preclinical pharmacology in phase I clinical trials. Cancer Treat Rep 70:73–80, 1986

35. Forrest A, Conley BA, Egorin MJ, et al: Adaptive control of hexamethylene bisacetamide pharmacodynamics (Abstr.) Proc Am Soc Clin Oncol 7:61, 1988

36. Borsi JD, Moe PJ: Systemic clearance of methotrexate in the prognosis of acute lymphoblastic leukemia in children. Cancer 60:3020–3024, 1987

37. Rodman JH, Sunderland M, Kanavagh RL, et al: Continuous infusion of methotrexate and teniposide for pediatric acute lymphocytic leukemia. Systemic pharmacokinetics and dosage regimen adjustment (Abstr.). Pharmacotherapy 8:137, 1988

38. Jain RK: Determinants of tumor blood flow: A review. Cancer Res 48:2641–2658, 1988

39. Jain RK: Transport of molecules in the tumor interstitium: A review. Cancer Res 47:3039–3051, 1987

40. Riordan JR, Ling V: Genetic and biochemical characterization of multidrug resistance. Pharmac Ther 28:51–75, 1985

41. Yalowich JC, Ross WE: Verapamil-induced augmentation of etoposide accumulation in L1210 cells in vitro. Cancer Res 45:1651–1656, 1985

42. Cairo MS, Siegel S, Anas N, Sender LK: Clinical trial of continuous infusion verapamil, bolus vinblastine, and continuous infusion of VP-16 in relapsed pediatric tumors: Modulation of drug resistance and cytotoxicity (Abstr.). Proc Am Assoc Cancer Res 29:223, 1988

43. Preisler HD, Rustum Y, Priore RL: Relationship between leukemic cell retention of cytosine arabinoside triphosphate and the duration of remission in patients with acute non-lymphocytic leukemia. Eur J Cancer Clin Oncol 21:23–30, 1985

44. Estey E, Plunkett W, Dixon D, et al: Variables predicting response to high dose cytosine arabinoside therapy in patients with refractory acute leukemia. Leukemia 1:580–583, 1987

45. Plunkett W, Iacoboni S, Estey E, et al: Pharmacologically directed ara-C therapy for refractory leukemia. Semin Oncol 12(suppl 3):20–30, 1985

46. Kramer RA, Zakher J, Kim G: Role of the glutathione redox cycle in acquired and de novo multidrug resistance. Science 241:694–696, 1988

47. Champlin R, Gale RP: Bone marrow transplantation for acute leukemia: Recent advances and comparison with alternative therapies. Semin Hematol 24:55–67, 1987

48. Hartmann O, Benhamou E, Beaujean F, et al: Repeated high-dose chemotherapy followed by purged autologous bone marrow transplantation as consolidation therapy in metastatic neuroblastoma. J Clin Oncol 5:1205–1211, 1987

49. Applebaum FR, Storb R, Ramberg RE, et al: Allogenic marrow transplantation in the treatment of preleukemia. Ann Intern Med 100:689–693, 1984

50. Hartmann PO, Biron P, Cahn JY, et al: High-dose therapy and

autologous bone marrow transplantation in partial remission after first-line induction therapy for diffuse non-Hodgkin's lymphoma. J Clin Oncol 6:1118–1124, 1988

51. Fox FC (ed): Progress in bone marrow transplantation. UCLA symposia on molecular and cellular biology. New York, Alan R Liss, 1986

52. Thompson JA, Lee DJ, Cox WW, et al: Recombinant interleukin 2 toxicity, pharmacokinetics, and immunomodulatory effects in a phase I trial. Cancer Res 47:4202–4207, 1987

53. Goldstein D, Laszlo J: Interferon therapy in cancer: From imaginon to interferon. Cancer Res 46:4315–4329, 1986

54. Schlom J: Basic principles and applications of monoclonal antibodies in the management of carcinomas: The Richard and Hinda Rosenthal Foundation Award Lecture. Cancer Res 46:3225–3238, 1986

55. Yarbro JW: Toxicity of chemotherapy. Semin Oncol 11:1–143, 1982

56. Morstyn G, Burgess AW: Hemopoietic growth factors: A review. Cancer Res 48:5624–5637, 1988

57. Morstyn G, Souza LM, Keech J, et al: Effect of granulocyte colony stimulating factor on neutropenia induced by cytotoxic chemotherapy. Lancet 1:667–672, 1988.

58. Gabrilove JL, Jakubowski A, Scher H, et al: Effect of granulocyte colony-stimulating factor on neutropenia and associated morbidity due to chemotherapy for transitional-cell carcinoma of the urothelium. N Engl J Med 318:1414–1422, 1988

59. Brandt S, Peters WP, Atwater SK, et al: Effect of recombinant human granulocyte-macrophage colony-stimulating factor on hematopoietic reconstitution after high-dose chemotherapy and autologous bone marrow transplantation. N Engl J Med 318:869–876, 1988

60. von Hoff DD, Rozencweig M, Layard M, et al: Daunomycin-induced cardiotoxicity in children and adults—A review of 110 cases. Am J Med 62:200–208, 1977

61. McHaney VA, Thibadoux G, Hayes FA, Green AA: Hearing loss in children receiving cisplatin chemotherapy. J Pediatr 102:314–317, 1983

62. Woods WG, O'Leary M, Nesbit ME: Life-threatening neuropathy and hepatotoxicity in infants during induction therapy for acute lymphoblastic leukemia. J Pediatr 98:642–645, 1981

63. Evans WE, Relling MV, deGraaf S, et al: Hepatic drug clearance in children: Studies with indocyanine green as a model substrate. J Pharm Sci (in press)

64. Jones B, Breslow NE, Takashima J: Toxic deaths in the second national Wilms' tumor study. J Clin Oncol 2:1028–1033, 1984

65. Rivkees SA, Crawford JD. The relationship of gonadal activity and chemotherapy-induced gonadal damage. JAMA 259:2123–2125, 1988

66. Dorr RT, Fritz WL (eds): Cancer Chemotherapy Handbook. New York, Elsevier, 1980

67. Gilman AG, Goodman LS, Gilman A (eds): The Pharmacological Basis of Therapeutics. New York, Macmillan, 1985

68. Bleyer WA: Antineoplastic drugs, in Yaffe SJ (ed): Pediatric Pharmacology: Therapeutic Principles in Practice. New York, Grune & Stratton, 1980, pp 349–377

69. Dinarello CA, Mier JW: Lymphokines. N Engl J Med 317:940–945, 1987

70. Clark SC, Kamen R: The human hematopoietic colony-stimulating factors. Science 236:1229–1237, 1987

37

ANALGESIC AGENTS

BERNARD P. SCHACHTEL

Of all objectives of pediatric care, none signifies a higher ideal than to provide comfort to the child in pain. Whether the source of pain is acute and self-limited or chronic and recurrent, the practitioner seeks to place the child on medication in amounts appropriate to the condition, the degree of pain, and the pharmacology of the drug. The medication should also be given when needed and should be within acceptable limits of tolerance and toxicity. Having made the determinations that the child's pain requires pharmacologic intervention and that treating pain will not obfuscate a correct diagnosis or mask a more serious disease, the pediatric caregiver must decide which medication and which dosage is appropriate to the level of pain the child is experiencing. As in other areas of pediatric medicine, this proper titration of drug to patient should be accomplished on a scientific basis as well as from practical experience.

Nevertheless, many will acknowledge, somewhat abashedly, that pain is a "new" subject to formal pediatric education and pediatric pharmacology.[1-3] Ironically, many who treated young children, especially infants,[4-6] did not consider pain a pediatric experience until the last decade and tended to undertreat children with pain.[7] The controversy over neonatal circumcision,[8-15] the infrequency of the administration of analgesic agents to postoperative pediatric patients compared to adult patients,[16-19] and the relative paucity of space devoted to the subjects of children's pain and its treatment in textbooks on pediatrics highlight this formerly prevailing point of view. The calling of pediatrics reveals a different attitude among its practitioners, however. Though not founded on scientific evidence, pediatric practice relies regularly upon clinical observation techniques to detect pain in children of different ages, cognitive levels, or sociofamilial and cultural backgrounds.[16,20-25] It is impossible to review here the inductive process that the practitioner employs before determining the need for an analgesic agent. Nor is it the purpose of this chapter to describe the emerging research techniques that are being utilized and tested by nursing, psychologic, pediatric, and phar-

macologic investigators (from smiley-face and pain thermometer rating scales to categorical relief and visual analog pain intensity scales).[26-37]

Nonpharmacologic interventions, of course, are routinely employed in alleviating a child's pain. In some situations these may comprise the entire intervention; in other situations they may constitute important ancillary measures. These nonmedicinal techniques (such as preparation for the painful experience; touching, smiling, and caring; biofeedback, distraction, relaxation, and art therapy; transcutaneous electrical nerve stimulation (TENS); and individual, group, and family counseling) have been comprehensively discussed in other sources.[31,38,39] For some of the practical aspects of administering local anesthetics (topical, regional, etc.), the reader is referred to other up-to-date reviews.[40-44] These and other therapeutic interventions, such as the use of sedatives, often comprise important adjunctive measures coordinated by a pediatric pain team[38,45] when analgesics must be employed.

SYSTEMIC ANALGESIC AGENTS
(References 46–49)

Pediatricians should be aware of current changes in adult analgesiology (the study of the causes, mechanisms, and treatment of pain). Like other specialties in clinical pharmacology, this branch of adult medicine will affect pediatric clinical pharmacology. In particular, one should note that the terms describing pain as "mild-to-moderate," "moderately severe," or "severe" are being abandoned by analgesiologists.[50] This change of categorization has occurred for at least two cogent reasons. First, the terms are also used to grade the intensity of pain, regardless of the condition. Thus, the child with a sprained ankle and the child awakening from anesthesia after orthopedic surgery may both have "severe" pain according to the clinician's and child's frame of reference, yet the conditions have been categorized (by pharmacologic convention) as mild-to-moderate, on the one hand, and severe, on the other. Avoiding these terms focuses the therapeutic decision on what is pertinent clinically, the patient's own level of pain.

These terms have been used in clinical pharmacology and drug regulatory arenas to serve another purpose: to create categories for the analgesic agents themselves indicative of their relative potency. Thus, for example, aspirin was identified as an analgesic for mild-to-moderate pain (a "mild" analgesic), acetaminophen with codeine as an analgesic for moderately severe pain, and morphine sulfate as an analgesic for severe pain (a "strong" analgesic). The drugs had become paramount, rather than the patient's experience and the practitioner's appraisal of it. Depending on the dosages of specific agents, however, and the conditions under which they are used, analgesic agents encompass a spectrum of use, not limited to one distinct category.

Eliminating these terms from the categorization of analgesic agents has overcome an inherent ambiguity, therefore, and broadened the clinician's armamentarium beyond these restrictive designations and indications. With direct comparisons of analgesic agents as they perform in different clinical trials (which are now appearing in the Clinical Pharmacology sections of FDA-approved package inserts for prescription drugs), the clinician will be able to use analgesics with greater confidence and precision in dosing. To decide which drug is best for the patient, the practitioner will review the results of clinical studies of analgesic agents when compared with placebo (negative control) and an active drug (positive control). The former control is important to assess the pharmacologic efficacy of the analgesic agent; the latter control is essential, from clinical and pharmacologic points of view, for comparing the new agent to the known activity of a standard drug (as well as ascertaining the sensitivity of the pain model). "Does it work?" is answered by the first ingredient of study design. "If so, how well?" is answered by the second.

Unfortunately, the scientific tools for assessing and measuring pain in children are in a developmental stage and are less refined than the investigative methods used in analgesic studies on adults. For the most part, placebo-controlled, double-blind trials that demonstrate the efficacy of analgesic agents in pediatric patients do not exist at the present time.[51-54] As a result, clinicians must rely on studies conducted on adults that compare the same active agents to placebo and to one another under double-blind conditions. This knowledge, fortified by experience with different analgesic agents and clinical observation of the child's response to them,[47] constitutes the current basis for selecting specific agents for use in treating the painful conditions that affect children.

NONOPIOID ANALGESIC AGENTS
(Reference 55)

By convention, drugs such as aspirin and acetaminophen have been called "peripheral analgesics." Their site of action is presumed to be at the painful stimulus,

peripheral to the central nervous system, that is, where the transmitted sensation is processed and interpreted as pain. While the mechanism of action of acetaminophen is not well defined, nonsteroidal anti-inflammatory agents (NSAIDs) are believed to provide analgesia by their reversible inhibition of the enzyme cyclo-oxygenase, thereby interfering with the production of tissue prostaglandins, especially PGE_1 and PGE_2. With diminished levels of prostaglandins at the site of injury, one theory holds that the afferent (sensory) neurons are relatively and briefly desensitized to the noxious stimulus, thereby blocking the uptake and subsequent transmission of the pain message to the central nervous system.[56]

Aspirin, or acetylsalicylic acid (ASA), and acetaminophen, or n-acetyl-para-amino-phenol (APAP), are well known to practitioners, having been available as nonprescription medications for several years.[57] They are regarded by clinical pharmacologists and regulatory authorities as equianalgesic,[55] but the anti-inflammatory superiority of aspirin clearly distinguishes it from acetaminophen when painful conditions with an inflammatory component require pharmacologic intervention. (Their pharmacology and safety are reviewed in Chapter 33, Antipyretics.)

Aspirin's analgesic efficacy has been demonstrated in several double-blind, randomized, placebo-controlled clinical trials on adults in a variety of pain models applicable to children and adolescents, such as the treatment of acute muscle-contraction headache,[58,59] dysmenorrhea,[60] dental pain,[61] musculoskeletal pain,[62] and acute sore throat.[63] For adults and for children 12 years of age and older, therefore, single dosages of 325 mg to 1 gm have been shown to be effective compared with placebo. For younger children with acute painful conditions, oral doses of 10–15 mg/kg may be given every 4 hours. This analgesic dosage is in contrast to the use of aspirin as an anti-inflammatory agent for juvenile rheumatoid arthritis, where higher doses may be administered. Some clinicians find aspirin particularly effective for children with pain of inflammatory origin (such as a sprained ankle treated over a few days on a p.r.n. basis), acute joint pain (as in tenosynovitis of the hip), or bone pain (after trauma, for example).

Another type of salicylate, choline-magnesium salicylate, has also been used in older children with chronic pain due to cancer or arthritis. The dose is 10–15 mg/kg t.i.d., which may provide less gastric irritation than aspirin and no interference with bleeding time, as suggested by one study in adults.[64]

One of the most widely used agents in children is acetaminophen, which, unlike aspirin, is stable in solution and thus is available in liquid as well as solid dosage forms. Like aspirin, its efficacy has been demonstrated in many placebo-controlled clinical trials on adults, such as models for acute muscle-contraction headache,[65] dental pain,[66] dysmenorrhea,[67] and acute sore throat,[63] establishing its role as an analgesic in single dosages of 325 mg to 1 gm for adults and children 12 years of age and older. In younger children, oral doses of 10–15 mg/kg may be given every 4 hours. In addition, infants may benefit from its postoperative use when given in single doses of 15–20 mg/kg rectally, although absorption by this route can vary.[68] Some clinicians have recommended higher doses: oral doses up to 15 mg/kg in older children or rectal doses up to 20 mg/kg in infants.[69]

Though not approved as analgesic agents for children (distinct from their approved indications for juvenile arthritis and, in the case of ibuprofen, juvenile pyrexia as well), the NSAIDs naproxen, tolmetin, and ibuprofen are prescribed by physicians for children with pain.[70] As in adults, children with bony metastases also appear to respond well to these agents, if bleeding is not a contraindication. (For a discussion of the clinical pharmacology and safety of ibuprofen, see Chapter 32, Antipyretics.) To date, there are three reports of randomized, placebo-controlled trials on ibuprofen for children with acute pain. In one study on 45 children (aged 5–12 years) following dental extractions,[51] aluminum ibuprofen 200 mg was shown to provide relief for 2 hours and overall when compared with placebo ($p < .05$). Another pediatric model, acute sore throat, has been recently tested in two studies:[53,54] a single dose of ibuprofen 10 mg/kg was shown to be effective ($p < .05$) when compared to placebo over a 6-hour treatment period in each study. In adults there are several clinical trials that establish the analgesic efficacy of ibuprofen when compared with placebo; some of these are in the same acute pain conditions frequently experienced by children and adolescents, such as acute muscle-contraction headache,[71] acute tonsillopharyngitis,[72] acute musculoskeletal trauma,[62] dental pain,[66,73] and dysmenorrhea.[67,74] For children 12 years of age and older, the nonprescription strength, 200 or 400 mg, at 4- to 6-hour intervals, up to 1200 mg/day, is recommended. For younger children, 3–10 mg/kg every 6–8 hours has been used.

Naproxen is a longer-acting NSAID that is also available in liquid and tablet formulations. Although there are no published studies of this agent used for nonrheumatic analgesic indications in children, the drug has been safely used in the treatment of acute pain at dosages of 3–7 mg/kg every 8–12 hours, confirming its proven efficacy in adults with acute pain.[75]

Experience in children treated with tolmetin is more limited, although the agent is prescribed by some physicians for children with pain refractory to the previously listed analgesics. Unlike ibuprofen and naproxen, tolmetin is not indicated for pain in adults, and it also differs from the other two NSAIDs in its pharmacokinetic profile, which is biphasic: an early phase with a half-life of about 1–2 hours and a later phase with a half-life of about 5 hours. Although there are no clinical trial data to support its use as an analgesic in adults or children, tolmetin can be used in an oral dose of 5–7 mg/kg every 6–8 hours.

Recommended doses of the nonopioid analgesics in children under 12 years of age are listed in Table 37–1.

OPIOID ANALGESICS (Reference 69)

The morphine-like or opioid analgesics have traditionally been the agents reserved for the most severe types and intensity of pain. Given the several misconceptions and biases that physicians have held about pain intensity in children, their tolerance of it, an unfounded fear of creating an addict (even by short-term use), and a general hesitation to "overtreat" in these circumstances, these agents tend to be underused[76] or, at best, inappropriately used.[17] There have been several excellent commentaries on this subject,[77,78] as recent investigations in this area have generated a more scientific and humane use of these agents in children whose pain requires such treatment.[79,80]

All of the agents classified as opioids are centrally acting analgesics.[81] Their binding to mu receptor sites throughout the central nervous system is thought to produce analgesia by reducing the sensation of pain (nociception) received from sensory neurons and by altering the affective, or emotional, component of the pain experience.[82] The pure-agonist opioids (morphine, hydromorphone, methadone, fentanyl) produce analgesia without a ceiling effect (increasing doses produce increasing analgesia). Their differential rates of binding to other sites (kappa and

TABLE 37–1. NONOPIOID ANALGESICS: RECOMMENDED DOSES IN CHILDREN UNDER AGE 12 YEARS

DRUG	DOSE	PEAK	DURATION	PRECAUTIONS	COMMENTS
Acetaminophen (APAP)	10–15 mg/kg P.O. 15–20 mg/kg P.R.	1–2 h	4 h	Larger doses may be hepatotoxic	Effective for mild pain
Aspirin (ASA)	10–15 mg/kg P.O.	1–2 h	4 h	Contraindicated in patients with bleeding disorders, GI hemorrhage	Anti-inflammatory dosages especially useful for musculoskeletal conditions
Choline-magnesium salicylate	10–15 mg/kg P.O.	1–2 h	6–8 h	Perhaps less risk for patients with bleeding disorders, GI hemorrhage	Especially useful for chronic pain.
Ibuprofen	3–10 mg/kg P.O.	1–2 h	6–8 h	Contraindicated in patients with GI hemorrhage.	Especially useful for moderate to severe pain
Naproxen	5–7 mg/kg P.O.	2–3 h	8–12 h	Contraindicated in patients with GI hemorrhage	Requires loading dose because of delayed onset
Tolmetin	5–7 mg/kg P.O.	1–2 h	6–8 h	Contraindicated in patients with GI hemorrhage	May be especially useful in refractory pain

TABLE 37–2. OPIOID ANALGESICS: RECOMMENDED STARTING DOSES IN CHILDREN

DRUG	DOSE	PEAK	DURATION	PRECAUTIONS	COMMENTS
Codeine	0.5–1.0 mg/kg P.O.	2 h	4–6 h	Nausea, constipation. Not for I.V. use	Used for mild to moderate pain
Fentanyl	0.5–2 μg/kg I.V.	3–5 min	1–2 h	Same precautions as morphine	Short duration. Less vasodilation and pruritus
Hydromorphone HCl (Dilaudid)	0.015 mg/kg I.V. 0.075 mg/kg P.O.	15 min 1 h	2–3 h 3–4 h	Same precautions as morphine	Quick onset of action. Available as high-potency solution 10 mg/ml for tolerant patients. Similar to heroin
Levorphanol (Levo-Dromoran)	0.02 mg/kg I.V. 0.04 mg/kg P.O.	15–30 min 2 h	3–4 h 4–5 h	Same precautions as morphine	Begin p.r.n. for 72 h to establish dose frequency and adverse effects; may then be given ATC
Meperidine (Demerol, Pethadol)	0.75 mg/kg I.V. 3.0 mg/kg P.O.	5–15 min 2 h	2–3 h 3–4 h	May cause CNS excitation (tremors and seizures) Contraindicated for patients with renal dysfunction and for chronic administration	Rapid onset, short duration
Methadone HCl (Dolophine)	0.1 mg/kg I.V. 0.2 mg/kg P.O.	15–30 min 2 h	3–4 h 4–5 h	Same precautions as morphine	Same as levorphanol
Morphine sulfate	0.1 mg/kg I.V. 0.05–0.06 mg/kg/h I.V. 0.3–0.6 mg/kg P.O.	15–30 min (Continuous infusion) 2 h	2–4 h 4–5 h	Contraindicated in patients with impaired ventilation, asthma, elevated intracranial pressure, liver failure	May cause oversedation, confusion, visual disturbance, urinary retention
Oxycodone (with aspirin— Percodan; with acetaminophen— Percocet)	0.3 mg/kg P.O.	1 h	3 hr	Same precautions as morphine	Short-acting. Available as oral solution
Oxymorphone (Numorphan)	0.01 mg/kg I.V. 1 mg/kg P.R.	15–30 min 2 h	3 hr 4–6 h	Same precautions as morphine	Not available P.O. Is available as 5-mg rectal suppository

Dosages are calculated using 0.1 mg/kg/dose of morphine as standard. (Adapted from Rogers,[69] with permission.)

sigma receptors) are believed to explain the different side effect profiles of these agents.

The adverse effects of opioids depend not only on the intrinsic properties of each opioid but also on the size of the dose and the route of administration. Unlike most peripheral analgesics, the centrally acting agents can be administered parenterally (intravenously, intramuscularly, subcutaneously, transdermally, intranasally) as well as through the epidural and subarachnoid routes. Regardless of the route of administration, most of the adverse effects of these agents (respiratory depression, nausea, constipation, transient paralytic ileus, urinary retention, suppressed cough reflex, biliary spasm, miosis, sedation, pruritus, vasodilation) can be avoided with proper titration of dose. The most serious of these adverse effects is respiratory depression, especially in infants under 3 months of age.[83] When the dosage and frequency of dosing are titrated according to each patient's needs, with side effects monitored as they occur and appropriate adjustments made in dose as indicated, most children can be safely and effectively treated with opioids.

Continuous intravenous or subcutaneous infusions[84–87] and patient-controlled analgesia (PCA)[88–93] have overcome the potential problems of overdosing and underdosing by providing near-steady-state plasma levels and a nearly constant state of analgesia. For example, severe sickle cell pain crises have been successfully treated with continuous intravenous infusion of morphine sulfate (0.15 mg/kg bolus followed by 0.07–0.10 mg/kg/h) or meperidine hydrochloride (1.0 mg/kg bolus followed by 0.5–0.7 mg/kg/h).[94] Alternate strategies include the administration of small, slow boluses of intermediate-duration opioids (morphine, meperidine) at 2- to 3-hour intervals or the administration of a long-acting agent (methadone) in small, slow boluses at 4- to 8-hour intervals or longer.[95] In addition, the worry of creating an addicted state during the treatment of acute pain is usually not a problem in short-term therapy[96] and is rare even in chronic therapy.[97] Beyond 2 weeks, however, physiologic dependence has been noted in some children,[98] but weaning the child over 5–7 days can overcome this situation comfortably.[99]

Doses of the pure-agonist opioids are listed in Table 37–2. Because all opioids are metabolized in the liver and the metabolites are excreted in the urine, patients with reduced hepatic or renal function should be monitored closely for evidence of toxicity.

Before stronger opioids are given, especially for children on an ambulatory basis, some physicians prescribe acetaminophen combined with codeine. This practice is based on the clinical impression of greater efficacy attributable to codeine. However, the observed effect may be sedation, rather than analgesia, and not desirable from a functional point of view. Indeed, codeine alone has a minimal analgesic effect in adults at 60 mg.[100] In clinical trials on adults with dental pain, no significantly greater analgesia was obtained by acetaminophen 600 mg with codeine 60 mg than by acetaminophen 600 mg,[101] and much greater analgesia was registered by ibuprofen 400 mg than by acetaminophen 600 mg with codeine 60 mg.[102] When a relatively mild opiate is desired for a child, codeine (with or without acetaminophen) can be administered in an oral dose of 0.5–1.0 mg/kg every 4 hours.

While their responsible use has increased in the treatment of children, especially for cancer-related pain, analgesic agents remain relative therapeutic orphans in pediatric clinical pharmacology. The guidelines presented in this chapter are predominantly experientially derived, not proven in children by using accepted analgesic assays. With the addition of promising new methods that are being developed for delivering analgesics to children (such as the transdermal fentanyl patch), and with the developing scientific methodology for evaluating them, the next decade should provide clinicians with more sound rationales for the choice of specific agents, dosages, and regimens, with improved relief for children in pain.

ACKNOWLEDGMENTS: From the Department of Epidemiology and Biostatistics, McGill University, Quebec, Canada.

REFERENCES

1. McGrath PJ, Unruh AM: The history of pain in childhood, in Pain in Children and Adolescents. Amsterdam, Elsevier, 1987, pp 1–46
2. Berlin CM Jr: Advances in pediatric pharmacology and toxicology. Adv Pediatr 36:431–460, 1989
3. Barr RG: Pain in children, in Wall PD, Melzack R (eds): Textbook of Pain. New York, Churchill Livingston, 1989, pp 568–588
4. Johnston CC: Pain assessment and management in infants. Pediatrician 16:16–23, 1989
5. Anand KJS, Aynsley-Green A: Does the newborn infant require potent anesthesia during surgery? Answers from a randomized trial of halothane anesthesia, in Dubner R, Gebhart GF, Bond MR (eds): Proceedings of the Vth World Congress on Pain. Amsterdam, Elsevier, 1988, pp 329–334
6. Porter F: Pain in the newborn. Clin Perinatol 16:549–564, 1989
7. Schechter NL, Hanson K, Allen D: Are we undertreating pain in children? (Abstr.). Washington, DC, Ambulatory Pediatrics Association, 1984
8. American Academy of Pediatrics Committee on the Fetus and Newborn: Standards and Recommendations for Hospital Care of Newborn Infants, 5th ed. Evanston, American Academy of Pediatrics, 1971, p. 110
9. Williamson PS, Williamson MN: Physiologic stress reduction by a local anesthetic during newborn circumcision. Pediatrics 71:36–40, 1983
10. Holve RL, Bromberger PJ, Gronerman HD, et al: Regional anesthesia during newborn circumcision: Effect on the pain response. Clin Pediatr 22:813–818, 1983
11. Porter FL, Miller RH, Marshall RE: Neonatal pain cries: Effect of circumcision on acoustic features and perceived urgency. Child Devel 57:790–802, 1986
12. Task Force on Circumcision: Report of the Task Force on Circumcision. Pediatrics 84:388–391, 1989
13. Maxwell LG, Yaster M, Wetzel RC, et al: Penile nerve block for newborn circumcision. Obstet Gynecol 70:415–418, 1987
14. Stang JH, Gunnar MR, Snellman L, et al: Local anesthesia for neonatal circumcision: Effects on distress and cortisol response. JAMA 259:1507–1511, 1988
15. Schoen, EJ: Sounding Board—The status of circumcision of newborns. N Engl J Med 322:1308–1312, 1990
16. Mather L, Mackie J: The incidence of postoperative pain in children. Pain 15:271–282, 1988
17. Eland J, Anderson J: The experience of pain in children, in Jacox A (ed): Pain: A Sourcebook for Nurses and Other Professionals. Boston, Little, Brown, 1977, pp 453–473
18. Beyer J, DeGood D, Ashley L, Russell G: Patterns of postoperative analgesic use with adults and children following cardiac surgery. Pain 17:71–81, 1983
19. Schechter NL, Allen DA, Hanson K: Status of pediatric pain control: A comparison of hospital analgesic usage in children and adults. Pediatrics 77:11–15, 1986
20. Craig KD, Gruneau RVE, Branson SM: Age-related aspects of pain: Pain in children, in Dubner R, Gebhart GF, Bond MR (eds): Proceedings of the Vth World Congress on Pain. Amsterdam, Elsevier, 1988, pp 317–328
21. Gaffney A: How children describe pain: A study of words and analogies used by 5–14 year olds, in Dubner R, Gebhart GF, Bond MR (eds): Proceedings of the Vth World Congress on Pain. Amsterdam, Elsevier, 1988, pp 341–347
22. Purcell-Jones G, Dorman F, Summer E: Paediatric anaesthetists' perceptions of neonatal and infant pain. Pain 33:181–187, 1988
23. McGrath PA: Evaluating a child's pain. J Pain Symptom Manage 4:198–214, 1989
24. Tesler M, Savedra M, Ward JA, et al: Children's language of pain, in Dubner R, Gebhart GF, Bond MR (eds): Proceedings of the Vth World Congress on Pain. Amsterdam, Elsevier, 1988, pp 348–352
25. Gaffney A, Duane EA: Developmental aspects of children's descriptions of pain. Pain 26:105–117, 1986
26. Abu-Saad H: Assessing children's responses to pain. Pain 19:163–171, 1984
27. Beyer J, Aradine C: Patterns of pediatric pain intensity: A methodological investigation of a self-report scale. Clin J Pain 3:130–141, 1987
28. Varni J, Thompson K, Hanson V: The Varni-Thompson Pediatric Pain Questionnaire. I. Chronic musculo-skeletal pain in juvenile rheumatoid arthritis. Pain 28:27–38, 1987
29. McGrath PJ, Johnson G, Goodman J, et al: The Children's Hospital of Eastern Ontario pain scale (CHEOPS): A behavioral scale for rating postoperative pain in children, in Fields LH, Dubner R, Cervero F (eds): Advances in Pain Research and Therapy, vol 9. Proceedings of the Fourth World Congress on Pain, Seattle. New York, Raven Press, 1985, pp 395–402
30. Maunuksela E-L, Olkkola KT, Korpela R: Measurement of pain in children with self-reporting and behavior assessment. Clin Pharmacol Ther 42:137–141, 1987
31. McGrath PJ, Unruh AM: The measurement and assessment of pain, in McGrath PJ, Unruh AM: Pain in Children and Adolescents. Amsterdam, Elsevier, 1987, pp. 73–104
32. Beyer JE, Wells N: The assessment of pain in children. Pediatr Clin No Am 36:837–854, 1989
33. Adams J: Pediatric pain assessment: Trends and research directions. J Pediatr Oncol Nurs 6:79–85, 1989
34. McGrath PA: An assessment of children's pain: A review of behavioral, physiological and direct scaling techniques. Pain 31:147–176, 1987

35. Beyer JE: The Oucher: A user's manual and technical report. University of Virginia Alumni Patent Foundation, Charlottesville, 1984
36. Rogers AG: The assessment of pain and pain relief in children with cancer. Pain 11(suppl 1):S11, 1981
37. Bieri D, Reeve RA, Champion GD, et al: The Faces Pain Scale for the self-assessment of the severity of pain experienced by children: Development, initial validation, and preliminary investigation for ratio scale properties. Pain 41:139–150, 1990
38. Berde CB, Lacostre PG, Mazek BJ, et al: Initial experience with a multidisciplinary pediatric pain treatment service. Pain (suppl 4):599, 1987, v. 31 p S599
39. Kuttner L: Management of young children's acute pain and anxiety during invasive medical procedures. Pediatrician 16:39–44, 1989
40. Berde CB, Sethna NF: Regional anesthetic approaches to postoperative pain in children and adolescents (Abstr.). Intensive Care Med 13:460, 1987
41. Berde CB, Sethna N, Anand KJS: Pediatric pain management, in Gregory GA (ed): Pediatric Anesthesia, 2nd ed. New York, Churchill Livingston, 1990
42. McIlvaine WB: Perioperative pain management in children: A review. J Pain Symptom Manage 4:215–229, 1989
43. Armitage EN: Regional anaesthesia in pediatrics. Clin Anaesth 3:553–568, 1985
44. Singler R: Pediatric regional anesthesia, in Gregory GA (ed): Pediatric Anesthesia. New York, Churchill Livingston, 1983, pp 481–518
45. Berde C, Sethna NR, Mazek B, et al: Pediatric pain clinics: Recommendations for their development. Pediatrician 16:94–102, 1989
46. Payne R: Principles of analgesic use in the treatment of acute pain and chronic cancer pain. Report of a committee to the American Pain Society. Washington, DC, American Pain Society, 1987
47. Schechter N: Pain and pain control in children. Curr Probl Pediatr 15:1–67, 1985
48. Yaster M, Deshpande JK, Maxwell LG: The pharmacologic management of pain in children. Compr Therap 15(10):14–26, 1989
49. Shannon M, Berde CB: Pharmacologic management of pain in children and adolescents. Pediatr Clin No Am 36:855–871, 1989
50. American Society for Clinical Pharmacology and Therapeutics. Proposed Revisions to Guidelines for the Clinical Evaluation of Analgesic Drugs. American Society for Clinical Pharmacology and Therapeutics, 1990
51. Moore PA, Acs G, Hargreaves JA: Postextraction pain relief in children: A clinical trial of liquid analgesics. Int J Clin Pharmacol Ther Toxicol 23:573–577, 1985
52. Maunuksela EL, Korpela R, Olkkola KO: Intravenous indomethacin as postoperative analgesic for children (Abstr.). Pain (suppl 4):S99, 1987, v. 31
53. Schachtel BP, King SA, Thoden WR: Pain relief in children: A placebo-controlled model. Clin Pharmacol Ther (manuscript in preparation)
54. Schachtel BP, Paull BR, Thoden WR: Sore throat pain model for the evaluation of analgesics in children (Abstr.). Montreal, 2nd International Symposium on Pediatric Pain, 1991
55. Beaver WT: Mild analgesics: A review of their clinical pharmacology. Am J Med Sci 251:576–599, 1966
56. Perl ER: Sensitization of receptors and its relation to sensation, in Bonica JJ, Albe-Fessard DG (eds): Advances in Pain Research and Therapy, vol 1. New York, Raven Press, 1976, pp 17–34
57. Rumack BH: Aspirin versus acetaminophen: A comparative view. Pediatrics 62:943–946, 1978
58. Murray WJ: Evaluation of aspirin in the treatment of headache. Clin Pharmacol Ther 5:21–25, 1964
59. Graffenried BV, Hill RC, Nuesch E: Headache as a model for assessing mild analgesic drugs. J Clin Pharmacol 20:298–302, 1980
60. Klein JR, Litt IF, Rosenberg A, Udall L: The effect of aspirin on dysmenorrhea in adolescents. J Pediatr 98:987–990, 1981
61. Cooper SA, Beaver WT: A model to evaluate mild analgesics in oral surgery outpatients. Clin Pharmacol Ther 20:241–250, 1976
62. Muckle DS: Comparative study of ibuprofen and aspirin in soft-tissue injuries. Rheumatol Rehab 13:141–147, 1974
63. Schachtel BP, Fillingim JM, Beiter DS, et al: Rating scales for analgesics in sore throat. Clin Pharmacol Ther 36:151–156, 1984
64. Danesh BJ, Saniabadi AR, Russell RI, Lowe GD: Therapeutic potential of choline magnesium salicylate as an alternative to aspirin for patients with bleeding tendencies. Scott Med J 32:167–168, 1987
65. Peters BH, Fraim CJ, Masel BE: Comparison of 650 mg aspirin and 1000 mg acetaminophen with each other and with placebo in moderately severe headache. Am J Med 74:36–42, 1983
66. Cooper SA, Schachtel BP, Goldman E, et al: Ibuprofen and acetaminophen in the relief of acute pain: A randomized, double-blind placebo-controlled study. J Clin Pharmacol 29:1026–1030, 1989
67. Molla AL, Donald JF: A comparative study of ibuprofen and paracetamol in primary dysmenorrhea. J Int Med Res 2:395–399, 1974
68. Gaudreault P, Guay J, Nicol O, Dupuis C: Pharmacokinetics and clinical efficacy of intrarectal solution of acetaminophen. Can J Anaesthesiol 35:149–152, 1988
69. Rogers AG: Analgesics: The physician's partner in effective pain management. Va Med 116(suppl 4):164–170, 1989
70. Stiehm ER: Nonsteroidal anti-inflammatory drugs in pediatric patients. Am J Dis Child 142:1281–1282, 1988
71. Schachtel BP, Thoden WR: Onset of action of ibuprofen in the treatment of muscle-contraction headache. Headache 28:471–474, 1988
72. Schachtel BP, Fillingim JM, Thoden WR, Lane AC, Baybutt RI: Sore throat pain in the evaluation of mild analgesics. Clin Pharmacol Ther 44:704–711, 1988
73. Beaver WT, Forbes JA, Barkoszi BA, Ragland RN, Hankle JJ: An evaluation of ibuprofen and acetaminophen in postoperative oral surgery pain (Abstr.). Clin Pharmacol Ther 41:180, 1987
74. Chan WY, Dawood MY, Fuchs F: Relief of dysmenorrhea with the prostaglandin synthetase inhibitor ibuprofen: Effect on prostaglandin levels in menstrual fluid. Am J Obstet Gynecol 135:102–108, 1979
75. Sevelius H, Runkel R, Segre E, et al: Bioavailability of naproxen sodium and its relationship to clinical analgesic effects. Br J Clin Pharmacol 10:259–263, 1980
76. Schechter NL: The undertreatment of pain in children: An overview. Pediatr Clin No Am 36:781–794, 1989
77. Angell M: The quality of mercy. N Engl J Med 306: 98–99, 1982
78. Newman RG: Sounding Board—The need to redefine "addiction." N Engl J Med 308:1096–1098, 1983
79. Yaster M, Deshpande JK: Management of pediatric pain with opioid analgesics. J Pediatr 113:421–429, 1988
80. Olkkola KT, Maunuksela E-L, Korpela R: Kinetics and dynamics of postoperative intravenous morphine in children. Clin Pharmacol Ther 44:128–136, 1988
81. Martin WR: Pharmacology of opioids. Pharm Review 35:285–323, 1985
82. Mense S: Basic neurobiologic mechanisms of pain and analgesia. Am J Med 75:4–14, 1983
83. Hertzka RE, Fisher DM, Gauntlett IS, Spellman BS: Are infants sensitive to respiratory depression from fentanyl? (Abstr.) Anesthesiology 67(3A):A512, 1987
84. Bray RJ: Postoperative analgesia provided by morphine infusion in children. Anaesthesia 38:1075–1078, 1983
85. Cole TB, Sprinkle RH, Smith SJ, Buchangh GR: Intravenous narcotic therapy for children with severe sickle cell pain crisis. Am J Dis Child 140:1255–1259, 1986
86. Miser AW, Miser JS, Clerk BS: Continuous intravenous infusion of morphine sulfate for control of severe pain in children with terminal malignancy. J Pediatr 96:930–932, 1980
87. Miser AW, Davis DM, Hughes CS, et al: Continuous subcutaneous infusion of morphine in children with cancer. Am J Dis Child 137:383–385, 1983
88. Bennet RL, Batenhorst RL, Bivins BA, et al: Patient-controlled

analgesia: A new concept of postoperative pain relief. Ann Surg 195:700–705, 1981

89. Dodd E, Wang JM, Rauck RL: Patient controlled analgesia for post-surgical pediatric patients ages 6–16 years (Abstr.). Anesthesiology 69(3A):A372, 1988

90. Tyler DC: Patient controlled analgesia in adolescents (Abstr.). Pain (suppl 4):S236, 1987, v. 31

91. Rodgers B, Webb C, Stergius D, Newman B: Patient controlled analgesia in pediatric surgery. J Pediatr Surg 23:259–262, 1988

92. White PF: Use of patient-controlled analgesia for management of acute pain. JAMA 259:243–247, 1988

93. Gaukroger PB, Tomkins DP, Van der Walt JH: Patient-controlled analgesia in children. Anaesth Inten Care 17:264–268, 1989

94. Cole TB, Sprinkle RH, Smith JJ, et al: Intravenous narcotic therapy for children with severe sickle cell pain crisis. Am J Dis Child 140:1255–1259, 1986

95. Berde CB: Pharmacokinetics of methadone in children and adolescents in the perioperative period (Abstr.). Anaesth 67(suppl. 3A):A519, 1987

96. Kanner RM, Foley KM: Patterns of narcotic drug use in a cancer pain clinic. Ann NY Acad Sci 362:162–171, 1981

97. Portenoy RK, Foley KM: Chronic use of opioid analgesics in nonmalignant pain: Report on 38 cases. Pain 25:171–186, 1986

98. Miser AW, Chayt KJ, Sandlund JT, et al: Narcotic withdrawal syndrome in young adults after the therapeutic uses of opioids. Am J Dis Child 140:603–604, 1986

99. Tennant FS, Rawson RA: Outpatient treatment of prescription opioid dependence—Comparison of two methods. Arch Intern Med 142:1845–1847, 1982

100. Cooper SA, Engel J, Ladov M, et al: Analgesic efficacy of an ibuprofen-codeine combination. Pharmacother 2:162–167, 1982

101. Cooper SA: Five studies on ibuprofen for postsurgical dental pain. Am J Med 77(suppl 1A): 70–77, 1984

102. Schachtel BP, Fazio RG, Greene JJ: Ibuprofen 400 mg compared to acetaminophen 600 mg with codeine 60 mg for pain relief following periodontal surgery (Abstr.). J Clin Pharmacol 30:846, 1990

38

PSYCHOACTIVE AGENTS

MARKUS J. P. KRUESI *and* JUDITH L. RAPOPORT

Much more is known about the pharmacology of psychoactive agents used in childhood and adolescent disorders than was known when the first edition of this text was published. Historically, the absence of consistent diagnostic classification has hampered research,[1] and despite hopes that pediatric psychopharmacology might contribute to the validity of child psychiatric nomenclature,[2] few methodologically sound pharmacologic studies have been conducted to examine the validity of diagnostic classifications in pediatric populations. It is already clear, however, that DSM-III and DSM-III-R greatly facilitate communication for pediatric psychopharmacology.[3] In addition, reluctance (and emotion) surrounding blood sampling in children impedes rational studies. The blood volume required for particular assays can present realistic limitations for repeated sampling in younger age groups. For example, the large blood volume requirement was an impediment in obtaining pharmacokinetic data on methylphenidate in children.[4] Techniques depending on measurements in body fluids other than blood have been sought, using, for example, saliva as a less invasive, more acceptable fluid to sample. However, inconsistencies in saliva-to-plasma ratios of many drugs render their measurement in saliva uninformative.[5] One source of variability for salivary concentrations of compounds that are weak bases (including many psychotropics) is salivary pH.[6] So far, salivary measures do not appear useful in pediatric psychopharmacology, although they may be useful as compliance checks.

This chapter reviews the pharmacokinetics and pharmacodynamics of psychoactive agents with known efficacy in children and adolescents, resorting to data from adults where none are available from pediatric age groups. One caveat regarding generalizing from the data: unlike adults, for whom data on normal volunteers are available, children and adolescents in these studies are almost always patients with psychopathology. Children with different disorders might have different responses to a given psychotropic agent.

General considerations regarding the prescription of psychoactive agents for children and adolescents are covered first. Indications for treatment are listed in Table 38–1. Effects of psychoactive agents on learning and cognition are a special concern in these age groups and are discussed as a separate topic. Then the pharmacology of medications in clinical use is presented by type of agent.

GENERAL CONSIDERATIONS

The stepwise process of psychopharmacologic treatment in children has been described as follows[7]:

1. Diagnostic evaluation
2. Symptom measurement
3. Risk/benefit ratio analysis
4. Establishment of a contract of therapy
5. Periodic reevaluation
6. Termination or tapered drug withdrawal.

Compliance appears to be pervasively inadequate in general pediatric medicine, and until recently little was known about compliance in child psychiatric patients. A study of compliance with methylphenidate and cognitive treatments in 58 children with attention deficit disorder offers a disturbing perspective.[8] Pill counts of medications remaining revealed that 25 percent less medication was consumed than prescribed. Parental reports underestimated noncompliance. This is not surprising, given that children may not like taking stimulants and parents are often conflicted about administering the medication. Interestingly, the number of sessions canceled and rescheduled did not correlate with the number of pills missed. Children from lower-socioeconomic-status homes were more likely not to take their medicine. Problems with stimulant compliance are not limited to prepubertal age groups, as investigators of stimulant treatment in adolescents report similar compliance problems.[9]

413

TABLE 38–1. DSM-III-R PSYCHIATRIC DISORDERS AND PSYCHOPHARMACOLOGIC AGENTS: INDICATIONS AND DEMONSTRATED BENEFIT

	MEDICATION	EFFICACY	COMMENTS
Disorders Usually First Appearing in Infancy, Childhood, or Adolescence			
Mental retardation	None		Use of agents for secondary symptoms can be useful
Pervasive developmental disorders Autistic disorder and others	Neuroleptics	+ +	Studies focus on autism
	Fenfluramine	+/−	
	Opiate antagonists	?	
Specific developmental disorders Academic skills disorders	Stimulants	?	Treat coexisting ADHD
Language and speech disorders	None		
Disruptive behavioral disorders Attention deficit hyperactivity disorder	Stimulants	+ + + +	Evidence less clear for adolescents
	Antidepressants	+ + +	
	Clonidine	+	
Conduct disorder	Lithium	+	
	Stimulants	+	
	Neuroleptics	+	
Oppositional defiant			Same agents as for other disruptive disorders
Anxiety disorders	Antidepressants	+	
	Benzodiazepines	?	
Eating disorders Anorexia Nervosa Bulimia	Antidepressants	+?	
Gender identity disorders	None known		
Tic disorders Gilles de la Tourette's disorder	Neuroleptics	+ +	Good evidence for efficacy in Gilles de la Tourette's Disorder
Elimination disorders Encopresis	Lithium	?	See ref. 92
Enuresis	Tricyclic antidepressants	+ +	
Other Disorders			
Mood disorders Bipolar disorders	Lithium	+?	
	Anticonvulsants	+?	
Depressive disorders	Antidepressants	+/−	Superiority over placebo not clear
Anxiety disorders Obsessive-compulsive disorder	Clomipramine	+ + +	Only available in U.S. under Treatment IND
	Fluoxetine	+?	
Schizophrenia	Neuroleptics	+?	
Impulse control disorders Trichotillomania	Clomipramine	+	
Intermittent explosive disorder	Lithium	+?	
	β-blockers	+?	
	Anticonvulsants	+?	
Sleep disorders	?		

EFFECTS OF PSYCHOACTIVE AGENTS ON LEARNING AND COGNITION

As John Werry stressed, "Studying the effect of drugs on learning is important, because the work of childhood is learning, and the use of these drugs is widespread in disturbed and handicapped children[10,11] who have particular difficulties learning anyway."[12]

Psychoactive agents may affect academic skills and/or laboratory-measured cognitive functions: both therapeutic benefits and negative side effects have been studied in some detail, particularly for stimulant drugs. Traditionally, these effects have been assessed by laboratory measures, which are often drug-sensitive but do not answer the more complex and important question of whether a drug affects "real world" school learning.[12,13]

As earlier reviews by Barkley[14] and Aman[15] indicate, evidence for enhanced learning with stimulant medication is not convincing. More recently, some positive effects on classroom learning by hyperactive children have been reported.[13] However, stimulants may not be beneficial for all students. Nonhyperactive reading-disabled students, for example, did not show a benefit from stimulants above and beyond that provided by remedial tutoring.[16]

An important and provocative single study[17] found lower methylphenidate (e.g., 0.3 mg/kg) doses better for cognition, but larger doses (e.g., 1 mg/kg) better for behavioral improvement. Since then, three studies[18–20] have noted improvements in cognition as well as behavior with increasing dosages. However, none of these three used doses at or above the 1 mg/kg dose that impaired cognitive performance in the Sprague and Sleator[17] study mentioned above; it may also be that the effect is selective for the somewhat idiosyncratic matching-to-sample task used in the initial study.

Fenfluramine, a little-used stimulant, was observed to improve cognitive functioning in autistic subjects in some studies. However, no effect was seen in hyperactive children,[21] and in one study of autistics, a detrimental effect on learning was noted.[22]

The cognitive effects of tricyclics appear to be similar to but weaker than those of stimulant medications. Both clomipramine and desipramine decreased errors on the matching-familiar-figures test.[23] Imipramine decreased commission errors during the continuous performance test.[24]

Neuroleptic effects on cognition are unclear, for a variety of reasons. There are few studies, and some of the few published studies in the mentally retarded have been called into question and/or authors have retracted.[25] Despite suggestions that neuroleptics may cause cognitive impairment,[26] some evidence exists to the contrary. Low doses of haloperidol resulted in cognitive improvement in autistic children.[27]

Lithium worsened cognitive functions in children with conduct disorder[28] but improved cognitive functions in autistic children.[27] Given the increased use of lithium in adolescents with affective disorders, it is unfortunate that data from that group of patients are not available.

The cognitive effects of anticonvulsants are beginning to be studied.[29] Sodium valproate caused dose-related decrements in cognitive functions in a study of epileptic children.[30]

State-dependent learning has been defined by the observation that the retrieval of a learning episode is enhanced when the circumstances of the initial conditioning prevail.[31] One clinical example of this is the alcoholic who can remember what he did during a previous "blackout" when similarly intoxicated but is amnestic for the episode when sober.[32] One study reported state-dependent learning in hyperactive children treated with stimulants,[33] but numerous recent studies have not supported that finding.[34–37]

STIMULANTS

Methylphenidate, amphetamine, and pemoline are the agents most commonly used in the treatment of attention deficit hyperactivity disorder in children. This disorder was formerly referred to as minimal brain dysfunction, attention deficit disorder, or simply "hyperactivity." Treatment of hyperactivity with stimulants is the best-described and most extensively studied area of pediatric psychopharmacology.[38]

Pharmacologic Actions

Amphetamine is the prototypic compound of this class. However, these three compounds are not exactly interchangeable. In rodents amphetamine is about twice as potent a stimulator of motor activity but about 10 times as potent a stimulator of sterotypies as methylphenidate.[39] Pretreatment with resperpine does not block amphetamine-induced behaviors in rats but does block methylphenidate-induced behaviors.[40,41] The pattern of urinary catecholamine metabolite excretion seen in children differs between the two stimulants.[42] Given the evidence for differential behavioral effects and pharmacologic actions, direct comparisons in children of the two most often prescribed stimulants are surprisingly limited. Preliminary data suggest that the two compounds have different behavioral effects and that clinically it may be useful to try both. (Borcherding, personal communication.)

Stimulant drug effects are presumed to be mediated via increased neurotransmitter activity at catecholaminergic receptors in the central nervous system.[43] Amphetamine has consistently been shown to decrease norepinephrine and dopamine concentration in tissue slices and synaptosomes, although questions about the relative roles of release versus blockade of reuptake remain.[43] Additionally, in mice brain monoamine oxidase has been shown to be weakly inhibited by amphetamine.[44] Amphetamine, when given in the dose range used for hyperactivity, also increases the synthesis of dopamine.[43] Similarly, the increase in norepinephrine following amphetamine[45] is likely due to the drug's ability to increase norepinephrine release, block norepinephrine reuptake, and/or inhibit the action of monoamine oxidase.[43]

Both methylphenidate and amphetamine were found to increase growth hormone release in most[46–49] but not all[50] studies of hyperactive children and adolescents. Both acute and chronic treatment with methylphenidate appear to increase growth hormone release, but perhaps only acute amphetamine has this action.[51]

Several metabolic pathways, including para-hydroxylation, N-demethylation, deamination, and conjugation in the liver, take part in the disposal of amphetamine; however, a substantial fraction is excreted unchanged in the urine.[52] Acidification of the urine hastens excretion, as renal elimination of amphetamine is highly dependent on urinary pH.[53]

Pharmacokinetic studies of all three stimulants have been carried out in hyperactive children. The elimination half-life of amphetamine in hyperactive children is just under 7 hours.[54] Tablet and sustained-release preparations (0.5 mg/kg dose) result in similar peak plasma concentrations of 60–63 ng/ml.[54,55] Although the peak plasma level remains elevated for a longer time with the sustained-release preparation, an increased period of behavioral response was not seen.

Importantly, in both the tablet and sustained-release studies,[54,55] the effect of the drug in ameliorating behavioral symptoms was most pronounced during the absorption phase. This is consistent with a clockwise hysteresis curve. A hysteresis curve is a mathematical model that attempts to describe the relationship between drug concentration and effect over time (Figure 38–1).[56] Although kinetically inexplicable, clockwise hysteresis is often found in the study of psychotropic agents.[56] The same concentration of the drug in the plasma compartment produces different effects at different times; thus, a pharmacodynamic rather than a pharmacokinetic explanation must be sought. Tolerance is one possible pharmacodynamic explanation.

Methylphenidate is easily absorbed after oral administration and then is deesterified to ritalinic acid, which is the predominant compound excreted in the urine.[57] The pharmacologic actions of methylphenidate in humans appear solely attributable to the parent compound.[58]

Methylphenidate pharmacokinetics appear similar in children and adults, with a half-life of about 2½ hours.[59,60]

Mean saliva concentrations of methylphenidate were over twice as high with the regular preparation as with the sustained-release preparation.[61] Although saliva concentrations did not correlate significantly with plasma concentrations, saliva measurement may prove a helpful noninvasive compliance check.

Plasma concentrations of methylphenidate neither differentiate responders from nonresponders[62] nor provide additional information over that provided by the oral dose.[63] Thus, plasma concentrations have not, to date, proved clinically useful.[58]

Studies of pemoline pharmacokinetics in hyperactive children found an average half-life of 7–8 one-half hours.[64,65] As with the other stimulants used for treatment of hyperactivity, substantial interindividual variation in serum concentration is seen.

Indications and Efficacy

The short-term (1 year or less) efficacy of stimulants in ameliorating the symptoms of attention deficit hyperactivity disorder has been overwhelmingly clearly documented by literally hundreds of studies.[66–68]

As unresolved issue is how long stimulant treatment should be continued. A placebo-controlled trial of stimulants in adolescents with a childhood history and continued symptoms of attention deficit disorder found improvement with drug treatment.[9] However, while improvement was noted at home by parents, teacher ratings did not consistently evidence improvement. The authors of the trial acknowledge that "despite the evidence of effectiveness of stimulant therapy in adolescence, it is clear that additional modalities are required." Two studies of adults with attention deficit disorder symptoms offer conflicting results; one[69] found no benefit from stimulant treatment, and another[70] reported stimulants to be beneficial in the residual state of attention deficit disorder.

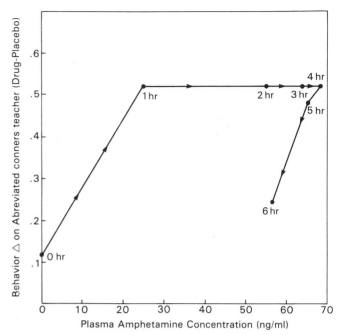

FIGURE 38–1. Example of clockwise hysteresis curve: relationship between plasma amphetamine concentration and behavior change over time. (Data from Brown et al.,[54] with permission.)

Side Effects and Drug Interactions

Anorexia and insomnia are the most common short-term adverse effects, with weight loss, headache, and abdominal pain less common. These side effects are usually transient but necessitate discontinuation of medication in perhaps 5 percent of pediatric patients. Many, if not most, alleged "nonresponders" are actually children for whom one of these side effects is not tolerable. Two potentially significant adverse consequences of stimulant treatment have received recent attention: suppression or retardation of growth, and impaired social functioning.

Growth (height and weight) suppression has been noted in short-term treatment studies (see reference 71 for a review). Longer-term studies have also noted decreases in height and weight percentiles. However, children from one of the longer-duration studies no longer evidenced a decrement when followed up into adolescence.[71] Similarly, children who had been treated with methylphenidate for 3 years did not differ in height from normal children or hyperactives who did not receive stimulants.[72] Height over the long term appears unaltered; however, none of the children were continued on stimulants into adulthood. Additionally, the long-term observations are confined to methylphenidate. Thus, questions remain about the long-term effects of continued treatment, particularly with amphetamine or pemoline.

As reviewed by Klein,[71] the earlier fear that stimulant treatment impairs social functioning has been examined, and no major negative effects were seen in a number of studies. A recent study from the United Kingdom,[73] where stimulants are far less commonly prescribed, adds additional confirmation. It is true, however, that some children may look overly serious or sad on stimulants and seem less socially interactive. These effects usually can be reversed by lowering the dose.

Clinical Administration

A thorough clinical assessment should always precede stimulant drug administration. Because of the potential hepatotoxicity of pemoline, baseline liver functions should be obtained if that medication is to be used. Dosage is started at low levels: for example, for children age 6 or older, 5 mg of methylphenidate b.i.d., or 5 mg of amphetamine (q.d. or b.i.d.), or 37.5 mg of pemoline q.d. The dose is adjusted upward every 3 days, titrating to the best ratio of clinical benefit to side effects. Dosages range from 0.15 to 0.5 mg/kg for amphetamine, 0.3 to 1.0 mg/kg for methylphenidate, and 0.5 to 2.0 mg/kg for pemoline. Drug doses need to be reevaluated over time as the child develops, and drug holidays should be enforced once a year to assess continuing need for the medication. The conventional wisdom that stimulants should be given to hyperactive children on an empty stomach because food could impair absorption has been disproved, at least in the case of methylphenidate. No difference in behavioral or cognitive effects is seen whether the drug is taken fasting or following breakfast, and the presence of food actually decreased time to peak plasma concentration of methylphenidate.[60,74]

TRICYCLIC ANTIDEPRESSANTS

The efficacy of tricyclic antidepressant drugs (TCAs) in depressed children and adolescents is open to question. However, several studies have documented their efficacy in enuresis and attention deficit disorder, and therefore they are included in this chapter. Knowledge of the pharmacologic properties of these compounds is useful in any event for understanding side effects and interactions with other compounds. This section focuses on TCAs because they are the most frequently prescribed type of antidepressant for children and adolescents.

Richelson[75] summarized the pharmacologic properties of antidepressant drugs other than monoamine oxidase inhibitors as follows: (1) blockade of norepinephrine, serotonin, and dopamine uptake at nerve endings; (2) blockade of histamine H_1, muscarinic, α_1- and α_2-adrenergic, dopamine D_2, and serotonin S_2 receptors. Importantly, the receptor blockade data have been obtained from human brain.

The mechanism of action in enuresis is also not understood. Speculation that anticholinergic properties of tricyclics were responsible for amelioration of enuresis ceased following a negative trial of methscopolamine, a peripheral anticholinergic agent that does not cross the blood–brain barrier.[76] Furthermore, desipramine and the more anticholinergic compound imipramine did not differ in their clinical effect on enuresis.[76]

The mechanism of action of clomipramine in obsessive-compulsive disorder (a disorder surprisingly prevalent in adolescents) is assumed to be related to its specific potency in blocking serotonin reuptake.[77] Support for this idea comes from the efficacy in adults of other serotonin reuptake blockers, fluoxetine[78] and fluvoxamine.[79] Importantly, clomipramine has been shown superior to placebo[80] and to desipramine[81] in children and adolescents with obsessive-compulsive disorder. This is all the more significant when one considers that tricyclic treatment of prepubertal and/or adolescent depressions has not been found superior to placebo.

Indications and Efficacy

The indications for use of TCAs in children and adolescents are attention deficit hyperactivity disorder, anxiety disorders, obsessive-compulsive disorder, and enuresis. (As noted above, depression in children and adolescents may not be an indication for TCAs.)

As reviewed by Pliszka,[82] tricyclics are superior to placebo in treatment of hyperactivity but are less effective than stimulants. However, there may be a subgroup of children characterized by higher levels of anxiety and/or depression for whom tricyclics are preferable. There is certainly a group of children for whom tics or other side effects make stimulants unworkable; these constitute the major treatment group of hyperactive children for whom TCAs are indicated.

Imipramine is more efficacious than placebo in ameliorating enuresis in short-term studies.[83] Adequate dosage appears necessary to see a response. Two groups found positive relationships between imipramine plus desipramine plasma concentrations and antienuretic response.[76,84] Where no relationship was seen between plasma concentration and efficacy,[85] the average level was low (18.1 ng/ml). However, relapse has been seen in some children despite drug concentrations at or above those that were previously effective.[76]

The therapeutic effectiveness of clomipramine in pediatric obsessive-compulsive disorder has been established in two double-blind controlled trials.[80,81] The delay of 2 or more weeks before symptomatic relief occurs parallels the time course of the antidepressants, but reductions in obsessive-compulsive disorder symptoms have been independent of depressive symptoms. While there is certainty about the short-term benefit from clomipramine in pediatric obsessive-compulsive disorder cases, the effects of long-term maintenance with this drug are not yet clear. Clomipramine is only available in the United States through an Investigational New Drug (IND) treatment from CIBA-Geigy, its manufacturer.

Imipramine's superiority over placebo in a controlled trial of school phobic children[86] is confirmation of its efficacy in anxiety disorders in pediatric age groups.

Both followup studies and family studies indicate that the diagnostic criteria applied to adults for depressive disorders can be used for children. Given the well-established efficacy of TCAs in adults, it is puzzling that no study, thus far, has demonstrated a clear-cut difference between drug and placebo in a double-blind trial in prepubertal or adolescent subjects. Interpretation of these studies is complicated by high (e.g., 68 percent) placebo response rates. Because imipramine responders have been shown generally to have higher serum concentrations than nonresponders, questions of adequacy of dose have been raised. However, recent trials in adolescents utilizing doses that are efficacious in adults did not find a drug–placebo difference.[87,88]

The risk/benefit ratio with TCAs makes their use for most cases of enuresis questionable. In addition to possible cardiac toxicity, a new side effect of tricyclic therapy has been identified for children and adolescents. A Scandinavian report comparing enuretics who received tricyclics with enuretics who were not medicated and with control children who were not bed wetters found dental caries increased in the tricyclic group.[89]

LITHIUM

The mechanism of lithium's action in psychiatric disorders is unknown. However, multiple actions have been described.[90] Lithium inhibits release of norepinephrine and dopamine, but not serotonin, from nerve terminals. Lithium also affects the inositol-based second messenger system. By inhibiting the hydrolysis of myoinositol-1-phosphate, lithium decreases the content of phosphatidylinositides of cells that are stimulated.

Lithium ions are easily absorbed from the gastrointestinal tract. Lithium is eliminated almost entirely via the urine, although about 5 percent can be eliminated via sweat.

There are now several conditions for which lithium is being tried in child and adolescent psychiatry.[91] Bipolar affective disorder and conduct disorder, undersocialized aggressive type, are the most common for adolescent subjects. As with adults, not all manic-depressive patients respond to lithium. On long-term followup, two-thirds of bipolar children and adolescents appeared to respond.[92]

Dosage requirements of lithium per kilogram of body weight are said to be relatively higher for children than for adults, perhaps due to higher renal clearance of this ion by children.[91] Lithium as well as haloperidol was found significantly better than placebo in decreasing behavioral symptoms in conduct disorder. Serum and salivary lithium levels correlated highly ($r = .83$).[93]

NEUROLEPTICS

During the early 1960s, it was recognized that clinically effective neuroleptics all had the ability to inhibit stereotyped behaviors in rats that are mediated by dopamine.[94] Subsequent studies showed that their clinical efficacy is correlated with their potency for dopamine receptor blockade.

Most neuroleptics used in children produce varying degrees of α-adrenergic blockade and histamine blockade, as well as having anticholinergic properties. As with TCAs, the relative strengths of histamine and α-adrenergic blockade are primary determinants for the side effects of sedation and orthostatic hypotension, respectively.[94] Some of these compounds have greater potency at sites other than dopamine receptors. For example, thioridazine and chlorpromazine are preferential 5-HT receptor blockers.[95] Pimozide, a neuroleptic of the diphenylbutylpiperidine type, is a recent addition to the therapeutic list and the first drug approved by the Federal Food, Drug, and Cosmetic Act's Orphan Drug Amendments (for its efficacy in Gilles de la Tourette's syndrome). It has calcium channel–blocking activity[96] in addition to dopamine receptor–blocking properties.

The absorption, metabolism, and excretion of these drugs have been summarized by Baldessarini.[90] Most are erratic and unpredictable in their absorption, particularly when taken orally (the usual route). The metabolism of antipsychotic drugs is by oxidative processes largely mediated by liver microsomal and other enzymes, and to a lesser extent by conjugation to glucuronides. The more hydrophilic metabolites are excreted in the urine and, to a lesser degree, in the bile.

Only limited information is available on the pharmacokinetics of neuroleptics in children; most of it has been obtained in autistic subjects.[97] In another study of children and adolescents,[98] haloperidol plasma concentrations, particularly concentrations greater than 6 ng/ml, were found to be significantly related to side effects but not to the weight-adjusted daily dose. Pimozide pharmacokinetics showed considerable intersubject variation in 5 children with Gilles de la Tourette's disorder[99]; half-lives ranged from 24 to 142 hours.

Indications and Efficacy

Aggressivity occurs as a symptom in diverse childhood and adolescent disorders, including conduct disorder and autism. Pimozide,[100] haloperidol,[93] molindone, and thioridazine[101] all have been found to reduce aggressive behavior in pediatric psychiatric patients. The use of p.r.n. doses for agitation or aggressive outbursts is questionable, as a recent study of pediatric psychiatric inpatients[102] failed to demonstrate therapeutic benefit following the majority of administrations.

Low doses (0.5–4 mg/day) of haloperidol produced clinically (and statistically) significant improvement in sterotypies, withdrawal, hyperactivity, fidgetiness, and abnormal relations with people in a double-blind trial in autistic children.[97]

Schizophrenia is seen in late adolescent populations and rarely in prepubertal subjects.[103] Clinical experience suggests that prepubertal patients may be less responsive to neuroleptics.[104] Haloperidol and loxapine were more effective than placebo in one study with schizophrenic adolescents.[105] Thiothixene was more efficacious and had fewer side effects than thioridazine in adolescents with chronic schizophrenia.[106]

Gilles de la Tourette's disorder (chronic motor and vocal tics) has been found to benefit from haloperidol[107] and pimozide[108] in controlled clinical trials.

Adverse Effects

Movement disorders have thus far been the most extensively studied side effects in children. Acute dystonic reactions occur and are treated with diphenhydramine or anticholinergic agents.[109] Parksinsonian reactions appear rare in preschool children[27] but are more common in school-age or adolescent patients.[110] Because of the long biologic half-life of pimozide in some subjects, steady state may not be reached until a month after a stable daily intake, and extrapyramidal side effects may follow what appeared earlier to be a problem-free course of therapy.[99]

Tardive dyskinesia, abnormal involuntary movements typically of the face and/or tongue that persist despite neuroleptic medication, is a side effect risk of neuroleptic treatment. Most of the data on tardive dyskinesia in children and adolescents are from subjects with developmental disabilities.[104,111,112] Mentally retarded children are reported to have dyskinesia rates of 29–63 percent.[104,111–114] The cumulative neuroleptic dose has been associated with dyskinesia in one study, but not in another (see Campbell and Spencer[104] for references). However, the earlier study described much larger cumulative doses. This suggests that the cumulative dose is likely associated with tardive dyskinesia risk.

Commonly recognized side effects such as sedation, dizziness, confusion, and seizures can occur. Autonomic side effects such as dry mouth, constipation, and hypotension appear rare in children.[115]

Neuroleptic malignant syndrome, characterized by hyperthermia and extrapyramidal symptoms, is a rare but potentially fatal condition. A review[116] of 115 cases in the literature noted that 9.5 percent of cases were in individuals between 12 and 19 years of age.

An important psychologic side effect of neuroleptic treatment is the production of clinically significant anxious or depressed states in children.[117,118] Case reports of pediatric patients becoming aggressive with haldol or pimozide describe a threshold phenomenon, with disappearance of aggression when the neuroleptic dose was lowered.[118] Anxiety can take the form of school phobia. Behavioral toxicity is described as one of the earliest and most common side effects of excess dosage in children.[115]

ANTICONVULSANTS

Beneficial effects of anticonvulsants in a variety of psychiatric disorders are beginning to be documented. As these compounds are also discussed in Chapter 29, Anticonvulsants, only their psychoactive properties are discussed here. Carbamazepine has stimulated a great deal of interest because of its utility in adults with manic-depressive illness[119,120] or borderline personality disorder.[121] The therapeutic benefit appears to be prophylaxis against major losses of control. Although carbamazepine has received the most attention, other anticonvulsants, such as clonazepam and phenytoin, may also have utility in selected cases.

Carbamazepine

Carbamazepine has a tricyclic structure similar to that of the familiar TCAs. It also appears to have some antidepressant efficacy, at least in selected adult populations.[120]

The mechanism(s) of action of its behavioral effects remain to be clarified. However, multiple pharmacologic effects have been documented. Carbamazepine blocks norepinephrine reuptake.[122] Although carbamazepine is only one-quarter as potent as imipramine, the dosage used clinically is sufficient to make the two compounds equally potent.

Side effects of drowsiness, nausea, vertigo, ataxia, and blurred vision are usually mild, transient, and dose-related.[123] Plasma concentrations above 10 mg/liter are apt to be associated with side effects.[124]

A recent review[125] of studies of behavioral effects of carbamazepine in childhood behavioral disorders concludes that carbamazepine has a place in pediatric psychopharmacology, but that systematic, well-controlled studies are needed.

Phenytoin

There is a paucity of recent literature on the use of phenytoin in pediatric and adolescent behavior disorders. (See reference 126 for a bibliography.)

Clonazepam

See the following section on benzodiazepines.

BENZODIAZEPINES

Benzodiazepines are relatively unstudied as treatment agents for psychiatric disorders in childhood and adolescence. Although an extremely small percentage of benzodiazepine prescriptions is written for children in general,[127] some populations are more likely to receive these compounds: 3–4 percent of mentally retarded persons in a U.S. national survey were taking benzodiazepines.[128] Their uses as anticonvulsants or as sedatives for procedures are covered elsewhere in this volume.

Although anxiety (as a symptom or as the anxiety disorders) seems a logical indication for benzodiazepines, there are few systematic data on any pharmacologic treatments of anxiety disorders in pediatric populations and no satisfactorily controlled trials of the benzodiazepines. Clonazepam in doses of 0.5–3 mg was reported to decrease anxiety disorder symptoms in three prepubertal subjects.[129] No adverse effects were reported. Preliminary reports of a study of school phobics reported alprazolam (0.03 mg/kg) to be more effective than placebo.[130]

As reviewed by Nino-Murcia and Dement,[131] occasionally benzodiazepines have utility in the treatment of somnambulism and night terrors.

Benzodiazepines often cause undesirable effects in pediatric patients; disinhibited and more aggressive behavior was seen in as many as 25 percent of children treated with clonazepam.[132] However, review of the adult literature[133] yields estimates of the incidence of clinical aggressive dyscontrol of less than 1 percent. Is this a developmental pharmacodynamic change or a reflection of other differences in treatment populations? More and better data are needed before a definitive statement can be made.

FENFLURAMINE

Autism is a childhood disorder characterized by qualitative impairment in reciprocal social interaction and in communication and by a markedly restricted repertoire of activities and interests. These children can appear to lack an awareness of others and treat people as furniture. Impaired social relatedness and social functioning usually persist into adulthood. Serotonergic abnormalities, particularly elevated concentrations of serotonin or its metabolites, have been found in autistic as well as in other retarded subjects.[134] Psychopharmacologic treatment is prescribed for those patients whose behavioral symptoms have failed to respond to behavior modification or other psychosocial interventions. The targeted behaviors include aggressiveness directed against self and/or others, hyperactivity, temper tantrums, and stereotypies.

Considerable excitement followed the first report of therapeutic benefit in open trials of fenfluramine.[135] As is often the case, however, double-blind studies have not been convincing. A recent multicenter, placebo-controlled, double-blind study of 81 autistic patients reported that one-third of the subjects were considered to have behavior improvement and increases in IQ.[136] However, the study design has been criticized because of a lack of randomization in some centers. Two centers that did use randomized orders of drug presentation found no benefit compared to placebo. Similarly, placebo-controlled trials of fenfluramine in hyperactive and/or conduct disordered children have not shown therapeutic benefit.[137]

Fenfluramine, a structural analog of amphetamine, has complex actions on the serotonergic system. Early in a course of administration, it selectively releases serotonin from presynaptic terminals.[138] However, chronic administration leads to decreased brain serotonin content.[139] Decreased serotonin concentration following chronic fenfluramine has been a consistent finding in studies of autistic children (see reference 22 for a review). Fenfluramine is an anorectic that delays gastric emptying.[140]

Side effects from fenfluramine are similar to those reported in adults and seem to be dose-dependent.[141,142] Transient weight loss (or failure to gain), sedation, and increased irritability are among the most common. The weight loss is not permanent, and weight gain is reported following discontinuation of the drug. No changes in cardiovascular function were seen in children.[142,143]

OPIATE ANTAGONISTS

Opiate antagonists have their main clinical use in reversing opiate intoxication or overdose. Recently, two groups have reported some therapeutic benefit for autistics in open trials with naltrexone, a long-acting opiate antagonist.[104,144] Open trials have also occurred in bulimia.[145] As summarized by Crabtree,[146] naltrexone is rapidly absorbed from the gastrointestinal tract and then metabolized by the liver, largely via glucuronide conjugation.

CLONIDINE

Clonidine is an α-adrenergic agonist that has been given to pediatric patients for attention deficit disorder[147] as well as Gilles de la Tourette's disorder.[148] However, it is not a first choice for either disorder. Side effects seen in children include sedation, early morning awakening, and headache,[149] and there is as yet no published controlled trial demonstrating efficacy for Gilles de la Tourette's disorder.

In addition to α_2-agonist properties, a variety of other pharmacologic effects have been noted, including inhibition of serotonin and acetylcholine release, stimulation of prostaglandin synthesis, and enhancement of endorphinergic activity (see references 150 and 151).

REFERENCES

1. Combrinck-Graham L, Gursky EJ, Saccar CL: Psychoactive agents, in Yaffe SJ (ed): Pediatric Pharmacology. New York, Grune and Stratton, 1980, p 455–478
2. Gittelman R, Spitzer R, Cantwell D: Diagnostic classification and psychopharmacological indications, in Werry J (ed): Pediatric Psychopharmacology: The Use of Behavior Modifying Drugs in Children. New York, Brunner/Mazel, 1978, pp 136–167
3. Rapoport JL: Pediatric psychopharmacology: The last decade, in Meltzer HY (ed): Psychopharmacology: The Third Generation of Progress. New York, Raven Press, 1985, pp 1211–1214
4. Gualtieri CT, Hicks RE: Neuropharmacology of methylphenidate and a neural substrate for childhood hyperactivity. Psychiatr Clin No Am 8:875–892, 1985
5. Danhoff M, Breimer DD: Therapeutic drug monitoring in saliva. Clin Pharmacokinet 3:39–57, 1978
6. Narang PK, Carliner NH, Fisher ML, Crouthamel WG: Quinidine saliva concentrations: Absence of correlation with serum concentrations at steady state. Clin Pharmacol Ther 34:695–702, 1983
7. Rapoport JL, Kruesi MJP: Organic therapies, in Kaplan HI, Sadock BJ (eds): Comprehensive Textbook of Psychiatry IV. Baltimore, Williams and Wilkins, 1985, pp 1793–1802
8. Brown RT, Borden KA, Wynne ME, Spunt AL, Clingerman SR: Compliance with pharmacological and cognitive treatments for attention deficit disorder. J Am Acad Child Adol Psychiat 26:521–526, 1987
9. Klorman R, Coons HW, Borgstedt AD: Effects of methylphenidate on adolescents with a childhood history of attention deficit disorder; I. Clinical findings. J Am Acad Child Adol Psychiat 26:363–367, 1987
10. Lipman RS: Overview of research in psychopharmacological treatment of mentally ill/mentally retarded. Psychopharmacol Bull 22:1046–1054, 1986
11. Safer DJ, Krager JM: Prevalence of medication treatment for

hyperactive adolescents. Psychopharmacol Bull 21:212–215, 1985

12. Werry JS: Annotation: Drugs, learning and cognitive function in children—An update. J Child Psychol Psychiat 29:129–141, 1988

13. Douglas VI, Barr RG, O'Neill ME, Britton BG: Short term effects of methylphenidate on the cognitive, learning and academic performance of children with attention deficit disorder in the laboratory and the classroom. J Child Psychol Psychiat 27:191–211, 1986

14. Barkley RA, Cunningham CE: The effects of methylphenidate on the mother-child interactions of hyperactive children. Arch Gen Psychiat 36:201–208, 1979

15. Aman MG: Psychotropic drugs and learning problems—A selective review. J Learn Disabil 13:87–97, 1980

16. Gittleman R, Klein D, Feingold I: Children with reading disorders, II. Effects of methylphenidate in combination with reading remediation. J Child Psychol Psychiat 24:193–212, 1983

17. Sprague RL, Sleator EL: Methylphenidate in hyperkinetic children: Differences in dose effects on learning and social behavior. Science 198:1274–1276, 1977

18. Ballinger CT, Varley CK, Nolan PA: Effects of methylphenidate on reading in children with attention deficit disorder. Am J Psychiat 141:1590–1593, 1984

19. Rapport MD, Stoner G, DuPaul GJ, Birmingham BK, Tucker S: Methylphenidate in hyperactive children: Differential effects of dose on academic, learning and social behavior. J Abnorm Child Psychol 13:227–244, 1985

20. Schecter MD, Timmons GD: Objectively measured hyperactivity II. Caffeine and amphetamine effects. J Clin Pharmacol 25:276–280, 1985

21. Donnelly M, Rapoport JL, Potter WZ, Oliver J, Keysor CS, Murphy DL: Fenfluramine and amphetamine treatment of childhood hyperactivity: Clinical and biochemical findings. Arch Gen Psychiat 46:205–212, 1989

22. Campbell M: Fenfluramine treatment of autism. Annotation. J Child Psychol Psychiat 29:1–10, 1988

23. Garfinkel BD, Wender PH, Sloman L, O'Neill I: Tricyclic antidepressant and methylphenidate treatment of attention deficit disorder in children. J Am Acad Child Psychiat 22:343–348, 1983

24. Werry JS, Aman MG, Diamond E: Imipramine and methylphenidate in hyperactive children. J Child Psychol Psychiat 21:27–35, 1980

25. Letters to the Editor. Arch Gen Psychiatr 45:685–686, 1988

26. Aman MG, Singh NN: A critical appraisal of recent drug research in mental retardation: The Coldwater studies. J Ment Def Res 30:203–216, 1986

27. Anderson LT, Campbell M, Grega DM, Perry R, Small AM, Green WH: Haloperidol in the treatment of infantile autism: Effects on learning and behavioral symptoms. Am J Psychiat 141:1195–1202, 1984

28. Platt JE, Campbell M, Green WH, Grega DM: Cognitive effects of lithium carbonate and haloperidol in treatment-resistant aggressive children. Arch Gen Psychiat 41:657–662, 1984

29. Corbett JA, Trimble MR, Nichol TC: Behavioral and cognitive impairments in children with epilepsy: The long-term effects of anticonvulsant therapy. J Am Acad Child Psychiat 24:17–23, 1985

30. Aman MG, Werry JS, Paxton JW, Turbott SH: Effect of sodium valproate on psychomotor performance in children as a function of dose, fluctuations in concentration, and diagnosis. Epilepsia 28:115–124, 1987

31. Jarbe TUC: State dependent learning and drug discriminative control of behaviour: An overview. Acta Neurol Scand 109(suppl):37–59, 1986

32. Goodwin DW, Crane JB, Guze SB: Phenomenological aspects of the alcoholic "blackout." Br J Psychiat 115:1033–1038, 1969

33. Swanson JM, Kinsbourne M: Stimulant-related state-dependent learning in hyperactive children. Science 192:1354–1357, 1976

34. Steinhausen HC, Kreuzer EM: Learning in hyperactive children: Are there stimulant-related and state-dependent effects? Psychopharmacology 74:389–390, 1981

35. Gan J, Cantwell DP: Dosage effects of methylphenidate on paired

associated learning: Positive/negative placebo responders. J Am Acad Child Psychiat 21:237–242, 1982

36. Stephens RS, Pelham WE, Skinner R: State-dependent and main effects of methylphenidate and pemoline on paired-associate learning and spelling in hyperactive children. J Consult Clin Psychol 52:104–113, 1984

37. Becker-Mattes A, Mattes JA, Abikoff H, Brandt L: State-dependent learning in hyperactive children receiving methylphenidate. Am J Psychiat 142:455–459, 1985

38. Weiner JM: Summary and prospect, in Wiener JM (ed): Diagnosis and Psychopharmacology of Childhood and Adolescent Disorders. 2nd ed. New York, Wiley-Interscience, 1985, pp 336–343

39. Browne RG, Segal DS: Metabolic and experimental factors in the behavioral response to repeated amphetamine. Pharmacol Biochem Behav 6:545–552, 1977

40. Domonic JA, Moore KE: Supersensitivity to the central stimulant actions of adrenergic drugs following discontinuation of a chronic diet of α-methyltyrosine. Psychopharmacologia 15:96–101, 1969

41. Scheel-Kruger J: Comparative studies of various amphetamine analogues demonstrating different interactions with the metabolism of the catecholamines in the brain. Eur J Pharmacol 14:47–59, 1971

42. Zametkin AJ, Karoum F, Linnoila M: Stimulants, Urinary Catecholamines, and Indoleamines in Hyperactivity: A comparison of methylphenidate and dextroamphetamine. Arch Gen Psychiat 42:251–255, 1985

43. Kuczenski R: Biochemical actions of amphetamine and other stimulants, in Creese I (ed): Stimulants: Neurochemical, Behavioral and Clinical Perspective. New York, Raven Press, 1983, pp 31–61

44. Green A, El Hait M: A new approach to the assessment of the potency of reversible monoamine oxidase inhibitors in vivo, and its application to (+)-amphetamine, p-methoxyamphetamine and harmaline. Biochem Pharmacol 29:2781–2789, 1980

45. Starke K: Regulation of noradrenaline release by presynaptic receptor systems. Rev Physiol Biochem Pharmacol 77:1–124, 1977

46. Aarskog D, Fevang FO, Klove H, Stoa KF, Thorsen T: The effect of stimulant drugs, dextroamphetamine and methylphenidate on secretion of growth hormone in hyperactive children. J Pediatr 90:136–139, 1977

47. Gualtieri CT, Kanoy R, Hawk B, Koriath U, Schroeder S, Youngblood W, Breese GR, Prange A Jr: Growth hormone and prolactin secretion in adults and hyperactive children: Relation to methylphenidate serum levels. Psychoneuroendocrinology 6:331–339, 1981

48. Shaywitz SE, Hunt RD, Jatlow P, Cohen DJ, Young JG, Pierce RN, Anderson GM, Shaywitz BA: Psychopharmacology of attention deficit disorder: Pharmacokinetic, neuroendocrine, and behavioral measures following acute and chronic treatment with methylphenidate. Pediatrics 69:688–694, 1982

49. Garfinkel BD, Brown WA, Klee SH, Braden W, Beauchesne H, Shapiro SK: Neuroendocrine and cognitive responses to amphetamine in adolescents with a history of attention deficit disorder. J Am Acad Child Phychiat 25:503–508, 1986

50. Greenhill LL, Puig-Antich J, Chambers W, Rubinstein B, Halpern F, Sachar EJ: Growth hormone, prolactin, and growth responses in hyperkinetic males treated with d-amphetamine. J Am Acad Child Psychiat 20:84–103, 1981

51. Donnelly M, Rapoport JL: Attention deficit disorders, in Wiener JM (ed): Diagnosis and Psychopnarmacology of Childhood and Adolescent Disorders, 2nd ed. New York, Wiley-Interscience, 1985, pp 178–197

52. Weiner N: Norepinephrine, epinephrine, and the sympathomimetic amines, in Gilman AG, Goodman LS, Rall TW, Murad F (eds): Goodman and Gilman's The Pharmacological Basis of Therapeutics, 7th ed. New York, Macmillan, 1985, pp 145–180

53. Gunne LM, Anggard E: Pharmacokinetic studies with amphetamines—Relationship to neuropsychiatric disorders. J Pharmacokinet Biopharm 1:481–495, 1973

54. Brown GL, Hunt RD, Ebert MH, Bunney WE, Kopin IJ: Plasma

levels of D-amphetamine in hyperactive children. Psychopharmacology 62:133–140, 1979

55. Brown GL, Ebert MH, Mikkelsen EJ, Hunt RD: Behavior and motor activity response in hyperactive children and plasma amphetamine levels following a sustained release preparation. J Am Acad Child Psychiat 19:225–239, 1980

56. Galeazzi RL: Pharmacodynamics, pharmacokinetics, or both?, in Barnett G, Chiang CN (eds): Pharmacokinetics and Pharmacodynamics of Psychoactive Drugs. Forest City, California, Biomedical Publications, 1985, pp 169–184

57. Faraj BA, Israili ZH, Perel JM, Jenkins ML, Holtzman SG, Cucinell SA, Dayton PG: Metabolism and disposition of methylphenidate-^{14}C: Studies in man and animals. J Pharmacol Exp Ther 191:535–547, 1974

58. Patrick KS, Mueller RA, Gualtieri CT, Breese GR: Pharmacokinetics and actions of methylphenidate, in Meltzer HY (ed): Psychopharmacology: The Third Generation of Progress. New York, Raven Press, 1987, pp 1387–1395

59. Wargin W, Patrick K, Kilts C, Gualtieri CT, Ellington K, Mueller RA, Kraemer G, Breese GR: Pharmacokinetics of methylphenidate in man, rat and monkey. J Pharm Exp Ther 226:382–386, 1983

60. Chan YM, Swanson JM, Soldin SJ, Thiessen JJ, Macleod SM, Logham W: Methylphenidate hydrochloride given with or before breakfast: II. Effects on plasma concentration of methylphenidate and ritalinic acid. Pediatrics 72:56–59, 1983

61. Greenhill LL, Cooper T, Soloman M, Fried J, Cornblatt B: Methylphenidate salivary levels in children. Psychopharmacol Bull 23:115–119, 1987

62. Gualtieri CT, Wargin W, Kanoy R, Patrick K, Shen CD, Youngblood W, Mueller RAS, Breese GR: Clinical studies of methylphenidate serum levels in children and adults. J Am Acad Child Psychiat 21:19–26, 1982

63. Winsberg BG, Kupietz SS, Sverd J, Hungund BL, Young NL: Methylphenidate oral dose plasma concentrations and behavioral response in children. Psychopharmacology 76:329–332, 1982

64. Tomkins CP, Soldin SJ, Mac Leod SM, Rochofort JG, Swanson JM: Analysis of pemoline in serum by high performance liquid chromatography: Clinical application to optimize treatment of hyperactive children. Ther Drug Monit 2:255–260, 1980

65. Sallee FR, Stiller R, Perel J, Bates T: Oral pemoline kinetics in hyperactive children. Clin Pharm Ther 37:606–609, 1985

66. Collier CP, Soldin SJ, Swanson JM, Mac Leod SM, Weinberg F, Rochefort JG: Pemoline pharmacokinetics and longterm therapy in children with attention deficit disorder and hyperactivity. Clin Pharmacokinet 10:269–278, 1985

67. Barkley RA: A review of stimulant drug research with hyperactive children. J Child Psychol Psychiat 18:137–165, 1977

68. Rapoport JL: The use of drugs: Trends in research, in Rutter M (ed): Developmental Neuropsychiatry. New York, Guilford Press, 1983, pp 385–403

69. Mattes JA, Boswell L, Oliver H: Methylphenidate affects symptoms of attention deficit disorder in adults. Arch Gen Psychiat 1:1059–1063, 1984

70. Wender PH, Reimherr FW, Wood D, et al: A controlled study of methylphenidate in the treatment of attention deficit disorder with hyperactivity, residual type in adults. Am J Psychiat 142:547–552, 1985

71. Klein RG: Pharmacotherapy of childhood hyperactivity, an update, in Meltzer HY (ed): Psychopharmacology: The Third Generation of Progress. New York, Raven Press, 1987, pp 1215–1224

72. Hechtman L, Weiss G, Perlman T: Young adult outcome of hyperactive children who received long-term stimulant treatment. J Am Acad Child Psychiat 23:261–269, 1984

73. Taylor E, Schachar R, Thorley G, Wieseiberg HM, Everitt B, Rutter M: Which boys respond to stimulant medication? A controlled trial of methylphenidate in boys with disruptive behaviour. Psychol Med 17:121–143, 1987

74. Swanson JM, Sandman CA, Deutsch C, Baren M: Methylphenidate hydrocholoride given with or before breakfast: I. Behavioral, cognitive, and electrophysiologic effects. Pediatrics 72:49–55, 1983

75. Richelson E: Pharmacology of antidepressants. Psychopathology 20(suppl 1):1–12, 1987

76. Rapoport JL, Mikkelsen EJ, Zavadil A, Nee I, Gruenau C, Mendelson W, Gillin C: Childhood enuresis, II. Psychopathology, tricyclic concentration in plasma, and antienuretic effects. Arch Gen Psychiat 37:1146–1152, 1980

77. Leonard HL, Rapoport JL: Anxiety disorders in childhood and adolescence, in Tasman A (ed): American Psychiatric Association Annual Review, vol 8. Washington, DC, American Psychiatric Press, 1989, pp 162–179

78. Fontaine R, Chouinard G: An open clinical trial of fluoxetine in the treatment of obsessive-compulsive disorder. J Clin Psychopharmacol 2:98–101, 1986

79. Goodman WK, Price LH, Rasmussen SA, Heninger GR, Charney DS: Fluvoxamine as an Antiobsessional Agent. Psychopharmacol Bull 25(1):31–35, 1989

80. Flament MF, Rapoport JL, Berg CJ, et al: Clomipramine treatment of childhood obsessive-compulsive disorder: A double-blind controlled study. Arch Gen Psychiat 42:977–983, 1985

81. Leonard HL, Swedo S, Rapoport JL, et al: Treatment of childhood obsessive compulsive disorder with clomipramine and desmethylimipramine: A double-blind crossover comparison. Psychopharmacol Bull 24:93–95, 1988

82. Pliszka SR: Tricyclic antidepressants in the treatment of children with attention deficit disorder. J Am Acad Child Adol Psychiat 26:127–132, 1987

83. Fournier JP, Garfinkel BD, Bond A, Beauchesne H, Shapiro SK: Pharmacological and behavioral management of enuresis. J Am Acad Child Adol Psychiat 26:849–853, 1987

84. Jorgensen OS, Lober M, Christiansen J, Gram LF: Plasma concentration and clinical effect in imipramine treatment of childhood enuresis. Clin Pharmacokinet 5:386–393, 1980

85. DeVane CL, Walker RD, Sawyer WP, Wilson JA: Concentrations of imipramine and its metabolites during enuresis therapy. Pediatr Pharmacol 4:245–251, 1984

86. Gittleman-Klein R, Klein DF: Controlled imipramine treatment of school phobia. Arch Gen Psychiat 25:204–207, 1971

87. Ryan ND, Puig-Antich J, Cooper T, et al: Imipramine in adolescent major depression: Plasma level and clinical response. Acta Psychiat Scand 73:275–288, 1986

88. Geller B, Cooper TB, McCombs HG, Graham D, Wells J: Double-Bind, Placebo-Controlled Study of Nortriptyline in Depressed Children Using a Fixed Plasma Level Design. Psychopharmacol Bull 25(1):101–108, 1989

89. Von Knorring AL, Wahlin YB: Tricyclic antidepressants and dental caries in children. Neuropsychobiology 15:143–145, 1986

90. Baldessarini RJ: Drugs and the treatment of psychiatric disorders, in Gilman AG, Goodman LS, Rall TW, Murad F (eds): Goodman and Gilman's The Pharmacologic Basis of Therapeutics. New York, Macmillan, 1985, pp 387–445

91. Jefferson JW, Greist JH, Ackerman DL, Carroll JA: Lithium Encyclopedia for Clinical Practice, 2nd ed. Washington, DC American Psychiatric Press, 1987

92. Delong GR, Aldershof AL: Long-term experience with lithium treatment in childhood: Correlation with clinical diagnosis. J Am Acad Child Adol Psychiat 26:389–394, 1987

93. Campbell M, Small AM, Green WH, et al: Behavioral efficacy of haloperidol and lithium carbonate: A comparison in hospitalized aggressive children with conduct disorder. Arch Gen Psychiat 41:650–656, 1984

94. Delini-Stula A: Neuroanatomical, neuropharmacological and neurobiochemical target systems for antipsychotic activity of neuroleptics. Pharmacopsychiatry 19:134–139, 1986

95. Ortmann R, Bischoff S, Radeke E, Buch O, Delini-Stula A: Correlations between different measures of antiserotonin activity of drugs. Study with neuroleptics and serotonin receptor blockers. Naunyn Schmiedeber's Arch Pharmacol 321:265–270, 1982

96. Gould RJ, Murphy K, Reynolds I, et al: Antischizophrenic drugs of the diphenylbutylpiperidine type act as calcium channel antagonists. Proc Natl Acad Sci USA 80:5122–5125, 1983

97. Campbell M, Anderson LT, Cohen IL, Perry R, Small AM, Green WH, Anderson L, McCandless WH: Haloperidol in autistic

children: Effects on learning, behavior and abnormal involuntary movements. Psychopharmacol Bull 18:110–113, 1982

98. Dugas M, Zarifian E, LeHeuzey MF, Regnier N, Durand G, Bianchetti G, Morselli PL: Surveillance des taux plasmatiques de psychotropes chez l'enfant, I. Taux plasmatiques d'haloperidol. Nouv Press Med 11:2201–2204, 1982

99. Sallee FR, Pollock BG, Stiller RL, Stull S, Everett G, Perel JM: Pharmacokinetics of pimozide in adults and children with Tourette's syndrome. J Clin Pharmacol 27:776–781, 1987

100. Naruse H, Nagahata M, Nakane Y, Shirahashi K, Taesada M, Yamazaki K: A multicenter double-blind trial of pimozide (Orap), haloperidol and placebo in children with behavioral disorders, using crossover design. Acta Paedopsychiatr 48:173–184, 1982

101. Greenhill LL, Solomon M, Pleak R, Ambrosini P: Molindone hydrochloride treatment of hospitalized children with conduct disorder. J Clin Psychiat 46(8, sec 2):20–25, 1985

102. Vitiello B, Behar D, Wolfson S, et al: Panic disorder in prepubertal children. Am J Psychiat 144:525–526, 1987

103. Kydd RR, Werry JS: Schizophrenia in children under 16 years. J Autism Dev Disord 12:343–357, 1982

104. Campbell M, Spencer EK: Psychopharmacology in child and adolescent psychiatry: A review of the past five years. J Am Acad Child Adol Psychiat 27:269–279, 1988

105. Pool D, Bloom W, Mielke DH, Roniger JJ, Gallant DM: A controlled evaluation of loxitane in seventy-five adolescent schizophrenic patients. Curr Ther Res Clin Exp 19:99–104, 1976

106. Realmuto GM, Erickson WD, Yellin AM, Hopwood JH, Greenberg LM: Clinical comparison of thiothixene and thioridazine in schizophrenic adolescents. Am J Psychiat 141:440–442, 1984

107. Bruun RD: Gilles de la Tourette's syndrome: An overview of clinical experience. J Am Acad Child Psychiat 23:126–133, 1984

108. Shapiro AK, Shapiro E: Controlled study of pimozide vs. placebo in Tourette's syndrome. J Am Acad Child Psychiat 23:161–173, 1984

109. Campbell M: Schizophrenic disorders and pervasive developmental disorders/infantile autism, in Weiner JM (ed): Diagnosis and Psychopharmacology of Childhood and Adolescent Disorders. New York, Wiley-Interscience, 1985, pp 113–150

110. Keepers GA, Casey DE: Prediction of neuroleptic-induced dystonia. J Clin Psychopharmacol 7:342–345, 1987

111. Gualtieri CT, Quade D, Hicks RE, Mayo JP, Schroeder SR: Tardive dyskinesia and other clinical consequences of neuroleptic treatment in children and adolescents. Am J Psychiat 141:20–23, 1984

112. Gualtieri CT, Schroeder SR, Hicks RE, Quade D: Tardive dyskinesia in young mentally retarded individuals. Arch Gen Psychiat 43:335–340, 1986

113. Perry R, Green WH, et al: Neuroleptic-related dyskinesias in autistic children: A prospective study. Psychopharmacol Bull 21:140–143, 1985

114. Campbell M, Adams P, Perry R, Spencer EK, Overall JE: Tardive and withdrawal dyskinesia in autistic children: A prospective study. Psychopharmacol Bull 24:251–256, 1988

115. Campbell M, Green WH, Deutsch SI: Child and Adolescent Psychopharmacology. Beverly Hills, California, Sage Publications, 1985

116. Addonizio G, Susman VL, Roth, SD: Neuroleptic malignant syndrome: Review and analysis of 115 cases. Biol Psychiat 22:1004–1020, 1987

117. Mikkelsen EJ, Detlor J, Cohen DJ: School avoidance and social phobia triggered by haloperidol in patients with Tourette's disorder. Am J Psychiat 138:1572–1576, 1981

118. Bruun RD: Subtle and underrecognized side effects of neuroleptic treatment in children with Tourette's disorder. Am J Psychiat 145:621–624, 1988

119. Okuma I, Inanaga K, Otsuki S, et al: Comparison of the antimanic efficacy of carbamazepine and chlorpromazine: A double-blind controlled study. Psychopharmacology 66:211–217, 1979

120. Post RM, Uhde TW, Ballenger JC, et al: Carbamazepine and its 10,11-epoxide metabolite in plasma and CSF: Relationship to antidepressant response. Arch Gen Psychiat 40:673–676, 1983

121. Cowdry RW, Gardner DL: Pharmacotherapy of borderline personality disorder. Arch Gen Psychiat 45:111–119, 1988

122. Purdy RE, Julien RM, Fairhurst AS, Terry MD: Effect of carbamazepine on the in vitro uptake and release of norepinephrine in adrenergic nerves of rabbit aorta and in whole brain synaptosomes. Epilepsia 18:251–257, 1977

123. Schmidt D: Adverse Effects of Antiepileptics. New York, Raven Press, 1982

124. Levy RH, Kerr BM: Clinical pharmacokinetics of carbamazepine. J Clin Psychiat 49(suppl):58–61, 1988

125. Evans RW, Clay TH, Gualtieri CT: Carbamazepine in pediatric psychiatry. J Am Acad Child Adol Psychiat 26:2–8, 1987

126. Smith BH, Bogoch S, Dreyfus J: The Broad Range of Clinical Use of Phenytoin. New York, Dreyfus Medical Foundation, 1988

127. Woods JH, Katz JL, Winger G: Abuse liability of benzodiazepines. Pharmacol Rev 39:251–413, 1987

128. Hill BK, Balow EA, Bruininks RH: A national study of prescribed drugs in institutions and community residential facilities for mentally retarded people. Psychopharmacol Bull 21:279–284, 1985

129. Biederman J: Clonazepam in the treatment of prepubertal children with panic-like symptoms. J Clin Psychiat 48(suppl):38–42, 1987

130. Bernstein GA, Hughes JR, Mitchell JE, Thompson T: Effects of narcotic antagonists on self-injurious behavior: A single case study. J Am Acad Child Adol Psychiat 26:886–889, 1987

131. Nino-Murcia G, Dement WC: Psychophysiological and pharmacological aspects of somnambulism and night terrors in children, in Meltzer HY (ed): Psychopharmacology: The Third Generation of Progress. New York, Raven Press, 1987, pp 873–880

132. Browne TR: Clonazepam: A review of a new anticonvulsant drug. Arch Neurol 33:326–332, 1976

133. Dietch JT, Jennings RK: Aggressive dyscontrol in patients treated with benzodiazepines. J Clin Psychiat 49:184–188, 1988

134. Ciranello RD: Hyperserotonemia and early infantile autism. N Engl J Med 307:181–183, 1982

135. Geller E, Ritvo ER, Freeman BJ, Yuwiler A: Preliminary observations on the effects of fenfluramine on blood serotonin and symptoms in three autistic boys. N Engl J Med 307:165–169, 1982

136. Ritvo ER, Freeman BJ, Yuwiler A, Geller E, Schroth P, Yokota A, Mason-Brothers A, August GJ, Klykylo W, Leventhal B, Lewis K, Pigott L, Realmuto G, Stubbs EG, Umansky R: Fenfluramine treatment of autism: UCLA collaborative study of 81 patients at nine medical centers. Psychopharmacol Bull 22:133–140, 1986

137. Kruesi MJP, Linnoila M, Rapoport JL, Brown G, Petersen R: Carbohydrate craving, conduct disorder and low 5HIAA. Psychiat Res 16:83–86, 1985

138. Borroni E, Ceci A, Garattini S, Mennini T: Differences between d-fenfluramine and d-norfenfluramine in serotonin presynaptic mechanisms. J Neurochem 40:891–893, 1983

139. Clineschmidt B, Totaro J, McGuffin J, Pflueger A: Fenfluramine: Long-term reduction in brain serotonin (5-hydroxytryptamine). Eur J Pharmacol 35:211–214, 1976

140. Rowland N, Carlton J: Inhibition of gastric emptying by peripheral and central fenfluramine in rats: Correlation with anorexia. Life Sci 34:2495–2499, 1984

141. Piggott LR, Gdowski CL, Villanueva D, Fischoff J, Frohman CF: Side effects of fenfluramine in autistic children. J Am Acad Child Psychiat 25:287–289, 1986

142. Realmuto GM, Jensen J, Klykylo W, Piggott L, Stubbs B, Yuwiler A, Geller E, Freeman BJ, Ritvo E: Untoward effects of fenfluramine in autistic children. J Clin Psychopharmacol 6:350–355, 1986

143. Campbell M, Small AM, Paly M, Perry BB, Lukashok D, Anderson LT: The efficacy and safety of fenfluramine in autistic children: Preliminary analysis of a double-blind study. Psychopharmacol Bull 23:123–127, 1987

144. Herman BH, Hammock MK, Arthur-Smith A, et al: Effects of naltresone in autism: Correlation with plasma opioid concentrations, in Scientific Proceedings of the Annual Meeting,

II:11–12, American Academy of Child and Adolescent Psychiatry, 1986

145. Jonas JM, Gold MS: Treatment of antidepressant-resistant bulimia with naltrexone. Int J Psychiat Med 16:305–309, 1987

146. Campbell M, Adams P, Small M, Purdy RV, Tesch L, Curren EL: Naltrexone in infantile autism. Psychopharmacol Bull 24:135–139, 1988

147. Crabtree BL: Review of naltrexone, a long-acting opiate antagonist. Clin Pharm 3:273–280, 1984

148. Hunt RD, Minderaa RD, Cohen DJ: Clonidine benefits children with attention deficit disorder and hyperactivity: Report of a double-blind placebo-crossover therapeutic trial. J Am Acad Child Psychiat 24:617–629, 1985

149. Cohen DJ, Leckman JF, Shaywitz BA: The Tourette syndrome and other tics, in Shaffer, D, Ehrhardt AA, Greenhill LL (eds): The Clinical Guide to Child Psychiatry. New York, The Free Press, 1985, pp 3–28

150. Leckman JF, Detlor J, Harcherik D, Ort S, Shaywitz BA, Cohen DJ: Short and long term treatment of Tourette's syndrome with clonidine: A clinical perspective. Neurology 35:343–351, 1985

151. Jarrott B, Conway EL, Maccarron C, Lewis SJ: Clonidine: Understanding its disposition, sites and mechanism of action. Clin Exp Pharm Physiol 14:471–479, 1987

152. Sandyk R, Gillman MA, Iacono RP, Bamford CR: Clonidine in neuropsychiatric disorders: A review. Neuroscience 35:205–215, 1987

39

ANTIHYPERTENSIVE AGENTS

Therapeutic regimens for treatment of high blood pressure have changed dramatically over the past decade. In a review of the use of antihypertensive drugs in children published in 1978,[1] the major emphasis was placed on diuretic and vasodilator therapy. Propranolol had only recently been marketed for use in the United States, and other β-blockers were not yet approved by the Food and Drug Administration. A relatively large section of the review was devoted to methyldopa, guanethidine, and reserpine; there was very little clinical experience with prazosin or clonidine; and converting enzyme inhibitors and calcium channel blockers were not yet available.

Traditionally, recommendations for treatment of childhood hypertension have been patterned after recommendations made for adults. This is the consequence of (1) the manyfold greater prevalence of hypertension in adults and (2) the fact that almost all premarketing drug testing has been performed in adult patients. Unfortunately, the latter continues to be the prevailing approach to introduction of new antihypertensive agents, and the data from studies in adults are not always directly applicable to children.

There are a number of differences between childhood and adult hypertension[2]: (1) Normal blood pressure is lower in children than adults and does not begin to approach adult norms until the late teenage years. (2) As a consequence of the lower range of normal blood pressure distribution in children, the diagnosis of hypertension is made at levels of blood pressure considerably lower than the levels used to define hypertension in adults. (3) When blood pressure becomes high enough to require antihypertensive therapy, it is usually secondary to a specific pathophysiologic condition, e.g., renal disease. (4) Secondary hypertension is usually more difficult to treat than essential hypertension, and as a result, successful antihypertensive control in childhood often requires aggressive treatment with a variety of drugs. (5) Doses of antihypertensive drugs, whether based on absolute or weight-related criteria, differ considerably in children from adults. These differences suggest that recommen-

dations for antihypertensive therapy are likely to be most reliable when based on drug studies conducted in children.

Very few antihypertensive drugs were subjected to clinical testing in children prior to 1980. However, many of the newer antihypertensive agents, particularly the converting enzyme inhibitors and calcium channel blockers, are now being evaluated in this age group. Although practical and ethical considerations still preclude the use of invasive studies during drug evaluation in the majority of the childhood population, accurate pharmacokinetic data and dosing schedules are now being developed for many new drugs.

The present review will focus on the pharmacology and clinical application of antihypertensive drugs most commonly used in pediatric practice today. The final section summarizes current recommendations, taking into consideration changes that have evolved since the 1987 Task Force Report.[2]

CONVERTING ENZYME INHIBITORS

Converting enzyme inhibitors (CEIs) interfere with the enzymatic conversion of angiotensin I to the active angiotensin octapeptide angiotensin II (Figure 39–1), the major vasoconstrictor in most vascular beds.[3] As seen in Figure 39–1, converting enzyme also functions in a complementary fashion as kininase II to convert the vasodilating peptide bradykinin to its inactive metabolites. Although inhibition of converting enzyme in both the kinin and renin–angiotensin systems has an antihypertensive effect, the general consensus holds that its primary contribution is made through reduction in angiotensin II production.

In addition to its effect on vascular reactivity, angiotensin II influences blood pressure via an interaction with other systems. It is an important stimulus for aldosterone production. An increase in natriuresis occurs following CEI administration, but it is not clear whether this

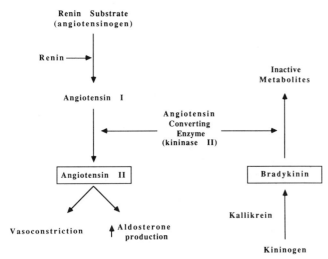

FIGURE 39-1. Action of converting enzyme in renin–angiotensin and kinin systems.

response is due to decreased levels of aldosterone or some other angiotensin-mediated effect.[4] Angiotensin II also stimulates norepinephrine release,[5] but its impact on vascular tone is relatively small and probably not as important as primary vasoconstriction.

The renin–angiotensin system initially was believed to be endocrine-like. Renin substrate produced by the liver is acted on by renin released from the renal juxtaglomerular cells to form angiotensin I; angiotensin I is enzymatically converted to angiotensin II during passage through the pulmonary circulation; and angiotensin II is delivered to its tissue sites of action. It is now clear that, in addition to this endocrine-like function, localized renin–angiotensin systems exist in a number of tissues intimately involved with blood pressure homeostasis. In particular, renin, angiotensin converting enzyme, and the angiotensins have each been identified in vascular beds,[6] cardiac tissue,[7] and the central nervous system.[7] Moreover, these local systems appear to be responsive to conditions known to modulate renin–angiotensin system activity and are susceptible to inhibition with CEIs.

It is generally conceded that the kidney plays a major, if not *the* major, role in the development of hypertension.[8] This is particularly true in pediatrics, where secondary forms of hypertension predominate, most commonly as a result of renal disease. The kidney is the primary source of circulating renin; the renal vasculature and glomerular structures[9] are highly responsive to angiotensin II; and renal control of sodium and water balance is a critical modulator of renin–angiotensin system activity. CEIs significantly affect renal perfusion and function[10,11] by reducing renal vascular resistance, increasing renal blood flow, and decreasing glomerular capillary pressure. Although the effects of these responses have not been sorted out with regard to etiologic influences on hypertension, administration of CEIs has been shown to reverse or prevent hypertension-related adverse effects on the kidney.[10]

Use of CEIs in the United States predominantly with captopril and enalapril[12] is also available and numerous other CEIs will soon follow.[13]

Captopril has been subjected to extensive pharmaco-

logic investigation in adults.[14] Approximately 70 percent of the drug is absorbed unchanged after an oral dose, but the bioavailability is reduced by 35–55 percent if the drug is given with a meal. Captopril undergoes both renal and hepatic metabolism. In healthy individuals almost the entire captopril dose is excreted via the urine, with approximately 40 percent excreted as the parent compound. The usual plasma half-life is 2 hours. As expected from the above, the plasma half-life increases in patients with renal failure, and dosage adjustments must be made. During hemodialysis, up to 35 percent of an oral dose can be recovered in the dialysate.

Captopril has been studied in children of all ages and under a variety of conditions, and it has proven to be a very effective antihypertensive agent.[15] Maximum drug concentrations are reached 1–2 hours after oral administration, and drug clearance is positively correlated with renal function.[15] The dose–response effect for CEIs is not graded, and there is very little change in blood pressure until converting enzyme has been inhibited by approximately 90 percent.[16] Thus, in older children dose–response studies have shown equivalent initial responses to 0.5, 1.0, or 2.0 mg/kg/dose.[17] It is recommended that therapy be started with a dose of 0.5 mg/kg/dose for children older than 6 months. This can be increased to 1.0 mg/kg/dose, but it is rare that a dose higher than this will improve blood pressure control. Captopril is usually administered on a t.i.d. basis, although twice-daily dosing has been successful. This may reflect recent data suggesting that CEI activity at tissue sites is relatively more important than reduction of circulating angiotensin II for blood pressure control. CEIs can be recovered from tissue for a considerable period of time after their disappearance from the plasma.[18]

CEI therapy is particularly useful in young infants and newborns. However, both the potency and the duration of action appear to be greater in this age group than in older children.[19] This may be related to the significantly higher renin–angiotensin system activity in the newborn or to the fact that the conditions associated with hypertension, i.e., renal emboli from umbilical artery catheters, glucocorticoid administration, and bronchopulmonary dysplasia, are reported to stimulate angiotensin formation.[10]

Blood pressure reduction as great as 60 percent below pretreatment levels and oliguria have been reported following administration of captopril doses of 0.3 mg/kg to prematures,[20] and normotensive blood pressure has been achieved with doses of 0.01 mg/kg to premature as well as full-term infants.[19] It is our practice to start treatment in this age group with a captopril dose of 0.01 mg/kg and increase rapidly over a 24- to 48-hour period until adequate blood pressure control is reached.

Enalapril is the first of a newer class of CEIs that differ from captopril in two important ways: (1) their molecular structure does not include a sulfhydryl group, believed to be an etiologic factor in the appearance of adverse effects; and (2) their plasma half-life is longer.

The clinical pharmacology of enalapril in adults has recently been reviewed.[21] Enalapril is a prodrug, i.e., an inactive drug that must be metabolically converted, in this case by deesterification to the active CEI drug enalaprilat.[21] This does not occur prior to absorption and takes place primarily in the liver, with only 6 percent of the prodrug converted to metabolites other than enalaprilat. This biologic conversion delays peak serum concentrations of enalaprilat until 3–4 hours after oral administration, limiting its usefulness when a rapid therapeutic response is desired. For long-term therapy, steady-state efficacy does not differ between captopril and enalapril, and use of the latter can improve compliance by reducing frequency of dosing. Enalapril and enalaprilat are excreted almost entirely by the kidney. Consequently, the dosage should be reduced in patients with renal failure. As is the case with captopril, approximately one-third of enalaprilat is cleared during hemodialysis.

A number of adverse effects have been reported in adults during CEI therapy.[22-24] Primary among these are rash, neutropenia, and loss of taste, each of which has been associated with other sulfhydryl-containing drugs in addition to captopril.[25] Thus, it is not surprising that the incidence of these adverse effects has been reported to be higher in patients treated with captopril than enalapril.[22] Other less common side effects are angioedema and a chronic, dry cough. The higher incidence of adverse effects with captopril appears to be dose-dependent, since it was established during the early years after captopril release, when extremely high doses of the drug were commonly used. More recently, a postmarketing surveillance study of 13,000 British patients reported that the incidence of adverse effects has decreased coincident with a decrease in the total daily dose of captopril and is not substantially different from the incidence reported for enalapril.[24] CEI-induced adverse effects usually respond to a reduction in dosage, but in some cases, it may be necessary to discontinue therapy.

The kidney can be particularly adversely affected during CEI therapy. Proteinuria has been reported in 2.5 percent of treated patients.[22] Membranous glomerulopathy has developed in the presence of a previously normal renal biopsy,[26] although it is approximately four times more common in patients with preexisting renal disease. Proteinuria is a known complication of treatment with other sulfhydryl-containing drugs but has been documented in patients treated with enalapril as well as captopril. CEI therapy may cause an increase in serum potassium secondary to a reduction in aldosterone production.[27,28] The degree of CEI-induced hyperkalemia is directly correlated with serum creatinine and can be severe in patients with end-stage renal disease.[28]

Renal function, in general, is maintained or improved during CEI therapy.[29,30] The compensatory homeostatic response to the reduction in renal mass and nephron loss in the diseased kidney is an increase in glomerular capillary flow and pressure. CEIs alter intrarenal hemodynamics to restore normal glomerular capillary pressure without a reduction in glomerular filtration rate.[30] Serum creatinine was shown to increase modestly, but significantly, during short-term CEI therapy in a group of children with renal transplant rejection,[17] but this was felt to be related to non-angiotensin-mediated effects.

The most dramatic adverse effect of CEIs on the kidney is a severe reduction in glomerular filtration in patients with bilateral renal artery stenosis or renal artery stenosis in a solitary or transplanted kidney.[10] As renal artery stenosis develops, there is a corresponding reduction in perfusion pressure in the renal afferent arteriole. The result is a fall in glomerular capillary, or hydrostatic, pressure and glomerular filtration. In severe renal artery stenosis, compensatory mechanisms maintain glomerular hydrostatic pressure via angiotensin II receptor–activated vasoconstriction in the efferent arteriole. CEI administration to these patients not only causes a further reduction in afferent arteriolar pressure as systemic blood pressure falls, but more importantly, it reverses the angiotensin II–dependent efferent arteriolar vasoconstriction. Because renal blood flow and renal perfusion are maintained during treatment with CEI despite the adverse effect on glomerular function, renal function returns to pretreatment levels when the drug is discontinued.

This pharmacologic effect forms the basis for using the captopril-modified 99m Tc-diethylenetriamine pentaacetic acid (DTPA) renogram for the diagnosis of renal artery stenosis.[31,32] DTPA is cleared by glomerular filtration. In the kidney with normal vasculature, a DTPA renogram will show the usual rapid uptake and excretion curve; when renal artery stenosis is present, the reduction in glomerular filtration by captopril will result in a normal uptake phase on the renogram but a flat (nonexcretory) pattern. Although this test tends to improve the reliability of the renogram in confirming the diagnosis of hemodynamically significant renal artery stenosis, there can be false positive results. We recently noted a classic positive study in a young severely hypertensive renal transplant patient treated with cyclosporine, a drug known to adversely affect the renal vasculature.[33]

Side effects similar to those described above for adults can occur in children, but the incidence and severity appear to be much lower.[34] In addition to those described above, we have seen one 4-year-old boy with enalapril-induced undefined anemia. The hemoglobin returned to pretreatment levels when the drug was discontinued.

CALCIUM CHANNEL BLOCKERS

The calcium channel blockers comprise a class of compounds first identified during the 1960s but only recently established as primary therapy for hypertension.[35] These drugs are also called "calcium antagonists" because their ultimate pharmacologic effect is an inhibition of calcium-mediated cellular events. However, the term "calcium channel blockers" seems to be a more specific description for these drugs because the reduction in cytosolic calcium concentration is the result of direct, dose-dependent inhibition of the inward flux of calcium via voltage-dependent slow channels in the cellular membrane (or sarcolemma).[36] The dose-dependent distinction deserves emphasis, since total calcium blockade is incompatible with cellular function.

Calcium is an integral component of mammalian cells and is particularly important for modulation of normal cellular functions such as stimulation–contraction coupling of myocardial and vascular smooth muscle.[37] It is not surprising, therefore, that the calcium channel blockers have been found to be exceptionally effective for treatment of cardiac arrhythmias and systemic hypertension.

The calcium channel blockers have been divided into two groups, based on their molecular structure and clinical application.[38] Type I drugs have a tertiary amine structure similar to verapamil. They are more effective in reducing atrioventricular nodal conduction[39] and reversing repetitive membrane depolarization,[40] and they are used primarily to treat cardiac arrhythmias. Type II drugs are characterized by a dihydropyridine nucleus similar to nifedipine and nitrendipine. They are less effective than type I drugs for treating cardiac arrhythmias but are more potent vasodilators. Consequently, the type II drugs are most effective as antihypertensive agents and for treatment of selected peripheral vascular diseases, such as Raynaud's phenomenon.[41]

At the present time, nifedipine has been the most widely used of the dihydropyridine analogs for the treatment of hypertension. However, a number of new agents are in various stages of research, development, and marketing (Table 39–1) and will be available for general clinical use sometime during the next decade.[42]

The pharmacokinetic properties of the dihydropyridine calcium channel blockers are similar.[42] Each undergoes considerable first-pass clearance, i.e., hepatic metabolism of drug after absorption from the gastrointestinal tract and prior to entering the systemic circulation. The result is a high degree of variability in bioavailability between drugs and between patients. These drugs are metabolized by the liver to inactive metabolites that are cleared primarily by the kidney. Thus, dosage modification is not required in renal failure.[43] The dihydropyridine drugs are poorly dialyzable.[50]

A number of studies have confirmed the antihypertensive effectiveness of the calcium channel blockers and their effects on a variety of physiologic systems (see references 45–48). As is usually the case with cardiovascular drugs, almost all studies have been performed in adults.

Adverse hemodynamic effects are limited to a brief period of time after initial drug administration.[49] Heart rate and cardiac output increase modestly but usually return to pretreatment levels within a few weeks, while peripheral resistance remains lower throughout therapy. Renal perfusion and function are maintained with calcium channel blockers.[50-52] Glomerular filtration rate

TABLE 39–1. CALCIUM CHANNEL BLOCKING DRUGS

Type 1
  Verapamil
  Diltiazem
  Tiapamil
Type II
  Nifedipine
  Nitrendipine
  Amlodipine
  Nisoldipine
  Nimodipine
  Nicardipine
  Isradipine
  Felodipine
  Nilvodipine

and renal plasma flow increase and renal vascular resistance decreases without any change in renin–angiotensin–aldosterone system activity. Nevertheless, these drugs seem to be most effective in patients with low-renin (i.e., volume-dependent) hypertension.[53] Sodium and water excretion may increase during the acute phase of drug administration,[54] but this is not maintained during long-term drug administration.[50,51]

The calcium channel blockers are remarkably free from other side effects. Hypotension and pedal edema have been reported in adults. Unlike the β-blockers and diuretics, calcium channel blockers do not adversely affect serum lipids, with clinical studies showing an increase in high-density lipoprotein cholesterol[55,56] and a decrease in low-density lipoprotein cholesterol.[56] Despite the integral role of calcium in normal hormonal and metabolic function, the calcium channel blockers have very little meaningful effect on these systems in humans.[57]

Nifedipine is widely used to treat hypertension in children and is the drug of choice in many medical centers for treatment of hypertensive emergencies.[58,59] It has a rapid onset of action after sublingual dosing and can be detected in the blood within 6 minutes after administration.[60] This has been the preferred route of administration. However, it is less well appreciated that nifedipine is also rapidly absorbed after oral administration, provided it is not taken with food,[61] and blood concentrations are significantly higher than after sublingual dosing.[60] The major disadvantage of nifedipine is its relatively short duration of action in many children and its failure to maintain an antihypertensive effect during chronic therapy. This is in contrast to the general experience in adults. It may be related to the fact that most hypertension in children requiring antihypertensive intervention is secondary in nature and relatively more severe than the essential hypertension usually seen in adults.

The newer dihydropyridine analogs have been designed to overcome some of these problems.[42] Although clinical data in children are not available for almost all of these new drugs, we have recently completed a clinical trial with nitrendipine. The drug was studied in 25 children ranging in age from 6 months to 16 years. All had severe hypertension, and the majority had renal disease. Significant reductions in blood pressure were noted within 24 hours, and the antihypertensive effect was sustained throughout the 12-week period of observation. Heart rate was minimally affected. Although nitrendipine is thought to require only once-daily or, at the most, twice-daily dosing, in this series of children more frequent dosing schedules (i.e., t.i.d. or q.i.d.) were necessary. Nevertheless, the duration of action and long-term effectiveness were felt to be substantially better than the response we have observed with nifedipine[61a] (T. G. Wells and A. R. Sinaiko, unpublished data).

DIURETICS

Diuretics continue to be an important component of antihypertensive therapy in adults[62] and children,[2] despite the availability of newer agents with a variety of specific actions. They are particularly useful in patients with renal disease because of the volume component of this form of hypertension. In general, our basic understanding of the antihypertensive effect of diuretics is not any greater today than it was in 1978.[1]

The antihypertensive response to thiazides, as well as other diuretics, appears to be dependent on their diuretic action, despite the vasodilating effect of the thiazide analog diazoxide. The immediate response to diuretics in the hypertensive patient is an increase in urine volume and sodium excretion, resulting in decreased extracellular and plasma volumes, body weight, and cardiac output.[63] Compensatory homeostatic mechanisms are activated to bring sodium loss into balance with sodium intake, and plasma volume and extracellular fluid volume return toward their pretreatment levels over a 6- to 12-month period.[64,65] However, the ultimate effect of diuretic therapy is a finite reduction in volume, a sustained decrease in peripheral vascular resistance, and a reduction in systemic blood pressure.[66,67]

Spironolactone is indicated for the treatment of hypertension secondary to disease characterized by mineralocorticoid excess. Its usefulness in other forms of hypertension has not been established. Although it was formerly recommended for patients with low-renin hypertension, on the presumption that renin suppression is caused by excessive mineralocorticoid production,[68] spironolactone has not been shown to be more effective in these patients than traditional diuretic therapy.[69,70]

Triamterene and amiloride are not considered primary therapeutic agents for hypertension. If there is a role for these drugs in hypertensive patients, it is to reduce urinary potassium excretion during diuretic therapy when other strategies for maintaining normal levels of serum potassium fail. Despite the recent reawakening to the potential importance of potassium balance in blood pressure homeostasis[71] and evidence that potassium repletion in hypertensive patients with diuretic-induced hypokalemia can result in a significant reduction in blood pressure,[72] the routine inclusion of potassium-sparing diuretics in antihypertensive regimens is to be discouraged.

DRUGS AFFECTING THE ADRENERGIC NERVOUS SYSTEM

The adrenergic (or sympathetic) nervous system has been a focus for therapeutic intervention since the earliest days of antihypertensive drug therapy. The adrenergic antihypertensive drugs form a diverse group with a variety of pharmacologic actions, but they share the common characteristic that their effects are mediated via specific adrenergic receptor sites.

Adrenergic neurons are found within the central and peripheral nervous systems. The primary adrenergic neurotransmitter, norepinephrine, is stored in the nerve ending until released into the synaptic cleft, the space between the nerve ending and the receptor sites on the effector tissue. Norepinephrine formation also takes place within the adrenal medulla, but through an additional biosynthetic step it is converted to epinephrine, which functions as a neurohormone after its release into the circulation. It is generally conceded that adrenergic function is mediated primarily via the autocoid function of norepinephrine, i.e., direct stimulation of the effector tissue following neuronal release into the synaptic cleft.

Norepinephrine interacts with adrenergic receptors located on either side of the synaptic cleft. The classic division of adrenergic receptors by Ahlquist[73] into alpha (α) and beta (β) components has been expanded to now include α_1- and α_2-receptors and β_1- and β_2-receptors.[74] In addition to their location at postsynaptic sites, i.e., on effector tissues, both α- and β-receptors have been identified at presynaptic sites located on the nerve endings themselves. The α_2-receptors appear to modulate neurotransmitter activity through a negative feedback mechanism, in which catecholamine release from the nerve ending is inhibited when these receptors are occupied by norepinephrine. In contrast, activation of presynaptic β_2-receptors appears to enhance norepinephrine secretion. Thus, the effect of adrenergic agents is a summation of the complex interaction at a variety of central and peripheral adrenergic receptor sites.

β-Adrenergic Blocking Drugs

β-adrenergic blocking drugs, as their name implies, act at the β-adrenergic receptor. Although they share this common characteristic, they differ from each other according to specific pharmacologic properties as follows (Table 39–2):

Cardioselectivity

Because cardiac β-adrenergic innervation is β_1 in type, drugs that are specific β_1-blockers have been termed "cardioselective." Selectivity is relevant only when low to moderate drug doses are used. At higher drug doses, such as those commonly used to treat systemic hypertension, a crossover effect is seen, and inhibition of β_2, in addition to β_1, responses occurs.

Lipid Solubility

The degree of partitioning of a drug between a mixture of water and an organic solvent determines its partition coefficient, the measure of lipid solubility. Lipid solubility is important because it is an estimate of the capacity of a drug to penetrate the central nervous system. Patients with well-controlled hypertension on a lipid-soluble β-blocker, but experiencing adverse central nervous system symptoms, can continue to be effectively treated by substituting a second, less lipid-soluble β-blocker.

Intrinsic Sympathomimetic Activity

The primary effect of the β-adrenergic blocking drugs is prevention of agonist access to β-adrenergic receptor sites, thus inhibiting the effector tissue response. The molecular

TABLE 39–2. PROPERTIES OF β-ADRENERGIC BLOCKING DRUGS

DRUG	CARDIOSELECTIVITY	INTRINSIC SYMPATHOMIMETIC ACTIVITY	LIPID SOLUBILITY	POTENCY	HALF-LIFE (h)	CLEARANCE
Propranolol	0	0	High	1.0	3–4	Hepatic
Acebutalol	+	+	Weak	0.3	3–4	Renal
Atenolol	+	0	Weak	1.0	6–9	Renal
Metoprolol	+	0	Moderate	1.0	3–4	Hepatic
Nadolol	0	0	Weak	1.0	14–24	Renal
Pindolol	0⁻	+	Moderate	6.0	3–4	Both
Timolol	0	0	Weak	6.0	4–5	Hepatic
Esmolol	+	0	Weak	–	0.15	Hepatic

configuration of some β-blockers is such that in addition to this inhibitory effect, they may also elicit a small, but significant, agonist response, known as intrinsic sympathomimetic activity. The partial agonist effect is much lower than that observed with pure agonists such as isoproterenol, and the effect on receptor blockade and antihypertensive response is not compromised. Although the clinical relevance of intrinsic sympathomimetic activity has not been established, the adverse effects of the agents possessing this property have been shown to be significantly milder for some responses, e.g., hypoglycemia and Raynaud's disease.[75]

Membrane-Stabilizing Effect

Some β-adrenergic blocking drugs possess a quinidine-like activity expressed as an alteration in cardiac electrochemical conduction.[76] This property appears to be an *in vitro* phenomenon, since it requires drug concentrations many times in excess of those observed in humans.

Potency

β-Adrenergic blocking potency is defined as the capacity of a drug to inhibit the tachycardic response to isoproterenol compared to inhibition by the reference β-blocker, propranolol. Although potency influences the amount of drug required to achieve an equivalent clinical response, it has little clinical significance, since less potent drugs can generally be administered in higher doses without increasing the incidence of adverse reactions.

The cardiovascular, renin–angiotensin, and central nervous systems are all thought to be involved in the β-blocker-mediated antihypertensive response. Although any one of these could predominate, it seems more likely that a combination of factors involving all of these systems determines the ultimate outcome. The cardiovascular system is affected immediately after the administration of β-blocking drugs, with a decrease in cardiac output and rate before any change in blood pressure is noted.[77] Peripheral vascular resistance increases as β-receptor-mediated peripheral vasodilation is inhibited, leaving the α-adrenergic vasoconstrictor response unopposed. With the continuation of β-blocker therapy, cardiac output and heart rate remain low and blood pressure begins to decrease, despite the persistence of peripheral vascular resistance at levels equal to or slightly above baseline lev-

els. The reduction in blood pressure is equivalent for β-blockers with and without intrinsic sympathomimetic activity.

Renin–angiotensin system activity is regulated, in part, by β-adrenergic-mediated stimulation of renin secretion.[78] Although plasma renin activity is generally lower in patients treated with β-blockers, pretreatment levels of plasma renin activity are not necessarily predictive of therapeutic success. While patients with high levels of plasma renin activity can be expected to respond to low or moderate doses of a β-blocker, even patients with low plasma renin activity, implying non-renin-mediated hypertension, can experience a reduction in blood pressure with β-blocker therapy.[79]

Propranolol penetrates the blood–brain barrier to become highly concentrated in brain tissue.[80] Evidence that propranolol has a direct central antihypertensive effect suggests that the central nervous system is the primary site for its antihypertensive action.[81,82] However, other β-blockers with low lipid solubility have equivalent antihypertensive effects, making it less likely that access to central adrenoceptors is the critical determinant for β-adrenergic blocker effectiveness.

β-blockers are well absorbed from the gastrointestinal tract after oral administration. Bioavailability may be severely limited by the first-pass phenomenon, in which a large percentage of drug is rapidly extracted from the portal circulation immediately after absorption and prior to reaching the systemic circulation. The result is a reduction of circulating plasma drug concentrations when compared to levels observed after intravenous administration. With continued oral dosing, hepatic extraction becomes saturated, leading to higher steady-state blood levels and a slightly prolonged half-life.[83]

Plasma β-blocker drug concentration and pharmacologic effect are poorly correlated, with the exception of the inhibitory response to isoproterenol- or exercise-induced tachycardia.[84] Therefore, levels of β-blocking drugs are rarely measured. Plasma concentrations as high as 700 ng/ml have been reported in children,[85] confirming the drug's high therapeutic index (i.e., the ratio between the drug concentration causing adverse effects and the drug concentration resulting in the desired therapeutic response). A starting dose equivalent to 0.5–1 mg/kg b.i.d. of propranolol is tolerated by almost all pediatric patients. The drugs can be titrated upward to achieve a satisfactory therapeutic response, and restricting maximal doses to 8 mg/kg/24 h will usually prevent excessive drug dosing.

The β-blockers are either excreted by the kidneys or

metabolized by the liver (Table 39–2). Propranolol is the only β-blocker to form an active metabolite, but this metabolite is of little clinical importance. The antihypertensive effect of the β-blockers is not well correlated with plasma concentration and exceeds the expected duration of drug action based on plasma half-life. Thus, even preparations with short half-lives usually can be administered on a twice-daily basis and may even be effective when given only once a day.

There are a number of potential adverse effects with the β-adrenergic blocking drugs (Table 39–3). Nevertheless, the reported incidence of side effects in children is exceptionally low, with the exception of patients with underlying cardiovascular, pulmonary, renal, or metabolic diseases. Resting bradycardia will be noted in children of all ages but is rarely severe enough to warrant withdrawal of therapy. Because these drugs act as competitive antagonists to norepinephrine, their effect can be overcome by an increase in endogenous sympathetic activity. Although exercise-induced tachycardia is inhibited, patients retain the capacity to increase their heart rate under conditions of stress.[86] As noted above, peripheral vasoconstriction may occur and can uncover or exacerbate Raynaud's disease in patients with collagen-vascular disease. Use of β-blockers with intrinsic sympathomimetic activity can attenuate this effect.

Bronchial dilation is mediated by activation of β_2-receptors. The use of β-adrenergic blocking drugs may be associated with an exacerbation of asthmatic symptoms or may aggravate pulmonary insufficiency in patients with chronic lung disease. Use of cardioselective (i.e., β_1) drugs in these patients may prevent pulmonary complications at low drug doses. However, when higher drug doses are used, cardioselective drugs can also affect β_2-sites, and administration of any of the β-blocking drugs to patients with obstructive forms of lung disease or asthma should be discouraged.

The chronic use of propranolol in adults has been associated with a reduction in glomerular filtration rate.[87,88] This effect is not observed in all treated patients and based on broad clinical experience, does not appear to be an important clinical problem in children.

Propranolol has been associated with a number of central nervous system side effects in adults, including nightmares, dreams, confusion, agitation, and depression. Similar findings appear to be infrequent in children and

TABLE 39–3. ADVERSE EFFECTS OF β-ADRENERGIC BLOCKING DRUGS

Bradycardia
Cardiac failure
Raynaud's disease
Bronchoconstriction
Reduction of glomerular filtration rate
Central nervous system effects
  Nightmares
  Confusion
  Agitation
  Depression
  Sleep disturbances
Hypoglycemia
Inhibition of symptoms of hypoglycemia
Altered serum lipoprotein concentrations

are more likely to present in the form of sleep disturbances. In patients with a good antihypertensive response to β-adrenergic blockade, changing to a less lipid-soluble drug may permit the continued use of a β-blocker when central nervous system effects appear.

β-Adrenergic blocking drugs adversely affect glucose[89] and lipid[90,91] metabolism. Patients with diabetes mellitus have an exaggerated hypoglycemic response and a reduction in the rate of rise of blood glucose after insulin administration. This is compounded by the concomitant inhibition in some patients of the systemic warning signs of hypoglycemia, i.e., tachycardia, palpitations, and hunger. β-Adrenergic blocking drugs also have an adverse effect on lipoprotein metabolism.[92] A variety of changes in serum lipoproteins, including elevation of triglycerides, reduction in high-density lipoproteins (HDLs), and an increase in the ratio of total cholesterol to HDL cholesterol have been reported and vary according to the specific β-blocker studied. These changes persist during long-term therapy and appear to be dependent on the pharmacologic characteristics of the β-blocker.

α-Adrenergic Agents

In contrast to β-adrenergic drug therapy, which is limited to agents possessing receptor antagonist properties, α-adrenergic agonists as well as antagonists have been used successfully to treat hypertension. At the present time, clinical experience is limited to a very few agents, and this section will be devoted to a discussion of those drugs.

The most widely used α-adrenergic blocker is prazosin, a selective α_1-blocker.[93] α_1-Receptors are located at postsynaptic sites, primarily within peripheral resistance vessels. Therefore, the antihypertensive action of prazosin is mediated through vascular smooth muscle relaxation, similar to the effect observed with direct vasodilators. Reflex sympathetic activity, expressed as an increase in heart rate, cardiac output, and renin secretion, does not occur. It is possible that this modifying effect on cardiac and other reflex-stimulated events results from the concomitant dilation of venous capacitance vessels which are also richly innervated with α_1-adrenergic receptors.

Prazosin is well absorbed after oral administration. It is metabolized by the liver, and dose adjustments in patients with renal failure on dialysis are not necessary. It has a relatively short plasma half-life, but its biologic effect is prolonged, and it can be administered on a twice-daily schedule.

Side effects with prazosin are minimal and are rarely a problem with children. Of particular importance is the so-called first-dose effect, in which severe orthostasis may occur in conjunction with the initial prazosin dose. The orthostatic effect almost always remits with ongoing prazosin therapy. A unique feature of prazosin is its capacity to alter lipoprotein metabolism and establish lipid profiles that are less atherogenic than those found in patients receiving β-adrenergic blockers.[92]

α-Agonists used in the treatment of hypertension act at α_2-receptor sites. The major antihypertensive effect of these drugs is mediated within the central nervous system, resulting in a reduction of electrical outflow activity along the sympathetic tract. The antihypertensive effect is also potentiated at peripheral sites by activation of presynaptic α_2-receptors, which reduces norepinephrine release from the nerve ending.

Clonidine is the principal α-agonist available for clinical use and is currently considered the reference drug for this class of centrally acting agents. It is metabolized primarily by the liver, with approximately one-third of the daily dose excreted by the kidney.[94] It has a half-life of 8 hours and can be used on a twice-daily dosing schedule. The clinical response to clonidine reflects the α_2-adrenoceptor activity. Shortly after administration, there is a rise in systemic blood pressure, resulting from the stimulation of synaptic α_2-adrenoceptors in resistant vessels. However, within a short time, there is a fall in blood pressure accompanied by suppression of cardiac activity and renin secretion, as the central inhibitory effects of clonidine become predominant.

Clonidine is associated with a high incidence of dry mouth and sedation. A critical adverse reaction with clonidine is rebound hypertension, occurring after the drug is precipitously withdrawn from patients on chronic therapy. This sudden increase in blood pressure to potentially malignant levels is apparently the result of a surge of adrenergic activity as central suppression of adrenergic nerve conduction remits.[95] This effect can be prevented by gradual withdrawal of the drug.

Drugs Acting at Both α- and β-Adrenergic Receptors

Labetalol is generally referred to as a primary β-adrenergic blocking agent with α-adrenergic blocking properties, because it is approximately eight times more potent in blocking β-receptors than α-receptors.[96] In addition to its adrenergic blocking properties, labetalol is also a selective β_2-agonist in the peripheral vasculature.[97]

Labetalol is well absorbed after oral administration and is extensively metabolized by the first-pass phenomenon. It is cleared from the body almost entirely by hepatic metabolism. The plasma half-life of labetalol is approximately 4 hours.

Labetalol is less potent than either α-adrenergic antagonists or β-blockers. It does not have intrinsic sympathomimetic activity or membrane-stabilizing activity and is weakly lipid-soluble. The side effects observed during treatment with other β-blockers can also occur with labetalol. A major therapeutic indication for labetalol is treatment of hypertensive crises.[98] The drug dose can be titrated during intravenous administration, with the result that blood pressure can be brought under control more gradually.

VASODILATING AGENTS

The two vasodilating agents currently available for clinical use, hydralazine and minoxidil, act directly on vascular smooth muscle to reduce vascular wall tension and peripheral vascular resistance. Because the major hemo-dynamic alteration in patients with established systemic hypertension is an increased peripheral vascular resistance, vasodilators might be expected to be among the most effective of the antihypertensive drugs. This has not proven to be the case. Hydralazine appears to be less effective than the newer agents, described earlier in this chapter, particularly in children with severe hypertension secondary to renal disease. Minoxidil, while probably the most potent of the antihypertensive drugs, has found limited use because of the associated high incidence of adverse effects.

The pharmacokinetics of hydralazine have recently been reviewed.[99] The drug is well absorbed from the gastrointestinal tract and undergoes a first-pass effect which may help to explain the clinical observation that intravenously administered hydralazine may be effective in reducing the blood pressure of patients refractory to similar doses administered by the oral route. The plasma half-life of hydralazine is poorly defined. Nevertheless, clinical studies have shown that the drug can be used effectively when administered in two daily divided doses.[100]

Hydralazine is eliminated primarily by acetylation in the liver. The rate of acetylation is genetically determined, and individuals are divided into either fast or slow acetylators. This distinction is important for two reasons: (1) bioavailability is lower in the fast-acetylator group, and (2) in patients with the genotype for slow acetylation, hydralazine may induce a systemic reaction similar to systemic lupus erythematosus (SLE).[101] Patients with the lupus-like syndrome have circulating antibodies to hydralazine and native DNA, but these disappear on drug withdrawal.[102] Other side effects associated with hydralazine are similar to those occurring with other vasodilators, including minoxidil. Generalized flushing and headache are regularly seen. Tachycardia, palpitations, and increased cardiac output also are extremely common and appear to be secondary to increased sympathetic nervous system activity.[103] Salt and water retention result from increased absorption in the renal proximal tubule secondary to a redistribution of renal blood flow.[104] This can be neutralized by the concurrent administration of a diuretic.

Minoxidil is many times more effective than hydralazine in reducing blood pressure and may be the most potent of all the antihypertensive agents. Minoxidil has been well studied in children.[105–107] Therapy should be started at a dose of 0.1–0.2 mg/kg/24 h that can be administered in two divided doses. Maximum dosages have not been determined, but doses as high as 1 mg/kg have been utilized safely.

Minoxidil shares the side effects common to all vasodilator agents, i.e., headache, flushing, tachycardia, palpitations, increased cardiac output, and salt and water retention. In all cases, a β-blocker and a loop diuretic should be started prior to the first dose of minoxidil, since the cardiovascular and sodium-retaining properties are particularly troublesome. A unique adverse effect of minoxidil is hypertrichosis, most prominent across the forehead, on all extremities, and over the trunk. This has been noted in every patient, beginning 2–3 weeks after the drug is started. A dose–response relationship for this phenomenon has not been identified. The hypertrichosis will remit within 3 months in every patient following cessation of minoxidil, regardless of duration of therapy. The hypertrichosis should not be minimized in discussing minoxidil therapy with patients and parents, because it can be the source of great anxiety to a degree sufficient to require discontinuation of the drug.

CURRENT RECOMMENDATIONS FOR ANTIHYPERTENSIVE THERAPY IN CHILDREN

Antihypertensive drug therapy should be started immediately in any patient presenting with symptomatic hypertension, i.e., severe hypertension with headache, eyeground changes, neurologic findings, or malignant renal disease. The goal in treatment of hypertensive emergencies is reduction of blood pressure to levels that eliminate the immediate risk of hypertension-related cardiovascular events, i.e., stroke, encephalopathy, or cardiac failure. Precipitous drops in blood pressure should be avoided because of the risk of hypotension-related adverse effects on the central nervous system.

A number of drugs are available for the treatment of hypertensive emergencies (Table 39–4). For patients without neurologic symptoms, we have found the calcium channel–blocking drug nifedipine to be very helpful because of its effectiveness in children of all ages,[108] ease of oral administration, rapid onset of action, and usual freedom from side effects. The highly variable duration of action and the fact that response seems to diminish with frequent administration, regardless of dose, are potential problems with nifedipine. Hydralazine is also a useful drug, but it may be less effective than nifedipine and must be used parenterally for a rapid effect. Repeated dosing with hydralazine is usually not tolerated because of flushing, tachycardia, headache, and nausea. Thus, if treatment is not successful with an initial dose followed by a second dose twice the amount of the first, it is best to select another drug.

Patients with severe symptoms or who fail to respond to the above drugs should receive intravenous therapy with more effective agents. Although clinical experience with labetalol in children is limited at the present time, it is very effective in treating hypertensive emergencies. However, some patients have a paradoxical increase in blood pressure. Diazoxide also remains a very effective antihypertensive agent because of its rapid clinical response. The use of a bolus injection may be associated

TABLE 39–4. ANTIHYPERTENSIVE DRUG THERAPY FOR HYPERTENSIVE EMERGENCIES

DRUG	DOSE
Nifedipine	0.25–0.5 mg/kg oral
Hydralazine	0.2–0.4 mg/kg I.V.
Labetolol	1–3 mg/kg I.V.
Diazoxide	2–5 mg/kg I.V.
Sodium nitroprusside	0.5–8 meq/kg/min I.V.
Minoxidil	0.1–0.2 mg/kg oral

TABLE 39–5. DRUGS USED FOR CHRONIC ANTIHYPERTENSIVE THERAPY

	DOSE (mg/kg/day)	
DRUG	Initial	Maximum
Captopril		
Neonates	0.03–0.15	2
Children	1.5	6
Enalapril	0.15	0.6
Nifedipine	0.25	3
Nitrendipine	0.25	2
Hydrochlorothiazide	1	2–3
Furosemide	1	12
Bumetanide	0.02–0.05	0.3
Metolazone	0.1	3
Spironolactone	1	3
Propranolol	1	8
Atenolol	1	8
Prazosin	0.65–0.1	0.5
Clonidine	?	?
Hydralazine	0.75	7.5
Minoxodil	0.1–0.2	1

with precipitous falls in blood pressure that can be avoided by using lower and slower infusion doses. The most reliable of the drugs currently available for hypertensive emergencies continues to be sodium nitroprusside. It must be administered by continuous intravenous infusion, but its onset of action occurs within 30 seconds, and its antihypertensive effect disappears almost as quickly when the drug dose is reduced or discontinued. The potential limiting side effect is tachycardia. Retention of thiocyanate or cyanide following nitroprusside metabolism is rarely a problem in patients with normal or moderately reduced renal function.

Recommendations for chronic antihypertensive drug therapy in children are based on the adult step-care model[62] in which therapy is started with a given drug and modified in a step-wise fashion depending upon response (Table 39–5). The step-care approach, as outlined in the Second Task Force Report,[2] is still recommended for children and adolescents. However, the order in which drugs are used has been modified in the brief period of time since this report was published as a result of broader clinical experience with newer antihypertensive agents.

In previous years, diuretics and β-adrenergic blocking drugs were recommended for first-line therapy. However, diuretic therapy is probably best reserved for patients with renal disease. Thiazide diuretics are effective until the glomerular filtration rate falls below 50 percent of normal, at which time a loop diuretic should be substituted. Aldactone may complement other diuretics in patients with diseases that increase aldosterone secretion, i.e., nephrotic syndrome, congestive heart failure, or liver failure, but is otherwise of limited benefit in children. β-Blocking drugs continue to be widely used. Choosing drugs with cardioselective or intrinsic sympathomimetic activity can minimize potential adverse effects, particularly increased serum lipids and hypoglycemia.

The major change taking place in antihypertensive drug therapy is the introduction of angiotensin converting enzyme inhibitors (CEIs) and calcium channel–blocking agents as first-line drugs. As noted earlier in this chapter, captopril and enalapril are both very effective in children. In contrast, there is far less information about the use of calcium channel blockers in children, with the exception of nifedipine. Unfortunately, nifedipine is less effective in chronic therapy because of its short duration of action. The newer calcium channel–blocking agents may be more useful. Experience in our institution with nitrendipine, a new dihydropyridine compound, suggests that this drug is effective in children during short- and long-term therapy, has a longer duration of action, and is remarkably free of side effects.[61a]

Agents acting on the α-adrenergic nervous system, i.e., prazosin and clonidine, are generally considered to be second-line drugs. The very effective vasodilator minoxidil is usually reserved for patients who are refractory to other antihypertensive therapies.

REFERENCES

1. Sinaiko AR, Mirkin BL: Clinical pharmacology of antihypertensive drugs in children. Pediatr Clin No Am 25:137–157, 1978
2. Task Force on Blood Pressure Control in Children: Report of the Second Task Force on Blood Pressure Control in Children—1987. Pediatrics 79:1–25, 1987
3. Cushman DW, Ondetti MA, Cheung HL, Antonaccio MJ, McCarthy VS, Rubin B: Inhibitors of angiotensin-converting enzyme, in Johnson JA, Anderson RR (eds): The Renin-Angiotensin System. New York, Plenum, 1980, pp 199–225.
4. Brunner HR, Waeber B, Nussberger J: Angiotensin converting enzyme inhibition and the normal kidney. Kid Internat 31(suppl 20):S-104–S-107, 1987
5. Zimmerman BG: Adrenergic facilitation by angiotensin: Does it serve a physiologic function? Clin Sci 60:343–348, 1981
6. Dzau VJ: Vascular renin–angiotensin system in hypertension: New insights into the mechanism of action of angiotensin converting enzyme inhibitors. Am J Med 84(suppl 4A):4–8, 1988
7. Jin M, Wilhelm MJ, Lang RE, Unger T, Lindpaintner K, Ganten D: Endogenous tissue renin–angiotensin systems: From molecular biology to therapy. Am J Med 84(suppl 3A):28–36, 1988
8. Guyton AC: The kidney in blood pressure control and hypertension, in Holliday MA, Barratt TM, Vernier RL (eds): Pediatric Nephrology. Baltimore, Williams and Wilkins, 1987, pp 729–737
9. Raij L, Keane WF: Glomerular mesangium: Its function and relationship to angiotensin II. Am J Med 79(suppl 3C):24–30, 1985
10. Hollenberg NC: Renal perfusion and function: The implications of converting enzyme inhibition. Am J Med 84(suppl 4A):9–14, 1988
11. Bauer JH, Reams GP: Hemodynamic and renal function in essential hypertension during treatment with enalapril. Am J Med 79(suppl 3C):10–13, 1985
12. Oparil S: Prinivil (Lisinopril) in the treatment of the older hypertensive patient. Am J Med 85(suppl 3B), 1988
13. Kostis JB: Angiotensin-converting enzyme inhibitors. Emerging differences and new compounds. Am J Hypertens 2:57–64, 1989
14. Duchin KL, McKinstry DN, Cohen AI, Migdalof BH: Pharmacokinetics of captopril in healthy subjects and in patients with cardiovascular diseases. Clin Pharmacokinet 14:241–259, 1988
15. Sinaiko AR, Mirkin BL, Hendrick DA, Green TP, O'Dea RF: Antihypertensive effect and elimination kinetics of captopril in hypertensive children with renal disease. J Pediatr 103:799–805, 1983
16. Belz GG, Kirch W, Kleinbloesem CH: Angiotensin-converting enzyme inhibitors: Relationship between pharmacodynamics and pharmacokinetics. Clin Pharmacokinet 15:295–318, 1988
17. Sinaiko AR, Kashtan CE, Mirkin BL: Antihypertensive drug therapy with captopril in children and adolescents. Clin Exp Hypertens A8:829–839, 1986
18. Unger T, Ganten D, Lang RE, Scholkens BA: Persistent tissue converting enzyme inhibition following chronic treatment with Hoe 498 and MK421 in spontaneously hypertensive rats. J Cardiovasc Pharmacol 7:36–41, 1985
19. O'Dea RF, Mirkin BL, Alward CT, Sinaiko AR: Treatment of neonatal hypertension with captopril. J Pediatr 113:403–406, 1988
20. Tack ED, Perlman JM: Renal failure in sick hypertensive premature infants receiving captopril therapy. J Pediatr 112:805–810, 1988
21. Riley LJ, Viasses PH, Ferguson RK: Clinical pharmacology and therapeutic applications of the new converting enzyme inhibitor, enalapril. Am Heart J 109:1085–1089, 1985
22. Weber MA: Safety issues during antihypertensive treatment with angiotensin converting enzyme inhibitors. Am J Med 84(suppl 4A):16–23, 1988
23. Gavras H, Gavras I: Angiotensin converting enzyme inhibitors: Properties and side effects. Hypertension 11(suppl II):II-37–II-41, 1988
24. Chalmers D, Dombey SL, Lawson DH: Post marketing surveillance of captopril (for hypertension): A preliminary report. Br J Clin Pharmacol 24:343–349, 1987
25. Jaffe IA: Adverse effects profile of sulfhydryl compounds in man. Am J Med 80:471–476, 1986
26. Sturgill BC, Shearlock KT: Membranous glomerulopathy and nephrotic syndrome after captopril therapy. JAMA 250:2343–2345, 1983
27. Textor SC, Bravo EL, Fouad FM, Tarazi RC: Hyperkalemia in azotemic patients during angiotension-converting enzyme inhibition and aldosterone reduction with captopril. Am J Med 73:719–725, 1982
28. Zanella MT, Mattei E, Draike SA, Kater CE, Aizen H: Inadequate aldosterone response to hyperkalemia during angiotensin converting enzyme inhibition in chronic renal failure. Clin Pharmacol Ther 38:613–617, 1985
29. Bauer JH, Reams GP, Lal SM: Renal protective effect of strict blood pressure control with enalapril therapy. Arch Int Med 147:1397–1400, 1987
30. Meyer TW, Anderson S, Rennke HG, Brenner BM: Converting enzyme inhibitor therapy limits progressive glomerular injury in rats with renal insufficiency. Am J Med 79(suppl 3C):31–36, 1985
31. Geyskes GG, Oei HY, Puylaert CBAJ, Mees EJD: Renovascular hypertension identified by captopril-induced changes in the renogram. Hypertension 9:451–458, 1987
32. Nally JV, Gupta BK, Clarke HS, Higgins JT, Potvin WJ, Gross M: Captopril renography for the detection of renovascular hypertension. Cleve J Med 55:311–318, 1988
33. Schrachter M: Cyclosporine A and hypertension. J Hypertens 6:51!–516, 1988
34. Mirkin BL, Nerman TJ: Efficacy and safety of captopril in the treatment of severe childhood hypertension: Report of the International Collaborative Study Group. Pediatrics 75:1091–1100, 1985
35. Fleckenstein A: History of calcium antagonists. Circ Res 52(suppl I):I-3–I-16, 1983
36. Janis RA, Scriabine A: Sites of action of Ca^{2+} channel inhibitor. Biochem Pharmacol 32:3499–3507, 1983
37. Braunwald E: Mechanism of action of calcium-channel-blocking agents. N Engl J Med 307:1618–1627, 1982
38. Sing BN: The mechanism of action of calcium antagonists relative to their clinical applications. Br J Clin Pharmacol 21:109S–121S, 1986
39. Rowland E, Evans T, Kirkler D: Effect of nifedipine on atrioventricular conduction as compared with verapamil. Br Heart J 42:124–127, 1979
40. Lee KS, Tsien RW: Mechanism of calcium channel blockade by verapamil, DTPA, diltiazem and nitrendipine in single dialysed heart cells. Nature 302:790–794, 1983
41. White CJ, Phillips WA, Abrahams LA, Watson TD, Singleton PT: Objective benefit of nifedipine in the treatment of Raynaud's phenomenon. Am J Med 80:623–625, 1986
42. Abernathy DR, Schwartz JB: Pharmacokinetics of calcium antagonists under development. Clin Pharmacokinet 15:1–14, 1988
43. Schran HF, Jaffe JM, Gonasun LM: Clinical pharmacokinetics of isradipine. Am J Med 84(suppl 3B):80–89, 1988

44. Kleinbloesem CH, van Brummelen P, Woittiez AJ, Foker H, Brimer DD: Influence of haemodialysis on the pharmacokinetics and haemodynamics of nifedipine during continuous intravenous infusion. Clin Pharmacokinet 11:316–322, 1986

45. Hansson L, Laragh JH (eds): Expanding role of calcium antagonists in cardiovascular therapy. Am J Med 84(suppl 3B), 1988

46. Hollenberg NK (ed): Calcium channel blockers: New insights into their role in the management of hypertension. Am J Med 82(suppl 3B), 1987

47. Chobanian AV (ed): Role of calcium channel blockers in the management of hypertension; and calcium channel blockers: Their evolving role in the management of hypertension. Am J Med 81(suppl 6A), 1986

48. Murphy MB, Dollery C (eds): Calcium antagonists in the treatment of hypertension. Hypertension 5(part II), 1983

49. Messerli FH, Oren S, Grossman E: Effects of calcium channel blockers on systemic hemodynamics in hypertension. Am J Med 84(suppl 3B), 8–12, 1988

50. Bauer JH, Reams G: Short- and long-term effects of calcium entry blockers on the kidney. Am J Cardiol 59:66A–71A, 1987

51. Romero JC, Raij L, Granger JP, Ruilope LM, Rodicio JL: Multiple effects of calcium entry blockers on renal function in hypertension. Hypertension 10:140–151, 1987

52. Reams GP, Hamory A, Lau A, Bauer JH: Effect of nifedipine on renal function in patients with essential hypertension. Hypertension 11:452–456, 1988

53. Resnick L: Calcium metabolism, renin activity and the antihypertensive effects of calcium channel blockade. Am J Med 81(suppl 6A), 1986

54. Luft FC, Aronoff GR, Fineberg NS, Weinberger MH: Effects of oral calcium, potassium, digoxin and nifedipine on natriuresis in normal humans. Am J Hypertens 2:14–19, 1989

55. Pool PE, Seagren SC, Salel AF: Effects of diltiazem on serum lipids, exercise performance, and blood pressure: Randomized, double-blind, placebo-controlled evaluation for systemic hypertension. Am J Cardiol 56:86H–91H, 1985

56. Ranramaa R, Taskinen E, Seppanen K, Rissanen V, Salonen R, Venalainen JM, Salonen JT: Effects of calcium antagonist treatment on blood pressure lipoproteins and prostaglandins. Am J Med 84(suppl 3B):93–98, 1988

57. Schoen RE, Frishman WH, Shamoon H: Hormonal and metabolic effects of calcium channel antagonists in man. Am J Med 84:492–504, 1988

58. Dilmen U, Caglor K, Senses A, Kinik EL: Nifedipine in hypertensive emergencies of children. Am J Dis Child 137:1162–1165, 1983

59. Siegler RL, Brewer ED: Effect of sublingual or oral nifedipine in the treatment of hypertension. J Pediatr 112:811–813, 1988

60. Raemsch KD, Sommer J: Pharmacokinetics and metabolism of nifedipine. Hypertension 5(suppl II):II-18–II-24, 1983

61. Reitberg DP, Love SJ, Quercie GT, Zinny MA: Effect of food on nifedipine pharmacokinetics. Clin Pharmacol Ther 42:72–75, 1987

61a. Wells TG, Sinaiko AR: (unpublished data)

62. The 1988 Report of the Joint National Committee on Detection, Evaluation, and Treatment of High Blood Pressure. Arch Intern Med 148:1023–1038, 1988

63. Frolich ED, Thurman AE, Pfeiffer MA: Altered vascular responsiveness: Initial hypotensive mechanism of thiazide diuretics. Proc Soc Exp Biol Med 14:1190–1196, 1972

64. Conway J, Lauwers P: Hemodynamics and hypotensive effects of long-term therapy with chlorothiazide. Circulation 21:21–27, 1960

65. Wilson IM, Freis ED: Relationship between plasma and extracellular fluid volume depletion and the antihypertensive effect of chlorothiazide. Circulation 20:1028–1036, 1959

66. Leth A: Changes in plasma and extracellular fluid volumes in patients with essential hypertension during long-term treatment with hydrochlorothiazide. Circulation 42:479–485, 1970

67. Tarazi RC, Dustan HP, Frohlich ED: Long-term thiazide therapy in essential hypertension: Evidence for persistent alteration in plasma volume and renin activity. Circulation 41:709–717, 1970

68. Spark RF, O'Hare CM, Regan RM: Low-renin hypertension. Restoration of normotension and renin responsiveness. Arch Intern Med 133:205–211, 1974

69. Douglas JG, Hollifield JW, Liddle GW: Treatment of low-renin essential hypertension: Comparison of spironolactone and hydrochlorothiazide-triamterene combination. JAMA 227:518–521, 1974

70. Ferguson RK, Turek DN, Rovner DR: Spironolactone and hydrochlorothiazide in normal-renin and low-renin essential hypertension. Clin Pharmacol Ther 21:62–69, 1977

71. MacGregor GA: Sodium and potassium intake and blood pressure. Hypertension 5(suppl III):III-79–III-84, 1983

72. Kaplan NM, Carnegie A, Raskin P, Heller JA, Simmons N: Potassium supplementation in hypertensive patients with diuretic-induced hypokalemia. N Engl J Med 312:746–749, 1985

73. Ahlquist RP: The study of the adrenotrophic receptors. Am J Physiol 153:556–600, 1948

74. Lefkowitz RJ, Carm MG, Stiles GL: Mechanisms of membrane-receptor regulation. N Engl J Med 310:1570–1579, 1984

75. Taylor SH: Intrinsic sympathomimetic activity: Clinical fact or fiction? Am J Cardiol 52:160–260, 1983

76. Williams EMV: Mode of action of beta receptor antagonists on cardiac muscle. Am J Cardiol 18:399–405, 1966

77. Frohlich ED, Dunn FG, Messerli FH: Pharmacologic and physiologic considerations of adrenoceptor blockade. Am J Med 75:9–14, 1983

78. Sinaiko AR: Influence of adrenergic nervous system on vasodilator-induced renin release in the conscious rat. Proc Soc Exp Biol Med 167:25–29, 1981

79. Hollifield JW, Sherman K, Vanderzwagg R, Shand DG: Proposed mechanisms of propranolol's antihypertensive effect in essential hypertension. N Engl J Med 295:68–73, 1976

80. Myers MG, Lewis PJ, Reid JL, Dollery CT: Brain concentration of propranolol in relation to hypotensive effect in the rabbit with observations on brain propranolol levels in man. J Pharmacol Exp Ther 92:327–335, 1975

81. Day MD, Roach AG: Central adrenoceptors and the control of arteriole blood pressure. Clin Exp Pharmacol Physiol 1:342–360, 1974

82. Reid JL, Lewis PJ, Myers MG: Cardiovascular effects of intracerebral vascular d-L-dl-propranolol in the conscious rabbit. J Pharmacol Exp Ther 188:394–399, 1974

83. Evans GH, Shand DG: Disposition of propranolol. Clin Pharmacol Ther 14:487–493, 1973

84. McDevitt DG, Shand DG: Plasma concentrations and the time-course of beta blockade due to propranolol. Clin Pharmacol Ther 18:708–713, 1975

85. Mirkin BL, Sinaiko AR: Clinical pharmacology and therapeutic utilization of antihypertensive agents in children, in New MI, Levine LS (eds): Juvenile Hypertension. New York, Raven Press, 1977, pp 195–217

86. Colfort DJ, Shand DG: Plasma propranolol levels in the quantitative assessment of beta-adrenergic blockade in man. Br Med J 3:731–734, 1970

87. Bauer JH, Brooks CS: The long-term effect of propranolol therapy on renal function. Am J Med 66:405–410, 1979

88. De Leeuw PW, Birkenheger WH: Renal response to propranolol treatment in hypertensive humans. Hypertension 4:125–131, 1982

89. Laper J, Blohme G, Smith U: Effect of cardio-selective blockade in hypoglycemic response in insulin-dependent diabetes. Lancet 1:458–462, 1979

90. Weidmann P, Uehlinger DE, Gerber A: Antihypertensive treatment and serum lipoproteins. J Hypertension 3:297–306, 1985

91. Weinberger MH: Antihypertensive therapy and lipids. Paradoxical influences on cardiovascular disease risks. Am J Med 80(suppl 2A):64–70, 1986

92. Ames RP: The effects of antihypertensive drugs on serum lipids and lipoproteins. II. Non-diuretic drugs. Drugs 32:335–357, 1986

93. Colucci WS: Alpha-adrenergic receptor blockade with prazosin. Ann Intern Med 97:67–77, 1982

94. Keranen A, Nykanen S, Taskinen J: Pharmacokinetics and side-effects of clonidine. Eur J Clin Pharmacol 13:97–101, 1978

95. Hansson L, Hunyor SN, Julius S, Hoobler SW: Blood pressure crisis following withdrawal of clonidine (Catapres, Catapresan), with special reference to arteriole and urinary catecholamine

levels, and suggestions for acute management. Am Heart J 85:605–610, 1973

96. Proceedings of the Symposium on Labetalol. Br J Clin Pharmacol 3(suppl 3):627–824, 1976

97. Baum T, Sybertz AJ: Pharmacology of labetalol in experimental animals. Am J Med 75:15–23, 1983

98. Blachakis ND, Marmde RF, Malory SW, Medakobic M, Kasseur N: Pharmacodynamics of intravenous labetalol follow-up therapy with oral labetalol. Clin Pharmacol Ther 38:503–508, 1985

99. Mulrow JP, Crawford MH: Clinical pharmacokinetics and therapeutic use of hydralazine in congestive heart failure. Clin Pharmacokinet 16:86–99, 1989

100. O'Malley K, Segal JL, Israeli ZH: Duration of hydralazine action in hypertension. Clin Pharmacol Ther 18:581–586, 1975

101. Perry HM: Late toxicity to hydralazine resembling systemic lupus erythematosus or rheumatoid arthritis. Am J Med 54:58–72, 1973

102. Hahn VH, Sharp GC, Ervin WS: Immune responses to hydralazine and nuclear antigens in hydralazine-induced lupus erythematosus. Ann Intern Med 76:365–374, 1972

103. Lin MS, McNay JL, Shepherd AMM, Musgrave GE, Keeton TK: Increased plasma norepinephrine accompanies persistent tachycardia after hydralazine. Hypertension 5:257–263, 1983

104. Zins GR: Alterations in renal function during vasodilator therapy, in Wesson LG, Fenalli GM Jr (eds): Recent Advances in Renal Physiology and Pharmacology. University Park Press, Baltimore, MD, 1974, pp 165–186

105. Sinaiko AR, Mirkin BL: Management of severe childhood hypertension with minoxidil: A controlled clinical study. J Pediatr 91:138–142, 1977

106. Sinaiko AR, O'Dea RF, Mirkin BL: Clinical response of hypertensive children to long-term minoxidil therapy. J Cardiovasc Pharmacol 2(suppl 2):S181–S188, 1980

107. Pennisi AJ, Takahashi M, Bernstein BH, Fine R: Minoxidil therapy in children with severe hypertension. J Pediatr 90:813–819, 1977

108. Siegler RL, Brewer ED: Effect of sublingual or oral nifedipine in the treatment of hypertension. J Pediatr 112:811–813, 1988

40

DRUGS USED TO MODULATE GASTROINTESTINAL FUNCTION

MICHAEL D. REED, JAMES L. SUTPHEN, *and* JEFFREY L. BLUMER

The alimentary tract, the largest organ system in the body, is a continuum which extends from the esophagus to the rectum. The gastrointestinal system is often divided into the upper and lower gastrointestinal tract. The upper gastrointestinal tract consists of the esophagus, stomach, and small intestine, which is subdivided into the duodenum, jejunum, and ileum. The lower gastrointestinal tract consists of the large intestine, comprising the cecum, ascending colon, transverse colon, descending colon, sigmoid colon, and rectum. The gastrointestinal tract serves numerous important physiologic functions:

1. As an interface between ingested elements from the external environment

2. As an organ for the delivery, processing, and absorption of fluids, electrolytes, and nutrients

3. For the final processing of nutrients and fluids with preparation, storage, and ultimate expulsion of waste materials

4. As an important component of overall host defense

5. As an important endocrine organ.[1-3]

The successful orchestration of these many and complex activities depends on the precise coordination of cellular and muscle function, which are directly influenced and controlled by a cadre of neurohumoral and local factors.[1-4]

Drugs, neurohumoral stimulation, pathogens, and toxins can alter gastrointestinal function[5] leading to disruption of the normal uptake, motility, and secretory processes of the gut. This chapter focuses on a select group of the many medications that can directly or indirectly influence gastrointestinal activity. The drug classes reviewed modulate secretion and motility and are often used in the management of gastrointestinal disorders in pediatrics. Unfortunately, as with many other classes of drugs, only limited data on the pharmacokinetics and pharmacodynamics of these drugs in infants and children exist. These data are presented in detail and hopefully will serve to stimulate future research with these and other compounds in the pediatric population.

PHARMACOKINETIC INTERFACE: DRUG ABSORPTION

From a pharmacologic perspective, the gastrointestinal tract serves an additional important function, i.e., regulation of the systemic absorption of orally[6,7] and rectally[8] administered drugs. The principles of drug absorption have been reviewed extensively[5-8] and will only be summarized here. In general, for drugs to distribute to and interact with their receptors, they must be absorbed into the systemic circulation. The majority of orally administered drugs are absorbed in the proximal portion of the small intestine. The physicochemical properties of a drug influence its rate and extent of absorption. Drugs for oral administration must be stable within the acid medium of the stomach and the more alkaline environment of the small intestine. Smaller molecules are generally absorbed more readily than larger molecules; the degree of lipophilicity and ionization under physiologic and pathophysiologic conditions directly influences a compound's extent of absorption. Other factors that influence the gastrointestinal absorption of a drug include product formulation and the presence and extent of disease.

Drugs must be liberated from their product formulation before becoming available for absorption. Solid dosage forms (tablets, capsules) contain many nontherapeutic ingredients used to form the solid unit as well as to provide shape, size, color, and possibly flavor. The quantity and constituency of these "binders" and "fillers" differ from drug to drug and manufacturer to manufacturer. As a result, the disintegration time of these dose formulations can differ depending on the specific manufacturer of the product. The rate of disintegration or dissolution and the resultant particle size markedly influence the bioavailability of a drug and are the primary basis of differences in bioavailability among different manufacturers' products of the same drug (multisource generic drug products).

Fewer data are available describing the influence of gastrointestinal disease on drug bioavailability.[6,7] From available data it is clear that the influence of gastrointestinal disease on drug bioavailability is highly variable and essentially unpredictable. Gastrointestinal disease may affect drug absorption due to changes in motility, changes in secretory function, and mucosal damage. The potential effects of these altered processes must be considered in the design of pharmacotherapeutic regimens and of pharmacokinetically and pharmacodynamically based monitoring strategies.

DRUGS THAT AFFECT GASTRIC ACID

Physiology of Gastric Acid Secretion

Although its presence has been recognized for decades, our understanding of the many physiologic roles of gastric acid remains incomplete.[9] One of the more important physiologic functions of gastric acid is to facilitate the digestion of foods and other substrates within the stomach. However, under certain physiologic and pathophysiologic conditions, gastric acid may damage gastroduodenal mucosa, leading to serious, potentially life-threatening complications. In children disorders associated with abnormally high rates of gastric acid secretion (duodenal ulcer, Zollinger-Ellison syndrome) are most common and serve as the focus of this overview.[10]

Gastric acid is produced and secreted by parietal cells that are located in the walls of the oxyntic glands in the fundus of the stomach.[9] The parietal cell contains a large number of mitochondria that fuel the energy-dependent "proton pump" responsible for the actual cellular secretion of hydrogen ion. This is catalyzed by a unique hydrogen–potassium ATPase[9] that exchanges hydrogen for potassium (Figure 40–1). Once stimulated, hydrogen ion is secreted into the stomach lumen, decreasing intragastric pH.

A number of clinical and environmental factors can influence the rate and amount of gastric acid secretion as well as the integrity of the intestinal mucosa. Cigarette smoking and excessive consumption of certain foods and beverages including coffee, cola beverages, and alcohol, as well as the use of certain medications such as salicylates and nonsteroidal anti-inflammatory drugs (NSAIDs), are associated with gastric acid secretion and peptic ulcer disease in adults. In children, on the other hand, ulcer disease or altered gastric acid secretion is more likely to be associated with drugs (including aspirin and NSAIDs), other diseases, and psychologic factors.[10]

As shown in Figure 40–1, specific secretagogues can stimulate the generation and secretion of hydrogen ion by the parietal cell. The three most important secretagogues are acetylcholine, histamine, and gastrin, which are also important targets for pharmacologic manipulation. Binding by any of these agonists to its specific receptor stimulates one of at least two second messenger pathways, resulting in increased intracellular concentrations of either cyclic AMP or cytosolic calcium. These increased intracellular concentrations of cyclic AMP (stimulated by histamine) or calcium (stimulated by gastrin and cholinergic agonists) activate cyclic AMP–dependent protein kinases which generate hydrogen ion for secretion into the gastric lumen by the hydrogen-potassium ATPase proton pump.[9]

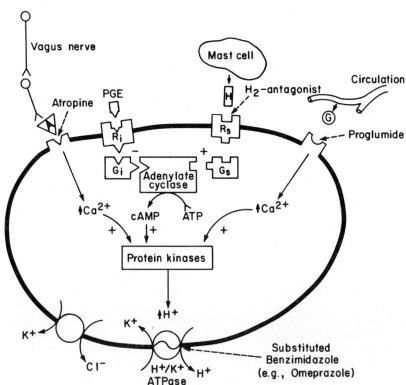

FIGURE 40–1. Schematic representation of a parietal cell, showing pathways by which secretagogues are believed to stimulate hydrogen ion secretion and sites of drug action. (From Wolfe and Soll,[9] with permission.)

**TABLE 40–1. COMPOSITION AND NEUTRALIZING CAPACITY OF
SELECTED ANTACID SUSPENSIONS***

PROPRIETARY PRODUCT	CONTENT (mg/5 ml)					ACID-NEUTRALIZING CAPACITY† (per 5 ml)
	Al (OH)$_3$	Mg (OH)$_2$	CaCO$_3$	Simethicone	Na	
MAALOX TC	600	300	0	0	0.8	27
MYLANTA-II	400	400	0	40	1.1	25
KUDROX DOUBLE STRENGTH	565	180	0	0	<15	25
GELUSIL-II	400	400	0	30	1.3	24
CAMALOX	225	200	250	0	1.2	18
DI-GEL	200	200	0	20	<5	–
ALTERNAGEL	600	0	0	–	<2.5	16
SILAIN-GEL	282	285	0	25	4.4	15
GELUSIL-M	300	200	0	25	1.2	15
Milk of magnesia (MOM)	0	390	0	0	0.12	14
MAALOX	225	200	0	0	1.4	13
MYLANTA	200	200	0	20	0.7	13
ALUDROX	307	103	0	–	2.3	12
GELUSIL	200	200	0	25	0.7	12
WINGEL	180	160	0	0	–	10
KOLANTYL GEL	150	150	0	0	<5	10
AMPHOJEL	320	0	0	–	<2.3	10

*Many of these preparations are also available in solid dosage forms. Although the composition of many of these forms is often similar to that of the suspension, variations exist.

†In milliequivalents. In some cases, a 60-minute rather than a 15-minute test was performed. Products listed in descending order of acid-neutralizing capacity.
Adapted from Derrida et al.,[16] with permission.

Antacids

Antacids have been used and abused by clinicians and consumers worldwide for decades. Despite the longstanding popularity of antacid use, controversy continues regarding their mechanism of pharmacologic action and their role in the management of gastrointestinal ulcer disease. The majority of the published experience with antacids emanates from their use in adults,[11–13] where the primary therapeutic goal has been to "neutralize" secreted gastric acid. This antacid-induced reduction in gastric fluid acid has, until recently, been considered their primary mechanism of drug action.[11–13] However, more recent data question acid neutralization as a primary mechanism[14,15] and suggest a cytoprotective effect on gastrointestinal mucosa by these drugs.

Antacids reduce the acidity of gastric fluid by neutralizing secreted gastric acid. Many compounds and antacid combinations are available for clinical use (see Individual Antacids); they vary in their potency to neutralize gastric acid and in associated adverse effects. Despite these differences, many early studies of antacid therapy neglected to control for the dose of antacid administered, making interpretation of these studies difficult.[11–13] Antacid doses were often described as volume (ml) administered and/or tolerated by the patient, with little attention paid to what was equipotent for the different products used. Moreover, the therapeutic end point of these studies, i.e., the targeted pH of gastric fluid or the amount of gastric acid neutralized, was also ill-defined. Fordtran and colleagues[11] in an elegant study defined clearly the marked variability in antacid potency, documenting that all antacids do not neutralize gastric acid equally at similar doses (i.e., volume of antacid in milliliters). Data derived from this study and others[16] defining the acid-neutralizing capacity relative to antacid dose are shown in Table 40–1. In addi-

tion, these authors described the more pronounced buffering effect of antacids (>3 hours) when they were administered after a meal when food was present in the stomach. These data have been used to support the now common antacid dosage recommendations of administration 1 hour after a meal.

In addition to dissimilarities in the dosage of antacid used, confusion persists relative to the optimal target pH of gastric fluid following antacid therapy. For decades the pharmacodynamics of antacids had been loosely correlated with their ability to neutralize gastric acid. Consistent with their presumed primary mechanism of action, limited experimental and clinical evidence is available defining a specific target hydrogen ion concentration of gastric fluid associated with symptomatic relief and ulcer cure.[12] Some authors have recommended 90 percent acid neutralization, whereas others have suggested 95 percent and even 99 percent reduction of available acid.[11,12] This lack of a defined target reduction in gastric acid concentration with antacid therapy compromises our ability to critically assess available data and to individualize antacid therapy for a specific patient. Despite a lack of consensus regarding an optimal target for reduction in gastric acid in the treatment of gastrointestinal ulcer disease or in the treatment or prophylaxis of stress ulcers, many authorities advocate antacid dosing directed at nearly complete neutralization of gastric acid, i.e. gastric pH ≥ 3.5.[17] Burget et al.[18] recently concluded that the degree and duration of acid suppression was most important for the healing of duodenal ulcers, but that acid suppression >pH 3.0 was not found to increase duodenal ulcer healing further. These data suggest that a relationship may exist between the degree of ulcer healing and the specific site of the ulcer. Many studies have described no effect of antacid therapy on healing rates of gastric and duodenal ulcers,[19–21] whereas others have demonstrated highly significant differences.[22,23] The lack of consistency in many of these studies with respect to antacid dose, targeted reduction in the amount of gastric acid, and duration of antacid therapy has led to confusion in the interpretation of individual studies, as well as these conflicting results for antacid efficacy. Today, most authorities agree that when administered in "adequate" doses, antacids promote ulcer healing.[11,12,21-24] Concern centers around the definition of adequate doses, and this issue was first addressed by Peterson et al.[22] who assessed the efficacy of high-dose or "intensive" antacid therapy for the treatment of duodenal ulcer. These investigators used a 30-ml antacid dose administered 1 and 3 hours after each meal and at bedtime (equivalent to 1008 mEq neutralizing capacity/day) for 28 days in the treatment of endoscopically proven duodenal ulcer disease in 74 adult patients. Ulcer healing was confirmed in 28 of 36 antacid-treated patients versus 17 of 38 patients who received placebo. Although intensive antacid therapy was superior to placebo in promoting ulcer healing, antacid was no more effective than placebo in relieving ulcer symptoms, a clinical finding reported by other investigators.[22] This and subsequent studies have been used to substantiate similar antacid dosage schedules for the treatment of gastric and duodenal ulcers. Unfortunately, additional studies addressing dose–response relationships for antacids have not been performed, primarily due to the availability of histamine H$_2$-receptor antagonists and the resultant enthusiasm for their use.

Prior to the availability of H$_2$-receptor antagonists, antacids were commonly used in children for the prevention and treatment of stress ulcers.[10] Like antacid therapy for the treatment of gastric and duodenal ulcers, the use of antacids for stress ulcer prophylaxis has also undergone a varied and convoluted history. The therapeutic goal of stress ulcer prophylaxis or treatment is the prevention of gastrointestinal bleeding. Stress ulcers are common in critically ill patients, most notably those suffering from multiple trauma, head trauma, shock, multiple organ failure, burns, and sepsis.[16,25] Accordingly, most patients admitted to the intensive care unit receive some form of antacid or gastric acid secretory therapy as a prophylactic measure.[25,26] Similar to gastric and duodenal ulcer therapy, studies support greater than 80 percent efficacy in preventing stress ulceration when gastric pH is consistently maintained above pH 3.5.[16,25,26]

Last, antacids provide prompt but temporary relief of the pain associated with gastroduodenal mucosal erosions. Many gastroenterologists use this clinical response as an important historical factor indicating peptic disease.

Individual Antacids

Sodium Bicarbonate

Sodium bicarbonate is one of the oldest antacid compounds used and is associated with a rapid onset and short duration of action. The chemical reaction of sodium bicarbonate and gastric acid results in the formation of sodium chloride, water, and carbon dioxide.[27] Following oral administration of sodium bicarbonate, sodium and

bicarbonate ions are readily absorbed into the systemic circulation, which can result in fluid retention and systemic alkalosis and the milk–alkali syndrome. For these reasons sodium bicarbonate is rarely used today as an antacid, and if it is used, prolonged or chronic therapy must be avoided.

Calcium Carbonate

Like sodium bicarbonate, calcium carbonate is a potent, rapid-acting antacid. The duration of action for calcium carbonate is much longer than for sodium bicarbonate. Although these two desirable pharmacologic characteristics would appear to support the use of calcium carbonate as an antacid of choice, adverse effects and concern relative to acid rebound have severely limited the use of this drug.[13]

Calcium carbonate reacts with gastric acid forming calcium chloride, water, and carbon dioxide. The majority of the calcium chloride formed is reconverted to insoluble calcium carbonate in the small intestine. However, approximately 10 percent of this formed calcium chloride is readily absorbed into the systemic circulation and, with chronic therapy, can result in substantial calcium absorption.[28] Sufficient calcium can be absorbed from calcium carbonate to lead to hypercalcemia, hypercalciuria, and calcium deposits in the kidney which can result in compromised renal function.[28]

In addition to the concern relative to systemic calcium absorption, a severe gastric hypersecretion or "acid rebound" has also been reported to be associated with calcium carbonate antacid use.[13] Studies have reported increased gastric acidity and volume of gastric juice following calcium carbonate therapy as compared to aluminum hydroxide, food ingestion,[29,30] or sodium bicarbonate[29] administration. This acid rebound associated with calcium carbonate appears to be the primary reason the drug is no longer used. Texter[13] recently reevaluated the data describing calcium carbonate–induced rebound and reviewed substantial amounts of data questioning whether this rebound phenomenon is unique to calcium carbonate. Texter clearly showed that all antacids or buffering substances, including food, can increase gastric acidity and that this increase is not unique to one or another antacid or to calcium. Moreover, he presented convincing evidence that much of this controversy stems from studies that compared nonequivalent doses of antacids relative to their gastric acid–neutralizing capacity. Thus, the interpretation of data on calcium carbonate-induced acid rebound is limited in a fashion similar to the studies assessing the effficacy of antacids in ulcer healing.[13] Nevertheless, these data suggest that calcium carbonate may be a viable antacid product, particularly for patients who would benefit from the additional systemic availability of calcium.

Magnesium Hydroxide

Many magnesium salts, including oxide, carbonate, hydroxide, and trisilicate, possess antacid properties. The hydroxide, carbonate, and oxide salts are more potent than the trisilicate salt in their ability to neutralize gastric acid. In general, their overall potencies are greater than that of aluminum-containing antacids but less than that of sodium bicarbonate or calcium carbonate. Magnesium-containing antacids react with acid forming magnesium chloride and water. Magnesium also forms insoluble salts which are responsible for the diarrhea often associated with magnesium-containing antacids. These magnesium salts produce catharsis osmotically without changing gastrointestinal motility.[31] In addition, portions of the administered magnesium are absorbed systemically from magnesium chloride and in general are rapidly eliminated from the body via the kidney in individuals with mature and competent renal function. In neonates and young infants, magnesium can accumulate, leading to systemic toxicity (see Adverse Effects of Antacids).

Aluminum

Like magnesium-containing antacids, many aluminum-containing salts are available as antacids, including hydroxide, carbonate, phosphate, and aminoacetate. Aluminum hydroxide is the most potent and most frequently used aluminum-containing antacid. Interaction with gastric acid yields aluminum trichloride, water, and insoluble aluminum phosphate.[27] Unlike magnesium-containing antacids, the primary adverse effect of aluminum antacids is constipation. For this reason it has been common practice to administer this antacid salt as a combination of magnesium- and aluminum-containing antacids. Aluminum binds with dietary phosphate, reducing the amount of phosphate available for systemic absorption. This effect is often used clinically in patients with chronic renal disease and associated hyperphosphatemia. However, chronic therapy with aluminum-containing antacids can lead to hypophosphatemia and resultant hypercalcemia.[32] Furthermore, although previous studies suggested that aluminum was not absorbed systemically, several studies have demonstrated elevated serum and/or bone concentrations of aluminum in patients receiving chronic therapy.[33,34] Aluminum is absorbed in the small intestine and small amounts are excreted daily in the urine.[35] In patients with immature or compromised renal function, aluminum accumulates in the body and can result in serious neurotoxicity.[33–37]

Adverse Effects of Antacids

Gastrointestinal complaints, including diarrhea and constipation, are the most common adverse effects associated with antacid therapy. As described above, magnesium salts are most often associated with a dose-related osmotic diarrhea, whereas aluminum and calcium salts are most often associated with constipation. Some authors have questioned this association with calcium carbonate administration, suggesting that the constipation may be a result of the ulcer rather than the calcium administration. Although attempts have been made to reduce the incidence of these effects on the gastrointesti-

nal tract by combining magnesium- and aluminum-containing antacids, diarrhea can occur with high, intensive doses of any antacid-containing combination. We have found diarrhea to be frequent when combination antacid doses (e.g., aluminum–magnesium hydroxide combination) exceeded 1 ml/kg/dose. Bezoar formation may also complicate antacid therapy, particularly in newborns.[38]

With the exception of aluminum phosphate, all aluminum-containing antacids form insoluble salts with phosphate present in the gastrointestinal tract.[32] This reaction reduces systemic phosphate absorption, and if the drug is taken for prolonged periods it can lead to hypophosphatemia requiring phosphate supplementation. This binding of dietary phosphate by aluminum-containing antacids is frequently used therapeutically in the treatment of hyperphosphatemia in patients with chronic compromised renal function.

Adverse effects associated with systemic absorption of antacid cations have only recently been critically assessed. Aluminum, calcium, and magnesium can all be absorbed following antacid administration.[32–37] Clinically important adverse effects associated with the absorption of these cations are most often observed in patients receiving prolonged high-dose therapy or with immature or compromised renal function. As a result, antacid administration must be used with caution in neonates and young infants because of their immature renal function.[36,37]

Drug interactions have also been associated with the use of antacids. The most common interaction involves the influence of antacids on the gastrointestinal absorption of concurrently administered medications.[39,40] The degree to which an antacid may interfere with the absorption of another drug depends on the specific antacid used, the dose, the time of administration, and the duration of therapy. Antacids may influence the absorption of other drugs by modifying gastric pH, which may alter the dissolution rate of the concurrently administered compound. Antacids may also adsorb coadministered compounds or lead to complex formation (e.g., with tetracycline). Although a large number of drugs have been shown to interact with antacids, and the potential for antacids to reduce the systemic absorption of drugs is great, this drug interaction is generally of limited clinical significance and can be avoided if the administration of the antacid is separated by 1–2 hours from that of other oral medications.[40]

Conclusion: Antacids

Despite limited published experience, antacids have been used frequently as adjunctive agents in the management of acid secretory disorders in infants and children.[10,36,37,41] Our understanding of how to dose antacids is derived almost entirely from studies performed in adults and guided by clinically defined but variable target gastric fluid pH values. The likelihood of additional research on the use of antacids in children is questionable, considering the clinical efficacy and nearly universal acceptance of the histamine H_2-receptor antagonists (see below). Nevertheless, some recommendations for the clinical use of antacids in infants and children can be developed from available data and experience. The smallest dose necessary (0.5–1 ml/kg liquid antacid in infants; 5–15 ml in older infants and children) up to a total single dose of 10–20 ml should be used to achieve a target pH of gastric fluid. Antacids should be administered after meals,[11,12] preferably 1 hour postprandially. Sutphen et al.[41] demonstrated pronounced as well as sustained buffering effects of antacids in infants when administered postprandially, consistent with earlier work in adults.[11,12] More importantly, postprandial antacid administration permitted a marked reduction in the dose required by these infants, with a concomitant decrease in the incidence of adverse effects.[41] Last, the chronic use of antacids (e.g., >2–4 weeks) in children should be approached cautiously, with appropriate monitoring for potential adverse effects including changes in stooling pattern, mineral metabolism,[32] and the possible accumulation of the antacid cations magnesium, aluminum, and calcium.[13,33–37]

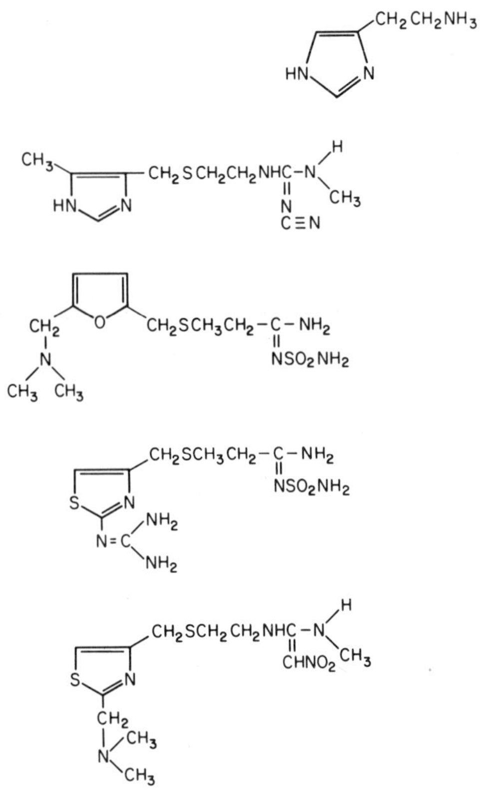

ANTISECRETORY MEDICATIONS

Histamine H$_2$-Receptor Antagonists

Histamine is a very effective and potent stimulator of gastric acid secretion by the parietal cell (Figure 40–1). The binding of histamine or other agonists, including acetylcholine and gastrin, to specific receptors residing on the parietal cell activates second messengers that stimulate cyclic AMP protein kinases; these kinases activate a specific hydrogen–potassium ATPase that exchanges hydrogen for potassium ions across the apical surface.[9]

Histamine possesses many important and varied pharmacologic effects that are mediated via histamine H$_1$ and H$_2$ receptors. Stimulation of the H$_1$ receptor results in the contraction of many smooth muscles, including those of the gut and bronchi, whereas histamine acting on the H$_2$ receptor is a potent stimulus to gastric acid secretion by the parietal cell. The effects of histamine on vascular tone (e.g., vasodilation) are mediated via both H$_1$ and H$_2$ receptors. Classic antihistamines used in cough and cold preparations and those used in the treatment of allergies (e.g., pyrilamine, chlorpheniramine) and in the treatment of acute allergic reactions (e.g., diphenhydramine) all competitively inhibit the effects of histamine at the H$_1$ receptor. Thus, these drugs do not influence the effect of histamine on gastric acid secretion, which is a result of H$_2$-receptor stimulation (Figure 40–1).

A large number of histamine H$_2$-receptor antagonists are now available for clinical use (Figure 40–2). These drugs are reversible competitive antagonists of the actions of histamine on the H$_2$ receptor. Their primary effect and the sole basis for their clinical use is the resultant decrease in histamine-mediated gastric acid secretion by the parietal cell (Figure 40–1). Available histamine H$_2$-receptor antagonists compete for binding only at the H$_2$ receptor and are without effects on other receptors, including the histamine H$_1$, muscarinic, nicotinic, or sympathomimetic α- or β-receptors.[9] However, although these drugs possess a very high specificity for the histamine H$_2$ receptor, they also decrease the acid secretory response of the

FIGURE 40–2. Chemical structures of histamine and selected histamine H$_2$-receptor antagonists.

parietal cell to cholinergic agents, gastrin, food, and vagal stimulation.[9] These extra-histamine H$_2$-receptor physiologic effects of these drugs are most likely a result of the important interdependency that exists between the effects of the neuroendocrine (acetylcholine), endocrine (gastrin), and paracrine (histamine) pathways on acid secretion by the parietal cell. Histamine H$_2$-receptor antagonists do not affect gastric motility, emptying times, tone at the lower esophageal sphincter, or exocrine pancreatic function.[42,43]

The clinical availability of the histamine H$_2$-receptor antagonists marked a new era in the pharmacotherapy of disorders of gastric acid secretion. These drugs provided a welcome therapeutic alternative to the unpleasant taste and adverse effects of antacids and the often common side effects associated with the use of anticholinergic medications. Major differences between the available H$_2$-receptor antagonists are their receptor specificity, potency, and resultant safety profile. A multitude of laboratory and clinical studies, controlled comparative evaluations, uncontrolled open evaluations, and clinical observations have been reported describing the effects of these drugs in the treatment and maintenance of gastric and duodenal ulcer and Zollinger-Ellison syndrome, as well as in the prophylaxis of stress ulcers.[43–48] Thus, it is not surprising that cimetidine and ranitidine are the most widely sold drugs in the world and that to date more than 1100 histamine H$_2$-receptor antagonists have been identified, resulting in approximately 250 drug patents with nearly 20 different compounds undergoing clinical investigation.[47]

The effectiveness of histamine H_2-receptor antagonists in promoting healing of duodenal ulcers ranges from 75 to 90 percent during a 4- to 6-week treatment period versus 30–60 percent healing rates with placebo. These rates are similar to those observed with high-dose antacid therapy and do not differ for different histamine antagonists when equipotent doses are used. Similarly, healing rates for gastric ulcer are approximately 70–80 percent at 6 weeks and 90+ percent with longer treatment regimens (e.g., 8 weeks) compared to an approximate healing rate of 35–40 percent with placebo.[43–46] In one of the single largest reported studies of H_2-receptor antagonist therapy in children, Tam and Saing[48] described their 20-year experience with the treatment of chronic peptic ulcer disease in children. A total of 78 children were aggressively managed: 46 children pre-histamine H_2 antagonist who received conventional antacid therapy, and 32 children who received the H_2-receptor antagonists cimetidine 20 mg/kg/day or ranitidine 6 mg/kg/day, both administered in three divided doses daily. The rate of ulcer healing associated with histamine H_2-receptor antagonist therapy (complete healing: 75.9 percent at 6 weeks, 91 percent at 8 weeks) is similar to that achieved in many adult series. Only one child who received an H_2-receptor antagonist failed therapy and required surgical intervention (1/32), whereas 16 failures (16/46) requiring surgery occurred in children receiving conventional antacid therapy. Tam and Saing[48] attributed the success of their therapy with H_2-receptor antagonists to an aggressive approach which included continued drug therapy until ulcer healing was confirmed endoscopically. Considering that individual differences among patients, drug dose requirements, and duration of therapy for ulcer disease can vary markedly, such an approach of documenting ulcer healing prior to discontinuation of pharmacologic therapy appears reasonable.

Cimetidine

Cimetidine was the first histamine H_2-receptor antagonist available for general clinical use. In 1977 the United States Food and Drug Administration approved the use of cimetidine for the treatment of duodenal ulcer disease, Zollinger-Ellison syndrome, and certain other gastric hypersecretory states.[44] Numerous publications describe the chemistry, pharmacology, efficacy, and safety profile of this drug in humans.[43–51] The majority of this literature describes experiences in adult subjects. Nevertheless, available data in pediatric subjects[48,52–59] permit an assessment of cimetidine pharmacology in children.

The pharmacokinetic characteristics of cimetidine in infants and children are shown in Table 40–2 and compared to adult controls in Table 40–3. Pharmacokinetic characteristics of cimetidine compared to other H_2-receptor antagonists in adults are outlined in Table 40–4.

Cimetidine is rapidly absorbed, with peak serum concentrations observed approximately 45–90 minutes after oral administration. Oral drug absorption appears linear over a dosage range of 200–800 mg.[47,49] The drug's bioavailability averages 60 percent, which does not appear to be influenced by coadministration with food.[60] Food may

TABLE 40–2. PHARMACOKINETICS OF CIMETIDINE IN INFANTS AND CHILDREN

PARAMETER	PREMATURE INFANT	INFANTS AND CHILDREN	CHILDREN
n	1	13	27
Age (years)	29 wks PCA*	5.9 (3.8)	9 (2.3)
$t_{1/2}$ (h)	2.6	1.4 (0.4)	1.4 (0.3)
V_d (liters/kg)	0.95	2.1 (0.6)	1.2 (0.5)
Cl (ml/min/kg)	4.4	14.2 (2.9)	10.4 (4)
Reference	54	53	57

n = Number of patients studied; $t_{1/2}$ = elimination half-life; V_d = apparent volume of distribution; Cl = total body clearance. Values expressed as mean ($\pm$S.D.).
*Age in weeks postconceptional age.

delay the time to peak serum concentration.[60] Concurrent administration of antacids may interfere with the absorption of cimetidine,[61] whereas concurrent sucralfate has no apparent effect.[62,63] Absorption following intramuscular injection is nearly complete (90–100 percent), with peak plasma concentrations occurring within 15 minutes of administration.[64] Approximately 20 percent of cimetidine is bound to plasma protein. Cimetidine crosses the placenta[65] and can achieve subpharmacologic concentrations in breast milk.[49]

In adults approximately 60–75 percent of the cimetidine dose is excreted unchanged in the urine, with approximately 25–40 percent undergoing hepatic metabolism and less than 2 percent being excreted via the bile.[49] Specific metabolite formation and their rates are ill defined in children. In adults, three metabolites have been identified. The sulfoxide is the predominant metabolite (10–15 percent of the dose), whereas the hydroxymethyl metabolite accounts for less than 5 percent of a given dose. A guanylurea metabolite that can be formed nonenzymatically and may represent an *in vitro* degradation product[66] accounts for less than 2 percent of a dose. A single study that evaluated the metabolic disposition of cimetidine in five cystic fibrosis patients aged 9.7–15.2 years revealed metabolite formation rates similar to that described in adult controls.[67]

The pharmacokinetics of cimetidine in children are shown in Tables 40–2 and 40–3. Only limited published experience is available describing the disposition of cimetidine in premature and newborn infants.[52–54] A single case report[54] revealed expected prolongation of the clearance of cimetidine in a 25-week-gestation, 29-week-postcon-

TABLE 40–3. PHARMACOKINETICS OF CIMETIDINE IN CHILDREN COMPARED TO ADULTS

PARAMETER	CHILDREN*	ADULTS†
n	13	8
Age (years)	1.3–12.4	21–35
$t_{1/2}$ (h)	1.4 (0.4)	1.5 (0.1)
V_d (liters/kg)	2.1 (0.6)	1.1 (0.1)
Cl (ml/min/kg)	14.2 (2.9)	9.2 (2.4)

Abbreviations as in Table 41–2.
*Critically ill children (data from Chin et al.[53]).
†Healthy adult volunteers (data from Lebert et al.[68]).

TABLE 40–4. COMPARISON OF PHARMACOKINETIC PARAMETER ESTIMATES FOR SELECTED HISTAMINE H$_2$-RECEPTOR ANTAGONISTS IN ADULTS

PARAMETER	HISTAMINE H$_2$-RECEPTOR ANTAGONIST (MEAN AND RANGE)			
	Cimetidine	Famotidine	Nizatidine	Ranitidine
F (%)	63–78	37–45	90–95	39–85
$t_{1/2}$ (h)	2	2.5–4	1–2	2–3
V_d (liters/kg)	0.8–1.2	1.1–1.4	0.8–1.6	1.2–1.9
C_p time (h)	1–2	1–3	0.5–3	1–3
Protein binding (%)	15–20	15–20	30–35	15–20
Cl (liters/h)	30–48	19–29	40–60	46
Cl$_R$ (liters/h)	24–36	15–27	30	24–32
% metabolized	25–40	30–35	7–10	6
Mean plasma conc (50%) (ng/ml)	500–1000	13	154	60–100

F = Oral bioavailability; $t_{1/2}$ = elimination half-life; V_d = apparent volume of distribution; C_p time = time to peak plasma concentration, oral dose; Cl = total body clearance; Cl$_R$ = renal clearance; mean plasma conc 50% = mean plasma drug concentration associated with 50% inhibition of stimulated gastric acid (estimate).
Data compiled from Berardi et al.,[43] Somogyi and Gugler,[49] Roberts,[87] and Smith.[102]

ceptional-age infant. In older infants and children (Tables 40–2 and 40–3), the data are highly suggestive of an increased volume of distribution and clearance as compared to adults.[53,57] Due to the lack of specifically controlled comparative studies, Table 40–3 compares cimetidine pharmacokinetic parameter estimates in children[53] and adults[68] in studies performed at different times but at the same institution by the same investigators. The reason for the increase in the volume of distribution and in body clearance in children as compared to adults for cimetidine is unclear. However, these observations support increased dosing for children on a weight basis, administered more frequently (i.e., every 4 hours versus every 6 hours). Similarly, patients with cystic fibrosis appear to have a higher body clearance as well as renal clearance of cimetidine than adults.[67]

Limited studies are available that specifically address the combined pharmacokinetics and pharmacodynamics of cimetidine in children. Lloyd and colleagues[57] studied a group of 27 critically ill children ranging in age from 4.1 to 15 years of age (Table 40–2). A large interindividual variation in cimetidine pharmacokinetics and pharmacodynamics was observed in this study population. Although these investigators did not identify any direct relationship between gastric pH and cimetidine concentrations in plasma or gastric fluid, they did note gastric pH values greater than 4 at 2 hours after the dose (cimetidine plasma concentrations greater than 1 mg/liter) and gastric fluid pH values less than 3 at 6 hours after the dose when the plasma cimetidine concentration fell below 1 mg/ liter. Similar serum cimetidine concentration relationships, though highly variable, have been described in adults (Table 40–4). The results of this study and others[47,49] support a dose of cimetidine of 20–30 mg/kg/ day administered intravenously in six divided doses daily. Subsequent dosing adjustments of cimetidine may be necessary due to the large interindividual variation in the drug's pharmacokinetic and pharmacodynamic profile, and these dosage adjustments should be guided by a predetermined target pH for gastric fluid. Such an approach to drug dosing has also been advocated by Tam et al.[48]

Numerous and varied adverse reactions have been

associated with the use of cimetidine.[45] The overall incidence of adverse reactions in patients receiving the drug has been estimated as approximately 4.5 percent, with gastrointestinal (2.1 percent) and central nervous system (1.2 percent) effects occurring most frequently. Central nervous system adverse reactions have included mental confusion, disorientation, agitation, hallucinations, and seizures.[45,69,70] These central nervous system reactions, although initially unexpected because animal studies suggested little cimetidine penetration across the blood–brain barrier, are most commonly observed in elderly or very young patients, patients receiving high-dose therapy, and patients with renal or liver disease or both. Schentag et al.[70] described increased cerebrospinal fluid/plasma cimetidine concentration ratios in adult patients with combined renal and hepatic dysfunction who experienced cimetidine-induced central nervous system toxicity. The mechanism of this adverse reaction is unknown, but it is believed to result from blockade of central histamine receptors or possibly other neuroendocrine mediators. Just as important in the use of this drug in pediatrics is the effect cimetidine may have on the endocrine system. Adverse endocrine effects associated with cimetidine therapy include gynecomastia, galactorrhea, impotence, and possibly a decrease in spermatogenesis.[45,71,72] The exact cause of these adverse endocrine effects is unknown, but they may be a result of the drug's antiandrogen action. The breast enlargement associated with cimetidine use may be unilateral, associated with local tenderness, and appears reversible upon discontinuation of cimetidine therapy. Last, cimetidine administration has been associated with increases in serum prolactin concentrations. Cimetidine-induced elevation in serum prolactin concentration is most commonly observed following intravenous administration and is unusual when the drug is administered orally. The reasons for this discrepancy relative to route of drug administration and the clinical significance of transient elevations in serum prolactin concentrations are unknown.

Among the presently available histamine H$_2$-receptor antagonists (Figure 40–2), cimetidine is a potent inhibitor of hepatic microsomal enzyme activity.[73–75] Concurrent

TABLE 40–5. INFLUENCE OF CIMETIDINE ON THE DISPOSITION OF SELECTED DRUGS

DRUG AFFECTED	PHARMACOKINETIC PARAMETER MEASURED (UNITS)	CHANGE	
		Before	After
Diazepam	Cl (ml/min)	19.9	11.4
Imipramine	$t_{1/2}$ (h)	10.8	22.7
Lidocaine	Cl (ml/min)	766	576
Meperidine	Cl (liters/kg/h)	0.6	0.47
Procainamide	$t_{1/2}$ (h)	2.9	3.7
Propranolol	AUC (µg/liter/h)	450	727
Theophylline	$t_{1/2}$ (h)	11.5	14.1
Triamterene	Renal Cl (ml/min)	71	27

$t_{1/2}$ = Elimination half-life; Cl = body clearance; AUC = area under the serum concentration–time curve.
Adapted from Reed et al.,[75] with permission.

cimetidine administration has been reported to inhibit the metabolism of over 25 different compounds (Table 40–5). In pediatrics one of the more important drug interactions involving cimetidine is its competitive interference with theophylline metabolism. Concurrent administration of cimetidine in children receiving theophylline will result in a prolongation of theophylline half-life and clearance with resulting accumulation of theophylline, which has been associated with an increased incidence of adverse effects and the development of seizures.[74,75] Dossing et al.[76] found that the inhibitory effect of cimetidine on microsomal enzyme activity occurred within 24 hours of initiating the drug and subsided within 2 days after the last dose. In rodents the inhibition of microsomal enzyme activity by cimetidine has been shown to decrease the hepatotoxicity of certain drugs,[74] including acetaminophen[77–79] and cocaine,[78] suggesting a possible therapeutic value for this metabolic interaction. However, the time course of the inhibitory effect of cimetidine on hepatic microsomes[76] would appear to limit its clinical utility as an adjunct in the treatment of acetaminophen intoxication. In addition, cimetidine, more than other histamine H_2-receptor antagonists, is capable of reducing hepatic blood flow, further compromising the metabolism of high-extraction-ratio drugs.[74]

Cimetidine has also been shown to decrease the renal clearance of a number of cationic drugs, including procainamide, n-acetyl procainamide, and triamterene, by inhibition of renal proximal tubular cationic secretion.[80,81] In contrast to cimetidine, clinically significant drug interactions with ranitidine, famotidine, or nizatidine are unusual,[47,74,82–85] involving only case reports. Although ranitidine has been shown to bind to cytochrome P-450,[47,74,86] its binding affinity is approximately 10-fold lower than that described for cimetidine.

Ranitidine

Unlike cimetidine, ranitidine contains an amino methyl furan moiety rather than an imidazole ring (Figure 40–2). This deviation from an imidazole ring structure resulted in the development of a drug with greater

potency and a longer duration of action.[46,87] In addition, the pharmacologic effectiveness of ranitidine demonstrated that an imidazole ring was not necessary for histamine H_2-receptor recognition and binding, and that the lack of this ring most likely decreases the type and incidence of associated systemic adverse effects.[46]

The pharmacokinetics of ranitidine in infants and children are shown in Table 40–6, and in adults compared to other available histamine H_2-receptor antagonists in Table 40–4. The bioavailability of ranitidine can be variable, ranging from 39 to 86 percent with an average of 50 percent.[87,88] Ranitidine concentrations in serum appear linear over the dosage range 50–400 mg. A second "peak" concentration has been observed in the serum ranitidine concentration–time profile by some[89] but not all[88] investigators. This biphasic character in the plot of serum drug concentration versus time has also been described for cimetidine[90] and has been observed in both fasting subjects and subjects permitted to eat 3 hours after dosing. This so-called double-peak phenomenon is blunted when these drugs are coadministered with food.[47,91] No biphasic character in the plot of ranitidine serum drug concentration versus time was observed in our study,[88] in which children were not permitted food within 6 hours of oral ranitidine dosing. The reason for this biphasic characteristic in the absorption profile for cimetidine and ranitidine (also for famotidine, see the next section) is yet to be determined, although its clinical importance would appear minimal.

The oral absorption of ranitidine may be decreased slightly when coadministered with antacids,[92] and conflicting data exist regarding an interaction with sucralfate. If sucralfate influences the oral absorption,[93] the effect occurs in the fasting state[94] and is most likely of limited clinical significance. Administration of propantheline concurrent with ranitidine delays the maximum ranitidine concentration and the time to maximum concentration by a probable decrease in gastric emptying time.[94] Again, this effect would be expected to be of little clinical significance. The absorption of ranitidine after intramuscular injection is virtually complete (90–100 percent). The plasma protein binding of ranitidine averages 15 percent,[95] and similar to cimetidine, ranitidine is found in breast milk in subpharmacologic concentrations.[96] The majority of a ranitidine dose (>70 percent) is eliminated unchanged via the urine.[47,87] The principal ranitidine

TABLE 40–6. PHARMACOKINETICS OF RANITIDINE IN INFANTS AND CHILDREN

PARAMETER	DATA EXPRESSED AS MEAN (± S.D.)		
	Infants	Children	Children
n	9	12	4
Age (years)	1 (0.5)	12.6 (3.7)	8.1 (1.8)
$t_{1/2}$ (h)	2.1 (1.3)	1.8 (0.3)	2.0 (0.7)
V_d (liters/kg)	1.6 (1.0)	2.3 (0.9)	1.5 (0.3)
Cl (ml/min/kg)	13.9 (10)	795 (334)*	9.5 (3.2)
Reference	98	88	97

Abbreviations as in Table 41–2.
*Cl expressed as ml/min/1.73 m.^{2}

metabolite found in the urine is the N-oxide, which constitutes approximately 4 percent of the dose. Other metabolites include the S-oxide and dimethyl ranitidine, at approximately 1 percent of the administered dose each. The remainder of the drug is eliminated via the feces with possibly some enterohepatic recycling.[87]

Table 40-6 shows the pharmacokinetics of ranitidine in infants and children.[88,97,98] No significant differences have been identified between the disposition of ranitidine in infants and children or between these populations and adults. In a preliminary abstract report by Leeder and colleagues,[97] no real differences in ranitidine half-life, volume of distribution, or body clearance were observed between a group of children 6–10 years of age ($n = 4$), a group of children 11–16 years of age ($n = 4$), and six disease-free adults of mean age 27 years ($n = 6$). Of interest, these investigators reported a central volume of distribution in the 6- to 10-year age group up to twice that observed in the older children and adults. These pharmacologic data support current initial ranitidine dosing recommendations in children: 2–4 mg/kg/day in two or three divided daily doses orally and 1–2 mg/kg/day in three or four divided daily doses intravenously.

The type and incidence of adverse effects associated with ranitidine appear to be much less than that reported during therapeutic courses of cimetidine.[46,82,83] Unlike cimetidine, ranitidine administration has not been associated with clinically significant effects on hepatic drug metabolism, endocrine function, the immune system, or the central nervous system.[46,47,85,99–101]

As described previously, the primary mechanism by which cimetidine interferes with the metabolism of most drugs is through its binding to cytochrome P-450 in the hepatic endoplasmic reticulum. Cimetidine avidly binds to cytochrome P-450, producing a stable cytochrome–substrate complex.[85] The binding of cimetidine to cytochrome P-450 prevents other drugs from having access to these drug-metabolizing enzymes, thus reducing their rate of metabolism. In contrast, ranitidine possesses far less affinity for cytochrome P-450, and whatever amount does bind forms a relatively labile complex.[99] Abernethy and colleagues[82] demonstrated a lack of effect of ranitidine on hepatic oxidative or conjugative metabolism using antipyrine, diazepam, and lorazepam as their study probes. Other investigators have reported similar noninteractions with ranitidine.[85]

Ranitidine therapy does not appear to be associated with any adverse effects on the endocrine system.[101] The drug does not raise basal concentrations of testosterone or cause an increase in prolactin secretion.[46] The drug seems to be devoid of any of the antiandrogen activity that has complicated therapy with cimetidine. Jensen and colleagues[72] described nine male patients treated with high-dose cimetidine for Zollinger-Ellison syndrome who developed impotence and gynecomastia. All nine patients were switched to equipotent doses of ranitidine and experienced control of their symptomatology, suppression of gastric acid secretion, and complete resolution of their impotence and gynecomastia. This lack of adverse effects on the endocrine system relative to cimetidine strongly supports the use of ranitidine in maturing infants and children.

Famotidine

Famotidine is a thiazole ring containing a histamine H_2-receptor antagonist (Figure 40-2). The drug is approximately 10–15 times more potent than ranitidine and 40–60 times more potent than cimetidine in inhibiting gastric acid secretion.[102] The efficacy and safety profile of famotidine appears similar to that of ranitidine.[43,103,104] However, due to its recent release into clinical medicine, much less reported experience is available with famotidine.[43]

Famotidine oral bioavailability ranges from 37 to 45 percent of the administered dose.[43] Like ranitidine, the bioavailability of famotidine may be slightly increased when it is administered with food and slightly decreased when it is coadministered with antacids.[105] Similarly, a second peak serum famotidine concentration has been described after oral[106] and parenteral[104] administration. As with ranitidine and cimetidine, the clinical significance of these observations is unknown. Approximately 15–20 percent of famotidine is bound to serum protein. Studies in lactating rodents suggest that famotidine is secreted into breast milk. Between 65 and 70 percent of famotidine is excreted unchanged via the urine.[47]

Pharmacokinetic data describing famotidine disposition in children are very limited. Kraus and colleagues[104] described the disposition of a single 0.3 mg/kg intravenous dose of famotidine in 10 children (2–7 years of age) following cardiac surgery. The average famotidine pharmacokinetic data obtained in this study (half-life, 3.3 hours; volume of distribution, 1.41 liters/kg; body clearance, 0.30 liter/h/kg) are very similar to values reported in healthy adults (Table 40-4). More importantly, a large variation was observed in the pharmacokinetics of famotidine in these children: approximately 55 percent coefficient of variation in half-life and clearance, and 70 percent in apparent volume of distribution. Although this variation in drug disposition may have occurred due to the altered physiologic status of their study subjects after cardiac surgery, similar variation has been observed in the pharmacokinetic data for ranitidine[98] in critically ill children. These data underscore the importance of titrating histamine H_2-receptor antagonist dosing to a predetermined pharmacodynamic target (e.g., gastric fluid pH) and therapeutic response. The results of this single famotidine pharmacokinetic-pharmacodynamic study suggest an intravenous dose of 0.3 mg/kg administered every 8 hours to maintain gastric fluid pH above 3.5 for the majority of the dosing interval. Our own preliminary experience supports a famotidine dose of 0.3–0.35 mg/kg administered every 8 hours. Oral dosing would need to be increased by approximately 60 percent to compensate for the drug's incomplete bioavailability. In a preliminary clinical evaluation of orally administered famotidine, Miyake et al.[103] successfully treated 17 severely handicapped bedridden children with reflux esophagitis using 1–2 mg famotidine/kg/day.

The primary advantage of famotidine as compared to ranitidine is the drug's increased potency and slightly longer elimination half-life, which may permit less frequent dosing (e.g., every 8–12 hours for famotidine versus every 6–12 hours for ranitidine). However, as for cimetidine and ranitidine, these recommended dosing intervals appear most appropriate for chronic acid suppression therapy in adults and possibly in children. Experience suggests that more frequent dosing of H_2-receptor antagonists is often required to achieve target gastric fluid pH in critically ill infants and children.[107-109] In contrast, sufficient experience is available[43,46] describing the efficacy of chronic H_2-receptor antagonist therapy for healing gastric and duodenal ulcers when administered to adults in larger single doses (e.g., ranitidine 300 mg) once daily at bedtime. Similar such studies in children are unavailable.

Proton Pump Inhibitors

Omeprazole

Omeprazole is the first agent representing a new class of very potent gastric acid antisecretory drugs.[110] The drug is a substituted benzimidazole which suppresses the secretion of gastric acid by competitively inhibiting the hydrogen–potassium ATPase present on the surface of the parietal cell (Figure 40–1). Based on this novel mechanism of action, this class of antisecretagogues is termed proton pump inhibitors.[110] At the time of this writing, no data on the use of omeprazole or other investigational proton pump inhibitors in children were available.

Omeprazole is administered orally as enteric-coated granules encased in a gelatin capsule to protect the drug from degradation by the acid medium of the stomach. As a result the bioavailability of omeprazole is variable, ranging from 30 to 40 percent upon initiation of therapy and increasing to 60 to 65 percent after chronic dosing once daily.[47,111,112] This increase in omeprazole bioavailability with chronic therapy may be due to a reduction in the amount of drug that is destroyed by gastric acid as the drug itself begins to suppress the amount of available gastric acid.[111] Decreased first-pass metabolism resulting from saturation of responsible hepatic enzymes may also contribute to this increase in bioavailability.[111] Food administered concurrently with omeprazole can decrease the rate but does not appear to influence the overall extent of drug absorption[47]; omeprazole absorption is unaffected by concurrent antacid administration.[113] Approximately 95 percent of the drug is bound to albumin.[111]

Omeprazole is extensively metabolized by the cytochrome P-450 drug-metabolizing enzyme system in the liver.[111,112,114] Three metabolites have been identified, none of which appear to be pharmacologically active in suppressing gastric acid secretion. Plasma concentrations of hydroxyomeprazole, a sulfide, and a sulfone derivative range from 30 to 50 percent, less than 1 percent and 15–20 percent of the plasma omeprazole concentration. In healthy volunteers, less than 0.1 percent of a dose is excreted as unchanged omeprazole in the urine.[111] The remainder of the drug (approximately 19 percent) is excreted in the feces.[112] The half-life of omeprazole ranges from 0.5 to 1.5 hours in individuals with normal liver function.[112-114] Preliminary studies suggest a minority of individuals (<5 percent) will be slow metabolizers of omeprazole. Slow metabolism of omeprazole has been correlated with the polymorphic hydroxylation of S-

mephenytoin.[115] In preliminary studies[115,116] of four slow and five rapid metabolizers of omeprazole and diazepam, the four slow omeprazole metabolizers were poor hydroxylators of S-mephenytoin. These data suggest that the metabolism of omeprazole and diazepam is associated with the S-mephenytoin hydroxylation polymorphism.[115,116]

Although the half-life of omeprazole is relatively short, its antisecretory effect on the parietal cell in adults persists for more than 24 hours. As a result, the drug is dosed once daily. This persistence of antisecretory effect appears to result from accumulation of the drug in the parietal cell.[110] A plateau in the amount of gastric acid suppression observed with repeated once-daily dosing of the same omeprazole dose is achieved by approximately day 4 of therapy.[110] Clinical pharmacology studies in adults reveal a reduction of approximately 80 percent each in basal acid output, peak acid output, and 24-hour acid secretion following repeated dosing of 20 mg omeprazole daily.[110]

The benzimidazole moiety of omeprazole predisposes the drug to numerous drug interactions due to interference with oxidative drug metabolism within the hepatic P-450 system. Interference with the activity of these enzymes by omeprazole is dose-dependent and has been shown to alter the clearance of diazepam, warfarin, and phenytoin,[110,117-120] whereas no effect has been demonstrated with concurrent omeprazole on the disposition of propranolol or theophylline.[110,121] Diaz et al.[122] recently demonstrated that omeprazole is an aryl hydrocarbon-like inducer of cytochrome P-450 in humans, i.e., cytochromes P-450 1A1 and P-450 1A2. Although no drug to date has been shown to be metabolized by P-450 1A1, P-450 1A2 has been characterized as the major phenacetin deethylase in humans responsible for the conversion of phenacetin to acetaminophen. Moreover, cytochromes P-450 1A1 and 1A2 have been shown to be responsible for the metabolic alteration of procarcinogenic moieties, including polycyclic hydrocarbons, aromatic amides, and amines, to reactive metabolites responsible for mutagenesis and chemical carcinogenesis.[122] The chemical relevance of these findings and their relationship, if any, to the possible association between omeprazole use and gastric carcinoid tumors (see later in text) is unknown. However, these preliminary data suggest that when the drug is administered in routine clinical doses (<40 mg/day in adults), omeprazole may not appreciably alter the metabolism of other hepatically metabolized drugs. The clinical significance, if any, of these and other potential drug interactions remains to be determined.

As mentioned above, no published experience exists with the use of omeprazole for the treatment of gastric acid secretory disorders in children. For adults, omeprazole has been shown to be equal or possibly superior to histamine H_2-receptor antagonists in the treatment of gastric ulcer,[110,123] duodenal ulcer,[110] and H_2-receptor-antagonist-resistant duodenal ulcers,[124] and in the management of patients with Zollinger-Ellison syndrome.[110,125] A primary concern with the use of omeprazole is the possible association with the development of gastric carcinoid tumors.[110] In preclinical studies, gastric carcinoid tumors were found in 23–40 percent of tested rats, predominantly females, who received 18–175 times the planned human dose of omeprazole.[110] Carcinoid tumors were not found in mouse or dog toxicity studies.[110] The cause of these tumors in rats is unknown, but they may be due to omeprazole-induced hypergastrinemia, which may exert atrophic effects on enterochromaffin-like cells of the gastric fundic mucosa, leading to the formation of carcinoids.[110] To date no carcinoids have been described in humans, and the true nature of this potential carcinogenic effect remains speculative.[110,122,125] Carefully controlled, long-term studies need to be undertaken to determine the carcinogenic potential of omeprazole in humans as well as the drug's influence, if any, on the metabolism of potentially carcinogenic xenobiotics. This possible adverse effect mandates the utmost caution in the use of omeprazole in pediatric patients.

Conclusion: Gastric Acid Antisecretory Drugs

The clinical availability of the histamine H₂-receptor antagonists has resulted in a clear change in the pharmacotherapeutic approach to disorders of gastric acid secretions.[43,46-48] This change in drug use is evident in their nearly universal acceptance in pediatrics. For infants and children, antacids are difficult to dose, and in particular, it is difficult to coerce as alert child to drink a dose of antacid liquid or chew an antacid tablet. As described above, the efficacy of the histamine H₂-receptor antagonists in the treatment of disorders of gastric acid secretion is excellent. Difficulties with the clinical use of H₂-receptor antagonists primarily involve adverse drug effects, drug interactions, or lack of clinical response, which is most likely due to either inappropriate drug dosing or the development of drug tolerance.

The question of tolerance to the pharmacodynamic effect of H₂-receptor antagonists has been raised since the mid-1970s,[126] soon after their release for clinical use. Though poorly studied, investigators have described a diminished effect of these drugs on pentagastrin- and meal-stimulated increases in gastric acid, as well as a diminished effect on basal acid output (BAO) after acute and chronic dosing.[126-129] The first study to address H₂-receptor antagonist tolerance in pediatrics[128] described five of six study infants who required weekly increases in daily ranitidine dose to achieve the same degree of suppression of BAO (<20 μmol/kg/h). Other investigators have reported similar findings.[129] Tolerance to H₂-receptor antagonists does not appear to be specific to any one antagonist or related to the route of drug administration or the number of doses administered per day, and it is not associated with any change in the drug's pharmacokinetic profile.[128,129] The development of tolerance appears to occur acutely[129] during the first week of therapy and persist. The reason for this tolerance is unknown but may reflect receptor up-regulation as a result of the hypergastrenemia that occurs with the use of all of these medications. More important, however, is the clinical significance of this drug tolerance for the chronic ambulatory therapy of gastric or duodenal ulcers. As discussed above,

the healing rate of these ulcers is significantly better with 6- to 8-week treatment courses of H₂-receptor antagonists than with placebo, despite the nearly universal development of tolerance.[129] The effect of acute tolerance on stress ulcer prophylaxis remains to be determined.

Of the histamine H₂-receptor antagonists available in 1990, the most pharmacokinetic and pharmacodynamic data in children are available for cimetidine[47,48,51-59] and ranitidine.[47,48,88,97,98,107,108] When dosed appropriately (cimetidine, 20-30 mg/kg/day divided into three to six equal doses; ranitidine, 2-4 mg/kg/day divided into two to four doses), both appear to be equally effective in children. Thus, due to the lack of serious adverse effects and, in particular, of endocrine disorders (e.g., gynecomastia, altered spermatogenesis) and drug interactions, it appears that ranitidine use in pediatrics should be favored. Clinical or metabolic advantages, if any, for the use of famotidine or nizatidine in children remain to be assessed. Similarly, at the time of this writing, the role of omeprazole and other proton pump inhibitors in pediatric practice is unclear. It appears that the use of these drugs in children should be reserved for those rare patients who fail more conventional therapies. Moreover, a clear understanding of the potential association between proton pump inhibitors and carcinoid tumors is needed before these agents can be recommended for therapy in infants and children.

As described above, much of the pharmacodynamic data with histamine H₂-receptor antagonists originates from published experience in adults. As a result, the present dosage recommendations for these drugs in pediatrics require continued refinement as our experience accumulates. At present it would appear desirable to define a specific target gastric fluid pH to serve as the initial therapeutic goal, which may change depending upon patient response and tolerance. This approach to therapy accounts for the marked variation observed in the pharmacokinetics of these drugs in children[57,88,98,104] and the development of drug tolerance[126-129] while maintaining constant the pharmacodynamic parameter most often associated with drug efficacy. Although optimal gastric fluid pH remains to be defined[17] and most likely varies according to therapeutic goal (i.e., gastric or duodenal ulcer treatment, stress ulcer prophylaxis), maintenance of gastric fluid pH above 3-3.5 for gastric and duodenal ulcer treatment and 3.5-4.0 for stress ulcer prophylaxis appears reasonable.[16,17,24,25]

Due to the tremendous variation in the pharmacokinetics of histamine H₂-receptor antagonists and the resultant variation in pharmacodynamic response in critically ill patients, many investigators have suggested the continuous intravenous infusion method for drug administration in these patients.[130-132] The true need for this method of drug administration remains to be defined.[132] Continuous intravenous infusion of H₂-receptor antagonists may provide a logistic benefit when comixed in parenteral nutrition solutions in some intensive care patients. However, it would appear that bolus or continuous intravenous infusion regimens are equivalent in therapeutic efficacy when either regimen maintains consistent control of gastric fluid pH equal to or greater than 3.0-4.0.[132]

PROKINETIC AGENTS

Introduction to Prokinetic Agents

Gastric hypomotility is a frequent component of many gastrointestinal disorders.[4] Drugs that can favorably influence gastrointestinal hypomotility have been termed prokinetic agents for their net effect on "forward motion."[133] In pediatrics gastroesophageal reflux disease and disorders of gastric emptying[4,134] are the conditions for which these drugs are used most frequently. However, those drugs which antagonize dopamine activity, e.g., metoclopramide, have become important agents in the adjunctive treatment of nausea and vomiting.[133]

Bethanechol

Bethanechol is a synthetic quaternary ammonium compound that is structurally and pharmacologically related to acetylcholine. The drug's effect appears to be selective for muscarinic receptors of cholinergic pathways. The metabolic fate of bethanechol is poorly understood,[135] but the drug is not metabolized by cholinesterases. No pharmacokinetic data for bethanechol in children are available,[136] which is most likely responsible for the diverse clinical responses described with the use of this drug in children.[136–139] Pharmacologic data in adults and children have been limited to the assessment of a pharmacodynamic response and the occurrence of undesirable effects. Bethanechol increases ureteral peristalsis and the tone of the detrusor muscle of the urinary bladder; increases the tone, amplitude of contractions, and peristaltic activity of the stomach and intestines; and can increase the pressure of the lower esophageal sphincter. The latter two effects of the drug have supported its use in the treatment of infants and children with gastroesophageal reflux.[136–139] Clinical studies have described an immediate effect of bethanechol in decreasing the mean duration of the reflux episode[137,139] and, with chronic therapy, a decrease in the frequency of reflux episodes.[136–138] Clinical studies in infants and children have shown expected differences in bethanechol pharmacodynamics relative to the route of drug administration. Sondheimer and Arnold[136] described an increase in lower esophageal sphincter pressure, beginning at their first 10-minute measurement point, which was "short lived" ($\leq$30 minutes) following subcutaneous administration of bethanechol. In contrast, Euler[137] reported initial effects beginning at 25 minutes and lasting for approximately 60–120 minutes after oral drug administration. These differences may merely reflect differences in the rate of systemic drug absorption that can occur following subcutaneous and oral dosing.

Sondheimer and Arnold[136] used two different bethanechol doses in their study, providing some insight into a dose–response effect for this drug. Increases in lower esophageal sphincter pressure occurred following a bethanechol dose of either 0.1 or 0.2 mg/kg administered subcutaneously; however, the musculature of the esophageal body, as measured by amplitude of esophageal contractions, increased with the higher dose only. More importantly, these data suggested a preferential effect on esophageal smooth muscle located in the mid- and distal portion rather than on the striated muscle located in the proximal portion of the esophagus. No effect of bethanechol was observed in the upper one-third of the esophagus, where the musculature is striated; the greatest effect was observed in the lower one-third, where the musculature is smooth; and only intermediate effects were observed in the middle segment of the esophagus, where the musculature is a mixture of smooth and striated muscle. Last, these limited data imply that bethanechol has the least effect on lower esophageal sphincter pressure and esophageal peristalsis in those infants and children with reduced resting lower esophageal sphincter pressure and esophagitis.[136] Obviously, specific pharmacokinetic and pharmacodynamic studies are needed to define optimal bethanechol dosing regimens in infants and children and to determine the true role this drug may have in gastroesophageal reflux disease and dysmotility disorders. Moreover, because many of the infants who are evaluated for gastroesophageal reflux disease also suffer from chronic pulmonary disease, bethanechol must be used cautiously due to its cholinergic effects on the lung.

Metoclopramide

Metoclopramide, 2-methoxy-5-chloro-procainamide, is a gastrointestinal prokinetic agent. Although structurally similar to procainamide, metoclopramide is without any appreciable anesthetic or antiarrhythmic properties. The exact mechanism of action of metoclopramide on the gastrointestinal tract is unknown, but it is believed to result from a combination of dopamine antagonism, most likely at the dopamine D_2 receptor, and augmentation of acetylcholine release from postganglionic nerve terminals.[133,140] The effect of metoclopramide on chlolinergic neurons is unlike that of bethanechol or other "cholinomimetic" agents, as metoclopramide does not increase gastric acid secretion, endogenous gastrin release, or salivation. Metoclopramide stimulates the release of acetylcholine but also appears to sensitize muscarinic receptors of gastrointestinal smooth muscle to acetylcholine.[141,142] Metoclopramide's effect on gastric emptying is unaffected by vagotomy,[143] but its effects on upper gastrointestinal smooth muscle may be reduced or abolished by atropine.[133] The gastrointestinal motility effects of metoclopramide appear unique to this drug class, promoting the coordination of gastric, pyloric, and duodenal motor function, which results in net aboral movement. This overall effect is due to the drug's coordination of accelerated gastric emptying by increasing gastric tone, increasing amplitude of antral contractions, and relaxation of the pylorus and duodenum, while increasing peristalsis of the jejunum, thus accelerating intestinal transit time from the duodenum to the ileocecal valve.[133]

Metoclopramide is rapidly absorbed following oral administration. Substantial interindividual variation has been observed in maximal serum concentrations following various doses, as well as in the drug's oral bioavailability (range 32–97 percent).[47,140] This variation is most likely due to first-pass drug metabolism.[144,145] Approximately 40 percent of metoclopramide is bound to plasma protein, primarily α_1-acid glycoprotein.[146] Limited data suggest ready distribution of metoclopramide into breast milk.[147,148] The majority of metoclopramide is metabolized by the liver to two primary metabolites: N-4-sulfate and the N-4-glucuronide, which account for 32–40 percent and less than 2 percent of the dose administered, respectively. Approximately 20 percent of the dose is excreted unchanged in the urine. The half-life of metoclopramide in adults ranges from 2.5 to 5 hours.[144,145]

Limited pharmacokinetic data are available on metoclopramide in children.[149,150] Bateman and colleagues[149] studied metoclopramide disposition in nine children aged 7–14 years who received the drug as prophylaxis for cytotoxic drug-induced vomiting (see below). Following an average dose of 0.35 mg/kg, the drug's half-life, apparent volume of distribution, and clearance averaged 3.7 ± 0.5 hours, 3 ± 0.4 liters/kg, and 0.56 ± 0.1 liter/kg/h, respectively. These pharmacokinetic parameter estimates are similar to those observed in healthy adults.[144] Kearns and colleagues[150] assessed the pharmacokinetics and pharmacodynamics of repeated-dose metoclopramide in six infants with gastroesophageal reflux disease. Pharmacokinetic evaluation was performed after the first and tenth dose of metoclopramide. The drug was rapidly absorbed following administration of the oral solution; half-life, apparent volume of distribution, and clearance averaged 5.1 hours, 4.9 liters/kg, and 0.66 liter/kg/h, respectively, after the first dose, and 4.2 hours, 4.4 liters/kg, and 0.67 liter/kg/h, respectively, after the tenth dose. These pharmacokinetic data from infants are very similar to those values described by Bateman et al. in older children[149] and adults.[145] The data of Kearns et al.[150] suggest a metoclopramide oral dose of 0.15 mg/kg administered every 6 hours in term infants between the ages of 1 and 6 months. This dose would also appear an appropriate starting dose for older infants and children.

Although metoclopramide can be an effective drug in the management of gastrointestinal dysmotility disorders and gastroesophageal reflux disease,[4,151–154] the drug also finds much of its use in children as an adjunct in the management of chemotherapy-induced nausea and vomiting.[155] Nausea and vomiting are well-known adverse effects associated with and complicating antineoplastic drug therapy. The mechanism by which antineoplastic chemotherapy induces emesis remains uncertain[156] but appears to involve stimulation of dopamine, histamine, serotonin, and muscarinic receptors within the central nervous system.[156–159] Emesis appears to be controlled by the vomiting center located in the lateral reticular formation of the medulla. The vomiting center does not appear to be directly sensitive to chemical stimuli but rather responds to impulses from the chemoreceptor trigger zone (CTZ) located in the area postrema, the vestibular center, afferent visceral nerves through the vagus and sympathetic system, and probably other centers within the cerebral cortex.[158,159] Thus, it is not difficult to appreciate the clinical use of combination antiemetic drug ther-

apy when considering these complex interrelationships involving different centers within organs and neurohumoral transmitters as they relate to drug-induced emesis.

Metoclopramide has been shown to be an important component of combination drug regimens used in the management of chemotherapy-induced nausea and vomiting.[156–161] However, the importance of metoclopramide in these treatment regimens was not fully realized until the late 1970s. Early studies employed usual therapeutic doses of metoclopramide (e.g., 0.15–0.3 mg/kg) and produced disappointing results,[155,156] suggesting the drug was ineffective as an antiemetic for chemotherapy-induced nausea and vomiting. Despite these discouraging results with low doses, animal studies and a positive benefit clinically in some patients suggested a dose-proportional effect with metoclopramide. These findings, combined with the proposed mechanism of action of metoclopramide, supported the undertaking of studies that employed higher doses, e.g., 1–3 mg/kg/dose. Based upon this hypothesis, numerous uncontrolled and controlled trials of metoclopramide were undertaken using high doses (e.g., 2–3 mg/kg) and established its importance as a useful agent in controlling nausea and vomiting associated with the use of chemotherapeutic agents, most notably cisplatin.[155,156] The efficacy of metoclopramide as an antiemetic at higher doses is most likely a result of the drug's ability to competitively antagonize dopamine and serotonin-3 (5HT-3) receptors in the CTZ combined with effects on gastrointestinal motility. Clinical pharmacology studies in patients receiving these higher doses of metoclopramide have revealed pharmacokinetic characteristics no different than those observed in patients receiving more conventional doses for the treatment of gastrointestinal dysmotility disorder.[162] In addition to drug dose, the timing of administration of antiemetic drug therapy relative to the administration of antineoplastic drug therapy has been determined to be a critical factor for pharmacotherapeutic efficacy. For the management of cisplatin-associated nausea and vomiting, metoclopramide should be administered 30 minutes before and 90 minutes after chemotherapy. For chemotherapy regimens involving cyclophosphamide or doxorubicin combinations, investigators have found metoclopramide administered every 2 hours for three doses, then every 4 hours for three more doses, to be an effective component of combination antiemetic therapy.[156]

Last, metoclopramide is also frequently used in pediatrics as an adjunctive measure to facilitate the passage of nasoenteric feeding tubes beyond the pylorus.[163] If stomach peristalsis is insufficient to move the tube along, premedication 10–20 minutes prior to tube placement with metoclopramide 0.1 mg/kg/dose is often helpful.

Adverse reactions are commonly associated with the use of metoclopramide, and their incidence appears to increase with increasing dose. The overall incidence of adverse effects approaches 20 percent,[133] with drowsiness, restlessness, dry mouth, lightheadedness, and diarrhea occurring most frequently. Extrapyramidal effects due to the drug's dopamine antagonism and augmentation of cholinergic pathways occur in approximately 1 percent of patients. These effects, which include opisthotonos, trismus, torticollis, and oculogyric reactions, may occur more commonly in children than adults[164–166] and occur more frequently with high-dose therapy. Early investigators speculated that the increased dystonic reactions with metoclopramide in children might have an underlying pharmacokinetic basis. However, the data of Bateman et al.[149] and Kearns et al.[150] refute this early belief, as the pharmacokinetic characteristics of metoclopramide are similar in infants, children, and adults. The reason for this apparent predilection for dystonic reactions in children is unknown. The occurrence of these reactions supports the routine concurrent administration of repeated-dose diphenhydramine or benzotropine as a component of high-dose metoclopramide antiemetic regimens. It would also appear prudent to avoid the use of other drugs with dopamine antagonist activity (e.g., phenothiazines) concurrent with metoclopramide. Other rare toxicities associated with metoclopramide have included methemoglobinemia[167] unmasking previously unrecognized seizure disorder, and the clinical consequences of elevated serum prolactin concentrations, including breast enlargement, nipple tenderness, galactorrhea, and menstrual irregularities.[133] Conversely, this metoclopramide-induced elevation in serum prolactin concentration may have therapeutic implications. Ehrenkranz and Ackerman[168] administered metoclopramide to 23 postpartum women who had delivered premature infants and were having difficulty maintaining milk production. In 15 of these women, metoclopramide therapy (10 mg every 8 hours for 7 days, tapered off over 2 days) was associated with the successful maintenance of lactation, with limited adverse effects in the mothers and none in the breast-feeding infants.

By enhancing gastric emptying and intestinal motility, metoclopramide has the potential to influence the oral bioavailability and resultant serum concentration relationships (e.g., C_{max}, t_{max}) of a multitude of drugs. Numerous studies[47] have been performed in an attempt to better define this possible drug interaction. The results of these studies have described variable and sometimes conflicting effects on the disposition of other drugs due to the concurrent administration of metoclopramide. Coadministered drugs studied, mostly in volunteer subjects, have included aspirin, acetaminophen, cimetidine, cyclosporine, diazepam, digitoxin, levodopa, maxilitine, morphine, and tetracycline, to mention a few.[47] Overall, the influence metoclopramide may have on the gastrointestinal absorption of concurrently administered drugs appears minimal and of limited clinical significance.

Other Prokinetic Agents

Other gastrointestinal prokinetic agents are available or currently under clinical investigation throughout the world, including domperidone and cisapride.[47,169,170] Both of these drugs are chemically related to metoclopramide and share very similar pharmacologic properties.

Domperidone is a benzimidazole derivative which is extensively metabolized by the liver. Like metoclopramide, domperidone is a dopaminergic antagonist that produces marked hyperprolactinemia. However, domperidone does not appear to possess any cholinergic activity, as atropine has no effect on the pharmacologic properties of this drug. The drug undergoes extensive hepatic first-pass metabolism following oral administration, with an oral bioavailability of approximately 15 percent. The majority of the drug and its metabolites are excreted in the feces. The plasma half-life of domperidone ranges from 7 to 8 hours in adults with normal liver function. Very little domperidone crosses into the central nervous system, which appears to explain the rare occurrence of extrapyramidal effects observed with this drug.[47] Possibly for similar reasons, domperidone may demonstrate less antiemetic activity than metoclopramide. Domperidone was clinically effective in decreasing symptoms associated with moderate to severe gastroesophageal reflux disease in 15 infants 3–13 months of age. Patients received 0.6 mg/kg three times daily 20 minutes before each meal and at bedtime.[171] Spontaneously resolving diarrhea, lasting 1–3 weeks, was the most common adverse effect noted in this study.

Cisapride is a benzamide derivative whose effects on stomach and small bowel motility appear very similar to those of metoclopramide and domperidone.[170] The mechanism of cisapride's gastrointestinal effects is poorly understood but is not due to dopamine receptor antagonism. Cisapride possesses no antidopamine effects, and as a result, the administration of the drug is not associated with increases in plasma prolactin concentration or extrapyramidal reactions. The drug appears to stimulate gastrointestinal motility indirectly by enhancing acetylcholine release from postganglionic nerves of the myenteric plexus.[47,170] Like metoclopramide and domperidone, cisapride demonstrates a hepatic first-pass effect following oral drug administration: oral bioavailability approximates 40–50 percent. The half-life of cisapride approximates 7–10 hours; less than 1 percent of an oral dose is excreted unchanged in the urine.[47] A reasonable initial starting dose of cisapride in children appears to be 0.2 mg/kg administered orally three or four times daily.

Older agents that have been evaluated for prokinetic properties include glucagon[172] and erythromycin.[173] Glucagon has been shown to relax segments of the gastrointestinal tract and has been used prior to radiographic studies and as adjunctive therapy to promote passage of foreign bodies.[172] The mechanism of the gastrointestinal effects of glucagon is unknown. The empirical dose of glucagon used by many clinicians for its effects on the gastrointestinal tract in children has been 1 mg. Preliminary data with erythromycin suggest this agent also may be effective in improving gastric emptying times and intestinal motility.[173] Doses have ranged from 20 to 250 mg/dose administered orally three times daily in adults. It is believed that erythromycin mimics the effects of the gastrointestinal polypeptide motilin.[173] Motilin stimulates interdigestive (between meals) but not postprandial intestinal motility. The clinical utility of glucagon appears to be due to its acute effects on the gastrointestinal tract, whereas erythromycin may be beneficial for more chronic therapy in patients with disorders of gastric emptying, e.g., diabetic gastroparesis.

Conclusion: Prokinetic Agents

Both bethanechol and metoclopramide have established roles in the treatment of specific gastrointestinal diseases, including gastroesophageal reflux disease and gastrointestinal dysmotility disorders. However, controversy continues regarding the most appropriate time to initiate the use of these drugs, which patients they will most benefit, and how best to optimize therapy. Much of the confusion with bethanechol appears to emanate from our lack of understanding of the drug's disposition characteristics in infants and children. A greater therapeutic response in the management of gastroesophageal reflux disease may be observed with more frequent daily dosing of this drug combined with greater attention to other therapeutic measures, including diet and positioning.[174] Clearly, more studies assessing the combined pharmacokinetics and pharmacodynamics of bethanechol in these patients are needed.

Metoclopramide is an effective prokinetic and antiemetic drug whose clinical use is associated with numerous and bothersome side effects. In pediatrics, extrapyramidal side effects, including dystonic reactions, are common and require close monitoring during initiation of metoclopramide therapy and dose escalation. These extrapyramidal reactions are a result of the drug's antidopaminergic activity and respond promptly to treatment with diphenhydramine or benztropine. Newer agents do not appear to offer any significant therapeutic advantages over metoclopramide, but they may be associated with a decreased incidence of extrapyramidal and other adverse drug reactions. The true role for these and other prokinetic agents in pediatrics remains to be determined.

DRUGS USED IN THE MANAGEMENT OF ACUTE DIARRHEA

Loose watery stools occur commonly in infancy and represent a major reason parents bring their children to the pediatrician. In developed countries, acute diarrheal disease in children is second only to respiratory illness as a cause of hopsitalization.[175] In underdeveloped countries, the median number of diarrheal episodes in children less than 3 years of age ranges from two to six per year; five million fatalities in children less than 5 years of age occur worldwide every year due to diarrhea.[175,176] The basis of successful therapy for these children is replacement and maintenance of fluid and electrolyte losses, adequate nutritional support, and resolution of the etiology of the diarrhea.[177] Previously, intravenous fluids were used as the first-line approach to the treatment of infants with acute diarrhea. However, it is now recognized that oral rehydration therapy offers an effective and highly viable alternative to parenteral rehydration therapy.[175-179] Drug therapy for the treatment of diarrhea in infants and children is uncommon, mostly because of its self-limiting nature, the desire of the clinician not to mask potential fluid losses within and from the bowel, and associated adverse drug effects.[175,177,180-182] Antidiarrheal drugs in children should be used cautiously and considered only as potential short-term adjuvants to optimal fluid and electrolyte therapy.[175,177] The majority of the available antidiarrheal agents alter gastrointestinal motility and thus treat the symptom rather than the cause of the disorder. More importantly, some data suggest equivocal efficacy of antidiarrheal drugs in children.[180] The reason for this finding with earlier drugs is unknown, but the results may actually reflect the use of inappropriate doses of these agents in the therapy of this disorder. Dose–effect studies with earlier drugs are essentially nonexistent; dose–effect relationships can only be extrapolated from very limited studies involving newer analogs.[182-184]

Adsorbents

Hundreds of antidiarrheal preparations, which contain one or more of 25 different ingredients, are available to the consumer for the self-medication of diarrhea.[185,186] Most of these products contain agents that nonspecifically adsorb ingredients present in the gastrointestinal tract, including nutrients, digestive enzymes, bacteria, and bacterial toxins. These agents are also capable of adsorbing drugs (e.g., lincomycin), leading to an important drug–drug interaction that decreases the systemic bioavailability of concurrently administered medications. The primary adsorbents used in antidiarrheal preparations are listed in Table 40–7. These agents have been used for centuries for symptomatic treatment of diarrhea and dysentery. Limited pharmacologic data are available with these agents alone or in combination, either in children or adults. Complications associated with these agents include bloating, abdominal cramping, constipation, and with excessive prolonged use, impaction. However, in general, these agents are inert, relatively nontoxic, and not absorbed into the systemic circulation.

Attapulgite is a naturally occurring hydrous magnesium aluminum silicate that exists as a three-layered crystalline structure that can adsorb eight times its weight in water.

Kaolin is a hydrated aluminum silicate.

Pectin is a purified carbohydrate extracted from the rind of citrus fruit or from apple pumice.

Antispasmodics

Drugs that possess anticholinergic activity have been used for the temporary treatment of diarrhea in an attempt to decrease the often associated hypermotility observed in these patients.[47,175,182,185,187] The so-called anticholinergic-antispasmodic agents include the naturally occurring belladonna alkaloids (e.g., atropine, scopolamine) and numerous other natural or synthetic quaternary ammonium (e.g., homatropine, clindinium bromide) or tertiary amine (e.g., dycyclomine) compounds. No controlled pharmacologic data exist assessing the combined pharmacokinetics and pharmacodynamics of these drugs in children. These drugs are rarely used today, mainly because of associated side effects that are fre-

TABLE 40–7. ADSORBENTS USED IN THE ADJUNCTIVE TREATMENT OF DIARRHEA

Activated charcoal
Aluminum hydroxide
Attapulgite
Bismuth subsalts
Kaolin
Magnesium trisilicate
Pectin

See text for details.

quently bothersome (e.g., dry mouth, urinary retention) but can be serious (e.g., anticholinergic psychosis, seizures). Specific individuals may benefit from careful dose titration of one of these drugs as an adjuvant in the treatment of certain bowel disorders, e.g., irritable bowel syndrome.[188]

Diphenoxylate

Diphenoxylate is chemically related to meperidine and for decades was the most frequently prescribed antidiarrheal medication.[47,180] The drug is usually available in combination with atropine. Diphenoxylate is extensively metabolized via ester hydrolysis to diphenoxylic acid, which is biologically active and represents the major metabolite found in the blood.[189] Less than 1 percent of the parent drug is excreted unchanged in the urine. The half-life of diphenoxylate in adults averages 7–8 hours.[47,189] Portions of the parent and/or its metabolites may undergo enterohepatic recycling.[189] Diphenoxylate and its active metabolite diphenoxylic acid are excreted in breast milk. Clinical experience with the use of diphenoxylate in pediatrics[180] suggests an initial starting dose of 0.3–0.4 mg/kg/day divided into three or four equal doses, with monitoring for changes in stooling pattern, consistency, and adverse effects.

Adverse effects with diphenoxylate include reactions associated with inappropriate, prolonged, or excessive doses of antidiarrheal agents as discussed above. Other frequent side effects of diphenoxylate are a result of the drug's weak opiate activity and include sedation and drowsiness. Most of the adverse effects of diphenoxylate in children have been described in children who have become acutely intoxicated with the drug following accidental ingestion.[190,191] Initial symptoms following overdose usually involve mild atropinism from the concurrent atropine in the Lomotil brand preparation. In moderate to severe overdose, opiate symptoms appear after approximately 2–3 hours and predominate. The symptoms include bradycardia, slow and depressed respiration, drowsiness, and lethargy and may progress to convulsions and coma. Opiate toxicity from diphenoxylate intoxication is readily reversible with naloxone.[190,191]

Loperamide

Loperamide is an α-diphenylbuteramide derivative that is used extensively for its properties as an antidiar-

rheal agent. This synthetic drug is structurally similar to diphenoxylate. However, unlike diphenoxylate, only limited amounts of loperamide following the usual clinical dosing penetrate into the central nervous system. This lack of penetration at least partially explains the drug's relative lack of central opiate-like adverse effects. Animal studies[192] and preliminary studies in humans[193] suggested that loperamide stimulated absorption rates or had a specific antisecretory effect on intestinal mucosa as its primary mechanism of antidiarrheal effect. Subsequent evaluations have demonstrated that loperamide exerts its antidiarrheal effect in a fashion similar to codeine and other like agents,[193] i.e., a change in motor function of the intestine with a decrease in the rate of fluid movement through the gut. Despite previous animal studies, the carefully controlled study of Schiller et al.[193] demonstrated that the antidiarrheal effect of loperamide was due primarily to a change in intestinal motor function rather than a change in the rate of absorption by intestinal mucosal cells. This effect on intestinal motility is most likely due to an inhibitory (slowing) effect on longitudinal and circular muscle activity.[194] The limited human pharmacokinetic data for loperamide[195] come from studies performed in adults. The drug's half-life ranges from 7 to 15 hours.[195]

Numerous uncontrolled and controlled studies have demonstrated the efficacy of loperamide in improving the time to recovery, decreasing the number of daily stools with improvement in stool consistency. Loperamide as an antidiarrheal drug has been shown to be superior to placebo and at least equivalent to appropriate doses of opioids (e.g., codeine) or diphenoxylate.[182–184,193,194,196,197] The Diarrhoeal Diseases Study Group (U.K.)[184] evaluated the efficacy of loperamide in 315 infants and children between the ages of 3 months and 3 years in a double-blind, placebo-controlled multicenter study. This collaborative study group found loperamide 0.8 mg/kg/day

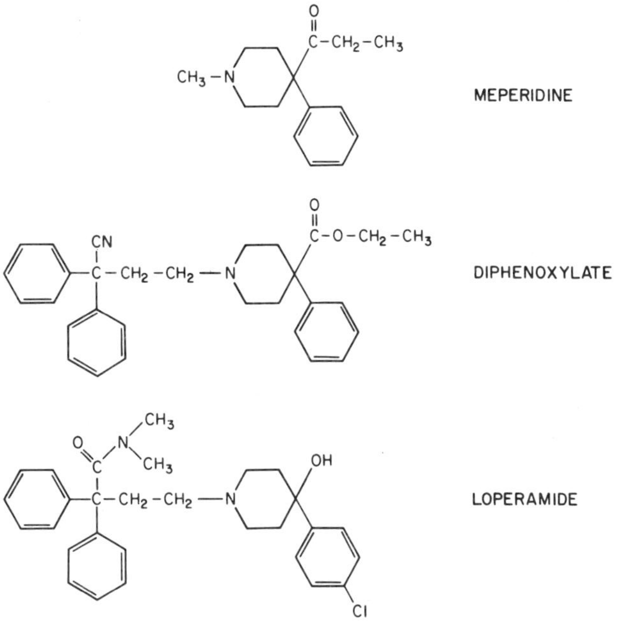

FIGURE 40–3. Chemical structures of meperidine, diphenoxylate, and loperamide.

administered in two divided doses daily along with oral rehydration therapy to be effective and superior to placebo plus oral rehydration therapy. The efficacy and relative lack of associated adverse effects led this study group to support the use of loperamide 0.4 mg/kg administered every 12 hours as adjunctive therapy with rehydration for acute diarrheal disease. Similar positive clinical results with loperamide 0.8 mg/kg/day administered in three divided doses per day as adjunctive treatment of infants with severe acute diarrheal illness were reported by Motala et al.[182] As discussed above, loperamide or any other antidiarrheal agent should not be used as monotherapy, and when it is used, the child's fluid and electrolyte status must be closely monitored.[175,184]

Adverse reactions associated with the use of loperamide in children and adults appear to be unusual. As commented previously, improper use of any antidiarrheal agent can lead to adverse effects on the gastrointestinal tract as well as fluid and electrolyte imbalances. According to pooled data from published studies, adverse reactions associated with loperamide do not appear to differ from those reported in patients receiving placebo. Adverse effects that have been associated with loperamide include central nervous system complaints such as dizziness, nervousness, somnolence, and headache, as well as constipation, vomiting, ileus, and rarely skin rash. The overall safety profile for loperamide led the United States Food and Drug Administration to approve it for use as a nonprescription medication in March 1988. Nevertheless, the potential for loperamide to cause serious adverse effects (ileus, toxic megacolon, etc.) suggests its prudent use in select patients under close medical supervision.

Bismuth

Bismuth-containing preparations have been used for the treatment of various abdominal disorders for over two centuries.[198,199] The primary bismuth-containing product in the United States, bismuth subsalicylate (Pepto-Bismol), is estimated to be in the medicine cabinets of approximately 60 percent of U.S. homes.[198] Despite this phenomenal worldwide product familiarity by health professionals and consumers alike, only recently have controlled evaluations of bismuth-containing products for diarrheal and ulcer disease been undertaken.[198-202] This rejuvenated interest in determining the pharmacokinetics and pharmacodynamics of bismuth salts under controlled conditions was most likely stimulated by the recent determination of the importance of *Helicobacter pylori* (previously *Campylobacter pylori*) in chronic gastritis and ulcer disease in children[199,203-205] and its "rediscovery" in adults.[199,202-206]

Regardless of the salt form administered, only limited amounts of bismuth are absorbed into the systemic circulation following the usual therapeutic doses.[202,207,208] Although earlier studies suggested no absorption of bismuth from oral preparations, these findings were most likely due to the presence of plasma bismuth concentrations that were below the limit of detection of early assay technology.[198,199,202] Atomic absorption spectrometry is now most often used to measure bismuth concentrations in biologic fluids. Froomes and colleagues[208] described the pharmacokinetics of bismuth in healthy adult volunteers and four patients under single- and multiple-dose conditions. The reported bismuth half-life of approximately 18 hours after the first dose was very different from the apparent half-life of 18–22 days determined after chronic doses of bismuth subcitrate for 4–8 weeks. These data underscore the complex disposition characteristics of bismuth that require further critical evaluation. Nevertheless, plasma bismuth concentrations obtained in this study, and in therapeutic evaluations using either subcitrate or subsalicylate salts, do not discourage the continued therapeutic use of these compounds (see later in text). Moreover, available data suggest that the efficacy of bismuth is due to its local concentration–effect relationship rather than concentrations in plasma.[198-202]

The most common bismuth salt used clinically is bismuth subcitrate (DE-NOL) which is available in most countries in the world but not in the United States. Bismuth subsalicylate (Pepto-Bismol) is available in the United States; each molecule contains 58 percent bismuth and 42 percent salicylate. At pH less than 4, bismuth from the subsalicylate or subcitrate salt is nearly completely hydrolyzed to form bismuth oxychloride and salicylic acid from the subsalicylate salt or bismuth citrate from the subcitrate salt. Bismuth and nondissociated bismuth adhere to the mucosal surface of the stomach and can penetrate gastrointestinal tract microvilli.[198] Bismuth appears to localize in ulcer craters, with only trace amounts found in surrounding normal mucosa.[202] The dissociation of bismuth from its salt occurs primarily in the stomach[202]; absorption of salicylate is believed to occur in the small intestine. Available salicylate from the bismuth subsalicylate salt is almost completely absorbed.[207,209] Bismuth reaching the small intestine will bind with bicarbonate and phosphate, forming insoluble bismuth subcarbonate and bismuth phosphate salts. Portions of these bismuth salts reaching the colon will react with hydrogen sulfide produced by anaerobic bacteria, forming insoluble bismuth sulfide which confers the characteristic darkened color of the stool in patients receiving bismuth salts.[198]

Bismuth salts have been used for decades for the symptomatic adjunctive treatment and patient self-management of diarrhea and other gastrointestinal disorders.[198] Soriano-Brucher et al.[201] demonstrated clear superiority of bismuth subsalicylate 100 mg/kg/day divided into five equal doses for 5 days compared to placebo in the treatment of acute diarrhea in children due to viral or bacterial causes. Both treatments (bismuth subsalicylate and placebo) were administered concurrently with appropriate hydration and progressive feeding. Infants and children who received bismuth subsalicylate had significantly lower stool weights sooner, had a decreased need for intravenous fluids, and demonstrated a more favorable clinical improvement more rapidly than patients who received placebo. These data suggest that bismuth salts may be a beneficial adjunctive therapeutic agent with appropriate fluid, electrolyte, and nutrition therapy for infants and children with acute diarrhea.

Similar beneficial clinical responses have been reported with the use of bismuth subsalicylate in children with chronic diarrhea.[200,210,211] Unlike acute diarrheal illness in children, which is usually a result of an enteric infection, chronic diarrhea in children often persists without any identifiable cause. A pathogenic role for bile acids in the etiology of chronic diarrhea has been proposed, since malabsorption of bile acids has been described in a number of these infants,[212,213] combined with a positive therapeutic effect following treatment with the bile acid–sequestering drug cholestyramine.[214] Gryboski and Kocohis[200] compared the effect of bismuth subsalicylate, $\frac{1}{2}$–1 teaspoon four times daily, and cholestyramine, 0.5 gm in two to four equal doses for 7 days, and found both agents to be equally effective in the treatment of children with chronic diarrhea who prior to therapy demonstrated elevated bile acid concentrations in their stool (green stools). Both cholestyramine and bismuth subsalicylate successfully decreased stool frequency, whereas bismuth subsalicylate was more effective in decreasing stool water content. These studies by Gryboski and colleagues[200,211] demonstrate the efficacy of bismuth subsalicylate in the treatment of chronic diarrhea in children as a less expensive alternative to cholestyramine therapy.

Interest in the therapeutic use of bismuth-containing salts in children has escalated with the recognition of the importance of *H. pylori* in the etiology of chronic gastritis and ulcer disease.[199,202–206] Glassman et al.[205] in a prospective evaluation identified *H. pylori* in 16 of their 95 studied children. All 16 of these children had evidence of acute and/or chronic gastritis. The bacterium appears to have a unique affinity for gastric mucosa, including sites of gastric metaplasia.[205] How the organism stimulates a gastric inflammatory response remains unknown. It has been demonstrated that *H. pylori* secretes a protease that can degrade gastric mucus glycoproteins and is also capable of synthesizing a urease that generates bicarbonate and ammonia.[205,216] This local bicarbonate production may protect these organisms from the bactericidal effects of gastric acid while potentiating enzymatic hydrolysis of mucosal glycoprotein. It is not known if invasion of the gastric mucosa by *H. pylori* is a primary event or whether the organism colonizes previously inflamed gastric mucosa.[205] Nevertheless, a definite link appears to exist between the presence of *H. pylori* and active antral gastritis and duodenitis,[202,205] underscoring the importance of drugs that are effective in inhibiting or eradicating this pathogen.[202,217,218] Thus, it would appear important to evaluate for the presence of *H. pylori* in all children with suspected gastric mucosal inflammatory lesions[205] and in particular, children who respond poorly to conventional therapy with antacids and/or histamine H_2-receptor antagonists.

The optimal antimicrobial regimen for eradication of *H. pylori* from gastrointestinal mucosa is yet to be determined. Furthermore, it is not known if antibiotic therapy is most effective when administered topically, systemically, or both. From available experience, it appears that antibiotic therapy is most efficacious in those individuals with documented gastric mucosal disease[205] as compared to those patients with colonization. A host of antibiotics have been used in combination with bismuth salts in the treatment of *H. pylori*-associated gastrointestinal disease, with the most common regimen being bismuth plus amoxicillin. More recent studies have begun to assess the therapeutic effect of combinations of bismuth with more poorly absorbed antibiotics such as furazolidone.[217] Conflicting data exist on the need for concurrent antimicrobial drugs as well as the dose and number of doses administered per day, making it difficult to develop sound recommendations for antimicrobial treatment of these patients. However, it is clear that bismuth salts are effective in the therapy of gastrointestinal diseases.[199,202] What combination antimicrobial, if any, and how it should be dosed concurrently with bismuth-containing salts remains to be determined.

Adverse effects associated with the therapeutic use of bismuth-containing salts are very unusual.[198,199,202] Patients and their family should be forewarned to expect blackened stools due to the fecal excretion of bismuth sulfide and the possible darkening of the tongue. Other side effects of bismuth, which appear uncommon, have included mild dizziness, headache, and constipation. In large doses administered chronically, and particularly in patients with diminished or compromised renal function, bismuth can accumulate causing neurotoxicity. Bismuth-associated neurotoxicity including mild ataxia, myoclonus, tremors, and convulsions has been described in several cases.[198,199,219] In addition, an apparent epidemic of neurotoxicity was described in approximately 1000 patients in France between the years 1973 and 1980.[198] The reason for this apparent epidemic is unknown and the epidemic has not recurred, but it appeared to occur in those patients who self-medicated with various bismuth salts for long periods (4 weeks to 30 years) with ingestion of large daily doses. Plasma bismuth concentrations in patients who have developed neurotoxicity are highly variable but appear to be greater than 150–300 μg/liter. Plasma bismuth concentrations following therapeutic doses, even for prolonged periods (e.g., greater than 8 weeks), have been reported to range between 50 and 70 μg/liter.[198,208]

The potential for bismuth salts to interfere with the absorption of other concurrently administered drugs has not been adequately studied. Preliminary data suggest decreased absorption of tetracycline, iron, and calcium when administered concurrently with bismuth salts.[202] Bismuth subsalicylate tablets (Pepto-Bismol brand), but not liquid, contain calcium carbonate as part of the formulation and thus may further decrease the absorption of tetracycline. Moreover, because Pepto-Bismol contains subsalicylate, this product should be used cautiously in patients receiving anticogulants (e.g., warfarin) or oral antidiabetic agents (e.g., sulfonylurea).[198] Last, it is important to recall that more than 90 percent of the salicylate administered with the bismuth subsalicylate formulation is absorbed systemically.[198,199,207,209] From the data of Soriano-Brucher et al.[201] using bismuth subsalicylate 100 mg/kg/day in children, plasma salicylate concentrations corresponded to those achieved with the usual doses of salicylate 50 mg/kg/day in children. To date we are unaware of any data describing an association between bismuth subsalicylate administration and the development of Reye's syndrome. However, because many of the infants and children who may receive bismuth subsalicylate will be suffering from a concurrent viral infection, caution should be exercised in the use of this drug in these patients.

Conclusion: Antidiarrheal Medications in Children

Antidiarrheal medications have been used and abused for decades, some for centuries. In pediatric practice the majority of these drugs find limited use on the advice of health care providers. However, parents may often give these drugs to their children on their own. The mainstay of therapy for acute diarrheal disease in pediatrics is appropriate fluid and electrolyte replacement and maintenance. Furthermore, due to the mechanism of action of systemically active antidiarrheal agents, i.e., decrease in gastrointestinal motility, caution must be exercised in their use in children. Use of these drugs can mask ongoing fluid losses; conversely, these agents can promote excessive fluid accumulation in the bowel, which can lead to fluid imbalances and abdominal distention extending to toxic megacolon. Nevertheless, antidiarrheal agents such as loperamide can hasten clinical improvement in infants and children when properly combined with rehydration therapy. The exact role and true need for such adjunctive therapy of acute diarrheal diseases in children remain to be defined.

For chronic diarrhea in childhood, a number of therapeutic approaches have been attempted, and the efficacy of drug therapy depends on the proposed etiology of the diarrhea. Adsorbents such as bismuth and possibly kaolin–pectin may be effective for bacterial toxin–associated diarrhea; cholestyramine and bismuth salts have been effective for chronic diarrhea associated with malabsorption of bile acids as well as disease associated with infection. Obviously, therapy must be individualized.

The rejuvenated interest in this group of drugs appears to reflect the recent excitement surrounding the therapeutic benefit of bismuth salts for both diarrhea and ulcer disease. As our understanding of the association between *H. pylori* and pediatric ulcer disease increases, the use of bismuth salts in pediatrics will also increase. Continued clinical monitoring of children for possible consequences of systemic bismuth absorption as well as the nearly complete absorption of salicylate from the bismuth subsalicylate preparation (Pepto-Bismol) will be necessary to ensure the safe use of these compounds both acutely and during chronic administration.

LAXATIVES

Primary and persistent constipation is a frequent clinical problem in pediatrics. A number of medications are common causes of constipation, some of which are outlined in Table 40–8. Constipation in children can result from defects in filling or emptying the rectum that may be caused by drug use (e.g., opiates) or disease (e.g., hypothyroidism), or from bowel obstruction or colonic stasis caused by a structural abnormality or by Hirschsprung's disease. Last, chronic constipation, often associated with

soiling of undergarments, can be a primary symptom associated with social and psychologic difficulties.

Laxatives are most commonly used in children for the management of occasional or chronic constipation. When constipation is severe laxatives are used to dislodge impacted stool. The usual course of laxative therapy for chronic severe constipation with impacted stool is 3–6 months. However, it is not uncommon for children to be maintained on regular laxatives for several years. The object of therapy is to allow the dilated megacolon to shrink in size and to diminish inappropriate external sphincter spasm associated with the passage of large, painful stools.[221]

In children, laxative use on the recommendation of health professionals is most commonly administered as part of a "bowel preparation" given to evacuate the bowel prior to gastrointestinal radiology or colonoscopy. Laxatives are also administered to children with accidental poisoning who have ingested a compound with a constipating effect. A host of laxative medications are available to the consuming public.

Dietary fiber and bulk-forming laxatives increase the water content, mass, and rate of transit of the stool. Bulk-forming laxatives are associated with very few adverse effects, with the exception of gas production by fermentable fiber. Although limited specific data are available, bulk-forming laxatives may decrease the intestinal absorption of some drugs via adsorption. Drugs that may demonstrate decreased absorption include digitalis glycosides, salicylates, and possibly coumarin derivatives.[220] The exact nature of this possible interaction is unknown, but the interaction suggests caution with concurrent coadministration of medication with these or any type of laxatives. Because these agents are capable of adsorbing large amounts of water in producing their bulk, they have also been used in patients with secretory diarrhea.

Docusates are anionic surfactants that are believed to promote hydration of stool, keeping it soft and thus easily passed through the colon. These drugs are often used to prevent "straining" that can be associated with defecation. Their time of onset of effect is usually slow (e.g., 2–4 days).

Stimulant laxatives are either anthraquinone derivatives (senna, cascara) or diphenylmethane derivatives (phenolphthalein, bisacodyl). These compounds exert their laxative effect by direct stimulation of nerves and effects on net fluid flux into the bowel lumen. The most bothersome side effect of this class of laxatives is excessive cramping. Senna compounds have been associated with

TABLE 40–8. MEDICATIONS THAT MAY CAUSE CONSTIPATION

Antacids (Ca- or Al-containing)
Anticholinergics (e.g., atropine)
Antihistamines, H$_1$ (e.g., diphenhydramine)
Cyclic antidepressants
Diuretics (hypokalemia)
Heavy metals (e.g., lead, iron)
Opiates
Phenothiazines (anticholinergic effects)
Polystyrene resins (e.g., cholestyramine)

Adapted from Breenton,[220] with permission.

melanosis coli, a presumably benign condition.[222] Phenolphthalein can cause severe allergic dermatologic side effects.[223] The recommended doses of these agents produce highly variable results in patients: the dose that may be therapeutic for one patient may result in severe abdominal cramping and diarrhea in another.

The saline cathartics are poorly absorbed and promote catharsis by their osmotic properties. Some preliminary data suggest that magnesium-containing salts may also stimulate intestinal fluid secretion and motility by increasing the duodenal secretion of cholecystokinin.[220]

Osmotic agents facilitate stooling by promoting water flux into the colon. The resultant luminal distention promotes peristalsis. Glycerin (used rectally only) and lactulose are examples of these agents. Lactulose is an unabsorbable sugar that can be fermented in the colon with resultant gas production. Occasionally, the gas production is severe enough to warrant discontinuing or decreasing the dose of the drug. A solution of polyethylene glycol and sodium and potassium salts is also available, which, if consumed in sufficient quantity at a rapid enough pace, can induce colonic lavage sufficient to cleanse the colon for radiographic or colonoscopic procedures. It has also been advocated by some clinicians as oral therapy for disimpactions. Its relative unpalatability often interferes with successful use.

Lubricant laxatives act by coating hard feces and facilitating passage. The possibility of aspiration limits use in patients with gastroesophageal reflux or swallowing difficulties. Palatability has been enhanced for some products by combining them with an emulsifying agent. Although concern has been voiced regarding possible interference with fat-soluble vitamin absorption, there are no prospective studies demonstrating this effect.

Enemas are used in the initial stages of management of fecal impaction. For children the Fleet's sodium biphosphate enema is most frequently used. Enemas are generally given at 12- 24-hour intervals to allow passage of impacted stools and prevent electrolyte imbalance.[224] Iatrogenic hyperphosphatemia, hypocalcemia, and hypernatremic dehydration have been reported with overly aggressive use. Mineral oil enemas given the night before a cleansing biphosphate enema may facilitate disimpaction. Saline enemas are most economical and, among all enema solutions, are least likely to induce abnormalities in rectal biopsy specimens obtained after enema administration.[225] Various exotic concoctions of milk, molasses, soapsuds, etc. are popular with selected grandmothers and clinicians the world over. Their advantages are unclear, at best, and some reports of rectal irritation have been described.

SALICYLATES USED IN GASTROINTESTINAL DISEASE

Sulfasalazine

Inflammatory bowel disease in children continues to pose important clinical and therapeutic challenges for the clinician. Inflammatory bowel disease includes two chronic disorders of unknown etiology, ulcerative colitis (UC) and Crohn's disease (CD),[226,227] and one probably self-limited form, nonspecific colitis. Accurate incidence and prevalence data for either UC or CD are unavailable, but estimates range from 4 to 6 cases per 100,000 for CD and from 3 to 13 per 100,000 for UC. Less than 10 percent of all inflammatory bowel disease occurs during the first decade of life. UC is a chronic nonspecific ulcerative process characterized by acute and chronic inflammation that is limited to colonic mucosa. The majority of UC cases involve the rectum with varying degrees of proximal extension. In contrast, CD is a chronic inflammatory disease that is characterized by transmural inflammation which often extends through the serosa, resulting in sinus tract, microabscess, and fistula formation; CD can involve any portion of the gastrointestinal tract.[226] Because the etiology of UC and CD is unknown, therapy has been directed by clinical experience, trial and error, and therapeutic approaches based on hypothetical etiologic targets. Sulfasalazine and corticosteroids are the mainstay of pharmacotherapy for inflammatory bowel disease involving the colon. Some data suggest a secondary role for immunosuppressive drugs (e.g., 6-mercaptopurine, azathioprine, or cyclosporine) and/or metronidazole in selected patients with CD.[226–228] Corticosteroids and immunosuppressant drugs are discussed elsewhere in this text (Chapter 41, page 466).

Sulfasalazine was first synthesized in 1938–1939 by the Scandinavian rheumatologist Nana Svartz[228,229] for use on her patients with rheumatoid arthritis. Though use of the drug in patients with rheumatoid arthritis was associated with variable clinical response, impressive results were obtained when the drug was tried with patients with colitis. Subsequently, sulfasalazine has become the most common drug used in the treatment of inflammatory bowel disease in both children and adults.[226,230,231] Sulfasalazine is a conjugate of 5-aminosalicylic acid and sulfapyridine linked by an azo bond.[228,231] Following oral administration, a portion (20–30 percent) of the compound is absorbed as sufasalazine from the proximal gastrointestinal tract. Peak plasma sulfasalazine concentrations have been described at 3–5 hours after a dose and have been highly variable. This variability is most likely the result of interindividual differences in absorption[231] rather than polymorphism in the metabolism of sulfapyridine.[231–234] The apparent half-life of sulfasalazine ranges from 5 to 16 hours, and the apparent volume of distribution is approximately >1 liter/kg.[47,232,235] Very little is absorbed as 5-aminosalicylic acid, and none appears to be converted systemically from sulfasalazine to sulfapyridine or 5-aminosalicylic acid.[232,235] Less than 10 percent of the administered dose is excreted in the urine unchanged as parent sulfasalazine. The majority of the absorbed drug is excreted via the bile and metabolized in the distal small intestine and colon.[231,232] Nearly 99 percent of sulfasalazine and absorbed sulfapyridine is bound to plasma proteins, primarily albumin.[236] Limited pharmacokinetic data in children suggest no differences in the disposition characteristics of sulfasalazine between children and adults.[47,234] Moreover, the disposition of sulfasalazine has been shown to be identical in healthy adult volunteers and in patients with inflammatory bowel disease.[235]

Unabsorbed sulfasalazine and systemically absorbed parent drug that is excreted in the bile back into the intestine are metabolized by colonic bacteria to sulfapyridine and 5-aminosalicylic acid. Intestinal bacteria present in the distal small intestine and colon reduce the azo bond, liberating sulfapyridine and 5-aminosalicylic acid. Metabolism studies in germ-free rats have demonstrated no evidence of sulfasalazine reduction.[237] Similarly, patients with ileostomies are unable to metabolize the compound, and most of the drug is excreted unchanged in the ileostomy effluent.[238] Further supporting the role of bacterial azoreductase in the metabolism of sulfasalazine was the lack of effect of concurrent phenobarbital on the drug's metabolism in these cholectomized patients with ileostomies.[238] Following reduction of the azo bond, nearly all sulfapyridine is absorbed from the colon, whereas only small amounts of 5-aminosalicylic acid are absorbed systemically (usual plasma 5-aminosalicylic acid concentrations <2 mg/liter). The majority of the sulfapyridine is excreted in the urine as free or metabolized sulfa, whereas the majority of the 5-aminosalicylic acid is recovered in the feces.

These metabolism data support the hypothesis that sulfasalazine is in fact a prodrug moiety that results in the deposition of 5-aminosalicylic acid within the colon where it remains essentially unabsorbed, producing a local therapeutic effect. Moreover, when sulfapyridine and 5-aminosalicylic acid are administered individually as separate agents via the oral route, both are absorbed into the systemic circulation from the proximal gastrointestinal tract and excreted as parent drug and metabolites in the urine.[231] These data, combined with experience with 5-aminosalicylic acid enemas and time-release product formulations,[230] further support the belief that 5-aminosalicylic acid is the primary pharmacologically active moiety.

The use of sulfasalazine is associated with a frequent occurrence of adverse reactions. Side effects are experienced by as many as 21 percent of children and adults who receive the drug.[230,233] The incidence and severity of adverse reactions appear to decrease (e.g., to less than 12 percent) with chronic therapy.[233] Most of these adverse drug effects are mild and include nausea, vomiting, anorexia, skin rash, headache, and less frequently, diarrhea and epigastric distress. Sulfasalazine-induced headache is particularly common and often limits the use of this drug in children. Many of these adverse effects have been shown to be dose-related and have supported initiating therapy at lower doses (e.g., 30 mg/kg/day), with slow escalation to currently recommended doses of 50–75 mg/kg/day. Experience with newer "locally acting anti-inflammatory" salicylates,[230] which do not contain the sulfa moiety, has demonstrated clearly that the majority of sulfasalazine adverse drug reactions are a result of absorbed sulfapyridine. Das and colleagues[233] described a close relationship between the incidence of sulfasalazine adverse reactions and serum concentrations of total sulfapyridine (i.e., parent plus metabolite concentrations of sulfapyridine) of 50 mg/liter. Those patients with elevated sulfapyridine concentrations were also identified as slow acetylator phenotypes.[233,234] Thus, considering that only approximately one-third of children are both rapid ace-

tylators and hydroxylators of sulfanilamide, slow dose titration appears prudent.

Other, more serious adverse effects associated with sulfasalazine include lupus-like reactions,[239] agranulocytosis,[240] and severe hepatotoxic reactions.[241,242] These reactions appear to be due to the sulfapyridine moiety of sulfasalazine. Adverse reactions of an allergic nature appear to occur early in the course of therapy (within the first month) and have been reported to respond to drug discontinuation or high-dose corticosteroid therapy. In patients with less severe allergic reactions, such as skin rash with or without fever, some of the investigators have suggested a desensitization protocol for sulfasalazine.[243] Despite the potential benefit of desensitization in some patients, the availability of sulfonamide-free 5-aminosalicylic acid preparations, such as 5-aminosalicylic acid enemas and newer congeners currently under investigation, would appear to negate the need for such a therapeutic approach. Overall, as many as 80–90 percent of patients intolerant of or allergic to sulfasalazine are able to tolerate topical 5-aminosalicylic acid.[230,244]

Very few drug interactions have been reported with sulfasalazine, suggesting that although the amount of sulfapyridine absorbed is capable of inducing adverse reactions, insufficient amounts are absorbed to interfere with protein binding or metabolism of other drugs or bilirubin. Sulfasalazine has been shown to impair the absorption of folic acid both in healthy subjects and in patients with inflammatory bowel disease. This interaction is most likely a result of sulfasalazine's competitive inhibition of the jejunal brush border enzyme folate conjugate which is responsible for hydrolysis of polyglutamate folate to the intestinally transported monoglutamate form.[231,245] In patients who require supplemental folic acid, it would appear prudent to monitor serum vitamin B_{12} concentrations to adequately assess for disease/drug-induced anemia that would be masked by folic acid therapy.

Concurrent cholestyramine, which may be used in some patients with CD, will decrease the azo reduction of sulfasalazine. This effect is most likely due to direct adsorption of sulfasalazine by cholestyramine.[231] Concurrent administration of broad-spectrum antibiotics may diminish the colonic metabolism of sulfasalazine, presumably by their effect on gut flora responsible for azo bond reduction. This potential drug interaction appears highly variable.[231] Sulfasalazine has also been shown to decrease the bioavailability of digoxin, as reflected by a decrease of approximately 25 percent in serum digoxin concentrations in volunteer studies.[246] A similar effect of sulfasalazine has been described with ferrous sulfate.[231] The clinical significance of these reported interactions with digoxin and ferrous sulfate is unknown, but they suggest that when needed in patients receiving sulfasalazine, their oral administration should be separated by 1–2 hours. Although sulfasalazine and sulfapyridine cross the placenta and are secreted in breast milk, both appear to be weak displacers of bilirubin.[231] Clinical studies evaluating sulfasalazine administration during pregnancy and in breast-feeding mothers have failed to describe any fetal effects.[231]

OTHER DRUGS USED IN THE TREATMENT OF GASTROINTESTINAL DISORDERS

Sucralfate

Sucralfate is a basic aluminum salt of sulfated sucrose formed from sucrose octasulfate and polyaluminum hydroxide. The drug is structurally related to heparin but contains no anticoagulant properties. At pH 4 or less, extensive polymerization of sucralfate occurs, resulting in the production of a very sticky, viscid, yellow-white gel. This gel appears to adhere preferentially to inflammatory or ulcer lesions of the gastrointestinal mucosa.[247] This substance may also act as a protective physical barrier against the action of gastric acid, pepsin, and bile acids on damaged or inflamed mucosal surfaces. In humans this pasty gel remains adherent to ulcerated epithelium for more than 6 hours and appears to be more adherent to duodenal than gastric ulcers. Sucralfate possesses no practical acid-neutralizing capacity. In addition to adhering to mucosal surfaces, some data have suggested that sucralfate locally stimulates the formation of prostaglandins by the gastric mucosa, thus exerting a cytoprotective effect.[247]

Very little if any sucralfate is absorbed from the gastrointestinal tract into the systemic circulation. However, as the drug continues to react with gastric acid, free aluminum ion is released. In adults plasma aluminum concentrations were doubled following a regimen of sucralfate 1 gm administered four times daily for 2 days.[47,247] As a result of this appreciable systemic absorption of aluminum, caution must be exercised in the use of sucralfate in infants and children with immature or impaired renal function.

Numerous studies have demonstrated the efficacy of sucralfate in the prophylaxis or treatment of gastric and duodenal ulcer disease, gastroesophageal reflux disease, and nonsteroidal anti-inflammatory drug (NSAID)-associated ulcer disease.[247-251] Sucralfate has been shown to be superior to placebo and at least as effective as histamine H_2-receptor antagonist therapy in the treatment of these patients. In these studies, drug administration before meals was found to be more effective than after meals. This meal-related influence on the therapeutic effect of sucralfate may merely be a result of the acid-buffering effect of food, increasing gastric pH to values above those which promote polymerization of the drug. Sucralfate has also been shown to be an effective agent for prophylaxis against stress-induced bleeding. Recent data have suggested that sucralfate may be more desirable as a stress ulcer prophylactic agent than antacids or histamine H_2-receptor antagonists in intubated patients, because sucralfate maintains the acid medium of the stomach, thus protecting against bacterial overgrowth which may predispose critically ill patients to potential aspiration pneumonia and/or systemic infection.[252]

Limited published experience with sucralfate use in pediatrics exists.[251-253] Arguelles-Martin and colleagues[251] demonstrated that sucralfate tablets 0.5 gm in children <6 years of age and 1.0 gm in children >6 years of age administered four times daily ½ hour before meals and at bedtime was equivalent to cimetidine in the treatment of reflux esophagitis in 75 children 3 months to 13 years of age. Sucralfate tablets were dissolved (not crushed) in water, and the drug was administered as a suspension. Preliminary data suggested efficacy of an oral sucralfate suspension in the therapy of chemotherapy-induced mucositis.[253,254] However, Schenep et al.[253] were unable to demonstrate any substantial effect of sucralfate in the prevention or treatment of chemotherapy-induced mucositis. These authors did find, like Driks et al.,[252] that sucralfate reduced colonization of the alimentary tract by potential pathogens. The mechanism of this effect is unknown. However, unlike the study of Driks et al.,[252] Schenep's patients were receiving placebo,[253] suggesting that factors other than gastric acid concentration were influencing alimentary colonization in patients receiving sucralfate.

Adverse reactions associated with sucralfate occur infrequently.[247,249] Constipation, dry mouth, diarrhea, nausea, gastric distress, and dizziness have been reported. Sucralfate has been shown to bind phosphate within the intestine, causing a decrease in plasma phosphate concentrations. As a result, serum phosphate concentrations should be monitored in patients receiving sucralfate. This effect on phosphate may be beneficial in patients with compromised renal function; however, caution must be exercised in the use of this drug in these patients due to the concurrent absorption of aluminum.

Conflicting data exist on the potential for sucralfate to decrease the absorption of simultaneously administered medications.[247] Recent studies in humans have demonstrated no significant effect of sucralfate on the bioavailability or disposition of chlorpropamide, digoxin, prednisone, theophylline, or NSAIDs.[247,255] Depending on the time of coadministration of sucralfate with another drug, some decrease (not statistically significant) in oral bioavailability as well as in the rate of absorption was observed. However, the clinical significance of these findings would appear to be minimal. Overall, these data suggest little or no effect of sucralfate on the bioavailability of most compounds. Garrelts and colleagues[256] recently described a significant decrease in the bioavailability of ciprofloxacin when this drug was coadministered with sucralfate 1 gm in eight healthy adult volunteers. Similar data has been reported for norfloxacin,[257] another fluoroquinolone, suggesting a possible propensity for this interaction with this class of antibiotics. Considering the variability of these findings, it would appear prudent to separate sucralfate administration from the administration of other drugs by a minimum of 1–2 hours. Last, since sucralfate is activated by acid present within the gastrointestinal tract, antacids should not be administered less than 30 minutes before or after sucralfate administration, nor should patients receive concurrent therapy with histamine H_2-receptor antagonists or proton pump inhibitors.

Misoprostol

Misoprostol is a synthetic analog of prostaglandin E_1 which has been shown to be effective in the prevention and treatment of gastrointestinal lesions due to NSAIDs and alcohol, in the treatment of gastric and duodenal ulcers, and as a prophylactic agent for the prevention of stress ulcers.[258,259] Prostaglandins are naturally occurring fatty acids that have been identified in most body tissues, fluids, and organs and that, depending on the series, possess varied pharmacologic properties. In the gastrointestinal tract, prostaglandin E_1 competitively inhibits basal and nocturnal acid secretion as well as histamine-, pentagastrin-, and coffee-stimulated gastric acid secretion by the parietal cell. These effects are very similar to those observed with histamine H_2-receptor antagonists. In addition, prostaglandin E_1 protects the gastrointestinal mucosa by stimulating mucus and bicarbonate secretion, thus increasing the natural mucus–bicarbonate barrier.[259] Misoprostol mimics the effects of prostaglandin E_1.

No data are available describing the pharmacokinetics of misoprostol in pediatrics. In adults the drug is rapidly absorbed following oral administration of the tablet formulation. The drug is rapidly and extensively metabolized (deesterified) to its free acid, which is its principal metabolite, is pharmacologically active, and is the only product measurable in plasma. The half-life of misoprostol free acid (SC-30695) ranges from 20 to 40 minutes.

Misoprostol has been shown to improve the activity of exogenous pancreatic enzyme supplementation in patients with cystic fibrosis.[260] The beneficial effect of misoprostol in improving fat absorption in cystic fibrosis patients was observed only in those patients who had absorption of <90 percent fat on standard enzyme therapy. Thus, misoprostol may improve fat absorption in cystic fibrosis patients who continue to malabsorb fat despite maximal pancreatic enzyme supplementation. The reason for this beneficial effect of misoprostol is unknown, but it may be due to the drug's effect on increasing duodenal bicarbonate and decreasing gastric acid concentrations. Both of these effects would decrease pancreatic enzyme destruction by acid and increase the amount of enzymes that reach the duodenum. Similar effects of protecting exogenously administered pancreatic enzymes from destruction by gastric acid have been described with the coadministration of histamine H_2-receptor antagonists. The efficacy of misoprostol for other gastrointestinal disorders in pediatrics in unknown and remains to be studied. The most common adverse effects during misoprostol therapy in adults have included diarrhea, abdominal pain, flatulence, and loose stools. The incidence of diarrhea appears to be minimized if the drug is administered with food. Due to the drug's uterotonic effects, misoprostol should not be used during pregancy.

REFERENCES

1. Lundgren O, Svanvik J, Jivegard L: Enteric nervous system I. physiology and pathophysiology of the intestinal tract. Dig Dis Sci 34:264–283, 1989
2. Isreal EJ, Walker WA: Host defense in gut and related disorders. Pediatr Clin No Am 35:1–15, 1988
3. Freier S, Lebenthal E: Neuroendocrine-immune interactions in the gut. J Pediatr Gastroenterol Nutr 9:4–12, 1989
4. Milla PJ: Gastrointestinal motility disorders in children. Pediatr Clin No Am 35:311–330, 1988
5. Burks TF: Gastrointestinal pharmacology. Annu Rev Pharmacol Ther 16:15–29, 1976
6. Gubbins PO, Bertch KE: Drug absorption in gastrointestinal disease and surgery. Pharmacotherapy 9:285–295, 1989
7. Van Hoogdalem EJ, de Boer AG, Breimer DD: Intestinal drug absorption enhancement: An overview. Pharmac Ther 44:407–443, 1989
8. deBoer AG, Moolenaar F, deLeede LGJ, Breimer DD: Rectal drug administration: Clinical pharmacokinetic considerations. Clin Pharmacokinet 7:285–311, 1982
9. Wolfe MM, Soll AH: The physiology of gastric acid secretion. N Engl J Med 319:1707–1715, 1989
10. Nord KS: Peptic ulcer disease in the pediatric population. Pediatr Clin No Am 35:117–140, 1988
11. Fordtran JS, Morawski SG, Richardson CT: In vivo and in vitro evaluation of liquid antacids. N Engl J Med 288:923–928, 1973
12. Morrissey JF, Barreras RF: Drug therapy: Antacid therapy. N Engl J Med 290:550–554, 1974
13. Texter EC Jr: A critical look at the clinical use of antacids in acid-peptic disease and gastric acid rebound. Am J Gastroenterol 84:97–108, 1989
14. Hollander D, Tarnawski A, Gergely H: Protection against alcohol-induced gastric mucosal injury by aluminum-containing compounds: Sucralfate, antacids and aluminum sulfate. Scand J Gastroenterol 1:151–153, 1986
15. Preclik G, Strange EF, Gerber K, Fetzer G, Horn H, Ditschuneit H: Stimulation of mucosal prostaglandin synthesis in human stomach and duodenum by antacid treatment. Gut 30:148–151, 1989
16. Brunton LL: Agents for control of gastric acidity and treatment of peptic ulcers, in Gilman AG, Rall TW, Nies AS, Taylor P (eds): Goodman and Gilmans: The Pharmacologic Basis of Therapeutics, 8th ed. New York, Pergamon Press, 1990, p 908
17. Derrida S, Nury B, Slama R, Marois F, Moreau R, Soupison T, Sicot C: Occult gastrointestinal bleeding in high-risk intensive care unit patients receiving antacid prophylaxis: Frequency and significance. Crit Care Med 17:122–125, 1989
18. Burget DW, Chiverton SG, Hunt RH: Is there an optimal degree of acid suppression for healing of duodenal ulcers? A model of the relationship between ulcer healing and acid suppression. Gastroenterology 99:345–351, 1990
19. Butler ML, Gersh H: Antacid vs placebo in hospitalized gastric ulcer patients: A controlled therapeutic study. Am J Dig Dis 20:803–807, 1975
20. Sturdevant RAL, Isenberg JI, Secrist D, Ansfield J: Antacid and placebo produced similar pain relief in duodenal ulcer patients. Gastroenterology 72:1–5, 1977
21. Littman A, Welch R, Fruin RC, Aronson AR: Controlled trials of aluminum hydroxide gels for peptic ulcer. Gastroenterology 73:6–10, 1977
22. Peterson WL, Sturdevant RAL, Frankl HD, Richardson CT, Isenberg JI, Elashoff JD, Jones JQ, Gross RA, McCallum RW, Fordtran JS: Healing of duodenal ulcer with an antacid regimen. N Engl J Med 297:341–345, 1977
23. Grossman MI, Kurata JH, Rotter JI, Meyer JH, Robert A, Richardson CT, Debas HT, Jensen DM: Peptic ulcer: New therapies, new diseases. Ann Intern Med 95:609–627, 1981
24. Morris T, Rhodes J: Progress report. Antacids and peptic ulcer—A reappraisal. Gut 20:538–545, 1979
25. Shuman RB, Schuster DP, Zuckerman GR: Prophylactic therapy for stress ulcer bleeding: A reappraisal. Ann Intern Med 106:562–567, 1987
26. Kleiman RL, Adair CG, Ephgrave KS: Stress ulcers: Current understanding of pathogenesis and prophylaxis. Drug Intell Clin Pharm 22:452–460, 1988
27. Malagelada JR, Carlson GL: Antacids and HCl. Scand J Gastroenterol 17(suppl 75):10–12, 1982
28. Stiel JN, Mitchell CA, Radcliff FJ, Peper DW: Hypercalcemia in patients with peptic ulceration receiving large doses of calcium carbonate. Gastroenterology 53:900–904, 1967
29. Fordtan JS: Acid rebound. N Engl J Med 279:900–905, 1968
30. Breuhaus H, Akre OH, Eyerly JB: Nocturnal gastric secretion in normal and duodenal ulcer patients on various forms of therapy. Gastroenterology 16:172–180, 1950
31. Erckenbrecht J, Kienle U, Zollner L, Wrenbeck M: Effects of high dose antacids on bowel motility. Digestion 25:244–247, 1982

32. Spencer H, Lender M: Adverse effects of aluminum containing antacids on mineral metabolism. Gastroenterology 76:603–606, 1979
33. Berlyne GM, Ben-Ari J, Pest D, Weinberger J, Stern M, Gilmore GR, Levine R: Hyperaluminemia from aluminum resins in renal failure. Lancet 2:494–496, 1970
34. Parsons V, Davies C, Goode C, Ogy C, Siddiqui J: Aluminum in bone from patients with renal failure. Br Med J 4:273–275, 1971
35. Kaehny WD, Hegg AP, Alfrey AC: Gastrointestinal absorption of aluminum from aluminum-containing antacids. N Engl J Med 296:1389–1390, 1977
36. Humphrey M, Kennon S, Pramanik A: Hypermagnesemia from antacid administration in a newborn infant. J Pediatr 98:313–314, 1981
37. Brand JM, Greer FR: Hypermagnesemia and intestinal perforation following antacid administration in a premature infant. Pediatrics 85:121–124, 1990
38. Portuguez-Malavasi A, Aranda J: Antacid bezoar in a newborn. Pediatrics 63:679–680, 1979
39. D'Arcy PF, McElnay JC: Drug-antacid interactions: Assessment of clinical importance. Drug Intell Clin Pharm 21:607–617, 1987
40. Gugler R, Allgayer H: Effects of antacids on the clinical pharmacokinetics of drugs: An update. Clin Pharmacokinet 18:210–219, 1990
41. Sutphen JL, Dillard VL, Pipan ME: Antacid and formula effects on gastric acidity in infants with gastroesophageal reflux. Pediatrics 78:55–57, 1986
42. Chremos AN: Pharmacodynamics of famotidine in humans. Am J Med 81(suppl 4B):3–7, 1986
43. Berardi RR, Tankanow RM, Nostrant TT: Comparison of famotidine with cimetidine and ranitidine. Clin Pharm 7:271–284, 1988
44. Feston JW: Cimetidine I. Developments, pharmacology and efficacy. Ann Intern Med 97:573–580, 1982
45. Freston JW: Cimetidine II. Adverse reactions and patterns of use. Ann Intern Med 97:728–734, 1982
46. Zeldis JB, Friedman LS, Isselbacher KJ: Ranitidine: A new H₂-receptor antagonist. N Engl J Med 309:1368–1373, 1983
47. Lauritsen K, Laursen LS, Rask-Madsen J: Clinical pharmacokinetics of drugs used in the treatment of gastrointestinal diseases. Clin Pharmacokinet 19(part I):11–31, (part II):94–125, 1990
48. Tam PKH, Saing H: The use of H₂-receptor antagonist in the treatment of peptic ulcer disease in children. J Pediatr Gastroenteral Nutr 8:41–46, 1989
49. Somogyi A, Gugler R: Clinical pharmacokinetics of cimetidine. Clin Pharmacokinet 8:463–495, 1983
50. Smith SR, Kendall MJ: Ranitidine versus cimetidine: A comparison of their potential to cause clinically important drug interactions. Clin Pharmacokinet 15:44–56, 1988
51. McCarthy DM: Ranitidine or cimetidine (editorial). Ann Intern Med 99:551–553, 1983
52. Chattiwalla Y, Colon AR, Scanlon JW: The use of cimetidine in the newborn. Pediatrics 65:301–302, 1980
53. Chin TWF, MacLeod SM, Fenje P, Baltodano A, Edmonds JF, Soldin SJ: Pharmacokinetics of cimetidine in critically ill children. Pediatr Pharmacol 2:285–292, 1982
54. Aranda JV, Outerbridge EW, Schentag JJ: Pharmacodynamics and kinetics of cimetidine in a premature newborn. Am J Dis Child 137:1207, 1983
55. Thomson RB, Attenburrow AA, Goel KM: Cimetidine in primary duodenal ulcer in children. Scott Med J 28:164–167, 1983
56. Martyn JAJ: Cimetidine and/or antacid for the control of gastric acidity in pediatric burn patients. Crit Care Med 13:1–3, 1985
57. Lloyd CW, Martin WJ, Taylor BD, Hauser AR: Pharmacokinetics and pharmacodynamics of cimetidine and metabolites in critically ill children. J Pediatr 107:295–300, 1985
58. Lacroix J, Infante-Rivard C, Gauthier M, Rousseau E, Van Doesburg N: Upper gastrointestinal tract bleeding acquired in a pediatric intensive care unit: Prophylaxis trial with cimetidine. J Pediatr 108:1015–1018, 1986
59. Murphy S, Eastham EJ, Nelson R, Jackson RH: Duodenal ulceration in 110 children (Abstr.) Arch Dis Child 61:628–629, 1986
60. Bodemar G, Norlander B, Fransson L, Walan A: The absorption of cimetidine before and during maintenance treatment with cimetidine and the influence of a meal on the absorption of cimetidine: Studies in patients with ulcer disease. Br J Clin Pharmacol 7:23–31, 1979
61. Gugler R, Brand M, Somogyi A: Impaired cimetidine absorption due to antacids and metoclopramide. Eur J Clin Pharmacol 20:225–228, 1981
62. Albin H, Vincon G, Lalague MC, Couzigou P, Amouretti M: Effect of sucralfate on the bioavailability of cimetidine. Eur J Clin Pharmacol 32:97–99, 1987
63. D'Angio R, Mayersohn M, Conrad KA, Bliss M: Cimetidine absorption in humans during sucralfate coadministration. Br J Clin Pharmacol 21:515–520, 1986
64. Walkenstein SS, Dubb JW, Randolph WC, Westlake WJ, Stote RM, Intoccia AP: Bioavailability of cimetidine in man. Gastroenterology 74:360–365, 1978
65. Schenker S, Dicke J, Johnson RF, Mor LL, Henderson GI: Human placental transport of cimetidine. J Clin Invest 80:1428–1434, 1987
66. Taylor DC, Cresswell PR, Bartlett DC: The metabolism and elimination of cimetidine, a histamine H₂-receptor antagonist in the rat, dog, and man. Drug Metab Dispos 6:21–30, 1978
67. Ziemniak JA, Assael BM, Padoan R, Schentag JJ: The bioavailability and pharmacokinetics of cimetidine and its metabolites in juvenile cystic fibrosis patients: Age related differences as compared to adults. Eur J Clin Pharmacol 26:183–189, 1984
68. Lebert PA, Mahon WA, MacLeod SM, Soldin SJ, Vandenberghe HM: Ranitidine kinetics and dynamics II. Intravenous dose studies and comparison with cimetidine. Clin Pharmacol Ther 30:545–550, 1981
69. Kimelblatt BJ, Cerra FB, Galleri G, Berg MJ, McMillen MA, Schentag JJ: Dose and serum concentration relationships in cimetidine-associated mental confusion. Gastroenterology 78:791–795, 1980
70. Schentag JJ, Cerra FB, Galleri G, DeGlopper E, Rose JQ, Bernhard H: Pharmacokinetic and clinical studies in patients with cimetidine-associated mental confusion. Lancet 1:177–181, 1979
71. Spence RW, Celestin LR: Gynecomastia associated with cimetidine. Gut 20:154–157, 1979
72. Jensen RT, Collen MJ, Pandol SJ, Allende HD, Raufman J-P, Bissonnette BM, Duncan WC, Durgin PL, Gillin JC, Gardner JD: Cimetidine-induced impotence and breast changes in patients with gastric hypersecretory states. N Engl J Med 308:883–887, 1983
73. Somogyi A, Muirhead M: Pharmacokinetic interactions of cimetidine. Clin Pharmacokinet 12:321–366, 1987
74. Powell JR, Donn KH: Histamine H₂ antagonist drug interactions in perspective: Mechanistic concepts and clinical implications. Am J Med 77(suppl 5B):57–84, 1984
75. Reed MD, Blumer JL: Drug-drug interactions, in Haddad LM, Winchester JF (eds): Clinical Management of Poisoning and Drug Overdose. 2d ed. Philadelphia, W.B. Saunders, 1990, pp 458–470
76. Dossing M, Pilsgoard H, Rasmussen B, Enghusen-Poulsen H: Time course of phenobarbital and cimetidine mediated changes in hepatic drug metabolism. Eur J Clin Pharmacol 25:215–222, 1983
77. Abernethy DR, Greenblatt DJ, Divoll M, Ameer B, Shader DI: Differential effect of cimetidine on drug oxidation (antipyrine and diazepam): Prevention of acetaminophen toxicity by cimetidine. J Pharmacol Exp Ther 224:508–513, 1983
78. Peterson FJ, Knodell RG, Lindemann NJ, Steele NM: Prevention of acetaminophen and cocaine hepatotoxicity in mice by cimetidine treatment. Gastroenterology 85:122–129, 1983
79. Speeg KV: Potential use of cimetidine for treatment of acetaminophen overdose. Pharmacotherapy 7(suppl):125S–133 S, 1987
80. Somogyi A, McLean A, Heinzon B: Cimetidine-procainamide pharmacokinetic interaction in man: Evidence of competition for tubular secretion of basic drugs. Eur J Clin Pharmacol 25:339–345, 1983
81. Van Crugten J, Bochner F, Keal J, Somogyi A: Selectivity of the cimetidine-induced alterations in the renal handling of organic substrates in humans. Studies with anionic, cationic, and zwitterionic drugs. J Pharmacol Exp Ther 236:481–487, 1986

82. Abernethy DR, Greenblatt DJ, Eshelman FN, Shader RI: Ranitidine does not impair oxidative or conjugative metabolism: Noninteraction with antipyrine, diazepam or lorazepam. Clin Pharmacol Ther 35:188–192, 1984

83. Kelly HW, Powell JR, Donohue JF: Ranitidine at very large doses does not inhibit theophylline elimination. Clin Pharmacol Ther 39:577–581, 1986

84. Kirch W, Hoensch H, Janisch HD: Interactions and non-interactions with ranitidine. Clin Pharmacokinet 9:493–510, 1984

85. Smith, SR, Kendall MJ: Ranitidine vs cimetidine. A comparison of their potential to cause clinically important drug interactions. Clin Pharmacokinet 15:44–56, 1988

86. Rendic S, Kajfez F, Ruf H-H: Characterization of cimetidine, ranitidine and other related structures interaction with cytochrome P450. Drug Metab Dispos 11:137–142, 1983

87. Roberts CJC: Clinical pharmacokinetics of ranitidine. Clin Pharmacokinet 9:211–221, 1984

88. Blumer JL, Rothstein FC, Kaplan BS, Yamashita TS, Eshelman FN, Myers CM, Reed MD: Pharmacokinetic determination of ranitidine pharmacodynamics in pediatric ulcer disease. J Pediatr 107:301–306, 1985

89. Miller R: Pharmacokinetics and bioavailability of ranitidine in humans. J Pharm Sci 73:1376–1379, 1984

90. Veng-Pedersen P, Miller R: Pharmacokinetics and bioavailability of cimetidine in man. J Pharm Sci 69:394–398, 1980

91. Bodemar G, Norlander B, Fransson L, Walan A: The absorption of cimetidine before and during maintenance treatment with cimetidine and the influence of a meal on the absorption of cimetidine: Studies in patients with ulcer disease. Br J Clin Pharmacol 7:23–31, 1979

92. Albin H, Vincon G, Begaud B, Bistue C, Perez P: Effect of aluminum phosphate on the bioavailability of ranitidine. Eur J Clin Pharmacol 32:97–99, 1987

93. Mullersman G, Gotz VP, Russell WL, Derendorf H: Lack of clinically significant in vitro and in vivo interactions betwen ranitidine and sucralfate. J Pharm Sci 75:995–998, 1986

94. Eshelman FN, Plachetka JR, Brown BCP: Effect of antacid and anticholinergic medication on ranitidine absorption (Abstr.). Clin Pharmacol Ther 33:216, 1983

95. Garg DC, Weidler DJ, Eshelman FN: Ranitidine bioavailability and kinetics in normal male subjects. Clin Pharmacol Ther 33:445–452, 1983

96. Kearns GL, McConnell RF, Trang JM, Kluza RB: Appearance of ranitidine in breast milk following multiple dosing. Clin Pharm 4:322–324, 1985

97. Leeder JS, Harding L, MacLeod SM: Ranitidine pharmacokinetics in children (Abstr.). Clin Pharmacol Ther 37:201, 1985

98. Wiest DB, O'Neal W, Reigart JR, Brundage RC, Gillette PC, Yost RL: Pharmacokinetics of ranitidine in critically ill infants. Dev Pharmcol Ther 12:7–12, 1989

99. Speeg KV Jr: Patwardhan RV, Avant GR, Mitchell MC, Schenker S: Inhibition of microsomal drug metabolism by histamine H₂-receptor antagonists studied in vivo and in vitro in rodents. Gastroenterology 82:89–96, 1982

100. Dunk AA, Jenkins WJ, Burroughs AK, Walt RP, Osuafor TOK, Sherlock S, Mackie S, Dick R: The effect of ranitidine on the plasma clearance and hepatic extraction of indocyanine green in patients with chronic liver disease. Br J Clin Pharmacol 16:117–120, 1983

101. Wang C, Wong KL, Lam KC, Lai CL: Ranitidine does not affect gonadal function in man. Br J Clin Pharmacol 16:430–432, 1983

102. Smith JL: Clinical pharmacology of famotidine. Digestion 32(suppl 1):15–23, 1985

103. Miyake S, Yamoda M, Iwamoto H, Yamashita S, Sugio Y: Effect of a new H₂-blocker; famotidine, in reflux esophagitis among severely handicapped children. Clin Ther 9:548–558, 1987

104. Kraus G, Krishna DR, Chmelarsch D, Schmid M, Klotz V: Famotidine pharmacokinetic properties and suppression of acid secretion in pediatric patients following cardiac surgery. Clin Pharmacokinet 18:77–81, 1990

105. Lin JH, Chremos AN, Kanovsky SM, Schwartz S, Yeh KC, Kann J: Effects of antacids and food on famotidine. Br J Clin Pharmacol 24:551–553, 1987

106. Kroemer H, Klotz V: Pharmacokinetics of famotidine in man. Int J Clin Pharm Ther Toxicol 25:458–463, 1987

107. Rosenthal M, Miller PW: Ranitidine in the newborn. Arch Dis Child 63:88–89, 1988

108. Sutphen JL, Dillard VL: Effect of ranitidine on twenty-four hour gastric acidity in infants. J Pediatr 114:472–474, 1989

109. Lopez-Herce J, Velasco LA, Codoceo R, Dominguez MAD, Jimenez E, Tarrio FR: Ranitidine prophylaxis in acute gastric mucosal damage in critically ill pediatric patients. Crit Care Med 16:591–593, 1988

110. Summary of the 34th meeting of the Food and Drug Administration Gastrointestinal Drugs Advisory Committee, March 15 and 16, 1989. Am J Gastroenterol 84:1351–1355, 1989

111. Regardh CG: Pharmacokinetics and metabolism of omeprazole in man. Scand J Gastroenterol 21(suppl 118):99–104, 1986

112. Regardh CG, Andersson T, Logerstrom PO, Lundborg P, Skanberg I: The pharmacokinetics of omeprazole in humans—A study of single intravenous and oral doses. Ther Drug Monitor 12:163–172, 1990

113. Pilbrant J, Cederberg C: Development of an oral formulation of omeprazole. Scand J Gastroenterol 20(suppl 108):113–120, 1985

114. Prichard PJ, Yeomans ND, Mihaly GW, Jones DB, Buckle PJ, Smallwood RA, Louis WJ: Omeprazole: A study of its inhibition of gastric pH and oral pharmacokinetics after morning or evening dosage. Gastroenterology 88:64–69, 1985

115. Anderson T, Cederberg C, Edvardsson G, Heggelund A, Lundborg P: Effect of omeprazole treatment on diazepam plasma levels in slow versus normal rapid metabolizers of omeprazole. Clin Pharmacol Ther 47:79–85, 1990

116. Andersson T, Regardh CG, Dahl-Pruustinen M-L, Bertilsson L: Slow omeprazole metabolizers are also poor S-mephenytoin hydroxylators. Ther Drug Monitor 12:415–416, 1990

117. Gugler R, Jensen JC: Omeprazole inhibits elimination of diazepam. Lancet 1:969, 1984

118. Gugler R, Jensen JC: Omeprazole inhibits oxidative drug metabolism. Gastroenterology 89:1235–1241, 1985

119. Prichard PJ, Walt RP, Kitchingham GK, Somerville KW, Langman MJS, Williams J, Richens A: Oral phenytoin pharmacokinetics during omeprazole therapy. Br J Clin Pharmacol 24:543–545, 1987

120. Andersson T, Lagerstrom P-O, Unge P: A study of the interaction between omeprazole and phenytoin in epileptic patients. Ther Drug Monitor 12:329–333, 1990

121. Henry D, Brent P, Whyte I, Mihaly G, Devenish-Meares S: Propranolol steady-state pharmacokinetics are unaltered by omeprazole. Eur J Clin Pharmacol 33:369–373, 1987

122. Diaz D, Fabre I, Daujat M, Saint Aubert B, Bories P, Michel H, Maurel P: Omeprazole is an aryl hydrocarbon-like inducer of human hepatic cytochrome P450. Gastroenterology 99:737–747, 1990

123. Walan A, Boder J-P, Classen M, Lambers CBHW, Piper DW, Rutgersson K, Ericksson S: Effect of omeprazole and ranitidine on ulcer healing and relapse rates in patients with benign gastric ulcer. N Engl J Med 320:69–75, 1989

124. Delchier J-C, Isal J-C, Eriksson S, Soule J-C: Double-blind multicentre comparison of omeprazole 20 mg once daily versus ranitidine 150 mg twice daily in the treatment of cimetidine or ranitidine resistant duodenal ulcers. Gut 30:1173–1178, 1989

125. Maton PN, Vinayek R, Frucht H, McArthur KA, Miller LS, Saeed ZA, Gardner JD, Jensen RT: Long-term efficacy and safety of omeprazole in patients with Zollinger-Ellison syndrome: A prospective study. Gastroenterology 97:827–836, 1989

126. Sewing KF, Hogie L, Ippoliti AF, Isenberg JI, Samloff IM, Sturdevant AL: Effect of one-month treatment with cimetidine on gastric secretion and serum gastrin and pepsinogen levels. Gastroenterology 74:376–379, 1978

127. Hyman PE, Garvey TQ, Harada T: Effect of ranitidine on gastric acid hypersecretion in an infant with short bowel syndrome. J Pediatr Gastro Nutr 4:316–319, 1985

128. Hyman PE, Garvey TQ, Abrams CE: Tolerance to intravenous ranitidine. J Pediatr 110:794–796, 1987

129. Wilder-Smith CH, Ernst T, Gennoni M, Zeyen B, Halter F, Merki HS: Tolerance of oral H₂ receptor antagonists. Dig Dis Sci 35:976–983, 1990

130. Ostro MJ, Russell JA, Soldin SJ, Mahon WA, Jeejeebhoy KN:

Control of gastric pH with cimetidine: Bolus versus primed infusions. Gastroenterology 89:532–537, 1985

131. Morris DL, Markham SJ, Beechey A, Hicks F, Summers K, Lewis P, Stannard V, Hutchinson A, Byrne AJ: Ranitidine-bolus or infusion prophylaxis for stress ulcer. Crit Care Med 16:229–232, 1988

132. Rovers JP, Souney PF: A critical review of continuous infusion H_2 receptor therapy. Crit Care Med 17:814–821, 1989

133. McCallum RW: Review of the current status of prokinetic agents in gastroenterology. Am J Gastroenterol 80:1008–1016, 1985

134. Sondheimer JM: Gastroesophageal reflux: Update on pathogenesis and diagnosis. Pediatr Clin No Am 35:103–116, 1988

135. Package Insert for Urecholine (bethanechol). Physicians Desk Reference, 43rd ed. Oradell, NJ, Medical Economics Co., 1989, pp 1402–1403

136. Sondheimer JM, Arnold GL: Early effects of bethanechol on the esophageal motor function of infants with gastroesophageal reflux. J Pediatr Gastroenterol Nutr 5:47–51, 1986

137. Euler AR: Use of bethanechol for the treatment of gastroesophageal reflux. J Pediatr 96:321–324, 1980

138. Strickland AD, Chang JHT: Results of treatment of gastroesophageal reflux with bethanenchol. J Pediatr 103:311–315, 1983

139. Sondheimer JM, Mintz HL, Michaels M: Bethanechol treatment of gastroesophageal reflux in infants: Effect on continuous esophageal pH records. J Pediatr 104:128–131, 1984

140. Cohen S, DiMarino AJ: Mechanism of action of metoclopramide on opossum lower esophageal sphincter muscle. Gastroenterology 71:996–998, 1976

141. Albibi R, McCallum RW: Metoclopramide: Pharmacology and clinical application. Ann Intern Med 98:86–95, 1983

142. Beani L, Bianchi C, Crema C: Effects of metoclopramide on isolated guinea pig colon. 1. Peripheral sensitization on acetylcholine. Eur J Pharmacol 12:320–331, 1970

143. Conell AM, George JD: Effect of metoclopramide on gastric function in man. Gut 10:678–680, 1969

144. Bateman DN: Clinical pharmacokinetics of metoclopramide. Clin Pharmacokinet 8:523–529, 1983

145. Ross-Lee L, Eadie MJ, Hooper WD, Bochner F: Single-dose pharmacokinetics of metoclopramide. Eur J Clin Pharmacol 20:465–471, 1981

146. Webb D, Buss DC, Fifield R, Bateman DN, Routledge PA: The plasma protein binding of metoclopramide in health and renal disease. Br J Clin Pharmacol 21:334–336, 1986

147. Lewis PJ, Devenish C, Kahn C: Controlled trial of metoclopramide in the initiation of breast feeding. Br J Clin Pharmacol 9:217–219, 1980

148. Kauppila A, Arvela P, Koivist M, Kivinen S, Ylikorkala O, Pelkonen O: Metoclopramide and breast feeding: Transfer into milk and the newborn. Eur J Clin Pharmacol 25:819–823, 1983

149. Bateman DN, Craft AW, Nicholson E, Pearson ADJ: Dystonic reaction and pharmacokinetics of metoclopramide in children. Br J Clin Pharmacol 15:560–563, 1983

150. Kearns GL, Butler HL, Lane JK, Carchman SH, Wright GJ: Metoclopramide pharmacokinetics and pharmacodynamics in infants with gastroesophageal reflux. J Pediatr Gastroenterol Nutr 7:823–829, 1988

151. Hyman PE, Abrams C, Dubois A: Effect of metoclopramide and bethanechol on gastric emptying in infants. Pediatr Res 19:1029–1032, 1985

152. Leung AKC, Lai PCW: Use of metoclopramide for the treatment of gastroesophageal reflux in infants and children. Curr Ther Res 36:911–915, 1984

153. Hyams JS, Leichtner AM, Zamett LD, Walter JK: Effect of metoclopramide on prolonged intraesophageal pH testing in infants with gastroesophageal reflux. J Pediatr Gastroenterol Nutr 5:716–720, 1986

154. Machida HM, Forbes DA, Gall DG, Scott RB: Metoclopramide in gastroesophageal reflux of infancy. J Pediatr 112:483–487, 1988

155. Gralla RJ: Metoclopramide, a review of antiemetic trials. Drugs 25(suppl 1):63–73, 1983

156. Gralla RJ, Tyson LB, Kris MG, Clark RA: The management of chemotherapy-induced nausea and vomiting. Med Clin No Am 71:289–301, 1987

157. Triozzi PL, Laszlo J: Optimum management of nausea and vomiting in cancer chemotherapy. Drugs 34:136–149, 1987

158. Edwards CM: Chemotherapy induced emesis—mechanisms and treatment: A review. J R Soc Med 81:658–662, 1988

159. Kobrinsky NL: Regulation of nausea and vomiting in cancer chemotherapy; a review with emphasis on opiate mediators. Am J Pediatr Hematol Oncol 10:209–213, 1988

160. Kris, MG, Gralla RJ, Tyson LB, Clark RA, Kelsen DP, Reilly LK, Groshen S, Bosl GJ, Kalman LA: Improved control of cisplatin-induced emesis with high-dose metoclopramide and with combinations of metoclopramide, dexamethasone and diphenhydramine. Results of consecutive trials in 255 patients. Cancer 55:527–534, 1985

161. Marshall G, Kerr S, Vowels M, O'Gorman-Hughes D, White L: Antiemetic therapy for chemotherapy-induced vomiting: Metoclopramide, benztropine, dexamethasone, and lorazepam regimen compared with chlorpromazine alone. J Pediatr 115:156–160, 1989

162. Havsteen H, Nielsen H, Kjaer M: Antiemetic effect and pharmacokinetics of high dose metoclopramide in cancer patients treated with cisplatin-containing chemotherapy regimens. Eur J Clin Pharmacol 31:33–40, 1986

163. Whatley K, Turner WW Jr, Dey M, Leonard J, Guthrie M: When does metoclopramide facilitate transpyloric intubation. J Parenteral Enteral Nutr 8:679–681, 1984

164. Casteels-van Daele M, Jaeken J, van Der Schueren P, Zimmerman A, van Den Bon P: Dystonic reactions in children caused by metoclopramide. Arch Dis Child 45:130–133, 1970

165. Kris MG, Tyson LB, Gralla RJ, Clark RA, Allen SC, Reilly LK: Extrapyramidal reactions with high-dose metoclopramide. N Engl J Med 309:433–434, 1983

166. Allen JC, Gralla R, Reilly L, Kellick M, Young C: Metoclopramide: Dose-related toxicity and preliminary antiemetic studies in children receiving cancer chemotherapy. J Clin Oncol 3:1136–1141, 1985

167. Kearns GL, Fiser DH: Metoclopramide-induced methemoglobinemia. Pediatrics 82:364–366, 1988

168. Ehrenkranz RA, Ackerman BA: Metoclopramide effect on faltering milk production by mothers of premature infants. Pediatrics 78:614–620, 1986

169. Grill BB, Hillemeier AG, Semeraro LA, McCallum RW, Gryboski JD: Effects of domperidone therapy on symptoms and upper gastrointestinal motility in infants with gastroesophageal reflux. J Pediatr 106:311–316, 1985

170. McCallum RW, Prakash C, Campoli-Richards DM, Goa KL: Cisapride a preliminary review of its pharmacodynamic and pharmacokinetic properties, and therapeutic use as a prokinetic agent in gastrointestinal motility disorders. Drugs 36:652–681, 1988

171. Grill BB, Hillemeier AC, Semeraro LA, McCallum RW, Gryboski JD: Effects of domperidone therapy on symptoms and upper gastrointestinal motility in infants with gastroesophageal reflux. J Pediatr 106:311–316, 1985

172. Monsein LH, Halpert RD, Harris ED, Feczko PJ: Retrograde ileography: Value of glucagon. Radiology 161:558–559, 1986

173. Janssens J, Peeters TL, Vantrappen G, Tack J, Urbain JL, DeRoo M, Muls E, Bouillon R: Improvement of gastric emptying in diabetic gastroparesis by erythromycin. Preliminary studies. N Engl J Med 322:1028–1031, 1990

174. Orenstein SR: Prone positioning in infant gastroesophageal reflux: Is elevation of the head worth the trouble? J Pediatr 117:184–187, 1990

175. Balistreri WF: Oral rehydration in acute infantile diarrhea. Am J Med 88(suppl 6A):30S–33S, 1990

176. Guandalini S: Overview of childhood acute diarrhoea in Europe: Implications for oral rehydration therapy. Acta Paediatr Scand 364(suppl):5–12, 1990

177. Avery ME, Snyder JD: Oral therapy for acute diarrhea. The underused simple solution. N Engl J Med 323:891–894, 1990

178. Santosham M, Daum RS, Dillman L, Rodriguez JL, Leique S, Russell R, Kourany M, Ryder RW, Bartlett AV, Rosenberg A, Benensen AS, Sack RB: Oral rehydration therapy of infantile diarrhea: A controlled study of well-nourished children hospitalized in the United States and Panama. N Engl J Med 306:1070–1076, 1982

179. Finberg L, Harper PA, Harrison HE, Sack RB: Oral rehydration for diarrhea. J Pediatr 101:497–499, 1982
180. Portnoy BL, DuPont HL, Pruitt D, Abdo JA, Rodriguez JT: Antidiarrheal agents in the treatment of acute diarrhea in children. JAMA 236:844–846, 1976
181. Choonara IA, Shoo EE, Owens GG: Prescribing habits for children with acute gastroenteritis: A comparison over 5 years. Br J Clin Pharmacol 23:362–364, 1987
182. Motala C, Hill ID, Mann MD, Bowie MD: Effect of loperamide on stool output and duration of acute infectious diarrhea in infants. J Pediatr 117:467–471, 1990
183. Sandhu BK, Trip JH, Milla PJ, Harries JT: Loperamide in severe protracted diarrhoea. Arch Dis Child 58:39–43, 1983
184. Diarrhoeal Diseases Study Group (UK): Loperamide in acute diarrhoea in childhood: Results of a double blind, placebo controlled multicentre clinical trial. Br Med J 289:1263–1267, 1984
185. Dukes GE: Over-the-counter antidiarrheal medications used for the self-treatment of acute non-specific diarrhea. Am J Med 88(suppl 6A):24S–26S, 1990
186. Antidiarrheal drug products for over-the-counter human use: Tentative final monograph. Fed Register 51:16138–16149, 1986.
187. Barkin RL, Stein ZLG: Drugs with anticholinergic side effects. So Med J 82:1547–1548, 1989
188. Ivy KJ: Are anticholinergics of use in irritable colon syndrome? Gastroenterology 68:1300–1307, 1975
189. Karem A, Ranney RE, Evensen KL, Clark ML: Pharmacokinetics and metabolism of diphenoxylate in man. Clin Pharmacol Ther 13:407–419, 1972
190. Rumack BH, Temple AR: Lomotil poisoning. Pediatrics 53:495–500, 1974
191. Curtis JA, Goel KM: Lomotil poisoning in children. Arch Dis Child 54:222–225, 1979
192. Nimegeers CJE, McGuire JL, Hegkants JJP, Janssen PAJ: Dissociation between opiate-like and antidiarrheal activities of antidiarrheal drugs. J Pharmacol Exp Ther 210:327–333, 1979
193. Schiller LR, Santa Ana CA, Morawski SG, Fordtran JS: Mechanism of antidiarrheal effect of loperamide. Gastroenterology 86:1475–1480, 1984
194. Summary of the 31st Meeting of the Food and Drug Administration Gastrointestinal Drugs Advisory Committee, December 8–9, 1986. Am J Gastroenterol 82:443–447, 1987
195. Killinger JM, Weintraub HS, Fuller BL: Human pharmacokinetics and comparative bioavailability of loperamide hydrochloride. J Clin Pharmacol 19:211–218, 1979
196. VanLoon FPL, Bennish ML, Speelman P, Butler C: Double blind trial of loperamide for treating acute watery diarrhea in expatriates in Bangladesh. Gut 30:492–495, 1989
197. Ericsson CD, Johnson PC: Safety and efficacy of loperamide. Am J Med 88(suppl 6A):10S–14S, 1990
198. Bierer DW: Bismuth subsalicylate: History, chemistry and safety. Rev Infect Dis 12(suppl 1):S3–S8, 1990
199. Gorbach SL: Bismuth therapy in gastrointestinal diseases. Gastroenterology 99:863–875, 1990
200. Gryboski JD, Kocohis S: Effect of bismuth subsalicylate on chronic diarrhea in childhood: A preliminary report. Rev Infect Dis 12(suppl 1):S36–S40, 1990
201. Soriano-Brucher HE, Avendano P, O'Ryan M, Soriano HA: Use of bismuth subsalicylate in acute diarrhea in children. Rev Infect Dis 12(suppl 1):S51–S56, 1990
202. Wagstaff AJ, Benfield P, Monk JP: Colloidal bismuth subcitrate. A review of its pharmacodynamic and pharmacokinetic properties, and its therapeutic use in peptic ulcer disease. Drugs 36:132–157, 1988
203. Drumm B, Sherman P, Cutz E, Karmali M: Association of Campylobacter pylori in the gastric mucosa with antral gastritis in children. N Engl J Med 316:1557–1561, 1987
204. Kilbridge PM, Dahms BB, Czinn SJ: Campylobacter pylori-associated gastritis and peptic ulcer disease in children. Am J Dis Child 142:1149–1152, 1988
205. Glassman MS, Schwarz SM, Medow MS, Beneck D, Halata M, Berezin S, Newman, LJ: Campylobacter pylori-related gastrointestinal disease in children. Incidence and clinical findings. Dig Dis Sci 34:1501–1504, 1989
206. Warren JR: Unidentified curved bacilli on gastric epithelium in active chronic gastritis. Lancet 1:1273, 1983
207. Pickering LK, Feldman S, Ericsson CD, Cleary TG: Absorption of salicylate and bismuth from a bismuth subsalicylate-containing compound (Pepto-Bismol). J Pediatr 99:654–656, 1981
208. Frooms PRA, Wan AT, Keech AC, McNeil JJ, McLean AJ: Absorption and elimination of bismuth from oral doses of tripotassium dicitrato bismuthate. Eur J Clin Pharmacol 37:533–536, 1989
209. Feldman S, Chen S-L, Pickering LK, Cleary TG, Ericsson CD, Hulse M: Salicylate absorption from a bismuth subsalicylate preparation. Clin Pharmacol Ther 29:788–792, 1981
210. Graham DY, Estes MK, Gentry LO: Double-blind comparison of bismuth subsalicylate and placebo in the prevention and treatment of endotoxigenic Escherichia coli-induced diarrhea in volunteers. Gastroenterology 85:1017–1022, 1983
211. Gryboski JD, Hillemeier AC, Grill B, Kocoshis S: Bismuth subsalicylate in the treatment of chronic diarrhea of childhood. Am J Gastroenterol 80:871–876, 1985
212. Balistreri WF, Partin JC, Schubert WK: Bile acid malabsorption—A consequence of terminal ileal dysfunction in protracted diarrhea of infancy. J Pediatr 90:21–28, 1977
213. Balistreri WF, Heubi JE, Suchy FJ: Bile acid metabolism: Relationship to bile acid malabsorption and diarrhea. J Pediatr Gastroenterol Nutr 2:105–121, 1983
214. Tamer MA, Santora TR, Sandberg DH: Cholestyramine therapy for intractable diarrhea. Pediatrics 53:217–220, 1974
215. Bowie MD: Antibiotics and cholestyramine in the treatment of persistent diarrhea in infants (editorial). J Pediatr Gastroenteral Nutr 8:425–429, 1989
216. Rosenthal LE, Mobley HLT, Cortesia MJ, Smoot D: Characterization of urease from Campylobacter pylori: Possible therapeutic role of urease inhibitors (Abstr.). Am J Gastroenterol 82:934, 1987
217. Graham DY, Klein PD, Opekum AR, Smith KE, Polasani RR, Evans DJ Jr, Evans DG, Alpert LC, Michaletz PA, Yoshimura HH, Adam E: In vitro susceptibility of Campylobacter pylori. Am J Gastroenterol 84:233–238, 1989
218. Manhart MD: In vitro antimicrobial activity of bismuth subsalicylate and other bismuth salts. Rev Infect Dis 12(suppl 1):S11–S15, 1990
219. Mendelowitz PC, Hoffman RS, Weber S: Bismuth absorption and myoclonic encephalopathy during bismuth subsalicylate therapy. Ann Intern Med 112:140–141, 1990
220 Breenton LL: Agents affecting gastrointestinal water flux and motility, digestants, and bile acids, in Gilman AG, Rall TW, Nies AS, Taylor P (eds): Goodman and Gilman's The Pharmacologic Basis of Therapeutics. 8th ed. New York, Pergamon Press, 1990, pp 914–932
221. Loening-Baucke VA, Younoszai MK: Effect of treatment on rectal and sigmoid motility in chronically constipated children. Pediatrics 73:199–205, 1984
222. Steer HW, Colin-Jones DG: Melanosis coli: Studies of the toxic effects of irritant purgatives. J Pathol 115:199–205, 1975
223. Wyatt E, Greaves M, Sondergaard J: Fixed drug eruption (phenolphthalein). Arch Dermatol 106:671–673, 1972
224. Davis RF, Eichner JM, Bleyer WA, Okamoto G: Hypocalcium, hyperphosphatemia, and dehydration following a single hypertonic phosphate enema. J Pediatr 90:484–485, 1977
225. Meisel JL, Bergman D, Graney D, Saunders DR, Rubin CE: Human rectal mucosa: Proctoscopic and morphological changes caused by laxatives. Gastroenterology 72:1274–1279, 1977
226. Kirschner BS: Inflammatory bowel disease in children. Pediatr Clin No Am 35:189–208, 1988
227. Ament ME: Inflammatory disease of the colon: Ulcerative colitis and Crohn's colitis. J Pediatr 86:322–334, 1975
228. Bachrach WH: Sulfasalazine I: An historical perspective. Am J Gastroenterol 83:487–496, 1988
229. Svartz N: Sulfasalazine II: Some notes on the discovery and development of salazopyrin. Am J Gastroenterol 83:497–503, 1988
230. Peppercorn MA: Advances in drug therapy for inflammatory bowel disease. Ann Intern Med 112:50–60, 1990
231. Peppercorn MA: Sulfasalazine pharmacology, clinical use, toxicity and related new drug development. Ann Intern Med 101:377–386, 1984

232. Schroder H, Campbell DE: Absorption, metabolism, and excretion of salicylazosulfapyridine in man. Clin Pharmacol Ther 13:539–551, 1972
233. Das KM, Eastwood MA, McManus JPA, Sircus W: Adverse reactions during salicylazosulfapyridine therapy and the relation with drug metabolism and acetylator phenotype. N Engl J Med 289:491–495, 1973
234. Goldstein PD, Alpers DH, Keating JP: Sulfapyridine metabolites in children with inflammatory bowel disease receiving sulfasalazine. J Pediatr 95:638–640, 1979
235. Azod Khan AK, Truelove SC, Aronson JK: The disposition and metabolism of sulphasalazine (salicylazosulfapyridine) in man. Br J Clin Pharmacol 13:523–528, 1982
236. Jansen JA: Kinetics of binding of salicylazosulfapyridine to human serum albumin. Acta Pharmacol Toxicol 41:401–416, 1977
237. Peppercorn MA, Goldman P: The role of intestinal bacteria in the metabolism of salicylazosulfapyridine. J Pharmacol Exp Ther 181:555–562, 1972
238. Schroder H, Lewkonia RM, Prince Evans DA: Metabolism of salicylazosulfapyridine in healthy subjects and in patients with ulcerative colitis. Effects of colectomy and phenobarbital. Clin Pharmacol Ther 14:802–809, 1973
239. Clementz GL, Dolin BJ: Sulfasalazine-induced lupus erythematosus. Am J Med 84:535–538, 1988
240. Derry CL, Schwinghammer TL: Agranulocytosis associated with sulfasalazine. Drug Intell Clin Pharm 22:139–142, 1988
241. Mihas AA, Goldenberg DJ, Slaughter RL: Sulfasalazine toxic reactions, hepatitis, fever and skin rash with hypocomplementemia and immune complexes. JAMA 239:2590–2591, 1978
242. Boyer DL, Li BU, Fyda JN, Friedman RA: Sulfasalazine-induced hepatotoxicity in children with inflammatory bowel disease. J Pediatr Gastroenterol Nutr 8:528–532, 1989
243. Purdy BH, Philips DM, Summers RW: Desensitization for sulfasalazine skin rash. Ann Intern Med 100:512–514, 1984
244. Rao SS, Cann PA, Holdsworth CD: Clinical experience of the tolerance of mesalazine and olsalazine in patients intolerant of sulphasalazine. Scand J Gastroenterol 22:332–336, 1987
245. Reisennauer AM, Halsted CM: Human jejunal brush border folate conjugate: Characteristics and inhibition by salicylazosulfapyridine. Biochim Biophys Acta 659:62–69, 1981
246. Juhl RP, Summers RW, Guillory JK, Blaug SM, Cheng FH, Brown DD: Effect of sulfasalazine on digoxin bioavailability. Clin Pharmacol Ther 20:387–394, 1976
247. Brogden RN, Heel RC, Speight TM, Avery GS: Sucralfate. A review of its pharmacodynamic properties and therapeutic use in peptic ulcer disease. Drugs 27:194–209, 1984
248. Herrereas-Gutierrez JM, Pardo L, Segu JL: Sucralfate vs ranitidine in the treatment of gastric ulcer. Randomized clinical results in short-term and maintenance therapy. Am J Med 86(suppl 6A):94–97, 1989
249. Smith CL: Sucralfate in the treatment of gastritis. A review. Am J Med 86(suppl 6A):70–72, 1989
250. Takemoto T, Namiki M, Ishikawa M, Tsuneoka K, Oshiba S, Kawai K, Ogawa N: Ranitidine and sucralfate as maintenance therapy for gastric ulcer disease: Endoscopic control and assessment of scoring. Gut 30:1692–1697, 1989
251. Arguelles-Martin F, Gonzalez-Fernandez F, Gentles MG: Sucralfate versus cimetidine in the treatment of reflux esophagitis in children. Am J Med 86(suppl 6A):73–76, 1989
252. Driks MR, Craven DE, Celli BR, Manning M, Burke RA, Garvin GM, Kunches LM, Farber HW, Wedel SA, McCabe WR: Nosocomial pneumonia in intubated patients given sucralfate as compared with antacids or histamine type 2 blockers. The role of gastric colonization. N Engl J Med 317:1376–1382, 1987
253. Shenep JJ, Kalwinsky DK, Hutson PR, George SL, Dodge RK, Blankenship KR, Thornton D: Efficacy of oral sucralfate suspension in prevention and treatment of chemotherapy-induced mucositis. J Pediatr 113:758–763, 1988
254. Solomon MA: Oral sucralfate suspension for mucositis. N Engl J Med 315:459–460, 1986
255. Caille G, Du Souich P, Besner JG, Gervais P, Vezina M: Effects of food and sucralfate on the pharmacokinetics of naproxen and ketoprofen in humans. Am J Med 86(suppl 6A):38–44, 1989
256. Garrelts JC, Godley PJ, Peterie JD, Gerlach EH, Yakshe CC: Sucralfate significantly reduces ciprofloxacin concentrations in serum. Antimicrob Agents Chemother 34:931–933, 1990
257. Parpia SH, Nix DE, Hejmanowski LG, Goldstein HR, Wilton JH, Schentag JJ: Sucralfate reduces the gastrointestinal absorption of norfloxacin. Antimicrob Agents Chemother 33:99–102, 1989
258. Charlet N, Gallo-Torres HE, Bounameaux Y, Willis RJ: Prostaglandins and the protection of gastrointestinal mucosa in humans: A critical review. J Clin Pharmacol 25:564–582, 1985
259. Collins PW, Poppo R, Dajani EZ: Chemistry and synthetic development of misoprostol. Dig Dis Sci 30(suppl):114S–117S, 1985
260. Robinson P, Sly PD: Placebo-controlled trial of misoprostol in cystic fibrosis. J Pediatr Gastroenterol Nutr 11:37–40, 1990

41
GLUCOCORTICOIDS

CHARIS LIAPI *and* GEORGE P. CHROUSOS

Glucocorticoids are steroid hormones produced and secreted into the systemic circulation by the adrenal glands. These glands lie on the superior pole of each kidney and are composed of two distinct parts, the cortex and the medulla. In the fetus the adrenal cortex divides into two zones: the outer *definitive zone* and the inner *fetal zone,* which makes up approximately 80 percent of the adrenal volume. After birth there is a rapid regression of the fetal zone during the first 2 weeks, and this zone disappears completely by the 3rd month of life. The definitive zone during infancy and childhood evolves into the adult adrenal cortex.[1] The adult adrenal cortex consists of three anatomic zones: the outer *zona glomerulosa,* the intermediate *zona fasciculata,* and the inner *zona reticularis.* The zona glomerulosa is responsible for the production of aldosterone, the zona fasciculata for the production of cortisol, and the zona reticularis for the production of adrenal androgens. The zona fasciculata secretes glucocorticoids in a circadian fashion or in response to stress. The adrenal medulla is functionally related to the sympathetic nervous system and secretes the hormones epinephrine and norepinephrine basally and in response to stress. The glucocorticoids have important effects on intermediary metabolism, cardiovascular function, behavior, and control of immune function; the major endogenous glucocorticoid in humans is cortisol. This steroid has some mineralocorticoid or salt-retaining activity.

SYNTHESIS

The major precursor of corticosteroids is cholesterol. Cholesterol is taken up by the adrenal cortex from plasma but can also be synthesized *de novo* in the gland from acetate. Cholesterol is converted in mitochondria to pregnenolone by side chain cleavage.[2-4] Pregnenolone is converted to the major corticosteroids cortisol and aldosterone by a series of subsequent reactions, most of

them hydroxylations, carried out in both microsomes and mitochondria by specific enzymes in the presence of NAD^+ or NADPH and O_2 (Figure 41-1).[5] During pregnancy maternal cortisol crosses the placenta, but most of it (approximately 80 percent) is converted to cortisone.[6,7] The rest contributes up to 25–50 percent of the fetal circulating cortisol.[6] The fetal adrenals synthesize cortisol from maternal and placental 17-OH-hydroxyprogesterone or *de novo*. Corticosteroids are four-ring molecules containing 21 carbons (Figure 41-2). The differences in activity among the various steroid compounds result from structural differences of the molecules. Cortisol synthesis and secretion is mainly regulated by adrenocorticotropic hormone (ACTH) secreted from the anterior pituitary gland. Aldosterone is regulated by four major factors: (1) the renin–angiotensin system (via angiotensin II and III), (2) plasma potassium, (3) sodium status (perhaps via atrial natriuretic factors), and (4) ACTH. The predominant regulator is angiotensin II, while ACTH perhaps modulates the circadian rhythm and contributes in states of stress. It should be noted that the fetal adrenal zone appears to be regulated by one or more placental factors in addition to ACTH.

Mode of Action

Glucocorticoids exert their effects by entering the cells, mostly by passive diffusion, and binding to their receptors. The binding of glucocorticoids to receptor conforms to a simple reversible equilibrium R + S ↔ RS, when examined in intact cells or in cell-free conditions.[8] The glucocorticoid receptor is a single, 777-amino-acid-long polypeptide chain with a molecular weight of approximately 90,000 daltons.[9,10] This receptor is widely distributed, being present in almost all mammalian cells.[11] The predominant receptor complementary DNA appears to arise from one receptor gene which is localized on chromosome 5.[12] The glucocorticoid receptor (Figure 41-3) is divided into three functional domains: (1) a carboxy-ter-

466

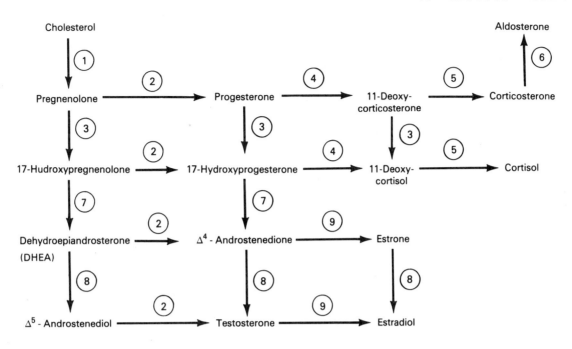

ENZYME NO.	ENZYMES AND COFACTORS OF ADRENAL STEROIDOGENESIS
1	Cholesterol desmolase system (20α-hydroxylase, 20,22-desmolase), NADPH, O_2
2	3β-Hydroxysteroid dehydrogenase-D5-D4-isomerase, NAD^+
3	17α-Hydroxylase, NADPH, O_2
4	21β-Hydroxylase, NADPH, O_2
5	11β-Hydroxylase, NADPH, O_2
6	Corticosterone methyloxidase types I and II
7	17,20-Desmolase
8	17-Ketosteroid reductase
9	Aromatase

FIGURE 41–1. Steroid biosynthesis pathway. Each enzyme is represented by a number.

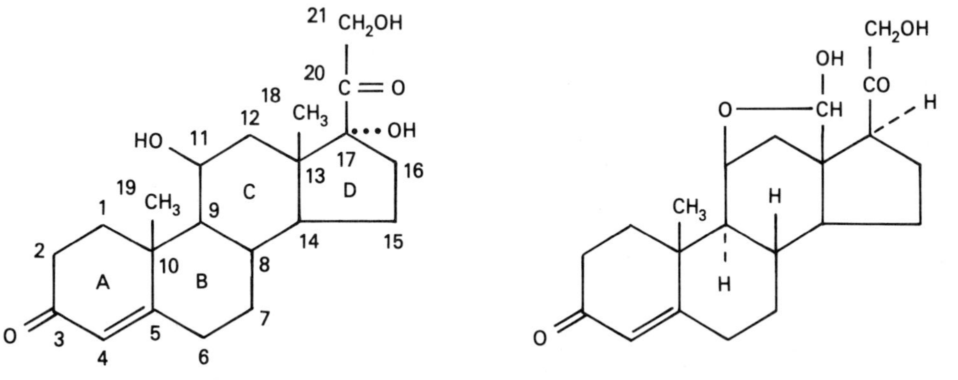

FIGURE 41–2. Structure of cortisol (I) and aldosterone (II).

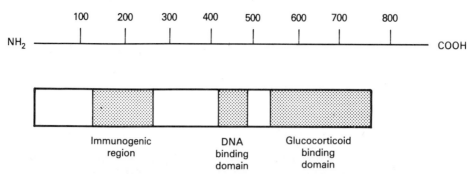

FIGURE 41–3. Modular structure of the human glucocorticoid receptor. The C-terminal steroidgenic-binding domain binds with glucocorticoid, the DNA-binding region recognizes the GREs, and the amino-terminal or immune domain is perhaps important in increasing the specificity of the complex. There are other smaller areas of the receptor which define binding to HSP 90, nuclear translocation, and dimerization.

minal steroid-binding domain; (2) a DNA-binding domain in the center of the molecule, which is highly homologous to the same domain of all steroid and thyroid hormone receptors as well as the erbA oncogene[13]; and (3) an amino-terminal domain of largely unknown function called the *immunogenic domain.*[14] This domain represents 45–50 percent of the amino acids of the receptor and may contribute to the specificity of glucocorticoid receptor–steroid complex effects on gene transcription.

Upon binding with the hormone, the glucocorticoid receptor–steroid complex undergoes a change called *transformation* or *activation.*[8,15] This involves dissociation of the receptor from heat shock protein 90 (HSP 90) and perhaps other intracellular proteins, dimerization of the complex, and translocation to the nucleus. The dimeric complex interacts with the chromatin of specific genes and modulates their transcription.[16] The DNA sequences in the regulatory region of glucocorticoid-responsive genes, with which the receptor–steroid complex interacts, are called *glucocorticoid-responsive elements* (GREs).[17] The specific effects of glucocorticoids on cellular functions are exerted by a final increase or decrease in protein synthesis.

SECRETION–METABOLISM

In normal individuals the secretion of glucocorticoids follows a diurnal pattern with peak levels between 6:00 and 8:00 AM and lowest concentrations around midnight.[18] This pattern of cortisol secretion is probably established early in life. The presence of a diurnal pattern, however, is not certain in neonates and young infants.[19] The cortisol production rate is approximately 12 mg/m²/day.[20] During the first hours of life, cortisol levels may be higher due to stress-induced secretion and/or transplacental cortisol passage from mother to fetus.[21] During the early neonatal period, there is a higher conversion of cortisol to cortisone due to increased 11-dehydrogenase activity in the neonate. The ratio of cortisone to cortisol is 2–3 at birth but decreases gradually to less than 0.7 after the first month of life.[22] Exogenous glucocorticoids are absorbed in the upper jejunum, and peak values are attained 30–100 minutes after oral administration.[23]

More than 90 percent of circulating cortisol, and to a lesser extent aldosterone, is bound tightly to a plasma glycoprotein[24] called *corticosteroid-binding globulin* (CBG) or *transcortin.* CBG is synthesized in the liver. The rest (10 percent) of the circulating cortisol is free or loosely bound to albumin. The free and albumin-bound fractions represent the active form of the hormone, while the CBG-bound represents the inactive form. When plasma cortisol levels exceed 20 μg/dl, CBG is saturated and most of the excess is in the free or albumin-bound forms. The synthesis of CBG is increased by estrogens and thyroid hormones, and the circulating concentration of the protein is elevated in pregnancy and in women taking oral contraceptives. In contrast, levels of CBG decrease by 20–50 percent in hypercortisolism. In hepatic disease, because of decreased synthesis, and in renal disease, because of protein loss in the urine, CBG levels may also be decreased. Increased or decreased concentrations of CBG do not alter the daily effect of cortisol, because the free fraction of the hormone is maintained normal by the complex feedback regulation of the hypothalamic–pituitary–adrenal (HPA) axis. Only 1 percent of the daily cortisol production is excreted in the urine as free cortisol. Corticosteroids are metabolized primarily in the liver by microsomal enzymes, mainly by reduction of the 4,5 double bond and the C-3 and C-20 keto groups. The hydroxy derivatives are conjugated with glucuronic acid to form water-soluble compounds that are excreted by the kidneys. The side chain (C-20 and C-21) is removed from about 5–10 percent of the cortisol, and the resulting keto compounds are further metabolized and excreted in urine as 11-oxyketosteroids.

METABOLIC EFFECTS

Glucocorticoids alter the regulation of many cellular processes, including enzyme synthesis and activity, membrane permeability, transport processes, hormone and receptor synthesis, and function and production of structural elements. They also have major effects on carbohydrate, protein, and fat metabolism. The effects of glucocorticoids can be categorized as *regulatory* or *permissive* (Table 41–1). The former participate primarily in the adaptive response to stress. The latter are necessary for several basal functions to take place. The permissive effects of glucocorticoids are unmasked only in states of glucocorticoid deficiency.

CLINICAL USES

Synthesis

Since the first successful therapeutic trial of cortisone in rheumatoid arthritis by Hench,[26] corticosteroids have been used in the therapy of a very broad spectrum of diseases. A large number of synthetic compounds with glucocorticoid activity have been developed. The differences among the various steroid compounds result from structural changes in rings A, B, C, and D. The structural changes of glucocorticoids can affect the affinity of the compound for the glucocorticoid and mineralocorticoid receptors,[27] the binding of the glucocorticoid receptor–steroid complex to the nucleus, the plasma half-life of the compound, and the metabolism of the compound in the liver, fat, or target tissues, as well as its gastrointestinal or parenteral absorption. Thus, a double bond between C-1 and C-2 increases glucocorticoid activity and at the same time decreases mineralocorticoid activity. Introduction

of an α-fluoro group at C-9 enhances, on the other hand, both glucocorticoid and mineralocorticoid activity. Addition of a hydroxyl or a methyl group at C-16 practically eliminates mineralocorticoid activity. Substitutions can also be introduced at C-6 instead of C-9. Dexamethasone, a synthetic compound that has a hydroxyl group at C-11, a fluoro group at C-9, and an α-methyl group at C-16, has 25–50 times the glucocorticoid potency of cortisol and a minimal mineralocorticoid effect. Certain structural modifications increase water solubility for parenteral administration or decrease water solubility to enhance topical potency. Introduction of a double bond between C-1 and C-2 results in slower metabolism of the steroid by liver and other tissues by stabilization of the A ring. Methylation at the C-2 or C-16 positions significantly prolongs plasma half-life. A keto group at C-11 is normally reduced by liver enzymes to an 11β-hydroxyl group, which is necessary for glucocorticoid activity. In contrast, an 11-C hydroxyl group is oxidized to a keto group in the kidney, minimizing the affinity of the compound for the mineralocorticoid receptor and its salt-retaining effect.

Methylprednisolone and dexamethasone are minimally bound to transcortin and mostly bound to albumin. The percentage bound to plasma proteins for these two glucocorticoids is thus constant, and since the protein binding is concentration-independent, their metabolic clearance remains constant regardless of dose.[28] Table 41–2 shows the properties of different glucocorticoids. The

TABLE 41–1. ACTIONS OF GLUCOCORTICOIDS IN THE RESTING AND STRESS STATES

RESTING STATE	STRESS STATE
Endocrine and Metabolic	
Negative feedback	Negative feedback
Maintenance of metabolic homeostasis (blood glucose levels, liver glycogen content, excretion of water load, effects on gluconeogenetic and lipolytic activities of hormones)	Adaptive changes in metabolic homeostasis [increased blood glucose and liver glycogen content (redirection of energy expenditure from growth or reproductive function to homeostasis), insulin resistance, stimulation of gluconeogenesis and ketogenesis (induction of tyrosine aminotransferase, tryptophan oxygenase, alanine aminotransferase), decreased growth factor action, decreased procollagen formation, suppression of fibroblast growth, decreased thyroid function and activation, gonadotropin suppression, and gonadal resistance to gonadotropins]
Cardiovascular System	
Maintenance of cardiovascular function	Questionable importance in cardiovascular function increase (increases of adenomedullary PMNT, plasma renin substrate)
Adequate heart function and blood vessel tone (permissive effects on inotropic, chronotropic, and pressor activities of hormones)	
Immune System	
Unknown importance of suppression on the immune system	Immunosuppression [thymolysis, altered leukocyte traffic, anti-inflammatory activity, suppression of inflammatory mediators (cytokines, prostanoids, kinins, serotonin, histamine, plasminogen activator, collagenase)]
Musculoskeletal System	
Maintenance of muscle work capacity	Unknown importance in increase of muscle work capacity (induction of enzymes increasing muscular metabolism)
Respiratory System	
Induction of fetal lung surfactant	Induction of fetal lung surfactant
Central Nervous System	
Unknown importance of effects on behavior	Behavioral activation (euphoria, alertness)
Scavenging Properties	
Unknown importance of maintaining adequate detoxification in the resting state	Detoxification of stress-induced toxic products (induction of glutamine synthetase, metallothionin, tyrosine aminotransferase, tryptophan oxygenase)

From Laue et al.,[25] with permission.

TABLE 41–2. GLUCOCORTICOID EQUIVALENCIES

	EQUIVALENT DOSE (mg)	GLUCOCORTICOID POTENCY	MINERALOCORTICOID POTENCY	PLASMA HALF-LIFE (min)	BIOLOGIC HALF-LIFE (h)	MAIN STRUCTURE MODIFICATIONS COMPARED TO CORTISOL			
						C-1–C-2	C-11	C-9	C-16
Glucocorticoids									
Short-acting									
Cortisol	20	1	2	90	8–12		−OH	−H	−H
Cortisone	25	0.8	2	80–118	8–12		=O	−H	−H
Intermediate-acting									
Prednisone	5	4	1	60	18–36	Double bond	=O	−H	−H
Prednisolone	5	4	1	115–200	18–36	Double bond	−OH	−H	−H
Triamcinolone	4	5	0	30	18–36	Double bond	−OH	−F	−OH
Methylprednisolone	4	5	0	180	18–36	Double bond	−OH	−H	−CH3
Long-acting									
Dexamethasone	0.5	25–50	0	200	36–54	Double bond	−OH	−F	−CH3
Betamethasone	0.6	25–50	0	300	36–54	Double bond	−OH	−F	−CH3
Mineralocorticoids									
Aldosterone		0.3	300	15–20	8–12		−O−	−H	−H
Fludrocortisone	2	15	150	200	18–36		=O	−F	−H
Desoxycorticosterone acetate	–	0	20	70	–		−H	−H	−H

biologic half-life of glucocorticoids is characterized as short-, intermediate-, or long-acting, based on the duration of ACTH suppression following a single dose of the compound.[29]

Therapeutic Indications and Side Effects

The therapeutic indications of glucocorticoids are broad and extend to different systems. In endocrinology they are used as substitution therapy in adrenal insufficiency (Table 41–3) or for suppression of adrenal androgen secretion in diseases characterized by androgen hypersecretion, such as congenital adrenal hyperplasia. Glucocorticoids are also employed in gastrointestinal, respiratory, nervous, autoimmune, collagen, renal, ophthalmic, and hematologic diseases. In addition, glucocorticoids are used in suppression of the host-versus-graft or graft-versus-host reaction in cases of tissue transplantation. Neoplastic disorders of the lymphoid system are also treated with glucocorticoids along with the appropriate chemotherapy.

Acute administration of glucocorticoids is necessary in a small number of diseases (Table 41–4), including acute adrenal insufficiency,[30,31] congenital adrenal hyperplasia,[32] neonatal hypoglycemia, malignant hyperthermia,[33,34] and

prevention of the respiratory distress syndrome when delivery is anticipated before the 34th week of gestation.[35] In the last case, treatment of the pregnant woman with 12 mg of betamethasone, followed by another 12 mg 18–24 hours later, stimulates the maturation of the fetal lungs.

Complications are unlikely with short-term treatment (less than 2 weeks) with moderate doses of glucocorticoids. Chronic treatment with glucocorticoids, on the other hand, has been associated with multiple side effects (Table 41–5).[36–47] These include the development of Cushing's syndrome during therapy and adrenal insufficiency after discontinuation of treatment. To avoid both complications, single daily doses of short-acting glucocorticoids or alternate-day administration of intermediate-acting glucocorticoids should be employed, when possible, in chronic therapy. Termination of chronic therapy (longer than 2 weeks) should be gradual both to prevent development of acute adrenal insufficiency and to avoid reactivation of the disease under therapy. The degree of cushingoid features or the chronicity of adrenal suppression depends on both the type and dose of the specific compound used, the duration of treatment, and the idiosyncrasy of the patient.[48,49]

Growth retardation is one of the major side effects of chronic glucocorticoid therapy in children. Normal growth, however, has been reported for up to 50 months on alternate-day administration of glucocorticoids.[50,51] Inhaled glucocorticoids are preferred for asthma, since

TABLE 41–3. TREATMENT OF CHRONIC ADRENAL INSUFFICIENCY

	DRUG	DOSE AND ROUTE OF ADMINISTRATION
Standard replacement	Hydrocortisone	10–15 mg/m^2/day P.O.
	Fludrocortisone or DOC pivalate	0.1–0.5 mg/day P.O. 1 mg/wk I.M.
Minor Surgery* (day of surgery) or febrile illness*	Hydrocortisone	X 2 std replacement dose (divided b.i.d.)
Major surgery* (day before surgery, day of surgery, postop day 1)	Hydrocortisone	X 5–10 std replacement dose (divided t.i.d.)

*Mineralocorticoid replacement continued unaltered.

TABLE 41–4. DISEASES IN WHICH ACUTE ADMINISTRATION OF GLUCOCORTICOIDS IS NECESSARY

DISEASE	DRUG	DOSE AND ROUTE OF ADMINISTRATION
Neonatal hypoglycemia	Glucose Hydrocortisone phosphate	2–5 mg/kg/24 h continuously I.V.
Malignant hyperthermia	Dexamethasone	8 mg I.V.
Acute adrenal insufficiency	(Fluids and electrolytes essential) Hydrocortisone phosphate Fludrocortisone or DOCA*	1–2 mg/kg I.V./6 h
Fetal lung distress	Betamethasone	12 mg × 2/24 h

*Not necessary if hydrocortisone phosphate is used because the latter provides sufficient salt-retaining activity.

TABLE 41–5. EFFECTS OF GLUCOCORTICOIDS DURING CHRONIC THERAPY

Endocrine and Metabolic Disorders
Suppression of HPA axis
Growth failure in children
Diabetes mellitus
 Hyperinsulinemia
 Insulin resistance
 Abnormal glucose tolerance test
 Ketoacidosis
Cushingoid features
 Moon facies, facial plethora
 Truncal obesity
 Supraclavicular fat collection
 Posterior cervical fat deposition (buffalo hump)
 Acne, hirsutism
 Thin and fragile skin, violaceous striae
Impotence, menstrual disorders
Decreased TSH and T_3
Hypokalemia, metabolic alkalosis

Gastrointestinal System
Peptic ulcer
Pancreatitis
Fatty infiltration of liver (hepatomegaly)

Hemopoietic System
Leukocytosis
 Neutrophilia
  Increased influx from bone marrow and
  Decreased migration from blood vessels
Monocytopenia
Lymphopenia
 Migration from blood vessels to lymphoid tissue
Eosinopenia

Immune System
Suppression of delayed hypersensitivity
 Inhibition of leukocytes and tissue macrophages migration
 Inhibition of cytokine secretion/action
Suppression of the primary antigen response

Musculoskeletal System
Osteoporosis, spontaneous fractures
Aseptic necrosis of femoral and humoral heads and other bones
Myopathy

Ophthalmic
Posterior subcapsular cataracts (more common in children)
Elevated intraocular pressure/glaucoma

Neuropsychiatric disorders (CNS)
Psychosis, depression, euphoria
Pseudotumor cerebri (benign increase of intracranial pressure)

From Laue,[25] with permission.

they have a lesser effect in suppressing growth.[52] Another complication, which seems to be frequent in children, is development of posterior subcapsular cataracts. Cataract deterioration ceases after discontinuation of treatment but is irreversible.[53,54]

Nonfluorinated glucocorticoids (cortisone, cortisol, prednisone, and prednisolone) cross the placenta poorly. Fluorinated steroids, on the other hand, cross the placenta readily and should be given cautiously in pregnancy. Maternal–fetal plasma concentration gradients are approximately 10 to 1 for cortisol or prednisolone,[55] 3 to 1 for betamethasone,[56] and 1 to 1 for dexamethasone. Newborns who have been exposed to high doses of synthetic fluorinated corticosteroids *in utero* should be checked for signs of adrenal insufficiency. Special precaution should be taken with premature infants, because some glucocorticoid preparations containing benzyl alcohol have been associated with a fatal "gasping" syndrome.

Most complications of glucocorticoid treatment are reversible after discontinuation of glucocorticoid administration, with the exception of posterior subcapsular cataracts and advanced bone necrosis.[57,58]

Adrenal Suppression

Recovery of the HPA axis can take as long as 12 months or even longer. Abrupt interruption of glucocorticoid treatment can precipitate an acute adrenal insufficiency crisis. The main symptoms are anorexia, fatigue, nausea, vomiting, dyspnea, fever, arthralgia, myalgia, orthostatic hypotension, dizziness, fainting, and circulatory collapse. Hypoglycemia is occasionally observed in children and thin individuals. Treatment should be immediate, primarily by administration of fluids and electrolytes and parenteral glucocorticoids (Table 41–4).

Diagnostic Uses

Dexamethasone has been used for diagnostic purposes primarily in the screening for, and the differential diagnosis of, Cushing's syndrome. Dexamethasone normally suppresses pituitary ACTH release and consequently adrenal cortisol secretion. In patients with Cushing's syndrome, in whom feedback control of ACTH by glucocorticoids is impaired, dexamethasone does not adequately suppress ACTH and cortisol secretion. Three different tests can be performed according to the suspected diagnosis (Table 41–6):

1.   Overnight 1 mg dexamethasone suppression test, in the screening of subjects suspected of having hypercortisolism.

2.   Overnight 8 mg dexamethasone suppression test in the differential diagnosis of Cushing's disease from ectopic ACTH and from primary adrenal Cushing's syndrome.

3.   Standard low- and high-dose dexamethasone suppression test (Liddle test[60]), for the differentiation of Cushing's disease from the ectopic ACTH syndrome or from cortisol-secreting tumors. The diagnostic accuracy of this test is approximately 85 percent.

Monitoring of Patients Under Chronic Treatment

Patients under chronic treatment with glucocorticoids should adhere to a diet with caloric restriction, high protein intake, and rich in potassium and low in sodium. For gastric problems they should take antacids or histamine 2 antagonists. Younger children (until age 2) should be monitored every 3 months and older ones every 6 months by measurement of body weight, length or height, blood pressure, 2-hour postprandial blood glucose, serum electrolytes, and bone maturation.

Concomitant Use of Glucocorticoids With Other Drugs

Special attention is required in the concomitant use of glucocorticoids with other drugs, because some of them

---

TABLE 41–6.   DEXAMETHASONE SUPPRESSION TESTS

Overnight 1-mg Dexamethasone Suppression Test
Method
1 mg dexamethasone (15 μg/kg in children) is given orally at 11:00 PM. A plasma sample for measurement of cortisol is drawn at 8:00 the following morning.

Interpretation
Suppression of basal plasma cortisol level to <5 μg/dl is defined as a normal suppression. A plasma cortisol level >5 μg/dl suggests hypercortisolism, and further evaluation to explore the possibility of Cushing's syndrome is required.

Uses
As a screening test for subjects suspected of having hypercortisolism

Problems
Technical errors such as failure to take the agent, poor sleeping, administration at the wrong time, and rapid or slow metabolism of dexamethasone. Pediatric standards have not been established, but the above dose is suggested.

Overnight 8-mg Dexamethasone Suppression Test
Method
Baseline plasma cortisol level is measured at 8:00 AM, and a single 8-mg (120 μg/kg in children) oral dose of dexamethasone is given at 11:00 PM. A plasma sample for measurement of cortisol is drawn at 8:00 the following morning.

Interpretation
Suppression of basal plasma cortisol to <50% of baseline the following morning suggests Cushing's disease. Failure of plasma cortisol to be suppressed indicates an ectopic source of ACTH or an adrenal cortisol-secreting tumor.

Uses
Differential diagnosis of Cushing's disease from other forms of Cushing's syndrome. Pediatric standards have not been established, but the above dose is suggested.

Standard Low- and High-Dose Dexamethasone Suppression Test (Liddle Test)
Method
The test begins with two baseline 24-hour urine collections for measurement of 17-hydroxycorticosteroids, free cortisol, and creatinine excretion. After the baseline period, dexamethasone is given orally at a dose of 0.5 mg every 6 hours for 2 days (2 mg/day in adults, 30 μg/kg/day in children). This is followed by administration of 2 mg of dexamethasone every 6 hours for 2 more days (8 mg/day in adults, initiation of 120 μg/kg/day in children). Blood for measurement of plasma cortisol and ACTH is obtained at 8:00 AM before and 24 and 48 hours after the low and/or high dose dexamethasone administration. Daily urine collections for measurements of 17-hydroxycorticosteroids, free cortisol, and creatinine are continued until the end of the test.

Interpretation
Low-dose
Suppression of urinary 17-hydroxycorticosteroids to <4 mg per day or to <2.5 mg/gm creatinine during the second day of dexamethasone indicates normal ACTH regulation. Suppression of urine free cortisol to >50% of baseline or a decrease in plasma cortisol to <5 μg/dl also suggests normal ACTH regulation.
High-dose
Suppression of urinary 17-hydroxycorticosteroids and cortisol to >50% and 90% of baseline levels, respectively, and suppression of plasma cortisol to <5 μg/dl suggests Cushing's disease.

Uses
Differential diagnosis of Cushing's disease from ectopic ACTH production or adrenal cortisol-secreting tumors

---

From Kamilaris and Chrousos,[59] with permission.

TABLE 41–7A. INTERACTIONS OF GLUCOCORTICOIDS WITH OTHER DRUGS

DRUG	SIDE EFFECT	COMMENTS
Amphotericin B	Hypokalemia	Monitor potassium levels frequently
Potassium-depleting diuretics	Hypokalemia	Monitor potassium levels frequently
Digitalis glycosides	Digitalis toxicity Hypokalemia	Monitor potassium levels frequently
Vaccines from live attenuated viruses	Severe allergic reactions or generalized infections	
Growth hormone	Ineffective	

TABLE 41–7B. EFFECT OF GLUCOCORTICOIDS ON BLOOD LEVELS OF OTHER DRUGS MAINLY DUE TO THEIR EFFECT ON THE METABOLISM AND CLEARANCE RATE OF THE DRUG

DRUG	DRUG BLOOD LEVELS	COMMENTS
Aspirin	Decreased	Increased metabolism or clearance Monitor salicylate levels
Coumarin anticoagulants	Decreased	Frequent control of prothrombin levels
Cyclophosphamide	Increased	Inhibition of hepatic metabolism Adjust the dose of the drug
Cyclosporine	Increased	Inhibition of hepatic metabolism
Insulin	Decreased	Adjust the dose of the drug
Isoniazid	Decreased	Increased metabolism and clearance
Oral hypoglycemic agents	Decreased	Adjust the dose of the drug

TABLE 41–7C. EFFECT OF DRUGS ON PLASMA GLUCOCORTICOID CONCENTRATIONS

DRUG	GLUCOCORTICOID BLOOD LEVELS	COMMENTS
Antacids	Decreased	Possible physical adsorption to antacid[61]
Carbamazepine	Decreased	Increased cytochrome P-450 activity[62–64]
Cholestyramine	Decreased	Decreased GI absorption of glucocorticoids
Colestipol	Decreased	Decreased GI absorption of glucocorticoids
Cyclosporine	Increased	Inhibition of hepatic metabolism
Ephedrine	Decreased	Probably increased metabolism[65]
Erythromycin	Increased	Impaired elimination[66]
Mitotane	Decreased	Adjust glucocorticoid levels
Oral contraceptives	Increased	Impaired elimination, increased protein binding[67]
Phenobarbital	Decreased	Increased cytochrome P-450 activity.[63,68] Adjust glucocorticoid dosage
Phenytoin	Decreased	Increased cytochrome P-450 activity.[63,68] Adjust glucocorticoid dosage
Rifampin	Decreased	Probably increased cytochrome P-450 activity.[69] Adjust glucocorticoid dosage
Troleandomycin	Increased	Partially due to impaired elimination[70–74]

may affect the metabolism of these steroids and may lead to a decreased or increased effect on their target tissues. Such interactions are shown in Table 41–7. Slight differences may exist among the various compounds.

Topical Glucocorticoids

Whereas most topical medications useful in dermatotherapy are odorous and may stain the skin, glucocorticoids are stable, colorless, and odorless drugs that, in addition, are nontoxic in the short term. The factors that determine local penetration are the structure of the steroid molecule, the vehicle, the basic additives,[75,76] occlusion versus open use,[77] normal skin versus diseased skin,[78-80] small areas versus large areas, localization of application,[81] and, in rare cases, the existence of another disease.

The complications of topical use of glucocorticoids can be local, including epidermal atrophy, telangiectasia, acne, folliculitis, and granuloma gluteale infantum,[82-85] or systemic, including Cushing's syndrome, retardation of growth in children, and adrenal suppression.[86] Systemic effects are increased in newborns and small children compared to adolescents and adults, because glucocorticoids penetrate the skin more easily and in larger proportional amounts in children due to higher permeability and relative surface area of the skin.[87] Systemic effects may also be increased in patients with renal and hepatic diseases.

REFERENCES

1. Benizschhke K: Adrenals in anencephaly and hydrocephaly. Obstet Gynecol 8:412, 1956
2. Constantopoulos G, Tchen TT: Cleavage of cholesterol side chain by adrenal cortex. JBC 236:65, 1961
3. Halkerston IDK, Eichorn J, Hechter O: A requirement for reduced triphosphopyridine nucleotide for cholesterol side chain cleavage by mitochondrial fractions of bovine adrenal cortex. JBC 236:374, 1961
4. Saba N, Hechter O, Stone D: The conversion of cholesterol to pregnenolone in bovine adrenal homogenates. J Am Chem Soc 76:3862, 1954
5. Mason HS: Mechanisms of oxygen metabolism. Adv Enzymol 19:79, 1957
6. Beitins IZ, Bayard F, Ances IG, Kowarski A, Migeon CJ: The metabolic clearance rate, blood production, interconversion and transplacental passage of cortisol and cortisone in pregnancy near term. Pediatr Res 7:509, 1973
7. Murphy BE, Clark SJ, Donald IR, Pinsky M, Vedaly D: Conversion of maternal cortisol to cortisone during placental transfer to the human fetus. Am J Obstet Gynecol 118:538, 1974
8. Rousseau GG, Baxter JD: Glucocorticoid receptors, in Baxter JD, Rousseau GG (eds): Monograph in Endocrinology. Berlin and New York, Springer-Verlag, 1979, pp 49–77
9. Baxter JD, Rousseau GG: Glucocorticoid hormone action: An overview, in Baxter JD, Rousseau GG (eds): Monograph in Endocrinology. Berlin and New York, Springer-Verlag, 1979, pp 1–24
10. Gustaffson JA, Carsteldt-Duke J, Poellinger L, Okret S, Wikstrom AC, Bronnegard M, Gillner M, Dong Y, Fuxe K, Cintra A, Agnati L: Biochemistry, molecular biology and physiology of glucocorticoid receptor. Endocr Rev 8:185, 1987
11. Ballard PL, Baxter JD, Rousseau GG, Higgins JJ, Tomkins GM: General presence of glucocorticoid receptors in responsive mammalian tissues. Endocrinology 94:998, 1974
12. Hollenberg SM, Weinberger C, Ong ES, Cerelli G, Oro A, Lebo R,

Thompson EB, Rosenfeld G, Evans RM: Primary structure and expression of a functional human glucocorticoid receptor cDNA. Nature 318:635, 1985
13. Weinberger C, Thompson CC, Ong ES, Lebo R, Grinol DJ, Evans RM: The c-erb A gene encodes a thyroid hormone receptor. Nature 324:641, 1986
14. Giguere V, Hollenberg SM, Rosenfeld MG, Evans RH: Functional domains of the human glucocorticoid receptor. Cell 46:645, 1986
15. Schmidt TJ, Litwak G: Activation of the glucocorticoid-receptor complex. Physiol Rev 62:1131, 1982
16. Yamamoto KRA: Steroid receptor regulated transcription of specific genes and gene networks. Rev Genet 19:209, 1985
17. Payvar F, De Franco D, Firestone GL, Edgar B, Wrange O, Gustaffson JA, Yamamoto KR: Sequence-specific binding of glucocorticoid receptor to MTV DNA at sites within and upstream of the transcribed region. Cell 35:38, 1983
18. Krieger DT, Allen W, Rizzo F, Krieger HP: Characterization of the normal temporal pattern of plasma corticosteroid levels. J Clin Endocrinol Metab 32:266, 1971
19. Franks RC: Diurnal variation of plasma 17-hydroxycorticosteroids in children. Clin Endocrinol Metab 27:75, 1967
20. Kenny FM, Richards C, Taylor FH: Reference standards for cortisol production and 17-hydroxycorticosteroid excretion during growth. Variation in the pattern of excretion of radiolabelled cortisol metabolites. Metabolism 19:28, 1970
21. Migeon CJ, Prystowsky H, Grumbach MM, et al: Placental passage of 17-hydroxycorticosteroids: Comparison of the levels in maternal and fetal plasma and effect of ACTH and hydrocortisone administration. J Clin Invest 35:488, 1956
22. Rokicki W, Bertrand J: The glucocorticoids in normal premature and small for dates newborn infants throughout the neonatal period, in Stern L, Salle B, Friis-Hansen B (eds): Intensive Care of the Newborn, II. New York, Masson, 1981, pp 325–342
23. Jamieson T: Corticosteroids for rheumatic disease. Postgrad Med 79:239, 1986
24. Lewis GP, Jusko WJ, Burke CW, et al: Prednisone side effects and serum protein levels. Lancet 2:778, 1971
25. Laue L, Kawai S, Udelsman R, Nieman LK, Brandon DD, Gallucci WT, Gold PW, Loriaux DL, Chrousos GP: Glucocorticoid antagonists: Pharmacological attributes of the prototype antiglucocorticoid RU486, in Lichtenstein LM, Claman H, Oronsky A, Schleimer RP (eds): Antiinflammatory Steroid Action: Basic and Clinical Aspects. New York, Academic Press, 1989, pp 303–329
26. Hench PS, Kendall EC, Slocumb CH, Polley H: The effect of a hormone of the adrenal cortex (17-hydroxy 11-dehydrocortisone): compound E and of pituitary adrenocorticotropic hormone on rheumatoid arthritis. Proc Staff Meet Mayo Clin 24:181, 1949
27. Rousseau GG, Baxter JD, Tomkins GP: Glucocorticoid receptor: Relation between steroid binding and biological effects. J Mol Biol 67:99, 1972
28. Szefler SJ, Ebling WF, Georgitis JW, Jusko WJ: Methylprednisolone versus prednisolone pharmacokinetics in relation to dose in adults. Eur J Clin Pharmacol 30:323, 1966
29. Harter JG: Corticosteroids: Their physiological use in allergic diseases. NY State J Med 66:827, 1966
30. Fass B: Glucocorticoid therapy for nonendocrine disorders: Withdrawal and coverage. Pediatr Clin Nor Am 26:251, 1974
31. Scott RS, Donald RA, Espiner EA: Plasma ACTH and cortisol profiles in Addisonian patients receiving conventional substitution therapy. Clin Endocrinol 9:571, 1978
32. Jones-Klingensmith G, Garcia SC, Jones HW Jr: Glucocorticoid treatment of girl with congenital adrenal hyperplasia: Effects on heights, sexual maturation and fertility. J Pediatr 90:996, 1977
33. Ellis FR, Clarke IMC, Appleyard TN, et al: Malignant hyperpyrexia induced by nitrous oxide and treated with dexamethasone. Br Med J 4:270, 1974
34. Raitt DG, Merrifield AJ: Dexamethasone in malignant hyperpyrexia. Br Med J 4:656, 1974
35. Collaborative group on antenatal steroid therapy: Effect of antenatal dexamethasone administration on the prevention of respiratory distress syndrome. Am J Obstet Gynecol 141:276, 1981
36. Bailin PL, Matkaluk RM: Cutaneous reactions to rheumatologic drugs. Clin Rheum Dis 8:493, 1982

37. Crews SJ: Adverse reactions to corticosteroid therapy in the eye. Proc R Soc Med 58:533, 1965

38. David DS, Grieco MH, Cushman P Jr: Adrenal glucocorticoids after twenty years—A review of their clinically relevant consequences. J Chron Dis 22:711, 1970

39. Gallant C, Kenny P: Oral glucocorticoids and their complications. J Am Acad Dermatol 14:161, 1986

40. Haanaes OC, Bergmann A: Tuberculosis emerging in patients treated with corticosteroids. Eur J Respir Dis 64:294, 1983

41. Hahn TJ: Corticosteroid-induced osteopenia. Arch Intern Med 138:882, 1978

42. Ivey KJ, Den Besten L: Pseudotumor cerebri associated with corticosteroid therapy in adult. JAMA 208:1698, 1969

43. Kjellstrand CM: Side effects of steroids and their treatment. Transplant Proc 7:123, 1975

44. Rimsza ME: Complications of corticosteroid therapy. Am J Dis Child 132:806, 1978

45. Rooklin AR, Lampert SI, Jaeger EA, et al: Posterior subcapsular cataracts in steroid-requiring asthmatic children. J Allergy Clin Immunol 63:383, 1979

46. Shiono H, Oonoshi M, Yamaguchi M: Posterior subcapsular cataracts associated with long term oral corticosteroid therapy. Clin Pediatr 16:726, 1977

47. Weisberg LA, Chutorian AM: Pseudotumor cerebri of childhood. Am J Dis Child 113:727, 1967

48. Conn HO, Blitzer BL: Non association of adrenocorticosteroid therapy and peptic ulcer. N Engl J Med 294:473, 1974

49. Messer J, Reitman D, Sacks HS, Smith H Jr, Chalmers TC: Association of adrenocorticosteroid therapy and peptic ulcer disease. N Engl J Med 309:21, 1983

50. Morris HG: Growth and skeletal maturation in asthmatic children: Effect of corticosteroid treatment. Pediatr Res 9:579, 1975

51. Sadeghi-Nejad A, Senior B: Adrenal function, growth and insulin in patients treated with corticoids on alternate days. Pediatrics 43:277, 1969

52. Soderberg-Warner M, Siegel S, Katz R, et al: Treatment of chronic childhood asthma with beclomethasone aerosols (BDA) IV. Long term effects on growth (Abstr.). J Allergy Clin Immunol 63:164, 1979

53. Kobayashi Y, Akaishi K, Nishio T, et al: Posterior subcapsular cataracts in nephrotic children receiving steroid therapy. Am Dis Child 128:671, 1974

54. Eitches RW, Rachelefsky GS, Katz RM, Mendoza GR, Siegel SC: Methylprednisolone and troleandomycin in treatment of steroid-dependent asthmatic children. Am J Dis Child 139:264, 1985

55. Beitins IZ, Bayard F, Ances IG, Kowarski A, Migeon CJ: The transplacental passage of prednisone and prednisolone in pregnancy near term. J Pediatr 81:936, 1972

56. Ballard PL, Grandberg P, Ballard RA: Glucocorticoid levels in maternal and cord serum after prenatal betamethasone therapy to prevent respiratory distress syndrome. J Clin Invest 56:1548, 1975

57. Richards JM, Santiago SM, Klaustermeyer WB: Aseptic necrosis of the femoral head in corticosteroid-treated pulmonary disease. Arch Intern Med XX:1473, 1980

58. Sutton RD, Benedek TG, Edwards GA: Aseptic bone necrosis and corticosteroid therapy. Arch Intern Med 112:594, 1963

59. Kamilaris TC, Chrousos GP: Adrenal diseases, in Moore T, Eastman R (eds): Diagnostic Endocrinology. Toronto, BC Decker, 1990, pp 79–109

60. Liddle GW: Tests of pituitary-adrenal suppressibility in the diagnosis of Cushing's syndrome. J Clin Endocrinol Metab 20:1539, 1960

61. Uribe M, Casian C, Rojas S, Sierra JG: Decreased bioavailability of prednisone due to antacids in patients with chronic active liver disease and in healthy volunteers. Gastroenterology 80:661, 1981

62. Bartoszeck M, Brenner AM, Szefler SJ: Prednisolone and methylprednisolone kinetics in children receiving anticonvulsant therapy. Clin Pharmacol Ther 42:424, 1987

63. Brooks SM, Werk EE, Ackerman SJ, Sullivan I, Thrasher K: Adverse effects of phenobarbital on corticosteroid metabolism in patients with bronchial asthma. N Engl J Med 286:1125, 1972

64. Stjenholm MR, Katz FH: Effects of diphenylhydantoin, phenobarbital and diazepam on the metabolism of methylprednisolone and its sodium succinate. J Clin Endocrinol Metab 41:887, 1975

65. Brooks SM, Sholiton LJ, Werk EE, Alten H: The effect of ephedrine and theophylline on dexamethasone metabolism in bronchial asthma. J Clin Pharmacol 17:308, 1977

66. LaForce CF, Szefler SJ, Miller MF, Ebling W, Brenner M: Inhibition of methylprednisolone elimination in the presence of erythromycin therapy. J Allergy Clin Immunol 72:34, 1983

67. Boekenoogen SZ, Szefler SJ, Jusko WJ: Prednisolone disposition and protein binding in oral contraceptives users. J Clin Endocrinol Metab 56:702, 1983

68. Haque N, Thrasher K, Werk EE, Knowles HC, Sholiton LJ: Studies on dexamethasone metabolism in man: Effect of diphenylhydantoin. J Clin Endocrinol Metab 34:44, 1972

69. Buffington GA, Dominguez JH, Piering WF, Herbert LA, Kauffman HM, Lemann J: Interaction of rifampin and glucocorticoids: Adverse effect on renal allograft function. JAMA 236:1958, 1976

70. Eitches RW, Rachelefsky GS, Katz RM, Mendora GR, Siegel SC: Methylprednisolone and troleandomycin in treatment of steroid dependent asthmatic children. Am J Dis Child 136:264, 1985

71. Spector SL, Katz F, Farr RS: Troleandomycin: Effectiveness in steroid dependent asthma and bronchitis. J Allergy Clin Immuncl 54:367, 1975

72. Szefler SJ, Rose JQ, Ellis EF, Spector SL, Green AW, Jusko WJ: The effect of troleandomycin on methylprednisolone elimination. J Allergy Clin Immunol 66:447, 1980

73. Szefler SJ, Brenner M, Jusko WJ, Spector SL, Flesher K, Ellis EF: Dose and time related effect of troleandomycin on methylprednisolone elimination. Clin Pharmacol Ther 32:166, 1982

74. Zeiger RS, Schatz M, Sperling W, Simon RA, Stevenson DD: Efficacy of troleandomycin in outpatients with severe, corticosteroid-dependent asthma. J Allergy Clin Immunol 66:438, 1980

75. Franz TJ: Kinetics of cutaneous drug penetration. Int J Dermatol 22:499, 1983

76. Wohlrab W: The influence of urea on the penetration kinetics of topically applied corticosteroids. Acta Dermatol Venerol 64:233, 1984

77. Weister RC, Maibach HI: Cutaneous pharmacokinetics: 10 steps to percutaneous absorption. Drug Metab Rev 14:169, 1983

78. Turpeinem M: Influence of age and severity of dermatitis on the percutaneous absorption of hydrocortisone in children. Br J Dermatol 118:517, 1988

79. Wester RC, Bucks DAW, Maibach HI: In vivo percutaneous absorption of hydrocortisone in psoriatic patients and normal volunteers. J Am Acad Dermatol 8:645, 1983

80. Wilson JE: Steroid atrophy—A histological appraisal. Dermatologica 152(suppl 1):107.1, 1976

81. Feldman R, Maibach HI: Regional variation in percutaneous penetration of ^{14}C-cortisol in man. J Invest Dermatol 103:39, 1970

82. Hogan DJ, Sibley JT, Lane PR: A case of osteoporosis and avascular necrosis of the hips following long-term use of clobetasol propionate ointment. J Am Acad Dermatol 15:515, 1986

83. Kligman AM, Frisb PJ: Steroid addiction. Int J Dermatol 18:23, 1980

84. Lee SS: Topical steroids. J Invest Dermatol 20:632, 1981

85. Smith JG, Sihr RF, Chalker DK: Corticosteroid induced atrophy and telangiectasia. Arch Dermatol 112:115, 1976

86. May P, Stein EJ, Ryter RJ, Levy P: Cushing's syndrome from percutaneous absorption of triamcinolone cream. Arch Intern Med 135:612, 1976

87. Munro DD: Topical corticosteroid therapy and its effect on the hypothalamic-pituitary-adrenal axis. Acta Dermatol 152(suppl 1):173, 1976

42

INSULIN AND DIABETES MELLITUS

ALICIA SCHIFFRIN *and* ELEANOR COLLE

In 1922 the glucose-lowering effects of pancreatic extracts were reported by Banting, Best, Collip, and MacLeod.[1] They named the active principle insulin. Since then, insulin has become one of the best-characterized of vertebrate hormones. It was the first protein to be completely sequenced[2] and chemically synthesized.[3] The structural details of the crystalline form are known.[4] The gene for insulin has been cloned[5] and localized, and a recombinant form has been utilized for treatment for several years. In addition, there is an enormous literature on the mechanism of action at the level of the cell, the organ, and the whole animal.

Insulin is the major anabolic hormone. It regulates the flow of nutrients across cell membranes and modulates the activities of enzymes that promote either utilization of these nutrients for energy needs or conversion of them to storage forms of energy. A deficiency of insulin, due either to failure of production or to interference with action, results in the complex metabolic disorders that comprise the diabetic syndromes.

SYNTHESIS, RELEASE, AND CIRCULATION IN BLOOD

Synthesis

Insulin is synthesized exclusively within the beta cells of the islets of Langerhans of the pancreas. These organelles, consisting of four types of endocrine cell, are embedded in the substance of the exocrine pancreas where they comprise about 1 percent of the mass of that organ. The beta cells are the predominant cell types of the islet and are located in the center of the islet surrounded by alpha cells that make glucagon, delta cells that make somatostatin, and cells that secrete pancreatic polypeptide.[6]

Insulin is derived from a precursor molecule, preproinsulin,[7] a 110-amino-acid peptide encoded by a single gene on human chromosome 11.[8] This presecretory hormone

is rapidly cleaved by microsomal peptidases. The resultant peptide, proinsulin, consists of 86 amino acid residues, of which 30 constitute the B chain of insulin, 21 the A chain, and 35 the connecting segment (C-peptide). The amino acid composition of the insulin molecule is highly conserved between species; porcine insulin differs from human insulin in only one amino acid in the B chain. However, there is considerable variation in the connecting peptide portion of the proinsulin molecule. The translated proinsulin chain undergoes folding and oxidation to the correct disulfide-bridged structure in the cisternae of the endoplasmic reticulum.

Conversion of labeled proinsulin to insulin normally begins after an approximately 20-minute delay associated with cellular transport of labeled proinsulin from the site of synthesis (rough endoplasmic reticulum) to the site of conversion (presumably the Golgi complex and secretory granules). Thereafter, conversion normally follows pseudo-first-order kinetics with a half-life of 36 minutes. Splitting of the proinsulin molecule results in 1 mole of the insulin molecule (now consisting of one A chain and one B chain linked by two disulfide bridges) and 1 mole of C-peptide. Since both are found within secretory granules, it is thought that packaging of proinsulin occurs before cleavage of the molecule.

The mature insulin molecule exists in a crystallized form within specific secretory granules that can be recognized by the characteristic appearance on electron microscopy and by staining with chemical or immunocytochemical methods. Two atoms of zinc are found to be present with six molecules of insulin in a spheroid unit.[9] The purified molecule has a biologic activity of approximately 25 units/mg. Insulin is relatively insoluble within the pH range of 4 to 7.

Release

The release of insulin occurs in response to a variety of stimuli. The secretory granules move to the plasma mem-

476

brane, a process probably related to the microtubular system. Here they fuse with the membrane and then rupture, freeing the granules.[10] Released mole for mole with insulin is the excised C-peptide. It has no biologic activity but is useful for following insulin release in individuals with anti-insulin antibodies that interfere with the usual immunoassays of insulin. A small amount of proinsulin which has escaped cleavage may also be released. It has a markedly reduced biologic activity.[11]

There is considerable evidence that there is more than one pool of insulin secretory granules. Grodsky[12] has suggested that certain secretory granules are "marked" for preferential secretion of newly synthesized insulin. Marking is regulated by the concentration of several secretagogues such as glucose and occurs only at a critical time when newly synthesized hormone is transiting the Golgi apparatus and new secretory granules are being formed. Basal release of insulin is pulsatile.[13] Pulses with periods of 11–13 minutes have been described. This is of some interest, since it has been reported that intravenous insulin administration is more effective in decreasing hepatic glucose output when given in a pulsatile fashion.[14]

Secretion

A variety of stimuli will lead to insulin release. Glucose elicits an immediate (within 2 minutes) increase in insulin release. If the concentration of glucose bathing the beta cell remains elevated, there is a continuous release of insulin. Since the acute release occurs so soon after elevation of glucose, it has been proposed that there is a glucose "sensor," the occupation of which permits immediate release. Matschinsky[15] has proposed that glucokinase is that sensor. The immediate effect is associated with closing of the ATP-sensitive K^+ channels and is dependent on calcium in the medium.[16] It is potentiated by any substance that increases cAMP release (glucagon, gastrin inhibitory peptide, acetylcholine, β-adrenergic stimulators) or decreases its degradation (methylxanthines). In insulin-producing cell lines, the sulfonylureas, alanine, and high K^+ release insulin in association with an increase in intracellular calcium influx via a voltage-dependent calcium channel. The second phase of insulin release may be dependent on the intracellular metabolism of glucose or other nutrients.

The observation that insulin levels are higher after oral glucose than after intravenous glucose suggested that factors in the gut may be contributing to insulin release. Three gut hormones, gastrin inhibitory peptide (GIP), cholecystokinin (CCPK), and glucagon-like peptide (GLP, 7-36),[17,20] have been shown to have such an effect. GIP increases intra-beta-cell cAMP, while it has been suggested that, at least in insulin-producing cell lines, CCPK may work through the inositol pathway to increase intracellular calcium.

Both parasympathetic and sympathetic nerve fibers impinge on the islets of Langerhans. Acetylcholine and β-adrenergic stimulators increase insulin release by increasing cAMP, whereas α-adrenergic stimulation inhibits insulin release.[21]

As indicated, there are also a variety of substances that inhibit insulin release. The delta cell of the islet of Langerhans contains somatostatin, a potent inhibitor of insulin release. Prostaglandin E_2 also inhibits insulin release, as do substances that bind to the α-adrenergic receptors.[22]

Overall, the release of insulin is under regulation at a number of levels. Within the cell, prostaglandins derived from breakdown of membrane lipids may amplify or dampen a stimulatory signal. Within the islet, paracrine mechanisms may potentiate (glucagon) or inhibit (somatostatin) release. Neural and catecholamine signals also provide the possibility of both up- and down-modulation. An enteropancreatic axis further tailors the insulin release to the presence of nutrient stimulants in the gut, and neurotransmitters and pituitary peptides suggest mechanisms whereby cephalic contributions to insulin release may occur.

Under normal physiologic conditions, the ingestion of a mixed meal results in release of insulin into the portal vein. The liver takes up about 50 percent of the plasma insulin, so that venous plasma levels are about one-half of those in the portal vein. Plasma levels peak between 30 and 60 minutes after an oral glucose challenge and return to baseline values by 2 hours.

During fetal life, the fetus is not exposed to variation in blood glucose and the islets of the fetus remain relatively nonreactive to changes in glucose concentration, although they do respond to amino acids and the compounds that inhibit cAMP breakdown. During the first few days of extrauterine life, plasma insulin levels are generally low and the infant exhibits a delayed insulin response to oral as well as to intravenous glucose loads.[23] Responsiveness with first-phase insulin release is usually present by the end of the first week. Infants of poorly controlled diabetic mothers exposed to higher ambient glucose concentrations in fetal life do show brisk first-phase insulin release immediately after birth.

The plasma levels of insulin that are necessary to maintain normoglycemia are generally lower in children than adults, both in the fasting and in the postabsorptive states. At puberty the levels of plasma insulin required to maintain euglycemia are increased. This has been attributed to changes in levels of growth hormone and gonadal steroids, which rise during this period.[24] Obese children at all ages have higher basal and higher postabsorptive levels than their lean peers.

MECHANISM OF ACTION

Insulin Receptor

Insulin is transported to its target tissue where it interacts with a specific receptor. This receptor consists of two alpha and two beta subunits. The alpha subunit is the site of binding of the insulin molecule. The beta subunit is an enzyme that specifically phosphorylates tyrosine residues, including the four on the beta subunit itself. It is thought that this phosphorylation is the initial step in the transduction of the insulin signal to the insulin-sensitive processes within the cell.[25] The insulin receptor is internalized within a short time following binding of the hormone, with the formation of an endosome which contains the insulin-bound hormone but allows the phosphorylated kinase opportunity to continue reaction with other intracellular structures.[26] Both *in vivo* and *in vitro* studies have suggested that in ketoacidosis there is a fall in the specific insulin binding.[27] Insulin is degraded after internalization. Insulin protease (E.C. 3.4.22.11, insulinase) is an important enzyme in this process.[28]

Tissue Targets

The maintenance of normoglycemia is only one manifestation of insulin's role in the regulation of the nutrient fuels used by the body as a source of energy. Overall, the postprandial surge of insulin promotes the storage of nutrients. As the levels of insulin fall, mobilization of energy from these insulin-sensitive storage sites proceeds under the influence of the counterregulatory hormones. The major sites of insulin action are the liver, the muscle, and the adipocyte. However, insulin receptors are found on virtually all cells of the body, and the hormone exerts its effects on all but the cells of the central nervous system and the mature red blood cell.

In the fasting (or low-insulin) state, these two non-insulin-dependent tissues account for the major portion of glucose uptake. Other tissues use free fatty acids or ketone bodies as energy substrates. Glucose is provided by the liver either by virtue of glycogen breakdown or by the formation of glucose from gluconeogenic precursors. The ingestion of food and the ensuing elevated insulin levels in plasma result in suppression of endogenous hepatic glucose production and increased hepatic uptake of glucose to be used for synthesis of glycogen and triglycerides. In humans the suppression of hepatic glucose output is more sensitive to insulin than is the stimulation of glucose utilization.[29] The liver is more sensitive to low concentrations of insulin than are the peripheral tissues. Furthermore, due to the anatomic relationship between the pancreas and the liver, the portal vein blood exposes the liver to insulin concentrations that are two- to fourfold higher than those found in peripheral tissue. In the patient being treated with insulin, the levels of insulin are higher in the peripheral than in the portal circulation, and hence the hepatic glucose output is not depressed to the same level as would be seen in a normal individual with a similar peripheral insulin level.[30]

In adipose tissue insulin increases glucose transport across cell membranes, favors esterification of triglycerides, and suppresses lipolysis. The suppression of lipolysis is more sensitive to insulin than either stimulation of glucose utilization[31] or suppression of hepatic glucose output.[32]

In muscle insulin increases the transport of glucose and amino acids into the cell. Exercised muscle is more sensitive to insulin action than rested muscle. Within the muscle insulin stimulates glycogen formation. In addition, insulin results in a net decrease in outflow of branched-chain fatty acids from skeletal muscle. Within the muscle cell, it stimulates protein synthesis and decreases protein breakdown (reviewed by Stevenson et al.[33]).

Finally, insulin is responsible for promoting growth of new tissues, either by acting through receptors for insulin-like growth factors (IGFs), particularly IGF-1,[34] or by stimulating production of these factors.

Administration of insulin is associated with a fall in plasma K^{+}[35] and phosphorus[36] levels.

INSULIN THERAPY

The manufacture of insulin from bovine and porcine sources was started soon after its discovery in 1922. Since that time major modifications have been introduced in the manufacturing processes that have substantially increased the efficacy and safety of insulin therapy. The primary structure of insulin was established by Sanger and coworkers[37] and reviewed by Sanger in 1959.[2]

Porcine insulin has a molecular weight of 5734. Bovine insulin contains alanine (instead of threonine) in position 8 and valine instead of isoleucine in position 10 of the A chain. Its molecular weight is 5778. The net charge of the insulin monomer is 0 at an approximate pH of 5.5. The solubility of insulin depends on the temperature, pH, concentration of salts and divalent ions, and nature of the solvent. In the absence of zinc, both porcine and bovine insulins are soluble at a pH below 4 and above 7.

Insulin purified solely by crystallization contains impurities identified as proinsulin, proinsulin intermediates, and a covalent insulin dimer.[38] Successive crystallization steps reduce the high-molecular-weight compounds (A component) but not the content of proinsulin and related substances (B component). Insulin itself is present in the C component, which also contains insulin-like components formed by hydrolysis and conversion of proinsulin and esterification of insulin during extraction.[39]

Because it was thought that these impurities resulted in the immunogenicity of insulin, insulin was further purified by anion exchange column chromatography in ethanolic solution, resulting in a preparation that contained less than 1 ppm of proinsulin-like immunoreactivity.[40]

Insulin Preparations

Single-peak insulins have been commercially available since 1972. The process of purification through gel filtration chromatography reduces the amount of proinsulin from 10,000 to 3,000 ppm. Further purification with ion exchange chromatography reduces the proinsulin to less than 50 ppm and even to less than 10 ppm, depending on the manufacturer (monocomponent). Changes from conventional insulins to highly purified insulins appear to produce less insulin allergy and lipodystrophy (hypertrophy or atrophy). Table 42–1 shows the characteristics of market insulins in simplified form. Durations of effect vary from subject to subject and, in the same subject, from time to time. With respect to promptness and duration of action, the order of the different insulins is regular (crystalline), semi-lente, isophane (NPH), lente, ultralente, and protamine zinc. Clinical experience has shown

TABLE 42–1. CHARACTERISTICS OF MARKET INSULINS
(APPROXIMATE FIGURES)

TYPE AND ACTION	APPEARANCE	PROTEIN	ZINC CONTENT (mg/100 UNITS)	BUFFER	ACTION (h)	
					Peak	Duration
Fast						
Regular	Clear	None	0.01–0.04	None	2–4	5–7
Semi-lente	Turbid	None	0.2–0.25	Acetate	2–8	8–16
Intermediate						
NPH	Turbid	Protamine	0.01–0.04	Phosphate	8–12	18–24
Lente	Turbid	None	0.2–0.25	Acetate	8–12	18–28
Slow						
Ultralente	Turbid	None	0.2–0.25	Acetate	16–18	20–36
Protamine zinc	Turbid	Protamine	0.2–0.25	Phosphate	16–20	24–36

that the NPH and lente are practically interchangeable. With the exception of regular insulin, all other insulins are modified to delay absorption and extend their duration of action by the addition of protamine, zinc, or both. The duration of effect and the hypoglycemic effect correlate with the size of the dose. Insulins are currently available in U40 and U100 strength (40 and 100 units/ml, respectively), depending on the country. Depending on the manufacturer, market animal insulins can be obtained from solely beef, solely pork, or combined beef and pork sources.

Regular insulin is a fast-acting preparation of neutral pH. The neutral solutions are better tolerated at the injection site, and in addition they have greater chemical stability and a greater miscibility with long-acting neutral preparations than the acid preparations. The addition of protamine prolongs the action of the regular insulins (protamine zinc insulin and NPH or isophane). The addition of zinc ions at neutral pH also protracts the action of insulin. Semi-lente insulin contains amorphous crystals, ultra-lente insulin contains crystalline insulin particles, and lente insulin contains a 3:7 mixture of amorphous and crystalline insulin particles.

When mixing short-acting and longer-acting preparations, it is important to take into account the physical compatibility of the preparations. The mixtures regular/NPH and regular/lente are not physically stable, as some of the soluble insulin binds to the protamine insulin crystals or precipitates with zinc, respectively. It has been shown that there is no problem when the mixtures are injected immediately after filling the syringe, but time lags of 5 minutes or more reduce the biologic action of the preparations.

In practice, all insulins are effective, and the selection of a given type or species depends on the patient's needs and the physician's judgment. For patients taking more than one type of insulin and more than one daily injection, the insulins must be of the same strength and type. To avoid errors, a single-scale insulin syringe should be used.

In addition to the purified insulins, human insulin is now available from two different sources.[41] Human insulin can be obtained by (a) an enzymatic procedure that replaces the alanine from the terminal position 30 in the B chain of purified pork insulin with threonine, or (b) inserting human gene sequences into plasmids of *Esche-*

richia coli. With this procedure there is separate production of A and B chains with two fermentations, and these are subsequently linked with sulfur by chemical means. An alternate method involves one fermentation that results in the production of proinsulin, which can be cleaved to provide proinsulin and C-peptide.

Numerous studies throughout the world indicate that biosynthetic insulin and recombinant DNA-produced human insulins are equivalent to pancreatic human insulin chemically and biologically. The synthetic insulins are free of other pancreatic peptides and bacterial contaminants. In their biologic effects they are similar to purified pork insulin, but they appear to have a faster and shorter duration of action. However, they may be useful for patients who present insulin allergy, insulin resistance, or lipodystrophy not controlled by pure pork insulin. At the present time there is no compelling evidence that human insulins are more advantageous than beef or pork insulins unless a shortage of cattle and swine pancreases develops. There is as yet no agreement as to whether insulin-dependent diabetic patients should be shifted to human insulins, especially if they are doing well with the other types.

MANAGEMENT OF CHILDHOOD DIABETES

Type I diabetes usually starts with polyphagia, weight loss, polydipsia, and polyuria. Symptoms caused by insulin deficiency may last from a few days to weeks before the diagnosis is made. In rare cases, usually in older children, symptoms may last for a few months. As insulin deficiency progresses, anorexia, vomiting, abdominal pain, fatigue, and irritability ensue. On occasion these symptoms may be attributed to a viral infection, and the early diagnosis may be missed if the physician does not have a high index of suspicion. Therefore, routine urine testing of glucose and ketones is warranted in a child with such complaints. At diagnosis dehydration and weight loss are the most obvious physical signs, and the blood glucose levels are generally markedly elevated. Ketonuria is almost always present, with or without acidosis.

After initiation of insulin therapy, many children with insulin-dependent diabetes mellitus (IDDM) have an amelioration of their disease, as reflected by decreasing insulin requirements and improvement of the hyperglycemia.[42,43] This phase (called honeymoon or remission) lasts for a few days to several weeks or months. It is characterized by variable endogenous insulin secretion indirectly measured by C-peptide radioimmunoassay in serum or urine.[44–46] In the majority of patients, the remission phase is followed by a progression to total insulin deficiency 2–5 years after the diagnosis.[47,48]

As soon as hyperglycemia or glucosuria is detected, immediate medical attention is needed because of the potential for rapid deterioration. Initial therapy will depend on how early the diagnosis is made and on the state of the child.

Insulin Treatment

Insulin treatment is usually initiated with a dose of 0.3–0.5 unit/kg/day. The insulin dose is adjusted to keep the glucose values between 4 and 8 mmol/liter. Children who are clinically well at the time of diagnosis may be started immediately on 0.3–0.5 unit/kg/day of a mixture of NPH/lente and regular insulin. Extra doses of regular insulin are added every 4 hours for blood glucose levels above the target. The sum of all the extra doses required during the previous day will give an approximation of the following day's requirements. Daily increases of insulin (depending on the degree of hyperglycemia and ketosis) are given until the blood glucose levels have approached the target values.

The child is fed three meals and three snacks per day, and the dietary intake of each day is used as a guide to the caloric adjustment for the following day. In the hospitalized child, treatment can be started with six doses of regular insulin given every 4 hours (before breakfast, lunch, supper, bedtime snack, midnight, and at 4:00 AM) for 1–2 days. The sum of the six doses administered during the previous 24-hour period will give an approximation of the following day's total insulin requirements. When the child is well and insulin requirements are stable (1–2 days), a mixture of intermediate-acting (NPH or lente) and short-acting (regular) insulin is given in one or two daily injections.

The first few days after diagnosis, blood glucose and urine ketones should be monitored every 4–6 hours to guide the insulin adjustments. Such testing is a useful teaching tool that helps the child and family learn the techniques of glucose monitoring as well as the action and duration of the insulin and the effects of activity and diet on glycemic control. Glucose self-monitoring technique should be supervised frequently so that the child and parents can compare the laboratory blood glucose results with their own measurements with reagent strips or reflectance meters. The education program should encompass urine and blood glucose self-testing, insulin administration, diet planning, dietary and insulin adjustments, and facts about the physiopathology of diabetes, insulin action, and insulin adjustments for exercise and illnesses.

Insulin requirements usually increase during the first week after diagnosis and decrease gradually after the second or third week. A progressive decrease in insulin requirements indicates the beginning of the remission period. During this period some patients show almost complete restoration of beta-cell function. The remission period lasts a few days to weeks in very young children, but in older adolescents it may last for a few months. As insulin deficiency progresses, insulin requirements increase toward 0.7–1.0 unit/kg/day.

Age and stage of sexual development, dietary intake, and potential adherence to the treatment should be taken into consideration when selecting the individual's insulin treatment. If insulin requirements and caloric intake are small (especially in the very young child), a single dose of a mixture of NPH and short-acting insulin given before breakfast, with a second dose of short-acting insulin before supper if the blood glucose values are high, is usually enough. Older children or children who are in the midst of the adolescent growth spurt may be started directly on a twice-daily injection regimen of a mixture of preferably NPH and regular insulin before breakfast and before supper. However, adolescents who are having difficulty accepting their condition may have to be started with only one daily injection instead of the more common twice-daily regimen until problems of acceptance are overcome. Some adolescents may have poor diabetic control because they tend to skip the second injection. The use of a single-dose regimen ensures they at least receive their necessary daily insulin requirement.

During the adolescent growth spurt, insulin requirements increase together with caloric requirements and may be as high as 1.5 units/kg/day. After full development has been achieved, diet and insulin dose should be decreased simultaneously to avoid overinsulinization and obesity. Blood glucose targets should take into consideration the frequency of blood glucose testing, the patient's ability to recognize hypoglycemia, and the patient's and family's ability or willingness to comply. Constancy in the timing of injections and meal intake is crucial for the success of any regimen. Insulin should be given at least 20–30 minutes before meals, or earlier if the prevailing blood glucose levels are well above the desired target.

Monitoring of Glycemic Control

Blood glucose self-monitoring is a relatively simple and practical method that facilitates insulin adjustment.[49]

Blood glucose or urine glucose tests should be performed regularly and the results charted in a logbook so that they can be discussed with the physician for insulin adjustments. Urine glucose can be monitored with the two-drop Clinitest method in second voided specimens or with sensitive methods that use reagent strips. Urine ketones should be tested at least once daily, preferably in the morning, but tests may be conducted more often if there is an intercurrent illness or stressful event. Blood glucose tests are preferred to urine glucose tests because they allow for the documentation of glycemic levels at home. Monitoring is recommended at least two to three times per day, before breakfast, supper, and bedtime.

Cation exchange chromatography separates hemoglobin A1 (HbA) into four minor components (hemoglobin

A_{1a1}, A_{1A2}, A_{1b}, and A_{1c}) which are referred to as hemoglobin A_1. The hemoglobin A_1 fraction is formed continuously within the red cell throughout its 120-day life span as a result of posttranslational nonenzymatic modification of the hemoglobin A. HbA_{1c}, the most abundant of these minor components, is increased in patients with diabetes mellitus.[50-52] Thus, glycosylated hemoglobin reflects the average blood glucose level to which the erythrocyte has been exposed during its life span and provides an objective assessment of long-term glycemic control.

Glycosylated hemoglobin can be measured with chromatographic methodologies that operate on the basis of charge (e.g., column chromatography, isoelectric focusing, high-pressure liquid chromatography, and the commercial microcolumn kits, all of which are sensitive to changes in buffer, pH, and temperature).[53,54] Chemical measurements of glycosylated hemoglobin have the advantage of being readily amenable to standardization and long-term quality control procedures because they are not influenced by the variables that may affect the chromatographic procedures.[55]

Adjustments of Insulin Dosage

Changes in insulin dose are made on the basis of recorded blood or urine glucose tests and are aimed at target values. If increments of insulin dosage are needed, these should not surpass 10 percent of the total daily dose and should be made only after 2 or 3 consecutive days of unexplained high blood or urine glucose tests. Decrements of insulin dosage in response to hypoglycemia not explained by exercise or missed meals should be done immediately and should be at least 15 percent of the relevant insulin dose. The first adjustment should be made in the overnight intermediate-acting insulin action. This is best made on the basis of 3:00–4:00 AM (targeted at above 4 mmol/liter) and fasting blood glucose values (targeted at 4–7 mmol/liter). Once the morning blood glucose is within the target range, adjustment of the premeal short-acting insulin doses can be made. If increments in the NPH or lente insulin necessary to achieve fasting tests within target result in nighttime hypoglycemia, the patient's bedtime snack should be increased to achieve bedtime blood glucose values above 7 mmol/liter. Dietary manipulations are usually necessary in patients taking one-dose regimens where insulin dosage changes can be implemented only once a day.

Single-Dose Regimen

Intermediate-acting insulins (NPH or lente) mixed with short-acting insulins are usually employed. Less frequently, long-acting (ultralente) insulins alone or in combination with regular insulin are used. Morning injections of intermediate-acting insulins provide higher plasma insulin levels during the day and can be used alone if there is enough endogenous insulin secretion during meals. Frequently, however, endogenous insulin secretion is inadequate, and regular insulin needs to be added to correct morning hyperglycemia. This single-dose regimen is usually effective only during the first few months after diagnosis in combination with a supplementary dose of short-acting insulin before supper if glucose tests are above the target. Ultralente insulins, which are absorbed very slowly from the injection site, may be less convenient to use, as necessary decreases in dosage cannot be made with short anticipation.

Short-acting insulin has major action between breakfast and early afternoon, and its effect is reflected in the noon and presupper glucose tests. The NPH insulin has major action between supper and nighttime, and its effect is reflected in the bedtime and fasting glucose values. Guidelines for adjustment of basic and temporary insulin doses for this regimen are outlined in Table 42–2.

Twice-Daily Regimen

The most frequent treatment regimen uses two daily mixtures of intermediate-acting and short-acting insulin. The morning short-acting insulin has major action between breakfast and lunch, and the intermediate-acting NPH or lente has major action between breakfast and supper. The evening short-acting insulin has major action between supper and bedtime, and its effect is reflected in the bedtime tests. The evening NPH or lente insulin has major action overnight, and its effect is reflected in the blood glucose level on arising the next morning. The theoretical advantages of this regimen are the reduction of

TABLE 42–2. INSULIN DOSE ADJUSTMENTS FOR ONCE DAILY INSULIN REGIMEN

- Increase the dose of NPH/lente by 10% if fasting blood glucose is above the target for 3 consecutive days. Repeat until blood glucose is within the target. (This modification can be made provided that the 3–4 AM blood glucose level is above 4 mmol/liter.)

- Decrease the dose of NPH/lente by 15% if fasting blood glucose is below the target for 2 consecutive days. Repeat until blood glucose increases to the target.

- Increase the dose of regular insulin by 10% if noon and supper blood glucose levels are above the target for 3 consecutive days. Repeat until blood glucose is within the target.

- Decrease the carbohydrate content of the afternoon snack if noon blood glucose is below or at the target and supper blood glucose is above the target for 3 consecutive days. Increases of the NPH/lente may result in night or early morning hypoglycemia.

- Use a supplementary dose of regular insulin (10% of total) when pre-supper blood glucose levels are higher than 10 mmol/liter).

- Test blood or urine glucose at bedtime every day and add an extra snack if blood glucose levels are below 7 mmol/liter or if second voided urine specimen for glucose is negative.

basal and postprandial hyperglycemia and the reduction of overnight and fasting glycemia. However, in some patients, attempts to achieve morning normoglycemia result in nocturnal hypoglycemia and early morning hyperglycemia. Guidelines for adjusting insulin dose with this regimen are shown in Table 42–3.

An alternative and more effective regimen for achieving normoglycemia is the administration of regular insulin before breakfast and lunch with a mixture of NPH or lente and regular insulin before supper. If fasting normoglycemia cannot be achieved without nocturnal hypoglycemia, the evening dose can be split so that regular insulin alone is given before supper and NPH or lente is given at bedtime. Studies have shown that treatment with multiple injections of regular insulin before each meal and NPH insulin at bedtime can be just as effective in normalizing blood glucose levels as the use of continuous subcutaneous insulin infusion (CSII).[56] An alternative regimen uses premeal doses of regular insulin plus long-acting insulin (ultralente) in the morning, or three daily injections of a mixture of ultralente and regular insulin in the morning and before supper, with regular insulin alone before lunch.

Compared with once- or twice-daily injection regimens, multiple injection regimens are demanding and therefore patient compliance has been poor. Devices that simplify the injection procedure are now available. These instruments, which look like fountain pens, have been shown to be very well accepted by adult diabetic patients. In children, however, the experience is as yet limited.[57]

Mechanical Devices for Continuous Insulin Administration

Devices for continuous insulin administration are used to normalize blood glucose levels throughout the day. Since insulin delivery is continuous, it can more or less mimic normal insulin secretion. Open-loop systems have been developed for ambulatory use that can use the intravenous, peritoneal, or subcutaneous route of insulin administration.[58] These relatively small and lightweight portable devices (insulin pumps) can be implanted subcutaneously or carried extracorporeally. The most widespread method is the continuous subcutaneous insulin infusion with a portable extracorporeal battery-driven pump.[59-62] There are now many types of devices on the market with different features such as alarms for low battery, pump runaway, and empty reservoir; variable basal rates; and preprogrammed boluses. This treatment is extremely effective in improving glucose control in diabetic patients. However, it should be restricted to very motivated and mature patients because it requires a high degree of cooperation. Although they have been used in children,[63] insulin pump use should be restricted in the pediatric population because of their severe potential complications.[64] The complications resulting from this therapy may be quite serious. Hypoglycemia, probably the most severe complication, could result in brain damage and even death.[65]

Strategies to reduce the risk of nocturnal hypoglycemia include increasing the target fasting blood glucose to above 7 mmol/liter, decreasing the basal rate if 3:00 AM blood glucose levels are below 4 mmol/liter, and daily measurements of blood glucose at bedtime followed by an extra snack if the values are less than or equal to 7 mmol/liter.[66]

Special Considerations

Adjustments for Exercise

In anticipation of exercise, caloric intake should be increased or insulin dose decreased to avoid hypoglycemic reactions. Hypoglycemia during or after exercise results from increased absorption of insulin, because exercise usually increases blood flow throughout the body. The intake of one carbohydrate exchange per every 30–45 minutes of moderate exercise may prevent hypoglycemia. For exercise anticipated to last longer than 1 hour, a decrease in the insulin dosage according to the intensity and duration of exercise may be effective in reducing the risk of hypoglycemia. Table 42–4 shows the guidelines for treatment in anticipation of exercise.

TABLE 42–3.   INSULIN DOSE ADJUSTMENTS FOR TWICE-DAILY INSULIN REGIMEN

Evening Dose
- Increase by 10% the dose of intermediate-acting insulin if the fasting blood glucose is above the target for 3 consecutive days. (This modification can be made with the provision that the 3–4 AM blood glucose is above 4 mmol/liter.)
- Reduce by 15% the evening dose of intermediate-acting insulin if 3–4 AM and/or fasting blood glucose are below 4 mmol/liter.
- Increase by 10% the evening dose of regular insulin if blood glucose 2 h after supper is above 10 mmol/liter for 3 consecutive days. (This modification can be made with the provision that blood glucose is above 7 mmol/liter after the bedtime snack.)
- The maneuvers should be repeated until blood glucose levels are within the target.

Morning Dose
- Increase by 10% the prebreakfast dose of regular insulin if blood glucose is above the target at midmorning or before lunch for 3 consecutive days.
- Increase by 10% the prebreakfast dose of intermediate-acting insulin if blood glucose is above the target before supper for more than 3 consecutive days.
- Reduce by 15% the morning dose of short-acting insulin if blood glucose after breakfast or before lunch is less than 4 mmol/liter.

TABLE 42–4. ADJUSTMENTS OF INSULIN DOSE FOR ANTICIPATED EXERCISE

Anticipated Exercise
Once-Daily Regimen
- Morning exercise lasting more than 45 minutes:
  Decrease regular insulin by 25% for mild to moderate activity
  Decrease regular insulin by 35% for moderate activity
  Decrease regular insulin by 50% for strenuous activity (athletes in training)

- Afternoon or evening exercise lasting more than 45 minutes:
  Decrease NPH/lente by 15% for mild to moderate activity
  Decrease NPH/lente by 20% for moderate activity
  Decrease NPH/lente by 25% for strenuous activity (athletes in training)

Twice-Daily Regimen

- Morning exercise lasting more than 45 minutes:
  Decrease morning regular insulin as above

- Early afternoon exercise lasting more than 45 minutes:
  Decrease morning NPH/lente insulin as above

- Evening exercise lasting more than 45 minutes:
  Decrease both supper NPH/lente and regular insulin as for once-daily insulin

Unanticipated Exercise

Adjustments of diet for unanticipated exercise (insulin doses cannot be modified, and thus hypoglycemia can be prevented by extra food)

- mild to moderate exercise—1 fruit exchange every 30 to 45 minutes

- moderate exercise—1 starch + 1 protein before exercise + 1 fruit every 30–45 minutes during exercise

- strenuous exercise—2 starches + 1 protein before exercise + 1 to 2 fruit(s) every 30–45 minutes during exercise

Management During Acute Illnesses or Stress

The increased secretion of counterregulatory hormones and decreased activity even in the face of reduced caloric intake or vomiting may increase insulin requirements. Blood glucose and urinary ketones should be tested every 4–6 hours. The physician should be contacted immediately for advice. The following guidelines, based on whether the patient is able to take food or liquids by mouth, are useful for managing a diabetic child during an illness.

An illness not accompanied by nausea or vomiting (e.g., minor infection or trauma requiring bed rest). If activity is normal, give the usual dose of NPH/lente plus extra regular insulin as per blood glucose or urine tests, i.e., 20 percent of the morning dose of regular every 4 hours if the blood glucose is above 12 mmol/liter and 30 percent if blood glucose is above 20 mmol/liter. If urine ketones are present in moderate to large amounts, 10 percent may be added above these recommendations.

If activity is reduced and the patient is confined to bed, the diet should be reduced by approximately one-third. The reduction in caloric intake compensates for the inactivity. The insulin adjustment is the same as for an illness without bed rest.

An illness accompanied by nausea, vomiting, or marked anorexia. The insulin dose must never be omitted, since this could lead to diabetic ketoacidosis. It is better to omit the NPH or lente insulin and replace it with injections of regular insulin every 4–6 hours according to the blood glucose tests and the presence or absence of ketones in the urine as follows: one-fourth of the total daily insulin dose for those patients on one daily injection or one-fourth of the total morning dose for those on two daily injections

for blood glucose levels above 12 mmol/liter, with an additional 10 percent of the total daily dose if urine ketones are moderate or large. The dose of insulin should be reduced if the blood glucose levels are lower. For a child who usually takes 5 units of short-acting insulin and 10 units of NPH or lente, 5 units for blood glucoses above 12 mmol/liter, 4 units for blood glucoses between 10 and 12 mmol/liter, 3 units for blood glucoses between 6 and 10 mmol/liter, and 2 units for blood glucoses below 6 mmol/liter. Add 1–2 units to the calculated dose if urine ketones are moderate to large. This is repeated at each testing until the child is able to eat or tolerate fluids well. If the child is well by noon, two-thirds of the usual total daily dose of NPH or lente is given together with regular insulin (one-half of the morning dose of NPH or lente for those on two daily injections). If the child is still unwell by supper time, regular insulin alone should be continued. At bedtime, one-fourth of the usual daily dose of NPH or lente should be given with a small dose of regular insulin. The diet should be replaced by regular soft drinks, fruit juice, or sweetened tea, 2–4 ounces every hour. As the child improves, light foods can be given as tolerated.

If vomiting occurs after the administration of the usual morning dose of insulin, sips of sugar-containing fluids should be given every 20–30 minutes to maintain blood glucoses between 6 and 10 mmol/liter. If vomiting persists and the blood glucose falls below 6 mmol/liter, the child should be taken to the hospital for intravenous glucose therapy. A subcutaneous injection of glucagon should be given at home before departing if the child lives at some distance from the hospital.

If the blood glucose is above 12 mmol/liter and the urine contains moderate to large amounts of ketones, the physician should be advised immediately because this could reflect diabetic ketoacidosis.

TABLE 42–5. INTRAVENOUS INFUSION REGIMEN

- Fluids: ½ normal saline in 10% dextrose at a rate to provide 100 cc/kg for first 10 kg of body weight plus 50 cc/kg for next 10 kg of body weight plus 20 cc/kg for above 20 kg of body weight. The total calculated fluids will be divided in 24 h and that result will be the maintenance infusion rate per hour.
- KCl 20 mEq/liter.
- Insulin/glucose ratio = 0.2 unit/gm. Insulin concentration 10 units/500 ml of 10% dextrose (2 units/100 ml). If the duration of diabetes is less than 3 years and the child requires less than 0.5 unit/kg/day, the starting dose of insulin should be halved.
- Start I.V. insulin when blood glucose is above 6 mmol/l.
- Increase insulin concentration by 0.25 U/100 ml/h if blood glucose is above 12 mmol/l.
- Decrease insulin concentration by 0.5 U/100 ml/h if blood glucose falls by more than 4 mmol/liter/h. If blood glucose falls below 6 mmol/liter, stop insulin infusion until blood glucose reaches 6 mmol/liter and then restart at 0.5 unit/100 ml/h.
- Discontinue insulin infusion and restart subcutaneous insulin treatment when patient is able to eat.

Management During Surgery

The treatment is aimed at maintaining metabolism as close to normal as possible by providing sufficient insulin and fluids. Using the regimen outlined in Tables 42–5 and 42–6, perioperative care is fairly flexible. Insulin and dextrose may be combined in the solution to minimize the risk of hypoglycemia and hyperglycemia due to changes in the glucose infusion rate. Alternatively, one-third to one-half of the morning NPH/lente dose the morning of surgery could be given together with a 10 percent dextrose solution, or short-acting insulin every 4 hours depending on blood glucose tests.

Treatment of Diabetes in the Infant

Symptomatic hyperglycemia can occur in newborn infants. These babies usually suffer from severe intrauterine malnutrition and therefore are small for their gestational age. They are hypoinsulinemic and fail to release insulin in response to any of the standard secretagogues; they must be treated with exogenous insulin with doses up to 1–2 units/kg/24 h in divided doses. Insulin requirements are best established by starting a continuous intravenous insulin infusion at rates to provide at least 0.5 unit/kg/24 h. Insulin treatment is simplified by using diluted insulins (we usually use a solution containing 10 units/ml) so that inadvertent overdoses do not occur. In most cases, beta-cell function develops sometime between the age of 6 and 12 weeks. It is thought that there is a delay in the development of normal beta-cell growth and differentiation. The children do well following the newborn period and do not appear to be at increased risk of developing type I diabetes at a later age.

Complications of Insulin Therapy

Diabetic Ketoacidosis

Diabetic ketoacidosis (DKA) results from severe insulin deficiency.[67] It is seen in 10–15 percent of newly diagnosed insulin-dependent diabetic children. In established diabetic children, it may be precipitated by factors that interfere with insulin action, such as the release of counterregulatory hormones during physical (infection, trauma) or emotional stress. Such factors may result in a failure to take extra insulin or psychologic disturbances leading to omission of the insulin treatment and/or lack of insulin adjustment because of infrequent blood glucose testing.

DKA is diagnosed when the pH is less than 7.3 and the plasma bicarbonate is less than 15 mEq/liter. DKA in the child is a life-threatening complication that requires careful supervision in an intensive care unit. Guidelines for clinical laboratory assessment are shown in Table 42–7.

Insulin deficiency causes progressive hyperglycemia,

TABLE 42–6. MANAGEMENT FOR ELECTIVE SURGERY

- Admit to hospital the day before surgery.
- One daily injection: decrease the morning NPH/lente by one-third and stabilize with extra regular insulin at noon, supper, and bedtime if necessary.
- Twice-daily injections: withhold the NPH or lente of the evening and administer regular insulin at 4-h intervals.
- Check blood glucose q4h.
- Start I.V. glucose–potassium–insulin infusion at bedtime if possible or very early the next morning.
- Schedule operation at 8 AM if I.V. insulin started the night before or after 10 AM if I.V. insulin started the morning of surgery.
- Omit breakfast and check fasting and hourly blood glucoses, and titrate insulin according to Table 43–5. Check potassium levels.
- Check blood glucose every 2–4 h and potassium every 6 h after surgery.
- Continue I.V. insulin until patient is able to eat.

TABLE 42–7. EVALUATION OF THE KETOACIDOTIC CHILD

1. Check vital signs and weigh. Monitor vital signs and sensorium continuously.

2. Assess dehydration, hyperventilation, acetone in breath, and search for infection.

3. Estimate glucose and acetone in blood and urine, blood gases, serum osmolality, BUN, electrolytes, CBC, ECG, urinalysis, and cultures if indicated. Repeat blood glucose every hour and electrolytes and blood gases every 2 hours.

4. Assess sensorium, need for nasogastric tube, bladder catheterization, O_2 (if patient is comatose).

unrestrained lipolysis, ketogenesis, systemic acidosis, and depletion of intracellular and extracellular water and electrolytes that if untreated may lead to coma and even death. Elevated levels of growth hormone, glucagon, cortisol, and catecholamines occur in response to the stress of DKA or as a consequence of volume depletion and acidosis.[68]

Rehydration should be started immediately with normal saline for the first 1–2 hours (since even the saline solution is hypotonic with respect to the patient's osmolality). Guidelines for rehydration are given in Table 42–8. Initial rehydration therapy is replaced by one-half normal saline with electrolytes (KCl and a mixture of KH_2PO_4-K_2HPO_4). Dextrose in a 10 percent solution is added as soon as the blood glucose levels decrease toward 12 mmol/liter to replenish the depleted glycogen stores. Hyperosmolarity should be corrected very slowly, because too rapid a decline may worsen the subclinical cerebral edema (usually present before treatment). Cerebral edema is now the major complication of DKA in children. Insulin replacement is usually started 1 hour after the commencement of fluid therapy through the intravenous route.[69] An initial bolus of 0.1 unit/kg is followed by a continuous infusion of 0.1 unit/kg/h, titrated according to blood glucose levels measured hourly. The rate of the intravenous infusion is then adjusted according to blood glucose levels. Potassium should be started as soon as the urine output is adequate, as the total body potassium is usually depleted and insulin treatment and correction of acidosis will shift potassium back to the intracellular compartment producing hypokalemia. Providing phosphate may promote the formation of 2,3-diphosphoglycerate and shift the oxygen dissociation curve to the right, releasing oxygen to the tissues and correcting acidosis. In addition, administration of potassium phosphate can reduce the inevitable chloride overload of the treatment of DKA, which may aggravate the acidosis.[70] The use of bicarbonate should be restricted to severe acidosis (pH < 7.0) where myocardial function may be impaired.[71] Use of bicarbonate may shift the oxygen dissociation curve to the left, accelerate the entry of potassium into the cells, and thus precipitate hypokalemia and worsen cerebral acidosis due to the rapid diffusion of CO_2 through the blood–brain barrier. When indicated, bicarbonate should be replaced slowly (over 1–2 hours) at a dose not exceeding 1–2 mEq/kg. The insulin infusion is usually maintained until acidosis is corrected (usually 12–

16 hours) and the patient is well enough to tolerate small amounts of oral fluids.

Hypoglycemia

Hypoglycemia is a very frequent complication of insulin therapy. Its symptoms result from adrenergic stimulation and neuroglycopenia. Hypoglycemia occurs when meals are skipped or delayed, during or after physical activity without increases of food or reductions of insulin dosage, and as a result of errors in the insulin dosage. Severe recurrent hypoglycemic episodes after the remission phase of diabetes may result from deliberate increases in the insulin dose that may indicate underlying psychologic problems. Education of the family, child, and all others involved in the care of diabetic children is critical to prevent and treat these episodes.

Local Reactions

Lipoatrophy and hypertrophy at the site of injection are the most common local complications of insulin therapy. The exact cause and incidence are not known. However, it appears that both occur less frequently with the use of purified insulins. Lipoatrophy improves with the injection of purified insulin directly in the area. In cases of local hypertrophy, rotation of injection sites with avoidance of the hypertrophic sites is recommended. Some patients may experience allergic reactions (burning, itching, rash, or hives) at the site of injection. Again, the cause is not known but the condition appears to improve when patients are switched to purified pork or human insulin.

TABLE 42–8. FLUID, ELECTROLYTE AND INSULIN INFUSION DURING DKA

1. If shock, use bolus of 10–20 cc/kg of 0.9% saline and repeat until blood pressure is normal.

2. If no shock, start 0.9% saline at an hourly rate depending on osmolality and dehydration. Total fluids are calculated (a) to correct the deficit (½ of the estimated deficit over 12 hours and the remainder of the deficit in 24–36 h); (b) to supply daily maintenance requirements; (c) to replace urinary losses until blood glucose levels decrease to 12 mmol/liter.

3. Switch to ½ normal saline after 1–2 h or when blood pressure is normal.

4. Add potassium (½ as KCl and ½ as KH_2PO_4-K_2HPO_4) 20 to 40 mEq/liter depending on serum levels as soon as urinary output is ensured.

5. Loading dose 0.1 unit/kg regular insulin by I.V. push (approximately 1 h after starting I.V. fluids) and 0.1 unit/kg/h with adjustments depending on blood glucose response. Blood glucose fall should not exceed 5 mmol/liter/h.

6. Add 5–10% dextrose when blood glucose falls to approximately 12 mmol/liter.

7. Continue I.V. insulin until acidosis is corrected. Titrate rate of infusion according to fall in blood glucose values.

8. Bicarbonate intravenously (not to exceed 1–2 mEq/kg over 1–2 h) only if pH < 7.0.

If symptoms persist, antihistamines may be given orally. A small percentage of patients may not respond to a change in insulin and may require desensitization.

Insulin resistance exists whenever there is interference with the action of insulin. This can occur because of abnormal degradation of insulin (usually for exogenous insulins), binding of insulin by high-capacity antibodies,[72] decreased binding of insulin to its receptor due either to decreased numbers of receptors (down-regulation) or to antagonists that block the binding, or interference with any of the postbinding steps by which the insulin signal is propagated intracellularly.[73]

REFERENCES

1. Bliss M: The Discovery of Insulin. Toronto, McClelland and Stewart, 1982
2. Sanger F: Chemistry of insulin. Science 129:1340–1344, 1959
3. Katsoyannis PG, Tometsko A, Fukuda K: Insulin peptides IX. The synthesis of the A-chain of insulin and its combination with natural B-chain to generate insulin activity. J Am Chem Soc 85:2863–2865, 1963
4. Hodgkin DC: The structure of insulin. Diabetes 21:1131, 1972
5. Bell GI, Pictet RL, Rutter WJ, Cordell B, Tischer E, Goodman HM: Sequence of the human insulin gene. Nature 284:26–32, 1980
6. Lacy P, Greider MH: Ultrastructural organization of mammalian pancreatic islets, in Stein DF, Freinkel N (eds): Handbook of Physiology, section 7: Endocrinology, vol 11: Endocrine Pancreas. American Physiological Society, Baltimore, Williams & Wilkins, 1972
7. Steiner DF: Insulin today. Diabetes 26:332–340, 1977
8. Owerbach D, Bell GI, Rutter WI, Brown JA, Shows TB: The insulin gene is located on the short arm of chromosome II. Diabetes 30:267–270, 1981
9. Kitabachi AE: Pro insulin and C-peptide: A review. Metabolism 26:547–587, 1977
10. Lacey PE, Finke EH, Codilla RC: Cinemicrographic studies of beta-cell granule movements in monolayers. Lab Invest 33:570, 1975
11. Freychet P: The interaction of proinsulin with insulin receptors on the plasma membrane of the liver. J Clin Invest 54:1020–1031, 1974
12. Gold G, Grodsky GM: Kinetic aspects of compartmental storage and secretion of insulin and zinc. Experimentia 40:1105, 1984
13. Lang DA, Matthews DR, Peto J, Turner RC: Cyclic oscillations of basal plasma glucose and insulin concentration in human beings. N Engl J Med 301:1023–1027, 1979
14. Bratusch-Marrain PR, Komjati M, Waldhausl WK: Efficacy of pulsatile versus continuous insulin administration on hepatic glucose production and glucose utilization in Type I diabetic humans. Diabetes 35:922–926, 1986
15. Bedoya FJ, Wilson JM, Ghosh AK, Finegold D, Matschinsky FM: The glucokinase glucose sensor in human pancreatic islet tissue. Diabetes 35:61–67, 1986
16. Cook DL, Satin LS, Ashford MLJ, Hales CN: ATP-sensitive K$^+$ channels in pancreatic B-cells. Diabetes 37:495–498, 1988
17. Andersen DK: Physiological effects of GIP in man, in Bloom SR, Polak JM (eds): Gut Hormones, 3rd ed. Edinburgh, Churchill Livingstone, 1981, pp 256–263
18. Hampton SM, Morgan LM, Tredget JA, Cramb R, Marks V: Insulin and C-peptide levels after oral and intravenous glucose: Contribution of enteroinsular axis to insulin secretion. Diabetes 35:612–616, 1986
19. Zwalich WS, Diaz VA: Prior cholecystokinin exposure sensitizes islets of Langerhans to glucose stimulation. Diabetes 36:118–122, 1987
20. Kreymann B, Williams G, Ghatei BA, Bloom SR: Glucagon-like peptide-1 7-36: A physiological incretion in man. Lancet 2:1300–1304, 1987
21. Loubatieres-Mariani MM, Chapal J, Alric R, Loubatieres A: Studies of the cholinergic receptors involved in the secretion of insulin using isolated perfused rat pancreas. Diabetologia 9:439–446, 1973
22. Robertson RP: Arachidonic acid metabolite regulation of insulin secretion. Diabetes Metab Rev 2:261–96, 1988
23. Milner RDG: Growth and development of the endocrine glands-endocrine pancreas, in Davis JA, Dibbing W (eds): Scientific Foundations of Paediatrics. London, W. Heinemann, 1974, pp 507–513
24. Amiel SA, Sherwin RS, Simonson DC, Lauritano AA, Tamborlane WV: Impaired insulin action in puberty. N Engl J Med 315:215–219, 1986
25. Rosen OM: After insulin binds. Science 237:1452–1458, 1987
26. Kahn MN, Sansoni PS, Bergeron JJ, Posner BI: Characterization of rat liver endosomal fractions. In vivo activation of insulin-stimulable receptor kinase in these structures. J Biol Chem 261:8462–8472, 1986
27. Pederson O, Beck-Nielsen H: Insulin resistance and insulin-dependent diabetes mellitus. Diabetes Care 10:516–523, 1987
28. Duckworth W, Kitabchi A: Insulin metabolism and degradation. Endocr Rev 2:210–232, 1981
29. Rizza R, Mandarino L, Gerich J: Dose-response characteristics for effects of insulin on production and utilization of glucose in man. Am J Physiol 240:E360–E639, 1981
30. Yki-Jarvinen H, Koivisto VA: Insulin sensitivity in newly diagnosed Type I diabetics after ketoacidosis and after three months of therapy. J Clin Endocrinol Metab 590:371–378, 1984
31. Miles JM, Rizza RA, Haymond MW, Gerich JE: Effects of acute insulin deficiency on glucose and ketone body turnover in man: Evidence for the primacy of overproduction of glucose and ketone bodies in the genesis of diabetic ketoacidosis. Diabetes 29:926–930, 1980
32. Nurjhan N, Campbell PJ, Kennedy FP, Miles JM, Gerich JE: Insulin dose-response characteristics for suppression of glycerol release and conversion to glucose in humans. Diabetes 35:1326–1331, 1986
33. Stevenson RW, Steiner KE, Abumrad NN, Cherringon AD: Insulin action in vivo, in Alberti KGMM, Krall LL (eds): The Diabetes Annual 1. Amsterdam, Elsevier, 1985, pp 418–445
34. Scheiwiller E, Guler HP, Merryweather J, Scandella C, Maerki W, Zapf J, Froesch ER: Growth restoration of insulin deficient diabetic rats by recombinant human insulin-like growth factor I. Nature 323:169–171, 1986
35. De Fronzo RA, Felig P, Ferrannini E, Wahren J: Effect of graded doses of insulin on splanchnic and peripheral potassium metabolism in man. Am J Physiol 238:E421–E427, 1980
36. Gertner JM, Tamborlane WV, Horst RL, Sherwin RS, Felig P, Genel M: Mineral metabolism in diabetes mellitus: Changes accompanying treatment with a portable subcutaneous insulin infusion system. J Clin Endocrinol Metab 50:862–866, 1980
37. Sanger F, Thompson EOP, Kitai R: The amide groups of insulin. Biochem J 59:509–518, 1955
38. Steiner DF, Hallund D, Rubenstein A, Cho S, Bayliss C: Isolation and properties of proinsulin, intermediate forms and other minor components from crystalline bovine insulin. Diabetes 17:725–736, 1968
39. Schlichtkrull J, Brange J, Christiansen A, Hallund O, Heding L, Jorgensen K: Clinical aspects of insulin-antigenicity. Diabetes 21(suppl 2):649–656, 1972
40. Schlichtkrull J, Brange J, Christiansen S, Hallund O, Heding L, Jorgensen K, Rasmussen SM, Sorensen E, Volund AS: Monocomponent insulin and its clinical implications. Horm Metab Res (Suppl Ser) 5:134–143, 1974
41. Skyler J: Symposium on human insulin of recombinant DNA origin. Diabetes Care 5(suppl 2):1–86, 1982
42. Baker L, Kaye R, Root A: The early partial remission of juvenile diabetes mellitus. J Pediatr 71:826–831, 1967
43. Park BN, Soeldner JS, Gleason RE: Diabetes in remission. Insulin secretory dynamics. Diabetes 23:616–623, 1974
44. Block MB, Rosenfield RL, Mako ME, Steiner DF, Rubenstein AH: Sequential changes in beta-cell function in insulin treated diabetic patients assessed by C-peptide immunoreactivity. N Engl J Med 288:1144–1148, 1973
45. Aurbach-Klipper J, Sharph-Dor R, Heding L, Karp M, Laron Z:

Residual B cell function in diabetic children as determined by urinary C-peptide. Diabetologia 24:88–90, 1983

46. Heding LG: Radioimmunological determination of human C-peptide in serum. Diabetologia 11:541–548, 1975
47. Heinze E, Beischer W, Keller L, Winkler G, Teller W, Pfeiffer E: C-peptide secretion during the remission phase of juvenile diabetes. Diabetes 27:670–676, 1978
48. Ludvigsson J, Heding LG, Larsson Y, Leander E: C-peptide in juvenile diabetics beyond the postinitial remission phase. Acta Paediatr Scand 66:177, 1987
49. Schiffrin A: Treatment of insulin-dependent diabetes with multiple subcutaneous insulin injections. Med Clin No Am 66:1251–1267, 1982
50. Bunn HF, Gabbay KH, Gallop PM: The glycosylation of hemoglobin: Relevance to diabetes mellitus. Science 200:21–27, 1978
51. Gabbay KH, Hasty K, Breslow JL, et al: Glycosylated hemoglobins and long-term blood glucose control in diabetes mellitus. J Clin Endocrinol Metab 44:859–864, 1977
52. Gabbay KH, Sosenko JM, Banuchi GA, et al: Glycosylated hemoglobins: Increased glycosylation of hemoglobin A in diabetic patients. Diabetes 28:337–340, 1979
53. Gallop PM, Fluckiger R, Hanneken A, et al: Chemical quantitation of hemoglobin glycosylation: Fluorometric detection of formaldehyde released upon periodate oxidation of glycoglobin. Anal Biochem 117:427–432, 1981
54. Garlick RL, Mazer JS, Higgins PJ, et al: Affinity chromatography: An improved method for measuring glycosylated hemoglobin. Clin Res 30:393A, 1981
55. Pecoraro RE, Graf RJ, Halter JB, et al: Comparison of a colorimetric assay for glycosylated hemoglobin with ion-exchange chromatography. Diabetes 28:1120–1125, 1979
56. Schiffrin A, Belmonte MM: Comparison between continuous subcutaneous insulin infusion and multiple injections of insulin. A one-year prospective study. Diabetes 31:255–290, 1982
57. Berger A, Saurbrey N, Kuhl C, Villumsen J: Clinical experience with a new device that will simplify insulin injections. Diabetes Care 8:73–76, 1985
58. Santiago JV, Clemens AH, Clarke WL, et al: Closed-loop and open-loop devices for blood glucose control in normal and diabetic subjects. Diabetes 38:71–84, 1979
59. Champion MD, Shepard GA, Rodger NW, et al: Continuous subcutaneous infusion of insulin in the management of diabetes mellitus. Diabetes 29:206–212, 1980
60. Pickup JC, Keen H, Parsons JA, et al: Continuous subcutaneous insulin infusion: An approach to achieving normoglycemia. Br Med J 1:204–207, 1978
61. Schiffrin A, Colle E, Belmonte MM: Improved control in diabetes with continuous subcutaneous insulin injections. Diabetes Care 3:643–649, 1980
62. Tamborlane WV, Sherwin RS, Genel M, Felig P: Reduction to normal of plasma glucose in juvenile diabetes by subcutaneous administration of insulin with a portable infusion pump. N Engl J Med 300:573–578, 1979
63. Bougneres PF, Landier F, Lemmel C, Mensire A, Chaussain JL: Insulin pump therapy in young children with Type I diabetes. J Pediatr 105:212–217, 1984
64. de Beaufort CE, Bruining GJ: Continuous subcutaneous insulin infusion in children. Diabetic Med 4:103–108, 1987
65. Teutsch SM, Herman WH, Dwyer DM, Lane JM: Mortality among diabetic patients using continuous subcutaneous insulin-infusion pumps. N Engl J Med 310:361–368, 1984
66. Schiffrin A, Suissa S: Predicting nocturnal hypoglycemia in Type I diabetics treated with continuous subcutaneous insulin infusion. Am J Med 82:1127–1132, 1987
67. Sperling M: Diabetic ketoacidosis. Pediatr Clin No Am 31:591–610, 1984
68. Foster D, McGarry D: The metabolic derangements and treatment of diabetic ketoacidosis. N Engl J Med 309:159–169, 1983
69. Alberti KGMM, Hockaday TDR: Diabetic coma: A reappraisal after five years. Clin Endocrinol Metab 6:421–455, 1977
70. Keller V, Berger W: Prevention of hypophosphatemia by phosphate infusion during treatment of diabetic ketoacidosis and hyperosmolar coma. Diabetes 29:87–95, 1980
71. Kaye R: Diabetic ketoacidosis: The bicarbonate controversy. J Pediatr 87:156–159, 1975
72. Davidson JK, De Bra DW: Immunologic insulin resistance. Diabetes 27:307–310, 1978
73. Kahn CR, Creitaz N: Insulin receptors and the molecular mechanism of insulin action. Diabetes Metab Rev 1:5–32, 1985

43

THYROID HORMONES

DELBERT A. FISHER

Thyroid hormones are critically important to normal growth and developmental during infancy, childhood, and adolescence. Thyroid hormone deficiency during infancy leads to mental retardation, and hypothyroidism during childhood and adolescence leads to growth and developmental retardation. In addition, there are significant effects of thyroid hormones on energy metabolism and on the metabolism of nutrients and inorganic ions, and these actions of the thyroid hormones are important in the maintenance of normal metabolic homeostasis. In the present chapter we review normal thyroid hormone physiology and pharmacology and the pharmacology of the drugs and chemicals used in the diagnosis and management of disorders of thyroid metabolism.

THYROID HORMONE SYNTHESIS AND RELEASE

The thyroid hormones and analogs are tyrosine derivatives. Their structures are summarized in Figure 43–1. The only source of thyroxine (tetraiodothyronine; T_4) is the thyroid gland. The major substrates for T_4 synthesis are iodide and tyrosine.[1,2] Tyrosine is not rate-limiting, but iodine is a trace element the limitation of which can severely impair thyroid hormone synthesis. The steps in thyroid hormone synthesis by the thyroid gland include (1) iodide trapping, (2) synthesis of thyroglobulin (TG), (3) organification of trapped iodide, (4) storage of iodinated TG in follicular colloid, (5) endocytosis and hydrolysis of TG to release thyroid hormones, and (6) deiodination of monoiodotyrosine (MIT) and diiodotyrosine (DIT) with intrathyroidal recycling of the iodide.[1,2] These steps are summarized in Figure 43–2.

The transport of iodide across the thyroid cell membrane is the first and rate-limiting step in thyroid hormone biosynthesis.[1-3] The salivary glands, gastric mucosa, uterus, mammary glands, small intestine, and placenta also are able to concentrate iodide; however, they are not capable of iodothyronine synthesis. Nor-

mally the thyroid follicular cell generates a thyroid/serum (T/S ratio) concentration gradient of 30- to 40-fold. This gradient increases markedly when stimulated by iodine deficiency, thyroid-stimulating hormone (thyrotropin; TSH), or thyroid-stimulating immunoglobins (TSI), or by drugs that impair the efficiency of hormone synthesis. Several inorganic anions are capable of competitively inhibiting iodide transport; these include bromide (Br^-), nitrate (NO_2^-), thiocyanate (SCN^-), and perchlorate (ClO_4^-).

The oxidation of iodide to an active intermediate is followed by iodination of TG-bound tyrosyl residues. The predominant protein in thyroid colloid is TG, and the thyroid gland normally contains 50–100 mg for every 1 gm of gland. The tyrosyl residues of TG, which are the iodine acceptors of TG, comprise about 3 percent of the weight of the protein, and about two-thirds of these are spatially oriented to be susceptible to iodination. Iodination of TG tyrosyl residues forms MIT and DIT. These iodotyrosines then couple to form the iodothyronines T_3 and T_4; DIT + DIT couple to form T_4 while MIT + DIT coupling forms T_3 (Figure 44–1). The relative proportions of T_3 and T_4 formed depend on the amount of available iodide and the extent of TG iodination. In the absence of iodine deficiency, about 30 percent of the iodoprotein is iodothyronine, with a T_4/T_3 ratio of 10:1 to 20:1.

The first step in thyroid hormone release is the endocytosis of stored colloid. The ingested colloid droplets fuse with proteolytic enzyme–containing lysosomes to form phagolysosomes. The enzymatic digestion of TG within the phagolysosomes releases free iodothyronines which are released into the cytoplasm and diffuse into the blood (Figure 43–2).

The MIT and DIT released during hydrolysis of TG are largely deiodinated under the influence of an iodotyrosine deiodinase.[1,2] The free iodide enters the intracellular iodide pool and is reutilized for new hormone synthesis (Figure 43–2). A defect in thyroidal iodotyrosine deiodinase leads to release of iodotyrosines into the circulation and their excretion in the urine. The loss from the thyroid gland of this normally recycled iodine, amounting to 70–

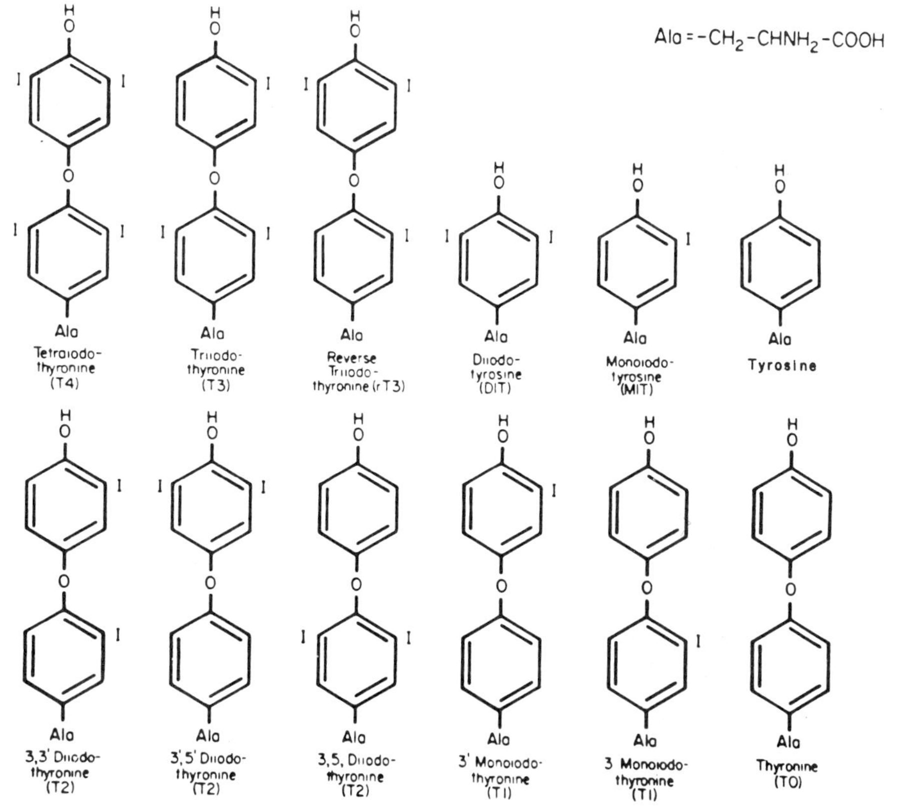

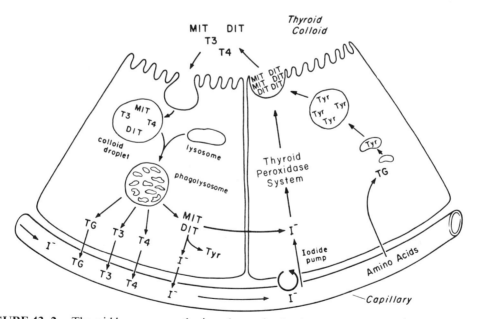

Ala = -CH₂-CHNH₂-COOH

FIGURE 43–1. Structure of the iodotyrosines and iodothyronines. The naturally occurring active thyroid hormones are thyroxine (tetraiodothyronine or T₄) and triiodothyronine (3,5,3′-triiodothyronine or T₃). In addition to progressive deiodination, T₄ is metabolized by degradation of the alanine side chain. See text for details.

FIGURE 43–2. Thyroid hormone synthesis and secretion by the thyroid follicular cell. The right-hand cell shows synthesis including iodide trapping and transport by the iodide pump, oxidation by the thyroid peroxidase system, and iodination of tyrosyl residues (Tyr) on thyroglobulin (TG). Monoiodotyrosine (MIT) and diiodotyrosine (DIT) couple to form thyroxine (T₄) or triiodothyronine (T₃). The left-hand cell summarizes secretion. Thyroid colloid is endocytosed as colloid droplets. These fuse with lysosomes to form phagolysosomes in which TG is degraded to release MIT, DIT, T₃, and T₄. MIT and DIT are largely deiodinated in the gland and the iodide reutilized for hormone synthesis. T₃ and T₄ are released into the bloodstream with some TG that has escaped degradation. See text for details. The cell separation of synthesis and secretion is for illustration only.

80 percent of the daily thyroidal iodine supply, can significantly compromise thyroid hormone synthesis.

Some TG escapes degradation in thyroid phagolysosomes and appears in serum in association with secreted iodothyronines.[1,4] There is good evidence that TG reaches the general circulation via thyroidal lymphatics. Circulating TG levels are high in premature infants during the first weeks of life, and values decrease with age throughout infancy and childhood.[5,6] Circulating TG concentrations in normal children range from <1 to 80 ng/ml.[6] Values increase after TSH administration and decrease during thyroid hormone administration.

REGULATION OF THYROID FUNCTION

Thyroid follicular cell function is regulated largely by circulating TSH and iodide levels.[1-3,7] TSH stimulates production of intracellular cyclic AMP (cAMP), and cAMP appears to mediate most of the effects of TSH on thyroid metabolism. TSH secretion is modulated by a negative feedback action of thyroid hormones (T_4 and T_3) on pituitary TSH synthesis. Increased thyroid hormone levels inhibit, and decreased concentrations stimulate, pituitary TSH synthesis. This feedback control is mediated via pituitary cell T_3 nuclear receptors that modulate TSH synthesis and pituitary cell membrane thyrotropin-releasing hormone (TRH) receptor binding.[8,9] TRH stimulates TSH release acutely and increases TSH synthesis as well as TSH glycosylation.[8,10,11] The rate of pituitary TSH release is the net effect of the stimulation by TRH and the inhibitory effect of T_3.

Hypothalamic TRH production is modulated by environmental temperature via both peripheral and central (hypothalamic) thermal receptors. Decreasing environmental and body temperature increases TRH production and increases the tonic level of TSH release. Thyroid hormone also modulates TRH synthesis within the hypothalamus.[12] Somatostatin (SRIF) and dopamine can inhibit TSH release, and these transmitters are thought to participate in central nervous system modulation of TSH release.[7] Norepinephrine and serotonin may inhibit TSH release, but their significance is not clear. Glucocorticoids inhibit TSH release at the hypothalamic level.[7]

The average level of plasma iodide also is an important factor in the control of thyroid gland function. Variation in iodine intake in the physiologic range modulates thyroid membrane iodide trapping and in pharmacologic doses will block thyroid hormone synthesis. At least one important mechanism for these effects is the inhibitory action of iodide on the stimulation of cAMP by TSH.

METABOLISM OF THYROID HORMONES

The thyroid gland is the sole source of T_4, but most of the T_3 in the blood is derived from nonglandular sources via monodeiodination of T_4 in peripheral tissues.[1,13] Both T_3 and T_4 in the blood are associated with plasma proteins; the binding affinities of these proteins are greater for T_4, so that the concentration of T_4 in human blood is 50 to 100 times greater than that of T_3. The concentrations of both are relatively constant in the steady state. The plasma half-life of T_4 in adult humans approximates 5 days; the half-life of T_3 approximates 1 day. The circulating thyroid hormone–binding proteins normally include T_4-binding interalpha globulin (TBG), T_4-binding prealbumin (TBPA), and albumin. TBG is the most important carrier protein for T_4; TBG and albumin seem equally important for T_3. The binding reactions are nearly complete, so that the euthyroid steady-state concentrations of free T_4 and free T_3 approximate 0.03 and 0.30 percent, respectively, of the total hormone concentrations. Absolute mean free T_4 and T_3 concentrations approximate 3.0 and 0.5 ng/dl, respectively. In adolescents and adults, the plasma concentrations of the several binding proteins are 1–4 mg/dl for TBG, 10–20 mg/dl for TBPA, and 2–5 gm/dl for albumin. TBG levels are higher in children than in adults and decrease progressively to adult levels during adolescence.

Two major extravascular pools of T_3 and T_4 probably exist, one in which plasma–tissue interchange is rapid (chiefly liver, kidney, and lung) and one in which exchange is slow (chiefly skeletal muscle and skin).[14] An additional pool, chiefly in gut and bone, with an intermediate exchange rate has been suggested. Peak T_4 concentrations after single-pulse doses of labeled hormone occur in these "pools" in minutes, hours, and days, respectively. Total body T_4 distribution in adults has been estimated as follows: about 20 percent in plasma, 30 percent in fast tissues, 45 percent in slow tissues, and 5 percent in intermediate tissues.

Deiodination is the major pathway of thyroid hormone metabolism in humans. The first step in T_4 metabolism is conversion either to T_3 or to reverse T_3 (Figure 43–1).[1,13,14] Monodeiodination of the beta or outer (hydroxyl) ring produces T_3, which has three to four times the metabolic potency of T_4. Monodeiodination of the alpha or inner ring produces rT_3, which is metabolically inactive. From 70 to 90 percent of circulating T_3 is derived from peripheral conversion and 10–25 percent from the thyroid gland; values for reverse T_3 probably are 96–98 percent and 2–4 percent, respectively. Progressive tissue monodeiodination reactions degrade T_3 and rT_3 to diiodo-, monoiodo-, and noniodinated thyronine (Figure 43–1).[1,13,14]

The alanine side chain of the inner ring of the hormones also is subject to degradative reactions, including transamination, deamination, and decarboxylation.[13,14] Pyruvic acid analogs and small amounts of a lactic acid analogs have been observed in urine and bile; these have minimal biologic activity. The extent of side chain cleavage reactions, relative to deiodination, has not been adequately quantified. Thyroid hormones are excreted in urine and stool in both free and conjugated forms. The conjugation reactions, which also inactivate the iodothyronines, involve both glucuronide and sulfoconjugation. T_4 is glucuronide-conjugated in the liver, and nearly all of this glucuronide is excreted in the bile; T_3 seems to be predominantly sulfoconjugated in kidney and other tissues.

Fecal excretion of thyroid hormones is somewhat variable, but usually 10–15 percent of T_3 or T_4 is excreted via the gut.

THYROID HORMONE ACTIONS

Thyroid hormones penetrate the cell membrane and bind to a specific nuclear, chromosomal, nonhistone receptor protein.[1,15] The thyroid receptors have significant homology with glucocorticoid receptors.[16,17] At least two human thyroid receptor genes have been characterized. One appears to be expressed predominantly in brain and to a lesser extent in several other tissues but excluding liver, and a second is expressed in placenta and other tissues including liver.[18,19] There may be other thyroid hormone receptor genes in the human genome, but the significance of these is not yet clear.[16]

T_3 binds to the nuclear receptors with 10 times the affinity of T_4. T_3 also binds to plasma membrane and mitochondrial receptors, but the major effects of thyroid hormones appear to be mediated via the nuclear T_3 receptors.[1,15] T_3 receptor binding modulates gene transcription and synthesis of messenger RNA and cytoplasmic proteins. Various tissues and cell functions are modified via varying patterns of genome activation and protein and receptor synthesis to account for the multiple physiologic actions of thyroid hormones. In addition to calorigenesis, these include stimulation of water and ion transport, acceleration of substrate turnover (including cholesterol) and amino acid and lipid metabolism, and stimulation of growth and development of various tissues at critical periods, including the central nervous system and skeleton.[1,15,20,21]

Thyroid hormone–dependent effects known to be mediated by stimulation and accumulation of mRNAs coding for specific proteins include synthesis of growth hormone (GH) in pituitary cells, selected enzymes and proteins in liver (including malic enzyme), α-myosin heavy chain in cardiac tissue, Na^+, K^+-ATPase in a variety of tissues, epidermal growth factor (EGF) in salivary gland and kidney, EGF receptors in liver, and uncoupling protein (thermogenin) in brown adipose tissue (BAT).[15,20–25] Thyroid hormones have been shown to inhibit the expression of other genes, including pituitary TSH and the β-myosin heavy chain in cardiac tissue.[20,21,26]

Thyroid hormones have important effects on other cell functions, although the mechanisms are not yet clear. They stimulate thermogenesis in most body cells, and this effect is associated with increases in mitochondrial RNA polymerase and α-glycerophosphate dehydrogenase.[15,27,28] It has been proposed that thyroid hormone–stimulated calorigenesis might be due to parallel enhancement of membrane Na^+, K^+ ATPase and mitochondrial α-glycerophosphate dehydrogenase activities coupling the augmented ADP production by Na^+, K^+ ATPase stimulation to increased mitochondrial ATP production.[29] Oppenheimer and colleagues[15] have shown that thyroid hormone stimulates S14 mRNA in BAT in association with a marked and proportional increase in BAT lipogenesis. They propose that thyroid hormone–stimulated fatty acid synthesis in BAT with cycling and oxidative degradation in liver could account for thyroid-stimulated thermogenesis. Thyroid hormone modulation of BAT thermogenesis may be mediated by modulation of BAT uncoupling protein.[25] Thyroid hormones also are known to modulate adrenergic receptor binding as well as postreceptor responsiveness.[30] The β-adrenergic-mediated effects of hyperthyroidism, such as tachycardia, tremor, and lid lag, can be blocked by propranolol, a β-receptor-blocking agent.

THYROID FUNCTION IN INFANCY AND CHILDHOOD

The thyroid gland is relatively hyperactive during infancy, and the oral replacement dose for T_4 decreases progressively from 10–15 μg/kg/day during the first year to 5 and 3 μg/kg/day at 5 and 15 years, respectively.[31–33] The latter approximates the adult dosage of 2–3 μg/kg/day. These changes correlate with a decreasing oxygen consumption rate with age, a decrease in percent labeled thyroid hormone appearing in plasma 24 hours after administration of a tracer dose of radioiodine, a decreasing serum TG concentration, and a decreasing T_4 degradation rate expressed as fraction of the extrathyroidal pool degraded daily (Figure 43–3).[31,34,35]

The serum TBG concentration falls with age to nadir values during adolescence.[36,37] There is a reciprocal change in TBPA levels.[37] These changes are mediated in part by gonadal steroids, but an age-dependent decrease in TBG is observed prior to puberty. The change in TBG is associated with corresponding decreases in serum T_4 and T_3 concentrations.[36] Recent results of Penny et al.[34] suggest a progressive fall in serum TSH concentrations in euthyroid children between 7 and 17 years of age.

RELATIVE EFFECTS OF THYROID HORMONES VERSUS AGE

Thyroid hormone actions also vary with age. Thyroid hormone deficiency during human fetal life has minimal untoward effects. Somatic growth and development and linear bone growth proceed normally in the athyroid fetus, and bone maturation is normal or minimally retarded (3–6 weeks).[38–40] Brain growth, as assessed by head circumference measurements, is not abnormal, and IQ measurements in athyroid children at 6–8 years of age are normal with early and adequate postnatal thyroid hormone replacement.[41–44] The reason(s) for the relative lack of thyroid hormone effect in the fetus are not clear. There is no deficiency of T_3 receptors; available data indicate an early appearance of nuclear thyroid receptors in human fetal tissues.[45,46] More likely explanations includes low levels of active thyroid hormone in fetal serum and tissues and/or immaturity of thyroid hormone receptor responsiveness at the transcription, translation, or action levels.[47]

The developmental effects of thyroid hormones are most obvious during infancy and early childhood.

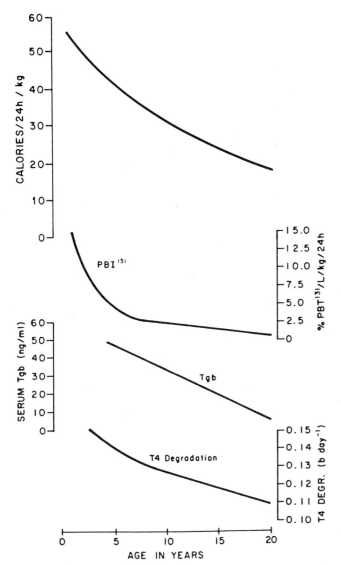

FIGURE 43–3. Changes in thyroid function parameters with increasing age in children and adolescents. The thyroid gland is quite active during infancy. The thyroxine (T4) production rate is high (10–15 μg/kg/day relative to the 20-year value of 2–3 ng/kg/day) and this is reflected in a progressive decrease in the T4 degradation rate expressed as a fraction of the extrathyroidal T4 pool cleared daily (bday^{-1}). The mean PBI[131] (protein-bound iodine[131]) turnover (percent dose administered appearing daily in plasma as PBI[131]) is high in infants and falls progressively with age. The serum thyroglobulin (Tgb) concentration also falls progressively. These changes are shown relative to the progressive decrease in metabolic rate expressed as calories/kg/24 h. (Data from Fisher and Dussault,[31] Penny et al.,[34] and Fisher.[6])

Somatic growth, bone growth and maturation, and tooth development and eruption are thyroid-dependent. In addition, 60–70 percent of postnatal brain growth and differentiation occurs during the first 2 years of life; and it is during this period that thyroid dependency is manifest.[48] Thyroid hormone replacement begun within 1–2 months after birth minimizes permanent brain damage.[43,44] After 3–4 years of age, thyroid hormone deficiency is not associated with mental retardation, but delayed somatic and linear bone growth and delayed eruption of permanent dentition are prominent. Bone maturation, measured as

bone age, also is delayed, diaphyseal bone growth is reduced, and epiphyseal growth and mineralization largely cease.[49–51]

Hypothalamic anterior pituitary function also may be abnormal in hypothyroid children. Although in most children thyroid hormone deficiency leads to delayed sexual development, occasional children manifest precocious sexual maturation with increased levels of circulating gonadotropins.[52–55] In females serum prolactin levels also tend to be increased, and galactorrhea may occur if serum estrogen levels are high enough to permit breast development and milk production. The mechanism of the precocious gonadotropin and prolactin hypersecretion is not clear. These changes seem to occur in children with high serum TSH levels, and enlargement of the sella turcica has been observed.

During childhood and adolescence and until epiphyseal closure, thyroid hormone deficiency leads to reduced somatic growth, reduced linear bone growth, and delayed bone maturation. In addition, epiphyseal dysgenesis is commonly observed.[56] The effects of thyroid hormone deficiency on dental development are less profound, but delay in eruption of second dentition may occur. Abnormalities of hypothalamic–pituitary function secondary to hypothyroidism also are common in adolescence. Puberty often is delayed or incomplete. In normal females menstrual cycles commonly are nonovulatory and bleeding may be irregular. This pattern usually is more prolonged in hypothyroid female adolescents. In addition, menorrhagia or hypomenorrhea may occur.

MECHANISMS OF THYROID ACTIONS ON GROWTH AND DEVELOPMENT

The effects of thyroid hormones on somatic and skeletal growth are mediated, at least in part, by stimulation of GH and somatomedin synthesis and action.[57] A synergism between GH and thyroid hormones with regard to growth has long been recognized. GH synthesis by pituitary cells is known to be thyroid hormone–dependent.[57–61] The growth effects of GH are thought to be mediated via somatomedins, a family of insulin-like hormones under GH control.[62] GH binding to liver and other cells stimulates somatomedin production, and somatomedins in turn stimulate growth effects, particularly in bone and muscle tissues.[62–67] T4 also has been shown to increase serum somatomedin activity in hypopituitary mice which are incapable of synthesizing GH.[65] Combined T3 and GH therapy of hypophysectomized rats is necessary to normalize growth as well as serum somatomedin levels.[65,68] In addition, there is evidence to suggest that thyroid hormones potentiate the actions of somatomedin on cartilage growth.[64]

The precise mechanism of T4 dependency of other growth processes is not so clear. There is suggestive evidence that other peptide growth factors, similarly to the somatomedins, mediate the thyroid hormone effects on specific target tissues. In the mouse the EGF content of various tissues has been show to be thyroid hormone–responsive,[69–72] and EGF has been shown to stimulate T_4-dependent eye opening and incisor eruption in hypothyroid neonatal mice.[71] T_4 also increases EGF receptor binding in selected tissues.[24,73] Erythropoietin synthesis by the kidney is known to be thyroid hormone–responsive, and there are known positive correlations between circulating erythropoietin levels, erythrocyte production, and hemoglobin concentrations in hypo- and hyperthyroidism.[57] Nerve growth factor (NGF) content of various tissues of the mouse is also thyroid hormone–responsive, and sympathetic nervous system development is known to be both thyroid hormone– and NGF-dependent.[57,74,75] NGF has been suggested to mediate the effects of thyroid hormone on sympathetic nervous system development. These observations have suggested the hypothesis that thyroid hormones exert their developmental effects, at least in part, via stimulation of the production and/or effect of various tissue-specific growth factors. The extent and significance of these pathways, however, are not clear.

THYROID HORMONE PREPARATIONS

The thyroid hormones as shown in Figure 43–1 are iodine-containing amino acid derivatives of thyronine. The structural requirements for bioactivity have been well defined. The two aromatic rings are essential, as is the ether linkage. The alanine side chain in position 1, halogen or methyl groups in positions 3, 5, and 3′, and the hydroxyl group in position 4 are all necessary for optimal activity. The natural hormones are levorotatory; the dextrorotatory isomers have 10 percent or less of the bioactivity of the l-isomers. The d-T_4 isomer has been utilized clinically as a cholesterol-lowering agent but has no role in replacement therapy. Triiodothyroacetic acid (TRIAC) binds to the thyroid hormone receptor as effectively as T_3 *in vitro* but has a much shorter half-life *in vivo*. It is not available for routine clinical use but has been proposed for treatment of TSH-dependent hyperthyroidism (pituitary T_3 resistance).

Several preparations of thyroid hormones are available, as summarized in Table 43–1. Na-l-thyroxine (T_4) and Na-l-triiodothyronine (T_3) are synthetic preparations of the natural hormones. These hormones also are available in combination in a 4:1 ratio of T_4 to T_3. Thyroid USP is a dried and powdered preparation of porcine or bovine thyroid gland. Thyroglobulin is a partially purified porcine preparation of the thyroid storage protein.

Na-l-thyroxine is the drug of choice for replacement therapy. It is more uniform in potency; it is easily measured in serum; and it provides physiologic serum T_3 levels, since most of the circulating T_3 normally is derived from T_4 by monodeiodination in the tissues. Most synthetic T_4 preparations have been reformulated since 1982 to guarantee specified hormone concentrations.[76] Absorption of the hormone is variable, ranging from 50 to 100 percent; average absorption approximates 80 percent.[76]

There is only limited application for Na-l-triiodothy-

TABLE 43–1. PREPARATIONS AND RELATIVE POTENCIES OF THYROID HORMONE PREPARATIONS

PREPARATION	SOURCE	EQUIVALENT DOSAGE
Na-l-thyroxine	Synthetic	100 μg
Na-l-triiodothyronine	Synthetic	25 μg
Na-l-thyroxine (80%) plus Na-l-triiodothyronine (20%)	Synthetic	50 + 12.5 μg
Thyroid (USP)	Natural	60 mg
Thyroglobulin	Natural	60 mg

ronine (T_3) in thyroid therapy. Absorption of T_3 is nearly complete after oral administration, but the serum half-life is short (1 day versus 5 days for T_4). Blood levels are more variable and more difficult to stabilize. T_3 may be useful in the early treatment of severe hypothyroidism or for short-term suppression studies. It may also be useful in management of TSH-dependent hyperthyroidism.

THERAPY WITH THYROID HORMONES

Congenital Hypothyroidism

Infants with congenital hypothyroidism (CH) usually have thyroid dysgenesis due to abnormal thyroid gland development. They may have agenesis or have a residual hypoplastic gland in the normal or an ectopic location. About 10 percent have an inborn abnormality in TSH secretion or response or in thyroid hormone synthesis. Less commonly, transient neonatal hypothyroidism can be caused by exposure to an antithyroid drug or chemical or an antithyroid antibody derived transplacentally from the mother.[77,78]

In infants with CH, institution of treatment with 10–15 μg/kg T_4 daily until 45 days of age usually is necessary to consistently normalize the serum T_4 concentration (to > 10 μg/dl) within 2–4 weeks (Table 43–2).[79] This amounts to an initial treatment dose of 50 μg daily in most term infants. It is now clear that the major source of brain cell T_3, the receptor-active hormone, is serum T_4. Some 70 percent of T_3 in the cerebral cortex of neonatal rats is derived from local monodeiodination of T_4.[80–82] Thus, institution of replacement T_4 in a dose adequate to rapidly

TABLE 43–2. DOSE OF ORAL THYROXINE FOR REPLACEMENT THERAPY OF INFANTS AND CHILDREN

AGE	ORAL DOSE	
	(μg/kg/day)	Range of Dose (μg)
1–6 months	7–15	30–50
6–12 months	4–8	50–100
1–5 years	5–6	75–150
5–10 years	3–4	100–200
10–20 years	1.5–3	100–250

normalize the serum T_4 concentration is essential to minimize the period of central nervous system T_4 deficiency and help ensure optimal brain development. Replacement therapy with T_3 or mixtures of T_4 and T_3 is not recommended.

Careful monitoring of individual infants and dosage adjustment are necessary during the early weeks and months of life to guarantee adequate treatment and prevent prolonged hyperthyroxinemia. Premature synostosis with and without brain dysfunction has been reported in association with neonatal thyrotoxicosis or with excessive thyroid hormone doses in the treatment of CH.[83-85] In the latter cases, the T_4 doses were in the 200–300 μg/day range throughout most of infancy.[85] The threshold and duration of T_4 secretion or dosage required to produce premature synostosis is not clear, but the modest doses recommended with careful monitoring produce little risk. It is useful to obtain serum 12–24 hours after the last T_4 dose to avoid transient and variable elevations of serum T_4 associated with acute and variable absorption. The T_4 dose can be altered during the first few months of treatment so that the adjusted serum T_4 (the free T_4 index) is in the 10–16 μg/dl range.

The serum TSH concentration may be inappropriately elevated in infants with CH and may not be suppressed to normal levels with treatment.[86-88] Adequate treatment probably should suppress serum TSH values to less than 15 μU/ml by 3–4 months, but more information is necessary to define the value and desirable range of serum TSH measurements during the first 3–4 months of life. Although the early weeks and months of treatment are critical for infants with CH, the central nervous system is thyroid hormone–dependent for 2–4 years, and growth is thyroid hormone–dependent during the first 2 decades of life. Thus, careful monitoring of treatment is required throughout childhood and adolescence. The total dosage of T_4 increases progressively to 200–300 μg daily in adolescence. The dosage on a kilogram body weight basis decreases progressively to the adult value of 1.5 μg/kg/day.

Adequacy of therapy is judged by clinical evidence of normal growth and development and lack of signs and symptoms of toxicity. Growth in length and weight should be plotted monthly during the first 3 months and at 2- to 3-month intervals thereafter during the first year. Bone age should be assessed at 3 months and at 6–12 months of treatment. Thereafter, 12- to 24-month evaluations will suffice. Measurements of circulating hormone concentrations are essential to assess adequacy of treatment. Measurements of T_4, TSH, and, on occasion, T_3 are helpful. Serum T_4 levels should be adjusted to the upper two-thirds of the normal range for age. At this time the serum TSH level should be normal or mildly increased and the serum T_3 concentration within the normal range for age.

If the hypothyroidism is secondary, due to hypothalamic–pituitary dysfunction, treatment with adrenal corticosteroids and GH is necessary if deficiencies of adrenocorticotropic hormone (ACTH) and GH are documented. Adrenal insufficiency may be manifest as failure to thrive and/or hypoglycemia in the neonatal period. GH deficiency also may contribute to hypoglycemia and may impair growth after 3–6 months.

Acquired Hypothyroidism

Acquired hypothyroidism before 5–6 years most commonly results from delayed failure of the thyroid remnant in infants with thyroid dysgenesis, but inborn defects in thyroid hormone synthesis, ingested goitrogens, chronic thyroiditis, or hypothalamic–pituitary disease may be involved. After 5–6 years, the same spectrum of etiologies is involved, but hypothyroidism most commonly is due to chronic lymphocytic (Hashimoto's) thyroiditis. Surgery or radioiodine treatment also can result in hypothyroidism.

Irreversible brain damage is not a likely result of hypothyroidism acquired after 2–3 years of age. By this time central nervous system growth is largely complete. Delayed growth, however, may be marked and most commonly is manifest as delayed tooth development and eruption, delayed skeletal growth and maturation, and linear growth retardation. Aberrations in pubertal development and menstrual irregularities are common. These manifestations are reversible with adequate replacement therapy. As in infants, the treatment of choice is oral Na-l-thyroxine. The replacement dose on a body weight basis decreases progressively with age (Table 43–1). The dosage should be adjusted at 2- to 4-week intervals to a level that maintains the serum T_4 concentration in the mid-range of normal together with normal T_3 and TSH concentrations. In contrast to adults, it is not necessary in most children with hypothyroidism to increase the dose of replacement T_4 gradually. Initial administration of the total daily estimated replacement dose will result in a gradual increase in serum T_4 concentrations over a 3- to 4-week period. If cardiac disease is suspected, more gradual replacement may be indicated.

Treatment of secondary hypothyroidism in childhood or adolescence may require simultaneous replacement with adrenal corticosteroids, GH, and gonadal steroid(s). Hashimoto's thyroiditis is the most common cause of acquired hypothyroidism.[89] It is an autoimmune disease associated with progressive autoimmune damage to thyroid follicular cells. The disease most frequently involves only the thyroid gland. Occasionally, however, Hashimoto's thyroiditis is associated with other endocrine gland autoimmune deficiencies.[90] These include diabetes mellitus, adrenal insufficiency, hypoparathyroidism, and, on rare occasions, hypogonadism. Autoimmune gastritis with pernicious anemia and cutaneous moniliasis are sometimes associated. Treatment of these other endocrine gland deficiencies may be necessary.

Hashimoto's thyroiditis presents early as a mild to moderate euthyroid goiter. The disease remits spontaneously in about one-third of children. The remainder gradually develop hypothyroidism. There is no specific therapy, but if the goiter is large, if the serum TSH concentration is elevated, or if the patient is clinically hypothyroid, replacement therapy with Na-l-thyroxine is indicated. Some physicians favor T_4 treatment of all children with Hashimoto's thyroiditis to avoid mild, undiagnosed hypothyroidism.

Nontoxic Diffuse Goiter

Nontoxic diffuse goiter in childhood often is referred to as simple colloid goiter.[77] It is most common during adolescence in females, where it has been referred to as adolescent goiter. These patients are euthyroid with mild to moderate goiters characterized histologically by large thyroid follicles rimmed by flattened epithelial cells. The glands usually are diffusely enlarged and of nearly normal consistency, but nodularity can occur. The etiology is unclear, but recent studies have shown the presence of thyroid growth–stimulating autoantibodies in the blood of affected individuals, suggesting that at least some of these patients have a variant form of autoimmune thyroid disease.[91,92] Systematic studies of treatment of these patients with T_4 to "suppress" the goiter have not been conducted. T_4 may suppress thyroid antigen production and reduce autoantibody titers.

Thyroid Nodules

Suppressive therapy with T_4 sometimes is used to differentiate benign from malignant thyroid nodules. Diagnostic procedures usually include thyroid scanning and/or fine-needle biopsy.[77] In the occasional patient with an inconclusive biopsy result, a trial of suppressive T_4 therapy may be useful. In this instance the end point is a decrease in size of the nodule or a failure of further growth over a period of 6–12 months. The dose of T_4 is adjusted to suppress serum TSH concentrations to the very low or undetectable level ($<0.02~\mu U/ml$) using a highly sensitive TSH assay method. This may require T_4 doses 30–50 percent higher than replacement doses. T_3 is not usually used for suppression because the half-life of serum levels is relatively short (1 day versus 5 days for T_4), and T_4 provides more reliable TSH suppression.

ANTITHYROID DRUGS

Many compounds and chemicals have been shown to inhibit the synthesis and/or metabolism of thyroid hormones. The most important of these are the thioureylenes, the iodinated organic radiographic contrast agents, iodide, and radioactive iodine.

The Thioureylenes

Astwood and colleagues[93,94] in the 1940s characterized a series of thioureylene drugs that inhibit thyroid hormone synthesis via a thiocarbamide group ($S=C-N$). Several compounds have been utilized for treatment of hyperthyroidism. These include thiourea, thiouracil, methylthiouracil, propylthiouracil (PTU), methimazole

(MMI), and carbimazole (CBI). The drugs currently used to treat hyperthyroidism include PTU, MMI, and CBI. CBI acts by conversion to MMI. The thioureylene drugs act by inhibiting the organification of iodine via inhibition of thyroid peroxidase activity.[95] Inhibition of hormone synthesis results in depletion of the thyroid stores of iodinated TG and a progressive decrease in thyroid hormone secretion from the thyroid gland. In addition to blocking hormone synthesis, PTU inhibits the peripheral conversion of T_4 to T_3; MMI does not share this action.[94] Effective amounts of the drugs are absorbed within 30–60 minutes after an oral dose. The half-life of PTU in plasma approximates 2 hours; that for MMI 6–13 hours.[94] The drugs are concentrated within the thyroid and metabolites are excreted largely in the urine. They cross the placenta and appear in breast milk.

There is a significant incidence of toxic reactions to all thioureylene drugs. The incidence of major and minor toxicities is summarized in Table 43–3. The most common minor reaction is a purpuric, papular rash which usually is mild and subsides spontaneously. Other minor reactions include nausea, headache, paresthesias, hair loss, and joint pain and stiffness. Agranulocytosis, the most serious reaction, is observed in 1 in 500 to 1 in 1000 cases. It usually develops during the first few months of treatment and may develop rapidly. Mild granulocytopenia may be due to thyrotoxicosis or may be an early sign of serious drug toxicity. Drug fever, hepatitis, nephritis, and a lupus-like reaction are rare complications.

A drug rash, if persistent, can be managed by substituting another thioureylene drug, since cross-sensitivity is not common. Should granulocytopenia be observed, frequent leukocyte counts are indicated to rule out serious drug toxicity. Routine blood counts are not helpful, since agranulocytosis can develop after several months and may appear rapidly. Patients should be instructed to report development of sore throat or fever which may herald agranulocytosis. Persistent neutropenia requires discontinuing drug treatment. Agranulocytosis usually reverses spontaneously, but intensive transient supportive treatment may be required if it is severe.

Sodium Ipodate or Iopanoate

These iodinated organic radiographic contrast agents have been shown to be effective antithyroid drugs.[96–99] They inhibit the enzymatic monodeiodination of T_4 to T_3 and produce a rapid reduction in serum T_3 concentrations.[96,97] In addition, they inhibit thyroid hormone secretion from the thyroid gland so that serum T_4 levels also fall.[96–100] Chronic treatment (6–12 months) has been successful in 50 to more than 90 percent of patients with Graves' disease.[96–98] Sodium ipodate may be more effective than sodium iopanoic acid, but data to date are limited in this regard.[97,98] Sodium ipodate has been used successfully in an infant with neonatal Graves' disease.[99]

No serious side effects have been observed to date, but experience is limited. Interestingly, in contrast to iodide, permanent blockade of thyroid function does not occur, and radioiodine treatment has been applied within 2–4

TABLE 43–3. CHARACTERISTICS OF COMMONLY USED THIOUREYLENE DRUGS

DRUG	BLOOD HALF-LIFE (h)	INITIAL DOSE (mg/kg/dose)	MAINTENANCE DOSE (mg/kg/day)	TOXIC MAJOR (%)	REACTIONS MINOR (%)
Propylthiouracil	2	5–8	1–3	0.9	2.2
Methimazole	6–13	0.5–0.7	0.1–0.3	1.4	4.5
Carbimazole	–	0.5–0.7	0.1–0.3	0.9	2.2

From Marchant et al.,[94] with permission.

weeks of discontinuing sodium ipodate therapy.[97] These agents may be very useful for treatment of patients who develop toxicity to thioureylene drugs. They may also be useful adjuncts to other antithyroid drug regimens and may be helpful in short-term preoperative or pre-radio-iodine treatment of severe thyrotoxicosis.

Iodide

Iodide is the oldest antithyroid drug. In large doses (> 0.1 mg/kg/day) it inhibits thyroid iodide transport, iodothyronine synthesis, and thyroid hormone release.[101] As a result there is a rapid fall in serum thyroid hormone levels that may persist several weeks. Eventually there is an "escape" from the thyroid iodide blockade mediated in part by the inhibition of thyroid cell membrane iodide transport and a reduction in intrathyroidal iodide concentrations. Thus, iodide usually is restricted to short-term therapy (several weeks). Iodide treatment has been used in the immediate preoperative period to prepare patients for thyroidectomy and for treatment of severe thyrotoxicosis or thyroid crisis in conjunction with thioureylene drugs.

Toxic reactions to iodide are observed occasionally.[101] Acute life-threatening angioedema and laryngeal edema may occur with or without a cutaneous hemorrhagic rash. Serum sickness-like manifestations also have been observed with fever, arthralgia, eosinophilia, and lymphadenopathy. Chronic intoxication (iodism) also is described, including soreness of the teeth and gums, increased salivation, nasal irritation, swelling of the eyes, headache, and chronic cough. Acneiform skin lesions, gastric irritation, and diarrhea may occur. These signs and symptoms disappear within a few days after discontinuing iodide ingestion.

Iodide preparations include Strong Iodine Solution (Lugol's solution) for oral use and sodium iodide for intravenous use. Lugol's solution is formulated as 5 percent iodine and 10 percent potassium iodide. The iodine is reduced to iodide in the intestine before absorption. Intravenous NaI is available as a 10 percent solution.

Radioactive Iodine

There are several clinically useful isotopes of radioiodine.[102] These include ^{131}I, ^{125}I, and ^{123}I. The half-lives are 8 days, 60 days, and 13 hours, respectively. Gamma ray-emitting isotopes are used for scanning, whereas beta radiation is desirable for tissue radiation treatment. All three iosotopes are gamma emitters and are used for thyroid scanning.[125]I and ^{123}I are preferred because they provide low thyroid radiation doses. ^{131}I is used for treatment because of its beta radiation. The average absorbed beta dose per gram tissue is approximately 10 rads/day/μCi. Other isotopes of iodine are not in general clinical use.

TREATMENT OF HYPERTHYROIDISM

Childhood Thyrotoxicosis

Hyperthyroidism in childhood usually is due to Graves' disease but can be secondary to Hashimoto's thyroiditis, hyperfunctioning thyroid nodule(s), or TSH hypersecretion. Treatment of the hyperthyroid state may be accomplished with antithyroid drugs, surgery, or radioiodine. Antithyroid drug treatment is considered the treatment of choice by most pediatric endocrinologists.[103–106] Both PTU and MMI (Tapazole) are effective drugs.

Initial therapy is instituted with PTU, 5–7 mg/kg/day, or MMI, 0.5–0.6 mg/kg/day, in three divided doses at about 8-hour intervals. The dose is increased if improvement is not observed within 2–3 weeks. Nearly all patients will respond to PTU in doses of 10–15 mg/kg/day or MMI in doses of 1–1.5 mg/kg/day. However, an occasional patient may require as much as 20 mg/kg/day for control. MMI has a longer half-life than PTU, and some patients will maintain effective blockade of thyroid hormone synthesis with once-daily drug administration, particularly after remission has been induced. PTU often can be given in two daily doses.

In patients with severe disease or distressing cardiovascular symptoms, propranolol is useful adjunctive therapy; 0.1–0.3 mg/kg I.V. followed by 2 mg/kg/day orally in divided doses, or oral therapy alone has been utilized. The dose of propranolol can be increased to 4–6 mg/kg/day.

Potassium iodide in large doses potentiates the action of thioureylene drugs. Therapeutic doses for hyperthyroidism range from 2 to 4 mg/kg/day, usually given as Strong Iodine Solution or a saturated solution of potassium iodide. The inhibitory effect on hormone synthesis and/or release usually persists 10–40 days. As indicated earlier, potassium iodide is most useful for short-term treatment of severe disease and for preoperative preparation of patients for surgery.

After the patient has become euthyroid, which usually

takes 30–90 days, the daily dose of medication can be reduced to 3–4 mg of PTU/kg or 0.3–0.4 mg of MMI/kg. Treatment must be monitored with measurements of serum T_4 concentrations to ensure an adequate drug effect and avoid hypothyroidism. Measurements of serum T_3 concentration often are useful when the clinical assessment and serum T_4 measurements are in disagreement; on occasion the antithyroid medication will be adequate to inhibit T_4 but not T_3 secretion, and the patient will appear euthyroid or even hyperthyroid, with low levels of serum T_4. Serum TSH measurements are helpful in assessing drug-induced hypothyroidism. Measurements of thyroid-stimulating antibody levels are useful in predicting remission.

Two approaches to long-term treatment have been used: (1) continue adjusting the antithyroid drug dose to maintain a euthyroid state, or (2) provide a blocking dose of drugs and treat the patient with exogenous T_4. The average remission rate for Graves' disease approximates 50 percent each 2–3 years. Some patients remit within 6–12 months, but these represent the minority. Effective drug management usually requires 2–5 years of continuous treatment. Markers for remission include disappearance of goiter and decreasing titers of thyroid-stimulating antibody.

If drug toxicity ensues, the drug becomes ineffective either for patient or for pharmacologic reasons, or if the goiter is large and unresponsive to a reasonable drug treatment regimen, alternative treatment may be considered. If an experienced thyroid surgeon is available, thyroidectomy may be preferable. Radioiodine is a viable alternative in the adolescent. It should be emphasized, however, that the physician threshold for abandoning medical therapy should be kept relatively high. These patients require frequent followup, support, and encouragement.

Radioiodine treatment has not been widely employed in children because of the concern about permanent hypothyroidism, radiation oncogenesis, and genetic damage. Late development of primary hypothyroidism after ^{131}I therapy has occurred in every series of patients studied, regardless of the dosage of radioiodine employed. Approximately 10–20 percent of patients treated with radioiodine are hypothyroid within 1 year, and the incidence of hypothyroidism is 3–5 percent per year thereafter. The fear of inducing leukemia and thyroid carcinoma in adult patients with radioiodine treatment has been largely alleviated. However, the thyroid glands of young animals are much more susceptible to induction of thyroid carcinoma by ionizing radiation than those of older animals, and radiation has been incriminated as an important cause of thyroid cancer in children.[107]

It has been the practice in most clinics to reserve the use of radioiodine for treatment of thyrotoxicosis in older adolescents who fail to follow a medical regimen and who cannot be adequately prepared for surgical thyroidectomy. However, the recent report by Hamburger[108] of the successful treatment of 191 children and adolescents with radioiodine over a 23-year period suggests that this approach may be safe enough to consider as initial treatment in some patients. In Hamburger's series one dose of radioiodine provided effective treatment in 85 percent of cases.

β-Adrenergic blocking drugs are useful to control the sympathetic hyperactivity. These drugs also have proven lifesaving in critically ill patients in thyroid storm, but they cannot be relied upon as the only therapy in such patients. β-Receptor blockade is potentially dangerous in patients with cardiac failure or arrhythmias.

Iodinated radiographic contrast agents (ipodate, iopanoic acid) may be useful in treatment of Graves' hyperthyroidism.[96–98] Doses of 0.01 μg/kg/day or 0.04–0.05 μg/kg every 3 days have been utilized successfully and have maintained remission for 6–8 months. There is only limited experience with their use in children.

Neonatal Thyrotoxicosis

Neonatal Graves' disease is rare, probably due to the low incidence of thyrotoxicosis in pregnancy (1–2 cases per 1000 pregnancies) and the fact that the neonatal disease occurs in only about 1 in 70 cases of thyrotoxic pregnancy.[99,109] In most cases the disease is due to transplacental passage of a thyroid-stimulating antibody from a mother with active or inactive Graves' disease or Hashimoto's thyroiditis.[109] Graves' disease in the newborn is manifested by irritability, flushing, tachycardia, hypertension, poor weight gain, thyroid enlargement, and exophthalmos. Thrombocytopenia, hepatosplenomegaly, jaundice, and hypoprothrombinemia also have been observed. Arrhythmias, cardiac failure, and death may occur if the thyrotoxicity is severe and the treatment is inadequate. Mortality approaches 25 percent in disease severe enough to be diagnosed.

The treatment of hyperthyroidism in the newborn includes sedatives and digitalization as necessary. Iodide or antithyroid drugs are administered to decrease thyroid hormone secretion.[110] These drugs have additive effects with regard to inhibition of hormone synthesis; in addition, iodide will rapidly inhibit hormone release. Lugol's solution (126 mg of iodine per milliliter) is given in doses of one drop (about 8 mg) three times daily. MMI, CBI, or PTU is administered in doses of 0.5–1 mg, 0.5–1 mg, or 5–10 mg, respectively, per kilogram daily in divided doses at 8-hour intervals. A therapeutic response should be observed within 24–48 hours. If a satisfactory response is not observed, the dose of antithyroid drug and iodide can be increased by 50 percent. Adrenal corticosteroids in anti-inflammatory dosage and propranolol (1–2 mg/kg/day) also may be helpful. Radiographic contrast agents also may be useful in treatment (100 mg/day or 0.5 gm every 3 days) either alone or more effectively in conjunction with antithyroid drug treatment.[99]

TSH-Dependent Hyperthyroidism

Hyperthyroidism with diffuse goiter and elevated serum levels of TSH has been reported in several patients without pituitary enlargement.[111–113] These patients manifest a defect in the feedback control of T_3 on TSH release such that a new set point is established with hypersecretion of TSH, hypersecretion of thyroid hormone, and mild to moderate tissue hyperthyroidism. In contrast to patients with TSH-secreting tumors, the TSH alpha sub-unit level is not elevated and the TSH response to TRH is augmented.[111]

Treatment is difficult and not generally satisfactory. Thyroid ablation controls the hyperthyroidism but aggravates the TSH hypersecretion and increases the risk of development of a pituitary adenoma. Suppression of TSH by exogenous thyroid hormone may aggravate the hyperthyroidism. However, this approach has been at least partially successful,[112,113] and treatment with TRIAC or long-acting SRIF has been proposed.[113,114] Both of the latter agents are experimental drugs.

Autonomous Nodular Hyperthyroidism

Autonomous functioning thyroid nodules are uncommon in childhood and adolescence. Rarely, single or multiple autonomously functioning nodules may be associated with clinical hyperthyroidism.[115–117] Such nodules are true follicular adenomas and nearly always are benign; the incidence of thyroid carcinoma in functioning nodules is less than 1 percent. It is generally felt that function in a thyroid nodule essentially excludes a diagnosis of thyroid carcinoma. Small functional nodules usually do not produce clinical thyrotoxicosis; large nodules (>3 cm diameter) are more likely to do so. Nodular autonomy usually is discerned by thyroid radioiodine scan and confirmed if the serum TSH concentration measured by a highly sensitive method is suppressed and/or is unresponsive to TRH stimulation.[115,116]

The natural history of functioning thyroid nodules in the individual patient is variable. Such patients, if euthyroid, usually will remain euthyroid, but there may be a gradual increase in thyroid hormone production with development of clinical evidence of hyperthyroidism. Nodule enlargement or thyrotoxic symptoms may create the need for ablative therapy. Functioning nodules producing clinical and chemical thyrotoxicosis require surgical removal. Radioiodine treatment now tends to be reserved for older patients (>40 years of age). Antithyroid drug therapy is considered only for short-term management.

THYROID NODULES AND CANCER

Thyroid Nodules

Thyroid nodules in children are significant for three reasons: they may herald underlying thyroid disease, they may be hyperfunctioning nodules and produce hyperthyroidism, or they may represent carcinoma. In the first instance, the approach is to the basic disease, often Hashimoto's thyroiditis. Functioning nodules producing clinical and chemical thyrotoxicosis require treatment, as indicated in the previous section. The likelihood of carcinoma in a cold nodule (one that does not concentrate radioiodine) in an otherwise normal thyroid gland is estimated to be 15–20 percent in children.[118] Most of these are thyroid follicular cell neoplasms, but about 5 percent

are medullary carcinomas secreting calcitonin and can be identified with a serum calcitonin measurement with or without stimulation testing.[119] Fine-needle biopsy is commonly employed in differential diagnosis. The result usually is reported as malignant, suspicious, or benign. Surgery is indicated if the needle biopsy indicates a malignant lesion. Many consider that surgery also is indicated if there is a prior history of therapeutic radiation to the head or neck, if the nodule is hard, if there is evidence of tracheal invasion (dysphagia, hoarseness, or cough) or vocal cord paralysis, if adjacent lymph nodes are involved, or if there are distant metastases.

T₄ Suppression

If the thyroid needle biopsy result is suspicious and no thyroid malignancy criteria is present, thyroid suppression with 0.2–0.3 mg of Na-l-T₄ daily can be employed. If over a period of 4–6 months the nodule grows, or if over a period of 12 months the nodule does not decrease in size, surgery is indicated. If the nodule decreases in size, longer followup is in order. It is important to remember that thyroid follicular cell carcinomas in children are rather indolent neoplasms and do not require urgent treatment.

Management of Thyroid Follicular Cancer: Use of Radioiodine

The initial approach is simple removal of the affected thyroid lobe. If frozen section reveals carcinoma, total lobectomy is indicated with as much of the contralateral lobe as possible, while attempting to preserve the parathyroid glands and recurrent laryngeal nerves. Regional lymph nodes are removed but mutilating neck dissection is contraindicated. Routine radioiodine treatment with ^{131}I is of questionable benefit in children with well-differentiated thyroid carcinoma and no evidence of metastases. In patients with lymph node metastases or distant metastases to bone or lungs, postoperative ^{131}I therapy is indicated (1) to ablate the residual thyroid tissue and (2) to ablate identifiable metastatic loci. A lower ^{131}I dose is given to accomplish the former goal, followed by a high-dose second metastatic treatment dose. Following surgery or surgery plus radioiodine, the patient is maintained on full suppression doses of exogenous T₄ to suppress endogenous TSH. Metastatic tumor growth is assessed by serial measurements of circulating TG. Recurrences usually are managed with repeat ^{131}I treatment.

Medullary Carcinoma

Medullary thyroid carcinoma (MTC) represents neoplasia of the parafollicular "C" cells and is associated with excessive secretion of calcitonin.[119] Other secretory products can include ACTH, melanocyte-stimulating hormone (MSH), histaminase, serotonin, prostaglandins, SRIF, and endorphin. Both familial and sporadic cases have been described. Familial cases are transmitted as an autosomal dominant trait and may be associated with multiple endocrine neoplasia (MEN) type II. In familial disease early diagnosis of small tumors is possible using calcium or pentagastrin stimulation tests.[119] Sporadic cases appear as non-iodide-concentrating (cold) thyroid nodule; the diagnosis is confirmed or suspected on the basis of needle biopsy or open biopsy. Thyroidectomy is the only current approach to treatment of medullary carcinoma, since "C" cells do not concentrate radioiodine.

THYROTROPIN-RELEASING HORMONE

TRH is the first hypothalamic peptide characterized and synthesized nearly simultaneously by Guillemin and coworkers[120] and Schally and coworkers.[121] It is a tripeptide (pyroglutamyl-histidyl-proline amide) secreted by the hypothalamus into the hypothalamic–pituitary portal vascular system to stimulate TSH release from anterior pituitary thyrotroph cells. TRH acts on these cells via a specific plasma membrane receptor. TRH stimulates prolactin release and in selected circumstances can evoke GH release.[122] TRH also is present in extrahypothalamic brain tissue and in extraneural tissues such as pancreas. TRH is synthesized as a 255-amino-acid precursor (preproTRH) containing five TRH progenitor sequences.[123] Processing of preproTRH results in cleavage of several larger peptides as well as TRH.[124] The significance of these is not clear.

TRH is metabolized via a pyroglutamyl amino peptidase to a cyclized metabolite, histadyl-proline diketopiperazine or cyclo (His-Pro).[122,125] Cyclo (His-Pro) also is widely distributed in brain tissue and appears to have unique bioactivities different from TRH. TRH also is deaminated and the free acid may have bioactivity.[122] The major bioactivity of TRH is the modulation, with T_3, of TSH release. However, a variety of other central nervous system actions have been described. It reverses the narcotic depression of barbiturate or ethanol, produces hyperthermia, suppresses eating and drinking, has antiopioid effects, and is mildly antidepressive.[122] Cyclo (His-Pro) has opposite effects to TRH, inhibiting prolactin release and causing hypothermia.

TRH is commercially available as a sterile, lyophilized powder (500-μg vials). The plasma half-life is very short (several minutes). The minimal intravenous dose required to evoke an increase in serum TSH is about 0.2 μg (200 ng)/kg. The TSH response increases progressively with increasing dose to plateau at 5–6 μg/kg. The peak rise in serum TSH is seen within 15–30 minutes; a secondary increase in serum T_3 levels occurs within 90–150 minutes.[122] TRH also is active orally, but doses 20 to 40 times greater are required.

TRH Testing

TRH is used for testing pituitary TSH reserve. An intravenous dose of TRH (7 μg/kg) is injected and measurements of serum TSH usually are conducted at 30 and 60 minutes. The TSH response, in general, is proportional to the basal TSH level. Thus, patients with primary hypothyroidism have augmented responses. Patients with hyperthyroidism have inhibited responses. The test usually is utilized (1) to confirm a diagnosis of thyrotoxicosis in patients with borderline serum T_4 and T_3 concentrations (an absent response to TSH supports a diagnosis of hyperthyroidism) and (2) to differentiate hypothalamic and pituitary etiologies for TSH deficiency in patients with hypothyroidism and low TSH levels. A normal TSH response to TRH indicates normal pituitary TSH secretory capacity and implies a hypothalamic TRH deficiency. An absent TSH response supports a diagnosis of pituitary TSH deficiency. Measurements of serum T_3 before and 4 hours after TRH administration provide information regarding thyroid gland responsiveness.

TRH has been injected intravenously in pregnant women to stimulate fetal thyroid function near term.[126] A dose of 400 μg induced a marked increase in cord blood TSH within 20 minutes and evoked significant increases in cord blood T_4 and T_3 levels as well. Maternal TRH administration with and without dexamethasone has been proposed to stimulate surfacant production in the premature fetus. TRH can be utilized to augment endogenous TSH production prior to radioiodine therapy of thyroid cancer. A definitive dosage regimen has not been defined, but a daily subcutaneous dose of 500 μg for 3 days probably is reasonable.

THYROID-STIMULATING HORMONE

Sterile, lypophilized TSH is available in vials of 10 international units. It is derived from animal pituitary glands (usually bovine) and is used to stimulate thyroid gland function for test purposes or to stimulate thyroid gland activity prior to administration of a treatment dose of radioiodine in patients with thyroid nodules or thyroid cancer. Daily injection of 10 units for 3–5 days has been effective in adults.

REFERENCES

1. Ingbar SH: The thyroid gland, in Wilson JD, Foster DW (eds): Textbook of Endocrinology. Philadelphia, WB Saunders, 1985, pp 682–815
2. Stanbury JB, Dumont JE: Familial goiter and related disorders, in Stanbury JB, et al (eds): The Metabolic Basis of Inherited Disease. 5th ed. New York, McGraw-Hill, 1983, pp 231–269
3. Wolff J: Congenital goiter with defective iodine transport. Endocrine Rev 4:240–254, 1983
4. Van Herle AJ, Vassart G, Dumont JE: Control of thyroglobulin synthesis and secretion. N Engl J Med 239:301–307, 1979
5. DeNayer PH, Cornette C, Van Dershuzeren M, Eggermont E, Devlieger H, Jaeken J, Beckers C: Serum thyroglobulin levels in preterm neonates. Clin Endocrinol 321:148–153, 1984
6. Fisher DA: Thyroid hormone and thyroglobulin synthesis and secretion, in Delange F, Fisher DA, Malvaux P (eds): Pediatric Thyroidology. Basel, Karger, 1985, pp 44–56
7. Morley JE: Neuroendocrine control of thyrotropin secretion. Endocrine Rev 2:326, 1981
8. Kourides IA, Gurr JA, Wolf O: The regulation and organization of thyroid stimulating hormone genes. Rec Prog Horm Res 40:79, 1984

9. Hinkle PM, Goh KBC: Regulation of thyrotropin releasing hormone receptors and responses by L-triiodothyronine in dispersed rat pituitary cell cultures. Endocrinology 110:1725, 1982

10. Gershengorn MC: Thyrotropin releasing hormone stimulation by pituitary hormone secretion. Annu Rev Physiol 48:515, 1986

11. Lippman SS, Amr S, Weintraub B: Discordant effects of thyrotropin (TSH)-releasing hormone in pre and post translational regulation of TSH biosynthesis in rat pituitary. Endocrinology 119:323, 1986

12. Segerson TP, Kauer J, Wolfe HC, Mobtaker H, Wu P, Jackson IMD, Lechan RM: Thyroid hormone regulates TRH biosynthesis in the paraventricular nucleus of the rat hypothalamus. Science 238:78, 1987

13. Engler D, Burger AG: The deiodination of iodothyronines and of their derivatives in man. Endocrine Rev 5:151, 1984

14. De Stefano JJ, Fisher DA: Peripheral distribution and metabolism of the thyroid hormones: A primarily quantitative assessment, in Hershman JM, Bray GA (eds): The Thyroid, Physiology and Treatment of Disease. Oxford, Pergamon Press, 1979, pp 47–82

15. Oppenheimer JH, Schwartz HL, Mariash CN, Kinlaw WB, Wong NCW, Freake HC: Advances in our understanding of thyroid hormone action at the cellular level. Endocrine Rev 8:288, 1987

16. Weinberger C, Thompson CC, Ong ES, Lebo R, Gruol GH, Evans RM: The c-erb A gene encodes a thyroid hormone receptor. Nature 324:641, 1986

17. Sap J, Munoz A, Damm K, Goldberg Y, Ghysdael J, Leutz A, Beng H, Vennstrom B: The c-erb A protein is a high affinity receptor for thyroid hormone. Nature 324:635, 1986

18. Thompson CC, Weinberger C, Lebo R, Evans RM: Identification of a novel thyroid hormone receptor expressed in the mammalian central nervous system. Science 237:1610, 1987

19. Benbrook D, Pfahl M: A novel thyroid hormone receptor encoded by a cDNA clone from a human testis library. Science 238:788, 1987

20. Samuels HH, Forman BM, Horwitz D, Ye ZS: Regulation of gene expression by thyroid hormone. J Clin Invest 81:957, 1988

21. Izumo S, Lompre AM, Matsuoka R, Koren G, Schwartz K, Nadal-Ginard B, Mahdavi V: Myosin heavy chain messenger RNA and protein isoform transitions between hemodynamic and thyroid hormone induced signals. J Clin Invest 79:970, 1987

22. Chaudhury S, Ismail-Beigi F, Glick GG, Levenson R, Edelman IS: Effect of thyroid hormone on the abundance of Na-K-adenosine triphosphatase alpha subunit messenger ribonucleic acid. Mol Endocrinol 1:83, 1987

23. Gubits RM, Shaw PA, Gresik EW, Onetti-Muda A, Barka T: Epidermal growth factor gene expression is regulated differently in mouse kidney and submandibular gland. Endocrinology 119:1382, 1986

24. Mukku VR: Regulation of epidermal growth factor receptor levels by thyroid hormones. J Biol Chem 254:6453, 1984

25. Bianca AC, Silva JE: Intracellular conversion of thyroxine to triiodothyronine is required for the optimal thermogenic function of brown adipose tissue. J Clin Invest 79:295, 1987

26. Shupnik MA, Chin WW, Habener JF, Ridgway EC: Transcriptional regulation of the thyrotropin subunit genes by thyroid hormone. J Biol Chem 260:2900, 1985

27. Barker SB, Klitgaard HM: Metabolism of tissues excised from thyroxine-injected rats. Am J Physiol 170:81, 1952

28. Martino G, Covello C, DeGiovanni R, Filippelli R, Pitrelli G: Direct in-vitro action of thyroid hormones on mitochondrial RNA-polymerase. Molec Biol Rep 11:205, 1986

29. Ismail-Beigi F, Edelman IS: Mechanism of thyroid calorigenesis. Role of active sodium transport. Proc Natl Acad Sci USA 67:1071, 1970

30. Stiles G, Caron MG, Lefkowitz RJ: Adrenergic receptors: Biochemical mechanisms of physiological regulation. Physiol Rev 64:661, 1984

31. Fisher DA, Dussault JH: Development of the mammalian thyroid gland, in Greer MA, Solomon DH (eds): Handbook of Physiology, Endocrinology III, The Thyroid, Chapter 3. Washington, DC, American Physiological Society, 1974, pp 143–166

32. Rezvani I, DiGeorge AM: Reassessment of the daily dose of oral thyroxine for replacement therapy of hypothyroid children. J Pediatrics 90:291, 1977

33. Abbassi V, Aldige C: Evaluation of sodium-l-thyroxine requirement in replacement. J Pediatrics 90:298, 1977

34. Penny R, Spencer CA, Frasier SD, Nicoloff JT: Thyroid stimulating hormone and thyroglobulin levels decrease with chronological age in children and adolescents. J Clin Endocrinol Metab 56:177, 1983

35. Oddie TH, Meade JH Jr, Fisher DA: An analysis of published data on thyroxine turnover in human subjects. J Clin Endocrinol Metab 26:425, 1966

36. Fisher DA, Sack J, Oddie TH, Pekary AE, Hershman JM, Lam RW, Parslow ME: Serum T4, TBG, T4 uptake, T3, reverse T3 and TSH concentrations in children 1 to 15 years of age. J Clin Endocrinol Metab 45:191, 1977

37. Braverman LW, Dawber NA, Ingbar SH: Observations concerning the binding of thyroid hormones in sera of normal subjects of varying ages. J Clin Invest 45:1273, 1966

38. Letarte J, Guyda H, Dussault JH: Clinical, biochemical and radiological features of neonatal hypothyroid infants, in Burrow GN, Dussault JH (eds): Neonatal Thyroid Screening. New York, Raven Press, 1980, pp 225–236.

39. Price DA, Ehrlich RM, Walfish PG: Congenital hypothyroidism, clinical and laboratory characteristics of infants detected by neonatal screening. Arch Dis Child 56:845, 1981

40. Letarte J, LaFranchi S: Clinical features of congenital hypothyroidism, in Walker P, Dussault JH (eds): Congenital Hypothyroidism. New York, Marcel Dekker, 1983, pp 351–383

41. Klein AH, Meltzer S, Kenny FN: Improved prognosis of congenital hypothyroidism treated before age 3 months. J Pediatrics 81:912, 1972

42. Raiti S, Newns GA: Cretinism: Early diagnosis and its relation to mental prognosis. Arch Dis Child 46:692–694, 1971

43. Glorieux J, Dussault JH, Morissette J, Dejardins M, Letarte J, Guyda H: Follow-up at ages 5 and 7 years on mental development in children with hypothyroidism detected by Quebec screening program. J Pediatrics 107:913, 1985

44. New England Congenital Hypothyroidism Collaborative: Neonatal hypothyroidism screening: status of patients at 6 years of age. J Pediatrics 107:915, 1985

45. Gonzales LW, Ballard PL: Identification and characterization of nuclear 3,5,3′ triiodothyronine binding sites in fetal human lung. J Clin Endocrinol Metab 53:21, 1981

46. Bernal J, Pekonen F: Ontogenesis of nuclear 3,5,3′ triiodothyronine receptor in human fetal brain. Endocrinology 114:677, 1984

47. Fisher DA: The unique endocrine milieu of the fetus. J Clin Invest 78:603, 1986

48. Dobbing J: The later growth of the brain and its vulnerability. J Pediatrics 53:2, 1974

49. Pickering DE, Fisher DA: Growth and metabolism following L-thyroxine administration in thyroid ablated infant rhesus monkeys. Am J Dis Child 86:147, 1953

50. Pickering DE, Fisher DA: Therapeutic concepts relating to hypothyroidism in childhood. J Chronic Dis 7:242, 1958

51. Andersen JH: Nongoitrous hypothyroidism, in Gardner LI (ed): Endocrine and Genetic Diseases of Childhood and Adolescence. Philadelphia, WB Saunders, 1975, pp 238–260

52. Van Wyk JJ, Grumbach MM: Syndrome of precocious menstruation and galactorrhea in juvenile hypothyroidism: An example of hormonal overlap in pituitary feedback. J Pediatrics 57:416, 1960

53. Costin G, Kershnar AK, Kogut MD, Turkington RW: Prolactin activity in juvenile hypothyroidism and precocious puberty. Pediatrics 50:881, 1972

54. Lee PA, Blizzard RM: Serum gonadotropins in hypothyroid girls with and without sexual precocity. J Hopkins Med J 135:55, 1974

55. Hemady ZS, Siler-Khodr TM, Najjar S: Precocious puberty in juvenile hypothyroidism. J Pediatrics 92:55, 1978

56. Reilly WA, Smyth FS: Cretinoid epiphyseal dysgenesis. J Pediatrics 11:786, 1937

57. Fisher DA, Hoath S, Lakshmanan J: The thyroid hormone effects on growth and development may be mediated by growth factors. Endocrinol Exper 16:259, 1982

58. Simpson ME, Asling CW, Evans HM: Some endocrine influences on skeletal growth and differentiation. Yale J Biol Med 23:1, 1950

59. Solomon J, Greep RD: The effect of alterations in thyroid function on the pituitary growth hormone content and acidophil cytology. Endocrinology 65:158, 1959

60. Samuels HH, Stanley F, Shapiro LE: Dose dependent depletion of nuclear receptors for L-triiodothyronine: Evidence for a role in induction of growth hormone synthesis in cultured GH cells. Proc Natl Acad Sci USA 73:3877, 1976

61. Baxter JD, Eberhardt NL, Apriletti JW, Johnson LK, Ivarie RD, Schacter BS, Morris JA, Seeburg PH, Goodman HM, Latham KR, Polansky JR, Martial JA: Thyroid hormone receptors and responses. Rec Prog Horm Res 35:97, 1979

62. Van Wyk JJ, Underwood LE, Hintz RL, Clemmons DR, Voina SJ, Weaver RP: The somatomedins: A family of insulin-like hormones under growth hormone control. Rec Prog Horm Res 30:259, 1974

63. Daughaday WH, Phillips LS, Muller MC: The effect of insulin and growth hormone on the release of somatomedin by the isolated rat liver. Endocrinology 98:1214, 1976

64. Froesch ER, Zapf J, Audhya TK, Ben Porath E, Segen BJ, Gibson KD: Nonsuppressible insulin-like activity and thyroid hormones: Major pituitary dependent sulfation factors for chick embryo cartilage. Proc Natl Acad Sci USA 73:2904, 1976

65. Holder AT, Wallis M: Actions of growth hormone, prolactin and thyroxine on serum somatomedin-like activity and growth in hypopituitary dwarf mice. J Endocrinol 74:223, 1977

66. Hughes JP: Identification and characterization of high and low affinity binding sites for growth hormone in rabbit liver. Endocrinology 105:414, 1979

67. Schalch DS, Udo EH, Draznin B, Johnson CF, Miller LL: Role of the liver in regulating somatomedin activity: Hormonal effects on the synthesis and release of insulin-like growth factor and its carrier protein by the isolated perfused rat liver. Endocrinology 104:1143, 1979

68. Glassock GF, Nicoll CS: Hormonal control of growth in the infant rat. Endocrinology 109:176, 1981

69. Walker P, Weichsel ME Jr, Hoath SB, Poland RE, Fisher DA: Effect of thyroxine, testosterone and corticosterone on nerve growth factor (NGF) and epidermal growth factor (EGF) concentrations in female mouse submaxillary gland. Dissociation of NGF and EGF responses. Endocrinology 109:582, 1981

70. Hoath SB, Lakshmanan J, Scott SM, Fisher DA: Effect of thyroid hormones on epidermal growth factor concentration in neonatal mouse skin. Endocrinology 112:308, 1983

71. Lakshmanan J, Perheentupa J, Hoath SB, Kim H, Grueters A, Odell C, Fisher DA: Epidermal growth factor in mouse ocular tissue: Effect of thyroxine and exogenous EGF. Pediatr Res 19:315, 1985

72. Perheentupa J, Lakshmanan J, Fisher DA: Epidermal growth factor in mouse urine: Maturative effect of thyroxine. Pediatr Res 18:1080, 1984

73. Hoath SB, Lakshmanan J, Fisher DA: Epidermal growth factor binding to neonatal mouse skin explants and membrane preparations; effect of triiodothyronine. Pediatr Res 19:277, 1985

74. Walker P, Weichsel ME Jr, Guo SM, Fisher DA, Fisher DA: Radioimmunoassay for mouse nerve growth factor (NGF), effect of thyroxine administration on tissue NGF levels. Brain Res 183:331, 1980

75. Lakshmanan J, Beri U, Perheentupa J, Grueters A, Kim H, Macaso T, Fisher DA: Acquisition of submandibular gland nerve growth factor responsiveness to thyroxine in neonatal mice. J Neurosci Res 12:71, 1984

76. Fish LH, Schwartz HL, Cavanaugh J, Steffes MW, Bantle JP, Oppenheimer JH: Replacement dose, metabolism and availability of levothyroxine in the treatment of hypothyroidism. N Engl J Med 316:764, 1987

77. Fisher DA: Thyroid disease in the neonate and child, in DeGroot LJ, Besser GM, Cahill GF, Marshall JC, Martini L, Nelson DH, Odell WD, Potts JT, Rubenstein AH, Steinberger E (eds): Endocrinology, vol II. New York, Grune and Stratton, 1990, Vol I, pp 733–745

78. Connors MH, Styne DH: Transient neonatal athyreosis resulting from thyrotropin inhibitory immunoglobulins. Pediatrics 78:287, 1986

79. Fisher DA, Foley B: Early treatment of congenital hypothyroidism. Pediatrics 83:785, 1989

80. Crantz FR, Silva JE, Larsen PR: An analysis of the sources and quantity of 3,5,3′ triiodothyronine specifically bound to nuclear receptor in rat cerebral cortex and cerebellum. Endocrinology 110:367, 1982

81. Silva JE, Larsen PR: Comparison of iodothyronine 5′ diiodinase and other thyroid hormone dependent enzyme activities in the cerebral cortex of hypothyroid neonatal rats. J Clin Invest 70:1110, 1982

82. Morreale De Escobar G, Obregon MJ, Ruiz De Ond C, Escobar Del Rey F: Transfer of thyroxine from the mother to the rat fetus near term: Effects on brain 3,5,3′-triiodothyronine deficiency. Endocrinology 122:1521, 1988

83. Daneman D, Howard NJ: Neonatal thyrotoxicosis, intellectual impairment and craniosynostosis in later years. J Pediatrics 97:257, 1980

84. Kapelman AE: Delayed cerebral development in twins with congenital hyperthyroidism. Am J Dis Child 137:842, 1983

85. Penfold JL, Simpson DA: Premature craniosynostosis, a complication of thyroid replacement therapy. J Pediatrics 86:360, 1975

86. Sato T, Suzuke Y, Taetani T, Ishigura K, Nakajima H: Age related change in the pituitary threshold for TSH release during thyroxine replacement therapy for cretinism. J Clin Endocrinol Metab 44:553, 1977

87. McCrossin RB, Sheffield LJ, Robertson EF: Persisting abnormality in the pituitary-thyroid axis in congenital hypothyroidism, in Nagataki S, Stockigt JHR (eds): Thyroid Research VIII. Canberra, Australian Academy of Sciences, 1980, pp 37–40

88. Schultz RM, Glassman MS, MacGillivray MH: Elevated threshold for thyrotropin suppression in congenital hypothyroidism. Am J Dis Child 134:19, 1980

89. Weetman AP, McGregor AM: Autoimmune thyroid disease: Developments in our understanding. Endocr Rev 5:309, 1984

90. Ahonen P, Koskimes S, Lokki ML, Tulikainen A, Perheentupa J: The expression of autoimmune polyglandular disease type I appears associated with several HLA-A antigens but not with HLA-DR. J Clin Endocr Metab 66:1152, 1988

91. Van der Gaag RG, Drexhage HA, Wiersinga WM, Brown RS, Docter R, Bottazzo GF, Doniach D: Further studies on thyroid growth stimulating immunoglobulins in euthyroid nonendemic goiter. J Clin Endocr Metab 60:972, 1985

92. Fisher DA, Pandian MR, Carlton E: Autoimmune thyroid disease, an expanding spectrum. Pediatr Clin No Am 34:907, 1987

93. Astwood EB, Bissell A, Hughes AM: Further studies on the chemical nature of compounds which inhibit the function of the thyroid gland. Endocrinology 37:456, 1945

94. Marchant B, Lees JFH, Alexander WD: Antithyroid drugs, in Hershman JE, Bray GA (eds): The Thyroid: Physiology and Treatment of Disease. Oxford, Pergamon Press, 1979, pp 209–252

95. Engler H, Taurog A, Nakashima T: Mechanism of inactivation of thyroid peroxidase by thioureylene drugs. Biochem Pharmacol 31:3801, 1982

96. Wu SY, Chopra IJ, Solomon DH, Johnson DE: The effect of repeated administration of ipodate (Orografin) in hyperthyroidism. J Clin Endocr Metab 47:1358, 1978

97. Shen DC, Wu SY, Chopra IJ, Huang HW, Shian LR, Bian TY, Jeng CY, Solomon DH: Long term treatment of Graves' hyperthyroidism with sodium ipodate. J Clin Endocr Metab 61:723, 1985

98. Wang YS, Tsou CT, Lin WH, Hershman JM: Long term treatment of Graves' disease with iopanoic acid (Telepaque). J Clin Endocr Metab 65:679, 1987

99. Karpman BA, Rappoport B, Filetti S, Fisher DA: Treatment of neonatal hyperthyroidism due to Grave's disease with sodium ipodate. J Clin Endocr Metab 64:119, 1987

100. Laurberg P: Multisite inhibitor by ipodate of iodothyronine secretion from perfused dog thyroid lobes. Endocrinology 117:1639, 1985

101. Haynes RC Jr, Murad F: Thyroid and antithyroid drugs, in Goodman LS, Gilman AG, Rall TW, Murad F (eds): The Pharmacological Basis of Therapeutics. 7th ed. New York, Macmillan, 1985, pp 1389–1411

102. Links JM, Wagner HN Jr: Radiation physics, in Ingbar SH, Braverman LE (eds): The Thyroid. 5th ed. New York, JB Lippincott, 1986, pp 417–431

103. Clayton GW: Thyrotoxicosis in children, in Kaplan SA (ed): Clinical Pediatric and Adolescent Endocrinology. Philadelphia, WB Saunders, 1982, pp 110–117

104. Barnes V, Blizzard RM: Antithyroid drug therapy for toxic diffuse goiter (Graves' disease): Thirty years experience in children and adolescents. J Pediatr 91:313, 1977

105. Maenpaa J, Kuusi A: Childhood hyperthyroidism. Acta Paediatr Scand 69:137, 1980

106. Collen RJ, Landau EM, Kaplan SA, Lippe PM: Remission rates of children and adolescents with thyrotoxicosis treated with antithyroid drugs. Pediatrics 65:550, 1980

107. Brill, AB, Becker DV: The safety of ^{131}I treatment of hyperthyroidism, in Van Middlesworth L, Givins JR (eds): The Thyroid, A Practical Clinical Treatise. Chicago, Year Book Publ., 1986, pp 347–362

108. Hamburger JI: Management of hyperthyroidism in children and adolescents. J Clin Endocrinol Metab 60:1019, 1985

109. Zakarija M, McKenzie JM, Hoffman WH: Prediction and therapy of intrauterine and late onset neonatal hyperthyroidism. J Clin Endocr Metab 62:368, 1986

110. Smallridge RC, Wartofsky L, Chopra IJ, Marinelli PV, Broughton RE, Dimond RC, Burman KD: Neonatal thyrotoxicosis: Alterations in serum concentrations of LATS protector, T_4, T_3, reverse T_3 and $3,3'T_2$. J Pediatr 93:118, 1978

111. Gershengorn MC, Weintraub BD: Thyrotropin induced hyperthyroidism caused by selective pituitary resistance to thyroid hormone: A new syndrome of inappropriate secretion of TSH. J Clin Invest 56:633, 1975

112. Rosler A, Litvin Y, Hoge C, Gross J, Cerasi E: Familial hyperthyroidism due to inappropriate thyrotropin secretion successfully treated with triiodothyronine. J Clin Endocr Metab 54:76, 1982

113. Beck Peccoz P, Piscitelli G, Cattaneo MG, et al: Successful treatment of hyperthyroidism due to non-neoplastic pituitary TSH secretion with $3,5,3'$ triiodothyroacetic acid (TRIAC). J Endocrinol Invest 6:217, 1983

114. Isales CM, Tamborlane W, Gertner JM, Genel M, Insogna KL: Effect of short-term somatostatin and long-term triiodothyronine administration to a child with nontumorous inappropriate thyrotropin secretion. Pediatrics 112:51, 1988

115. Abe K, Konno M, Sato T, Matsuura N: Hyperfunctioning thyroid nodules in children. Am J Dis Child 134:961, 1980

116. Osburne RC, Goren EN, Bybee DE, Johnsonbaugh RE: Autonomous thyroid nodules in adolescents: Clinical characteristics and results of TRH testing. J Pediatr 100:383, 1982

117. Fisher DA: Thyroid nodules in childhood and their management. J Pediatrics 84:866, 1982

118. Scott MD, Crawford JD: Solitary thyroid nodules in childhood: Is the incidence of thyroid carcinoma declining? Pediatrics 58:521, 1976

119. Melvin KEW: Familial medullary carcinoma of the thryoid, in Van Middlesworth L, Givens JR (eds): The Thyroid Gland, A Practical Clinical Treatise. Chicago, Year Book Publ., 1986, p 429

120. Guillemin R: Peptides in the brain: The new endocrinology of the neuron. Science 202:390, 1978

121. Schally AV: Aspects of the hypothalamic regulation of the pituitary gland: Its implications for the control of reproductive processes. Science 202:18, 1978

122. Jackson IMD: Thyrotropin releasing hormone. N Engl J Med 306:145, 1982

123. Lechan RM, Wu P, Jackson IMD, Wolf H, Cooperman S, Mandel G, Goodman RH: Thyrotropin releasing hormone precursor: Characterization in rat brain. Science 231:159, 1986

124. Wu P, Lechan RM, Jackson IMD: Identification and characterization of thyrotropin releasing hormone precursor peptides in rat brain. Endocrinology 121:108, 1986

125. Iruichijima T, Prasad C, Wilber JF, Jayaraman A, Rao JK, Robertson HJF, Rogers DJ: Thyrotropin releasing hormone and cyclo (His-Pro)-like immunoreactivities in the cerebrospinal fluids of normal infants and adults and patients with various neuropsychiatric and neurologic disorders. Life Sci 41:2419, 1987

126. Roti E, Gnudi A, Braverman LE: The placental transport, synthesis and metabolism of hormones and drugs which affect thyroid function. Endocr Rev 4:131, 1983

44
GROWTH HORMONE

SELNA L. KAPLAN

Human growth hormone (hGH) is the most abundant polypeptide synthesized and secreted by the acidophiles of the pituitary. Only hGH is biologically active in humans; bovine, ovine, and porcine GH are ineffective. Other mammalian pituitary hormones [adrenocorticotropic hormone (ACTH), thyroid-stimulating hormone (TSH), and gonadotropins] are less species-specific. Human GH is unique also in its intrinsic prolactin-like effects, a biologic action not shared by other mammalian growth hormones.[1]

The primary structure of hGH contains 191 amino acids with two intrachain disulfide bridges (MW 22,000 daltons). It shares a significant structural homology (87 percent) with the placental somatropic hormone (hCS, human chorionic somatomammotropin).[2] Chromosome 17 contains the locus for the five genes that comprise the GH–GS family; hGH 1 encodes pituitary GH, hGH-V is expressed in the placenta, hCS 1 and 2 encode this hormone in the placenta, and hCS 5 is a pseudogene. A variant 20,000-dalton pituitary hGH is the product of a deletion induced by alternative mRNA splicing.[3]

NEUROENDOCRINE REGULATION OF GROWTH HORMONE SECRETION

Neural regulation of GH secretion is mediated by the interaction of stimulatory [growth hormone-releasing hormone (GHRH)] and inhibitory [somatostatin (SRIH)] hypothalamic peptides. The GHRH-containing neurons are found principally in the arcuate nucleus and the ventromedial nucleus in the medial basal hypothalamus, and the SRIH neuronal cell bodies are located in the periventricular zone of the anterior hypothalamus.[4,5] The nerve fibers from both the GHRH and SRIH neurons project laterally to the median eminence.

Neurotransmitters of the monoaminergic neural pathways modulate GH secretion by integration of the tonic and pulsatile release of GHRH and SRIH. The dual action of neurotransmitters has been attributed to their effect on both GHRH and SRIH receptors and concordant interaction with other neuropeptides. The noradrenergic system predominates in the regulation of GH secretion; both α_1- and α_2-adrenergic receptors are present in the median eminence and arcuate and ventromedial nuclei. Their effects on GH secretion differ in that α_2-amine receptors are stimulatory and α_1- and β_2-amine receptors are inhibitory.[6] Activation of cholinergic transmitters induces the sleep-related release of GH and affects to a lesser extent the hypoglycemic stimulation of GH release.[7,8] Administration of cholinergic agonists enhances basal and GHRH-stimulated GH levels.[9] In the human dopaminergic involvement in GH release is still unclear and may be more inhibitory than stimulatory.[10] The action of γ-aminobutyric acid (GABA) on GH secretion appears to be mediated by stimulation of GHRH and to a lesser extent by suppression of somatostatin secretion.[11] The serotonergic and histaminergic systems are not involved in the regulation of GH release in humans.[12] Modulation of GH secretion may be controlled by an autofeedback system that suppresses GH release at the hypothalamic level by inhibition of GHRH release or stimulation of somatostatin secretion,[13] or at the pituitary level directly by GH or IGF-1.[14]

SECRETION OF GROWTH HORMONE

Multiple forms of pituitary GH are released into the circulation; the major fraction (78 percent) is monomeric 22,000-daltons, 18 percent is 20,000-daltons, and the remainder may be deamidated hGH. Human GH circulates in a bound form that represents 45 percent of the total concentration in plasma.[15] The bound form has a 10-fold slower disappearance rate than the free form. The major 51,000-dalton binding protein constitutes the extracellular portion of the GH receptor in the rat and in the human.[16]

As is true for other pituitary and hypothalamic hormones, GH is secreted in a pulsatile pattern with individual variations in pulse height and frequency. Evans et al.[17] have observed maximal peaks of GH with 5-minute sampling periods, but the mean peak height was similar when the range of sampling times was 10–30 minutes. The onset of deep sleep (stages 3–4) induces the greatest surge in GH release.[18] Lower levels of GH occur after meals, which may be the consequence of the suppressive effect of elevated free fatty acids and hyperglycemia.

Secretion of GH occurs by 6–8 weeks of gestation in the human fetus, with levels in the acromegalic range by midgestation (80–200 ng/ml). As hypothalamic maturation progresses, the imposition of regulatory mechanisms gradually decreases GH concentrations.[19] By birth, the serum concentration of GH is lower (33 ng/ml) and remains relatively elevated for the first few months of life. By 1–2 years of age, the surge in GH release when the onset of sleep occurs. During childhood, daytime random levels of GH are in the range of 1–5 ng/ml.[20]

PHARMACOKINETICS OF GROWTH HORMONE

The metabolic clearance rate (MCR) of hGH as determined by constant infusion studies with ^{131}I-pituitary hGH in normal adults correlates with the body surface area. The MCR in normal adults (112 ± 5 ml/min/m^2) is similar to that in GH-deficient children.[21,22] The estimated production rate is higher in normal adults (363 ± 105 ng/min/m^2) than in GH-deficient children (166 ± 22 ng/min/m^2). Studies utilizing monomeric biosynthetic hGH (BhGH) in GH-deficient subjects indicated a lower MCR of 86.4 ml/min/m^2.[23] The disappearance rate of pituitary hGH is multicompartmental, with an initial component of 15–25 minutes. The mean disappearance rate of BhGH was monoexponential during the first 30 minutes, with a $t_{1/2}$ of 21.1 minutes as described by Jorgensen and associates,[23] which is in accord with data reported by Faria et al.[24] Recent studies by Baumann et al.[25] demonstrated that bound GH has a slower MCR disappearance rate and degradation rate.

Assessment of Growth Hormone Function

Since random daytime levels of GH are low, pharmacologic agents have been used to provoke GH release. In general, their effect is mediated by stimulation of GHRH secretion either by activation of the adrenergic system (clonidine and L-dopa),[26-28] by hypoglycemia (insulin or deoxyglucose),[29] by suppression of somatostatin release (arginine),[30] or by exercise.[31] The individual variability in the response to these pharmacologic agents necessitates the use of two or more stimuli to assess the adequacy of hypothalamic–pituitary function.[32,33] Priming the individual with a β-agonist (propanolol or atenolol)[34] or with sex steroids magnifies the peak GH rise.[35,36]

In response to these stimuli, serum levels of GH increase to more than 7 ng/ml in normal children and 20 ng/ml or above in adults. The identification of children with severe GH deficiency can be made on the basis of a GH response of less than 3 ng/ml to several stimuli; a peak response of 3–7 ng/ml suggests partial GH deficiency.[32]

Serial sampling of GH at 20-minute intervals for a 24-hour period during normal activities has been proposed as a physiologic assessment of GH secretion.[37] There is considerable disagreement as to the discriminatory characteristics of this test for the assessment of GH function of short prepubertal children. As reported by Rose and associates,[38] the mean 24-hour GH is 1.0 ± 0.4 ng/ml in GH-deficient prepubertal children with decreased pulse frequency and amplitude and low 24-hour integrated GH secretion. The mean 24-hour GH was 2.8 ± 1.2 ng/ml in normal children, which is similar to the levels in short children. Short-statured children who have a normal response to provocative tests have a normal 24-hour GH concentration. In contrast, a significant correlation of height S.D. and height velocity with the integrated concentration of GH over a 24-hour period has been reported by Albertsson-Wikland and associates.[39] They conclude that short children secrete less GH than do tall children or children of normal stature. Bercu[40] has suggested a classification of neurosecretory dysfunction for short children who have a normal GH response to provocative tests but low 24-hour GH secretion. The basis for the discrepancies in interpretation among all these investigators remains unclear. An abnormality in the processing of GH in some children with short stature may explain the observed disparate GH responses. None of these tests provide discriminatory characteristics to ensure the beneficial effect of supplemental GH in children with non-GH-deficient short stature.[41]

Synthetic GHRH can establish the presence of functional somatotropes in patients with GH deficiency. The GH response to an intravenous bolus of 1–5 μg/kg is generally less in patients with GH deficiency than in normal children or adults.[42,43] Multiple doses of GHRH may be required in some GH-deficient children to induce release of GH.[44]

MEASUREMENT OF CIRCULATING GROWTH HORMONE

Radioimmunoassays that utilize radiolabeled hGH and specific polyclonal antisera directed against hGH are the principal methods for assay of serum hGH. Recently, single monoclonal or dual monoclonal assays have been utilized by commercial laboratories and in marketed kits. The absolute levels determined by the latter assays are in general 35–50 percent less than values obtained by the polyclonal assays.[45-47] The difference in absolute values may be attributable to their specificity for 22,000-dalton hGH, in contrast to the polyclonal assays which detect both 20,000- and 22,000-dalton hGH.[47] The detection of bound and free hGH is not consistent for either the polyclonal or monoclonal assays. Adequate age-related controls are essential. It must be recognized that all these assays determine the immunoreactive form of GH, which may not correlate with the biologic activity of GH in some children with short stature and poor growth.

Measurement by radioimmunoassay of urinary GH demonstrates levels of 0.27 ± 0.02 ng/kg/12 h in normal prepubertal children, 0.08 ± 0.02 ng/kg/12 h in GH-deficient children, and 0.17 ± 0.02 ng/kg/12 h in short-statured children.[48] The overlap in the urinary GH levels in these three groups of children limits the usefulness of this assay at present.

Bioassays for GH generally are less sensitive and require larger quantities of serum; included in this group are the tibia test in hypophysectomized rats[49] and the erythroid blast assay of Golde.[50] The biologic response of humans to administration of GH qualifies as a bioassay for hGH.

TREATMENT WITH HUMAN GROWTH HORMONE

Purified pituitary hGH was first used for the treatment of GH deficiency in 1958.[51] The use of pituitary hGH was discontinued in 1985 when the possibility of contamination of the pituitary preparations with a slow virus (Creutzfeldt-Jakob disease) was suggested. This decision was based on the demonstration of this disease in several young adults who had been treated with GH during childhood.[52] At present only biosynthetic hGH produced by recombinant DNA methods is available for therapeutic purposes.[53]

Administration of hGH induces an augmented rate of growth (7–12 cm/year) during the first year in GH-deficient children.[54,55] There is an inverse relationship of bone age to the magnitude of increment in height. The yearly growth rate is slightly less during subsequent years of therapy. The attainment of an appropriate height for population and/or familial pattern requires normalization of height before puberty.[56] Thus, initiation of therapy at an early age (<5 years) may be essential.

Synthetic GHRH stimulates an increase in growth rate in GH-deficient children.[57] However, the need for multiple daily doses has limited enthusiasm for its use as chronic therapy.

The increased availability of GH has led to studies of its effect in children with short stature not associated with GH deficiency. Short children who grow at a less than optimal rate for age despite a stimulated GH response of more than 7 ng/ml may show an improvement in growth rate on GH treatment.[58–60] However, an improvement in final height has yet to be demonstrated. Recent studies suggest an improved growth rate and final height in some patients with Turner's syndrome after multiple years of therapy with biosynthetic hGH.[61]

Prior studies by Frasier et al.[62] have established a relationship between the dose of hGH administered and the growth rate in GH-deficient individuals. Doses of less than 0.01 mg/kg are ineffective, and doses of 0.05–0.1 mg/kg induce a maximum effect on growth rate.

Administration of hGH by the intramuscular or the subcutaneous route achieves peak concentrations by 4 hours with undetectable levels by 16–24 hours in GH-deficient patients.[63–65] No difference in bioactivity or antibody formation has been observed.

Increased frequency of injections from three times a week to daily administration without a change in the total weekly dose improves the growth rate of GH-deficient children.[65,66]

ACTIONS OF GROWTH HORMONE

The biologic effects of GH may be mediated directly by its binding to GH receptors in tissues or by its induction of second messengers such as IGF-1. Preadipocytes, prechondrocytes, and fibroblast precursors, all of which have GH receptors, are cell types in which a direct action of GH has been demonstrated.[67,68] The principal action of GH is to promote protein accretion and synthesis either directly or via IGF-1 mediation. GH directly increases intracellular amino acid uptake and indirectly affects the synthesis of ribosomal and messenger RNA and incorporation of amino acids into protein. Recent evidence suggests that the effects of 22,000-dalton hGH on amino acid transport and protein synthesis are attributable to its insulin-like properties. In contrast, 20,000-dalton hGH manifests limited insulin-like effects and has no effect on protein synthesis or amino acid transport.[69] The administration of hGH to GH-deficient patients induces nitrogen and phosphorus retention, decreases serum urea nitrogen, increases serum alkaline phosphatase,[70,71] and promotes excretion of calcium, hydroxyproline, and procollagen peptide.[72,73] The stimulatory effect of GH on chondrocyte growth is induced by a paracrine effect of the local release and action of IGF-1.[74]

The lipolytic actions of GH are expressed by an increase in free fatty acids (FFA), oxidation of fat, and decreased conversion of glucose to triglycerides and FFA. During starvation or prolonged fasting, GH has a protein-sparing action and promotes the increased oxidation of fat.[75] GH-deficient patients have increased fat deposition, decreased fat mobilization, and increased levels of cholesterol and lipoprotein lipase.[74] FFA release is induced following administration of hGH.[76,77]

Both insulin-like and contra-insulin effects have been ascribed to GH. Decreased glucose utilization, diminished responsiveness of tissues to insulin, and decreased conversion of glucose to fat are contra-insulin actions.[75] GH-deficient patients have low fasting blood glucose levels, decreased hepatic glucose production, low insulin secretion, and increased sensitivity to insulin.[20]

It is still unclear whether the effects of GH on lipid and carbohydrate metabolism are direct or secondary to another GH-stimulated peptide. The insulin-like action is an acute effect demonstrable primarily in tissues depleted of GH or in hypophysectomized animals. These effects are of short duration followed by a prolonged refractory period. Thus, in normal individuals who secrete frequent pulses of GH, the insulin-like effect is variable. It has been suggested that this is an intrinsic function of hGH, but its physiologic significance is not established.[75]

GROWTH FACTORS IGF-1 AND IGF-2

These growth factors are the intracellular mediators of most of the biologic actions attributable to GH. GH stimulates the synthesis and release of IGF-1; IGF-2 is less GH-dependent. IGF-1 is a 70-amino-acid basic peptide which shares a 70 percent homology with IGF-2; both are structurally similar to proinsulin.[78,79] The IGF-1 receptor preferentially binds IGF-1 but binds insulin and IGF-2 less avidly. The IGF-2 receptor is not structurally similar to the IGF-1 or insulin receptor and has limited affinity for IGF-1 and none for insulin.[80] There is little free IGF-1 or IGF-2 in the circulation, both circulate bound to carrier proteins. Six IGF binding proteins have been identified; IGF-3 is the major binding protein in the child and adult. It is regulated in parallel with changes in serum GH. IGFBP-1 and 2 are present in higher concentrations during fetal life than in the postnatal period. IGFBP-1 is altered during fasting and the serum concentration varies inversely with that of insulin. Specific function of the other binding proteins has not been elucidated.[81]

The localization and sites of synthesis of IGF-1 are ubiquitous.[82] Similarly, its biologic effects are diverse, encompassing cellular proliferation, differentiation, and stimulation or potentiation of cellular hormonal release.[83]

Clinical Aspects of IGF-1 and IGF-2

The serum concentration of IGF-1 is age-dependent. Low levels are detected at birth and for the first 5 years of life. A gradual increase occurs during childhood, with peak levels attained during mid-puberty. The serum concentration in adults is lower than that of pubertal children.[84-86] The levels of IGF-2 are low in the infant but increase gradually through adolescence.[87]

Urinary IGF-1 expressed as milliunits per kilogram (mU/kg) is higher in normal children (28.4 ± 2.1) than in GH-deficient children (8.6 ± 1.3). Increased excretion occurs after administration of hGH.[88] Urinary IGF-1 levels correlate positively with urinary GH levels. Preterm and full-term infants have higher urinary IGF-1 levels than older children, whereas serum levels show the reverse pattern.[89] Whether this difference in IGF-1 in infants is related to immature renal function or rapid turnover is not established.

Deficient secretion of GH is associated with low levels of IGF-1 and lesser decreases in IGF-2 levels.[86,90] However, low levels of IGF-1 are not diagnostic for GH deficiency in short children.[90] Measurement of serum IGFBP-3 may be a more discriminating test than IGF-1 for abnormalities of GH secretion in children with short stature. Administration of GH induces a sharp rise in serum concentrations of IGF-1. Alterations in nutritional status, liver disease, and renal failure all result in decreased concentrations of IGF-1.[92,93] In patients with gigantism or acromegaly due to a GH-secreting pituitary tumor, the concentrations of IGF-1 are markedly elevated.[94]

Clinical syndromes in which IGF-1 concentrations are low despite measurable serum GH levels are rare. In the pygmy tribe, low IGF-1 and normal concentrations of serum GH and serum IGF-2 have been reported, but the precise defect has not been identified.[95] Laron dwarfism is an autosomal dominant abnormality due to the absence of the GH receptor.[96,97] Marked retardation in height, elevated serum GH, and low serum IGF-1 are the characteristics of this disease. Administration of hGH stimulates neither a rise in serum IGF-1 nor an increase in growth rate. Absence of feedback of IGF-1 on pituitary secretion of GH may lead to the elevated concentrations of serum GH. Studies of the biologic effectiveness of biosynthetic IGF-1 have demonstrated an insulin-like action, hypoglycemia, and suppression of FFA in patients with Laron dwarfism and in normal adults.[98,99] Nitrogen and phosphorous retention, increased creatinine clearance and suppression of serum IGF-2, GH, and C-peptide were observed following ten days of intravenous infusion of rIGF-1 in a child with GH insensitivity syndrome. Stimulation of growth occurs in GH-deficient mice treated long-term with biosynthetic IGF-1.[101] Its potential use as a therapeutic agent in children with Laron dwarfism and GH deficiency has not been assessed.

REFERENCES

1. Dixon JS, Li CH: Retention of the biological potency of human pituitary growth hormone after reduction and carbamidomethylation. Science 154:785–786, 1966
2. Goeddel DV, Heyreker HL, Hozumi T: Direct expression in Escherichia coli of a DNA sequence coding for human growth hormone. Nature 281:544–548, 1979
3. Denoto F, Moore DD, Goodman HM: Human growth hormone DNA sequence and mRNA structures: Possible alternative splicing. Nucleic Acids Res 9:3719, 1981
4. Bloch B, Gaillard RC, Brazeau P, Lin HD, Ling N: Topographical and ontogenetic study of the neurons producing growth hormone-releasing factor in human hypothalamus. Regul Pept 8:21–31, 1984
5. Hokfelt T, Efendic S, Hellerstrom C, Johansson O, Loft R, Arimura A: Cellular localization of somatostatin endocrine-like cells and neurons of the rat with special references to the A1-cells of the pancreatic islets and to the hypothalamus. Acta Endocrinol Suppl 200:4–41, 1975
6. Krulich L, Mayfield MA, Steele MK, McMillen BA, McCann SM, Koenig J: Differential effects of pharmacological manipulations of central α_1 and α_2 adrenergic receptors on the secretion of thyrotropin and growth hormone in male rats. Endocrinology 110:196–204, 1982
7. Blackard WG, Waddel CC: Cholinergic blockade and growth hormone responsiveness to insulin hypoglycemia. Proc Soc Exp Biol Med 131:192–196, 1969
8. Taylor BJ, Smith PJ, Brook CGD: Inhibition of physiological growth hormone secretion by atropine. Clin Endocrinol 22:497–501, 1985
9. Locatelli V, Torsello A, Redaelli M, Ghigo E, Massara F, Muller EE: Cholinergic agonists and antagonist drugs modulate in the rat the growth hormone response to growth hormone releasing hormone. Evidence for mediation by somatostatin. J Endocrinol 11:271–278, 1986
10. Bansal SA, Lee LA, Woolf PD: Dopaminergic stimulation and inhibition of growth hormone secretion in normal man; studies of pharmacologic specificity. J Clin Endocrinol Metab 53:1273–1277, 1981
11. Fioretti P, Melis GB, Paoletti AM, Parodo G, Caminiti F, Corsini GU, Martini L: Gamma-amino-β hydroxybutyric acid (GABA) stimulates prolactin and growth hormone release in normal women. J Clin Endocrinol Metab 47:1336–1341, 1978
12. Muller EE: Neural control of somatotropic function. Physiol Rev 67:962–1053, 1987
13. Tannenbaum GS: Evidence for autoregulation of growth hor-

mone secretion via the central nervous system. Endocrinology 107:2117–2120, 1980

14. Berelowitz M, Szabo M, Frohman LA, Firestone S, Chu L, Hintz RH: Somatomedin-C mediates growth hormone negative feedback by effects on both the hypothalamus and the pituitary. Science 212:1279–1281, 1981

15. Baumann G, Stolar MW: Molecular forms of human growth hormone secreted in vivo: Non-specificity of secretory stimuli. J Clin Endocrinol Metab 62:789–790, 1986

16. Leung DW, Spencer SA, Cachianes G, Hammonds RG, Collins C, Henzel WJ, Barnard R, Waters MJ, Wood WJ: Growth hormone receptor and serum binding protein: Purification, cloning and expression. Nature 330:537–543, 1987

17. Evans WS, Faria ACS, Christiansen E, et al: Impact of intensive venous sampling on characterization of pulsatile GH release in normal men. Am J Physiol 252:E549–556, 1987

18. Takahashi Y, Kipnis DM, Daughaday WH: Growth hormone secretion during sleep. J Clin Invest 47:2079–2090, 1968

19. Kaplan SL, Grumbach MM, Aubert ML: The ontogenesis of pituitary hormones and hypothalamic factors in the human fetus: Maturation of central nervous system regulation of anterior pituitary function. Rec Prog Horm Res 32:161–243, 1976

20. Kaplan SL, Abrams CAL, Bell JJ, Conte FA, Grumbach MM: Growth and growth hormone. I. Changes in serum level of growth hormone following hypoglycemia in 134 children with growth retardation. Pediatr Res 2:43–63, 1968

21. MacGillivray MH, Frohman LA, Doe J: Metabolic clearance and production rates of human growth hormone in subjects with normal and abnormal growth. J Clin Endocrinol Metab 30:632–638, 1970

22. Hendricks CM, Eastman RC, Takeda S, Asakawa K, Gorden P: Plasma clearance of intravenously administered pituitary human growth hormone: Gel filtration studies of heterogeneous components. J Clin Endocrinol Metab 60:864–869, 1985

23. Jorgensen JOL, Flyvbjerg A, Christiansen JS: The metabolic clearance rate, serum half-time and apparent distribution space of authentic biosynthetic human growth hormone in growth hormone-deficient patients. Acta Endocrinol 120:8–13, 1989

24. Faria ACS, Veldhuis TD, Thorner MO, Vance ML: Half time of endogenous growth hormone disappearance in normal man after stimulation of GH secretion by GH-releasing hormone and suppression with somatostatin. J Clin Endocrinol Metab 68:535–541, 1989

25. Baumann G, Amburn KD, Buchanan TA: The effect of circulating growth hormone-binding protein on metabolic clearance, distribution, and degradation of human growth hormone. J Clin Endocrinol Metab 64:657–660, 1987

26. Eden S, Eriksson, Martin JB, et al: Evidence for a growth hormone releasing factor mediating alpha-adrenergic influence on growth hormone secretion in the rat. Neuroendocrinology 33:24–27, 1981

27. Donnadieu M, Evain-Brion D, Tonon MC, Vaudry H, Job JC: Variations of plasma growth hormone (GH) releasing factor levels during GH stimulation tests in children. J Clin Endocrinol Metab 60:1132–1134, 1985

28. Chihara K, Kashio Y, Kita T, Okimura Y, Kaji H, Abe H, Fujita T: L-Dopa stimulates release of hypothalamic growth hormone-releasing hormone in humans. J Clin Endocrinol Metab 62:466–473, 1986

29. Kashio Y, Chihara K, Kita T, Okimura Y, Sato M, Kadowaki S, Fujita T: Effect of oral glucose administration on plasma growth hormone-releasing (GHRH)-like immunoreactivity levels in normal subjects and patients with idiopathic GH deficiency: Evidence that GHRH is released not only from the hypothalamus but also from extra hypothalamic tissue. J Clin Endocrinol Metab 64:92–97, 1987

30. Alba-Roth J, Muller OA, Schopohl J, Von Werder K: Arginine stimulates growth hormone secretion by suppressing endogenous somatostatin secretion. J Clin Endocrinol Metab 67:1186–1189, 1988

31. Casaneuva FF, Villaneuva L, Caranes JA, Cabezas-Cerrato J, Fernandez-Cruz A: Cholinergic mediation of growth hormone secretion elicited by arginine, clondine and physical exercise in man. J Clin Endocrinol Metab 59:526–530, 1984

32. Youlton R, Kaplan SL, Grumbach MM: Growth and growth hormone: IV. Limitations of the growth hormone response to insulin and arginine and of the immunoreactive insulin response to arginine in the assessment of growth hormone deficiency in children. Pediatrics 43:989–1004, 1969

33. Frasier SD: A review of growth hormone stimulation tests in children. Pediatrics 53:929–937, 1974

34. Massara F, Camanni F: Effect of various adrenergic receptor stimulating and blocking agents on human growth hormone secretion. J Endocrinol 54:195–206, 1972

35. Frantz AG, Rabkin MT: Effects of estrogen and sex difference on secretion of human growth hormone. J Clin Endocrinol Metab 25:1470–1480, 1965

36. Link K, Blizzard RM, Evans WS, Kaiser DL, Parker MW, Rogol AD: The effect of androgens on the pulsatile release and the twenty-four hour mean concentration of growth hormone in precocious pubertal males. J Clin Endocrinol Metab 62:159–164, 1986

37. Bercu BB, Shulman D, Root AW, Spiliotis BE: Growth hormone provocative testing frequently does not reflect endogenous growth hormone secretion. J Clin Endocrinol Metab 63:709–716, 1986

38. Rose SR, Ross JL, Uriarte M, Barns KM, Cassora FG, Cutler GB: The advantage of measuring stimulated as compared with spontaneous growth hormone levels in the diagnosis of growth hormone deficiency. N Engl J Med 319:201–207, 1988

39. Albertsson-Wikland K, Rosberg S: Analyses of 24 hour growth hormone profiles in children: Relation to growth. J Clin Endocrinol Metab 67:493–500, 1988

40. Spiliotis B, August G, Hung W, Sonis W, Mendelson W, Bercu BB: Growth hormone neurosecretory dysfunction: A treatable cause of short stature. JAMA 251:2223–2230, 1984

41. Kaplan SL, Grumbach MM: Long term treatment with growth hormone of children with non-growth hormone deficient short stature, in Isaksson O, et al (eds): Growth Hormone. Basic and Clinical Aspects. Amsterdam, Elsevier, 1987, pp 197–204

42. Borges JLC, Blizzard RM, Gelato MC, Furlanetto R, Rogol AD, Evans WS, Vance ML, Kaiser DL, MacLeod RM, Merriam CR, Loriaux DL, Spiess J, Rivier J, Vale W, Thorner MO: Effects of human pancreatic tumor growth hormone releasing factor on growth hormone and somatomedin C levels in patients with idiopathic growth hormone deficiency. Lancet 2:119–124, 1983

43. Schriock EA, Lustig RH, Rosenthal SM, Kaplan SL, Grumbach MM: Effect of growth hormone (GH)-releasing hormone (GHRH) on plasma GH in relation to magnitude and duration of GH deficiency in 26 children and adults with isolated GH deficiency or multiple pituitary hormone deficiencies: Evidence of hypothalamic GHRH deficiency. J Clin Endocrinol Metab 58:1043–1049, 1984

44. Schriock EA, Hulse JA, Harris DA, Kaplan SL, Grumbach MM: Evaluation of hypothalamic dysfunction in growth hormone (GH)-deficient patients using single versus multiple doses of GH-releasing hormone (GHRH-44) and evidence for diurnal variation in somatotroph responsiveness to GHRH in GH-deficient patients. J Clin Endocrinol Metab 65:1177–1182, 1987

45. Reiter EO, Morris AH, MacGillivray MH, Weber D: Variable estimates of serum growth hormone and concentrations by different radioassay systems. J Clin Endocrinol Metab 66:68–71, 1988

46. Levin PA, Chalew SA, Martin L, Kowarski AA: Comparison of assays for growth hormone using monoclonal or polyclonal antibodies for diagnosis of growth disorders. J Lab Clin Med 109:85–88, 1987

47. Celniker AC, Chen AB, Wert RM, Sherman BM: Variability in the quantitation of circulating growth hormone using commercial immunoassays. J Clin Endocrinol Metab 68:469–476, 1989

48. Albini CH, Quattrin T, Vandlen RL, MacGillivray MH: Quantitation of urinary growth hormone in children with normal and abnormal growth. Pediatr Res 23:89–92, 1988

49. Greenspan FS, Li CH, Simpson ME, Evans HM: Bioassay of hypophyseal growth hormone: The tibia test. Endocrinology 45:455–463, 1949

50. Golde DW, Bersch N, Li CH: Growth hormone modulation of

murine erythroleukemia cell growth in vitro. Proc Natl Acad Sci USA 75:3437–3439, 1978

51. Raben MS: Treatment of a pituitary dwarf with human growth hormone. J Clin Endocrinol 18:901–903, 1958

52. Brown P, Cathala F, Raubertas RF, Gajdusek DC, Castaigno P: The Epidemiology of Creutzfeldt-Jakob disease. Neurology 37:895–904, 1987

53. Kaplan SL, August GP, Blethen SL, Brown DR, Hintz RL, Johansen A, Plotnick LP, Underwood LE, Bell JJ, Blizzard RG, Van Wyk JJ: Clinical studies with recombinant-deficient children. Lancet 1:697–700, 1986

54. Goodman HG, Grumbach MM, Kaplan SL: Growth and growth hormone II. A comparison of isolated growth hormone deficiency and multiple pituitary-hormone deficiencies in 35 patients with idiopathic hypopituitary dwarfism. N Engl J Med 278:57–68, 1968

55. Frasier SD: Human pituitary growth hormone (hGH) therapy in growth hormone deficiency. Endocrine Rev 4:155–170, 1983

56. Burns EC, Tanner JM, Preece MA, Cameron N: Final height and pubertal development in 55 children with idiopathic growth hormone deficiency, treated for between 2 and 15 years with human growth hormone. Eur J Pediatr 137:155–164, 1981

57. Thorner MO, Resche J, Chitwood J, Rogol AD, Furlanetto R, Rivier J, Vale W, Blizzard RM: Acceleration of growth in two children treated with human growth hormone releasing factor. N Engl J Med 312:4–9, 1985

58. Van Vliet G, Styne DM, Kaplan SL, Grumbach MM: Growth hormone treatment for short stature. N Engl J Med 309:1016–1022, 1983

59. Grunt JA, Howard C, Daughaday WH: Comparison of growth and somatomedin C responses following growth hormone treatment in children with small-for-date short stature, significant idiopathic short stature and hypopituitarism. Acta Endocrinol 106:168–174, 1984

60. Gertner JM, Genel M, Granfredi SP, Hintz RL, Rosenfeld RG, Tamborlane WV: Prospective clinical trial of human growth hormone in short children without growth hormone deficiency. J Pediatr 104:172–176, 1984

61. Rosenfeld RG, Hintz RL, Johanson AJ, et al: Three year results of a randomized prospective trial of methionyl human growth hormone and oxandrolone in Turner Syndrome. Pediatrics 113:393–400, 1988

62. Frasier SD, Costin G, Lippe BM, Aceto T, Bunger BF: A dose response curve for human growth hormone. J Clin Endocrinol Metab 53:1213–1217, 1981

63. Russo L, Moore WV: A comparison of subcutaneous and intra muscular administration of human growth hormone in the therapy of growth hormone deficiency. J Clin Endocrinol Metab 55:1003–1006, 1982

64. Wilson DM, Baker B, Hintz RH, Rosenfeld RG: Subcutaneous versus intramuscular growth hormone therapy: Growth and acute somatomedin response. Pediatrics 76:361–364, 1985

65. Takano K, Shizume K, Hibi I: A comparison of subcutaneous and intramuscular administration of growth hormone (hGH) and increased growth rate by daily injection of hGH in GH deficient children. Endocrinol Japon 35:477–484, 1988

66. Albertsson-Wiklund K, Westphal O, Westgren U: Daily subcutaneous administration of human growth hormone in growth hormone deficient children. Acta Pediatr Scand 75:89–97, 1986

67. Green H, Morikawa M, Nixon T: A dual effector theory of growth hormone action. Differentiation 29:195–198, 1985

68. Mendelsohn LG: Minireview: Growth hormone receptors. Life Sci 43:1–5, 1988

69. Cameron CM, Kostyo JL, Adamafio NA, Brostedt P, Roos P, Skottner A, Forsman A, Fryklund L, Skoog B: The acute effects of growth hormone on amino acid transport and protein synthesis are due to its insulin-like action. Endocrinology 122:471–474, 1988

70. Raben MS, Matsuzaki F, Minton PR: Growth-promoting and metabolic effects of growth hormone. Metabolism 13:1102–1107, 1964

71. Prader A, Zachmann M, Poley JR, Illig R: The metabolic effect of a small uniform dose of human growth hormone in hypo-pituitary dwarfs and in control children. Acta Endocrinol 57:115–128, 1968

72. Trivedi P, Hindmarsh P, Risteli J, Ristell L, Mowat AP, Brook CGD: Growth velocity, growth hormone therapy and serum concentrations of the amino-terminal propeptide of type III procollagen. J Pediatr 114:225–230, 1989

73. Danne T, Gruters A, Sehuppan D, Quantas N, Enders I, Weber B: Relationship of procollagen type III propeptide-related antigens in serum to somatic growth in healthy children and patients with growth disorders. J Pediatr 114:257–260, 1989

74. Schlecter NL, Russell SM, Spencer EM, Nicoll CS: Evidence suggesting that the direct growth-promoting effect of growth hormone in cartilage in vivo is mediated by local production of somatomedin. Proc Natl Acad Sci USA 83:7932–7934, 1986

75. Davidson M: Effect of growth hormone on carbohydrate and lipid metabolism. Endocrine Rev 8:115–131, 1987

76. Beck JC, McGarry EE, Dyrenfurth I, Morgan EH: Primate growth hormone studies in man. Metabolism 9:699–751, 1960

77. Van Vliet G, Bosson D, Craen M, Du Caju MVL, Malvaux P, Vanderschueren-Lodeweyckx M: Comparative study of the lipolytic potencies of pituitary-derived and biosynthetic human growth hormone in hypopituitary children. J Clin Endocrinol Metab 65:876–879, 1987

78. Rinderknecht E, Humbel RE: The amino acid sequence of human insulin-like growth factor I and its structural homology with proinsulin. J Biol Chem 253:2769–2776, 1978

79. Zapf J, Schoenle E, Froesch ER: Insulin-like growth factors I and II: Some biological actions and receptor binding characteristics of two purified constituents of nonsuppressible insulin-like activity of human serum. Eur J Biochem 87:285–296, 1978

80. Rechler MM, Nissley SP: The nature and regulation of receptors for insulin-like growth factors. Annu Rev Physiol 47:425–442, 1985

81. Sara VR, Hall K: Insulin-like Growth Factors and Their Binding Proteins. Physiol Rev 70:591–614, 1990

82. Lund PK, Moats-Staats BM, Haynes MA, Simmons JG, Jansen M, D'Ercole AJ, Van Wyk JJ: Somatomedin/insulin-like growth factor-I and insulin-like growth factor-m RNAs in rat fetal and adult tissues. J Biol Chem 261:14539–14544, 1986

83. Van Wyk JJ, Trippel SB: Endocrine, paracrine, and autocrine effects of the somatomedins/insulin-like growth factors, in Isaksson O, et al (eds): Growth Hormone. Basic and Clinical Aspects. Amsterdam, Elsevier, 1987, pp 337–354

84. Luna AM, Wilson DM, Wibbelsman CJ, Brown RC, Nagashima RJ, Hintz RL, Rosenfeld RG: Somatomedins in adolescence: A cross-sectional study of the effect of puberty on insulin-like growth factor I and II levels. J Clin Endocrinol Metab 57:268–271, 1983

85. Bala RM, Lopatka J, Leung A, McCoy E, McArthur RG: Serum immunoreactive somatomedin levels in normal adults, pregnant women at term, children at various ages and children with constitutionally delayed growth. J Clin Endocrinol Metab 52:508–512, 1981

86. Zapf J, Walter H, Froesch ER: Radioimmunological determination of insulin-like growth factors I and II in normal subjects and in patients with growth disorders and extra pancreatic tumor hypoglycemia. J Clin Invest 68:1321–1330, 1981

87. Kaplowitz PB, D'Ercole AJ, Van Wyk JJ, et al: Plasma somatomedin-C during the first year of life. J Pediatr 100:932–934, 1982

88. Quattrin T, Albini CH, Vandlen RL, MacGillivray MH: Quantitation of urinary somatomedin-C in children with normal and abnormal growth. J Clin Endocrinol Metab 65:1168–1171, 1987

89. Quattrin T, Albini CH, Cara JF, Vandlen RL, Mills BJ, MacGillivray MH: Quantitation of urinary somatomedin-C and growth hormone in preterm and fullterm infants and normal children. J Clin Endocrinol Metab 66:792–797, 1989

90. Blum WF, Ranke MB: Insulin-like Growth Factor Binding Proteins (IGFBPs) with Special Reference to IGFBP-3. Acta Ped Scand (suppl) 367:55–62, 1989

91. Rosenfeld RG, Wilson DM, Lee PDK, Hintz RL: Insulin-like growth factors I and II in evaluation of growth retardation. J Pediatr 109:428–433, 1986

92. Clemmons DR, Klibanski A, Underwood LE: Reduction of immunoreactive somatomedin-C during fasting in humans. J Clin Endocrinol Metab 53:1247–1250, 1981

93. Powell DR, Rosenfeld RG, Baker BK, Liu F, Hintz RL: Serum somatomedin levels in adults with chronic renal failure: The importance of measuring insulin-like growth factor I (IGF-I) and IGF-II in acid chromatographed uremic serum. J Clin Endocrinol Metab 63:1186–1192, 1986

94. Clemmons DR, Van Wyk JJ, Ridgway EC, Kliman B, Jellberg RN, Underwood LE: Evaluation of acromegaly by radioimmunoassay of somatomedin-C. N Engl J Med 301:1138–1142, 1979

95. van Buul-Offers S, Hoogerbrugge CM, Branger J, Feijibrief M, Van den Brande JL: Growth stimulating effects of somatomedin-C/insulin-like peptides in Snell dwarf mice. Hormone Res 29:229–236, 1988

96. Eshet R, Laron Z, Petzelan A, Dintzman M: Defect of human growth hormone receptors in the liver of two patients with Laron-type dwarfism. Isr J Med Sci 20:8–11, 1984

97. Daughaday WH, Trivedi B: Absence of serum growth hormone binding protein in patients with growth hormone receptor deficiency (Laron dwarfism). Proc Natl Acad Sci USA 84:4636–4640, 1987

98. Guler HP, Zapf J, Froesch ER: Short-term metabolic effects of recombinant human insulin-like growth factor I in healthy adults. N Engl J Med 317:137–140, 1987

99. Laron Z, Erster B, Klinger B, Anin S: Effect of acute administration of insulin-like growth factor I in patients with Laron-type dwarfism. Lancet 2:1170–1172, 1988

100. Walker JL, Ginalska-Malinowska M, Romer TE, Pucilowska JB, Underwood LE: The effect of Infusion of Insulin-like Growth Hormone Factor-I in a child with Growth Hormone Insensitivity Syndrome. New Engl J Med 324:1483–1488, 1991

101. Merimee TJ, Zapf J, Froesch ER: Insulin-like growth factors (IGFs) in pygmy trait characterization of the metabolic actions of IGF I and IGF II in man. J Clin Endocrinol Metab 55:1081–1088, 1982

45

THERAPEUTIC AGENTS AND THE KIDNEY: Pharmacokinetics and Complications

LAWRENCE S. MILNER, MOHAMMED AL-MUGEIREN, *and* BERNARD S. KAPLAN

Many of the most useful modern therapeutic agents (drugs) have created formidable health problems.[1] Many of the unwanted effects or drug reactions occur because a reduction in renal function precludes normal excretion of the drug or its metabolites. Paradoxically, many of the drugs most often used by nephrologists are among the most potent known nephrotoxic agents. These problems have given rise to a body of literature so vast that it is impossible to cover every aspect of drugs and the kidneys within the limits of a chapter or even a book; we have therefore chosen to deal with a number of aspects of relevance to pediatricians. These include the pharmacokinetics of drugs in renal failure, modifications of drug doses in patients with renal disease, a summary of nephrotoxic syndromes, and the nephrotoxic effects of amphotericin B, the aminoglycosides, cisplatin, and cyclosporine A. Unwanted nephrotoxic complications have been reported with a large number of therapeutic agents, but a great deal remains to be learned about the prevalence of these complications, especially in neonates, infants, and children. Furthermore, it cannot always be established clearly whether or not it is the drug or the disease itself that is responsible for a particular clinico-pathologic finding. The development, for example, of acute or chronic tubulointerstitial disease in a patient with lupus nephritis who is being treated with hydrochlorothiazide could theoretically be the result of the disease, the drug, or an interaction between the two. A list of excellent references has been provided for more detailed information on some of these topics.

PRINCIPLES OF PHARMACOKINETICS IN RENAL DISEASE

Drug Clearance (See References 2–5)

Although the excretion of a drug depends on more factors than does the excretion of creatinine, the renal clear-

ance of a drug or its metabolites can be determined in a similar manner. In general, the process of drug excretion by the kidneys depends on glomerular filtration, plasma protein binding of the drug, renal tubular reabsorption, and tubular secretion. Drugs are also metabolized by the liver and, to a lesser extent, the lungs, and their metabolites may then be excreted via the intestine and/or kidneys. Eventually most drugs and their metabolites are excreted, although the duration of their sojourn within the body varies enormously from one drug to another in healthy individuals. Compromised renal function delays the excretion of drugs that are eliminated mainly by the kidneys in a fairly predictable fashion, despite the complexities involved in the handling of the drug.

Body clearance is the sum of the individual clearances (renal + hepatic + pulmonary). Body clearance is the elimination rate divided by the midpoint plasma concentration of the drug. Body clearance can be determined by measuring the area under a curve of the plasma concentration versus the time that has elapsed after intravenous administration of a single dose of the drug (AUC): body clearance = dose/AUC.

The body clearance can also be determined by obtaining a steady-state concentration in plasma (C_{ss}) by infusing the drug at a constant rate (R): body clearance = R/C_{ss}.

Rearrangement of the equation shows the effect of a change in body clearance on the steady-state concentration of a drug in plasma: $C_{ss} = R/$body clearance.

This equation also applied to oral administration of a drug: $C_{ss} = f_{dose}/r/$body clearance (f is the fraction of the dose that enters the general circulation, and r is the interval between doses).

Half-Life

Drugs with first-order kinetics have an exponential decrease in concentration that is greatest when the serum level is highest.[2,4] Under these circumstances, the half-life connotes the time during which there is a 50 percent

510

reduction in serum concentration. The elimination rate constant (K_e) reflects the amount of drug removed per unit time. K_e has an inverse relationship to half-life expressed as: $t_{1/2} = 0.7/K_e$. The appropriate interval for prescribing maintenance doses in renal failure is determined mainly by the half-life of a drug, which in turn is influenced by clearance and volume of distribution.

Volume of Distribution

This reflects the relationship between the blood concentration of a drug and its amount in the body. The tissue distribution of a drug depends on protein binding and its ability to enter cells. The volume of distribution (V) = V plasma + V extracellular water $\times$ f/ft, where f is the unbound plasma fraction and f_t is the unbound tissue fraction.[2,4]

Uremia and hypoalbuminemia alter the protein binding of drugs and therefore may affect the volume of distribution.[6,7] The relationship among body clearance, half-life, and volume of distribution is $t_{1/2} = V \times 0.7/K_e$.

Renal Excretion of Drugs

This occurs by glomerular filtration, tubular secretion, or both mechanisms.[3] Adjustments of doses are mandated in any form of renal failure irrespective of the mechanism of renal elimination of a particular drug. Furthermore, special considerations are needed for drug modification in prematures and neonates because of the immaturity of their glomerular filtration rates and tubular secretory mechanisms.[8-11] Filtration of a drug is governed by the patient's glomerular filtration rate and the molecular weight and degree of protein binding of the drug. Tubular secretion occurs in the proximal tubule at the basolateral membrane in the case of anionic drugs and at the brush border in the case of cationic drugs.[12-14] Examples of anionic (acidic) drugs include thiazides, furosemide, ethacrynic acid, probenecid, penicillins, cephalosporins, spironolactone, salicylates, and methotrexate. Transport of an anionic drug such as penicillin can be blocked by probenecid. Examples of cationic (basic) drugs are dopamine, histamine, neostigmine, procaine, and cimetidine. Cimetidine may block cationic transport and it has been shown to cause accumulation of procainamide.

Route of Elimination

This may be exclusively renal (class A), exclusively hepatic (class B), or both renal and hepatic (class C). The route of elimination depends in part on whether the drug is water- or lipid-soluble. Lipid-soluble drugs tend to be excreted by the liver, and water-soluble substances are excreted by the kidneys.[15] If 50 percent of a drug is eliminated by the kidneys, then the half-life will be prolonged by renal insufficiency.[15] Although the pharmacokinetics of many drugs have been established in renal failure, this may not apply to newer agents. However, it can be

assumed that their doses will need to be altered as well. The modification of doses will depend on the major route of elimination of the particular drug.

Modification of Doses of Drugs in Renal Insufficiency

There is a curvilinear relationship between the reduction in glomerular filtration rate and the half-life of a drug. In adults the drug half-life increases significantly when the glomerular filtration rate falls below 20 ml/min. The principles of drug modification depend on the elimination rate constant (K_e), the volume of distribution, and the renal and nonrenal clearances of the drug. Nomograms[16-18] derived from studies in adults must be used with discretion as guides to the adjustment of doses in children and infants. The half-life of a drug can, however, be calculated by determining the elimination rate constant (K_e) for the degree of renal impairment.[19]

1. The estimated renal clearance of a drug in reduced renal function = normal drug clearance $\times$

$$\frac{\text{patient's GFR}}{\text{normal GFR for age}}$$

GFR is the glomerular filtration rate as determined for these purposes usually by creatinine clearance. This method of determining the GFR is, however, fraught with many difficulties.[20] Furthermore, a number of drugs may produce falsely elevated serum creatinine concentrations, either by inhibiting tubular secretion of creatinine (e.g., triamterene, spironolactone, amiloride, cimetidine, and trimethoprim[21]) or by affecting the measurement of serum creatinine (e.g., cephalosporins, vitamin C, and flucytosine[22]).

2. Body clearance = renal + nonrenal clearance, or body clearance = $K_e \times$ volume of distribution.

3. K_e (renal impairment) = K_e (normal) $\times$

$$\frac{\text{body clearance (renal impairment)}}{\text{body clearance (normal)}}$$

The K_e (normal) and the K_e (renal impairment) of a drug can therefore be calculated if its volume of distribution and clearances are known. K_e can be expressed as the amount of the drug eliminated per unit time, or as the percentage of the drug removed from its volume of distribution. Since

$$K_e \text{ (renal impairment)} = \frac{0.7}{t_{1/2}}$$

therefore

$$t_{1/2} \text{ (renal impairment)} = \frac{t_{1/2}}{K_e \text{ (renal impairment)}}$$

The half-life of drugs may also be determined from equations and nomograms based on known pharmacokinetic data of their elimination constants in individuals with normal renal function or in anephric patients.[17,18,23,24] In patients with unstable renal function, calculations of a new half-life that corresponds to changes in creatinine clearances should be made for drugs excreted by the kidneys. These formulas are theoretically acceptable provided that a number of assumptions are made: that the volumes of distribution in a normal person and in a patient with renal failure are similar; that renal function is stable; that the patient is not malnourished; and that the biotransformation of drugs is the same in patients as in normal people. In practice, these caveats have led to the development of fairly reliable assays for many drugs, so that the determination of half-lives is becoming redundant. Therapeutic levels may, however, be achieved by decreasing the maintenance dose,[15–18,23,25] by increasing the dosing intervals, or by changing both. In general, the loading dose in a patient with renal impairment should equal that in a patient with normal kidney function.

Loading dose = volume of distribution
$\times$ desired peak blood level.

Example: 10-kg child treated with amikacin.

Loading dose = volume of distribution (L/kg)
$\times$ peak blood level desired (mg/L)
= (0.3 $\times$ 10) $\times$ 25
= 75 mg
= 7.5 mg/kg

Drug Dosing in Peritoneal Dialysis

The dialyzability of a drug correlates to some extent with the normal renal clearance of that agent. However, drugs with greater than 20 percent protein binding or a large volume of distribution tend to be dialyzed poorly.[26–28] The doses of drugs such as the aminoglycosides, certain cephalosporins (e.g., ceftazidime), and vancomycin must be modified in patients treated with any mode of peritoneal dialysis (acute, chronic ambulatory, or continuous cycling) because there is substantial peritoneal clearance of these drugs. The movement of some drugs is bidirectional (e.g., penicillin), and therefore systemic infection can be treated by adding the antibiotic to the peritoneal fluid. On the other hand, peritonitis can be treated parenterally. The dialyzability of some frequently used drugs and the recommended dose adjustments are summarized in Table 45–1. The loading doses in children on peritoneal dialysis are the same as in those with normal

renal function. The maintenance dose needs to be adjusted according to known pharmacokinetic data derived for a particular drug in the context of peritoneal dialysis. Adequate blood levels can be maintained in the case of drugs with bidirectional transport by intraperitoneal instillation (amikacin, aminoglycosides, cefotaxime).

Similar principles can be employed in patients with peritonitis, a frequent complication of peritoneal dialysis. Vancomycin is often used because *Staphylococcus epidermidis* is a frequent cause. The loading dose may be given parenterally or intraperitoneally; this is followed by doses given intravenously at intervals relative to the drug's calculated half-life, or by doses given intraperitoneally in order to achieve a desired therapeutic level.

Drug Dosing in Hemodialysis

The clearance of a drug by hemodialysis is determined by properties of the apparatus as well as those of the drug.[29,30] The surface area of the dialysis membrane relative to the patient's surface area, the porosity of the dialysis membrane, the blood and dialysate flow rates, and the length of time on dialysis all affect the clearance of a drug. Drugs that are poorly cleared by hemodialysis include those with large molecular weights (e.g., vancomycin, 1800 daltons), with greater than 20 percent protein binding, with a large volume of distribution (e.g., digoxin, greater than 2 liters/kg), with mainly nonrenal excretion (e.g., paracetamol), and with lipid solubility (e.g., cyclosporine). The $t_{1/2}$ of a drug that is very dialyzable (e.g., the aminoglycosides) will be reduced by hemodialysis. Therefore an additional dose must be given at the end of dialysis. The amount should equal that removed during dialysis. Data are available for predicting this value.[31]

The clearance of a drug in a patient on hemodialysis is expressed as:

Total body clearance = dialysis clearance
+ residual renal clearance + nonrenal clearance

Clearance of a drug by hemodialysis must increase total body clearance by 30 percent or produce subtherapeutic levels for it to be meaningful clinically. Maintenance doses of drugs that are substantially removed by dialysis should be given at the end of the period of dialysis.

TABLE 45–1. FACTORS THAT AFFECT THE NEPHROTOXIC POTENTIAL OF A DRUG

1. Administration of large doses of a nephrotoxic drug.
2. Administration of reasonable doses over a long period of time.
3. Prior administration of the same drug.
4. Prior administration of another drug with nephrotoxic potential.
5. Concomitant administration of two potentially nephrotoxic drugs with a cumulative effect.
6. Concomitant administration of a potentially nephrotoxic drug with a diuretic.
7. Patients with a single kidney may be at greater risk for nephrotoxic injury.
8. Prior injury to the kidney may render it at greater risk for drug-induced injury.

DRUG DOSE MODIFICATION IN RENAL FAILURE

A number of principles that govern the nephrotoxic potential of a drug are summarized in Table 45–1.

Penicillins

The nephrotoxic side effects of penicillins include glomerular injury, tubulointerstitial disease, and electrolyte

TABLE 45–2. PHARMACOLOGIC FEATURES OF THE EXTENDED-SPECTRUM PENICILLINS[37]

	HALF-LIFE (h)	RENAL EXCRETION (%)	REMOVAL BY HEMODIALYSIS
Carbenicillin	1.1	95	Yes
Ticarcillin	1.2	80	Yes
Azlocillin	0.8	50–70	Yes
Mezlocillin	0.8	55	Yes
Piperacillin	0.9	70	Yes

disturbances. Methicillin is the most nephrotoxic member of the penicillin family. Penicillin or methicillin nephropathy is characterized by fever, eosinophilia, rash, urinary abnormalities (including proteinuria), azotemia, and histologic evidence of tubular injury with interstitial nephritis. Penicilloyl hapten has been demonstrated along tubular basement membranes.[32,33] The nephropathy does not seem to be related to dose or duration of treatment but may be a hypersensitivity reaction. Remission of the abnormalities usually occurs following withdrawal of the drug.[34] Ampicillin, especially if given in very large doses, has been associated with a syndrome of fever, rash, polydipsia, polyuria, eosinophilia, and acute interstitial nephritis.[35,36]

Penicillins are eliminated by tubular secretion and glomerular filtration. Penicillin and ampicillin have a short half-life of 30 minutes, which increases to 12 hours in anephric patients. Children with impaired renal function need only a modest reduction in dose. The half-life of cloxacillin normally is also 30 minutes, and although it may increase to 2 hours in renal failure, the dose need not require modification. Penicillin and ampicillin are substantially cleared by hemodialysis, and therefore the doses must be increased. Peritoneal clearance of penicillin and ampicillin is minimal, but up to 75 percent of intraperitoneal ampicillin can be absorbed. The dose of carbenicillin must be reduced in renal failure because its half-life may range from 1 to 16 hours in patients with renal impairment. The prolonged half-life can be reduced by hemodialysis but not by peritoneal dialysis. Aminoglycosides may be inactivated by extended-spectrum penicillins (e.g., carbenicillin, ticarcillin) when given together in patients with renal failure.[37] The doses of piperacillin also must be modified similarly (Table 45–2).[37–39]

Cephalosporins

The cephalosporins have been associated with an elevation of the serum creatinine as well as with interstitial nephritis and subsequent acute or chronic renal failure. These antibiotics are eliminated by glomerular filtration and tubular secretion, and therefore their doses must be modified in patients with impaired renal function. Their half-life may be shortened in patients on peritoneal dialysis, but because peritoneal clearance is poor, oral doses of cephalexin and cephradine are the same as for patients with end-stage renal disease.[40,41] Plasma levels in the therapeutic range can, however, be obtained after intraperitoneal administration of cefazolin and cefuroxime, which are absorbed slowly from the peritoneal cavity, and therefore an intravenous loading dose should be given in addition to intraperitoneal instillations. Cefazolin,[42] cefotaxime,[43,44] and ceftazidime[45–47] are easily cleared by peritoneal dialysis and by hemodialysis. Cefotaxime and ceftazidime can be used to treat systemic infections when given intraperitoneally; intravenous loading doses may have to be given in order to achieve therapeutic blood levels rapidly.

Ceftriaxone is eliminated mainly by biliary secretion, although renal excretion can account for about 50 percent in infants and 70 percent in neonates.[48] The normal half-life of 8 hours is prolonged 2.5 times in end-stage renal failure. Reduced doses are indicated mainly for patients with severe renal insufficiency.[49] The half-life is unaltered by hemodialysis or peritoneal dialysis,[50,51] and yet adequate blood levels can be achieved following intraperitoneal administration (Table 45–3).[52]

Vancomycin

The only route of elimination of vancomycin is by the kidneys. Consequently, the normal half-life of 2–3 hours in children[53] may be extended up to 200 hours in end-stage renal failure in adults. Nomograms may be used to adjust maintenance doses or dosage intervals for creatinine clearances.[54,55] The transfer of vancomycin is predominantly unidirectional from the peritoneum to the blood.[56,57] Because there is virtually no removal of vancomycin during hemodialysis, a loading dose of 10–15 mg/kg will be sufficient for as long as 7 days. The treat-

TABLE 45–3. PHARMACOLOGIC FEATURES OF THE THIRD-GENERATION CEPHALOSPORINS[37]

	MOXALACTAM	CEFOTAXIME	CEFTIZOXIME	CEFTRIAXONE	CEFOPERAZONE	CEFTAZIDIME
Half-life (h)	2.2	1.0	1.7	8.0	2.0	1.8
Renal excretion (%)	70	60	80	50	25	80
Hemodialysis (% reduction in serum concentration)	50	80	50	0	0	80
Peritoneal dialysis						
Dose removed (%)	N.D.	6	15	N.D.	N.D.	7
I.P. dose absorbed (%)	50	50–90	80–90	70	70–90	50

N.D. = not determined; IP = intraperitoneal.

ment of peritonitis in a patient on chronic peritoneal dialysis requires a similar intravenous dose. If instilled intraperitoneally, the loading dose would be 30 mg/kg followed by 1.5 mg/kg every 6 hours.[53]

Trimethoprim/Sulfamethoxazole (TMP/SMZ)

TMP/SMZ is a potentially nephrotoxic agent, especially in patients with compromised renal function or underlying renal injury in whom it has been associated with acute interstitial nephritis. There have been very few reports, however, in children.[58] Approximately 50 percent of TMP is excreted unchanged by the kidneys in children (80 percent in adults).[59] The half-life of TMP/SMZ in children with end-stage renal failure is prolonged from the normal 4–5 hours to 20 hours.[60] A 50–75 percent reduction in the dose of TMP is recommended in patients with severe renal impairment, and a similar reduction is suggested in the dose of SMZ in those with moderate impairment. In addition, the dosage interval should be prolonged. Patients with residual renal function must be treated with caution because of the possibility of crystalluria leading to further deterioration in function. Removal by peritoneal clearance is negligible.[61] Removal by hemodialysis may be efficient enought to warrant supplemental doses.

Erythromycin

Erythromycin does not seem to be a cause of renal injury. Doses should be modified in patients with renal failure because of the possibility of causing ototoxicity in these circumstances.[62] Both oral and parenteral doses result in abnormally high blood levels of erythromycin in uremic adults. This drug is not excreted by the kidneys. The high blood levels are therefore due either to a decrease in its volume of distribution or to an increase in its bioavailability.[62] The daily dose of eythromycin should not exceed 1.5 gm in adults on hemodialysis.[62]

Antifungal Agents

Amphotericin B, miconazole, and ketoconazole are not eliminated substantially by the kidneys.[63,64] Amphotericin B is a potent nephrotoxic agent and can cause acute and chronic renal failure, distal renal tubular acidosis, hypokalemia, hyposthenuria, nephrocalcinosis, and renal wasting of sodium, potassium, and magnesium.[65,66] It has been suggested that the dose of amphotericin B used in children should be based on the amount needed to treat an infection rather than on data derived from studies in adults.[67] Nevertheless, the nephrotoxic potential of this drug remains a serious problem, which, however, may be alleviated by salt repletion.[68] The dose of amphotericin B may need to be modified in a patient with renal insufficiency because of its nephrotoxic potential.

The doses of flucytosine do have to be modified because it is excreted by the kidneys. In patients with a GFR under 10 ml/min the daily dose is reduced to 25–50 mg/kg, and in patients with mild to moderate renal failure the dose is 25–50 mg/kg given twice a day.[63] Supplemental doses of flucytosine are needed in patients on peritoneal dialysis or hemodialysis because its clearance by these may be substantial. Treatment of fungal peritonitis with miconazole or ketoconazole requires that they be instilled intraperitoneally. On the other hand, fungemia must be treated by intravenous injections of these agents.

Acyclovir

Acyclovir can cause a reduction in GFR, hematuria, and cylinduria possibly by deposition of crystals in the tubules.[69] The clearance of acyclovir is low in infants but reaches adult values by 12 months.[70] Complications may be prevented by maintaining good hydration, by dissolving the drug in 100 ml of 5 percent dextrose water, and by infusing the drug over a 1-hour period if the dose exceeds 5 mg/kg.[71] The normal half-life of acyclovir in children of 2.5–4 hours is lengthened to 20 hours in end-stage renal failure because 60–80 percent is normally excreted by the kidneys.[72] Doses are modified in moderate to severe impairment by increasing the interval between doses. Acyclovir is not cleared as well with peritoneal dialysis as with hemodialysis.[73] The usual daily dose or supplemental doses are required after hemodialysis.

Ciprofloxacin

Ciprofloxacin, a quinolone antibiotic, is rapidly absorbed, widely distributed, and excreted partially by filtration and tubular secretion and partially by hepatic metabolism. In severe renal failure the half-life is twice normal and the dose must be reduced by 50 percent.[74] The drug is not cleared by peritoneal dialysis,[75] and clearance by hemodialysis is minimal.[76]

Metronidazole

The alcohol and acid metabolites of metronidazole are excreted in urine and feces.[77] Dosage does not need to be modified in mild to moderate renal insufficiency. Metronidazole and its metabolites are cleared sufficiently during hemodialysis so that the dose need not be modified.[78] The clearance of the drug and its metabolites is low during peritoneal dialysis; the doses must therefore be reduced in patients on continuous peritoneal dialysis.[79]

Digoxin

Digoxin is eliminated from the body mainly by the kidneys. The volume of distribution is large, the half-life is long, and protein binding is minimal. These pharmacokinetic parameters vary according to the age of a normal child: premature neonates have lower body clearance values, smaller volumes of distribution, and longer half-lives when compared with older children.[80] The half-life ranges from about 55 hours in 500-gm premature infants to 35 hours in full-term neonates and older children. The half-life of digoxin is prolonged in renal insufficiency, the volume of distribution is smaller, and therefore the loading dose must be reduced by 50–75 percent of the standard loading dose.[81] Maintenance doses must be modified according to the degree of renal impairment, but because the toxic–therapeutic range is so narrow, nomograms have been developed for treatment of adults with renal failure.[81,82] For patients with severely impaired renal function, 50 percent of the usual maintenance dose should be given.

Serum digoxin levels should be measured at least 6 hours after administration in the postdistributive phase. The desired levels should be between 1.0 and 2.0 ng/ml.[80] Ideally, the doses need to be monitored by measuring the serum levels as well as by using nomograms and formulas. Each method has its problems. The levels of digoxin may be falsely elevated in renal failure, especially in neonates,[83] because of cross-reactivity with endogenous digoxin-like substances. Spironolactone may also be a cause of falsely elevated serum digoxin levels. Digoxin cannot be dialyzed to any significant extent. Because of all the potential problems with digoxin in patients with renal failure, digitoxin may be preferable; its route of elimination is mainly nonrenal and it is highly bound to protein.

Antihypertensives

The half-lives of propranolol and metoprolol are unaffected by renal insufficiency, peritoneal dialysis, or hemodialysis.[86] The half-life of atenolol is prolonged significantly from a normal of 6 hours in adults with compromised renal function (and may be cumulative) because its main route of elimination is by the kidneys. The half-life of the drug is normal in patients on hemodialysis and prolonged fourfold in those treated with chronic peritoneal dialysis.[84]

Hydrallazine, prazocin, and minoxidil have large volumes of distribution, are not eliminated by the kidneys, and do not require adjustments of doses in patients in renal failure, whether or not they are on hemodialysis or peritoneal dialysis.[85]

The renal side effects of the angiotensin-converting enzyme (ACE) inhibitors captopril and enalapril have included hyperkalemia, acute renal failure, and possibly proteinuria. Administration of an ACE inhibitor can reduce the GFR of a kidney with renal artery stenosis. This is usually reversible.[86] Proteinuria with membranous nephropathy can occur in patients treated with high doses of captopril, but this is a rare side effect if the maximum daily dose in an adult is less than 150 mg.[87] There is no convincing evidence that progressive renal damage occurs in patients who become proteinuric while being treated with captopril.[88] Interstitial nephritis has been ascribed to, but not proven to be caused by, ACE inhibitors.[87] Unpredictable decreases in blood pressure have been observed in infants while being treated with captopril.[89] These infants had hypertension associated with elevated peripheral renin values, evidence of renal artery thrombosis,

and/or renal parenchymal disease.[89] These episodes were accompanied by oliguria, azotemia, and neurologic signs.

ACE inhibitors are mainly eliminated by the kidneys. The half-life of captopril is prolonged from 3.5 hours in patients with mild renal insufficiency to as long as 20 hours in those with severe insufficiency.[90] The action of the drug may be prolonged in renal failure, and therefore starting doses should be as low as 0.1 mg/kg/dose with gradual increments in dosage until control of blood pressure has been achieved. Care must be taken to monitor the serum potassium concentrations because of the possibility of the side effect of hyperkalemia. Enalapril is converted to an active antihypertensive metabolite enalaprilat. The normal half-life of enalaprilat in adults is 11 hours, and this is prolonged in renal failure.[91] Both captopril and enalapril are cleared by hemodialysis, and this may offset their toxic side effects.[92,93]

Anticonvulsants

Phenobarbital displays linear kinetics, has a long half-life, and 30–50 percent is excreted by the kidneys.[94,95] The doses need to be decreased in renal failure to prevent accumulation. The safest approach is to give a standard loading dose of 10 mg/kg and to monitor the blood levels. Phenobarbital is cleared by dialysis. The kinetics of carbemazepine are also linear, 70–80 percent is protein-bound, it is metabolized in the liver, and the epoxide is partly excreted by the kidneys. A 25 percent reduction of the dose is recommended in children with severe renal failure.

Neither phenytoin nor sodium valproate is eliminated by the kidneys, and modifications in dosage regimens are not required for either.[95]

NEPHROTOXIC AGENTS

Although a large number of drugs (including those discussed above) have been incriminated as causes of renal injury (Table 45–4), several caveats are warranted.[96] The actual number of cases of drug-induced nephropathy is relatively small in comparison to the large numbers of patients using a particular drug. The evidence for a drug-induced nephropathy is often circumstantial. Concurrent drugs are often being given. The underlying illness for which the drug is being given may be the cause of the untoward reaction or may contribute to it.

Despite these caveats, however, there are some drugs that unequivocally have been associated with nephrotoxic injury. Some of these are extremely important and essential therapeutic agents and will therefore be discussed in more detail. Included among these in pediatric practice are gentamicin, cisplatin, and cyclosporine. Long-term administration of furosemide is becoming an important cause of nephrocalcinosis in neonates with bronchopulmonary dysplasia. This is discussed in detail in Chapter 46. Sulfonamides were an important cause of renal injury in the past but now tend to be used infrequently except as

TABLE 45–4. DRUG-INDUCED NEPHROTOXIC SYNDROMES

PROTEINURIA-NEPHROTIC SYNDROME
Penicillin
Gold
Trimethadone
Paramethadone
Dapsone
Penicillamine
Probenecid
Mercurial diuretics
Tolbutamide
Perchlorate
Phenindione
Rifampin
Adriamycin
Doxorubicin
Fenoprofen

FANCONI'S SYNDROME
Salicylates
Gentamicin
Tetracycline
Ifosfamide

DISTAL RENAL TUBULAR ACIDOSIS
Amphotericin B
Penicillin
Lithium
Toluene

NEPHROGENIC DIABETES INSIPIDUS
Demethylchlortetracycline
Methoxyflurane
Lithium
Diphenylhydantoin

SYNDROME OF INAPPROPRIATE SECRETION OF ADH
Vincristine

DILUTIONAL HYPONATREMIA
Cyclophosphamide
Hydrochlorothiazide

PAPILLARY NECROSIS
Salicylates
Phenacetin
Phenylbutazone

ACUTE INTERSTITIAL NEPHRITIS
β-Lactam Antibiotics
  Cephalosporins
    Cefotaxime
    Cephradine
    Cephalexin
    Cephalothin
  Penicillins
    Penicillin G
  Synthetic penicillins
    Amoxicillin
    Ampicillin
    Carbenicillin
    Methicillin
    Nafcillin
    Oxacillin

Non-β-Lactam Antibiotics
  Aminoglycosides
    Gentamicin
  Antitubercular agents
    p-Aminosalicylic acid
    Ethambutol
    Isoniazid
    Rifampin
  Polymyxins
    Polymyxin B
    Colistin
  Tetracyclines
    Minocycline

  Urinary anti-infectants
    Nitrofurantoin
Sulfonamide Derivatives
  Diuretics
    Amiloride
    Chlothalidone
    Furosemide
    Thiazides
    Ticrynafen
  Sulfonamides
    Cotrimoxazole
    Sulfonamide
  Uricosuric agents
    Probenecid
    Sulfinpyrazone

Nonsteroidal Anti-Inflammatory Agents
  Carboxylic acids
    Aspirin
    Diflunisal
  Acetic acids
    Fenclofenac
  Carboheterocyclic acids
    Indomethacin
    Sulindac
    Tolmetin
    Zomepirac
  Propionic acids
    Benoxaprofen
    Ibuprofen
    Naproxen
  Fenamic acids
    Mefenamic acid
    Meclofenamate
  Enolic acids
    Apazone
    Dipyrone
    Oxyphenbutazone
    Phenylbutazone
    Piroxicam

Miscellaneous Groups of Agents
  Analgesics
    Glafenin
  Anticoagulants
    Phenindione
  Anticonvulsants
    Carbamazepine
    Phenobarbital
    Phenytoin
  ACE inhibitors
    Allopurinol
    Captopril
  H$_2$ blockers
    Cimetidine
  Immunosuppressants
    Azathioprine
    Cyclosporine
    Interferon
  Sympathomimetics
    Amphetamine
    Phenylpropanolamine
  Clofibrate
  Methyldopa
  Propranolol

CHRONIC TUBULOINTERSTITIAL NEPHRITIS
Phenacetin
Acetaminophen
Salicylates
Cisplatin
Phenindione
Rifampin
Carmustine

TABLE 45–4. DRUG-INDUCED NEPHROTOXIC SYNDROMES *Continued*

Lomustine	Aminoglycosides
Lithium	Cephalosporins
Cyclosporine	Tetracyclines
Gold	Amphotericin B
Nonsteroidal anti-inflammatory agents	Polymyxin
Methoxyflurane	Contrast media
	Cisplatin
NEPHROCALCINOSIS	Bismuth compounds
Furosemide	Methotrexate
	Epsilon amino caproic acid
HEMORRHAGIC CYSTITIS	Diphenylhydantoin
Cephalosporins	Phenindione
Penicillin G	Propranalol
Methicillin	Dextran
Ticarcillin	Tolazaline
Carbenicillin	Captopril
Piperacillin	Acyclovir
Ifosphamide	Pentamidine
Cyclophosphamide	
Busulfan	**CHRONIC RENAL FAILURE**
Isoniazid	Analgesics
Acyclovir	Aminoglycosides
	Cisplatin
HEMOLYTIC UREMIC SYNDROME	Contrast media
Cyclosporine A	Cyclosporine A
Mitomycin C	Methoxyfluorane
Oral contraceptives	Nitrosureas
	Tetracycline
ACUTE RENAL FAILURE–REDUCED GFR	Vancomycin
Aspirin	
Indomethacin	
Phenylbutazone	

the trimethoprim/sulfamethoxazole combination. Nonsteroidal anti-inflammatory agents are an extremely important cause of renal injury in adults but have only occasionally been incriminated as a cause of renal damage in children.

The Aminoglycosides

Mechanism of Action

The aminoglycosides (gentamicin, tobramycin, amikacin, netilmicin, kanamycin, streptomycin, and neomycin) consist of two or more amino sugars joined in glycosidic linkage to a hexose nucleus. They inhibit protein biosynthesis by interfering with the attachment of mRNA to the 30S ribosome. Gentamicin is the most widely used and studied aminoglycoside.

Pharmacology (See Reference 97)

The aminoglycosides are polycations that are almost incapable of being absorbed from the gastrointestinal tract. Peak plasma concentrations are reached 30 minutes after an infusion. Estimates of binding to plasma proteins have ranged from zero to 30 percent. The volume of distribution is about 25 percent of the lean body mass and approximates the volume of the extracellular fluid. The serum half-life of gentamicin in patients with normal renal function is about 2 hours. Gentamicin is not metabolized and is excreted mainly by glomerular filtration.[98]

Both net secretion and reabsorption by proximal renal tubules have been demonstrated in experimental studies.[99] After a single intravenous dose, 40–65 percent can be recovered in the urine within 24 hours, and 90 percent is eventually excreted.[100] Gentamicin accumulates within renal cells, and renal cortical concentrations are much greater than plasma levels.[101,102] Gentamicin may be recovered from the urine 20 days after treatment for 1 week.[103]

Risk Factors for Nephrotoxicity

The potential for nephrotoxic side effects of aminoglycosides is the result of their low therapeutic index, widespread use, and dependence on the kidneys for excretion. Additional risk factors include elevated initial 1-hour postdose trough levels, advanced age, volume depletion, shock, and liver disease. Increased gentamicin nephrotoxicity is produced in rats that are on a low-sodium diet, are volume-depleted, or are potassium-depleted.[104,105] Patients with renal insufficiency from any cause have a greater prevalence of aminoglycoside nephrotoxicity because of an increased load of drug per functioning nephron. The dose of the drug is the most important factor that results in renal injury. Large doses and/or prolonged administration result in more rapid achievement of toxic concentrations in the renal parenchyma. There is a relationship among the plasma levels, the parenchymal concentration, and the toxic potential for any of the aminoglycosides. This toxic potential is also a function of the total quantity of aminoglycoside given during separate courses over a period of time.

Older patients are at greater risk for aminoglycoside nephrotoxic injury than are infants and children. This may be related in part to the fact that doses are often based on the serum creatinine concentration, which may reflect a much lower GFR because of reduced creatinine production in someone with decreased muscle mass. Inappropriately high doses may therefore inadvertently be given. In addition, the potential to induce renal injury seems to depend on the weight of the kidneys relative to total body weight. In rats the weight of the kidneys relative to total body weight is much less in the neonate than in the mature animal.[106] Aminoglycosides do not seem to cause permanent renal damage in the newborn. Renal failure, when it does occur in the neonate, is usually mild, transient, and associated with treatment for more than 10 days or with the administration of large doses, and manifests mainly as diminished postnatal maturation of renal function.[107]

Aminoglycosides with six ionizable amino groups (e.g., neomycin) tend to be more toxic than those with fewer of these groups. This is not the only determinant of toxicity, because gentamicin and tobramycin each have five ionizable amino groups but have different toxic potentials. Tobramycin is three to four times less toxic than gentamicin in rats. Many of the drugs that are often given together with an aminoglycoside have an additive effect with respect to the nephrotoxic potential of the aminoglycoside. These include cisplatin, amphotericin B, clindamycin, the cephalosporins, vancomycin, and furosemide.

Clinical Features of Aminoglycoside Nephrotoxicity

Histologic studies have revealed features of acute tubular necrosis. Ultrastructural studies have demonstrated the presence of myeloid bodies in the epithelial cells. These consist of concentric laminated whorls in the lysosomes and have been seen in kidneys from patients with and without clinical evidence of aminoglycoside nephrotoxicity, and with other nephrotoxins.

Enzymuria is the earliest demonstrable renal manifestation of aminoglycoside-induced injury. Increased amounts of several brush border enzymes may be detected in the urine as early as 24 hours after a single dose, and the concentrations then rise progressively with continuing treatment. Further injury to the proximal tubule may result in glycosuria, aminoaciduria, excretion of β-microglobulins, and other features of Fanconi's syndrome. Selective effects on the renal handling of the intracellular cations may result in magnesium and potassium wasting.

Mild proteinuria and cylinduria are early findings that may occur before the decline in renal function. The most serious complication is a reduction in GFR that may range from a modest decrement to complete cessation of filtration with consequent renal failure. Patients may have an acute reduction in renal function or they may have nonoliguric renal failure.

Nephrogenic diabetes insipidus with polyuria may occur early in the course of aminoglycoside nephrotoxi-

TABLE 45–5. GUIDELINES FOR THE PREVENTION OF AMINOGLYCOSIDE-INDUCED NEPHROTOXICITY

1. Be aware of the possibility.
2. Provide optimal hydration and perfusion.
3. Avoid hyponatremia, hypokalemia, hypomagnesemia.
4. Limit treatment to less than 16 days.
5. Monitor plasma concentrations.
6. Adjust doses according to GFR.
7. Avoid, if possible, concurrent use of potentially nephrotoxic drugs.
8. Be especially careful if the patient has been treated previously with an aminoglycoside or any other potentially nephrotoxic agent.

city. A number of mechanisms have been suggested to account for acquired nephrogenic diabetes insipidus. These include an inability to maintain the hypertonic medullary gradient secondary to tubulointerstitial injury, inhibition of the action of antidiuretic hormone (ADH) via adenylate cyclase, or possibly a direct effect of aminoglycosides on important membrane-bound enzymes.

Dose Modification in Renal Impairment

Aminoglycosides have a narrow therapeutic–toxic range and a normal half-life of 2 hours, which may be prolonged to 60 hours in anephric patients. There is a close correlation between the half-life and the degree of renal impairment.[108,109] In infants and children under 8 years, the prolonged half-life approximates the serum creatinine concentration multiplied by 4 ($t_{1/2}$ = serum creatinine in mg/dl × 4).[108] The loading dose in renal failure is the same as in normal renal function. Ideally the dosing regimen should be individualized[110,111] by calculating the half-life from the serum concentrations over time, or from the peak serum concentration.

Individualizing the dose may also be beneficial for children on hemodialysis in whom the clearances for the intra- and interdialytic periods can be calculated.[112] There may be substantial clearances by hemodialysis and by peritoneal dialysis but less so with the latter.[113] Intraperitoneal administration of 8 mg of gentamicin/liter of dialysate can produce a serum level of about 5–8.0 mg/liter. The corresponding figure for tobramycin is 8 mg/liter and for amikacin 20 mg/liter. For systemic infections the intraperitoneal loading doses are 1.5–2 mg/kg for gentamicin and tobramycin and 7.5 mg/kg for amikacin.[114] Table 45–5 summarizes guidelines for the prevention of aminoglycoside-induced nephrotoxicity.

RENAL DISEASES INDUCED BY ANTINEOPLASTIC AGENTS

Renal disease is a not infrequent complication in patients with malignancies. Renal involvement may be caused by the malignant disease itself (for example, Hodgkin's disease and the nephrotic syndrome), by products released by a malignant tumor as a result of its treatment (for example, the cell lysis syndrome), by a drug used for treatment of the tumor (for example cisplatin, ifospamide), by a drug used for treatment of infections that often occur in patients with malignancies (gentamicin, amphotericin B), or by a combination of factors. A particular drug may cause a variety of nephrotoxic syndromes. This is particularly evident in the case of cisplatin, which has been incriminated as a cause of acute renal failure, chronic renal failure, and magnesium wasting (Table 45–6). Acute renal failure, chronic renal failure, electrolyte disturbances, and hypertension, alone or in combination, are often encountered in patients who have had bone marrow transplants. The propensity of these patients to develop renal impairment is probably enhanced by the fact that their malignancy has been treated prior to transplant with potentially nephrotoxic agents; they may then be treated posttransplant with agents such as cyclosporine A, amphotericin B, and gentamicin. Cisplatin will be discussed in more detail because although it is one of the most useful antineoplastic agents, it is also one of the most nephrotoxic.

Cis-Diamminedichloroplatinum (II) (Cisplatin)

Mechanism of Action

The toxic effects seem to be the consequence of inhibition of DNA synthesis by alteration of the DNA template. Intrastrand cross-links are formed, mainly between guanine–guanine groups. The drug has synergistic cytotoxicity with radiation, 5-azacytidine, and cytarabine.

Pharmacology (See Reference 115)

Cisplatin is administered intravenously every 3–4 weeks, usually 50–120 mg/m^2 as a single dose or in divided doses for 5 days. It is diluted in physiologic saline because it is unstable and more toxic when chloride ions are not present. When chloride groups are exchanged for hydroxyl groups or water, a positively charged compound is formed that reacts with DNA. When this occurs *in vitro,* the positively charged compounds have difficulty entering the cytoplasm. Furthermore, platinum compound trimers and dimers, which seem to cause organ toxicity, are formed. After intravenous injection there is a triphasic plasma half-life decay at 0.3, 1.0, and 24 hours; the drug distributes in three compartments: unbound, protein-bound, and bound to erythrocytes. The plasma clearance of cisplatin is rapid after intravenous injection; 23–70 percent is excreted by the kidneys at 24 hours, and 90 percent is excreted within a few days. The half-life is prolonged in patients with renal failure and in those with ascites, as the latter may act as a reservoir for cisplatin.

Nephrotoxicity

Despite adequate hydration, GFR and renal plasma flow may be reduced even though the serum creatinine concentration remains unaltered.[116] GFRs have been measured in children receiving cisplatin by the plasma clearance of ^{51}Cr-EDTA method. The degree of cisplatin-induced reduction in GFR varied widely, and neither plasma creatinine concentrations nor creatinine clearances were found to be reliable guides to the GFR.[117] The precise cause of the reduced GFR is unknown, but it may be due in part to reduced renal blood flow and lowered effective filtration pressure.[118] The early changes in GFR in rats are partially reversible, but differences in renal vascular resistance and effective filtration pressure persist despite plasma volume expansion.[118] Urinary albumin and lysozyme to creatinine concentrations remain within the normal range.[117] Histologic studies reveal changes in the pars recta of the proximal tubule, in the distal tubule, and in the collecting duct.[119]

Hypomagnesemia was found in 21 of 37 patients during treatment and in 8 after cessation of cisplatin.[120] Seventy-six percent of patients became hypomagnesemic, and as many as 50 percent remained so for as long as 3 years after cessation of treatment.[120] This was associated with inappropriate renal wasting of magnesium. In cisplatin-induced hypomagnesemia in rats, abnormalities of magnesium metabolism involving kidney (abnormal excretion of magnesium) and intestine (reduced fractional intestinal absorption of magnesium), and a significant decrease in body magnesium and phosphorus stores were found.[121]

Hypomagnesemia may be accompanied by hypokalemia and hypocalcemia. Some patients may have a syn-

TABLE 45–6. RENAL DISEASES INDUCED BY ANTINEOPLASTIC AGENTS

ACUTE RENAL FAILURE
Cisplatin
Streptozotocin
Methotrexate
Mithramycin
Doxorubicin
Ifosphamide

CHRONIC RENAL FAILURE
Cisplatin
Lomustine (CCNU)
Semustine (Methyl CCNU)
Mitomycin

HEMORRHAGIC CYSTITIS
Cyclophosphamide
Ifosphamide

FANCONI'S SYNDROME
Ifosphamide

SIADH
Vincristine

TUBULAR DEFECTS
Phosphate Wasting
  Streptozotocin
Magnesium Wasting
  Cisplatin
Dilutional Hyponatremia
  Cyclophosphamide

drome of panhypoelectrolytemia.[122] Rats can develop polyuria despite reduced GFR; this is associated with decreased concentrations of sodium and urea in the renal papilla as a result of abnormal function of the collecting duct or pars recta of the proximal tubule.[123]

Mannitol, diuretics, variations in dosage schedule and, above all, adequate pretreatment hydration reduce the incidence and severity of the renal complications.[124] Cisplatin nephrotoxicity may be less common in children than in adults.[125] Identical total doses (mg/kg) caused less marked reductions in GFR and effective renal plasma flow (ERPF) in young than in adult rats. This may be due to the comparatively larger renal mass resulting in lower renal concentrations of cisplatin in younger animals.[126] Both captopril and verapamil[127] have been used in an attempt to prevent cisplatin-induced nephrotoxicity, but neither has been able to prevent the ultimate reduction in GFR.

The many other complications of cisplatin (hypersensitivity reactions, nausea, vomiting, bone marrow depression, neurotoxicity, ototoxicity, and Raynaud's phenomenon) must be kept in mind but have not been discussed in this chapter.

CYCLOSPORINE

The introduction of cyclosporine,[128] a potent immunosuppressive agent, has had an important influence on the survival of allografts. It is also being used in the treatment of diabetes mellitus type I and other conditions in which abnormalities of T-cell function seem to be important in their pathogenesis. Cyclosporine is a metabolite of the soil fungi *Cylindrocarpum lucidum* Booth and *Tolypocladium inflatum* Gams. It is a cyclic endecapeptide with a molecular weight of 1203. Cyclosporine depresses T-helper/inducer cell function, inhibits interleukin-2 production by T-helper cells, abrogates cytotoxic T-cell proliferation and development, and spares T-suppressor subpopulations.[129]

Cyclosporine is metabolized by the liver and excreted via the bile. About 10 percent of the total metabolites of the agent are excreted by the kidneys.[130] Rifampin, diphenylhydantoin, and intravenous trimethoprim–sulfadimidine reduce cyclosporine levels, whereas ketoconazole, cimetidine, and large doses of methylprednisolone may cause increased levels.

TABLE 45–8. NEPHROLOGIC COMPLICATIONS OF DRUGS USED IN THE TREATMENT OF NEPHROLOGIC PROBLEMS

DRUG	COMPLICATIONS
Aluminum	Bone disease
Cyclosporine A	Hemolytic uremic syndrome Chronic renal failure Magnesium wasting
Cyclophosphamide	Hemorrhagic cystitis Hyponatremia
Corticosteroids	Hypertension
Captopril	Acute renal failure ? Nephrotic syndrome
Furosemide	Nephrocalcinosis Metabolic alkalosis
Gentamicin	Acute renal failure Chronic renal failure Renal tubular dysfunctions
Hydrochlothiazide	Hypokalemia Hyperuricemia

Cyclosporine-induced nephrotoxic effects are very common and include mild and reversible renal insufficiency, acute nephrotoxic injury, and chronic nephrotoxicity with chronic renal failure.[96] A functional and reversible effect on the kidney is evidenced by the observation that the GFR may decrease soon after administration of cyclosporine and then return to normal after its discontinuation. The histopathologic findings of acute nephrotoxicity include no obvious changes, proximal tubular degeneration, tubular cell necrosis, tubular microcalcifications, mild interstitial lymphocyte infiltration without edema, and acute cyclosporine-associated arteriolopathy. Acute nephrotoxicity may be difficult to differentiate from acute rejection of the allograft and may be potentiated by other factors that can occur in association with renal transplantation. Chronic changes include segmental or diffuse fibrosis, tubular atrophy, and arteriolopathy. Chronic nephrotoxicity may be indistinguishable from chronic renal allograft rejection. Clinical features associated with cyclosporine nephrotoxicity include hyperkalemia, renal tubular acidosis, hypertension, and oliguria with low urine sodium excretion. Hyperuricemia without renal failure has been reported.[131] Factors that may enhance cyclosporine nephrotoxicity include increased bioavailability, increased blood hematocrit, pretransplant factors (hypotension in the donor, an older donor, a preservation time over 48 hours, previous treatment with cyclosporine), and posttransplant acute renal failure. Suggested optimal cyclosporine concentrations are shown in Table 45–7.

SELECTED REVIEWS

Adelman RA, Sinaiko AR: Drugs and the kidney, in Holliday M, Barratt TM, Vernier R (eds): 2nd ed. Williams and Wilkins, Baltimore, 1987, pp 252–271

Bennett WB, Muther RS, Parker RA, Feig P, Morrison G, Golper TA, Singer I: Drug therapy in renal failure: Dosing guidelines for adults. Ann Intern Med 93:286–325, 1980

TABLE 45–7. SUGGESTED OPTIMUM CONCENTRATIONS OF CYCLOSPORINE (μg/liter)[95]

ASSAY	EARLY POST-Tx PERIOD, 1–3 MONTHS	LATE POST-Tx PERIOD, 1>3 MONTHS
Serum RIA	150–300	50–150
Whole blood RIA	250–800	150–450
Whole blood HPLC	100–500	

RIA = radioimmunoassay; HPLC = high-performance liquid chromatography.

Levy G: Pharmacokinetics in renal disease. Am J Med 62:461–465, 1977

Relling MV, Schunk JE: Drug-induced hemorrhagic cystitis. Clin Pharmacol 5:590–597, 1986

Rieselbach RJ, Garnick MB: Renal diseases induced by antineoplastic agents, in Schrier RW, Gottschalk CW (eds): Diseases of The Kidney. 4th ed. Boston, Little, Brown and Co., 1988, pp 1275–1299

Roxe DM: Toxic nephropathy from diagnostic and therapeutic agents. Review and commentary. Am J Med 69:759–766, 1980

Trompeter RS: A review of drug prescribing in children with end-stage renal failure. Pediatr Nephrol 1:183–194, 1987

REFERENCES

1. Melmon KL: Preventable drug reactions-Causes and cures. N Engl J Med 284:1361–1368, 1971
2. Freed CR: Clinical pharmacology for the clinician, in Anderson RJ, Schrier RW (eds): Clinical Use of Drugs in Patients with Kidney and Liver Disease. Philadelphia, WB Saunders, 1981, pp 1–15
3. Bekersky I: Renal excretion. J Clin Pharmacol 27:447–449, 1987
4. Levy RH, Bauer LA: Basic pharmacokinetics: Therapeutic drug monitoring. Ther Drug Monit 8:47–58, 1986
5. Gibaldi M: The basic concept: Clearance. J Clin Pharmacol 26:330–331, 1986
6. Gibaldi M: Drug distribution in renal failure. Am J Med 62:471–474, 1977
7. Tiula E, Neuvonen PJ: Effect of total drug concentration on the free fraction in uremic sera. Ther Drug Monit 8:27–31, 1986
8. Braunlich H: Excretion of drugs during perinatal development. Pharmacol Ther 12:299–320, 1981
9. Morselli PL, Franco-Morselli R, Bossi L: Clinical pharmacokinetics in newborns and infants. Clin Pharmacokinet 5:485–527, 1980
10. Stewart CF, Hampton EM: Effect of maturation on drug disposition in pediatric patients. Clin Pharm 6:548–558, 1987
11. Warner A: Drug use in neonate: Interrelationships of pharmacokinetics, toxicity and biochemical maturity. Clin Chem 32:721–727, 1986
12. Somogyi A: New insights into the renal secretion of drugs. Trends Pharmacol Sci 8:354–357, 1987
13. Ross CR, Holohan PD: Transport of organic anions and cations in isolated renal plasma membranes. Annu Rev Pharmacol Toxicol 23:65–85, 1983
14. Cafruny EJ: Renal tubular handling of drugs. Am J Med 62:490–496, 1977
15. Mawer GE: Dosage adjustment in renal insufficiency. Br J Clin Pharmacol 13:145–153, 1982
16. Tozer TN: Nomogram for modification of dosage regimens in patients with chronic renal functional impairment. J Biopharmacokinet Biopharm 2:13–28, 1974
17. Dettli L: Individualization of drug dosage in patients with renal disease. Med Clin No Am 58:977–985, 1974
18. Dettli L: Drug dosage in renal disease. Clin Pharmacokinet 1:126–134, 1976
19. Levy G: Pharmacokinetics in renal disease. Am J Med 62:461–465, 1977
20. Kassirer JP, Harrington JT: Laboratory evaluation of renal function, in Schrier RW, Gottschalk CW (eds): Diseases of the Kidney, 4th ed, vol 1. Boston, Little, Brown and Co., 1988, pp 393–441
21. Kampmann JP, Hansen JM: Glomerular filtration rate and creatinine clearance. Br J Pharmacol 12:7, 1981
22. Herrington D, Drusano G, Smalls U, Standford HC: False elevation in serum creatinine levels. JAMA 252:2962, 1984
23. Dettli L: Drug dosage in patients with renal disease. Clin Pharm Ther 16:274–280, 1974
24. Chow MSS: Half-life prediction in unstable renal function: Its utility in therapeutic drug monitoring and theoretical and practical considerations. Ther Drug Monit 6:148–152, 1984
25. Fabre J, Balant L: Renal failure, drug pharmacokinetics and drug action. Clin Pharmacokinet 1:99–120, 1976
26. Manuel MA, Paton TW, Cornish WR: Perit Dial Bull 3:117–125, 1983
27. Maher JF: Influence of continuous ambulatory peritoneal dialysis on elimination of drugs. Perit Dial Bull 7:159–167, 1987
28. Paton TW, Cornish WR, Manuel MA, et al: Drug therapy in patients undergoing peritoneal dialysis. Clinical pharmacokinetic considerations. Clin Pharmacokinet 10:404–426, 1985
29. Lee CC, Marbury TC: Drug therapy in patients undergoing hemodialysis. Clinical pharmacokinetic considerations. Clin Pharmacokinet 9:42–66, 1984
30. Gibson TP: Principles of drug dose adjustment during hemodialysis. Am J Kid Dis 3:111–113, 1983
31. Keller F, Offerman F, Lode H: Supplementary dose after hemodialysis. Nephron 30:220–227, 1982
32. Baldwin DS, Levine BB, McCluskey RT, Gallo GR: Renal failure and interstitial nephritis due to penicillin and methicillin. N Engl J Med 279:1245–1252, 1968
33. Lehman DH, Egan JD, Sass HJ, Glode JE, Wilson CB: Antitubular basement-membrane antibodies in methicillin-associated interstitial nephritis. N Engl J Med 291:381–384, 1974
34. Sanjad SA, Haddad GG, Nassar VH: Nephropathy, an underestimated complication of methicillin therapy. J Pediatr 84:873–877, 1974
35. Tannenberg AM, Wicher KJ, Rose NR: Ampicillin nephropathy. JAMA 218:449, 1971
36. Ruley EJ, Lisi LM: Interstitial nephritis and renal failure due to ampicillin. J Pediatr 84:878–881, 1974
37. Donowitz GR, Mandell GL: Beta-lactam antibiotics. N Engl J Med 318:419–426, 1988
38. Wilson CB, Koup JR: Clinical pharmacology of extended-spectrum penicillins in infants and children. J Pediatr 106:1049–1056, 1985
39. Wellington PG, Craig WA, Bundtzen RW, et al: Pharmacokinetics of piperacillin in subjects with various degrees of renal failure. Antimicrob Agents Chemother 23:881–887, 1983
40. Bunke CM, Aronoff GR, Brier BS, et al: Cefazolin and cephalexin kinetics in continuous ambulatory peritoneal dialysis. Clin Pharmacol Ther 33:66–72, 1983
41. Johnson CA, Welling PG, Zimmerman SW: Pharmacokinetics of oral cephradine in continuous ambulatory peritoneal dialysis patients. Nephron 38:57–61, 1984
42. Hiner LB, Baluarte J, Polinsky MS, et al: Cefazolin in children with renal insufficiency. J Pediatr 6:335–339, 1980
43. Albin HC, Demotes-Mainard FM, Bouchet JL, et al: Pharmacokinetics of intravenous and intraperitoneal cefotaxime in chronic ambulatory peritoneal dialysis. Clin Pharmacol Ther 38:285–289, 1985
44. Heim KL, Halstenson CE, Comty CM, et al: Disposition of cefotaxime and desacyl cefotaxime during continuous ambulatory peritoneal dialysis. Antimicrob Agents Chemother 30:15–19, 1986
45. Ohkawa M, Nakashima T, Shoda R, et al: Pharmacokinetics of ceftazidime in patients with renal insufficiency and in those undergoing hemodialysis. Chemotherapy 31:410–416, 1985
46. Nikolaides P, Tourkantonis A: Effect of hemodialysis on ceftazidime pharmacokinetics. Clin Nephrol 24:142–146, 1985
47. Tourkantonis A, Nicolaides P: Pharmacokinetics of ceftazidime in patients undergoing peritoneal dialysis. J Antimicrob Chemother 12(suppl A):263–267, 1983
48. Martin E, Koup JR, Paravicini U, et al: Pharmacokinetics of ceftriaxone in neonates and infants with meningitis. J Pediatr 105:475–481, 1984
49. Kowalsky SF, Echols RM, Parker MA: Pharmacokinetics of ceftriaxone in subjects with renal insufficiency. Clin Pharm 4:177–181, 1985
50. Ti T-Y, Fortin L, Kreeft JH, et al: Kinetic disposition of intravenous ceftriaxone in normal subjects and patients with renal failure on hemodialysis or peritoneal dialysis. Antimicrob Agents Chemother 25:83–87, 1984
51. Cohen D, Appel GB, Scully B, et al: Pharmacokinetics of ceftriaxone in patients with renal failure and in those undergoing hemodialysis. Antimicrob Agents Chemother 24:529–532, 1983
52. Albin H, Demotes-Mainard F, Vincon G, et al: Pharmacokinetics

of antibiotics in chronic ambulatory peritoneal dialysis (Abstr.). Acta Pharmacol Toxicol 195:1222, 1986

53. Scaad UB, McCracken GH, Nelson JD: Clinical pharmacology and efficiency of vancomycin in pediatric patients. J Pediatr 96:119–126, 1980

54. Moellering RC, Krogstad DJ, Greenblatt DJ: Vancomycin therapy in patients with impaired renal function: A nomogram for dosage. Ann Intern Med 94:343–346, 1981

55. Matzke GR, McCrory RW, Hastenson CE, et al: Pharmacokinetics of vancomycin in patients with varying degrees of renal function. Antimicrob Agents Chemother 25:433–437, 1984

56. Bunke CM, Aronoff GR, Brier ME, et al: Vancomycin kinetics during continuous ambulatory peritoneal dialysis. Clin Pharmacol Ther 34:631–637, 1983

57. Morse GD, Faroling DF, Apicella MA, et al: Comparative study of intraperitoneal and intravenous pharmacokinetics during continuous ambulatory peritoneal dialysis. Antimicrob Agents Chemother 31:173–177, 1987

58. Kraemer MJ, Kendall R, Hickman RO, Haas JE, Bierman CW: A generalized allergic reaction with acute interstitial nephritis following trimethoprim-sulfamethoxazole use. Ann Allergy 49:323–325, 1982

59. Hoppu K: Age differences in trimethoprim pharmacokinetics: need for revised dosing in children. Clin Pharmacol Ther 41:336–343, 1987

60. Hoppu K, Koskimies O, Tuomisto J: Trimethoprim pharmacokinetics in children with renal insufficiency. Clin Pharmacol Ther 42:181–186, 1987

61. Halstenson CE, Blevins RB, Salem NG, et al: Trimethoprim-sulfamethoxazole pharmacokinetics during chronic ambulatory peritoneal dialysis. Clin Nephrol 22:239–243, 1984

62. Kanfer A, Stamatakis G, Torlotin G, et al: Changes in erythromycin pharmacokinetics induced by renal failure. Clin Nephrol 27:147–150, 1987

63. Daneshmend TK, Warnock DW: Clinical pharmacokinetics of systemic antifungal drugs. Clin Pharmacokinet 8:17–42, 1983

64. Morgan DJ, Ching MS, Raymond K, et al: Elimination of amphotericin B in impaired renal function. Clin Pharmacol Ther 34:248–253, 1983

65. McCurdy DK, Frederic M, Elkinton JR: Renal tubular acidosis due to amphotericin B. N Engl J Med 278:124–131, 1968

66. Barton CM, Pahl M, Vaziri MD, et al: Renal magnesium wasting associated with amphotericin B therapy. Am J Med 77:471–474, 1984

67. Cherry JD, Lloyd CA, Quilty JF, Laskowski LF: Amphotericin B therapy in children. A review of the literature and a case report. J Pediatr 75:1063–1069, 1969

68. Heidemann HT, Gerkens JF, Spickard WA, Jackson EK, Branch RA: Amphotericin B nephrotoxicity in humans decreased by salt repletion. Am J Med 75:476–481, 1983

69. Bean B, Aeppli D: Adverse effects of high-dose intravenous acyclovir in ambulatory patients with acute herpes zoster. J Infect Dis 151:362–365, 1985

70. Blum MR, Liao SHT, De Miranda P: Overview of acyclovir disposition in adults and children. Am J Med 73:186–192, 1982

71. Peterslund NA, Black FT, Tauris P: Impaired renal function after bolus injection of acyclovir. Lancet 1:243–244, 1983

72. Deeter RG, Khanderia U: Recent advances in antiviral therapy. Clin Pharm 5:961–976, 1986

73. Boelaert J, Schurgers M, Daneels R, et al: Multiple dose pharmacokinetics of intravenous acyclovir in patients on continuous ambulatory peritoneal dialysis. J Antimicrob Chemother 20:69–76, 1987

74. Gasser TC, Ebert SC, Graverson PH, et al: Ciprofloxacin pharmacokinetics in patients with normal and impaired renal function. Antimicrob Agents Chemother 31:709–712, 1987

75. Shalit I, Greenwood RB, Marks MI, et al: Pharmacokinetics of single-dose oral ciprofloxacin in patients undergoing chronic ambulatory peritoneal dialysis. Antimicrob Agents Chemother 30:152–156, 1986

76. Boelart J, Valke Y, Daneels R, et al: The pharmacokinetics of ciprofloxacin in patients with impaired renal function. J Antimicrob Ther 31:87–93, 1985

77. Ralph ED: Clinical pharmacokinetics of metronidazole. Clin Pharmacokinet 8:43–62, 1982

78. Roux AF, Moirot E, Delhotal B, et al: Metronidazole kinetics in patients with acute renal failure on dialysis: A cumulative study. Clin Pharmacol Ther 36:363–368, 1984

79. Guay DR, Meatherall RC, Baxter H, et al: Pharmacokinetics of metronidazole in patients undergoing continuous ambulatory peritoneal dialysis. Antimicrob Agents Chemother 25:306–310, 1984

80. Hastreiter AR, van der Horst RL, Voda C, et al: Maintenance digoxin dosage and steady-state plasma concentration in infants and children. J Pediatr 107:140–146, 1985

81. Gault MH, Jeffrey JF, Chirito E, et al: Studies of digoxin dosage, kinetics and serum concentrations in renal failure and review of the literature. Nephron 17:161–187, 1976

82. Jellife RW, Brooker B: A nomogram for digoxin therapy. Am J Med 57:63–68, 1974

83. Valdez R, Groves SW, Brown BA, et al: Endogenous substance in newborn infants causing false positive digoxin measurements. J Pediatr 102:947–950, 1983

84. Campese VM, Feinstein EI, Gura V, et al: Pharmacokinetics of atenelol in patients treated with chronic hemodialysis or peritoneal dialysis. J Clin Pharmacol 25:393–395, 1985

85. Maher JF: Pharmacokinetics in patients with renal failure. Clin Nephrol 21:39–46, 1984

86. Wenting GT, Tan-Tjiong HL, Derkx FH, et al: Split renal function after captopril in renal artery stenosis. Br Med J 288:886–890, 1980

87. Donker AJM: Nephrotoxicity of angiotensin converting enzyme inhibition. Kidney Int 31(suppl 20):S132–S137, 1986

88. Lewis EJ: Glomerular abnormalities in patients receiving angiotensin converting enzyme inhibitor therapy. Kidney Int 31(suppl 20):S138–S142, 1987

89. Tack ED, Perlman JM: Renal failure in sick hypertensive premature infants receiving captopril therapy. J Pediatr 112:805–810, 1988

90. Duchin KL, Pierides AM, Heald A, et al: Elimination kinetics of captopril in patients with renal failure. Kidney Int 25:942–947, 1984

91. Vlasses PH, Larijani GE, Conner DP, et al: Enalapril, a non-sulfhydryl angiotensin-converting enzyme inhibitor. Clin Pharm 4:27–40, 1985

92. Lowenthal DT, Irvin JD, Merrill D, et al: The effect of renal function on enalapril kinetics. Clin Pharmacol Ther 38:661–666, 1985

93. Hirakata H, Onoyama K, Iseki K, et al: Captopril (SQ14225) clearance during hemodialysis treatment. Clin Nephrol 16:321–323, 1981

94. Dodson WE: Antiepileptic drug utilization in pediatric patients. Epilepsia 23(suppl):132–139, 1984

95. Asconape JJ, Penry JK: Use of antiepileptic drugs in the presence of liver and kidney diseases: A review. Epilepsia 23(suppl):65–79, 1982

96. Nogueira HJ, Hammond PG, Cutler RE, Foeland SC: Drugs and the kidney, in Gonick HC (ed): Current Nephrology, vol 10. Chicago, Year Book Medical Publ., 1987, pp 291–323

97. Appel GB, Neu HC: Gentamicin in 1978. Ann Intern Med 89:528–538, 1978

98. Kaloyanides GJ, Pastoriza-Munoz E: Aminonucleoside nephrotoxicity. Kidney Int 18:571–582, 1980

99. Pastoriza-Munoz E, Bowman RC, Kaloyanides GJ: Renal tubular transport of gentamicin in the rat. Kidney Int 16:440–450, 1979

100. Wilson TW, Mahon WA, Inaba T, et al: Elimination of tritiated gentamicin in normal human subjects and in patients with severely impaired renal function. Clin Pharmacol Ther 14:815–822, 1973

101. Luft FC, Kleit SA: Renal parenchymal accumulation of aminoglycoside antibiotics in rats. J Infect Dis 130:656–659, 1974

102. Edwards CQ, Smith CR, Baughman KL, et al: Concentrations of gentamicin and amikacin in human kidneys. Antimicrob Agents Chemother 9:925–927, 1976

103. Schentag JJ, Jusko WJ: Renal clearance and accumulation of gentamicin. Clin Pharmacol Ther 22:364–370, 1977

104. Klotman PE, Boatman JE, Volpp BD, et al: Captopril enhances aminoglycoside nephrotoxicity in potassium-depleted rats. Kidney Int 28:118–, 1985
105. Bennett WM, Hartnett MN, Gilbert D, et al: Effect of sodium intake on gentamicin nephrotoxicity in the rat. Proc Soc Exp Biol Med 151:736–, 1976
106. Provost AP, Adejuyigbe O, Wolff ED: Nephrotoxicity of aminoglycosides in young and adult rats. Pediatr Res 19:191–196, 1985
107. Adelman RD, Wirth F, Rubio T: A controlled trial of the nephrotoxicity of mezlocillin and gentamicin plus ampicillin in the neonate. J Pediatr 111:888–893, 1987
108. Sirinavin S, McCracken GH, Nelson JD: Determining gentamicin dosage in infants and children with renal failure. J Pediatr 96:331–334, 1980
109. Pijck J, Hallynck T, Baert SL, et al: Pharmacokinetics of amikacin in patients with renal insufficiency: Relation of half-life and creatinine clearance. J Infect Dis 134S:331–341, 1976
110. Cipolle RJ, Seifert RD, Zaske DE, et al: Systematically individualizing tobramycin dosage regimens. J Clin Pharm 20:570–580, 1980
111. Lesar TS, Rotschafer JC, Stroud LM, et al: Gentamicin dosing errors with four commonly used nomograms. JAMA 248:1190–1193, 1982
112. Melby MJ, Heissler JF, Grochowski EC, et al: Predicting serum gentamicin concentrations in patients undergoing hemodialysis. Clin Pharm 4:74–76, 1985
113. Bunke MC, Aronoff GR, Brier ME, et al: Tobramycin kinetics during continuous ambulatory peritoneal dialysis. Clin Pharmacol Ther 34:110–116, 1983
114. Smeltzer BD, Schwartzman MS, Bertino JS: Amikacin pharmacokinetics during continuous ambulatory peritoneal dialysis. Antimicrob Agents Chemother 32:236–240, 1988
115. Loehrer PJ, Einhorn LH: Cisplatin. Ann Intern Med 100:704–713, 1984
116. Meijer S, Sleijfer DT, Mulder NH, et al: Some effects of combination chemotherapy with cisplatinum on renal function in patients with nonseminomatous testicular carcinoma. Cancer 51:2035–2040, 1983
117. Womer RB, Pritchard J, Barratt TM: Renal toxicity of cisplatin in children. J Pediatr 106:659–663, 1985
118. Winston JA, Safirstein R: Reduced renal blood flow in early cisplatin-induced acute renal failure in the rat. Am J Physiol 249:F490–496, 1985
119. Dentino M, Luft FC, Yum MN, et al: Long-term effects of cisdiamminedichloride platinum (CDDP) on renal structure and function in man. Cancer 41:1274–1281, 1978
120. Schilsky RL, Anderson T: Hypomagnesemia and renal magnesium wasting in patients receiving cisplatin. Ann Intern Med 90:929–931, 1979
121. Mavichak V, Wong NLM, Quamme GA, et al: Studies on the pathogenesis of cisplatin-induced hypomagnesemia in rats. Kidney Int 28:914–921, 1985
122. Giaccone G, Donadio M, Ferrati P, et al: Disorders of serum electrolytes and renal function in patients treated with cis-Platinum on an outpatient basis. Eur J Clin Oncol 21:433–437, 1985
123. Safirstein R, Miller P, Dikman S, et al: Cisplatin nephrotoxicity in rats: Defect in papillary hypertonicity. Am J Physiol 241:F175–185, 1981
124. Weiss RB, Poster DS: The renal toxicity of cancer chemotherapeutic agents. Cancer Treat Rev 9:37–56, 1982
125. Kamalakar P, Freeman AI, Higby DJ, et al: Clinical response and toxicity with cis-Dichlorodiammine platinum (II) in children. Cancer Treat Rep 61:835–839, 1977
126. Jongejan HTM, Provoost AP, Wolff ED, et al: Nephrotoxicity of cis-platin comparing young and adult rats. Pediatr Res 29:9–14, 1986
127. Offerman JJG, Mulder NH, Sleijfer DT, et al: Influence of captopril on cis-Diamminedichloroplatinum-induced renal toxicity. Am J Nephrol 5:433–436, 1985
128. Borel JF, Feurer C, Gubler HU, et al: Biological effects of cyclosporin A: A new antilymphocyte agent. Agents Actions 6:648–675, 1976
129. Cohen DJ, Loertscher R, Rubin MF, et al: Cyclosporine: A new immunosuppressive agent for organ transplantation. Ann Intern Med 101:667–682, 1984
130. Wood AJ, Maurer G, Niederberger WW, et al: Cyclosporine: Pharmacokinetics, metabolism and drug interactions. Transplant Proc 15:2409–2415, 1983
131. von Graffenried B, Harrison WB: Renal function in patients with autoimmune diseases treated with cyclosporine. Transplant Proc 17(suppl 1):215–231, 1985

46

DIURETICS

JOSEPH R. SHERBOTIE *and* BERNARD S. KAPLAN

Attention to fluid and electrolyte balance has traditionally been a major part of caring for sick children. Despite such attention, situations arise in which fluid and biochemical balances become problems and may give rise to serious consequences. Diuretics, initially utilized to treat heart failure, have become widely used in numerous other situations in clinical medicine. As with any other medication, therapeutic benefits are accompanied by side effects, and because diuretics are among the most used, they have also become among the most abused medications in medical practice. Compounding the problem in pediatrics is the dearth of objective knowledge concerning their pharmacokinetics and pharmacodynamics in children. These problems are amplified by the fact that the child is developing physiologically, so considerations of specific age-appropriate approaches need to be taken if these medications are to be used rationally. Given the major voids in knowledge of the biodynamics of diuretics in children, the clinician needs guidelines to utilize diuretics correctly in infants and children. By understanding the basic mechanisms of action of these agents and the stages of physiologic development (particularly of the kidney), the usual regimens of diuretic use in children can be reviewed, and the medications may then be used in an enlightened manner.

The changes in renal function with age are reviewed because the kidneys are the major anticipated target organ of diuretics, and renal function plays a significant role in their peak effects and disposition. Renal physiology as it pertains to the effects of diuretics is reviewed as it is currently understood. The major classes of diuretic agents are discussed in relation to age-specific estimates of bioavailability, dosing, duration of action, metabolism, and significant side effects. Drug interactions that may be clinically important are noted. The appropriate selection of an agent in specific clinical situations is examined in light of known mechanisms of action and anticipated toxic complications.

DEVELOPMENT OF RENAL FUNCTION

Although diuretics have numerous systemic effects, natriuresis and increased urine flow are the most important. Differential effects of diuretics based on the level of renal maturity have not been studied in detail. A knowledge of the basic processes inherent to the maturing kidney is essential for judicious choice and use of diuretics. Much of the data on early renal functional development is based on studies in fetal and young animals, so extrapolation of this information to humans must be done with caution.

Renal development begins by the 3rd week of gestation and proceeds through three stages: pronephros, mesonephros, and metanephros. Only remnants of the first two stages contribute to the developed genitourinary system while the metanephros forms one functioning kidney. Nephron development proceeds centripetally from the juxtamedullary area to the cortex. This continues until all of the nephrons are finally formed anatomically at about 34 weeks of gestation. Functional maturity, however, takes longer. Blood flow and filtration rate gradually increase but remain quite low throughout prenatal and perinatal life. Prior to 34 weeks of gestation, renal blood flow and glomerular filtration rate (GFR) increase in direct proportion to increasing renal mass. Significant increases in renal blood flow and GFR occur only after 34 weeks of gestation. Renal blood flow and GFR increase dramatically in term infants within the first 4–7 days of life, with a longer lag period in the premature infant. GFR reaches mature levels earlier than tubular functions. This is exemplified by a higher fractional excretion of sodium, a decreased capacity for glucose reabsorption, tubular proteinuria, and a relative metabolic acidosis with a decreased threshold for bicarbonate reabsorption and reduced net acid excretion in the neonate compared to the adult. These functions mature at different rates, with maximum renal functional capacity occurring at 1–2 years of age. The immature kidney has maximal diluting capacity, but a decreased GFR makes it less able to promptly excrete a fluid and solute load. The concentrating ability of the neonatal kidney is much less than that of the older child or adult (700–800 mOsm/kg compared to 1200–1400 mOsm/kg).[1]

The kidneys play a pivotal role in acid–base homeostasis. This involves reclamation of filtered bicarbonate in the proximal tubule and to a lesser extent in more distal nephron segments, and net acid excretion by the collecting ducts. The renal tubular threshold for bicarbonate reabsorption corresponds to serum levels of approximately 20–21 mEq/liter in infants, possibly because of the heterogeneity of nephrons; lower values are seen in premature infants. Ammoniogenesis is decreased in the immature kidney and correlates positively with gestational age, so that net acid excretion is low. The newborn has little reserve to withstand additional stresses on the ability to excrete acid, and severe acidosis is commonly seen in critically ill neonates.[1,2] Agents with the potential for interfering with this delicate balance, such as carbonic anhydrase inhibitors, should not be used in neonates except in special circumstances.

PHARMACOKINETICS

Changes in body composition occur as the child matures. Additional factors affecting drug handling include alterations in gastrointestinal motility and absorptive capacity, hepatic blood flow and microsomal enzymatic activity, and renal functional changes.[3] These may all influence drug disposition in maturing individuals.

After absorption, biodisposition is affected by volume of distribution. Since children have relatively more total body and extracellular water, drugs that are water-soluble may have a larger volume of distribution and may have decreased peak plasma levels and possibly prolonged half-lives. Young children, especially neonates, have lower serum albumin levels and higher fatty acid concentrations, rendering a drug more or less available for metabolism, action, and/or excretion.[3] Indirect factors may affect drug distribution and bioavailability, as exemplified by competition for albumin binding between bilirubin and sulfa-based therapeutic agents. This increases the possibility of the toxic effects of diuretics in the neonate.

Infant hepatic microsomal enzyme systems, serum esterases, and overall synthetic capacity available to metabolize drugs are often less optimally induced than in the adult. The hepatic microsomal enzymes may be inducible and result in changes in metabolism of drugs and compounds handled in a similar manner.[3]

Excretion of administered agents depends on all routes of clearance. Renal clearance is important, even if it is not always the major mode of elimination. Because of low GFRs in the neonate, drugs eliminated by filtration may have longer half-lives. Paradoxically, however, gentamicin, which is excreted by glomerular filtration, can be

given in larger doses to neonates than to adults. Filtration is therefore not the sole factor influencing the dose, clearance, and likelihood of toxicity of gentamicin. Aminoglycosides are thought to be concentrated in cortical nephrons in mature individuals where they may cause toxic effects. Cortical nephrons are the youngest population in the neonatal kidney and have relatively less blood flow. Because of this, aminoglycosides do not effectively concentrate in these nephrons, and renal damage is therefore less likely. This formulation is being questioned because methods commonly used to detect decrements in renal function (e.g., serum creatinine measurements) are not sensitive enough to reveal functional impairment in neonates. This example serves to demonstrate that the clearances and potential toxicities of medications, especially in neonates, may be complex, and are dependent on interactions of numerous developing physiologic processes (e.g., differential blood flow, organogenesis). Dosing of many medications in neonates is likely to be based on clinical experience as well as the application of developmental principles. The possibility of drug toxicity or, alternatively, inadequate treatment should be kept in mind even after giving the "usual" neonatal dose, as the handling of drugs in neonates is not simple and may not be uniform. Measurements of drug serum levels compared to therapeutic levels adjusted for age, when known, and close monitoring of clinical and laboratory parameters where toxicity is possible are essential.

MECHANISMS OF SODIUM AND WATER TRANSPORT: POSSIBLE SITES OF DIURETIC ACTION

A classification of diuretic agents based on structural similarities is confusing. Drugs with similar structural characteristics may have very different potencies and mechanisms of action, while structurally diverse drugs may be equally potent and produce effects by similar mechanisms. The most useful classification system for diuretics is based on the site or mechanism of action, and this correlates with clinical potency and degree of natriuresis (Table 46–1).[4]

Diuretics require access to the luminal side of the tubule. This may be partially accomplished by filtration but occurs to a greater extent by tubular secretion. Most agents are secreted by proximal tubular cells, often via transport systems used to secrete organic acids. In the proximal tubule, solute (sodium) is absorbed actively with water following passively. This results in net reabsorption of about 70 percent of filtered volume and an isotonic filtrate. Sodium reabsorption is accomplished by coupling with a proton antiporter at the apical membrane. Intracellular sodium concentration is maintained at a low level by the Na^+, K^+-ATPase system at the basolateral membrane. A favorable gradient for sodium transport from lumen to cell is thereby produced. There is less of a proton gradient from lumen to cell, and this is maintained by the action of carbonic anhydrase (CA). Protons excreted into the luminal fluid are buffered by filtered bicarbonate. The

TABLE 46–1. CLASSIFICATION OF DIURETICS

TYPE	PRIMARY SITE OF ACTION	MAXIMAL FRACTIONAL SODIUM EXCRETION
Carbonic anhydrase inhibitor	Proximal tubule	Minimal
Loop	Thick ascending limb, loop of Henle	25%
Thiazide	Distal tubule	5–8%
Potassium-sparing	Cortical collecting tubule	3%
Osmotic	Variable (may affect many nephron segments)	Variable
Filtration	Glomerular (increase GFR)	Variable

carbonic acid so formed is converted to water and carbon dioxide by apical CA. The intracellular supply of protons is partially produced by the action of intracellular CA, combining CO_2 with H_2O to form H^+ and HCO_3^- within the tubular cell. This results in the reclamation of bicarbonate which would otherwise be lost in the filtrate with no net loss or gain of protons.[4,5] Several diuretics inhibit sodium (and water) reabsorption in the proximal tubule by inhibition of CA. Agents that inhibit the sodium–proton antiporter system may produce marked toxicity because of the importance of this transport system throughout the body. Additional sodium transport in the proximal tubule is coupled with organic acid, amino acid, and glucose transport, and, possibly, simultaneous chloride–bicarbonate and sodium–proton exchange.[4]

Water is removed from the filtrate as it proceeds into the deep medullary nephrons in the descending limb of the loop of Henle. Sodium is reabsorbed in the thick ascending limb of the loop of Henle (TAH) by an electroneutral cotransport system on the apical membrane with potassium and two chloride ions. A favorable sodium gradient is again maintained by a basolateral Na^+, K^+-ATPase which ensures a low intracellular sodium concentration.[5] Potassium and chloride ions must both have some way of exiting from the intracellular fluid. The basolateral membrane possesses an electroneutral potassium–chloride cotransport system which transports both ions into the peritubular fluid. The basolateral membrane also has a high conductance for chloride, which encourages its exit. Potassium ion exits into the tubular lumen via a high-conductance pathway at the apical membrane. Diuretic agents, by inhibiting sodium reabsorption in the TAH, increase the distal delivery of solute and therefore overwhelm the sodium reabsorptive capacity of more distal nephron segments, thus producing natriuresis. Drugs could act on the apical membrane, inhibiting the electroneutral Na-K-2Cl cotransport system or the potassium conductance channel. Possible sites of action on the basolateral membrane include the potassium–chloride cotransport system, the chloride conductance channel, or less likely, the Na^+, K^+-ATPase.[6]

In the distal convoluted tubule, a different electroneutral sodium–chloride cotransport system is probably located on the luminal side of the cell. Na^+, K^+-ATPase is responsible for active transport on the basolateral membrane. Inhibition of the sodium–chloride cotransport system in the distal convoluted tubule results in natriuresis.[6]

The cortical collecting tubule is composed of several morphologically and functionally distinct cell types with interspecies variation. The principal cell in this nephron segment is responsible for sodium reabsorption. The apical membrane allows the sodium ion to enter through conductive channels. Sodium is actively pumped out of the cell by a basolateral Na^+, K^+-ATPase, which also pumps potassium into the cell. Potassium exits the cell driven by higher intracellular potassium concentration via potassium conductance channels on the basolateral and the apical membranes. Because potassium conductance is greater on the apical membrane, net potassium excretion into the lumen (urine) occurs. Weak diuretic agents can inhibit the apical sodium conductance channel and/or the Na^+, K^+-ATPase.[6]

Inhibition of sodium absorption in the proximal segments, loop of Henle, and early distal tubule can result in increased concentrations of sodium delivered to the collecting tubule, with increased sodium absorption in this segment and consequent potassium and proton loss. Transport of NaCl from lumen to interstitium in the medullary segments of the TAH is crucial to generating a hypertonic interstitium, allowing urinary concentration to occur in the collecting tubules under the permissive influence of antidiuretic hormone (ADH). ADH increases the permeability of the deep distal nephron segments to water, but movement of water out of the tubule is dependent on a hypertonic surrounding extracellular milieu. Because of difficulties in studying deep nephron segments in intact kidneys using micropuncture techniques, diuretic effects on the concentrating and diluting capabilities of the kidneys under conditions of relative dehydration or water loading can provide valuable information on the site(s) of action.[4,7] Isolated single nephron perfusion techniques also have provided more direct evidence for the mechanisms of action.[4,5] Specific sites and modes of action will be discussed with each class of diuretic. Advantages of several classes of diuretics are listed in Table 46–2. Complications of diuretic use are shown in Table 46–3 and are explained within the text.

TABLE 46–2. ADVANTAGES OF EACH CLASS OF DIURETIC

Loop
  Very potent
  Efficacy with low GFR
  Redistribution of renal blood flow
  Oral and parenteral routes
  Calciuric

Thiazide
  Moderately potent
  Extensive clinical experience
  Hypocalciuric
  Oral route

Potassium-sparing
  Decrease in urinary potassium losses
  Decrease in production of aqueous humor, CSF

TABLE 46–3. COMPLICATIONS OF DIURETICS

	LOOP	THIAZIDE	POTASSIUM-SPARING	OSMOTIC	CA INHIBITOR
Volume depletion	+++	++	+	+++	−
Hypokalemia	+++	++	−	++	+
Hyperkalemia	−	−	++	−	−
Hyponatremia	++	+++	−	++	−
Hypercalciuria	++	−	−	+	−
Hypercalcemia	−	++	−	−	−
Hyperuricemia	++	++	−	−	−
Hypomagnesemia	+	+	−	+	−
Hypophosphatemia	+	+	−	+	−
Worsened glycemic control (preexisting diabetes mellitus)	−	+	±	−	−
Hyperlipidemia	−	+	−	−	−
Alkalosis	++	++	−	+	−
Acidosis	−	−	+	+	++

CARBONIC ANHYDRASE INHIBITORS

These agents are weak diuretics. Drugs with the sulfonamide nucleus are capable of varying degrees of CA inhibition and include acetazolamide, furosemide, and some thiazides. The noncompetitive inhibition of CA results in a decrease of available intracellular proton. Decreased proton availability will prevent coupled sodium reabsorption because the reabsorption of filtered sodium is active and is coupled to proton excretion. Filtered bicarbonate ions remain in the tubular fluid, since protons (hydrogen ions) are not available to combine with them and bicarbonate acts as a nonreabsorbable anion. Delivery of bicarbonate to more distal nephron segments is increased above their capacity for reabsorption. Bicarbonate is excreted and exchange of sodium for potassium in the cortical collecting duct is increased with concomitant potassium wasting.[5,6] CA inhibitors produce a hyperchloremic metabolic acidosis, which may be self-limited after a new steady state for bicarbonate reabsorption has occurred. They are utilized for specific inhibitory effects on the production of isolated body fluids. They are used for the treatment of glaucoma and in childhood hydrocephalus[6] because they decrease the production of bicarbonate-rich aqueous humor and cerebrospinal fluid (CSF). Transient increases in central nervous system pressure may occur early in the course of treatment with acetazolamide, perhaps because of increased cerebral blood flow prior to the inhibitory effects on the production of CSF by the choroid plexus. Their efficacy in the treatment of posthemorrhagic hydrocephalus is unclear, as varied results have been obtained.[8] Acetazolamide has been used in combination with serial lumbar punctures and/or furosemide in several of these studies. CA inhibitors may also be used prophylactically in hyper- and hypokalemic periodic paralysis, to prevent acute mountain sickness, and to treat volume-expanded alkalotic patients.[6] Isolated successes in the treatment of some seizure disorders have been reported, possibly related to systemic acidosis and/or nebulous central nervous system effects.[8]

Acetazolamide[4] is rapidly absorbed and reaches peak levels in 2 hours, is secreted into the tubular lumen, and binds to CA. The drug undergoes no known significant metabolic changes. It is excreted by the kidneys and is not detectable in the serum of adults after 24 hours. The usual starting dosage is 5 mg/kg/dose given orally every 6–8 hours, with the maximum dose 25 mg/kg/dose. The activity of renal CA must be almost totally inhibited before a clinical effect can be observed. Because the infant has less intrinsic CA activity, lower doses are usually sufficient in this age group, and unnecessarily high doses should be avoided.[6,8] Specific pharmacokinetic data are not available for neonates.

The acidosis produced may, at least theoretically, adversely affect growth in children. Base supplements can be administered, but this may blunt some of the therapeutic benefits that may depend on the acidosis. Severe metabolic acidosis has been reported with the combination of CA inhibitors and salicylates.[9] The mechanism of this interaction may be related to decreased availability of carbon dioxide when high salicylate levels produce hypocapnia. This provides less substrate for the production of bicarbonate (independent of CA activity), thus interfering with the mechanism limiting the degree of acidosis. Use of CA inhibitors in the presence of renal failure may also result in severe acidosis because of the inability of damaged tubules to reabsorb bicarbonate distally. High doses may result in paresthesias and drowsiness, and occasional side effects in adults have included bone marrow suppression, fever, rash, and interstitial nephritis. Caution is warranted when acetazolamide is used in liver disease[6] because decreased luminal availability of protons may result in a loss of ammonia-trapping capacity.

LOOP DIURETICS

The fortuitous discovery in 1919 of the natriuretic effects of organomercurial compounds provided an impetus to search for agents that would have the same effects on renal salt and water loss but would avoid toxicity and the necessity for parenteral administration. It was only in the mid-1960s that two drugs, ethacrynic acid and furosemide, were introduced almost simultaneously. Since that time, several additional agents have been developed.[4]

The loop or "high ceiling" diuretics are the most potent

diuretic agents available. As a group, they are six to eight times more potent than thiazide diuretics. Each drug has its own peculiar site(s) of action in the tubule in addition to the major site common to the group. Na–K–2Cl cotransport in the cortical and medullary TAH, which is generally responsible for production of hypotonic tubular fluid, is blocked.[4-6] In addition to this interference with urine dilution, decreased NaCl transport to the medullary interstitium decreases medullary tonicity. This prevents maximal urinary concentration and decreases free water reabsorption, even in the presence of ADH. The ability of more distal nephron segments to reabsorb tubular sodium is overcome, and up to 20–25 percent of filtered sodium may be excreted. Loop diuretics increase renal medullary blood flow in part by stimulating production of vasodilatory prostaglandins. They are effective even in significant renal insufficiency with GFRs less than 25 percent of normal.[6,8]

Furosemide is the most frequently used diuretic. The pharmacodynamics of its diuretic effect(s) in children have only recently been examined.[10,11] Furosemide is a sulfonamide derivative. Both oral and intravenous administration result in a predictable diuresis. The usual effective dose is 1 mg/kg. The maximum recommended dose is 2 mg/kg/dose parenterally or 6 mg/kg/dose orally,[8] although higher doses may occasionally be given parenterally to a patient with renal failure in an attempt to promote diuresis when significant volume overload is present or to convert an oliguric into a more easily manageable nonoliguric form of renal failure. Its bioavailability after an oral dose appears to decrease in renal failure: approximately 45 percent of the administered dose in renal failure compared to 65 percent in individuals with normal renal function.[8] The drug must be transported to the tubular lumen to exert its effects. Binding to serum albumin is important for promoting uptake into renal tubular cells.[12] Volume-expanded and hypoalbuminemic patients generally have higher total plasma clearance of furosemide and higher volumes of distribution. These factors often result in prolonged half-lives and prolonged duration of action, which may be 40 minutes in normal adults and 8–20 hours in young or volume-expanded patients who have relatively decreased GFRs. The dosing interval can be determined by the observed duration of the diuretic effect in a patient, taking a 6- to 8-hour interval as a starting point. Dosing in neonates is discussed later in this chapter. The diuretic effect generally begins within 30 minutes of administration and peaks at 1–2 hours. Furosemide is tightly bound to plasma proteins (98 percent).[6] The drug is excreted primarily via the proximal tubule organic acid transport system, and to a lesser extent by filtration. In the presence of decreased GFR and/or tubular dysfunction, glucuronide conjugation by the liver and intestine becomes more prominent and the half-life is prolonged. Furosemide produces a 10- to 35-fold increase in sodium excretion and a 10-fold increase in urine flow rate in infants.[3] ADH administration does not prevent furosemide's ability to increase free water clearance.[7] Explanations for this effect include interference with the action of ADH in the collecting duct, the high tubular flow rate preventing equilibration with the relatively

hypertonic medullary interstitium, and CA inhibition resulting in increased urinary bicarbonate excretion.

Ethacrynic acid is used less frequently than furosemide, but its pharmacokinetics in adults and effects on urine flow are similar. There are few studies in children. It may be given orally or intravenously, usually at 1 mg/kg/dose. The onset of action after an oral dose is approximately 15–30 minutes, with peak action occurring after 30–60 minutes. The time to onset and peak of action using intravenous dosing is about half that of an oral dose, with a proportional decrease in duration of action. Ethacrynic acid is more lipid-soluble than the other loop diuretics, but more than 90 percent is bound to plasma proteins. Although some is filtered, it is mainly secreted by probenecid-sensitive proximal tubule organic acid transport systems. The ethacrynic acid–cysteine complex is the active product in the tubular lumen. Ethacrynic acid does not have detectable anti-CA activity and does not increase free water clearance. It may increase or redistribute renal blood flow with shunting away from superficial cortical to deeper nephrons, but it has not been shown to change cardiopulmonary hemodynamics independently of its diuretic effects.[6,8] Ethacrynic acid has been used after apparent furosemide resistance in the belief that ethacrynic acid is more toxic and that it may be effective in situations in which furosemide is ineffective. This view has not been validated in a carefully conducted study (Chemtob et al., unpublished communication). Gastrointestinal irritation is greater using ethacrynic acid, but other toxic effects at conventional doses have not been convincingly greater. However, it has become the practice to document a lack of response to furosemide before using ethacrynic acid in infants.

Bumetanide, a metanilamide derivative, may be less dependent on active tubular secretion, gaining access to the tubular lumen by diffusing across tubular cells by virtue of its lipid solubility. Most is transported by the same organic acid transport system as the other loop diuretics. Approximately 96 percent of bumetanide is tightly bound to plasma proteins. An equipotent oral dose of bumetanide is 1/40 that of furosemide, suggesting an oral dose of 0.01–0.02 mg/kg/dose. Its pharmacokinetics have been studied in infants under 6 months of age with congenital heart disease and volume overload.[3] Significant extrarenal metabolism or clearance occurs, with the renal clearance accounting for 30 percent of total plasma clearance. The half-life is variable and ranges from 1 to 5 hours. The dose used in children is an extrapolation from adult data, because studies in which the doses in pediatric patients have been determined have not been published.[6-8]

The loop diuretics indacrinone, L-ozolinone, and muzolimine have not been used in children. These drugs, and to some extent ethacrynic acid, may act at least partially on the basolateral surface of the tubular cells in the TAH by inhibiting potassium–chloride cotransport. Furosemide has this effect only with very high serum concentrations.[6]

Furosemide has been used in the management of respiratory distress syndrome (RDS) in neonates and bronchopulmonary dysplasia (BPD) in infants.[13,14] Its use in these conditions rapidly improves the clinical status before there is an observable effect on urine output.[15] Hypercapnia and the work of breathing are reduced, possibly as a consequence of hemodynamic changes and mobilization of pulmonary interstitial edema.[13,16–20] Furosemide selectively and rapidly favors water movement from interstitial to intracellular compartments following parenteral administration to infants with chronic lung disease.[21] All these beneficial effects occur despite an absence of improvement in arterial pO_2, a consistent reduction in alveolar to arterial O_2 gradient, or closure of a patent ductus arteriosus.[16,22] The improvement in lung compliance has not been sustained for longer than 4 hours after a dose,[19] despite much longer half-lives. Loop diuretics increase venous capacitance independently of their diuretic effects on the kidney. This results in decreased preload by lessening venous return to the heart and thereby reduces pulmonary edema.[6] A decrease of transvascular migration of fluid into the pulmonary interstitium has been observed in animals, but the changes in pulmonary lymph flow have been inconsistent.[19] Despite all these observations, three caveats are warranted: a nondiuretic action of furosemide in neonates with pulmonary edema has not been proven,[19,22] there is no reduction in the prevalence of BPD in infants with RDS treated with furosemide, nor is there a decreased mortality rate.[22]

Interpretation of studies on the use of furosemide in BPD is difficult, as the criteria for inclusion of neonates with chronic lung disease, choice of the parameters that are monitored, specific dosage regimens, and time after dosing chosen to study pulmonary effects have been variable. Pulmonary mechanics and gas exchange have been measured as early as 20 minutes after a single intravenous dose of furosemide.[17] Some investigators have used the onset of diuresis to determine the adequacy of doses of furosemide for subsequent pulmonary studies.[23] Comparison of furosemide with a combination of spironolactone and a thiazide diuretic, after 7 days of therapy, suggested that despite similar increases in urine output in both groups, only the furosemide group exhibited significant improvement in pulmonary mechanics.[15] Most studies have dealt with short-term parenteral therapy of less than 7 days. Longer durations of therapy have been studied in which thiazides and antikaliuretic agents have been used.[24,25] The general effects of furosemide use in BPD are increased pulmonary dynamic compliance[16–18,23,26] and decreased airway resistance.[16,18,20] In one study, airway resistance decreased but improvement in pulmonary compliance was not significant.[20] Improvements in pO_2 are not consistent findings.[16,20,26] Reports of improvement in venous admixtures suggest better matching of ventilation and perfusion.[23]

An improvement in the overall outcome of BPD and a sustained improvement of gas exchange is not at all clear.[27] Dose–response effects have not been properly examined, and perhaps much lower doses of loop diuretics may be as effective as doses currently employed in BPD. In addition, other therapeutic agents may have the same pulmonary effects without the adverse reactions of loop diuretics if the pulmonary effects can indeed be separated from the diuresis. Further investigations are indicated. At present, the use of loop diuretics in BPD must be accompanied by conscientious monitoring to avoid toxic effects, especially nephrocalcinosis and renal calculus formation. Concomitant use of thiazide anticalciuric agents may be beneficial for avoiding or minimizing hypercalciuria, but these carry the possibility of their own complications. The lowest effective dose of an agent to produce the specific desired effect(s) should be used, with the end point being improvement of pulmonary status rather than the onset of diuresis. Prolonged furosemide administration to this group of young patients has resulted in secondary hyperparathyroidism,[28] nephrocalcinosis,[29–33] hypercalciuria, and bone demineralization. Several of these adverse effects may have detrimental effects on growth. Marked chloride depletion and metabolic alkalosis in infants with severe BPD treated with diuretics, particularly furosemide, has been associated with increased morbidity. An increased incidence of hypertension, hypoventilation, weakness, and poor head growth was noted in the infants with the most severe metabolic abnormalities.[34]

Reabsorption of the divalent cations calcium and magnesium relies on luminal membrane positivity, and therefore the inhibition of chloride anion resorption by loop diuretics results in urinary calcium and magnesium losses. This may have beneficial effects in the treatment of hypercalcemia or may produce unwanted negative calcium or magnesium balance. Of particular importance is the increased prevalence of nephrolithiasis and nephrocalcinosis in neonates treated with loop diuretics for BPD.[29–33] This may be dose-dependent, with an association with doses of more than 2 mg/kg/day for more than 12 days.[31] More sensitive screening methods suggest that a lower dose will produce similar problems.[33] The etiology is likely to be multifactorial, with high calcium intake, low phosphorus intake, vitamin D supplementation, corticosteroid therapy, immature renal acidification mechanisms, and other issues contributing to promote renal calcification,[29] but furosemide use appears to be present in most cases. Furosemide may decrease the excretion of urinary inhibitors of calcification,[35] but this is not documented. Although the total excretion of urinary citrate is normal in this group of premature infants, the molar concentration of citrate and its relationship to concentrations of stone-promoting substances have not been examined. Retrospective study in preterm neonates has suggested that renal calcification generally improves with time if precipitating factors are eliminated, but a degree of diminished renal function may persist in some patients.[29]

Urinary calcium excretion in neonates relative to GFR normally may be greater than in older patients, and their urinary calcium-to-creatinine ratio may be increased.[36] Others have found similar values in adults and in neonates.[37] This increase in urinary calcium excretion is potentiated by a low phosphorus intake.[38] Phosphorus depletion may result in increased vitamin D–dependent absorption of calcium in the gut in the absence of sufficient enteral phosphorus. The use of a calciuric loop diuretic may potentiate these effects, resulting in decreased substrates available for proper bone mineralization.

Furosemide has been shown to keep the ductus arteriosus patent in patients with RDS, possibly by stimulating prostaglandin E_2, a potent dilator of ductal tissue.[39] Intravascular volume and lung water may decrease with furosemide treatment, but the patent ductus arteriosus may persist. Indomethacin has been used successfully to constrict or close the ductus. Furosemide has been combined with indomethacin in order to protect the kidneys from the effects of indomethacin, which may decrease GFR by reducing renal blood flow or by preventing the potentiation of vasopressin action, without affecting patent ductus arteriosus closure.[40,41]

The mechanism for the induction of gallstones or cholecystitis in patients treated with parenteral alimentation and furosemide is not understood.[42]

The most common adverse effects of loop diuretics are volume and potassium depletion.[6,8] The latter is related to increased distal nephron sodium delivery in the face of aldosterone release with resultant nonstoichiometric exchange for potassium. Hypokalemia may become more dangerous in patients receiving cardiac glycosides. Treatment with either potassium-sparing diuretics or potassium supplements is reasonable, but in general one should avoid using both. Increasing potassium administration to a patient with a decreased GFR should be done very cautiously. Volume depletion can be avoided by the judicious use of loop diuretics, paying attention to the patient's weight, volume status, and coexisting conditions that might increase extrarenal fluid and electrolyte losses. In addition, concomitant therapy with diuretic agents from another class, particularly thiazides, can result in markedly decreased intravascular volume and also hyponatremia.

Hearing loss is a major potential complication of toxic levels of loop diuretics. The prolonged half-life of the drug in premature infants may allow toxic levels to be reached inadvertently. The half-life of furosemide is inversely related to postconceptional age in neonates. Doses given every 12 hours to neonates less than 29 weeks postconceptional age produced potentially ototoxic plasma levels. Furosemide half-life fell with increasing postconceptional age. Furosemide is mainly excreted by the kidneys in neonates and depends on mature GFR and tubular secretory mechanisms. Dosing every 24 hours or using even longer intervals is necessary in order to avoid potentially toxic plasma levels of furosemide from accumulating in neonates less than 31 weeks postconceptional age. Longer dosage intervals of 12 hours are recommended for older preterm neonates.[10] The combination of loop diuretics with other ototoxic agents, particularly aminoglycoside antibiotics, potentiates ototoxicity, and these combinations should be used cautiously.[43]

Interstitial nephritis and serum sickness have been reported following the use of loop diuretics, particularly furosemide.[6,44,45]

THIAZIDE DIURETICS

The discovery in the mid- to late 1950s of the diuretic properties of the sulfonamides was the first major breakthrough in diuretic therapy since the discovery of the diuretic properties of the relatively toxic organomercurials.[4] These agents are today known as thiazide diuretics. Despite extensive clinical use, their precise mechanisms of action remain unclear. The maximal potency of these agents is less than loop diuretics in that they prevent 5–7 percent of filtered sodium from being reabsorbed. Although doses among agents vary widely, all thiazides have the same maximal diuretic effect. They are incompletely absorbed from the gastrointestinal tract, begin to act within 60 minutes of administration, and require access to the renal tubular fluid to exert their natriuretic effects. This is accomplished by a probenicid-sensitive organic acid transport pathway in the proximal straight tubule.[6]

The thiazides are potent inhibitors of coupled electroneutral sodium–chloride transport. This information is derived from data in which decreased free water clearance was found without effects on free water reabsorption. The most likely site of action is in the cortical diluting segment, or more specifically, the proximal portion of the distal tubule.[3,6]

The half-lives of different thiazides depend on lipid solubility and are longer in the more lipid-soluble drugs, which also have greater volumes of distribution. *Hydrochlorothiazide* and *chlorothiazide* are the most widely used thiazide diuretics in infants and children. Suggested dosages for hydrochlorothiazide are 1–3 mg/kg/day orally in children (adult dose 25–100 mg/day orally) divided every 12 hours. Chlorothiazide is given orally in a dose of 10–20 mg/kg/day divided every 12 hours (adult dose 250–500 mg/day orally).[3,6,8]

More recently developed thiazides include chlorthalidone, metolazone, and indapamide.[6] *Metolazone* is a thiazide-like diuretic with some proximal tubular effects. It is indicated in children because of its ability to produce a diuresis despite a decreased GFR, whereas the other thiazides are generally ineffective with a GFR under 35 ml/min/1.73 m². Despite this effect, the same proportion of filtered sodium (5–8 percent) is excreted.[3] The half-life of metolazone is prolonged in adults (8 hours), with diuretic effects lasting for more than 24 hours. Metolazone is approximately 95 percent bound to plasma proteins in adults. It is also filtered, but more importantly, secreted into the lumen of the proximal tubule, and there is evidence of enterohepatic recirculation. Some studies have suggested that there is less potassium wasting than with other thiazide diuretics. Metolazone possesses no significant CA inhibitory activity and does not promote bicarbonate loss. Significant changes in renal blood flow have not been demonstrated.[8] It has a synergistic effect when combined with furosemide, which can be beneficial, but it may induce unwanted volume depletion in combination.[46] Pharmacokinetic studies of metolazone in children are not available. Dosage in adults is 2.5–20 mg/day orally as a single dose. Appropriate pediatric doses have not been firmly established, but 0.1–0.4 mg/kg/day orally has been used.[46]

Thiazides decrease systemic blood pressure, but this mechanism is poorly understood. This effect may be the result of a decrease in intravascular volume, but thiazides also produce a sustained decrease in peripheral vascular resistance. Of particular importance is knowledge of the fact that antihypertensive effects are seen at low doses, and prolonged administration for months is necessary before a true steady state is reached.[6] Additional therapy for hypertensive patients therefore may be required initially. Low doses may be appropriate for blood pressure control to avoid possible dose-dependent adverse effects of thiazide therapy.[4]

The use of thiazides for the treatment of edema is most successful in patients with mild to moderate congestive heart failure,[6] and they are the drugs of choice for the initiation of diuretic therapy in this setting. Thiazides have also been used to produce a diuresis in infants with BPD.[24,25] Patients with the nephrotic syndrome tend to respond poorly to thiazides, but they may be efficacious in selected patients. Other than metolazone, thiazides do not produce a diuresis in the presence of significantly impaired renal function.

The remarkable urine volumes produced in patients with nephrogenic diabetes insipidus may be decreased with thiazides.[6] This apparently paradoxical response may be secondary to volume contraction producing increased proximal sodium and water reabsorption. These effects can be enhanced by decreasing dietary sodium. The acidosis of proximal renal tubular acidosis may be partially ameliorated in patients refractory to large quantities of base supplementation by treatment with thiazides.[6] Decreased intravascular volume results in a reduced filtered load, and a greater proportion of fluid and solute is therefore reabsorbed proximally.

Unlike loop diuretics, thiazides can decrease renal calcium excretion and have been used in the treatment of selected patients with idiopathic hypercalciuria.[6] The patterns of sodium and calcium reabsorption are very similar in different accessible nephron segments. This suggests that both cations may be handled by the kidney in a similar manner, though manipulations with parathyroid hormone (PTH) or thiazide diuretics can selectively affect fractional excretion of either cation. Induction of natriuresis in distal nephron segments using thiazides does not produce an analogous calciuresis, and PTH decreases urinary calcium excretion while concomitantly increasing urinary sodium losses. It appears that these differences are most pronounced in distal nephron segments.[6]

Thiazide-induced extracellular fluid volume depletion results in enhanced proximal tubular reabsorption of sodium and calcium.[47] Also, thiazide-induced decreased negativity of distal tubular fluid may promote calcium reabsorption and decrease passive calcium secretion.[6] Intact parathyroid function or appropriate supplementation with vitamin D may be necessary for thiazide diuretics to exert their anticalciuric effects.[47] When thiazides are used for the treatment of the renal leak form of hypercalciuria, sodium intake must be restricted to avoid overwhelming the renal calcium-absorbing mechanism.[48] Calcium balance has been variable when studied in patients taking thiazide diuretics, and possible negative calcium balance in growing children may be a concern. Measurements of renal calcium excretion in neonates receiving thiazides have been variable, and hypercalciuria may be seen in some of these premature infants. This may be related to immaturity of renal tubule functions, altera-

tions in parathyroid function, or typically high sodium and calcium intakes.[48] The criteria for thiazide treatment of hypercalciuria are imprecise and controversial at present, and the decision to use these agents in children must not be made casually, because long-term use is mandated. The occurrence of urolithiasis in the presence of hypercalciuria has been supported by some and challenged by other studies. Issues such as a past history of calcium-containing stones, a strong family history of nephrolithiasis, the possible embarrassment of renal function secondary to stones or calcium deposition, and the inability of more conservative attempts to decrease hypercalciuria or stone formation in these patients may be indications for administering thiazides.

There are many side effects of thiazides. Hypokalemia is often seen with thiazides when they are used for extended periods, especially in adults. Increased delivery of sodium to the distal nephron results in nonstoichiometric exchange of this cation for potassium and hydrogen. The effects of mild hypokalemia are controversial, but marked potassium depletion can occur and the levels must be monitored regularly.[4,6]

Excessive use of thiazides can result in volume depletion and possibly prerenal azotemia.[3,5,6] Hyponatremia may develop within days of beginning therapy in susceptible patients.[3,5,6,49,50] The postulated mechanism for the development of hyponatremia includes hypotonic fluid intake in the presence of hypovolemia because of increased thirst, with resultant stimulation of ADH release and increased water reabsorption. Free water clearance is decreased, and potassium depletion[50] may contribute as well because of a shift of sodium into cells to preserve their osmolal concentration when intracellular potassium deficit exists. Simultaneous administration of a thiazide and a loop diuretic can produce marked hyponatremia and volume depletion by these mechanisms and by decreasing urea transport to the medullary interstitium. This may occur by decreasing the transport of sodium, and therefore water, from the cortical distal tubule lumen. This prevents the usual increase in tubular urea concentration which normally serves to favor urea movement into the interstitium in the more distal urea-permeable segment of the collecting duct. By interfering with sodium and urea transport into the medullary interstitium, water reabsorption is decreased even in the presence of maximal ADH, and fluid losses are increased.

Thiazides may aggravate hyperuricemia, a potential problem for patients prone to complications of elevated uric acid levels.[3,5] Mechanisms include the competition for tubular secretion, and increased fractional reabsorption in the proximal tubule in the face of thiazide-induced volume contraction.[6]

Magnesium depletion may be related to the effects of elevated aldosterone. Urinary magnesium losses are increased. Magnesium depletion is important in the presence of hypokalemia, as the magnesium-dependent Na^+, K^+-ATPase is necessary to normalize intracellular potassium.[6]

Some patients develop hypercalcemia when taking thiazides as a consequence of a reduction in renal calcium excretion.[3,5,6] Contraindications for thiazide use include prolonged immobilization, vitamin D administration, hyperparathyroidism, and hypercalcemia because of a malignancy.

A metabolic alkalosis can be produced and maintained with thiazides.[3,5,6] This may be secondary to unreplaced chloride losses which enhance distal exchange of chloride for bicarbonate, increased proximal reabsorption of bicarbonate with volume depletion, and coexisting hypokalemia.

Carbohydrate intolerance may be worsened in patients with diabetes mellitus treated with thiazide diuretics, but their effects in individuals with normal glucose metabolism remain controversial. Hypokalemia associated with thiazide use has been shown to blunt insulin release, but the exact mechanism(s) remain unclear.[5,6]

Short-term use of thiazides often results in hyperlipidemia with effects on triglycerides and cholesterol. Elevations of low-density lipoprotein (LDL) and not high-density lipoprotein (HDL) cholesterol have been noted. This hyperlipidemia may partially resolve with continued use of thiazides.[6] Modulation of lipid profiles by thiazides should be kept in mind when considering diuretic therapy in patients already prone to lipid abnormalities or premature atherosclerosis. The mechanism whereby this occurs is not understood.

Associations of thiazides with pancreatitis, acute hepatitis, cholecystitis, and impotence have been reported.[6]

Thiazides can produce hypersensitivity reactions including dermatitis, vasculitis, interstitial nephritis, and occasionally bone marrow suppression.[6,44,45] They are contraindicated in patients with known reactions to sulfonamides.

In summary, thiazide diuretics can produce a moderate natriuresis, and additional systemic effects can be utilized in a variety of situations. It is prudent to utilize the smallest effective dose in a clinical situation to avoid toxicity, and appropriate monitoring of mineral levels is necessary. Potassium depletion occurs frequently and can be treated with supplements. Further depletion may be prevented or decreased with adjuvant use of antikaliuretic diuretic agents after repletion. These agents may also correct coexisting magnesium depletion. Angiotensin-converting enzyme (ACE) inhibitors may also result in decreased aldosterone stimulation, with resultant decreased losses of magnesium and potassium, though the potential for volume depletion and a markedly decreased GFR using this combination must be kept in mind.

POTASSIUM-SPARING DIURETICS

Potassium-sparing diuretics, first introduced in the 1950s,[4] are not particularly effective in producing a natriuresis or a diuresis and only inhibit the resorption of less than 2 percent of filtered sodium. The major use of these drugs is to prevent urinary potassium losses induced by other diuretics. Spironolactone is a competitive aldosterone antagonist, and triamterene and amiloride are noncompetitive inhibitors of potassium transport in the distal nephron.[5,6]

Spironolactone has a steroid-like molecule which competes with aldosterone for its binding site, primarily in the principal cell of the cortical collecting tubule (CCT). Aldosterone effectively promotes potassium secretion by increasing intracellular potassium concentration. Aldosterone stimulates the basolateral Na^+, K^+-ATPase, thereby producing a favorable concentration gradient for potassium to move out of the cell and into the tubular lumen. Aldosterone also further increases the negative potential on the luminal aspect of the tubule cells, providing a favorable gradient for potassium secretion. Aldosterone increases the number of apical membrane potassium conductance channels, allowing more potassium to move across the membrane into the tubular fluid of the CCT. All of these functions are inhibited when spironolactone displaces aldosterone from its binding site. Delivery of sodium to the lumen of the CCT also affects potassium excretion, because movement of luminal sodium into the CCT cell results in depolarization of the luminal membrane, thereby allowing potassium movement to occur more easily. Low intraluminal sodium concentrations limit potassium excretion, and low urine flow rates in this nephron segment also limit potassium excretion because of a less favorable concentration gradient.[6]

Spironolactone and salt restriction are used to treat patients with hepatic cirrhosis. Spironolactone is given orally (although an intravenous preparation of a metabolite, canrenoate, is produced, which has a half-life of about 20 hours) and is well absorbed, but gastrointestinal distress may occur. Spironolactone and its metabolite canrenone are 90 percent bound to plasma proteins. Significant clinical effects are seen only after several days of administration because aldosterone-induced protein synthesis remains active for 48 hours. Doses are 1.0–3.0 mg/kg/day divided into two to four doses. The maximum dose in adults is 200 mg/day. Spironolactone also decreases aldosterone synthesis and induces hepatic cytochrome microsomal enzymes. Spironolactone is useful in states where clinical signs are directly related to an excess of mineralcorticoids or their metabolites. These include some forms of hypertensive congenital adrenal hyperplasia, adjuvant therapy of primary and secondary hyperaldosteronism, adrenal tumors, and adrenocorticotropic hormone (ACTH)-producing adenoma. Because of the decreased urinary potassium excretion, the use of spironolactone in renal failure must be avoided if possible. Potassium supplements should be used with caution and with careful monitoring of electrolytes. Some ganglionic blocking agents may have prolonged effects in the presence of spironolactone.[6,8]

Triamterene, a nonsteroidal compound, is a noncompetitive inhibitor of distal nephron potassium secretion. It acts by inhibiting apical sodium conductance (absorbance) in the CCT. About 70–80 percent of an oral dose is absorbed and 50 percent is bound to plasma proteins. The drug is metabolized mainly in the liver by hydroxylation and sulfate conjugation. Conjugated metabolites, some of which are active, may accumulate in renal failure. Doses are 2–4 mg/kg/day once daily or divided into two or three doses and taken after meals. Maximum daily dose is 300 mg. Complications of triamterene use include hyperkalemia, potentiation of neuromuscular blockade by nondepolarizing agents, worsening of glycemic control, potentiation of lithium toxicity, crystallization of the drug in the urine, and reversible acute renal failure when used with nonsteroidal anti-inflammatory agents.[6,8,51]

Amiloride is another noncompetitive inhibitor of distal nephron potassium secretion with a similar mechanism of action to triamterene. Reports of use in children are scant. Amiloride is taken on an empty stomach; absorption is 50 percent. The drug is excreted mainly by the kidneys and is not significantly metabolized.[6]

In summary, antikaliuretic agents have poor natriuretic effects. Their major clinical use is in combination with other classes of diuretics that promote renal potassium losses. The site of action is in the CCT. Additional clinical uses include antagonism to aldosterone and in patients with hepatic cirrhosis in whom initially mild diuresis and natriuresis are needed to avoid problems associated with excessive volume loss. The major adverse effect of potassium-sparing diuretics is hyperkalemia. This occurs most frequently in the setting of decreased GFR, volume depletion with low urine flow rates and enhanced proximal tubule sodium reabsorption, and concomitant potassium replacement.

OSMOTIC DIURETICS

The glomerulus filters some small molecules that the tubule is incapable of reabsorbing. *Mannitol* is such an agent. Its molecules are osmotically active and proximal tubule fluid reabsorption is therefore inhibited. This results in increased urinary flow rates that prevent effective reabsorption of large quantities of electrolytes. Mannitol is also osmotically active intravascularly and consequently increases intravascular volume at the expense of extravascular volume. The increase in circulating plasma volume contributes to increased urine flow rates by increasing GFR. Mannitol increases renal vasodilation. Mannitol can be used to decrease intracellular fluid volume in patients with increased intracerebral pressure secondary to cerebral edema. It is also used to increase urine flow rates in patients with prerenal azotemia, and to prevent renal failure in the tumor lysis syndrome and in patients who are to be placed on cardiopulmonary bypass for cardiac surgery. In these situations it is usually given along with furosemide. The usual dose of mannitol is 0.25–2.0 gm/kg/dose given intravenously. Use of this agent in the face of existing intravascular volume overload, or increasing the potential for such in the face of a decreased ability to excrete mannitol, such as in patients with diminished renal function, is very likely to have adverse hemodynamic and/or pulmonary effects. Continued use will result in marked depletion of virtually all filtered electrolytes and minerals unless they are properly monitored and appropriately replaced. Administration of mannitol to premature infants may be detrimental, with abrupt changes in serum osmolality contributing to the incidence of intraventricular hemorrhage.[3,5,8]

Prolonged administration of mannitol and its possible effects on renal function are controversial. Anatomic changes of vacuolization and endocytosis occur in tubular cells, but their relationship to functional impairment is unclear.

FILTRATION DIURETICS

Glucocorticoids and *theophylline* are capable of increasing GFR. Positive inotropes which improve cardiac output and consequently improve renal blood flow are often used in an intensive care unit. *Dopamine* in low doses directly improves renal blood flow. One benefit of increased GFR is enhanced delivery of filtrate and possibly increased water and electrolyte excretion.

REFERENCES

1. Yared A, Kon V, Ichikawa I: Functional development of the kidney, in (Tune BM, Mendoza SA, Brenner BM, Stein JH) (eds:) Pediatric Nephrology. Contemporary Issues in Nephrology, vol 12. New York, Churchill Livingstone, 1984, pp 61–84
2. Arant BS: Renal disorders of the newborn infant, in Tune BM, Mendoza SA, Brenner BM, Stein JH (eds): Pediatric Nephrology. Contemporary Issues in Nephrology, vol 12. New York, Churchill Livingstone, 1984, pp 111–135
3. Witte MK, Stork JE, Blumer JL: Diuretic therapeutics in the pediatric patient. Am J Cardiol 57:44A–53A, 1986
4. Lant A: Diuretics: The current basis for use. Drugs 31(suppl 4):40–55, 1986
5. Anderson RJ, Schrier RW: Renal sodium excretion, edematous disorders, and diuretic use, in Schrier RW (ed): Renal and Electrolyte Disorders. Boston, Little, Brown & Co, 1986, pp 79–139
6. Jacobson HR: Diuretics: Mechanisms of action and uses. Hosp Pract 22(12):107–134, 1987
7. McNabb WR, Noormohamed FH, Brooks BA, Lant AF: Renal actions of piretanide and three other "loop" diuretics. Clin Pharmacol Ther. 35:328–337, 1984
8. Roberts RJ: Diuretics, in Drug Therapy in Infants: Pharmacologic Principles and Clinical Experience. Philadelphia, WB Saunders, 1984, pp 226–249
9. Cowan RA, Hartnell GG, Lowdell CP, Baird IM, Leak AM: Metabolic acidosis induced by carbonic anhydrase inhibitors and salicylates in patients with normal renal function. Br Med J 289:347–348, 1984
10. Mirochnick MH, Miceli JJ, Kramer PA, Chapron DJ, Raye JR: Furosemide pharmacokinetics in very low birth weight infants. J Pediatr 112:653–657, 1988
11. Prandota J: Pharmacodynamic determinants of furosemide diuretic effect in children. Dev Pharmacol Ther 9:88–101, 1986
12. Inoue M, Okajima K, Itoh K, Ando Y, Watanabe N, Yasaka T, Nagase S, Morino Y: Mechanism of furosemide resistance in analbuminemic rats and hypoalbuminemic patients. Kid Int 32:198–203, 1987
13. Bancalari E, Gerhardt T: Bronchopulmonary dysplasia. Pediatr Clin No Am 33:1–23, 1986
14. Costarino A, Baumgart S: Modern fluid and electrolyte management of the critically ill premature infant. Pediatr Clin No Am 33:153–178, 1986
15. Hazinski TA, Engelhardt B, Rush MG: Diuresis does not explain why furosemide improves lung function in infants with BPD. Pediatr Res 23(4) part 2:509A, 1988
16. Engelhardt B, Hazinski TA: What is the objective of furosemide therapy in infants with chronic lung disease? Pediatr Res 19:403A, 1985
17. Graff M, Novo R, Smith C, Hiatt IM, Hegyi T: The effect of furosemide on compliance (CDYN) in acute and chronic pulmonary failure. Pediatr Res 19:405A, 1985
18. Kao LC, Warburton D, Sargent CW, Platzker ACG, Keens TG: Furosemide acutely decreases airways resistance in chronic bronchopulmonary dysplasia. J Pediatr 103:624–629, 1983
19. Najak ZB, Harris EM, Lazzara A Jr, Pruitt AW: Pulmonary effects of furosemide in preterm infants with lung disease. J Pediatr 102:758–763, 1983
20. Tapia JL, Gerhardt T, Goldberg RN, Gomez-del-Rio M, Hehre D, Bancalari E: Furosemide and lung function in neonates with chronic lung disease (CLD). Pediatr Res 17:338A, 1983
21. O'Donovan BH, Bell EF: Furosemide acutely decreases interstitial

water but not cell water or blood volume of infants with bronchopulmonary dysplasia. Pediatr Res 23(4) part 2:420A, 1988

22. Yeh TF, Shilbli A, Leu ST, Raval D, Pildes RS: Early furosemide therapy in premature infants (≤2000 gm) with respiratory distress syndrome: A randomized controlled trial. J Pediatr 105:603–609, 1984

23. McCann EM, Lewis K, Deming DD, Donovan MJ, Brady JP: Controlled trial of furosemide therapy in infants with chronic lung disease. J Pediatr 106:957–962, 1985

24. Albersheim S, Sharma A, Solimano A, Smyth J, Rotschild A: A randomized double-blind controlled trial of long-term diuretic therapy in bronchopulmonary dysplasia (BPD). Pediatr Res 23(4) part 2:497A, 1988

25. Kao LC, Warburton D, Cheng MH, Cedeno C, Platzker ACG, Keens TG: Effect of oral diuretics on pulmonary mechanics in infants with chronic bronchopulmonary dysplasia: Results of a double-blind crossover sequential trial. Pediatrics 74:37–44, 1984

26. Singhal N, McMillan DD, Rademaker AW: Furosemide improves lung compliance in infants with bronchopulmonary dysplasia. Pediatr Res 17:336A, 1983

27. Aranda JV, Chemtob S, Laudignon N, Sasyniuk BI: Furosemide and vitamin E: Two problem drugs in neonatology. Pediatr Clin No Am 33:583–602, 1986

28. Venkataraman PS, Han BK, Tsang RC, Daugherty CC: Secondary hyperparathyroidism and bone disease in infants receiving long-term furosemide therapy. Am J Dis Child 137:1157–1161, 1983

29. Ezzedeen F, Adelman RD, Ahlfors CE: Renal calcification in preterm infants: Pathophysiology and long-term sequelae. J Pediatr 113:532–539, 1988

30. Gilsanz V, Fernal W, Reid BS, Stanley P, Ramos A: Nephrolithiasis in premature infants. Radiology 154:107–110, 1985

31. Hufnagle KG, Khan SN, Penn D, Cacciarelli A, Williams P: Renal calcifications: A complication of long-term furosemide therapy in preterm infants. Pediatrics 70:360–363, 1982

32. Jacinto JS, Modanlou HD, Crade M, Strauss AA, Bosu SK: Renal calcification incidence in very low birth weight infants. Pediatrics 81:31–35, 1988

33. Myracle MR, McGahan JP, Goetzman BW, Adelman RD: Ultrasound diagnosis of renal calcification in infants on chronic furosemide therapy. J Clin Ultrasound 14:281–287, 1986

34. Perlman JM, Moore V, Siegel MJ, Dawson J: Is chloride depletion an important contributing cause of death in infants with bronchopulmonary dysplasia? Pediatrics 77:212–216, 1986

35. Adams ND, Rowe JC, Liu RX, Swahney R, Lazar AM, Condren TB: Premature infants treated with furosemide (F) do not have reduced urinary citrate excretion (UcitV). Pediatr Res 23(4) part 2:530A, 1988

36. Karlen J, Aperia A, Zetterstrom R: Renal excretion of calcium and phosphate in preterm and term infants. J Pediatr 106:814–819, 1985

37. Arant BS: Renal handling of calcium and phosphorus in normal human neonates. Semin Nephrol 3:94–99, 1983

38. Rowe J, Rowe D, Horak E, Spackman T, Saltzman R, Robinson S, Phillips A, Raye J: Hypophosphatemia and hypercalciuria in small premature infants fed human milk: Evidence for inadequate dietary phosphorus. J Pediatr 104:112–117, 1984

39. Green TP, Thompson TR, Johnson DE, Lock JE: Furosemide promotes patent ductus arteriosus in premature infants with the respiratory distress-syndrome. N Engl J Med 308:743–748, 1983

40. Gouyon JB, Guignard J.P: Drugs and acute renal insufficiency in the neonate. Biol Neonate 50:177–181, 1986

41. Yeh TF, Wilks A, Singh J, Betkerur M, Lilien L, Pildes RS: Furosemide prevents the renal side effects of indomethacin therapy in premature infants with patent ductus arteriosus. J Pediatr 101:433–437, 1982

42. Bunyapen C, Howell CG, Kanto WP: Cholecystitis in a preterm infant. Clin Pediatr 25:96–97, 1986

43. Lynn AM, Redding GJ, Morray JP, Tyler DC: Isolated deafness following recovery from neurologic injury and adult respiratory distress syndrome: A sequela of intercurrent aminoglycoside and diuretic use. Am J Dis Child 139:464–466, 1985

44. Cotran RS: Tubulointerstitial nephropathies. Hosp Pract January:79–92, 1982

45. Linton AL, Clark WF, Driedger AA, Turnbull DI, Lindsay RM: Acute interstitial nephritis due to drugs. Ann Intern Med 93:735–741, 1980

46. Arnold WC: Efficacy of metolazone and furosemide in children with furosemide resistant edema. Pediatrics 74:872–875, 1984

47. Brickman AS, Massry SG, Coburn JW: Changes in serum and urinary calcium during treatment with hydrochlorothiazide: Studies on mechanisms. J Clin Invest 51:945–954, 1972

48. Atkinson SA, Shah JK, McGee C, Steele BT: Mineral excretion in premature infants receiving various diuretic therapies. J Pediatr 113:540–545, 1988

49. Ashraf N, Locksley R, Arieff AI: Thiazide-induced hyponatremia associated with death or neurologic damage in outpatients. Am J Med 70:1163–1168, 1981

50. Fichman MP, Vorherr H, Kleeman CR, Telfer N: Diuretic-induced hyponatremia. Ann Intern Med 75:853–863, 1971

51. Favre L, Blasson P, Vallotton MB: Reversible acute renal failure from combined triamterene and indomethacin. Ann Intern Med 96:317–320, 1982

47

VITAMIN A SUPPLEMENTATION IN THE VERY-LOW-BIRTH-WEIGHT INFANT

JAYANT P. SHENAI

Vitamin A (retinol) is a fat-soluble micronutrient recognized since 1912 as a constituent of the diet essential for promotion of growth.[1,2] The chemical structure of the active form of vitamin A, all-trans-retinol, was determined in 1931.[3] Vitamin A is transported in the plasma as the lipid alcohol retinol bound to a specific carrier protein, retinol-binding protein (RBP). The isolation and partial characterization of RBP was first reported in 1968.[4] The human RBP molecule consists of a single polypeptide chain with a molecular weight of approximately 21,000 and a single binding site for one molecule of retinol.[5,6] RBP interacts with another protein, transthyretin, and normally circulates in plasma as a 1:1 molar RBP–transthyretin complex.[7]

Vitamin A influences orderly growth and differentiation of epithelial cells, and its deficiency affects various organ systems, including the lung.[8] The characteristic histopathologic changes in the respiratory system generally precede other consequences of vitamin A deficiency.[8] The role of vitamin A in promotion of normal epithelial cell differentiation and function in the developing lung makes it an important nutrient during the perinatal period. This chapter focuses on the effects of vitamin A deficiency on lung injury and healing in very-low-birth-weight (VLBW) neonates and, more specifically, examines the role of vitamin A supplementation in these VLBW infants who are at risk for chronic lung disease.

RATIONALE FOR VITAMIN A SUPPLEMENTATION

Vitamin A deficiency results in a predictable sequence of progressive changes in the epithelial lining of the pulmonary conducting airways.[8-10] These changes are described as necrotizing tracheobronchitis in the early stages and squamous metaplasia in more advanced stages of the deficiency. The pathophysiologic consequences of these changes include: (1) loss of normal secretions of gob-let cells and of other secretory cells, (2) loss of normal water homeostasis across the tracheobronchial epithelium, (3) loss of cilia and resultant inability to move the mucous blanket in which bacteria or inhaled foreign particles may be trapped, and (4) probably some narrowing of lumen and loss of distensibility of airways with resultant increase in airway resistance and work of breathing. The histopathologic changes seen in vitamin A deficiency are reversible with restoration of normal vitamin A status.[11,12]

Examination of the tracheobronchial tree in VLBW infants who, after neonatal pulmonary insults such as hyaline membrane disease, undergo an abnormally protracted healing phase and subsequently die reveals the sequential epithelial changes classically described as bronchopulmonary dysplasia (BPD).[13] These changes also consist of necrotizing tracheobronchitis in the early stages and squamous metaplasia in more advanced stages of the disease. These changes in human infants with BPD and those in animals with vitamin A deficiency appear to be remarkably similar. Many of the clinical manifestations, such as recurrent atelectasis and airway infection typically seen in infants with BPD and in children with vitamin A deficiency, can be explained on the basis of the functional alterations caused by the histopathologic changes in the lung and the tracheobronchial tree.

BPD occurs commonly in VLBW infants susceptible to acute, subacute, and chronic lung injury.[13] The development of BPD in these infants is believed to be influenced by factors promoting tissue injury and healing involving the lung and the tracheobronchial tree. VLBW neonates are susceptible to repeated lung injury from such insults as hyaline membrane disease, prolonged and high inspired oxygen concentrations, barotrauma from mechanical ventilation, and secondary infection common with prolonged tracheal intubation, all occurring against the background of lung immaturity.[14] It is hypothesized that if vitamin A deficiency were present at the same time as injury, normal healing would not occur, resulting in worsening lung disease. Conversely, the

535

potential role of vitamin A in influencing normal differentiation of regenerating airways could have a favorable effect on the healing process, resulting in reduced pulmonary morbidity. To test this hypothesis, a series of clinical studies was performed to evaluate vitamin A status and its influence on lung disease in VLBW infants.

CLINICAL STUDIES ON VITAMIN A

Plasma Vitamin A Status at Birth

Plasma concentrations of vitamin A and RBP were measured in cord blood samples from newborn infants of various gestational ages.[15] The mean ($\pm$ SD) plasma concentration of vitamin A was significantly lower in infants born prematurely ($n = 39$) than in infants of term gestation ($n = 32$) (16.0 ± 6.2 versus 23.9 ± 10.2 μg/dl, respectively) ($p < .001$). Whereas normal plasma concentrations of vitamin A range from 20 to 80 μg/dl in healthy children and adults,[16] a high percentage (82 percent) of preterm neonates in this study had values of plasma vitamin A that were < 20 μg/dl. A plasma vitamin A concentration < 20 μg/dl is generally considered to be indicative of vitamin A deficiency.[16] Brandt et al.[17] have published similar values for cord blood concentrations of vitamin A. The mean ($\pm$ SD) plasma concentration of RBP was also significantly lower in infants born prematurely than in infants of term gestation (2.8 ± 1.2 versus 3.6 ± 1.1 mg/dl, respectively) ($p < .001$).[15] The normal plasma concentration of RBP (mean $\pm$ SD) in healthy human adults is 4.6 ± 1.0 mg/dl.[18] Plasma concentrations of RBP in children are approximately 60 percent of the adult values.[19] A plasma RBP concentration < 3.0 mg/dl is generally considered to be indicative of vitamin A deficiency.[20] A high percentage (77 percent) of preterm neonates in this study[15] had values of plasma RBP that were < 3.0 mg/dl. Bhatia and Ziegler[21] have published similar values for cord blood concentrations of RBP. These studies have shown that most VLBW infants are born with low plasma concentrations of vitamin A and RBP. It is possible that these infants are vitamin A deficient because of deprivation of transplacental vitamin A supply resulting from their delivery at an early gestational age.

Liver Vitamin A Reserve at Birth

Inasmuch as 90 percent of the total body reserve of vitamin A is found in the liver, measurement of liver vitamin A concentration gives an accurate indication of the vitamin A status of an individual.[22] The normal liver concentrations of vitamin A range from 100 to 300 μg/gm in healthy human adults.[23] The liver vitamin A concentrations in children vary with age, being low during infancy relative to later childhood, adolescence, and young adulthood.[24,25] A liver vitamin A concentration < 40 μg/gm is generally considered to be indicative of low vitamin A reserve, and < 20 μg/gm is generally considered as deficient.[22,24,25] The liver vitamin A reserve at birth was assessed in a group of VLBW neonates ($n = 25$) dying

within 24 hours of birth, prior to possible changes in vitamin A status induced by postnatal intervention.[26] The mean ($\pm$ SD) liver vitamin A concentration was 30 ± 13 μg/gm (range: 2–49 μg/gm). A high percentage (76 percent) of VLBW neonates in this study had values of liver vitamin A that were < 40 μg/gm, and approximately 37 percent of those infants had values < 20 μg/gm. Others[25,27–29] have published similar values for liver concentrations of vitamin A. These studies have shown that most VLBW infants are born with limited liver reserve of vitamin A. The potential ability of these infants to offset an inadequate vitamin A intake in the postnatal period is therefore limited.

Vitamin A Status in Bronchopulmonary Dysplasia

A prospective study was performed involving the assessment and comparison of the vitamin A status of two groups of VLBW infants (< 1500 gm birth weight, < 32 weeks gestational age). One group had clinical and radiographic evidence of BPD ($n = 10$), and the other (control) had no significant lung disease ($n = 8$).[30] The mean plasma vitamin A concentrations in infants with BPD were significantly lower than those of controls at four sampling times in the first postnatal month. In contrast to controls, the infants with BPD showed a substantial decline in their plasma vitamin A concentrations from the initial values. The lowest plasma vitamin A concentrations were seen at 3–5 weeks postnatal age and were markedly below the optimal level. Although a gradual increase in plasma vitamin A concentrations was seen in a majority of these infants during the subsequent 4-week period, a high percentage (88 percent) of individual values of plasma vitamin A continued to remain < 20 μg/dl during the 8-week postnatal period of observation. Delayed establishment of enteral feeding and a lower vitamin A intake in these infants relative to controls might have contributed to their low vitamin A status. The vitamin A status of infants with BPD in this study showed a typical biphasic pattern (Figure 47–1). During the initial phase of declining plasma vitamin A concentrations, the average vitamin A intake was < 700 IU/kg/day, and the mode of feeding was predominantly intravenous. During the subsequent period of increasing plasma vitamin A concentrations, the average vitamin A intake was > 1500 IU/kg/day, and the mode of feeding was predominantly by the enteral route. This study has shown that most VLBW infants with development of BPD manifest clinical, biochemical, and histopathologic evidence of vitamin A deficiency. Hustead et al.[31] have shown a similar association between vitamin A deficiency and BPD in their preterm infant population.

Clinical Trial of Vitamin A Supplementation

A randomized, blinded, controlled clinical trial was conducted to determine whether vitamin A supplementation from early postnatal life could reduce the morbid-

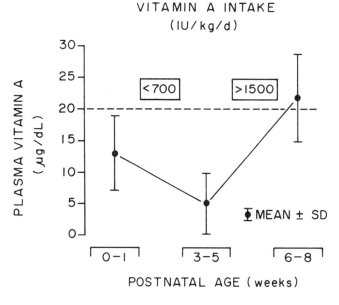

FIGURE 47–1. Biphasic pattern of plasma vitamin A concentrations in VLBW infants with BPD. Figures in boxes indicate average daily vitamin A intake during each phase. Plasma vitamin A concentration < 20 µg/dl is indicative of vitamin A deficiency.[16] (Adapted from Shenai et al.,[30] with permission.)

ity associated with BPD in VLBW infants.[32] Forty VLBW neonates (700–1300 gm birth weight, 26–30 weeks gestational age), who required supplemental oxygen and mechanical ventilation for at least 72 hours after birth, were given by the intramuscular route either supplemental vitamin A (retinyl palmitate 2000 IU) or 0.9 percent saline solution on postnatal day 4 and on alternate days thereafter for a total of 14 injections over 28 days. The study groups were comparable in gestational maturity, clinical characteristics, initial lung disease, and vitamin A status at entry into the trial. Vitamin A administration resulted in significantly higher mean plasma concentrations of vitamin A and RBP in treated infants when compared to controls. BPD was diagnosed in 9 of 20 infants given vitamin A supplement versus 17 of 20 control infants ($p < .008$). The need for supplemental oxygen, mechanical ventilation, and intensive care was reduced in infants given vitamin A supplement when compared to controls. Airway infection and retinopathy of prematurity were less frequent in the vitamin A group. The reduced incidence of retinopathy of prematurity in vitamin A–treated infants might have been related to their reduced exposure to prolonged and high concentrations of supplemental oxygen. This study has shown that vitamin A supplementation resulting in a total vitamin A intake between 1500 and 2800 IU/kg/day in VLBW infants not only improves their vitamin A status but also appears to promote regenerative healing from lung injury, as evidenced by decreased incidence and morbidity of BPD. Additional studies will be important in assessing the value of this therapeutic approach in the management of VLBW infants at risk for BPD.

PROTOCOL FOR VITAMIN A SUPPLEMENTATION

The beneficial effect of vitamin A supplementation shown in the clinical trial[32] has led to implementation in the neonatal intensive care unit at Vanderbilt Medical Center of routine vitamin A supplementation in VLBW infants at risk for BPD. According to the protocol, all infants meeting the following criteria are eligible for supplementation: (1) birth weight < 1300 gm, (2) gestational age < 31 weeks, (3) appropriate growth for gestational age, (4) no major congenital anomalies, and (5) requirement for supplemental oxygen ($FiO_2 > 0.3$) and mechanical ventilation for at least 24 hours after birth. These criteria are similar to those proposed by Bancalari et al.[33] to prospectively identify infants at risk for BPD. In addition to routine vitamin A intake from parenteral and enteral nutrition, these infants receive 2000 IU supplemental vitamin A by intramuscular injection on postnatal day 1 and on alternate days thereafter for a total of 14 injections over 28 days or until establishment of full enteral feeding. Full enteral feeding is considered established when energy intake by the enteral route exceeds 75 percent of total energy intake and when enteral multivitamin supplementation is initiated. A water-miscible preparation containing vitamin A in the form of retinyl palmitate is used for supplementation. Each unit dose of this preparation (2000 IU vitamin A) is dispensed by the pharmacy in a glass tuberculin syringe placed in a container shielding the solution from light and is administered within 30 minutes to the infant by the nursery staff. The site of intramuscular injection is rotated, and the appropriate standard of care related to intramuscular administration of a medication is followed.

Plasma concentrations of vitamin A are monitored before the first dose of supplemental vitamin A and at weekly intervals thereafter throughout the period of supplementation. The dose of supplemental vitamin A is adjusted based on these weekly plasma vitamin A concentrations. The target range of plasma vitamin A concentrations is 30–60 µg/dl. If the plasma vitamin A concentration is < 30 µg/dl, the dose of supplemental vitamin A is increased by 500 IU. If the plasma vitamin A concentration is 60–80 µg/dl, the dose of supplemental vitamin A is decreased by 500 IU. If the plasma vitamin A concentration is > 80 µg/dl, the remainder of the supplemental doses for the week are discontinued until a repeat measurement of plasma vitamin A concentration is performed the following week. All infants are monitored for evidence of toxicity, as described in the section on Vitamin A Toxicity.

VITAMIN A ADMINISTRATION

Nutritional management of VLBW infants is often complicated by difficulties in the establishment of enteral feeding. Vitamin A supplementation by the enteral route may therefore be precluded, particularly in early postnatal life. Vitamin A in human milk, infant formulas, and enteral multivitamin supplements is largely in the form of retinyl esters. Digestion and absorption of dietary fat and retinyl esters in VLBW infants may be limited by factors such as low pancreatic lipase activity,[34] reduced bile acid pool size,[35,36] and low concentrations of gut-specific cellular RBP (type two).[37] Transpyloric infusion is often used for feeding VLBW infants with lung disease, particularly those requiring mechanical ventilation or administration of continuous distending airway pressure. Bypassing the stomach, which is inherent in this method of feeding, may preclude intragastric dispersion and emulsification of dietary fat,[38] limiting absorption of retinyl esters. Several studies[39–43] have shown that the absorption of vitamin A by the enteral route is inefficient in preterm infants. Woodruff et al.[44] have made similar observations in formula-fed VLBW infants receiving enteral multivitamin supplementation.

VLBW infants experiencing difficulties with enteral feeding are often sustained exclusively with intravenous nutrition for prolonged periods. A protein–dextrose solution and a lipid emulsion are commonly used for parenteral nutrition. Various nutrients, including vitamins, are generally administered through the protein–dextrose solution. Vitamin A is subject to photodegradation[45] and also binds to intravenous tubing,[46] both potential sources of loss of the vitamin in transit from solution bottle to infant. The efficiency of vitamin A administration in parenteral nutrition solution was examined in an *in vitro* system.[47] A typical curve based on measurements of vitamin A concentrations in aliquots of the parenteral nutrition solution from the bottle and the effluent from one *in vitro* experiment is shown in Figure 47–2. If the expected delivery of vitamin A, based on a constant infusion rate and a fixed vitamin A concentration in the parenteral nutrition solution, was expressed as a 100 percent value, the mean (± SD) loss of vitamin A from photodegradation was 16 ± 9 percent and that from adsorption to intravenous tubing was 59 ± 9 percent. The net loss ranged from 62 to 89 percent, suggesting that even under optimal conditions, less than 38 percent of the expected amount of vitamin A was actually being delivered through the intravenous route. Gillis et al.[48] have made similar observations. These studies have shown that intravenous administration of vitamin A is inefficient because of substantial photodegradative and adsorptive losses of the vitamin. It is suggested that fat-soluble vitamins, including vitamin A, might be incorporated into the micellar phase of lipid emulsions and would therefore be potentially protected

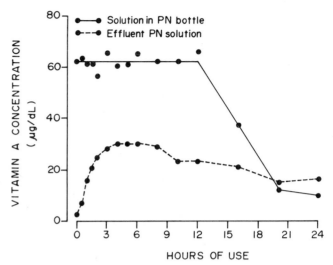

FIGURE 47–2. Concentrations of vitamin A in aliquots of parenteral nutrition (PN) solution from bottle and effluent under routine conditions of intravenous administration. (From Shenai et al.,[47] with permission.)

from losses caused by photodegradation and adsorption to intravenous tubing.[49] A clinical trial is required to determine whether the lipid emulsion is a more suitable vehicle than the protein–dextrose solution for administration of supplemental vitamins in intravenously nourished VLBW infants. There is also a need to develop and evaluate other intravenous tubing material that can appreciably decrease or eliminate the adsorptive losses of vitamin A. Until such material becomes available, alternative methods of vitamin A administration, such as the intramuscular route, may be necessary to optimize the vitamin A status of VLBW infants.

VITAMIN A REQUIREMENT

The precise requirement of vitamin A in VLBW infants is still undefined. Vitamin A values of diets are expressed in international units (IU) or as retinol equivalents (RE).[16] One IU of vitamin A is equivalent to 0.3 μg preformed retinol; one RE of vitamin A is equivalent to 1.0 μg retinol. The recommended dietary intake of vitamin A for term newborn infants is 100 RE/kg/day or approximately 333 IU/kg/day.[50] This recommendation does not seem applicable to prematurely born newborns. The previous study[30] in VLBW infants has shown that plasma concentrations of vitamin A decline to low levels when the vitamin A intake is < 700 IU/kg/day. The correlation between the change in serial plasma vitamin A concentrations and the average daily vitamin A intake in this study has shown that an intake of at least 700 IU/kg/day is required to raise the plasma concentrations of vitamin A in these infants (Figure 47–3). Normalization of plasma concentrations of vitamin A and RBP in VLBW infants can be achieved with a vitamin A intake > 1500 IU/kg/day.[32,51] The lack of clinical and biochemical evidence of toxicity in any of the vitamin A-supplemented infants and the observation that the plasma vitamin A concentra-

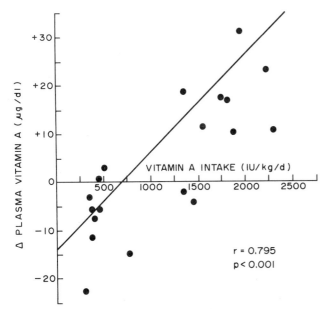

FIGURE 47–3. Correlation between the change in serial plasma vitamin A concentrations (Δplasma vitamin A) and the average daily vitamin A intake ($r = .795$, $p < .001$). (Adapted from Shenai et al.,[30] with permission.)

tions did not exceed 80 μg/dl in these studies suggest that a total vitamin A intake in the range of 1500 to 2800 IU/kg/day is safe for VLBW infants.[32,51] Further systematic evaluation of vitamin A needs of VLBW infants is required to determine the optimal daily intake of the vitamin that would provide maximal therapeutic benefits and minimal risk of toxicity.

VITAMIN A ASSESSMENT

Long-term vitamin A supplementation in VLBW infants raises the need for monitoring of their vitamin A status. Serial measurements of plasma concentrations of vitamin A and RBP and of plasma retinol/RBP molar ratios are useful for such monitoring. Plasma vitamin A concentrations in the normal range of 20 to 80 μg/dl[16] can be achieved with vitamin A supplementation in VLBW infants (Figure 47–4).[32,51] Likewise, plasma RBP concentrations > 2.5 mg/dl can be achieved with vitamin A supplementation in these infants (Figure 47–4).[32,51] Plasma retinol/RBP molar ratio is calculated from the values of plasma concentrations, assuming that the molecular weights of retinol and RBP are 286 and 21,000, respectively.[52] In vitamin A–sufficient individuals, RBP is saturated with vitamin A in plasma, and consequently the plasma retinol/RBP molar ratio is approximately 1.0.[18] The reported mean plasma retinol/RBP molar ratio in normal adults is 0.82,[19] whereas the mean ratio at birth in term neonates is 0.51[15,53] and that in preterm neonates is 0.39.[15] Plasma retinol/RBP molar ratios ranging from 0.9 to 1.1 can be achieved with vitamin A supplementation in VLBW infants (Figure 47–4).[51]

Although they are useful indices of vitamin A status, the plasma vitamin A concentrations do not always cor-

relate with liver vitamin A concentrations.[26,54] The plasma RBP concentrations and plasma retinol/RBP molar ratios can be potentially altered in severe protein malnutrition[55] and other disease states.[18] Although liver vitamin A concentrations are more accurate indicators of vitamin A status,[22] these measurements cannot be used for monitoring. Thus there is a need for a diagnostic test that is simple to perform, clinically applicable, and a predictive indicator of vitamin A status.

Plasma RBP response to vitamin A administration has recently been shown to be a useful functional test of vitamin A status in VLBW infants.[51] This test is based on the varied response of RBP secretion from liver into plasma after vitamin A administration observed in animals with varying degrees of vitamin A sufficiency. Normally, RBP is synthesized in the liver and secreted into the plasma as the retinol–RBP complex.[7] In vitamin A–deficient animals, RBP secretion is blocked, leading to its accumulation in the liver and resulting in high liver and low plasma concentrations of RBP.[56,57] When these animals are given vitamin A, mobilization of RBP from the liver occurs, which leads to a rapid decrease in the liver RBP concentration and a concomitant increase in the plasma RBP

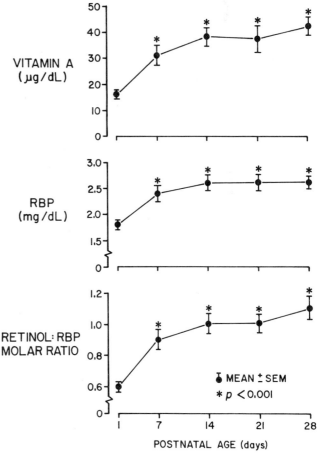

FIGURE 47–4. Plasma concentrations of vitamin A and RBP, and plasma retinol/RBP molar ratios in VLBW infants. Mean values on day 1 reflect values before vitamin A supplementation. All mean values marked with asterisk on days 7, 14, 21, and 28 are significantly higher than those on day 1 ($p < .001$). (From Shenai et al.,[51] with permission.)

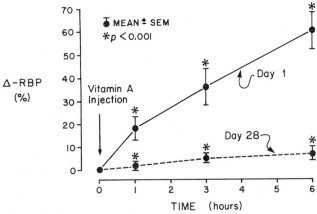

FIGURE 47–5. Plasma RBP response to vitamin A administration in VLBW infants. ΔRBP is calculated as percentage of increase in plasma RBP concentration from baseline value at 1, 3, and 6 hours after intramuscular injection of vitamin A (2000 IU/kg retinyl palmitate). All mean values marked with asterisk reflecting plasma RBP response on day 1 are significantly higher than those on day 28 ($p < .001$). (From Shenai et al.,[51] with permission.)

concentration.[56] In vitamin A-sufficient animals, on the other hand, RBP does not accumulate in the liver, and minimal or no change in plasma RBP concentration is seen after vitamin A administration.[56] These observations led to the hypothesis that changes in plasma RBP concentration in response to vitamin A administration might be a useful test for evaluating the functional vitamin A status in VLBW infants.[51] This test involves measurement of plasma RBP concentrations in sequentially obtained blood samples just before (baseline) and 1, 3, and 6 hours after an intramuscular injection of vitamin A (2000 IU/kg retinyl palmitate). The percent increase in the plasma RBP concentration (ΔRBP) from its baseline value is calculated by the following equation: ΔRBP (percent) = [RBP (maximum) − RBP (baseline)]/RBP (baseline) × 100. The lowest ΔRBP value assigned is zero if there is no change or if there is a decrease in the plasma RBP concentration from the baseline value. The dose of vitamin A used in this test is based on previous observations of vitamin A supplementation in VLBW infants.[32] The timing of blood samples is based on kinetic studies of RBP secretion in human adults[58] and in rats.[57]

Plasma RBP response to vitamin A administration was evaluated in 24 VLBW infants at risk for BPD, studied shortly after birth and again after a 28-day period of vitamin A supplementation.[51] The ΔRBP was high (mean ± SD: 61 ± 37 percent) (Figure 47–5) and the plasma vitamin A and RBP concentrations were low on postnatal day 1, indicating vitamin A deficiency. Supplemental vitamin A improved the vitamin A status of all infants, as shown by low ΔRBP values (mean ± SD: 8 ± 9 percent) (Figure 47–5) and normal plasma vitamin A and RBP concentrations on postnatal day 28. There was a significant negative correlation between the ΔRBP values and the plasma concentrations of vitamin A ($r = .70$; $p < .001$) (Figure 47–6). BPD was diagnosed in 12 of 24 infants. Infants with BPD had a higher mean (± SD) ΔRBP on postnatal

day 28 than those without BPD (13 ± 10 percent versus 3 ± 3 percent, $p < .01$) (Figure 47–7), indicative of the persistence of low vitamin A status despite supplementation in infants with lung disease. The individual ΔRBP values on postnatal day 28 exceeded 8 percent in 9 of 12 infants with BPD, compared to none from the group without BPD (Figure 47–7). This study has shown that the plasma RBP response to vitamin A administration is a useful indicator of the functional vitamin A status in VLBW infants. Although vitamin A supplementation resulting in a total vitamin A intake of approximately 2000 IU/kg/day normalizes conventional plasma indices of vitamin A in VLBW infants, the plasma RBP response to vitamin A administration may continue to reflect persistence of low vitamin A status in the more immature infants with significant lung disease.

Plasma RBP response to vitamin A administration, as reported in this study,[51] is simple to assess. The dose of vitamin A (2000 IU/kg retinyl palmitate) used in this test is within the range that has been reported to be safe for VLBW infants.[32,51] The intramuscular route of administration avoids the potential difficulties associated with variable absorption after enteral administration and with variable losses in the delivery system after intravenous administration of vitamin A. The blood volume required for testing is within the range commonly used for biochemical monitoring of VLBW infants. More important, the test provides information that may be useful for identification of infants with persistence of low vitamin A status despite supplementation and possibly with increased risk for BPD.

Loerch et al.[59] have reported a relative dose–response test in which the increase in plasma concentration of vitamin A 5 hours after an oral dose of retinyl acetate was determined and correlated over a wide range of levels of plasma and liver vitamin A values in rats. This approach has been evaluated in adults with alcoholic hepatic cirrhosis,[60] adults undergoing abdominal surgery,[61] and children subjected to liver biopsy.[62] A variation of the relative

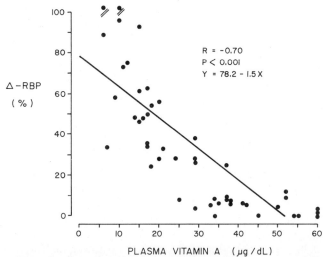

FIGURE 47–6. Correlation between ΔRBP values and plasma vitamin A concentrations ($r = -.70$; $p < .001$). (Adapted from Shenai et al.,[51] with permission.)

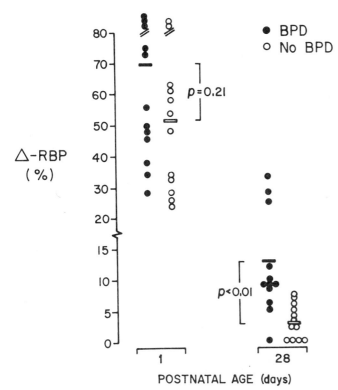

FIGURE 47-7. Individual ΔRBP values on day 1 and 28 in VLBW infants with BPD (*n* = 12) and without BPD (*n* = 12). Mean ΔRBP on day 28 is significantly higher in infants with BPD than in those without BPD (*p* < .01). (Adapted from Shenai et al.,[51] with permission.)

dose–response test has been performed in preterm infants to determine their vitamin A status at discharge from the hospital.[63] No information is available, however, regarding the usefulness of this test as a reliable indicator of vitamin A status in VLBW infants.

VITAMIN A TOXICITY

Hypervitaminosis A may develop from acute intoxication or from chronic ingestion of vitamin A. In infants, acute intoxication may occur when a single massive dose of vitamin A in excess of 100,000 IU is administered.[16] Clinical manifestations of acute hypervitaminosis A include symptoms and signs of increased intracranial pressure. Long-term ingestion of vitamin A in excess of 25,000 IU/day may cause chronic intoxication in children and adults.[16,64,65] Clinical manifestations of chronic hypervitaminosis A include symptoms and signs of increased intracranial pressure, bone and joint pains, and mucocutaneous lesions. Hepatomegaly and hepatic injury, hypercalcemia, and hematologic abnormalities are variably seen.[66] Radiographic findings in infants younger than 6 months include widened metaphyses, especially of the distal ulna, and radiolucent zones in the radius proximal to the metaphysis.[67] Cortical hyperostosis of multiple long bones and soft tissue changes are typically seen in infants older than 6 months.[67] In hypervita-

minosis A, the plasma concentrations of vitamin A are generally well in excess of 100 μg/dl, and the ratio of retinyl ester to free retinol in plasma is elevated.[68] The plasma concentrations of RBP usually remain normal.[68] Hypervitaminosis A is generally reversible with restriction of vitamin A intake. Infusion of 2-hydroxypropyl-β-cyclodextrin as a means of solubilizing retinoids and enhancing their urinary excretion has occasionally been used as adjunctive therapy.[69]

The potential toxicity of vitamin A in newborn infants has not been systematically studied. Whether the threshold for acute and chronic intoxication is lower in neonates when compared to older infants and children remains unknown. Careful physical examination for evidence of mucocutaneous lesions and bone and joint abnormalities, periodic monitoring of blood chemistry profiles including liver function tests, periodic monitoring of hematologic indices, and serial measurements of plasma concentrations of vitamin A and RBP are important in management of VLBW infants receiving long-term vitamin A supplementation. Ultrasonographic scanning of the brain for evidence of intracranial hemorrhage and assessment of intracranial pressure by noninvasive methods such as fontanel tonometry are also important.

SUMMARY

Most VLBW infants are born with low plasma concentrations of vitamin A and RBP and with limited liver reserve of vitamin A. VLBW infants who progress to develop BPD often manifest clinical, biochemical, and histopathologic evidence of vitamin A deficiency. Vitamin A supplementation from early postnatal life in these infants not only improves their vitamin A status but also appears to promote regenerative healing from lung injury, as evidenced by decreased incidence and morbidity of BPD. Until further studies are conducted, intramuscular administration may remain the preferable route of vitamin A supplementation. Normalization of conventional plasma indices of vitamin A is possible with a total vitamin A intake in the range of 1500 to 2800 IU/kg/day in VLBW infants. Plasma RBP response to vitamin A administration appears to be a useful functional test of vitamin A status that may allow identification of infants with persistence of low vitamin A status despite supplementation and possibly with increased risk for BPD. Careful monitoring for evidence of toxicity is indicated in all infants receiving long-term vitamin A supplementation. Additional studies will be important in assessing the value of these diagnostic and therapeutic approaches in the management of VLBW infants at risk for severe complications of lung immaturity.

ACKNOWLEDGMENTS: This work was supported by Research Grants HL 14214 and HD 09195 from the National Institutes of Health. The author gratefully acknowledges Mildred T. Stahlman, M.D., for her advice and encouragement, and Frank Chytil, Ph.D., for sharing his expertise in vitamin A metabolism.

REFERENCES

1. Hopkins FG: Feeding experiments illustrating the importance of accessory factors in normal dietaries. J Physiol 44:425–460, 1912
2. McCollum EV, Davis M: The influence of certain vegetable fats on growth. J Biol Chem 21:179–182, 1915
3. Karrer P, Morf R, Schopp K: Zur Kenntnis des vitamines-A aus fischtranen II. Helv Chim Acta 14:1431–1437, 1931
4. Kanai M, Raz A, Goodman DS: Retinol-binding protein: The transport protein for vitamin A in human plasma. J Clin Invest 47:2025–2044, 1968
5. Rask L, Anundi H, Bohme J, et al: Structural and functional studies of vitamin A-binding proteins. Ann NY Acad Sci 359:79–90, 1981
6. Raz A, Shiratori T, Goodman DS: Studies on the protein–protein and protein–ligand interactions involved in retinol transport in plasma. J Biol Chem 245:1903–1912, 1970
7. Goodman DS: Plasma retinol-binding protein, in Sporn MB, Roberts AB, Goodman DS (eds): The Retinoids, vol 2. Orlando, Academic Press, 1984, pp 41–88
8. Wolbach SB, Howe PR: Tissue changes following deprivation of fat-soluble vitamin A. J Exp Med 42:753–777, 1925
9. Wong YC, Buck RC: An electron microscopic study of metaplasia of the rat tracheal epithelium in vitamin A deficiency. Lab Invest 24:55–66, 1971
10. McDowell EM, Keenan KP, Huang M: Effects of vitamin A-deprivation on hamster tracheal epithelium. A quantitative morphologic study. Virchows Arch (Cell Pathol) 45:197–219, 1984
11. Wolbach SB, Howe PR: Epithelial repair in recovery from vitamin A deficiency. J Exp Med 57:511–526, 1933
12. McDowell EM, Keenan KP, Huang M: Restoration of mucociliary tracheal epithelium following deprivation of vitamin A. A quantitative morphologic study. Virchows Arch (Cell Pathol) 45:221–240, 1984
13. Northway WH Jr, Rosan RC, Porter DY: Pulmonary disease following respirator therapy of hyaline-membrane disease: Bronchopulmonary dysplasia. N Engl J Med 276:357–368, 1967
14. Stahlman MT, Cheatham W, Gray ME: The role of air dissection in bronchopulmonary dysplasia. J Pediatr 95:878–882, 1979
15. Shenai JP, Chytil F, Jhaveri A, et al: Plasma vitamin A and retinol-binding protein in premature and term neonates. J Pediatr 99:302–305, 1981
16. Underwood BA: Vitamin A in animal and human nutrition, in Sporn MB, Roberts AB, Goodman DS (eds): The Retinoids, vol 1. Orlando, Academic Press, 1984, pp 281–392
17. Brandt RB, Mueller DG, Schroeder JR, et al: Serum vitamin A in premature and term neonates. J Pediatr 92:101–104, 1978
18. Smith FR, Goodman DS: The effects of diseases of the liver, thyroid, and kidneys on the transport of vitamin A in human plasma. J Clin Invest 1971; 50:2426–2436, 1971
19. Vahlquist A, Rask L, Peterson PA, et al: The concentrations of retinol-binding protein, prealbumin, and transferrin in sera of newly delivered mothers and children of various ages. Scand J Clin Lab Invest 35:569–575, 1975
20. Vahlquist A, Sjolund K, Norden A, et al: Plasma vitamin A transport and visual dark adaptation in diseases of the intestine and liver. Scand J Clin Lab Invest 38:301–308, 1978
21. Bhatia J, Ziegler EE: Retinol-binding protein and prealbumin in cord blood of term and preterm infants. Early Hum Dev 8:129–133, 1983
22. Olson JA: Evaluation of vitamin A status in children. World Rev Nutr Diet 31:130–134, 1978
23. Pearson WN: Blood and urinary vitamin levels as potential indices of body stores. Am J Clin Nutr 20:514–525, 1967
24. Huque T: A survey of human liver reserves of retinol in London. Br J Nutr 47:165–172, 1982
25. Olson JA, Gunning DB, Tilton RA: Liver concentrations of vitamin A and carotenoids, as a function of age and other parameters, of American children who died of various causes. Am J Clin Nutr 39:903–910, 1984
26. Shenai JP, Chytil F, Stahlman MT: Liver vitamin A reserves of very low birth weight neonates. Pediatr Res 19:892–893, 1985
27. Iyengar L, Apte SV: Nutrient stores in human foetal livers. Br J Nutr 27:313–317, 1972
28. Olson JA: Liver vitamin A reserves of neonates, preschool children and adults dying of various causes in Salvador, Brazil. Arch Latinoam Nutr 26:992–997, 1979
29. Montreewasuwat N, Olson JA: Serum and liver concentrations of vitamin A in Thai fetuses as a function of gestational age. Am J Clin Nutr 32:601–606, 1979
30. Shenai JP, Chytil F, Stahlman MT: Vitamin A status of neonates with bronchopulmonary dysplasia. Pediatr Res 19:185–188, 1985
31. Hustead VA, Gutcher GA, Anderson SA, et al: Relationship of vitamin A (retinol) status to lung disease in the preterm infant. J Pediatr 105:610–615, 1984
32. Shenai JP, Kennedy KA, Chytil F, et al: Clinical trial of vitamin A supplementation in infants susceptible to bronchopulmonary dysplasia. J Pediatr 111:269–277, 1987
33. Bancalari E, Abdenour GE, Feller R, et al: Bronchopulmonary dysplasia: Clinical presentation. J Pediatr 95:819–823, 1979
34. Lebenthal E, Lee PC: Development of functional response in human exocrine pancreas. Pediatrics 66:556–560, 1980
35. Norman A, Strandvik B, Ojamae O: Bile acids and pancreatic enzymes during absorption in the newborn. Acta Paediatr Scand 61:571–576, 1972
36. Watkins JB, Ingall D, Szczepanik P, et al: Bile-salt metabolism in the newborn. Measurement of pool size and synthesis by stable isotope technic. N Engl J Med 288:431–434, 1973
37. Ong DE: A novel retinol-binding protein from rat. Purification and partial characterization. J Biol Chem, 259:1476–1482, 1984
38. Roy RN, Pollinitz RP, Hamilton JR, et al: Impaired assimilation of nasojejunal feeds in healthy low-birth-weight newborn infants. J Pediatr 90:431–434, 1977
39. Henley TH, Dann M, Golden WRC: Reserves, absorption and plasma levels of vitamin A in premature infants. Am J Dis Child 68:257–264, 1944
40. Lewis JM, Bodansky O, Birmingham J, et al: Comparative absorption, excretion, and storage of oily and aqueous preparations of vitamin A. J Pediatr 31:496–508, 1947
41. Sobel AE, Besman L, Kramer B: Vitamin A absorption in the newborn. Am J Dis Child 77:576–591, 1949
42. Kahan J: The vitamin absorption test. I. Studies on children and adults without disorders in the alimentary tract. Scand J Gastroenterol 4:313–324, 1969
43. Norman A, Strandvik B, Zetterstrom R: Test-meal in the diagnosis of malabsorption in infancy. Tolerance tests using simultaneous oral administration of glucose, D-xylose, cream and vitamin A. Acta Paediatr Scand 60:165–172, 1971
44. Woodruff CW, Latham CB, James EP, et al: Vitamin A status of preterm infants: The influence of feeding and vitamin supplements. Am J Clin Nutr 44:384–389, 1986
45. Howard L, Chu R, Feman S, et al: Vitamin A deficiency from long-term parenteral nutrition. Ann Intern Med 93:576–577, 1980
46. Hartline JV, Zachman RD: Vitamin A delivery in total parenteral nutrition solution. Pediatrics 58:448–451, 1976
47. Shenai JP, Stahlman MT, Chytil F: Vitamin A delivery from parenteral alimentation solution. J Pediatrics 99:661–663, 1981
48. Gillis J, Jones G, Pencharz P: Delivery of vitamins A, D, and E in total parenteral nutrition solutions. J Parenter Enteral Nutr 7:11–14, 1983
49. Green HL, Phillips BL, Franck L, et al: Persistently low blood retinol levels during and after parenteral feeding of very low birth weight infants: Examination of losses into intravenous administration sets and a method of prevention by addition to a lipid emulsion. Pediatrics 79:894–900, 1987
50. Food and Agriculture Organization/World Health Organization: Requirements of vitamin A, thiamine, riboflavin and niacin. Report of a Joint FAO/WHO Expert Group. FAO/WHO, Geneva. Tech Rep Ser 1967:362
51. Shenai JP, Rush MG, Stahlman MT, et al: Plasma retinol-binding protein response to vitamin A administration in infants susceptible to bronchopulmonary dysplasia. J Pediatr 116:607–614, 1990
52. Smith JE, Goodman DS: Retinol-binding protein and the regulation of vitamin A transport. Fed Proc 38:2504–2509, 1979
53. Jansson L, Nilsson B: Serum retinol and retinol-binding protein in mothers and infants at delivery. Biol Neonate 43:269–271, 1983

54. Meyer KA, Popper H, Steigmann F, et al: Comparison of vitamin A of liver biopsy specimens with plasma vitamin A in man. Proc Soc Exp Biol Med 49:589–591, 1942

55. Ingenbleek Y, Van Den Schrieck HG, De Nayer P, et al: The role of retinol-binding protein in protein-calorie malnutrition. Metabolism 24:633–641, 1975

56. Muto Y, Smith JD, Milch PO, et al: Regulation of retinol-binding protein metabolism by vitamin A status in the rat. J Biol Chem 247:2542–2550, 1972

57. Smith JE, Muto Y, Milch PO, et al: The effects of chylomicron vitamin A on the metabolism of retinol-binding protein in the rat. J Biol Chem, 248:1544–1549, 1973

58. Vahlquist A, Peterson PA, Wibell L: Metabolism of the vitamin A transporting protein complex. I. Turnover studies in normal persons and in patients with chronic renal failure. Eur J Clin Invest 3:352–362, 1973

59. Loerch JD, Underwood BA, Lewis KC: Response of plasma levels of vitamin A to a dose of vitamin A as an indicator of hepatic vitamin A reserves in rats. J Nutr 109:778–786, 1979

60. Mobarhan S, Russell RM, Underwood BA, et al: Evaluation of the relative dose response test for vitamin A nutriture in cirrhotics. Am J Clin Nutr 34:2264–2270, 1981

61. Amedee-Manesme O, Anderson D, Olson JA: Relation of the relative dose response to liver concentrations of vitamin A in generally well-nourished surgical patients. Am J Clin Nutr 39:898–902, 1984

62. Amedee-Manesme O, Mourey MS, Hanck A, et al: Vitamin A relative dose response test: Validation by intravenous injection in children with liver disease. Am J Clin Nutr 46:286–289, 1987

63. Woodruff CW, Latham CB, Mactier H, et al: Vitamin A status of preterm infants: Correlation between plasma retinol concentration and retinol dose response. Am J Clin Nutr 46:985–988, 1987

64. Mahoney CP, Margolis MT, Knauss TA, et al: Chronic vitamin A intoxication in infants fed chicken liver. Pediatrics 65:893–896, 1980

65. Farris WA, Erdman JW Jr: Protracted hypervitaminosis A following long-term, low-level intake. JAMA 247:1317–1318, 1982

66. Goodman DS: Vitamin A and retinoids in health and disease. N Engl J Med 310:1023–1031, 1984

67. Persson B, Tunell R, Ekengren K: Chronic vitamin A intoxication during the first half year of life. Description of 5 cases. Acta Paediatr Scand 54:49–60, 1965

68. Smith FR, Goodman DS: Vitamin A transport in human vitamin A toxicity. N Engl J Med 294:805–808, 1976

69. Carpenter TO, Pettifor JM, Russell RM, et al: Severe hypervitaminosis A in siblings: Evidence of variable tolerance to retinol intake. J Pediatr 111:507–512, 1987

SECTION V

ADVERSE
DRUG EFFECTS

48

ADVERSE DRUG EFFECTS AND DRUG EPIDEMIOLOGY

ALLEN A. MITCHELL

It is well-accepted that the practice of rational drug therapy requires one to weigh the benefits expected from the use of a given drug against its hazards. Unfortunately, this ideal circumstance is rarely achieved, because no matter how much we know about a drug's benefit, we usually have an inadequate understanding about the frequency and severity of its adverse effects.

This deficiency in our knowledge is a direct consequence of the process by which drugs become available for use. In the United States, the mandate of the Food and Drug Administration requires that the agency ensure that a drug is safe and effective before it is released to the general market. Premarketing studies are carried out according to a specified sequence: Phase I studies evaluate a drug's biologic effects, pharmacology, and safe dosage range in small numbers of normal human volunteers; phase II studies evaluate the drug in the treatment or prevention of a specific disease in limited numbers of patients; in phase III, the drug is evaluated in selected human populations by means of clinical trials (usually randomized, double-blind studies). In the phase III studies, the drug must be shown not only to be safe, but also effective in terms of some intended use. These studies are necessarily limited in size (usually involving a total of a few hundred to a few thousand subjects).

Such trials may be sufficiently large to evaluate efficacy, but they are inadequate to describe the full range of adverse reactions attributable to a given agent. In particular, they are unlikely to detect adverse reactions that are uncommon (occurring in as few as 1 in 100 or 1 in 1000 drug users), and even less likely to detect reactions that occur less frequently (e.g., 1 in 10,000). In addition, because the duration of phase III studies tends to be quite limited, they will fail to identify those adverse effects that manifest only after a latent interval between exposure and onset as well as those effects that become manifest only after long periods of use. Many types of patients who will ultimately be treated with the drug of interest are excluded from phase III studies; for example, such trials tend to exclude patients with diseases other than the one

under evaluation and patients concurrently using other medications.

These limitations reduce the likelihood that phase III studies will detect adverse drug effects that may later be identified in various patient populations. From the pediatrician's perspective, however, premarketing studies suffer from an additional major deficiency: they rarely evaluate a drug in pediatric populations. Even when studies are conducted among children, they tend to include only very small numbers of patients and rarely, if ever, evaluate the drug throughout the spectrum of age that concerns the pediatrician, from the premature newborn to the adolescent. As a result, drugs are often released to the market without the benefit of even limited experience in pediatric age groups, and adverse drug reactions that occur uniquely or more frequently in infants and children will necessarily go undetected. Examples of such reactions are numerous: sulfonamide-induced kernicterus in premature infants,[1] tetracycline-induced tooth staining,[2] and the chloramphenicol-induced "gray syndrome."[3,4]

Even after we have accumulated decades of experience with a given drug in the pediatric population, there is no assurance that a far more complete understanding of the drug's adverse effects will have emerged. For example, although phenytoin (Dilantin and others) has been widely used as an anticonvulsant for almost 50 years, over 3 decades of use elapsed before it was recognized that the drug may be responsible for movement disorders.[5] Rash, on the other hand, has been a known adverse effect of this drug since the original studies of phenytoin were published in 1938. However, the frequency with which rash occurs is unclear; the often-quoted 5 percent rash rate in exposed patients can ultimately be traced to the original studies that involved a very heterogeneous and poorly described population of 200 adult and pediatric patients.[6] Not only are we left with a poor understanding of the rate of rash among exposed patients, we have virtually no understanding of factors that may make some patients more likely to develop a rash than others.

If neither premarketing studies nor decades of experience provide the prescriber with sufficient information on the adverse effects of the drug, are there other approaches that can? Before responding to that question, let us explore the issue of adverse drug reactions in greater depth.

THEORETICAL CONSIDERATIONS

Whether from the clinical or epidemiologic perspective, three broad areas of information must be considered in the study of adverse drug effects: the drug of interest (i.e., the "exposure"), the adverse reaction to that drug (i.e., the "outcome"), and the nature of the patients who experience these effects (i.e., the "population").

Exposure

Though the concept of exposure is straightforward, the definitions of what constitutes a drug and what constitutes an exposure to that drug are not always apparent. For example, few would quarrel with including in the definition oral or parenteral exposure to an antibiotic, but does "exposure" also include intravenous fluids, vitamins, electrolytes, and dextrose? Does the route of exposure affect the definition? For example, what about topically applied drugs, or drugs given by inhalation (is supplemental oxygen a drug)? Three studies describing drug use in the newborn intensive care nursery differed with respect to the average number of drugs used in patients, ranging from 3.4 to 10.4.[7–9] These substantial differences can be largely explained by the definitions of a drug that were used in each study (of interest, the latter two studies were drawn from the same population). Variations in the definition of what constitutes an exposure will clearly affect not only estimates of drug use, but also the observed rates of adverse drug reactions in these patients.

Pediatricians must also consider another kind of drug exposure—the so-called inactive ingredients. These agents are included in a variety of medications to increase stability, solubility, shelf life, and the like. While it is well recognized that certain ingredients, such as sulfites and tartrazine, can produce adverse effects in sensitive individuals, observations from neonatal intensive care units have revealed that patients may suffer serious and even fatal reactions from such "inactive" ingredients as benzyl alcohol and propylene glycol.[10,11] Unfortunately, agents added to active pharmaceuticals vary over time and manufacturer, and pharmacists, nurses, and physicians alike are usually unaware of the number and nature of "inactive" ingredients they are administering to patients. Obviously, our ignorance about such exposures limits the likelihood of our detecting their adverse effects.

Outcomes

What outcomes are considered to be adverse drug reactions (often abbreviated as ADRs)? Much of the debate

(and confusion) in the study of adverse drug effects centers around the definition of the term "adverse drug reaction." The World Health Organization (WHO), for example, defines an adverse reaction as one that is noxious and unintended and that occurs at doses used in humans for prophylaxis, diagnosis, or therapy.[12] This definition does not exclude events that may be associated with a patient's disease state, though other definitions may make such an exclusion.

Most definitions include noxious or pathologic signs and symptoms,[13] but do they also consider, for example, abnormalities in laboratory values in the absence of signs and symptoms? Would asymptomatic hyperkalemia be considered an adverse reaction to potassium supplements? Many question whether certain signs and symptoms should be included as adverse reactions, particularly where they may be common, trivial, or unavoidable consequences of a drug's pharmacologic action (e.g., drowsiness with antihistamines, mild diarrhea with ampicillin, and leukopenia with cytotoxic drugs, respectively). Some would consider as adverse drug reactions only those outcomes requiring a change in drug therapy.

We prefer a broad definition of adverse drug reaction (as long as one does not give undue importance to the "*total* ADR rate" derived from such a definition), since it facilitates study of the spectrum of drug-related events. However, since few studies use a common definition of an adverse drug reaction, one should be wary about making comparisons among different studies.

Another source of confusion results from failure to make clear distinctions between effects of drugs that become manifest after short-term use and effects that become apparent only after long-term use. Acute effects following short-term exposure often involve allergic reactions (e.g., urticaria due to ampicillin), idiosyncratic responses (e.g., extrapyramidal signs due to phenothiazines), or extensions of a drug's known pharmacology (e.g., arrhythmias due to digitalis). Effects following long-term administration can occur in a precipitate manner (e.g., gastrointestinal bleeding with aspirin) or can have a more insidious onset (e.g., cataract with corticosteroids); some effects may involve a latent interval, becoming apparent long after the drug exposure has ceased (e.g., adenocarcinoma of the vagina in adolescent females exposed *in utero* to diethylstilbestrol). A classification based on the temporal relation between duration of therapy and onset of adverse effect is particularly useful in considering various strategies for evaluating the full spectrum of adverse drug reactions.

Few adverse drug reactions represent unique clinical events. As a result, signs or symptoms that might be attributed to drug therapy by one observer might as easily be attributed to the patient's underlying disease state by another. As examples, rash occurring in association with amoxicillin treatment of otitis media may be attributed either to amoxicillin or to a presumed viral etiology of the otitis; marked lethargy in a patient with recurrent seizures may be attributed to the anticonvulsant used to control the seizures or to the patient's postictal state. While the interpretation of clinical events occurring in drug-treated patients poses difficulties, even healthy individuals who are receiving no medications will frequently report symptoms that are commonly considered side effects of drugs, such as fatigue, headache, and rash.[14]

Reports in the mid-1970s described the difficulties inherent in attempts to establish valid and reproducible systems for implicating a particular drug in a specific adverse event.[15,16] More recently, a number of researchers devised various schemes (algorithms) to formally assess causality in suspected adverse drug reactions.[17,18] Unfortunately, these approaches rely heavily on current information about a drug and its side effects, and they are therefore unlikely to facilitate discovery of new, previously unrecognized adverse effects of a drug; in fact, by relying on current knowledge about a drug's effects, some schemes may tend to discourage such discovery. Further, effective use of the algorithms requires the availability of information (such as the results of dechallenge and rechallenge) that is often unavailable in the usual context of clinical practice. Critical assessment of specific algorithms has suggested that they have very limited utility for their stated purpose,[19,20] and it is unlikely that these approaches will have major value in furthering our understanding of diverse adverse drug reactions.

On the other hand, algorithms do identify the kinds of questions that must be answered in order to assess causality, and for this reason various algorithms can indeed prove helpful by highlighting appropriate questions in the clinician's assessment of a particular adverse event in a particular patient.

Population

The third area of information needed for the study of adverse drug reactions concerns the population of patients being treated. Such information provides critical insight into both the nature of the adverse drug reactions and the risk factors for their occurrence. For example, age is especially important in pediatrics, as it may affect the risk of particular reactions; it is uninformative to describe the risk of sulfonamide-induced kernicterus in the entire pediatric age range, since this particular outcome is limited to newborn infants. The diseases for which patients receive drugs also affect the risk of experiencing an adverse drug reaction; patients with cancer are far more likely to receive life-threatening drugs, and therefore have life-threatening adverse reactions, than are other patients with less serious illnesses. Additional factors to consider in adverse drug reaction assessments are body weight, surface area, sex, blood pressure, cigarette smoking (active and passive), laboratory values, allergy, and prior and concurrent exposure to other medications (both prescribed and over-the-counter).

Proper assessment of drug–effect relationships invariably requires other information related to patient characteristics, but identification of the specific factors relevant to a given assessment requires a more detailed understanding of the drug and outcome under consideration. For example, in a study of aspirin and Reye's syndrome, one would be interested in the preceding illnesses (e.g., influenza) that might distinguish those adversely affected by the exposure from those who were not. In a study of valproate-associated hepatotoxicity, one would

wish to know if valproate-treated epileptic patients differed from those who were treated with alternative drugs; for example, if valproate is the drug of "last resort," it may preferentially be administered to those who suffered ADRs on other anticonvulsants and who, therefore, may also be at increased risk for ADRs on valproate.

RATES

One of the most important aspects of adverse drug reactions is the frequency, or rate, with which they occur. *Rate* is expressed as a fraction, and in epidemiologic terms refers to the number of people with the outcome of interest (numerator) divided by the population at risk (denominator), over a specified time. When applied to the study of adverse drug reactions, the numerator is the number of patients with reactions to a given drug, and the denominator is the number of patients exposed to that drug. The importance of denominator information is often overlooked: if penicillin-induced anaphylaxis is observed in 10 patients, the rate of this event cannot be determined unless the number of patients exposed to penicillin is also known.

In statements reflecting rates of adverse drug reactions, the time reference is often implied, and commonly refers to the period of drug exposure (for example, the number of cases of anaphylaxis occurring during the course of penicillin therapy). However, for reactions that may occur after drug exposure has ceased (e.g., Stevens-Johnson syndrome), one must be particularly cautious that the time periods are appropriate in both the numerator and denominator.

Finally, recall that the definition of the denominator refers to the population *at risk* for the reaction. Thus, although all penicillin-exposed patients might constitute an appropriate denominator in a consideration of anaphylaxis, since all exposed patients are at risk for anaphylaxis, the denominator for consideration of cyclophosphamide (Cytoxan)-induced azoospermia would not be all patients, since only pubescent and postpubescent males are at risk for azoospermia.

ESTIMATING THE RATE (AND RISK) OF ADVERSE DRUG REACTIONS

Consider a hypothetical clinical trial in which 50 patients with pneumonia are treated with oral amoxicillin, and 15 of these patients develop a rash immediately following initiation of drug therapy. The rash rate is then 15/50, or 30 percent. We cannot conclude, however, that this rate is related entirely (or even partially) to amoxicillin until we compare it to the rate that would be expected among similar patients who did not receive amoxicillin. For example, assume that among a comparable group of 50 patients, one observes five rashes in the absence of amoxicillin exposure (rate = 10 percent). The observed differences in rate (30 versus 10 percent) may reflect differences associated with the drug exposure or they may merely represent a chance occurrence. To help distinguish between chance and nonchance differences, we use statistical testing. By convention, we usually state that a difference is statistically significant when the probability that the observation is due to chance is 5 percent or less ($p \leq .05$); that is, we are 95 percent confident that the observation is due to factor(s) other than chance. It is important to keep in mind, however, that statistical testing is based solely on probability assessments to which we attach arbitrary cut points—it does not entirely rule out chance. Thus, if the amoxicillin–rash association is significant at $p = .05$, there remains a 5 percent probability that the observed difference in rate *is* due to chance, and that the apparent association between amoxicillin exposure and an increased rate of rash is nothing more than a "statistical fluke." This type of error is called a "type I" or "alpha" error; it is equivalent to the "false positive" conclusion in the evaluation of diagnostic tests. The magnitude of the alpha (false positive) error is equal to the p value that one uses to define "statistically significant" and, as noted above, is usually set at 5 percent. In our example, the likelihood that the observed difference (15/50 versus 5/50) is due to chance is less than 5 percent ($\chi^2 = 5.6$). Thus, if we accept a 5 percent chance of making a wrong call, we can state that in this trial we have detected a significantly higher than expected rate of rash among amoxicillin recipients.

In the above example, the rash rate among the amoxicillin-exposed patients was 30 percent, but this frequency took on clinical importance only when the rash rate in the nonexposed (the "baseline" rate) was considered. A statistic that takes into account the rate in the nonexposed is the "relative risk." In the context of adverse drug reactions, relative risk (RR) is defined as the rate of the adverse event in the exposed individuals divided by the rate in the nonexposed:

$$RR = \frac{\text{rate of occurrence in exposed}}{\text{rate of occurrence in nonexposed}}$$

In the above example, the relative risk would be expressed as follows:

$$RR = \frac{0.30}{0.10} = 3.0$$

In other words, rash occurred three times more commonly in the exposed individuals than in those not exposed. If rash occurred with equal frequency in both groups, the relative risk would equal 1.

Since adverse reactions to a given drug occur more frequently among exposed patients than among nonexposed patients (by definition), it follows that in detecting adverse reactions, we seek to identify relative risks greater than 1. In the present example, we identified a relative risk of 3 for rash among amoxicillin-exposed patients, but this risk statement in itself does not provide information on statistical significance. As our testing of statistical significance already revealed, we are 95 percent confident that this relative risk is not due to chance (i.e., $p \leq .05$). Put another way, we are 95 percent confident that the observed relative risk of 3 is different from 1. To express this "confi-

dence," most would prefer to use "confidence intervals" (rather than p values), since these intervals not only convey the information on statistical significance, but they also provide, at the same time, the magnitude of the difference in rates between the two groups that is compatible with the observed level of significance. Thus, the 95 percent confidence intervals calculated for this example range from relative risks of 1.2 (the lower bound) to 7.5 (the upper bound). That the lower 95 percent confidence bound (1.2) excludes a risk of 1.0 reflects the p value of < .05; the range of the confidence interval provides the additional information that (according to our assumptions) we are 95 percent confident that the true relative risk lies between 1.2 and 7.5. Confidence bounds provide an additional benefit: statistical perspective. For a given risk estimate (e.g., RR = 4), p will be "<.05" whether the lower bound is 1.1 or 3.0 (since both bounds exclude 1.0); however, the values of the respective lower bounds should prompt the observer to recognize the more tentative (less stable) nature of the former estimate.

What if our clinical trial revealed not 15 rashes, but 10? The relative risk would decrease to 2 (10/50 divided by 5/50), so we must again estimate whether this observation is due to chance. For this example, the 95 percent confidence interval (0.6, 6.7) *includes* a relative risk of 1.0 (a 95 percent confidence interval that includes a relative risk of 1 is equivalent to a p value >.05). Thus, the observed difference in rash rates between patients exposed and not exposed to amoxicillin is (by our definition of significance) consistent with a chance observation.

What if our clinical trial revealed only five rashes among the amoxicillin-exposed patients? In this case, the rash rates are equal in both groups, and the relative risk is 1 (5/50 divided by 5/50). Statistical testing would of course lead us to conclude that, as in the preceding example, there is no evidence of a difference in rash rates between the two groups. Were these findings to be reported, it would not be unusual to see a conclusion such as: "Because there was no increased rate of adverse reactions among amoxicillin recipients, this drug appears safe." This statement is not justified, yet the frequency with which such statements are made serves as evidence of the failure to appreciate the very important distinction between "lack of evidence" of an association between a drug and adverse effect and "evidence of no association." In the first example (RR = 3), there was evidence of an association between amoxicillin and rash. In the second (RR = 2), the evidence was inconclusive, and in the third (RR = 1), there was no evidence of an association between amoxicillin and rash. Even though no association was *observed* in the last example, however, one cannot (in these circumstances) confidently rule out its existence. For example, this study of only 50 patients could easily have failed to detect a true rate of drug-related rash of 1 in 50 exposures (which, when added to the baseline rash rate of 5/50, yields a total rash rate among exposed patients of 6/50, versus the expected rate of 5/50 among nonexposed); it would almost certainly have missed the association if the true rate were 1 in 5000 exposures.

Thus, the detection of adverse drug reactions requires that we not only consider the possibility of falsely identifying an association between a drug and outcome where in reality none exists (type I, or alpha error), but that we also consider the possibility of failing to observe an association when one actually exists. This type of error is called a "type II" or "beta" error, and is comparable to the "false negative" conclusion in the evaluation of diagnostic tests. If, for example, we set beta = 0.20, we are then willing to accept a 20 percent chance of failing to detect a real association. In other words, we have an 80 percent chance (1 − beta) of detecting an association where one does exist. This latter estimate (1 − beta) is called the "power" of a test.

In summary, when statistical testing of rates is used in the detection of adverse drug effects, we must keep in mind two possible errors: First, are we incorrectly stating that an effect (i.e., difference in rates) exists, where in fact none exists (alpha error)? Second, are we failing to detect adverse reactions (i.e., differences in rates) where they truly exist (beta error)?

SAMPLE SIZE CONSIDERATIONS

It is useful to consider the number of exposed patients one would have to observe in order to detect various rates of adverse drug reactions. For example, Table 48–1 presents the number of drug users needed to detect relative risks from 2 to 4 for adverse events that occur among nonexposed patients with varying frequencies. It assumes a 5 percent chance of "identifying" effects that do not exist (alpha = 0.05), and it assumes a 20 percent chance of failing to identify effects that do exist (beta = 0.20); the power of the test, therefore, is 80 percent. Thus, if a drug is associated with a fourfold increase in an adverse effect, and the rate of the effect in the nonexposed (i.e., the "expected") is 1 in 50, the effect can be detected in a sample of only 184 exposed patients. On the other hand, to detect a relative risk of the same magnitude (RR = 4) where the "baseline" rate of the adverse event is 1 in 10,000, 38,000 exposed patients would have to be studied; if the exposed patients have only a doubled risk (RR = 2) of the adverse effect, its detection will require studying 230,000 patients exposed to the drug.

A WORD ABOUT DRUG SAFETY

While the detection of adverse reactions involves identifying relative risks greater than one, evaluations intended to provide assurance that there is no effect of a drug, that is, assurances of safety, require evidence that the relative risk equals 1. Rather than settling for *no evidence of association* (as noted above), providing assurances of safety requires that we seek *evidence of no association.* The theoretical demonstration of *absolutely* no difference in rates of adverse events between exposed and nonexposed patients requires a sample of infinite size. Since we can never demonstrate "no effect" with absolute confidence, we settle for a specified relative risk that we

TABLE 48–1. NUMBER OF DRUG USERS NEEDED TO DETECT A RELATIVE RISK OF 2–4 FOR FREQUENCIES OF ADVERSE EVENTS IN THE NONEXPOSED OF 1/50 TO 1/10,000

FREQUENCY IN NONEXPOSED	SAMPLE SIZE OF EXPOSED		
	RR = 2	RR = 3	RR = 4
1/50	1,100	350	184
1/100	2,200	710	377
1/500	11,000	3,600	1,900
1/1,000	23,000	7,200	3,800
1/10,000	230,000	72,000	38,000

Assumptions: α = .05; 1 − β = .80; frequencies in nonexposed are known.

wish to rule out. For example, we may want to assure ourselves that a drug produces less than a doubling of the risk of a reaction. We can then identify the size of the patient population required to rule out a relative risk of 2 or greater (given an estimated relative risk of 1.0 and an upper confidence interval of 1.9), recognizing that the study sample will not be large enough to identify (with statistical stability) relative risks of less than 2.

It should be noted that in our examples we have carefully waffled about whether amoxicillin "caused" the observed rashes. Even when we observed increased rates of rash among amoxicillin-exposed children in the various examples, it would have been premature to conclude from the information available that amoxicillin *caused* the higher rate of rash. As noted above, to reach such a conclusion we would require more information on the characteristics of the study population; in particular, we would require assurance that amoxicillin exposure was the only relevant difference between the two study groups. If, for example, those exposed to amoxicillin more commonly had otitis media, the etiology of which might include viruses, one might wonder whether the excess rash rate among amoxicillin recipients reflects an excess of viral exanthems among the drug-treated patients.

This caution is intended to highlight a common misunderstanding in the assessment of drug-related complications. That a drug is *associated* with a given outcome simply reflects the fact that, by statistical testing, we have determined that the observed rate of occurrence of the outcome is higher among exposed patients than would be expected by chance. Such a conclusion does not mean that the drug *caused* the increased rate of complication (with one exception: we generally accept a causal inference from significantly increased complication rates occurring in rigorous clinical trials where study groups are identical except for the drug administered). Statistical significance is directly a function of both the magnitude of the differences in rates and the number of subjects under study. In our example of amoxicillin-treated children, the same difference in rates would gain statistical significance as the study size became larger; however, the increase in statistical significance does not point to causality, since it would not alter the underlying fact that the amoxicillin-treated children may have had higher rates of viral exanthems. As described below, attributing causality to a given exposure is far more complex than the mere finding of statistical significance.

APPROACHES TO THE STUDY OF ADVERSE DRUG REACTIONS

At the present time, qualitative and quantitative information on adverse drug reactions in children is provided by spontaneous reporting, registries, studies focused on specific drugs or reactions, and epidemiologic surveillance programs.

Spontaneous Reporting

Spontaneous reporting of adverse drug effects is the oldest and, to date, the most productive source of information regarding adverse drug reactions. It requires that one observe an event, recognize it as a potential adverse drug effect, and report it. Such reports may be sent to drug manufacturers, regulatory agencies, or medical journals where they appear as letters to the editor, case reports, or small case series.

Spontaneous reports have two major deficiencies. First, they are subject to the various biases of the observers. For example, physicians are more likely to report an "adverse effect" once others have; on the other hand, as the effect becomes known, they tend to stop reporting its occurrence (this practice is encouraged by editors who view continued publication of such reports as unnecessary). Second, spontaneous reports provide no estimates of the number of patients exposed (the denominator) to the drug in question. Because spontaneous reports identify only a fraction of all adverse drug reactions, they provide poor numerator estimates as well. As a result, estimates of the rate of adverse events cannot be derived and therefore cannot be compared to "baseline" rates to determine if patients exposed to a drug are indeed at increased risk for an adverse effect.

Despite these deficiencies, there are circumstances where adverse drug effects can be identified by spontaneous reporting; in fact, under certain circumstances, spontaneous reporting offers the most efficient mechanism for identification of new adverse drug reactions. The most likely setting for such discovery is where the relative risk of a reaction is high, the drug is widely used, and it produces an effect that is immediate, rare, dramatic, and unrelated to the disease under treatment. For example, deafness shortly following the administration of furosemide fulfills these criteria, and such a reaction is likely to be recognized by spontaneous reports. When any one of these criteria is absent, however, discovery may be delayed substantially. For example, the relative risk for thalidomide-induced phocomelia is extremely high, the drug was in reasonably wide use in certain countries, and the effect was very rare, dramatic, and unrelated to the disease under treatment (maternal anxiety or insomnia). However, because of the lag between exposure to the drug in early pregnancy and appearance of the malformed child at delivery, over 6000 babies were affected before spontaneous reporting identified the association. In addition to the time lag between exposure and outcome, the likelihood that spontaneous reporting will identify adverse drug effects diminishes if the relative risk is small, if use of the drug is not widespread, if the adverse event is relatively common and not dramatic, or if the effect may be related to the disease under treatment. For example, if penicillin increased the risk of coughing by 50 percent ($RR = 1.5$) in patients with pneumonia, it is highly unlikely that spontaneous reports would identify this adverse effect. The possibility of detecting an adverse effect by spontaneous reporting becomes even more remote if the effect appears long after the exposure began, and especially if it appears long after the exposure ceased.

Because of the theoretical usefulness and demonstrated value of spontaneous reports, it is important that practitioners remain sensitive to the possibility that an unusual event represents a previously unrecognized adverse drug reaction and that such events be reported. A number of similar independent observations, spontaneously reported by other health professionals, will stimulate formal studies to further evaluate apparent relationships. Despite the development of sophisticated approaches for detecting adverse drug reactions (described later in text), spontaneous reports by physicians and others will continue to generate a major proportion of clinically relevant questions regarding adverse drug effects in children.

Registries

Registries represent attempts to centralize and formalize spontaneous reports of adverse drug reactions. In 1960, stimulated by concern about chloramphenicol-related aplastic anemia, the American Medical Association established a registry of blood dyscrasias, which evolved into a broader registry of adverse drug reactions. In 1962, the Food and Drug Administration (FDA) developed a registry for spontaneous adverse drug reaction reports, which eventually evolved into the FDA's Division of Drug Experience. This office coordinates the major registries of adverse drug reactions in the United States. The problems inherent in registries are similar to those described for spontaneous reporting—for example, no denominator data are available, so that estimates of adverse drug reaction rates cannot be developed. Because of these problems, registries cannot *systematically* identify previously unsuspected effects of drugs.

However, like spontaneous reports, registries have particular value in identifying strong and/or unusual associations between drugs and adverse effects. For example, as a result of a few spontaneous reports to the FDA registry regarding central nervous system disturbance following application of gamma benzene hexachloride (Kwell and others), the FDA was able to alert practitioners to this newly discovered adverse effect.[21] By periodic review and publication of registry data, the FDA provides a formal mechanism for stimulating research aimed at clarifying potential adverse drug reactions.[22]

Specific Studies

Adverse drug reaction information can also be provided by specific studies. Some adverse effects are identified by traditional laboratory, animal, and human studies that precede the approval and marketing of a given drug. More recent work has suggested methods by which specific reactions to specific drugs may be predicted; researchers have demonstrated that the risks for certain hypersensitivity reactions, such as hepatotoxicity or Stevens-Johnson syndrome, are directly related to the offending drug's metabolism, which in turn is affected by genetically determined pathways (pharmacogenetic polymorphisms) by which subpopulations of patients handle such drugs.[23] For example, these workers have shown that lymphocytes from patients with hepatotoxic reactions to phenytoin or Stevens-Johnson syndrome to sulfonamides respond differently when challenged with metabolites of the offending drugs than do exposed lymphocytes from unaffected patients.[24,25] As understanding of drug metabolism and related pharmacogenetic polymorphisms increases, it is likely that one will be able to predict which drugs will cause certain rare reactions before such drugs come into widespread use; similarly, one may be able to identify, in advance of their exposure, those patients who are pharmacogenetically at risk for such reactions.

Historically, and at least for the foreseeable future, the majority of adverse drug effects have been and are likely to continue to be identified in the postmarketing period, either by case reports or by specific studies. The latter are usually controlled clinical trials directed to a specific question, such as the efficacy of the drug for a new indication, or its use in an age group not previously considered (often infants or children). When the design includes patients receiving a placebo or a drug other than the one under study, such trials can and do provide useful information on adverse reactions. As with premarketing evaluations, however, these studies tend to be limited in both numbers of patients and duration of observation, and even though in the aggregate clinical trials may evaluate large numbers of patients exposed to a given drug, it is unlikely that such efforts will identify adverse drug reactions that are rare, previously unsuspected, or occur only after long-term exposure to the drug.

Occasionally, pediatric investigators will focus more specifically on adverse drug reactions to a given drug, utilizing "cohort" or "case-control" approaches.[26] In the former, a group of patients exposed to a drug (a cohort) is observed for the development of adverse events that may be related to the exposure. Ampicillin has been the subject of a number of such studies, leading to our current understanding of the rates of rash and diarrhea attributable to this agent.[27-30] Cohort studies have a number of advantages,[26] including the availability of valid information on the exposure and (usually) the outcome of interest. Because cohort studies identify a defined population of exposed patients, such approaches permit one to estimate population-based rates of adverse drug reactions; however, they are generally inefficient for the detection of rare events. Because cohort studies tend to involve followup of particular populations over some period of time, they tend to require relatively long-term involvement on the part of investigators and substantial financial support.

Investigators may also use the case-control approach to study adverse reactions in the pediatric population.[26] In this approach, patients with and without a given adverse event ("cases" and "controls," respectively) are identified, and the frequency of exposure to the drug in question is ascertained to determine if exposure is more common in patients with the effect than in those without it. For example, one might identify newborn patients with cardiorespiratory collapse and patients without collapse and then ascertain exposure to benzyl alcohol–containing infusions.[10] Because the case-control approach begins with the outcome, that information is usually well documented and therefore valid; however, valid information on the exposure may not be readily available. Unlike cohort studies, which provide rates of adverse reactions, estimation of absolute adverse drug reaction rates from case-control studies is somewhat more complicated. Case-control studies are generally inefficient for the assessment of rare exposures. Whereas cohort studies tend to represent long-term efforts involving considerable cost, case-control studies are more likely to be conducted relatively quickly and inexpensively.

The cohort and case-control approaches have their respective strengths and weaknesses, and proper attention to the design and conduct of a study using either approach can yield equivalently valid findings. Why, then, do some view the cohort approach as the scientifically more rigorous study design? Such a perception, we believe, reflects less the inherent qualities of the two designs, and more their respective "track records." Because it is relatively easy to mount a case-control study, inexperienced and unskilled investigators can, without much thought to issues of design or analysis, assemble cases and controls, and then seek information on exposure. By contrast, the logistics involved in most cohort studies tend to attract investigators who will commit substantial effort to the study over a relatively long time, and who can design a protocol that will pass scientific and funding reviews. Given these considerations, it is not surprising that "quick and dirty" studies are more likely to be conducted with the case-control than with the cohort approach (most often, the "dirty" reflects unrecognized or uncontrolled bias). This experience reinforces the importance of understanding that the efficiencies in time and cost inherent in the case-control approach in no way diminish the need for experience and scientific rigor on the part of the investigators.

Although specific studies can and do offer useful information relating to adverse drug effects in the pediatric population, they generally do not provide a comprehensive evaluation of drug use and effects. For example, most such studies do not consider the potential effects of the concurrent use of additional drugs, the patient's disease state, and other factors that are likely to affect the risk of adverse reactions. Most importantly, however, case reports and most specific studies do not offer a mechanism for the systematic discovery of previously unsuspected adverse drug effects.

Data Bases

As third parties have become more involved in the financing of medical care, record keeping related to medical encounters has become more common. Insurance plans (e.g., Medicaid) and health maintenance organizations, for example, have developed data files containing information on drug exposures, outcomes, and population variables. As a result, much attention in recent years has been devoted to utilizing such preexisting data bases for the purposes of assessing drug effects. In a recent critical review, Shapiro[31] cited several factors which at present limit the validity of assessments drawn from such approaches. The problem with automated data bases is directly related to their attractiveness: They are inexpensive because they were developed for other purposes (e.g., billing); because they were developed for other purposes, the information available is often inadequate to meet the needs of an epidemiologically rigorous assessment of the risks and safety of drug exposures. Though others take issue with some of the points expressed by Shapiro,[32] his critique serves as an excellent basis for considering the potential utility of various preexisting automated data resources.

Surveillance Systems

Approaches to the systematic discovery of adverse drug reactions vary greatly, as do the terms used to describe them. "Drug monitoring" was an early name for such activities, but it has now come to be associated with the assessment of drug levels in patients (therapeutic drug monitoring). More recently, the term "postmarketing surveillance" (PMS) has become popular; while properly reflecting the increasing focus on the identification of adverse drug reactions once a drug has come onto the general market, this term encompasses the broad range of approaches, from spontaneous case reports, to specific studies designed to test hypotheses, to efforts designed to discover previously unrecognized adverse drug reactions. For reasons of history and personal taste, we believe "drug surveillance" is the most appropriate and established term for systematic efforts designed specifically to test and generate hypotheses regarding the effects of drugs.

The theoretical basis for drug surveillance was proposed in 1965 by Finney[33] as "any systematic collection and analysis of information pertaining to adverse effects or other idiosyncratic phenomena associated with the normal use of drugs." At approximately the same time, Cluff and colleagues[34] described their in-hospital drug surveillance system at Johns Hopkins (which was continued at the University of Florida in Gainesville), and shortly thereafter Slone, Jick, and coworkers described their program in Boston, which evolved into the Boston Collaborative Drug Surveillance Program (BCDSP).[35] Surveillance efforts were also undertaken by other investigators in the mid-1960s, but the Gainesville and Boston programs were the largest efforts and are generally considered models for the conduct of drug surveillance.

Both programs focused primarily on acutely ill hospitalized adults and were intensive systems (by "intensive" we mean the collection of detailed information relating to the period of hospitalization). Information regarding drug exposure, outcome, and population characteristics was gathered by monitors employed by the programs. Cluff utilized pharmacists, who obtained information on drug

exposures and selected patient variables (age, sex, weight, diagnosis, hospital stay) from the patient record. Possible adverse drug reactions were identified by review of drug orders for changes in therapy, review of the patient record, and discussions with ward physicians. Between 1969 and 1975, Cluff and colleagues[36] monitored 14,457 patients in Gainesville. During 1971, 658 pediatric patients were monitored as part of this larger program, and 3556 pediatric patients were monitored for adverse drug reactions that led to hospitalization.[37,38]

The BCDSP used nurses as monitors; they were assigned to specific wards where they collected detailed information on variables of interest. Data relating to drug exposures were abstracted from doctors' orders, and included the indication for use and the reason for stopping each order. Monitors identified potential adverse reactions by detailed review of the patient record, attendance at ward rounds, and discussions with the ward physician. Information on patient variables (in addition to that collected by Cluff) included allergy history, history of previous reactions, and detailed descriptions of other exposures (e.g., smoking, coffee consumption).[39] Over 35,000 patients were intensively monitored by the BCDSP in a number of hospitals both in North America and abroad. In 1969 the BCDSP conducted a pilot pediatric surveillance effort; using adult-oriented data collection forms, the BCDSP monitored 361 pediatric admissions.[40]

Neither pediatric study was designed primarily to monitor drug effects in children, and both were small and short-lived. In the mid-1970s, two drug surveillance efforts were developed that focused specifically on hospitalized pediatric populations. One, developed by Aranda in Montreal, was concerned exclusively with newborn infants hospitalized in a newborn intensive care unit. That effort monitored 1200 infants between 1977 and 1981 and produced useful information on the epidemiology of adverse drug reactions in this setting.[41,42]

The Pediatric Drug Surveillance (PeDS) Program was established in 1974 at the Children's Hospital in Boston in collaboration with the Drug Epidemiology Unit (now the Slone Epidemiology Unit) of Boston University School of Medicine.[8] The PeDS Program intensively monitored over 11,500 pediatric patients, from premature newborns to adolescents. The methods used by this program generally followed those of the adult-oriented BCDSP and have been described in detail.[8] As was noted earlier in this chapter, an assessment of drug effects requires information on exposures, outcomes, and the population under study. To obtain data in these three categories, the PeDS Program employed specially trained pediatric nurses who were stationed on specific wards where they collected the following detailed information on a sample of patients admitted for more than 24 hours: (a) drug exposures, including indication, dose, route, frequency, duration, dates, and reason for stopping; (b) outcomes, including the discharge diagnoses and the occurrences of any of a list of specified clinical (or laboratory) "events" (e.g., rash, gastrointestinal bleed, renal failure, hyperglycemia, convulsions); all instances of these events were recorded, whether they were attributed by the staff to drug therapy (i.e., an "adverse drug reaction") or considered a part of the patient's underlying illness; (c) population characteristics, including demographic data, medications used prior to admission, and results of admission laboratory analyses. Standard computer programs were used to describe and evaluate the data, and *ad hoc* analyses were conducted to address specific issues.

The accumulated data can be used to provide descriptions of various aspects of drug therapy, such as rates and trends in drug exposure[9] and reported rates of adverse drug reactions[43] and clinical events; such data can be derived for both teaching and community hospitals.[44] Known risk factors for certain reactions can be quantified (e.g., $D_{10}W$-induced hyperglycemia in the newborn.[45] Finally, a unique feature of drug surveillance efforts is the ability to generate hypotheses related to previously unrecognized ADRs. As one example, the PeDS Program identified, in low-birth-weight infants, an unexpected association between intracranial hemorrhage and low doses of heparin given to maintain the patency of intraarterial infusion lines.[46]

Few have attempted to apply drug surveillance to the outpatient pediatric setting. One study in a general pediatric group practice monitored prescription and nonprescription drug therapy over a 1-year period.[47] A researcher interviewed parents at the time of the doctor's visit; all patients who received drugs were followed by telephone a few days later and were asked about the occurrence of a variety of symptoms. The study involved 3181 children and provided useful information on patterns of drug use in the population. Information on adverse reactions was based on parental observation, which may have been biased; since assessments of causality were made by means of an algorithm (an issue discussed earlier in this chapter), the study design did not provide for the detection of previously unrecognized adverse reactions to drugs used in the pediatric outpatient population.

While intensive drug surveillance has clear advantages over other approaches, it also has limitations. Programs are expensive to develop and maintain, and require multidisciplinary expertise and facilities (pediatrics, epidemiology, biostatistics, computer science) that are available in few centers. Because of the detail accumulated on each patient monitored in the in-hospital setting, only a few hundred patients each year can be monitored by one nurse, so accumulation of sufficient data takes many years to accomplish. This concern is particularly problematic in pediatrics, since the marked differences in drug effects among neonates, infants, toddlers, and older children require that large numbers be monitored in each age category. Further, drug surveillance programs are inefficient for the purposes of identifying relatively rare reactions, particularly if the drug involved is used infrequently.

SUMMARY

To develop meaningful information on rates of adverse drug reactions and their associated risk factors, we need valid information on the exposure, outcome, and population under study. No single design can be expected to provide answers to all questions; rather, we need a variety of methods which, in the aggregate, will lead to much needed improvements in our understanding of the nature, causes, and prevention of adverse drug reactions in children.

ACKNOWLEDGMENTS: This work was supported in part by grant HD 17958-10 from the National Institute of Child Health and Human Development and by grant MCJ-250484 from the Division of Maternal and Child Health, Bureau of Health Care Delivery and Assistance.

REFERENCES

1. Silverman WA, Andersen D, Blanc WA, et al: A difference in mortality rate and incidence of kernicterus among premature infants allotted to two prophylactic antibacterial regimes. Pediatrics 18:614, 1956
2. Conchie JM, Munroe JT, Anderson DO: The incidence of staining of permanent teeth by the tetracyclines. Can Med Assoc J 103:351, 1970
3. Burns LE, Hodgman JE, Cass A: Fatal circulatory collapse in premature infants receiving chloramphenicol. N Engl J Med 261:1318, 1959
4. Lischner H, Seligman SJ, Krammer A, et al: An outbreak of neonatal deaths among term infants associated with administration of chloramphenicol. J Pediatr 59:21, 1961
5. Chalhub E, DeVivo D, Volpe JJ: Phenytoin-induced dystonia and choreoathetosis in two retarded epileptic children. Neurology 26:494, 1976
6. Merritt HH, Putnam JJ: Sodium diphenylhydantoinate in the treatment of convulsive disorders. JAMA 3:1068, 1938
7. Aranda JV, Cohen S, Neims AH: Drug utilization in a newborn intensive care unit. J Pediatr 89:315, 1976
8. Mitchell AA, Goldman P, Shapiro S, et al: Drug utilization and reported adverse reactions in hospitalized children. Am J Epidemiol 110:196, 1979
9. Lesko S, Epstein MF, Mitchell AA: Recent patterns of drug use in newborn intensive care. J Pediatr 116:985, 1990
10. Gershanik J, Boecler D, Ensley H, et al: The gasping syndrome and benzyl alcohol poisoning. N Engl J Med 307:1384, 1982
11. Glasgow AM, Boeck RL, Miller MK, et al: Hyperosmolality in small infants due to propylene glycol. Pediatrics 72:353, 1983
12. World Health Organization: International drug monitoring—The role of the hospital. Drug Intell Clin Pharmacol 4:101, 1970
13. Davies EM: Textbook of Adverse Drug Reactions. Oxford, Oxford University Press, 1977
14. Reidenberg MM, Lowenthal DT: Adverse nondrug reactions. N Engl J Med 279:678, 1968
15. Koch-Weser J: Validation of ADRs, in Gross FH, Inman WHW (eds): Drug Monitoring. New York, Academic Press, 1977
16. Karch FE, Smith CL, Kerzner B, et al: Adverse drug reactions—A matter of opinion. Clin Pharmacol Ther 19:489, 1976
17. Karch FE, Lasagna L: Toward the operational identification of adverse drug reactions. Clin Pharmacol Ther 21:247, 1977
18. Naranjo CA, Busto U, Sellers EM, et al: A method for estimating the probability of adverse reactions. Clin Pharmacol Ther 30:239, 1981
19. Louik C, Lacouture PG, Mitchell AA, et al: A study of adverse reaction algorithms in a drug surveillance program. Clin Pharmacol Ther 38:183, 1985
20. Pere JC, Begaud B, Haramburu F, Albin H: Computerized comparisons of six adverse drug reaction assessment procedures. Clin Pharmacol Ther 40:451, 1986
21. FDA Drug Bulletin 1976; 6:28, and 1977; 7:10
22. Faich GA: Adverse-drug-reaction monitoring. N Engl J Med 314:1589, 1986
23. Spielberg SP: Pharmacogenetics, in MacLeod SM, Radde IC (eds): Textbook of Pediatric Clinical Pharmacology Littleton, MA, PSG-Wright, 1985
24. Rieder J, Uetrecht J, Shear NH, et al: Diagnosis of sulfonamide

hypersensitivity reactions by in vitro "re-challenge" with hydroxylamine metabolites. Ann Intern Med 110:286, 1989

25. Shear NH, Spielberg SP: Anticonvulsant hypersensitivity syndrome: In vitro assessment of risk. J Clin Invest 82:1826, 1988
26. McMahon B, Pugh TF: Epidemiology—Principles and Methods. Boston, Little, Brown, 1970, pp 207–282
27. Bass JW, Crowley DM, Steele RW, et al: Adverse effects of orally administered ampicillin. J Pediatr 83:106, 1973
28. Boston Collaborative Drug Surveillance Program: Ampicillin rashes. Arch Dermatol 107:74, 1972
29. Caldwell JR, Cluff LE: Adverse reactions to antimicrobial agents. JAMA 230:77, 1974
30. Collaborative Study Group: Prospective study of ampicillin rash. Br Med J 1:7, 1973
31. Shapiro S: The role of automated record linkage in the postmarketing surveillance of drug safety: A critique. Clin Pharmacol Ther 46:371, 1989
32. Faich GA, Stadel BV, Strom BL, Carson JL, Shapiro S: The future of automated record linkage for postmarketing surveillance: A response to Shapiro. Clin Pharmacol Ther 46:387–398, 1989
33. Finney DJ: The design and logic of a monitor of drug use. J Chron Dis 18:77, 1965
34. Seidel LG, Thornton GF, Smith JW, et al: Studies on the epidemiology of adverse drug reactions. Bull Johns Hopkins Hosp 119:299, 1966
35. Slone D, Jick H, Borda I, et al: Drug surveillance utilizing nurse-monitors—An epidemiologic approach. Lancet 2:901, 1966
36. Stewart RB, Cluff LE, Philip JR: Drug Monitoring: A Requirement for Responsible Drug Use. Baltimore, Williams and Wilkins, 1977
37. McKenzie MW, Stewart RB, Weiss CF, et al: A pharmacist-based study of the epidemiology of adverse drug reactions in pediatric medicine patients. Am J Hosp Pharm 30:898, 1973
38. McKenzie NW, Marchall GL, Netzloff ML, et al: Adverse drug reactions leading to a hospitalization in children. J Pediatr 89:487, 1976
39. Miller RR, Greenblatt DJ (eds): Drug Effects in Hospitalized Patients. New York, Wiley, 1976
40. Lawson DH, Shapiro S, Slone D, et al: Drug surveillance—Problems and challenges. Pediatr Clin North Am 19:117, 1972
41. Aranda JV, Portuguez-Malavasi A, Collinge JM, et al: Epidemiology of adverse drug reactions in the newborn. Dev Pharmacol Ther 5:173, 1982
42. Aranda JV: Factors associated with adverse drug reactions in the newborn. Pediatr Pharmacol 3:245, 1983
43. Mitchell AA, Louik C, Lacouture PG, et al: Risks to children from computed tomographic scan pre-medication. JAMA 247:2385, 1982
44. Mitchell AA, Lacouture PG, Sheehan J, et al: Adverse drug reactions in children leading to hospital admission. Pediatrics 82:24, 1988
45. Louik C, Mitchell AA, Epstein MF, Shapiro S: Risk factors for neonatal hyperglycemia. Am J Dis Child 139:783, 1985
46. Lesko SM, Mitchell AA, Epstein MF, et al: Heparin use as a risk factor for intraventricular hemorrhage in low-birth-weight infants. N Engl J Med 314:1156, 1986
47. Kramer MS, Hutchinson TA, Flegel KM, et al: Adverse drug reactions in general pediatric outpatients. J Pediatr 106:305, 1985

49

DRUG UTILIZATION IN NON-HOSPITALIZED NEWBORNS, INFANTS, AND CHILDREN

INGRID MATHESON

The decision on when, where and how to use a certain drug is the final and crucial step in the therapeutic decision chain. No matter how accurate the diagnostic and therapeutic considerations might have been in the prescribing process, the outcome will finally be determined by the behavior of the user. This in turn reflects fundamental attitudes of the individual and the society to drugs and health, as well as life-style preferences (Figure 49–1).[1]

Drugs are often used in children for self-limiting disorders and for symptoms for which drug efficacy has not been established. The World Health Organization (WHO) has claimed that as much as two-thirds of all drugs used by children may have little or no value.[2] Large differences exist between less developed and more developed countries. Some children receive drugs that they do not need, whereas others do not receive drugs that they need. Drug utilization studies focusing on medicine use in children are thus necessary in order to improve health and ensure optimal use of drugs.

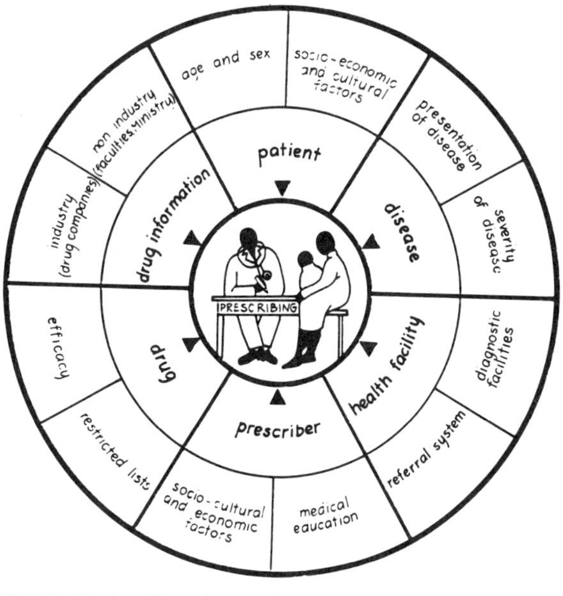

Drug utilization has been defined by WHO as "the marketing, distribution, prescription and use of drugs in a society, with special emphasis on the resulting medical, social and economic consequences" (WHO Technical Report Series No. 615, Geneva). Additionally, nonpharmacologic factors such as anthropologic, behavioral, and economic factors influence drug taking. This new emerging discipline is also termed "pharmaco-epidemiology" because it aims to describe, explain, control, and predict the effects and uses of pharmacologic treatment in a defined time, space and population.[3,4] The objectives of drug utilization studies are to:

1. Describe patterns of drug therapeutic practice in various populations and at various levels of the health care system
2. Make estimates of the number of individuals exposed to appropriate and inappropriate drug use
3. Diminish the gap between therapeutic practice as recommended and current clinical practice
4. Measure the effects of informative, educational, and regulatory efforts, and thus provide a basis for intervention strategies aimed at improving prescription behavior
5. Analyze the clinical, social, ecologic, and economic consequences of drug use in a society.

FIGURE 49–1. The circle of prescribing. Some of the factors which influence drug prescribing. (From Diwan and Tomson,[1] with permission.)

NEWBORNS

Healthy newborns usually receive few drugs directly after they are born, whereas quite extensive indirect drug exposure via placenta and breast milk has been reported.[5,6] Therapeutic routines immediately after birth will inevitably vary with economy, culture, and the dis-

557

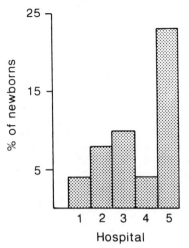

FIGURE 49–2. Proportion of newborns (*n* = 978) who received a drug during their stay in the maternity wards of five university hospitals in Norway.

ease pattern in different parts of the world. Very few surveys have reported the use of drugs in apparently healthy newborns,[7] whereas infants treated in intensive care units or referred to special care nurseries have been found to be given numerous drugs.[8] Recently, drug exposure in the perinatal period has been associated with long-term effects such as cancer.[9]

In Scotland 2–5 percent of maternity ward babies received a mean of 1.2 drugs, most often topical chloramphenicol and systemic antibiotics (penicillin and ampicillin). However, among the babies referred to special care units, 17 percent received drugs.[7] The majority were given antimicrobial combination therapy, as broad-spectrum cover was often necessary. A survey of five university hospitals in Norway[10] found that on average 10 percent of the newborns lying in with their mothers received drugs directly (Figure 49–2). One hospital, in particular, gave naloxone routinely to babies exposed to maternal pethidine analgesia, without awaiting symptoms of respiratory depression. This questionable routine[11] was eventually changed as a result of discussions following the presentation of the drug survey. Other routines

such as the administration of silver nitrate solution (Credé prophylaxis) to prevent gonococcal eye infection, are still practiced in some countries. However, the latter practice has been abandoned in many countries, such as the United Kingdom and Scandinavia.[12]

As a result of *in utero* exposure, some newborns are affected by drugs for many days, e.g., phenobarbitone and metabolites of diazepam and pethidine may be present for weeks in infant blood. The possibility of passive drug exposure in newborns as a result of drugs in breast milk may be estimated by looking at the drug utilization patterns of puerperal mothers (Table 49–1). Whereas breast-feeding rates varied from 98[10] to 36[13] percent, or were not mentioned,[14–16] the percentage of mothers who received drugs during their stay varied from 67 to 99 percent, excluding iron and vitamins. In brief, large variations in the use of hypnotics, analgesics, laxatives, and uterine-contracting agents, with apparently little attention to selection of drugs with minimal excretion in breast milk, were found in these studies.

In general, harmful effects of drugs ingested through breast milk may occur in the newborn, but they have seldom been reported unless repeated doses of a slowly eliminated drug were ingested or maternal drug was still present in the newborn after birth.[17]

INFANTS

Based on several studies including children from 0 to 14 years, drug exposure seems to have a peak at approximately 1 year of age. Thus, the greatest number of prescribed medications was documented at ½–1 year of age in Baltimore,[18] 0–1 year in Norway,[19] 0–2 years in Sweden,[20] and 0–2 years in Spain.[21] The youngest age group received from 2.5 to 10 times more prescriptions than the age group 10–14 years.[19,20] However, age-related prescribing to children has not been found in all studies.[22]

Data from a cross-sectional sample of Swedish children show that the average rate of prescriptions per child was around 2.5 during both the first and the second year of

TABLE 49–1. DRUG UTILIZATION STUDIES IN POSTPARTUM WOMEN IN VARIOUS COUNTRIES

YEAR	COUNTRY	METHOD, PATIENTS	APPROACH	RATE OF DRUG USE PER 100 WOMEN	REF.
1978	U.S.A.	Drug administration sheets (*n* = 168)	Most frequent drugs	78	14
1980	U.K.	Prescriptions (*n* = 308)	Most frequent drugs and indications		15
1981	Ireland	Charts	Most frequent drugs	67	16
1984	U.K.	Charts (*n* = 2004)	Most frequent drugs Focus drugs and BF	99	13
1989	Norway	Charts, 5 hosp. (*n* = 970)	Most frequent drugs Focus drugs and BF	>95	10
1990	WHO (20 countries)	Charts + interviews (*n* = 14,421)	Most frequent drugs and indications in BF women	80	*

BF = Breast-feeding.
*Bonati et al. (not yet published).

life.[20] Longitudinal data from a cohort of 1497 Swedish infants showed that half of them had received a prescribed drug by the age of 6 months and 70 percent by one year.[23]

In the first three months of life, the proportion of Australian infants who had received a drug, according to postal questionnaires, was 65 percent.[24] This agrees with Norwegian, Yugoslavian, and Swedish findings where 58, 55, and 32 percent of infants, respectively, were exposed to drugs excluding vitamins during the first 4 months of life.[25] Questions about who recommended the medication to the parents indicated that 75–85 percent of the drugs were advised by health personnel, possibly reflecting the good access to health services for this age group and the insecurity of the parents.[26]

How often are medicines used in the daily life of an infant? Interviews have been carried out with parents, usually the mother. In Oslo, Norway, 12% of 4-month-old infants received at least one drug (excluding vitamins) during a 2-week period, according to questionnaires and interviews.[27] About 80 percent of English children 0–2 years old received at least one drug (prescribed or nonprescribed) during a period of 2 weeks according to household interviews in 1970,[28] whereas much lower rates were found in a diary study conducted in Birmingham, England, in 1985.[29] Prospective studies based on the diary method suggest that drugs were given on 25 and 10 percent, respectively, of all days in Swedish[30] and English infants.[29] Topical decongestants, ointments, and antibiotics ranked highest in the Swedish survey, whereas vitamins and expectorants were most common among the youngest age group in Birmingham. Interviews about any medicine intake during the last 2 days revealed that one-third and one-half, respectively, of the youngest children in both Finnish[31] and American[32] families had received drugs. Thirteen percent of the Finnish children and 30 percent of the American children received prescription drugs.

The reasons that drug treatment was initiated, according to the mothers of the Norwegian and Swedish infants, were most often respiratory tract disorders such as common cold and blocked nose.[26,27] It should be noted that slightly different wording of symptoms, e.g., diarrhea versus loose stools, resulted in different rates of treatment. One of the most difficult therapeutic problems in this age group is infantile colic, which frequently affects the entire family. Colic symptoms (excessive crying in normal babies more than 2–3 hours a day at least 4 days a week) were treated with drugs in 98 and 68 percent of the cases in Norway and Sweden respectively. Furthermore, Norwegian as well as Australian studies showed that anticolic drugs were given to more than one-third of all babies. In contrast, only one-tenth of Yugoslavian and Swedish infants[25] received these drugs. This possibly reflects differences in perceived disease, therapeutic traditions, and use of nonpharmacologic measures in colic therapy. However, it should be emphasized that in some parts of the world infantile colic seems to be a more or less unknown phenomenon.[33]

Factors that predict high drug use at this early age have also been investigated. The number of illnesses reported or the mother's perception of having a problem with the infant usually explained most of the variance in drug use.[24,27] The type of day care and the birth order in the family also played a role, particularly for older infants.[34]

The question has also been raised whether breast-fed infants receive more drugs than bottle-fed ones, or alternatively, whether breast feeding protects against some of the direct use of medicine. According to recent results in Norway,[27] neither of these hypotheses is supported, but studies should also be performed in other areas where the health benefit of breast feeding is more substantial. In terms of doses, direct and indirect drug exposure via breast milk during a 2-week period corresponded to an average of 10 and 1.7 percent respectively of the infant population using one infant DDD (Defined Daily Dose)* per day.[27]

Most studies in this section document quite extensive drug exposure in infancy, a period of rapid growth and development. During the first year, some receptor systems, such as the dopaminergic, are very sensitive to early pharmacologic effects. Later alterations in behavior and learning may in some cases be attributed to drugs,[35–37] analogously to behavioral teratogenicity in animals. However, as is known for toxic environmental substances such as alcohol and nicotine, this type of study is extremely difficult to accomplish.

CHILDREN

Most drug utilization studies in children have focused on the issue of unnecessary or inappropriate prescription of drugs. Thus, 73 percent of presumably healthy children visiting the doctor for a routine checkup in Tenerife, Spain, received at least one drug, and more than three drugs were prescribed for 40 percent of them. The drugs most often prescribed were antiflatulents; calcium, potassium, and mineral supplements; spasmolytics; anabolic hormones; and appetite stimulants.[21] In Australia it was reported that 53 percent of the children had received medication, although their mothers described them as being perfectly well.[24]

An audit of prescriptions to Italian children showed that an average of two drugs were prescribed per consultation, several of which were potentially harmful drugs such as aminophenasone, tetracycline, dihydrostreptomycin, and chloramphenicol. Moreover, 80 percent of the drugs given to children were judged unacceptable based on their inefficacy, toxicity, or undue cost.[38] Children in Nigeria and Indonesia received an average of 4.7 and 3.8 drugs per consultation, respectively.[39,40] In Sri Lanka the corresponding figure was 2.7.[22] Sanz[21] found 2.3 drugs per prescription, whereas in Norway and Sweden the figures were 1.3 and 1.4, respectively.[19]

Several studies indicate a tendency to overmedicate children in both rich and poor societies. The authors argue that the psychosocial consequences may be that

---

*The defined daily dose (DDD) is a technical unit for comparison of drug use. It has been established on the basis of average dose/day for the main indication in adults. It may be divided by 10 to obtain the newborn or infant DDD.

children are brought up to believe that drugs are the solution to most health problems.[22,24,41] It is reasonable to think that their future medicine use will resemble their early behavior patterns. Therefore, children's perceptions of what medicines do to their bodies are important to investigate.[41] Moreover, the child receiving a drug may think that he or she is "permitted to be sick."

In the following sections drug utilization data for different categories of drugs are discussed.

ANTIMICROBIALS

The most frequent category of drugs prescribed to children is the anti-infective agents. They account for one-third of all drugs prescribed to children in outpatient surveys from several countries, despite differences in methodology.[19,21,42–44] The prescribing of antibiotics to children aged 4 years and under has been substantial and increasing.[20,45,46] This is a matter of concern, since the reasons for and the effects of the increased prescribing are insufficiently known.

First, increased anti-infective prescribing could reflect a real increase in infectious illness among young children, a phenomenon that might be a function of the growing numbers of children attending day-care centers or other unrecognized factors. Children attending day-care centers are known to be at increased risk for acquiring respiratory, gastrointestinal, and skin infections, and they are recognized as having an important role in transmission of disease to household members and the community.[34,47]

Second, sick children who formerly would have been hospitalized for their illness may today be treated on an outpatient basis, possibly as a result of improved oral anti-infective therapy, hospital cost, or improved outpatient medical care. Finally, anti-infectives might be increasingly used inappropriately to treat viral illness.

The increase in the prescription rate of antibiotics in Sweden was due to the prescribing of second-line drugs.[20] An increasing prevalence of *Haemophilus influenzae* with reduced susceptibility to erythromycin has paralleled the increased use of this drug.[48] Erythromycin has also gained undeserved popularity among children in, for example, Norway,[19,27] Sweden,[49] and Yugoslavia,[50] presumably because of successful marketing, the overstated risk of penicillin allergy, and a better taste.

Penicillin V was the most commonly prescribed antibiotic to children in Sweden as well as in Sri Lanka. Throughout 1977–1988 the prescription rate per child of penicillin V was stable in Sweden[20] compared with other countries. In the United States[45] the use of penicillin in children declined by 68 percent from 1977 to 1986, as the use of broad-spectrum penicillins and sulfonamide combinations increased by 40 and 430 percent, respectively (Figure 49–3). Costly cephalosporins have steadily increased their share of antibiotic prescriptions to children during the last decade.[45]

It is discouraging that tetracycline is still prescribed to children[38,40,50] and that tetracycline in syrup formulations is still on the market in some countries. Prescription of tetracyclines to children below 8 years of age has been sug-

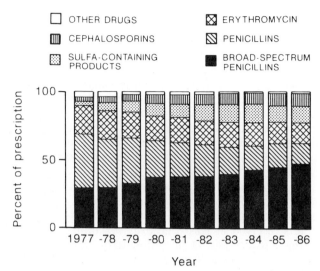

FIGURE 49–3. Distribution of outpatient systemic antiinfective prescriptions by subgroups for children 3 to 9 years old, by year 1977–1986 in the United States. (From Nelson et al.,[45] with permission.)

gested as an indicator of inappropriate prescribing.[22] In fact, the most common antimicrobial among Indonesian children was oxytetracycline. In Indonesia 27 percent of the pediatric outpatients were prescribed tetracycline,[22,40] compared to only 0.5 percent in Sri Lanka.

It was found that educational visits conducted in the office of practicing doctors by a clinical pharmacist[51] or by a specially trained physician counselor[52] reduced inappropriate prescribing of cephalosporins. In the latter study, the improvement persisted for 2 years after the educational visit.[53]

RESPIRATORY DRUGS

An increase in the use of antiasthmatics has been noticeable during the last decade.[20,29,54] Thus, the β_2-adrenoreceptor agonist salbutamol was the drug most commonly taken by English children, followed by vitamins.[29] Swedish cumulative drug data showed that by the fifth birthday one or more bronchodilators had been purchased for 47 percent of the children, while only 3 percent had made consultations concerning asthma (Figure 49–4). Moreover, 44 percent had purchased antitussives or expectorants before age 5.[23] The efficacy of cough remedies has been questioned, and since 1984 they have not been prescribed in Sweden under the drug benefit scheme. Together with the nonapproved use of β_2-agonists against common cold symptoms, a change toward a more intense drug therapy in asthma has also contributed to the increase in the annual number of antiasthmatic prescriptions to children.[20] In Norway the higher use of antiasthmatics among boys than girls was documented (Figure 49–5).[19]

An extensive use of systemic decongestants developed

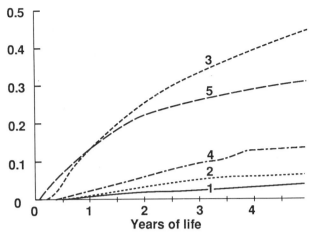

FIGURE 49–4. Cumulative proportions of children with at least one physician visit at Tierp health center, Sweden, for wheezy bronchitis or bronchial asthma (1), atopic dermatitis (2), and cumulative proportions with at least one purchase of bronchodilators (3), systemic antihistamines (4), or dermatological corticosteroids (5). (From Rasmussen and Smedby,[23] with permission.)

in many countries during the 1970s.[20,42] The efficacy of these compounds in middle ear infections was eventually questioned.[1,55] Systemic decongestants in Scandinavia have gradually been substituted by topical decongestants, mostly sold over the counter.[19,20] In many countries antihistamines, either alone or in combination with decongestants, are among the most popular remedies for the common cold, unfortunately. In fact, antihistamines were the most commonly prescribed drugs for children in Sri Lanka.[22]

ANALGESICS

Analgesics are increasingly used by adolescents, especially females.[44,56] Still, prescriptions for analgesics are

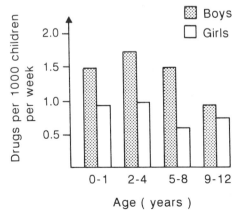

FIGURE 49–5. Rate of antiasthmatic prescriptions in Norway in 1986 according to age and sex. (From Andrew and Toverud,[19] with permission.)

four times more frequent in the age group 0–4 years than in the group 10–14 years in Sweden,[20] due to fever therapy.

In many countries acetaminophen (paracetamol) strongly dominates the prescribing of analgesics/antipyretics to children,[19,20,22,27,56] but this was not the case in the Birmingham study.[29] In contrast to the situation in the United States, acetaminophen gained its dominant position in Scandinavia before Reye's syndrome was noticed.[20]

ANTIDIARRHEALS

The treatment of diarrhea in Indonesia followed the pattern of multiple drug use. Antibiotics were used twice as frequently as and vitamins were used more frequently than oral rehydration solution (ORS), and an average of four drugs were prescribed per case.[22]

In response to the presentation of a fictitious infant with diarrhea, only 16 of 75 pharmacies in Bangladesh, Sri Lanka, and Yemen gave the appropriate recommendation: ORS or consultation with a health worker. Combination antibiotics were frequently dispensed, but the most frequent remedies sold were kaolin and pectin.[57] It was concluded that appropriate training of pharmacy attendants is a formidable task if health care is to be improved in the private sector in these countries.

A therapeutic scheme for treating acute diarrhea was evaluated in two family medicine clinics in Mexico City.[58] The use of oral rehydration and nonrestrictive diets was increased, and there was a "modest" decrease in the use of antimicrobial drugs (from 75 to 40 percent of the cases). This study, like many others, demonstrated that the therapeutic behavior of the physician was not changed by written information. However, attendance (by random selection) in an educational workshop of an active participating nature showed a clear relationship with the modified habits.

PSYCHOTROPIC DRUGS

The prescribing of psychotropic drugs for children has been criticized by many, including pediatric pharmacologists and the lay press. Frightening figures about the consumption of psychotropic drugs by children and allegations of "a medicalization of deviant behavior" have been published in Germany.[59] However, based on a national data base on drug prescriptions, it has been calculated that children under 6 years receive an average of only 1.1 DDDs of psychotropic agents per year, and that children over 6 years receive an average of 0.6 DDDs per year.[59] In the youngest age group (0–5 years), homeopathics/herbal pharmaceutics, neuroleptics, and benzodiazepines were most prevalent. The prevalence of methylphenidate treatment was 100–300 times more frequent in America than in Germany, according to data from Elliger et al.[59] and Quinn.[60]

Data indicate that the proportion of children who are prescribed psychotropics is 3–4 percent per year up to the age of puberty.[44,61] Sedatives were the drugs most frequently prescribed, usually for fever, nausea, and allergy in Finland and respiratory disease in North America.

In Sweden 1 in 10 children had received a neuroleptic drug before they were 5 years old.[23] Alimemazine (trimeprazine), which has sedative as well as antihistaminic effects and is classified as a neuroleptic, was the psychotropic most often prescribed to children in Scandinavia, usually for sleeping problems,[19,20] whereas promethazine is more popular in North America.[61] However, both these phenothiazines have been associated with sudden infant death syndrome (SIDS)[62] and should not be prescribed to those below age 1.[2]

The dominant reason for prescribing tricyclic antidepressants to children is enuresis. Imipramine prescriptions peaked at age 8 and were higher for males than females, whose use started to increase after age 12.[44] The use of antidepressants in the treatment of bed wetting has been criticized with regard to side effects and poor treatment results, especially in comparison with those achieved when using urine alarm devices.[63]

NONPRESCRIBED MEDICINE AND SELF CARE

The first response in 50–70 percent of illnesses is a nonprescribed medicine.[64,65] This fact emphasizes the importance of physicians inquiring into self-medication provided by the parents. In a community survey in upstate New York, it was found that 1 in 5 children was on some nonprescribed medication.[32] Well-off families were found to use more kinds of nonprescribed medicine and spend more money on them,[64,65] reflecting the impact of economy on drug use. During a 2-week period, as many as 75 percent of those in the household less than 2 years old had been given nonprescription drugs.[28]

Alternative treatment is frequently sought as a supplement to drugs. A recent Danish survey found that nearly one-third of the patients attending a pediatric outpatient clinic had received alternative therapy, including osteopathy, zone therapy, and homeopathy.[66] It is noteworthy that asthma and allergy accounted for half the treatment causes.

An English study[67] examined the benefits of a mail-distributed health education booklet describing how to handle six common symptoms. Fewer consultations were made for preschool children of families receiving the booklet as compared with a control group. It did not, however, lead to any increase in knowledge among the parents receiving it. A similar study in Sweden showed that the proneness to follow the recommendations in the booklet was higher among readers than nonreaders. However, participation in the educational session did not seem to improve their hypothetical behavior with regard to children's symptoms.[68]

Casey et al.[69] reported that misuse of antipyretic drugs and inappropriate calls to the physician for minor transient febrile illnesses among young children of well-educated American parents were reduced by an educational interview reinforced by a printed information sheet. However, no significant effects of a self-care booklet were found on the number of physician visits made during 6- and 12-month study periods by middle-class American families enrolled in a prepaid insurance plan.[70]

DRUG UTILIZATION AND DEMOGRAPHIC VARIABLES

Age and Sex

Cross-sectional studies from Finland since 1964 indicate that medication has increased relatively more in children than in adults.[31] The reasons could be the higher prevalence of chronic diseases such as asthma and chronic bronchitis in childhood, better diagnostic tools, or more extensive medicalization due to a lower tolerance of minor illnesses, since many families have two parents working outside the home.

Useful information on the distribution of prescriptions according to age, sex, and therapeutic group can be found in annual sales statistics, e.g., in Sweden[20]. All drug use should be adjusted for population statistics. Thus, young boys use an average of 23–37 percent more prescribed drugs than girls.[19,28,29] In particular, more respiratory, nutritional, psychotropic, and anticonvulsant medications are used by boys.[29] By puberty, females use more prescribed drugs than males, and their higher use continues up to the pension age when sex differences seem to decline. However, when factors associated with women's reproductive role are statistically controlled, sex differences in drug use are claimed to be substantially reduced,[71] while others have found that the explanation is much more complicated.

Bush and Rabin[65] claim that the use of nonprescribed medicine may be a learned response to symptoms that is more acceptable for whites and females. The learned behavior may begin early: almost one-fourth of female children less than 2 years old were given an illness-related nonprescribed medicine compared to 14 percent of the males. Dahlquist et al.[72] claim that the strikingly high frequency of nonprescribed medication, especially among small children, calls for further studies, as the harmlessness of this habit cannot be judged at present.

Ray[44] found that girls at puberty received more psychotropics and analgesics than boys did. Controlling for more physician visits made by girls than boys, females still received more prescriptions than males with similar diagnoses. Possibly there might have been an excess of minor gynecologic or menses-related disorders secondary to the presenting complaint in many of these patients, but physician sex stereotyping cannot be ruled out.

Social Class and Education

Half the drug use in children refers to prescribed medicines, which are often reimbursed and thus quite evenly distributed.[28] An association between high family income and high drug use, including over-the-counter drugs, was found in children in Finland[31] and Birmingham, England.[29] More medicines are bought and kept in the home among the higher than the lower social classes.[28,73] It was apparent that with increasing income and education, the use of antacids, pain remedies, dermatologicals, and vitamins increased, but remedies for constipation, diarrhea, and cough decreased.[73] Dunnel and Cartwright[28] found that the children of manual workers received fewer drugs than the children of nonmanual workers. In fact, several studies have found a high proneness to use professional care in those who have a high to intermediate socioeconomic status.

Partially in agreement with the Australian study,[24] we found a positive correlation between length of maternal education and number of drugs per infant in Oslo (Figure 49–6).[27] In concordance with these findings, a positive association between education or income and health care utilization was demonstrated in several studies,[31,74,75] but not in all of them.

Family Characteristics

Households with children appear to keep more prescribed and nonprescribed medicines than those without children.[28] First-born children and only children had more symptoms reported and received more medicines. An inverse relationship between family size and medicine use has been predicted.[76] Our study among 4-month-old infants did not find any association between parity and drug use.[27] On the other hand, Rasmussen[68] found that antibiotics were more often prescribed to children with older siblings than to those who were first-borns without siblings. Contacts outside the family, e.g., in day-care centers, have an important impact on the utilization of drugs, especially antimicrobials.

Significant associations between mothers' and infants' use of drugs as well as physician visits have been documented[27,34,65,74] Families vary considerably with respect to their proneness to use medical services for young children's health problems. The proneness to seek

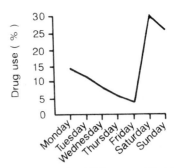

FIGURE 49–7. Drug use in children aged 0–16 related to day of the week. Based on weekly questionnaires filled in by parents. (From Rylance et al.,[29] with permission.)

medical attention is influenced by the type and severity of the illness, the perceived vulnerability of the infant, and the general tendency to interpret problems as illnesses[32,73,74,77]

Our studies in Oslo[27] suggested that maternal drug use was associated with the number of disorders reported, her own as well as the infant's. The association between high education and infant drug use in that study and between occupational status and proneness to medicate the baby in the Australian study was strong in mothers who worked outside the home (whereas a negative, but not significant, association was seen in Oslo housewives). This may be a characteristic of employed women which needs further analysis. However, this contention was apparently not consistent with data from Birmingham,[29] where drug use increased during weekends (Figure 49–7) when the family presumably was together and parents' awareness of children's symptoms increased. Another explanation of this finding is that chronic medication was more often forgotten on weekdays.

CONCLUSIONS

The aim of this chapter is to demonstrate the extent of children's drug use and the role of pharmaceuticals in children's illnesses. The studies indicate a confidence in the effect of drugs that is hardly consistent with their actual pharmacotherapeutic efficacy. In fact, drug efficacy and safety in children are often extrapolated from data in adults.

It may be concluded from these studies that young children receive more drugs than older children, that boys below the age of 10 receive more than girls at the same age, that children born into well-off, educated families receive more medicine than those with a less favorable background, and that children in the undeveloped world receive less adequate drug treatment than those in the developed world. There are, however, large international differences in medicine use due to variations in attitudes, traditions, drug availability, economy, and disease.

Drug utilization studies are considered as a tool to change inappropriate drug use. Unfortunately, it is not yet known to what degree the quoted studies have had that effect. The introduction of essential or limited lists of drugs as well as extensive educational programs for health

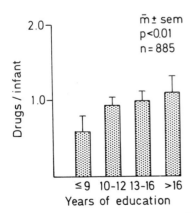

FIGURE 49–6. Correlation between maternal length of education and average number of drugs per infant recorded in a 4-month period in Oslo, Norway. (From Matheson et al.,[27] with permission.)

personnel and parents may give some promise for a better pharmacotherapy in the future.

ACKNOWLEDGMENTS I wish to thank my colleagues Marit Andrew and Else-Lydia Toverud for valuable comments on this chapter.

REFERENCES

1. Diwan VK, Tomson G: The complexity of drug prescribing. Mimeo IHCAR, Stockholm, Department of Health Care Research, Karolinska Institute, 1989
2. WHO, Rylance G (ed): Drugs for children. Copenhagen, WHO Regional Office for Europe, 1987, pp 11–19
3. Lunde PKM, Baksaas I: Epidemiology of drug utilization—Basic concepts and methodology. Act Med Scand(suppl 712):7–11, 1988
4. Porta SM, Hartzema AG: The contribution of epidemiology to the study of drugs. Drug Intell Clin Pharm 21:741–747, 1987
5. Bonati M, Bortolus R, Marchetti F, Romero M, Tognoni G: Drug use in pregnancy: An overview of epidemiological drug utilization studies. Eur J Clin Pharmacol 38:325–328, 1990
6. Matheson I: Drugs taken by mothers in the puerperium. Br Med J 290:1588–1589, 1985
7. Rylance GW, Moreland TA: Drug use in the newborn. J Clin Pharmacol 4:95–100, 1979
8. Aranda JV, Cohen S, Neims AH: Drug utilization in a newborn intensive care unit. J Pediatr 89:315–317, 1976
9. Golding J, Paterson M, Kinlen LJ: Factors associated with childhood cancer in a national cohort study. Br J Cancer 62:304–308, 1990
10. Matheson I: Drugs to mother and infant in the maternity ward. A survey at five university hospitals in Norway (in Norwegian). Tidsskr Nor Lægeforen 109:2118–2122, 1989
11. Welles B, Belfrage P, de Chateau P: Effects of naloxone on newborn infants' behavior after maternal analgesia with pethidine during labor. Acta Obstet Gynecol Scand 63:617–619, 1984
12. Wahlberg V: Reconsideration of Credé prophylaxis. Acta Paediatr Scand (suppl) 295, 1982
13. Passmore CM, McElnay JC, D'Arcy P: Drugs taken by mothers in the puerperium: In-patient survey in Northern Ireland. Br Med J 289:1593–1596, 1984
14. Doering PL, Stewart RB: The extent and character of drug consumption during pregnancy. JAMA 239:843–846, 1978
15. Lewis PJ, Boylan P, Bulpitt CI: An audit of prescribing in an obstetric service. Br J Obstet Gynaecol 87:1043–1046, 1980
16. Treacy V, McDonald D: Drug utilization in antenatal and postnatal wards. Ir Med J 74:159–160, 1981
17. Bennett PN, WHO Working Group (eds): Drugs and human lactation. Amsterdam, Elsevier, 1988
18. Fosarelli P, Wilson M, DeAngelis C: Prescription medications in infancy and early childhood. Am J Dis Child 141:772, 1987
19. Andrew M, Toverud E-L: Drug prescriptions to Norwegian children, age 0–12 years (in Norwegian). Tidsskr Nor Lægeforen 110:3215–3219, 1990
20. Wessling A, Söderman P. Boëthius G: Monitoring of drug prescriptions for children in the county of Jämtland and Sweden as a whole 1977–1987. Eur J Clin Pharmacol 38:329–334, 1990
21. Sanz EJ, Boada J: Drug utilization in pediatric outpatients in Tenerife (Canary Islands). Eur J Clin Pharmacol 134:495–499, 1988
22. Tomson G: Drug utilization studies in Sri Lanka. Towards an understanding of medicines in society. Dissertation, Department of International Health Care Research, Karolinska Institutet, Stockholm, 1990
23. Rasmussen F, Smedby B: Life table methods applied to use of medical care and prescription drugs in early childhood. J Epidemiol Com Health 43:140–146, 1989
24. Cockington RA, Don N, Gilbert L: Use of medications in infancy. Aust Paediatr J 17:216–217, 1981
25. Sabo A, Söderman P, Matheson I: Disorders and drug use in
26. mother/infant-pairs during breast-feeding in regions in Yugoslavia, Sweden and Norway. Meeting of the WHO Drug Utilisation Research Group, Netherlands, June 1989. Pharm Weekbl (Sci) 11(suppl):F12, 1989
26. Blomquist HK, Söderman P: Prevalence and treatment of symptoms in Swedish infants and their mothers. Scand J Primary Health Care, 1990 (in press)
27. Matheson I, Kristensen K, Lunde PKM: Disorders and drug use in infants. Does breast-feeding have an impact? (in Norwegian). Tidsskr Nor Lægeforen 109:2123–2128, 1989
28. Dunnell K, Cartwright A: Medicine takers, prescribers and hoarders. London, Routledge & Kegan Paul, 1972
29. Rylance GW, Woods CG, Cullen RE, Rylance ME: Use of drugs by children. Br Med J 27:445–447, 1988
30. Höjer B, Sterky G, Widlund G: Acute illnesses in young children and family response. Acta Paediatr Scand 76:624–630, 1987
31. Klaukka T, Marti J: Drug utilization in Finland 1964–1987. Publications of the Social Insurance Institution, M:71, Helsinki, 1990
32. Haggerty RJ, Roghmann KJ: Noncompliance and self medication. Two neglected aspects of pediatric pharmacology. Pediatr Clin North Am 19:101–115, 1972
33. Illingworth RS: Infantile colic revisited. Arch Dis Child 60:981–985, 1985
34. Rasmussen F, Smedby B: Physician visits and prescribed drugs among young children and their mothers. Scand J Prim Health Care 5:225–231, 1987
35. Farwell JR, Young JL, Hirtz DG, et al: Phenobarbital for febrile seizures: Effects on intelligence and seizure recurrence. N Engl J Med 322:364–369, 1990
36. Little RE, Anderson KW, Ervin CH, Worthington-Roberts B, Clarren SK: Maternal alcohol use during breast-feeding and infant mental and motor development at one year. N Engl J Med 321:425–430, 1989
37. Benesova O: Perinatal pharmacotherapy and brain development. Int J Prenatal Perinatal Stud 1:417–435, 1989
38. Franzosi MG, Tognoni G: Problemi de uso di farmaci nella practica pediatrica extra-ospedaliera. Riv Ital Ped 5:21–36, 1979
39. Isenalumhe AE, Oviawe O: Polypharmacy: Its cost burden and barrier to medical care in a drug-oriented health care system. Int J Health Serv 18:335–342, 1988
40. Anonymous: Where does the teracycline go? Health centre prescribing and child survival in East Java and West Kalimantan, Indonesia. Management Sciences for Health, Boston, in collaboration with Ministry of Health, Indonesia and Yavasean Indonesia Sejahtena, 1989
41. Trakas D, Sachs L: Socialization of the sick role: The use of medicines for children's illness episodes (Abstr). Pharm Weekbl (Sci) 11(suppl):F5, 1989
42. Kennedy DL, Forbes MB: Drug therapy for ambulatory pediatric patients in 1979. Pediatrics 70:26–29, 1982
43. Buchanan N, Mashigo S: Problems in prescribing for ambulatory black children. South Afr Med J 52:227–229, 1977
44. Ray WA, Schaffner W, Federspiel CF: Differences between female and male children in the receipt of prescribed psychotropic and controlled-analgesic drugs. Med Care 24:801–813, 1986
45. Nelson WL, Kennedy DL, Chang SL, Kuritsky JN: Outpatient systemic antiinfective use by children in the United States, 1977 to 1986. Pediatr Infect Dis J 7:505–509, 1988
46. Stolley PD, Becker MH, Mcevilla JD, et al: Drug prescribing and use in an American community. Ann Intern Med 76:537–540, 1972
47. Pickering LK, Evans DG, DuPont HL, et al: Diarrhea caused by Shigella, rotavirus, and Giardia in day care centers: A prospective study. J Pediatr 99:51–55, 1986
48. Ringertz S, Kronvall G: Increased use of erythromycin causes resistance in Haemophilus influenzae. Scand J Infect Dis 19:247–256, 1987
49. Sanz EJ, Bergman U, Dahlstrøm M: Paediatric drug prescribing. A comparison of Tenerife (Canary Islands, Spain) and Sweden. Eur J Clin Pharmacol 37:65–68, 1989
50. Stanulovic M, Milosev M, Jakocljevic V, Roncevic N: Epidemiological evaluation of anti-infective drug prescribing for children in outpatient practice. Dev Pharmacol Ther 10:278–291, 1987

51. Avorn J, Soumerai SB: Improving drug-therapy decisions through educational outreach: A randomized controlled trial of academically based "detailing." N Engl J Med 308:1457, 1983
52. Schaffner W, Ray WA, Federspiel CF, et al: Improving antibiotic prescribing in office practice: A controlled trial of three educational methods. JAMA 250:1728, 1983
53. Ray WA, Schaffner W, Federspiel CF: Persistence of improved antibiotic prescribing in office practice. JAMA 253:1774, 1985
54. Sinclair BL, Clark DWJ, Facoory BD, Silva PA: Medication use in nine year olds: types of medicines used and recall of advice given. N Zeal Med J 103:263–265, 1990
55. Olson AL, Klein SW, Charney E, MacWhinney JB, McInerny TK, Miller RL, Nazarian LF, Cunningham D: Prevention and therapy of serious otitis media by oral decongestants. A double-blind study in pediatric practice. Pediatrics 61:679–683, 1978
56. Olubadewo JO, Ikponmwamba SA: Profile of prescription medication in a pediatric population. Drug Intell Clin Pharm 22:999, 1988
57. Tomson G, Sterky G: Self-prescribing by way of pharmacies in three Asian developing countries. Lancet 2:620–622, 1986
58. Gutierrez G, Guiscafre H, Munoz O: Conclusions and research perspectives. Arch Invest Med (Mexico) 19:437–443, 1988
59. Elliger TJ, Trott G-E, Nissen G: Prevalence of psychotropic medication in childhood and adolescence in the federal republic of Germany. Pharmacopsychiatry 23:38–44, 1990
60. Quinn DMP: Prevalence of psychoactive medication in children and adolescents. Can J Psychiatr 31:575–580, 1986
61. Kreula E, Hemminki E: Frequency of psychotropic drug prescribing for children in Tampere, Finland. Acta Paediatr Scand 67:449–452, 1978
62. Hickson GB, Altemeier WA, Clayton EW: Should promethazine in liquid form be available without prescription? Pediatrics 86:221–225, 1990
63. Foxman B, Valdes B, Brook R: Childhood enuresis: Prevalence, perceived impact and prescribed treatments. Pediatrics 77:482–487, 1986
64. Knapp DA, Knapp DE: Decision-making and self-medication: Preliminary findings. Am J Hosp Pharm 29:1004, 1972
65. Bush PJ, Rabin DL: Who's using nonprescribed medicines? in Wertheimer AI, Smith MC (eds): Pharmacy Practice: Social and Behavioral Aspects. 3rd ed. Baltimore, Williams & Wilkins, 1988, pp 212–222
66. Wolthers OD: Employment of alternative forms of treatment by patients attending a paediatric outpatient clinic. A questionnarie investigation (in Danish). Ugeskr Læg 151:87–90. 1989
67. Anderson JE, Morrell DC, Avery AJ, Watkins CJ: Evaluation of a patient education manual. Br Med J 281:924–926, 1980
68. Rasmussen F: Self-care, medical care and prescription drugs in early childhood. Uppsala, University of Uppsala, 1988. 55 pp. (Acta Universitatis Upsaliensis. Comprehensive Summaries of Uppsala Dissertations from the Faculty of Medicine, no. 178) Stockholm, Almquist & Wiksell, 1988
69. Casey R, McMahon F, McCormick MC, Pasquariello PS, Zavod W, King FH: Fever therapy: An educational intervention for parents. Pediatrics 73:600–605, 1984
70. Moore SH, LoGerfo J, Inui TS: Effect of a self-care book on physician visits. A randomized trial. JAMA 243:2317–2320, 1980
71. Svarstad BL, Cleary PD, Mechanic D, Robers PA: Gender differences in the acquisition of prescribed drugs: An epidemiological study. Med Care 25:1089–1098, 1987
72. Dahlquist G, Sterky G, Ivarsson J-I, Tengvald K, Wall S: Health problems and care in young families. Scand J Prim Health Care 5:79–86, 1987
73. Maiman LA, Becker MH, Cummings KM, Drachman RH, O'Connor PA: Effects of sociodemographic and attitudinal factors on mother-initiated medication behaviour for children. Public Health Reports 97:140–149, 1982
74. Starfield B, Hankin J, Steinwachs D, et al: Utilization and morbidity. Random or tandem? Pediatrics 75:241–247, 1985
75. Cafferata GL, Kasper JD: Family structure and children's use of ambulatory physician services. Med Care 23:350–360, 1985
76. Tessler R: Birth order, family size and children's use of physician services. Health Serv Res 15:55–62, 1980
77. Jackson JD, Smith MC, Sharpe TR, Freeman RA, Hy R: An investigation of prescribed and nonprescribed medicine use behavior within the household context. Soc Sci Med 16:2009–2015, 1982

PHARMACOKINETICALLY BASED DRUG INTERACTIONS IN THE PEDIATRIC PATIENT

SUSAN L. HOGUE *and* STEPHANIE J. PHELPS

INTRODUCTION

Although thousands of drug interactions have been described, relatively few are clinically significant. Nonetheless, their importance cannot be overstated, since the adverse effects associated with a clinically significant drug interaction are almost always preventable. It is also essential that a possible drug interaction be distinguished from an adverse drug reaction (ADR) or an exacerbation of disease. For these reasons, practitioners must understand the mechanisms of drug–drug interactions so that they can be anticipated and recognized.

Drugs may interact by a number of different mechanisms that are generally classified as pharmaceutic, pharmacodynamic, or pharmacokinetic in nature. Pharmaceutic interactions result from drug inactivation when two compounds are physically mixed. For example, the inactivation of aminoglycosides by certain β-lactam antibiotics represents one of the more common examples of a pharmaceutic interaction.[1] Pharmacodynamic interactions involve two drugs that compete for the same receptor or physiologic system, thereby altering a patient's response to drug therapy. In many instances, drug interactions have a pharmocokinetic rather than a pharmaceutic or pharmacodynamic basis. While pharmacokinetic drug interactions may occur by a variety of complex mechanisms, they usually involve an alteration in the rate or extent of the absorption, distribution, metabolism, or elimination of a drug. These alterations result in differences in drug concentration within the body, which ultimately may affect clinical response. A number of texts[2,3] and review articles[4–12] have been published on the subject of drug interactions. The purpose of this chapter is to review the general principles or mechanisms of pharmacokinetically based drug interactions and to provide the reader with a summary of clinically important interactions that may occur in pediatric patients.

EPIDEMIOLOGY

It is common for pediatric patients to receive two or more medications concomitantly. Kennedy and Forbes[13]

reported that patients <14 years of age accounted for 12 percent of all prescriptions filled in 1979. Fosarelli et al.[14] reported that the average number of different medications in 222 children <5 years of age was 5.18 per child and ranged as high as 20. Recently, Lesko et al.[15] reported on patterns of drug use in a neonatal intensive care unit. Among the 2690 infants studied, the median number of medications per patient treated was eight. A number of epidemiologic studies have clearly demonstrated that the incidence of ADRs increases as the number of simultaneously prescribed drugs increases.[4,16,17]

In 1972 the Boston Collaborative Drug Surveillance Program[18] reported that 3600 ADRs occurred in 9900 patients and that 6.5 percent of reactions occurred secondary to a drug interaction. Borda et al.[19] noted that 22 percent of ADRs occurring on medical wards were the result of a drug interaction. Mitchell and colleagues[20] studied the incidence of ADRs that required hospitalization in pediatric patients. Although data from 10,297 admissions were reviewed, only 2.85 percent were attributed to an ADR, and only two reactions proved fatal. Although the authors did not distinguish drug interactions from ADRs, it is interesting to note that one of the two deaths was attributed to theophylline toxicity that occurred following an interaction between erythromycin and theophylline.[20,21]

PRINCIPLES OF PHARMACOKINETIC DRUG INTERACTIONS

Absorption Interactions

Absorption is defined as the translocation of a drug from its site of administration into the systemic circulation. Following oral administration, drug absorption is affected by a variety of patient factors, including gastric pH, gastric emptying time, intestinal transit time, and blood perfusion of the gastrointestinal tract. Administration of a drug that significantly alters any of these factors may affect either the rate or extent of absorption of a second drug. Although the total amount of drug absorbed is unchanged, a decrease in the rate of absorption may result in failure to achieve a "therapeutic" concentration. Although they are potentially significant, the majority of interactions that affect the bioavailability of medications can be avoided by administering interacting drugs at least 2 hours apart.

Following oral administration, drug absorption is dependent on the gastric and duodenal pH. Although extensive absorption of several weakly acidic and weakly basic drugs may occur in the stomach, the small intestine is the most important gastrointestinal site for drug absorption. The pH of the stomach and small intestine determines the degree of ionization of a drug moiety. A low pH favors absorption of acidic drugs, since the drug will remain largely un-ionized in this environment. Conversely, a high pH will enhance the diffusion of basic drugs across the lipid cell membranes of the gut wall and will impair the transport of acidic medications. For example, the administration of H_2 antagonists or antacids that increase the gastric pH may result in enhanced absorption of weakly basic drugs such as nafcillin, penicillin G, and sulfonamides, while decreasing the absorption of phenobarbital, aspirin, or ketoconazole.[12,22,23] Changes in pH also affect the dissolution rate of a drug. For example, enteric-coated medications (e.g., erythromycin, aspirin) undergo degradation in the stomach instead of the small intestine when the gastric pH is basic.[12]

Because most orally administered medications are absorbed in the small intestine, the rate and extent of absorption are dependent on gastric emptying time. If the rate of gastric emptying is prolonged or enhanced (shortened), the rate of intestinal drug absorption may also be affected. Thus, absorption is related to gastric emptying time and to intestinal transit time. Medications that prolong (e.g., propantheline, antacids, codeine) or enhance (e.g., metoclopramide) a patient's gastric emptying or intestinal transit time can significantly alter a drug's absorption profile. For example, propantheline has been reported to significantly reduce the absorption of sulfamethoxazole[24] while increasing the absorption of hydrochlorothiazide,[25] nitrofurantoin,[26] and digoxin.[27] Intramuscular administration of meperidine causes a delay in gastric emptying and thus a delay in the absorption of acetaminophen.[28] Conversely, metoclopramide increases the rate of acetaminophen absorption[29] and increases the extent of tetracycline absorption.[30] Accelerated intestinal transit time caused by laxatives, such as bisacodyl, decreases the azo reduction of sulfasalazine to 5-amino salicylic acid and sulfapyridine in the colon, thereby reducing the affectiveness of this agent.[31]

Blood perfusing the gastrointestinal tract is another determinant of drug absorption.[32] Although the absorption of most drugs is dependent on intestinal blood flow, a substantial and sustained decrease in mesenteric blood flow is required to produce a significant change in the rate of absorption. Recently, Van Bell and colleagues[33] reported that a single intravenous dose of indomethacin produced an immediate, sustained, and significant reduction in superior mesenteric artery blood flow in infants. While the effect of this reduction in mesenteric blood flow on drug absorption remains to be investigated, it may pose the possibility of a drug interaction in patients receiving concurrent oral medications.

Drug absorption is also affected by specific physicochemical drug properties that allow for adsorption, complexation, or drug–metal ion chelation. Numerous studies have demonstrated a decrease in bioavailability due to adsorption of one drug to another. This interaction results in decreased absorption of the adsorbed agent; thus, lower serum concentrations are achieved. Adsorption of a variety of drugs (e.g., tetracycline) commonly occurs following coadministration of antidiarrheal agents (e.g., kaolin-pectin, bismuth subsalicylate) or after administration of antacids to adults.[34,35] Brown et al.[36] noted a 40 percent reduction in digoxin absorption following coadministration with kaolin–pectin. Although adsorption can significantly alter the efficacy of several medications, this interaction is not always detrimental. For instance, activated charcoal is routinely used to decrease the absorption or enhance the systemic clearance of several drugs in the intoxicated patient.[37,38]

Complexation or chelation reactions are also common types of drug interactions that decrease the bioavailability of select drugs. Cholestyramine, an ion exchange resin, may decrease absorption of anticoagulants[39] or thyroxine[40] via complexation. Chelation reactions commonly occur between drugs and di- and trivalent metals such as calcium, iron, aluminum, and magnesium. The aluminum in sucralfate and the calcium in various products may bind with tetracycline, causing a reduction in the bioavailability of the antibiotic.[23] Likewise, iron salts may decrease the bioavailability of various tetracyclines by the same mechanism.[41]

Finally, certain drugs are biotransformed to inactive metabolites by the bacterial flora in the intestines. Antibiotics that alter the intestinal flora may limit the metabolism and ultimate bioavailability of slow-release or immediate-release products, respectively. For example, digoxin serum concentrations increased 43–116 percent following therapy with tetracycline or erythromycin, respectively.[42] Conversely, concomitant therapy with neomycin[43] or sulfasalazine[44] reduced the bioavailability of digoxin.

Distribution Interactions

Drug distribution is the movement of drug or active metabolite from the systemic circulation into various body compartments or tissues. The pharmacokinetic parameter that attempts to describe the relationship between the amount of drug in the body and the drug's serum concentration is the apparent volume of distribution. The distribution of a drug is dependent on its blood-to-tissue partition coefficient, the extent of plasma protein or tissue binding, and the regional blood flow.

The most common type of drug interaction that involves distribution is an alteration in the plasma protein binding of a drug. These alterations most commonly result from the displacement of drug from circulating endogenous plasma proteins such as albumin, globulins, or α_1-acid glycoprotein. Anionic medications (e.g., β-lactam antibiotics) and weak acids (e.g., phenytoin) are primarily bound to albumin. Cationic drugs (e.g., lidocaine) and weak bases (e.g., carbamazepine) are predominantly bound to α_1-acid glycoprotein.[45,47]

Because the free or unbound fraction of a drug is the pharmacologically active moiety, any change in the unbound fraction can lead to a change in the amount of drug available for interaction with a receptor. Thus, in order for a drug to exert its effect, it must not be bound to plasma proteins. The extent of protein binding may depend on the presence of other drugs that are bound to the same protein, the drug serum concentration, the protein concentration, and the presence of endogenous competitors. When two or more highly protein-bound drugs (>90 percent) are administered simultaneously, competitive binding or displacement may increase the unbound or free fraction, thereby resulting in an altered pharmacologic effect. Any change in protein binding that results in an increase in the amount of unbound drug may increase the quantity of drug available to interact with the drug's site of action.

Although many examples of competitive binding with displacement between drugs have been reported in the literature, the majority of these interactions are rarely of clinical significance.[48] In order for such reactions to be clinically important, both compounds must be >80–90 percent bound to the same type of protein. Increasing the amount of unbound drug will concurrently increase the amount of drug available for metabolism or excretion. Therefore, the total serum concentration of the affected drug will initially decrease, while the free or unbound concentration increases. Once a new steady-state concentration is achieved, the total serum concentration will be lower; however, the unbound concentration at steady state will be the same as the unbound concentration before initiation of the displacing drug. The elevated unbound drug concentration that occurs during the transition period to a new steady-state concentration could cause a transient and temporary increase in the pharmacologic effect that may result in toxicity. Although protein-binding interactions are rarely clinically important, it is still prudent to exercise caution when concomitantly administering two drugs that are highly protein-bound. In patients who experience signs or symptoms of toxicity, a temporary reduction in dose may be required.

The displacement of dicumarol-like oral anticoagulants (e.g., warfarin) from albumin binding sites by other highly protein-bound compounds (e.g., aspirin, sulfa drugs, phenylbutazone) represents a classic example of this type of drug interaction.[49] Salicylic acid, sulfisoxazole, and phenylbutazone displace methotrexate,[50] phenytoin,[50–52] and valproic acid.[53]

Alterations in tissue binding are also rare and are best exemplified by the interaction between digoxin and quinidine in adults.[54,55] A decrease in the volume of distribution of digoxin and a simultaneous increase in serum digoxin concentration is thought to occur when quinidine displaces digoxin from tissue binding sites.

Metabolism Interactions

Most of the clinically important drug interactions involve an alteration in drug metabolism. Although the

adrenals, kidneys, lungs, placenta, and gut are capable of metabolizing drugs, the liver is the primary organ involved in metabolism. Hepatic biotransformation of a drug may be affected by liver blood flow, protein binding, or intrinsic clearance and by the affinity of the drug for hepatic extraction.

Biotransformation of most drugs occurs primarily in the smooth endoplasmic reticulum of the liver hepatocyte, where hundreds of enzyme systems are involved in the metabolism of compounds. The physical and chemical properties of a drug determine the degree to which the liver removes or extracts the drug from the bloodstream. Since drugs with a low hepatic extraction ratio (e.g., theophylline, phenytoin, warfarin, valproic acid) undergo little to no hepatic first-pass metabolism, they have a low systemic clearance. Drugs with a high extraction ratio (e.g., propranolol, lidocaine) tend to be less available to the systemic circulation. Hepatic clearance of compounds with a low extraction ratio is dependent on intrinsic clearance and the free fraction of drug in the plasma and is independent of hepatic blood flow. In contrast, high-extraction drugs are dependent primarily on liver blood flow for metabolism.

A number of drugs and environmental agents are capable of inhibiting or inducing certain enzymatic pathways in the mixed-function oxidase system (MFO). Inducers are generally lipophilic, bind to MFO enzymes, and have relatively long half-lives.[6] Enzyme induction results in increased intrinsic clearance, which leads to decreased serum concentrations and reduced efficacy of coadministered drugs that are metabolized by these enzymatic pathways. Induction of MFO enzyme pathways occurs following the administration of a variety of medications including rifampin,[56–58] phenobarbital,[59–62] phenytoin,[59–61,63] and carbamazepine.[60,63–65] Patients treated with mono- or polyanticonvulsant therapy have an increased ability to metabolize many drugs, which often necessitates an increase in drug dose. Significant interactions of this type include reduced serum chloramphenicol concentrations following rifampin administration[58] and breakthrough seizures due to decreased phenytoin or phenobarbital serum concentrations[62] The time course for induction varies with the inducing agent. However, induction requires generation of new enzymes; thus, the time to onset of effect may be delayed when compared to drugs that inhibit enzymes. Rifampin has been reported to cause induction as early as the second day of therapy.[58] Induction by phenobarbital has been reported to occur following 1[66] to 3[59] weeks of therapy, with effects still evident for up to 4 weeks after discontinuation of phenobarbital in adults.[67]

Inhibition of an MFO pathway typically results in elevated serum concentrations and associated toxicities of the second drug. Typically, inhibition occurs sooner than induction. Enzyme inhibition is a competitive interaction; therefore, it theoretically begins as soon as the inhibitor is in the blood. The duration of inhibition following discontinuation of the drug is dependent upon the elimination of the drug from the body. Examples of inhibitors include cimetidine,[68–72] erythromycin,[73–75] valproic acid,[76,77] and chloramphenicol.[78–79] Numerous studies have demonstrated elevated serum concentrations of agents, such as theophylline, when administered either concomitantly with, or after, cimetidine[68,80] or erythromycin.[73,81] Complications, such as seizures, have occurred in adults due to chloramphenicol inhibition of hepatic enzymes, resulting in elevated phenytoin concentrations.[78]

Lastly, the bile represents an additional means of elimination for a number of drugs. Parent compounds or their metabolites that are excreted via the bile may be reabsorbed or absorbed into the systemic circulation from the intestines. This process of enterohepatic recycling is important for drugs such as phenothiazines, phenobarbital, and carbamezepine. Interfering with this elimination process may be advantageous in the intoxicated patient. For example, repeat-dose activated charcoal has become routine therapy to enhance elimination of compounds that undergo substantial enterohepatic circulation.[37,38]

Excretion Interactions

Renal excretion of drugs and drug metabolites involves glomerular filtration, active tubular secretion, or both. Drugs that alter renal blood flow will alter glomerular filtration rate (GFR) and may influence renal elimination. For drug interactions that affect renal elimination to be clinically important, the removal of active drug or metabolites from the body must be dependent on renal elimination. Changes in the GFR following administration of various drugs may result in altered handling of coadministered medications that are eliminated via filtration. For example, drugs such as the nonsteroidal anti-inflammatory agents (e.g., ibuprofen, indomethacin) can significantly decrease a patient's GFR.[82,83] A decrease in the GFR could reduce filtration and renal clearance of select drugs or metabolites and thereby increase serum concentrations of agents such as the aminoglycosides[11,84,85] or digoxin.[85,86] In contrast, dopamine has been reported to increase GFR in dogs, which in turn increases the renal clearance of the aminoglycosides and digoxin and results in decreased serum concentrations.[87]

The majority of significant drug interactions that result from an alteration in renal clearance occur secondary to alterations in tubular function. Two transport systems are responsible for the elimination of organic acids (e.g., penicillin, salicylates, probenecid) and organic bases (e.g., cimetidine, procainamide).[7,11] Competition for secretion can occur following concomitant administration of agents that are actively secreted. For instance, probenecid competitively inhibits proximal tubular secretion of a wide variety of acidic compounds (e.g., penicillins, aspirin), resulting in an increase in their serum concentrations. On occasion this interaction has been used advantageously to produce higher penicillin serum concentrations required for the treatment of uncomplicated gonorrhea in adults.

Alterations in urinary pH or flow can significantly affect the passive distal tubular reabsorption of various drugs. The pH of the urine will affect the degree of ionization and the extent of passive reabsorption or excretion of weak acids and weak bases.[6,7,9] For example, an alkaline urine following large doses of antacids or administration

of sodium bicarbonate will cause increased ionization of a weakly acidic drug (e.g., phenobarbital), resulting in increased urinary excretion. Occasionally, alkalinization or acidification of the urine may be an effective method of enhancing excretion of agents in an overdose situation. On the other hand, acidic urine following large systemic doses of aspirin would enhance tubular reabsorption of an acidic agent such as phenobarbital, thereby increasing its half-life. A basic drug such as quinidine would become more ionized and therefore would have enhanced excretion in the presence of an acidic urine.

DRUG–DRUG INTERACTIONS

A variety of clinically significant pharamacokinetically based drug–drug interactions have been reported. The vast majority of these reports originate from anecdotal case histories, studies of normal volunteers, or single-dose studies. Several prospective, controlled, multiple-dose studies have been conducted in adult volunteers and patients. However, very few trials have been performed in the pediatric population. Although limited data are available in neonates, infants, and children, it is reasonable to expect that interactions noted in adults will also occur in the pediatric patients. In fact, the incidence and severity of concentration-dependent interactions may be enhanced in certain patient populations (e.g., neonates, infants) where protein binding, metabolism, or elimination are not fully developed.

Although numerous drug interactions have been reported, the following drugs were selected for review because they are commonly prescribed in pediatric patients and interactions associated with their use are generally considered clinically significant. Obviously, new research and experiences will lead to the identification of additional clinically significant interactions; therefore, the clinician must maintain a high index of suspicion whenever a new drug is added to or deleted from an existing regimen and the patient develops symptoms of drug toxicity or has exacerbation of disease.

Anticonvulsants

Carbamazepine

Cimetidine–Carbamazepine

Because cimetidine inhibits the metabolism of carbamazepine, concomitant administration of these two medications may result in elevations in serum carbamazepine concentrations. Symptoms of carbamazepine toxicity were manifested following 2 days of concurrent cimetidine therapy in a patient who had received carbamazepine for 20 years.[88] Dalton and colleagues[89] demonstrated a 17 percent increase in carbamazepine steady-state serum concentrations 2 days after the addition of cimetidine in eight healthy adults; however, the increase was transient and carbamazepine concentrations returned to pre-cimetidine values within 7 days.

The clinical significance of this interaction is probably time-dependent. It also appears that the magnitude of the increase in carbamazepine concentration may be greater when carbamazepine autoinduction is not complete or when patients have not reached steady-state on a dose of carbamazepine. Thus, an initial reduction in carbamazepine dose should be based on an individual's serum carbamazepine concentration as well as the duration of the carbamazepine regimen. Serum concentrations should be monitored prior to initiation of cimetidine and within 7 days of the time that cimetidine is begun. During this time, parents and/or patients should be reminded of the symptoms of carbamazepine toxicity. Because ranitidine has an approximately 10-fold lower binding affinity for the cytochrome P-450 enzyme systems than does cimetidine, the potential for ranitidine to cause inhibition and thus drug interactions is low.[90] For this reason, it may be preferred in patients receiving carbamazepine who require an H_2 antagonist.

Erythromycin–Carbamazepine

A clinically significant drug interaction has been reported between carbamazepine and erythromycin in both adults and children.[74,91–95] Erythromycin appears to inhibit the epoxide–diol metabolic pathway of carbamazepine, resulting in reduced clearance and elevation of serum carbamazepine concentrations.[92] This interaction typically occurs within 3–5 days following administration of erythromycin[74,91,95] and is readily reversed within 48 hours after erythromycin discontinuation.[95] However, Goulden et al.[93] reported signs of carbamazepine toxicity, including ataxia, nystagmus, and drowsiness, 8–12 hours after initiation of erythromycin in six pediatric patients. Miles et al.[92] suggested that the severity of toxicity is correlated with the carbamazepine clearance rate and speculated that symptoms in their population might have been more severe if autoinduction had been complete. The most significant report of toxicity occurred in a 10-year-old on chronic carbamazepine therapy who suffered sinus arrest and subsequent A-V block 5 days after erythromycin was added to his regimen.[91]

A carbamazepine concentration should be obtained prior to beginning erythromycin therapy. If the concentration is already at the upper end of the therapeutic range, dosage should empirically be decreased by approximately 30–40 percent. Serum carbamazepine concentrations should also be obtained 3–5 days into therapy and 48 hours after discontinuation of erythromycin.

Phenobarbital

Chloramphenicol–Phenobarbital

Koup[79] demonstrated an apparent inhibition of phenobarbital following administration of chloramphenicol. Symptoms of toxicity were noted 1 day after chloramphenicol was begun in an adult patient receiving chronic anticonvulsant therapy. Clearance of phenobarbital decreased during chloramphenicol by approximately 50 percent, necessitating a 30 percent reduction in phenobarbital dose. Three days after discontinuing chloramphenicol, preantibiotic phenobarbital dosage was resumed.

It is also interesting to note that phenobarbital has been reported to significantly increase the clearance of chloramphenicol in pediatric patients.[96–98] Krasinski and colleagues[97] noted that concurrent administration of intravenous chloramphenicol succinate and phenobarbital resulted in reduced chloramphenicol peak and trough concentrations when compared to children receiving only chloramphenicol succinate. Likewise, Windofer et al.[98] noted significantly lower chloramphenicol concentrations in a group of premature and full-term neonates who received phenobarbital plus chloramphenicol versus patients receiving chloramphenicol alone.[98] For these reasons, the dose of chloramphenicol may require adjustment in patients receiving phenobarbital.

A serum phenobarbital concentration should be obtained prior to initiating chloramphenicol. Followup phenobarbital concentrations should be obtained 5–6 days into chloramphenicol treatment. Phenobarbital dose may need to be reduced by approximately 30 percent in patients who experience sedation. Phenobarbital doses will require further adjustment upon discontinuation of chloramphenicol.

Valproic Acid–Phenobarbital

Several studies have demonstrated a reduction in phenobarbital clearance with a resultant elevation of serum phenobarbital concentrations in pediatric and adult patients.[99–103] Valproic acid appears to inhibit the p-hydroxylation pathway responsible for conversion of phenobarbital to hydroxyphenylphenobarbital.[100,101] A reduction (mean = 46 percent) of phenobarbital dosage was required to maintain nontoxic phenobarbital concentrations in a group of 13 pediatric and adult patients receiving valproic acid.[99] The authors speculated that a reduction in renal clearance of phenobarbital is the mechanism of the interaction. However, Patel[101] demonstrated a reduction of both total body clearance and metabolic clearance of approximately 30 and 40 percent, respectively, but no reduction in renal clearance in adult patients. Suganuma and colleagues[103] investigated the effect of concomitant phenobarbital and valproic acid in approximately 100 pediatric neurology patients. They noted that phenobarbital serum concentrations to dosage ratios were significantly higher in patients receiving concurrent valproic acid when compared to patients receiving phenobarbital alone. Serum concentration/dose ratio has been elevated in children by as much as 112 percent, compared to only a 50 percent increase in adults, leading some to speculate that age may be an important factor in this interaction.[102]

Serum phenobarbital concentrations should be evaluated prior to initiating valproic acid. Patel[102] noted a significant elevation of serum phenobarbital concentrations after 72 hours of concurrent valproic acid; thus, phenobarbital serum concentrations should be obtained 2–3 days into valproic acid therapy, with appropriate dosage adjustments at this time. A 30–40 percent reduction in phenobarbital dose may be warranted in patients receiving valproic acid therapy.

Phenytoin

Chloramphenicol–Phenytoin

Chloramphenicol, a known MFO inhibitor, significantly decreases phenytoin clearance, resulting in phenytoin toxicity.[61,78,79,97,104,105] Christensen et al.[105] reported considerable elevation of phenytoin half-life following chloramphenicol in three adult patients. Pre-chloramphenicol phenytoin half-life ranged from 10 to 16 hours, while post-chloramphenicol half-life ranged from 23 to 38 hours.[105] Ballek et al.[104] also noted significant alterations in phenytoin parameters, reporting that serum phenytoin concentrations rose from 7 μg/ml prior to chloramphenicol to 24 μg/ml after 6 days of antibiotic therapy in adults. Koup[79] reported a similar interaction in a patient with cystic fibrosis on chronic phenytoin therapy after 6 days of oral chloramphenicol. Phenytoin clearance decreased from 38.2 to 18.9 ml/min and symptoms of toxicity occurred when serum phenytoin concentrations exceeded 20 μg/ml. The apparent inhibition continued until 3 days after discontinuation of chloramphenicol.

Phenytoin may also affect serum concentrations of chloramphenicol. Powell and colleagues[61] reported a 74–96 percent reduction in peak and trough serum chloramphenicol concentrations following the addition of phenytoin in a 7-year-old. Conversely, Krasinski et al.[97] reported toxic serum chloramphenicol concentrations in 11 pediatric patients receiving concomitant chloramphenicol and phenytoin.

Patients who require both phenytoin and chloramphenicol may experience toxicity significant enough to warrant a reduction in phenytoin dose. Baseline and 4- to 6-day phenytoin concentrations should be obtained. It is also imperative that serum chloramphenicol concentrations be monitored in patients receiving phenytoin.

Cimetidine–Phenytoin

Several studies have demonstrated a significant drug interaction between cimetidine and phenytoin.[106–111] Conversely, this interaction has not been shown to occur to the same extent with ranitidine.[109] The proposed mechanism of this interaction is cimetidine inhibition of the MFO enzymes responsible for the biotransformation of phenytoin.[106,108,111] This interaction has been shown to occur as early as 48 hours after initiation of cimetidine.[107,110] However, serum phenytoin concentrations 2 weeks after cessation of cimetidine were not significantly different from baseline.[106,108]

Mean increases in serum phenytoin concentrations of 60 and 70 percent have been reported in patients receiving cimetidine therapy.[106,109] However, serum concentration increases as large as 280 percent have been reported.[109] As with cimetidine and theophylline, a dose- or concentration-dependent cimetidine inhibition has been reported.[107] Serum phenytoin concentrations increased from controls by 141.2 percent in volunteers given 2.4 gm/day versus 70.6 percent in individuals receiving 1.2 gm/day.[107]

Substantial interpatient variability in phenytoin clearance has been reported following cimetidine administration; thus, predosing and 48-hour phenytoin serum concentrations should be obtained. If the initial phenytoin concentration is between the middle and the upper end of the "therapeutic" range, an initial 30–40 percent decrease in phenytoin dose should be made at the time cimetidine is initiated. Phenytoin concentrations should be monitored once a new phenytoin steady-state concentration is obtained (e.g., approximately 1 week after dosage adjustment), or sooner in patients who exhibit evidence of toxicity. Because ranitidine binds with an approximately 10-fold lower affinity than does cimetidine, the potential for ranitidine to cause inhibition and thus drug interactions is low.[90] For this reason ranitidine may be preferred in patients receiving phenytoin who require an H₂ antagonist.

Phenobarbital–Phenytoin

The results of studies evaluating the interaction of concomitantly administered phenytoin and phenobarbital are conflicting. Booker et al.[112] demonstrated no effect on phenytoin parameters following 19 days of concomitant phenobarbital and phenytoin in children and adults. In contrast, Lambie et al.[113] reported elevated serum phenobarbital concentrations during concomitant administration with phenytoin in adults, and Buchanan et al.[62] noted reduction of serum phenytoin concentrations after 28 days of phenobarbital in five children.

The effect of coadministration of these two drugs is difficult to predict. Concomitant administration of these agents should be preceded by evaluation of phenytoin serum concentration. Dosage adjustments should be made based on followup phenytoin and phenobarbital serum concentrations that are obtained during the first 2 weeks of therapy.

Valproic Acid–Phenytoin

The effect of valproic acid on phenytoin is variable. Some authors report a reduction in total phenytoin serum concentrations, while others have reported an elevation.[76,77,114–118] Like phenytoin, valproic acid is highly bound (>90 percent) to serum albumin. It has been postulated that valproic acid competitively displaces phenytoin from plasma protein binding sites.[76,77] Perucca et al.[76] speculated that displacement from tissue binding sites reduces phenytoin's volume of distribution and results in an increase in systemic clearance of total phenytoin. In this same adult population, valproic acid also appeared to inhibit hepatic metabolism of free drug, which has resulted in clinical toxicity.[76] Windorfer et al.[116] reported an interaction in five pediatric patients receiving phenytoin and valproic acid. Although these patients experienced a 2- to 3-fold increase in serum phenytoin concentration following the addition of valproic acid, concentrations returned to baseline values within 1–3 months.

Phenytoin may also affect valproic acid. De Wolff and

colleagues[118] noted that children receiving both phenytoin and valproic acid had significantly lower (50 percent) serum valproic acid concentrations than controls receiving similar doses of valproic acid monotherapy.

Transient phenytoin toxicity may occur in patients when valproic acid therapy is added to a regimen. It is imperative to remember that total phenytoin may be within the therapeutic range, while unbound or free concentrations are elevated. Therefore, if signs or symptoms of phenytoin toxicity are present, a free phenytoin concentration should be obtained. Once a new steady-state phenytoin concentration is achieved, the dose may need to be increased.

Cyclosporine

Calcium Channel Blockers—Cyclosporine

The calcium channel antagonists (e.g., diltiazem and verapamil) have been implicated as agents responsible for a significant elevation in cyclosporine concentrations in adults and children.[119–122] Because cyclosporine undergoes extensive oxidation and N-demethylation metabolism, inhibition of hepatic enzymes can cause significant elevations in cyclosporine concentrations.[119,123] The proposed mechanism for the cyclosporine–diltiazem interaction is interference of diltiazem with cyclosporine hepatic N-demethylation metabolism.[120,124] Pochet and Pirson[120] demonstrated a significant increase in cyclosporine concentrations after 3 days of diltiazem therapy, and Lindholm and Henricsson[121] reported a significant elevation of cyclosporine concentration after 1 week of verapamil therapy in adults. Ogborn and colleagues[122] reported cases involving two pediatric renal transplant patients receiving cyclosporine and verapamil. Initially the patients had been maintained on nifedipine and cyclosporine without problem. However, after changing to verapamil, both patients experienced a reduction in cyclosporine clearance that necessitated a 40 and 50 percent reduction in cyclosporine dosage in the two patients, respectively. Several authors have speculated that verapamil also has a synergistic immunosuppressive effect when given in combination with cyclosporine[119,124]; however, no clinical data are available to substantiate this hypothesis. Cyclosporine concentrations returned to baseline within 1 week following the discontinuation of verapamil or diltiazem.

Cyclosporine concentrations should be monitored prior to the use of verapamil or diltiazem. Most patients will require a reduction in dose within the first week of therapy. Because nifedipine has little effect on the hepatic MFO system, it may be an alternative calcium channel blocker provided it offers the desired pharmacologic effect.[125]

Erythromycin–Cyclosporine

Several cases of cyclosporine toxicity secondary to erythromycin have been reported.[75,119,126,127] Martell et al.[127] demonstrated a mean elevation in cyclosporine concentrations from 130 ng/ml at baseline to 630 ng/ml following addition of erythromycin in pediatric patients. The increase in cyclosporine concentrations was noted over a 72-hour period.[112] Ben-Ari and colleagues[75] reported two pediatric patients with substantial elevations of cyclosporine A serum concentrations 5–14 days after beginning concurrent erythromycin therapy. Upon addition of erythromycin, cyclosporine concentrations rose from 30–45 to 192 ng/ml in the first patient and from 73 to 373 ng/ml in the second patient. The cyclosporine concentrations returned to baseline 5–10 days after the discontinuation of erythromycin. However, Menta et al.[119] and Ptachcinski et al.[126] reported an elevation in cyclosporine concentration as early as 24 hours after the initiation of erythromycin therapy in adults. The area under the concentration-time curve has been reported to increase by as much as 156 percent during erythromycin therapy in adults.[119] Administration of erythromycin during cyclosporine therapy should be done cautiously, since renal toxicities have been associated with elevated cyclosporine concentrations. Renal function and cyclosporine concentrations should be monitored, and doses should be individualized based on response.

Ketoconazole–Cyclosporine

An interaction has also been reported between cyclosporine and the antifungal agent ketoconazole.[128,129] Ferguson[129] demonstrated a 255 percent increase in cyclosporine concentrations over a 7-day period during ketoconazole therapy. The magnitude and time to largest increase in concentration were consistent with that reported by Morganstern.[128] The proposed mechanism for this interaction is unknown. Close monitoring of renal function and cyclosporine concentrations is essential when ketoconazole is added to a cyclosporine regimen. Cyclosporine serum concentration will likely decrease when ketoconazole is discontinued; thus, cyclosporine dose will require adjustment.

Metoclopramide–Cyclosporine

Cyclosporine absorption occurs in the small intestine and is slow and incomplete. Mean bioavailability following oral administration approximates only 30 percent[119,130] Coadministration of cyclosporine and metoclopramide resulted in an increase in cyclosporine bioavailability, reflected by a mean increase of 29 percent in the area under the blood concentration versus time curve in adults.[130] No toxicity was noted in the study. Metoclopramide is known to enhance gastric emptying times; therefore, it has been postulated that gastric emptying is the rate-limiting factor in cyclosporine absorption. During concurrent therapy with metoclopramide, cyclosporine concentrations should be monitored and the dose decreased as necessary.

Phenytoin–Cyclosporine

Induction of the hepatic MFO systems has been suggested as the mechanism responsible for the reduction of cyclosporine concentrations following the administration of phenytoin in adults and children.[119,131–133] A decrease in cyclosporine concentrations was apparent after 48 hours of phenytoin, and cyclosporine concentrations returned to baseline 1 week after phenytoin was discontinued.[132] Freeman et al.[131] demonstrated a 50 percent reduction in the area under the cyclosporine concentration-time curve after 9 days of phenytoin. Doses of cyclosporine had to be increased by as much as 100 percent in order to maintain baseline cyclosporine concentrations.[131,132]

In light of the significant reductions in cyclosporine concentration following administration of phenytoin, cyclosporine concentrations should be closely monitored to prevent organ rejection. Concentrations should be monitored 2–3 days and 7–10 days after phenytoin is begun.

Digoxin

Increased Bioavailability

Several cases of antibiotic-associated digoxin toxicity have been noted following administration of erythromycin or tetracycline in adults.[134–136] Approximately 10 percent of patients receiving digoxin metabolize on average 40 percent of a total dose to inactive digoxin reduction products (DRPs), e.g., dihydrodigoxin, dihydrodigoxigenin.[42] These DRPs are produced when *Eubacterium lentum,* an anaerobic gram-positive rod that is part of the normal colonic flora, metabolizes digoxin.[42,136,137] Alterations in the normal intestinal flora following administration of broad-spectrum antibiotics such as tetracycline or erythromycin can result in decreased intestinal reduction of digoxin, resulting in increased availability of parent digoxin for absorption. This increase in bioavailability in patients who are DRP "excretors" can result in digoxin toxicity.[42,135]

In normal adult volunteers who were DRP excretors, Lindenbaum et al.[42] reported that serum digoxin concentrations were increased by 75–115 percent following 5 days of erythromycin and by 42 percent following 7 days of tetracycline. Other investigators[136,138] have reported serum concentration increases of 104–174 percent following a 4- to 6-day course of erythromycin. Friedman[134] also reported a 73 percent increase in serum digoxin concentrations following only four doses (24-hour period) of erythromycin in adults. It may be important to note that the greatest increases in digoxin serum concentrations have occurred in patients receiving digoxin tablets, which have limited bioavailability compared to products with standard dissolution rates or encapsulated liquid.[139]

If a patient metabolizes substantial amounts of digoxin in the gut, administration of an antibiotic that inhibits metabolism may cause digoxin serum concentrations to increase to the point where clinical toxicity occurs. Serum digoxin concentrations should be monitored and dose adjusted as needed. Patients with symptoms of toxicity should have a digoxin concentration obtained as soon as possible.

Decreased Bioavailability

Adsorption of digoxin commonly occurs following the coadministration of digoxin with kaolin–pectin or antacids.[36,140,141] For instance, Brown et al.[36] demonstrated a significant reduction (42 percent) in digoxin absorption following coadministration with kaolin–pectin in adults. The authors also noted a 29 percent decrease in absorption following concomitant digoxin and normal doses of magnesium trisilicate. A decrease in the serum digoxin concentration is also associated with concomitant cholestyramine therapy and is related to complexation of digoxin by the resin.[36] In adults, metoclopramide has been shown to decrease serum digoxin concentrations by increasing gastric motility and shortening the digoxin dissolution time.[27] A 36 percent decrease in serum digoxin concentration has been demonstrated following 10 days of metoclopramide therapy.[27] Although the mechanism of the interactions has not been fully elucidated, both sulfasalazine[44] and neomycin[43] have been shown to affect digoxin serum concentrations. In a single-dose study in adults, a 24 percent decrease in the mean area under the concentration-time curve of digoxin was demonstrated following sulfasalazine,[44] whereas neomycin was found to decrease steady-state digoxin concentrations by 28 percent.[43]

Although these interactions may result in a significant alteration in bioavailability, the majority of these can be avoided by separating the administration times by 2–3 hours.

Amiodarone–Digoxin

Several cases of amiodarone-associated digoxin toxicity have been reported in infants, children, and adults.[142–144] Digoxin serum concentrations increased up to 70 percent over a 7-day period[142] and up to 90 percent in a 5-day period[144] following initiation of amiodarone. In the pediatric population, serum concentrations have been reported to increase by 68–800 percent, suggesting that the magnitude of the interaction may be greater in children than in adults.[143]

Moysey et al.[142] postulated that the increase in digoxin concentration was due to digoxin tissue-binding displacement by amiodarone. Koren et al.[143] demonstrated that children who had an elevation of digoxin concentrations secondary to amiodarone had a reduction in the apparent volume of distribution of digoxin. Conversely, several investigators[143–145] have demonstrated that the increase was secondary to a reduction in both renal and nonrenal digoxin clearance and that volume of distribution remained unchanged.

Any patient receiving digoxin will require close monitoring when amiodarone is instituted or discontinued. Because the interaction has been noted after several days to weeks of amiodarone therapy,[142] serum concentrations should be periodically obtained during the first few weeks of therapy. A digoxin concentration should be obtained as soon as possible in any patient with symptoms of digoxin toxicity.

Calcium Channel Antagonists–Digoxin

Verapamil has been reported to interact with digoxin, resulting in up to a 70 percent increase in the serum digoxin concentrations in virtually all patients studied.[146–149] However, reports evaluating the effects of diltiazem[147,150–152] or nifedipine[152,153] on digoxin kinetics are inconsistent. Diltiazem may increase the digoxin concentration by approximately 20 percent in some patients,[150–152] while nifedipine does not appear to increase the digoxin concentration.[152,153]

A variety of theories have been suggested to explain the mechanism of verapamil–digoxin interaction, including a reduction in the volume of distribution,[148] nonrenal clearance,[148] and renal clearance[146,148] of digoxin following verapamil. In contrast, Rodin et al.[149] could not attribute a 42 percent increase in serum digoxin concentration to an inhibition of renal elimination. Although the mechanism of this interaction is not fully elucidated, it does appear to be related to the dose/serum concentration of the calcium channel blocker.[147] Maximum digoxin concentrations generally occur within 1–2 weeks following addition of verapamil. Careful monitoring of digoxin serum concentrations must occur when the two agents are used concomitantly.

Indomethacin–Digoxin

Finch et al.[154] demonstrated no effect on digoxin clearance, half-life, or volume of distribution following maintenance oral indomethacin in six healthy adult volunteers. However, the authors speculated that a significant digoxin–indomethacin interaction could occur in patients with renal function abnormalities. The proposed mechanism is a reduction of renal blood flow and subsequent decrease in GFR that results from a potentiation of angiotensin II vasoconstriction directly related to indomethacin-induced inhibition of prostaglandin synthesis.[154] A significant interaction has been reported in premature infants due to indomethacin-induced renal insufficiency.[82,152–156] A mean elevation of serum digoxin concentration of 50 percent following concomitant administration of indomethacin has been reported.[155] Decreased urine output following indomethacin was also noted. Digoxin concentrations, renal function, and urine output should be closely monitored in neonates receiving concurrent digoxin and indomethacin therapy. Digoxin doses may require a reduction of as much as 50 percent in these patients.

Quinidine–Digoxin

Approximately 25–90 percent of patients who receive concomitant digoxin and quinidine experience an interaction.[157] Typically, this drug–drug interaction causes a decrease in digoxin clearance and an elevation in serum digoxin concentrations. The magnitude of the quinidine-induced effect is variable, ranging from a 20 percent to a 330 percent increase in digoxin concentration. However, most adult and pediatric patients experience a two- to threefold increase in digoxin serum concentration.[54,155,157–163] This increase can be apparent within 6–18 hours after quinidine is started.[157,164] The time required for full manifestation of the interaction is variable, but many investigators feel that the maximum effect is complete after 4,[161] 7,[165] or 9[166] days of quinidine therapy. Leahey and colleagues[158] reported that digoxin concentrations doubled within 24 hours when a quinidine loading dose was given. Thus, it appears that the interaction is dependent on the serum concentration of quinidine[162,165] and has little to do with the pre-quinidine digoxin concentration.[162] Koren et al.[155] noted a twofold increase in the serum digoxin concentration of 8 of 11 infants and children receiving concomitant digoxin and quinidine. Of interest was the fact that three newborn infants experienced no change in serum digoxin concentration following the addition of quinidine.

A variety of mechanisms have been postulated for the digoxin–quinidine interaction. Quinidine has been reported to increase the rate and extent of digoxin absorption.[167] Quinidine has also been shown to decrease the apparent volume of distribution of digoxin by 20–40 percent[55,158,160] Hager et al.[55] initially speculated that the decrease might be due to displacement of digoxin from tissue binding sites. Dahlqvist and colleagues[164] demonstrated continued elevation of digoxin concentrations for up to 36 hours following discontinuation of digoxin, further leading to the conclusion that quinidine may displace digoxin from tissue binding sites. However, others have not noted a decrease in digoxin's volume of distribution.[168,169]

Quinidine has also been shown to significantly decrease the renal elimination of digoxin.[55,159,160,166,169] Both total body clearance and renal clearance of digoxin have been shown to decrease by 30–50 percent and by 30–72 percent, respectively, following quinidine administration.[55,160,164] Hager et al.[55] found that creatinine clearance remained constant during quinidine–digoxin therapy, suggesting that tubular secretion is inhibited and glomerular filtration is unaffected. Others have also noted that quinidine reduces the nonrenal clearance of digoxin.[55,160]

The combination of digoxin redistribution and reduced renal and nonrenal elimination is most likely responsible for the elevation in digoxin serum concentrations following quinidine use. Some authors have suggested that the digoxin dose be empirically reduced by 50 percent when quinidine is instituted.[170] Because the interaction may occur within hours, the digoxin dose may be held on the day that quinidine is begun. This may be especially important if a loading dose of quinidine is given. Close monitoring of digoxin serum concentrations is essential whenever digoxin and quinidine are used concomitantly.

If the dose of digoxin is not reduced, a serum digoxin concentration should be obtained within 24–48 hours of beginning quinidine. A steady-state digoxin concentration should also be obtained in approximately 4–7 days. A digoxin concentration should be assessed as soon as possible in any patient who exhibits signs or symptoms of digoxin toxicity.

Theophylline

Carbamazepine–Theophylline

Decreased theophylline half-life and increased theophylline clearance have been reported following carbamazepine.[171,172] It is thought that the mechanism responsible for this interaction is induction of hepatic enzyme pathways by carbamazepine. Although induction can be seen as early as 1–4 days, the time to maximum induction is approximately 3 weeks.[60] Reed and Schwartz[171] demonstrated significant changes in theophylline clearance in a nonsmoking adult who had received carbamazepine for 2 years. On two separate occasions theophylline clearance was 0.139 and 0.093 liter/kg/h versus 0.069 liter/kg/h when the patient was receiving theophylline alone.[171] A significant carbamazepine–theophylline interaction has also been reported in a pediatric patient.[172] After several months of theophylline therapy (23 mg/kg/day) and 3 weeks of carbamazepine, theophylline half-life was found to be decreased by 48 percent.[172] This increase in clearance resulted in a subtherapeutic theophylline concentration and exacerbation of the patient's asthma.

When carbamazepine is added to or deleted from the therapeutic regimen of a patient receiving theophylline, the practitioner should ensure that "therapeutic" theophylline concentrations are maintained. Patients receiving carbamazepine prior to initiation of theophylline may require larger than normal maintenance doses of theophylline.

Erythromycin–Theophylline

Although some investigators have demonstrated no alteration of theophylline parameters after erythromycin therapy,[173–175] a significant alteration in theophylline clearance has been demonstrated by the vast majority of investigators.[21,73,176–179] The lack of an interaction in some studies may have resulted from a short duration of erythromycin therapy[173] or a low erythromycin dose.[174,176] The proposed mechanism of the theophylline–erythromycin interaction is inhibition of the hepatic MFO system.[21,73,177] No change in the volume of distribution of theophylline has been noted.[73,177]

Following erythromycin therapy, the average decrease in theophylline clearance is approximately 25–30 percent, but reported decreases have been as large as 75 percent.[73] The theophylline concentration generally begins to increase within the first 24 hours of erythromycin therapy and reaches maximal concentrations following 3–5 days

of treatment.[21,177,180] Although the interaction has been described after administration of all forms of oral erythromycin salts (e.g., estolate, sterate, ethyl succinate), the magnitude of the effect may be greater in patients who receive erythromycin salts that produce high serum concentrations. The theophylline–erythromycin interaction has also been documented in pediatric patients.[20,21,81,180,181] LaForce and colleagues[21] documented a 40 percent elevation of steady-state serum theophylline concentrations due to a 25 percent reduction in theophylline clearance following 1 week of erythromycin in 15 children with asthma. The authors noted that patients with the highest initial theophylline clearance rates tended to be affected the most by erythromycin. It should be noted that a fatality has been reported in a child that was attributed to this interaction.[20,21]

Careful monitoring of theophylline serum concentrations is necessary prior to, during, and after concomitant use of erythromycin and theophylline. If the peak serum theophylline concentration is <10 μg/ml, no adjustment in dose may be needed. However, a 25 percent reduction in total daily theophylline dose is warranted if the patient's theophylline concentration is ≥10 μg/ml. A 40–50 percent reduction in theophylline concentration has been reported 7 days following discontinuation of erythromycin; thus, serum theophylline concentration should be monitored and the dose titrated upwards after discontinuation of erythromycin.

H₂ Antagonists–Theophylline

The H_2 antagonists (e.g., cimetidine, ranitidine, etc.) are known inhibitors of the hepatic MFO enzyme system.[69–72] It has been shown that both cimetidine and ranitidine bind at the cytochrome P-450 sites; however, cimetidine binding is much stronger.[90] Ranitidine binds with an approximately 10-fold lower affinity than does cimetidine[90]; thus, the potential for ranitidine drug interactions due to inhibition of hepatic enzymes is low. The significant decrease in theophylline clearance, increased half-life, and increased serum theophylline concentrations following cimetidine therapy result from inhibition of hepatic metabolism.[69–72]

Following 2–9 days· of oral cimetidine therapy in healthy adult volunteers, mean reduction in clearance ranged from 18.5 to 39 percent.[69–72] Reitberg et al.[69] demonstrated an 18.5 and 30 percent decrease in theophylline clearance after 1 and 8 days of cimetidine, respectively. Powell et al.[72] were unable to document a dose-dependent cimetidine inhibition in healthy volunteers given either 1.2 or 2.4 gm/day of cimetidine for 4 days prior to administration of theophylline. Conversely, Krstenansky et al.[182] noted that the interaction was dependent on the serum cimetidine concentration and that patients receiving continuous infusion of cimetidine did not experience a clinically significant increase in serum theophylline concentration. In contrast, recent studies noted that theophylline clearance was not different in patients receiving a continuous versus intermittent infusion of cimetidine.[183]

A decrease in theophylline clearance has been documented in the pediatric population following administration of cimetidine.[68,80] Serum theophylline concentrations increased by 35 percent in a 15-year-old outpatient given cimetidine and theophylline.[68] Two patients <2 years of age at steady state on continuous infusion theophylline developed serum concentrations in excess of 20 mg/ml within 8–12 hours of the initiation of intravenous cimetidine.[80]

Conflicting results evaluating the effect of ranitidine on theophylline metabolism and clearance have been published. Several cases of theophylline toxicity have been attributed to ranitidine inhibition of the hepatic MFO system,[184] while others have found no alteration in theophylline clearance following the use of ranitidine.[72,185,186]

As with other agents that inhibit theophylline metabolism, concomitant administration of cimetidine should be approached with caution. If an H_2 antagonist must be used, ranitidine may be preferred over cimetidine in patients receiving theophylline. If the serum theophylline concentration is <10 μg/ml, no adjustment in dose may be needed. However, a 30 percent reduction in total daily theophylline dose is warranted if the patient's theophylline concentration is ≥10 μg/ml. Upon discontinuation of cimetidine, an increase in the theophylline dosage will likely be required.

Isoproterenol–Theophylline

Isoproterenol, a pure β-agonist catecholamine, has been used as adjunct therapy in combination with theophylline in severe cases of status asthmaticus.[187–189] Isoproterenol significantly increases theophylline clearance and may necessitate substantial increases in the maintenance dose of theophylline. Hemstreet and colleagues[188] reported a significant alteration in theophylline clearance following the addition of a continuous infusion of isoproterenol in six pediatric patients at steady state on a continuous aminophylline infusion. The mean increase in theophylline clearance was 19 percent; however, two of the six patients had increases in excess of 30 percent. The authors found a significant correlation between percent change in clearance and the rate/dose of isoproterenol infusion. O'Rourke and Crone[189] described a group of 12 patients receiving both isoproterenol and theophylline. In this series of patients, theophylline requirements increased by approximately 36 percent. Griffith et al.[187] also demonstrated a significant elevation in theophylline clearance following administration of continuous isoproterenol in a 14-year-old. Maintenance theophylline infusion increased from 0.4 to 4.8 mg/kg/h (115 mg/kg/day theophylline) with an increase in clearance of 354 percent (0.085–0.386 liter/kg/h) upon administration of 0.1 μg/kg/min of isoproterenol. The patient was a smoker and was also receiving concurrent medications known to increase theophylline clearance.

The mechanism of the isoproterenol–theophylline interaction has not been fully elucidated. Proposed mechanisms include induction of the hepatic MFO pathways and increased hepatic blood flow. It is important to recognize that theophylline is a low-extraction drug; thus, liver blood flow should not affect its clearance. Because

the interaction has been noted within hours of beginning isoproterenol, it is questionable whether the effect is solely related to hepatic enzyme induction. Serum theophylline concentrations should be obtained prior to initiating isoproterenol, and daily thereafter until isoproterenol has been discontinued. Because the interaction may be noted as early as 2 hours after isoproterenol is begun, a serum theophylline concentration should be obtained within 6 hours. Increased theophylline needs should be anticipated during the isoproterenol infusion, and subsequent reductions in theophylline dose should be made following discontinuation of isoproterenol.

Phenobarbital–Theophylline

Phenobarbital, a known enzyme inducer, has been shown to affect the metabolism of theophylline in both adults and children[67,190–192] Following 4 weeks of phenobarbital in healthy adult volunteers, theophylline clearance increased by 34 percent.[67] Four weeks after discontinuation of phenobarbital, theophylline clearance values had returned to pre-phenobarbital values. This is in agreement with results published by Jusko et al.[190] involving a survey of 100 hospitalized patients receiving theophylline. Those patients receiving concurrent barbiturate therapy had an increase in theophylline clearance. In contrast, Piafsky et al.[193] concluded there was no significant change (17 percent increase) in theophylline clearance following 14 days of phenobarbital in six volunteers.

Following addition of phenobarbital, a significant difference was noted in theophylline dosage requirements in nine premature infants receiving theophylline for apnea.[191] The authors noted a significant difference in pre- and post phenobarbital theophylline requirements. Pre-phenobarbital mean theophylline dosage requirements were not different for this group when compared to controls receiving only theophylline. Yazdan et al.[192] noted a 30 percent decrease in theophylline concentrations in seven children following 19 days of phenobarbital therapy. Theophylline clearance increased from 0.077 l/kg/h pre-phenobarbital to 0.107 l/kg/h following phenobarbital therapy.

Serum theophylline concentrations should be monitored before and after phenobarbital induction occurs. Increased theophylline doses should be anticipated and adjusted based on serum theophylline concentrations that are obtained 1–2 weeks after initiation of phenobarbital.

Phenytoin–Theophylline

Phenytoin is capable of inducing the metabolism of theophylline, which may result in an increase in the total daily dose of theophylline. Marquis and colleagues[194] demonstrated significant increases in theophylline clearance during concomitant phenytoin administration in 10 nonsmoking volunteers and one patient. The patient had a 60 percent increase in theophylline clearance, while the volunteers had a 72 percent increase in clearance. Reed and Schwartz[171] reported substantially elevated theophylline clearance (i.e., 26–53 percent) following phenytoin use in two adult patients, and Sklar et al.[195] reported a two-to threefold increase in theophylline clearance in two adult patients on concomitant phenytoin. Theophylline clearance began to increase on day 4 and reached a maximum value on day 5 in one patient and on day 9 in another.[195]

Close monitoring of theophylline serum concentrations is necessary to maintain "therapeutic" theophylline concentrations. Dosage alterations in response to phenytoin induction may be necessary during the first or second week of concomitant use.

Quinolones–Theophylline

Several case reports in adults[196,197] and normal adult volunteer studies[198–200] have noted a significant elevation in serum theophylline concentration in individuals that received theophylline and quinolone antibiotics (e.g., ciprofloxacin, enoxacin, or norfloxacin). Interaction between theophylline and the quinolone derivatives is commonly associated with a twofold or greater increase in theophylline concentrations.[196,197] Schwartz and colleagues[199] reported a 23 and 31 percent decrease in theophylline clearance after 2 and 4 days of ciprofloxacin–theophylline therapy, respectively. Likewise, a 30 percent reduction in theophylline clearance was found by Wijnands,[198] while Thomson[196] and Raoof[200] demonstrated decreases in theophylline clearance of approximately 60 percent. It is unlikely that the parent quinolone derivatives are responsible for the interaction, since they are structurally dissimilar. Wijnands et al.[198] speculated that the 4-oxoquinolone metabolite competitively inhibits theophylline demethylation. Serum theophylline concentrations tend to increase after approximately 2 days of ciprofloxacin,[196,197,199] and maximum concentrations generally occur following 5 days of therapy.[199]

Although contraindicated in children, quinolones are occasionally used in patients with cystic fibrosis who may also receive theophylline. Because the average change in theophylline clearance is decreased by approximately 30 percent, patients may not require an automatic reduction in theophylline dose when a quinolone derivative is begun. However, if the patient's theophylline concentration is ≥ 10 μg/ml prior to quinolone therapy, an initial 25–30 percent reduction in dose may be prudent. If the patient's theophylline dose is not decreased prior to initiation of quinolone therapy, the parents and/or patients should be educated on symptoms of theophylline toxicity and serum concentrations should be monitored within 3–5 days. Theophylline dosage requirements generally return to normal within 2–3 weeks following discontinuation of ciprofloxacin.[196]

Warfarin

Erythromycin–Warfarin

All salt forms of erythromycin have been shown to decrease the clearance of warfarin, presumably secondary to inhibition of the hepatic MFO pathways.[201–203] This interaction can result in significant hemorrhagic toxicities

as a result of elevation of warfarin serum concentrations. Bachmann et al.[201] demonstrated a 14 percent reduction in warfarin clearance in a group of healthy volunteers receiving erythromycin base for 8 days. Serum warfarin concentrations increased by a mean of 9.4 percent, with the most pronounced effects seen in those patients who initially had slow warfarin clearance rates. A 9.9 percent increase in prothrombin time (PT) was noted in patients receiving chronic warfarin therapy when erythromycin base was given.[202] PT should be monitored prior to initiating erythromycin therapy and within the first 3 days of coadministration. During and after erythromycin therapy, warfarin dosage alterations should be individualized according to patient response.

H₂ Antagonists–Warfarin

Several cases of cimetidine-related warfarin toxicity have been published.[204,205] Hetzel et al.[204] reported elevations of PT of 40–50 percent in a patient chronically anticoagulated following 800–1000 mg of cimetidine daily. In the same patient, a dose of 400 mg daily resulted in only a 10 percent increase in PT, suggesting the existence of a dose-dependent response. The author postulated that inhibition of warfarin metabolism was the mechanism of this interaction.

Serlin et al.[205] evaluated both normal volunteers and patients, demonstrating prolongation of PT and elevated serum warfarin concentrations following doses of 1000 mg/day of cimetidine. The authors speculated that the mechanism of this interaction was inhibition of warfarin metabolism or a reduction of warfarin volume of distribution. In a later study, no alteration in warfarin metabolism or response was noted following 14 days of ranitidine therapy in five volunteers.[206]

PT should be monitored prior to initiating cimetidine and over the first few days of cimetidine therapy. Warfarin doses should be adjusted based on individual patient response. Because ranitidine binds with an approximately 10-fold lower affinity than does cimetidine, the potential for ranitidine to cause inhibition and thus drug interactions is low.[90] For this reason it may be preferred in patients receiving warfarin who require an H₂ antagonist.

Metronidazole–Warfarin

Coadministration of metronidazole and warfarin results in a significant hypoprothrombinemic effect.[207–209] It would appear that the S(−) enantiomorph of warfarin is primarily affected by this drug interaction.[207] In a study involving healthy volunteers, warfarin half-life increased from 35 to 46 hours and the area under the concentration–time curve increased by 42 percent following a 14-day course of metronidazole.[207] Dean and Talbert[209] reported that PT was elevated at 75 seconds compared to a control value of 12 seconds after 6 days of concurrent administration. Kazmier[208] also noted that PT was 147 seconds (control 17–19 seconds) after 10 days of concomitant metronidazole in a patient receiving warfarin. PT should be monitored prior to initiating metronidazole and closely over the first 7–10 days of therapy. Alterations in warfarin doses should be individualized based on the patient's response when beginning or discontinuing metronidazole.

Rifampin–Warfarin

Concomitant administration of rifampin with warfarin has resulted in suboptimal anticoagulation.[210–212] Rifampin is a potent inducer of hepatic enzymes and has been shown to increase the clearance of warfarin R(+) and S(−) isomers two- to threefold, respectively.[212] Warfarin dosage may increase by as much as two to three times prerifampin requirements.[211] This interaction reportedly occurs within 5–7 days following initiation of rifampin.[211] PT should be monitored prior to initiation of rifampin therapy and within 5–7 days of beginning therapy. Dosage adjustments should be determined by individual response.

Sulfamethoxazole/Trimethoprim–Warfarin

An interaction between warfarin and sulfamethoxazole/trimethoprim (SMX/TMP) has been reported.[213,214] Barnett and Hancock[213] noted that only during a period of coadministration of SMX/TMP were the pharmacologic effects of warfarin apparent in a patient who was relatively resistant to the anticoagulant effects of warfarin. The authors speculated that the mechanism for this interaction was antibiotic-induced inhibition of warfarin metabolism.[213] O'Reilly[214] noted significant prolongation of PT in healthy volunteers after 8 days of SMX/TMP. In a later study evaluating the stereoselective interaction between SMX/TMP and racemic warfarin, O'Reilly[214] demonstrated a significant elevation in the area under the curve for the S(−) warfarin enantiomorph and a prolongation of PT from 40 to 67 seconds. As with erythromycin, PT should be monitored prior to initiating therapy and within the first 3 days of coadministration. Any dosage reduction during SMX/TMP therapy should be individualized according to patient response.

REFERENCES

1. Pickering LK, Rutherford I: Effect of concentration and time upon inactivation of tobramycin, gentamicin, metilmicin, and amikacin by azlocillin, carbenicillin, mecillinam, and piperacillin. J Pharmacol Exp Ther 217:345–349, 1981
2. Hansten PD, Horn JR: Drug Interactions: Clinical Significance of Drug–Drug Interactions, 6th ed. Philadelphia, Lea and Febiger, 1989
3. Olin BR (ed): Facts and Comparisons: Loose Leaf Drug Information Service. St. Louis, JB Lippincott, 1990
4. Robinson DS: The application of basic principles of drug interaction to clinical practice. J Urol 113:101–107, 1975
5. Gillette JR, Pang KS: Theoretical aspects of drug interactions. Clin Pharmacol Ther 22:623–639, 1977
6. Aarons L: Kinetics of drug–drug interactions. Pharmacol Ther 14:321–344, 1981
7. Kosoglou T, Valasses PH: Drug interactions involving renal transport mechanisms: An overview. DICP, Ann Pharmacother 23:116–122, 1989
8. Welling PG: Interactions affecting drug absorption. Clin Pharmacokinet 9:404–434, 1984
9. Levy G: Pharmacokinetic approaches to the study of drug interactions. Ann NY Acad Sci 281:24–39, 1976
10. Gillette JR: Overview of factors affecting drug interactions. Ann NY Acad Sci 281:136–150, 1976
11. Offerhaus L: Drug interactions at excretory mechanisms. Pharmac Ther 15:69–78, 1981
12. Chudzik GM, Yaffe S: Drug interactions—an important consideration for rational pediatric therapy. Pediatr Clin N Am 19:131–140, 1972
13. Kennedy D, Forbes M: Drug therapy for ambulatory pediatric patients in 1979. Pediatrics 70:26–29, 1982
14. Fosarelli P, Wilson M, DeAngelis C: Prescription medications in infancy and early childhood. Am J Dis Child 141:772–775, 1987
15. Lesko SM, Epstein MF, Mitchell AA: Recent patterns of drug use in a newborn intensive care. J Pediatr 116:985–990, 1990
16. McInnes GT, Brodie MJ: Drug interactions that matter. A clinical reappraisal. Drugs 36:83–110, 1988
17. Smith JW, Seidi LC, Cluff LE: Studies on the epidemiology of adverse interactions. V. clinical factors influencing susceptibility. Ann Intern Med 65:629–640, 1977
18. Boston Collaborative Drug Surveillance Program: Adverse drug interactions. JAMA 220:1238–1239, 1972
19. Borda IT, Slone D, Hick H: Assessment of adverse reactions within a drug surveillance program. JAMA 205:645–647, 1968
20. Mitchell AA, Lacouture PG, Sheehan JE, et al: Adverse drug reactions in children leading to hospital admission. Pediatrics 82:24–29, 1988
21. LaFarce CF, Miller MF, Chai H: Effect of erythromycin on theophylline clearance in asthmatic children. J Pediatr 99:153–156, 1981
22. Van der Meer JWM, Scheijground HW, Heykants J, et al: The influence of gastric acidity on the bioavailability of ketoconazole. J Antimicrob Chemother 6:552–554, 1980
23. Griffin JP: Drug interactions occurring during absorption from gastrointestinal tract. Pharmac Ther 15:79–88, 1981
24. Antonioli JA, Schelling JL, Steiniger E, et al: Effect of gastrectomy and of an anticholinergic drug on the gastrointestinal absorption of sulfonamide in man. Int J Clin Pharmacol 5:212–215, 1971
25. Beermann B, Groschinsky-Grind M: Enhancement of the gastrointestinal absorption of hydrochlorothiazide by propantheline. Eur J Clin Pharmacol 13:385–387, 1978
26. Jaffe JM: Effect of propantheline on nitrofurantoin absorption. J Pharm Sci 64:1729–1730, 1975
27. Manninen V, Apajalahti A, Melvin J, et al: Altered absorption of digoxin in patients given propantheline and metoclopramide. Lancet 1:398–400, 1973
28. Nimmo WS, Heading RC, Wilson J, et al: Inhibition of gastric emptying and drug absorption by narcotic analgesics. Br J Clin Pharmacol 2:509–513, 1975
29. Nimmo J, Heading RC, Tothill P, et al: Pharmacological modification of gastric emptying: Effects of propantheline and metoclopramide on paracetamol absorption. Br Med J 1:587–589, 1973
30. Nimmo J: The influence of metoclopramide on drug absorption. Postgrad Med J 49:25–29, 1973
31. VanHees PA, Tuinte JH, van Rossum JM, van Tongeren JH: Influence of intestinal transit time on azo-reduction of salicyazosulphapyridine. Gut 20:300–304, 1979
32. Winne D: Influence of blood flow on intestinal absorption of xenobiotics. Pharmacology 21:1–15, 1980
33. Van Bel F, Van Zoeren D, Schipper J, et al: Effect of indomethacin on superior mesenteric artery blood flow velocity in preterm infants. J Pediatr 116:965–970, 1990
34. Albert KS, Welch RD, DeSante KA, DiSanto AR: Decreased tetracycline bioavailability caused by a bismuth subsalicylate antidiarrheal mixture. J Pharm Sci 68:586–588, 1979
35. Ericsson CD, Feldman S, Pickering LK, Cleary YG: Influence of subsalicylate bismuth on absorption of doxycycline. JAMA 247:2266–2267, 1982

36. Brown DD, Juhl RP: Decreased bioavailability of digoxin due to antacids and kaolin-pectin. N Engl J Med 295:1034–1037, 1976
37. Berlinger WG, Spector R, Goldberg MJ, et al: Enhancement of theophylline clearance by oral activated charcoal. Clin Pharmacol Ther 33:351–354, 1983
38. Berg MJ, Berlinger WG, Goldberg MJ, et al: Acceleration of the body clearance of phenobarbital by oral activated charcoal. N Engl J Med 307:642–644, 1982
39. Robinson DS, Benjamin DM, McCormack JJ: Interaction of warfarin and nonsystemic gastrointestinal drugs. Clin Pharmacol Ther 12:491–495, 1971
40. Northcutt RC, Stiel JN, Hollifield JW, et al: The influence of cholestyramine on thyroxine absorption. JAMA 208:1857, 1969
41. Neuvonen PJ, Gothoni G, Hackman R, Bjorksten K: Interference of iron with the absorption of tetracyclines in man. Br Med J 4:532–534, 1970
42. Lindenbaum J, Rund DG, Butler VP, et al: Inactivation of digoxin by gut flora; reversal by antibiotic therapy. N Engl J Med 305:789–794, 1981
43. Lindenbaum J, Maulitz RM, Butler VP: Inhibition of digoxin absorption by neomycin. Gastroenterology 71:399–404, 1976
44. Juhl RP, Summers RW, Guillory JK, et al: Effect of sulfasalazine on digoxin bioavailability. Clin Pharmacol Ther 20:387–394, 1976
45. Meyer MC, Guttman DE: The binding of drugs by plasma proteins. J Pharm Sci 57:895–918, 1968
46. Piafsky KM: Disease induced changes in the plasma binding of basic drugs. Clin Pharmacokinet 5:246–262, 1980
47. Svensson CK, Woodruff MN, Baxter JG, et al: Free drug concentration monitoring in clinical practice: Rationale and current status. Clin Pharmacokinet 11:450–469, 1986
48. Sellers EM: Plasma protein displacement interactions are rarely of clinical significance. Pharmacology 18:225–227, 1979
49. Aggeler PM, O'Reilly RA, Leong L, et al: Potentiation of anticoagulant effect of warfarin by phenylbutazone. N Engl J Med 276:496–501, 1967
50. Fraser DG, Ludden TM, Evens RP, Sutherland EW: Displacement of phenytoin from plasma protein binding sites by salicylates. Clin Pharmacol Ther 27:166–169, 1980
51. Friel PN, Leal KW, Wilensky AJ: Valproic acid-phenytoin interactions. Ther Drug Monit 1:243–248, 1979
52. Frigo GM, Lecchini S, Gatti G, et al: Modification of phenytoin clearance by valproic acid in normal subjects. Br J Clin Pharmacol 8:553–556, 1979
53. Orr JM, Abbott FS, Farrell K, et al: Interaction between valproic acid and aspirin in epileptic children: Serum protein binding and metabolic effects. Clin Pharmacol Ther 31:642–649, 1982
54. Schenck-Gustafsson K, Jogestrand T, Nordlander R, Dahlqvist R: Effect of quinidine on digoxin concentration in skeletal muscle and serum in patients with atrial fibrillation: Effect of reduced binding of digoxin in muscle. N Engl J Med 305:209–211, 1981
55. Hager WD, Mayersohn M, Graves PE: Digoxin bioavailability during quinidine administration. Clin Pharmacol Ther 30:594–599, 1981
56. Baciewicz AM, Self TH: Rifampin drug interactions. Arch Int Med 144:1667–1671, 1984
57. Baciewicz AM, Self TH, Bekemeyer WB: Update on rifampin drug interactions. Arch Int Med 147:565–568, 1987
58. Prober C: Effect of rifampin on chloramphenicol levels. N Engl J Med 312:788–789, 1985
59. Breckenridge AM, Orme MLE: Clinical implications of enzyme induction. Ann NY Acad Sci 179:421–431, 1971
60. Park BK, Breckenridge AM: Clinical implications of enzyme induction and inhibition. Clin Pharmacokinet 6:1–24, 1981
61. Powell DA, Nahata MC, Durrell DC, Glazer JP, Hilty MD: Interaction among chloramphenicol, phenytoin, and phenobarbital in a pediatric patient. J Pediatr 98:1001–1003, 1981
62. Buchanan RA, Heffelfinger JC, Weiss CF: The effect of phenobarbital on diphenylhydantoin metabolism in children. Pediatrics 43:114–116, 1969
63. Perucca E: Pharmacokinetic interactions with antiepileptic drugs. Clin Pharmacokinet 7:57–84, 1982
64. Pitlick WH, Levy RH, Troupin S, Green JR: Pharmacokinetic

65. Rosenberry KR, Defusco CJ, Mansmann HC, McGeady SJ: Reduced theophylline half-life induced by carbamazepine therapy. J Pediatr 102:472–474, 1983
66. Dossing M, Pilsgaard H, Rasmussen B, Poulsen HE: Time course of phenobarbital and cimetidine mediated changes in hepatic drug metabolism. Eur J Clin Pharmacol 25:215–222, 1983
67. Landay RA, Gonzalez MA, Taylor JC: Effect of phenobarbital on theophylline disposition. J Allergy Clin Immunol 62:27–29, 1978
68. Weinberger MM, Smith G, Milavetz G, Hendeles L: Decreased theophylline clearance due to cimetidine. N Engl J Med 103:672, 1981
69. Reitberg DP, Bernhard H, Schentag JJ: Alteration of theophylline clearance and half-life by cimetidine in normal volunteers. Ann Intern Med 95:582–585, 1981
70. Roberts RK, Grice J, Wood L, et al: Cimetidine impairs the elimination of theophylline and antipyrine. Gastroenterology 81:19–21, 1981
71. Jackson JE, Powell JR, Wandell M, et al: Cimetidine decreases theophylline clearance. Am Rev Resp Dis 123:615–617, 1981
72. Powell JR, Rogers JF, Wargin WA, et al: Inhibition of theophylline clearance by cimetidine but not ranitidine. Arch Intern Med 144:44–46, 1984
73. Renton KW, Gray JD, Hung OR: Depression of theophylline elimination by erythromycin. Clin Pharmacol Ther 30:422–426, 1981
74. Hedrick R, Williams F, Morin R, et al: Carbamazepine–erythromycin interaction leading to carbamazepine toxicity in four epileptic children. Ther Drug Monit 5:405–407, 1983
75. Ben-Ari J, Eisenstein B, Davidovites M, et al: Effect of erythromycin on blood cyclosporine concentrations in kidney transplant patients. J Pediatr 112:992–993, 1988
76. Perucca E, Hebdige S, Frigo GM, Gatti G, Lecchini S, Crema A: Interaction between phenytoin and valproic acid: Plasma protein binding and metabolic effects. Clin Pharmacol Ther 28:779–789, 1980
77. Bruni J, Wilder BJ, Willmore LJ, Barbour B: Valproic acid and plasma levels of phenytoin. Neurology 29:904–905, 1979
78. Zarfin Y, Koren G, Maresky D, et al: Possible indomethacin aminoglycoside interaction in preterm infants. J Pediatr 106:511–513, 1985
79. Rose JQ, Chio HK, Schentag JJ, et al: Intoxication caused by interaction of chloramphenicol and phenytoin. JAMA 237:2630–2631, 1977
80. Koup JR, Gibaldi M, McNamara P, et al: Interaction of chloramphenicol with phenytoin and phenobarbital. Clin Pharmacol Ther 24:571–575, 1978
81. Fenje PC, Isles AF, Baltodano A, et al: Interaction of cimetidine and theophylline in two infants. CMA J 126:1178, 1982
82. Cummins LH, Kozak PP, Gillman SA: Erythromycin's effect on theophylline blood levels. Pediatrics 59:144–145, 1977
83. Dunn MJ: Nonsteroidal anti-inflammatory drugs and renal function. Ann Rev Med 35:411–428, 1984
84. Cifuentes RF, Olley PM, Balfe JW, et al: Indomethacin and renal function in premature infants with persistent patent ductus arteriosus. J Pediatr 95:583–587, 1979
85. Tilstone WJ, Semple PF, Lawson DH, Boyles JA: Effects of furosemide on glomerular filtration rate and clearance of practolol, digoxin, cephaloridine, and gentamicin. Clin Pharmacol Ther 22:389–394, 1977
86. Schimmel MS, Onwood RJ, Eidelman AI: Toxic digitalis levels associated with indomethacin therapy in a neonate. Clin Pediatr 19:768–769, 1980
87. Kirby MG, Dasta JF, Armstrong DK, Tallman R Jr: Effect of low-dose dopamine on the pharmacokinetics of tobramycin in dogs. Antimicrob Agents Chemother 29:168–170, 1986
88. Tellerman-Toppet N, Duret ME, Coers C: Cimetidine interaction with carbamazepine. Ann Intern Med 94:544, 1981
89. Dalton MJ, Powell JR, Messenheimer JA Jr, Clark J: Cimetidine and carbamazepine: A complex drug interaction. Epilepsia 27:553–558, 1986
90. Mitchard M, Harris A, Mullinger BM: Ranitidine drug interac-

tions—A literature review. Pharmacol Ther 32:2923–2925, 1987

91. Macnab AJ, Robinson JL, Adderly RJ, D'Orsogna L: Heart block secondary to erythromycin-induced carbamazepine toxicity. Pediatrics 80:951–953, 1987

92. Miles MV, Tennison MB: Erythromycin effects on multiple-dose carbamazepine kinetics. Ther Drug Monitor 11:47–52, 1989

93. Goulden KJ, Camfield P, Dooley JM, Fraser A, et al: severe carbamazepine intoxication after coadministration of erythromycin. J Pediatr 109:135–138, 1986

94. Wroblewski BA, Singer WD, Whyte J: Carbamazepine–erythromycin interaction case studies and clinical significance. JAMA 255:1165–1167, 1986

95. Pippenger CE: Clinically significant carbamazepine drug interactions: An overview. Epilepsia 28(suppl 3):S71-S76, 1987

96. Bloxham RA, Durbin GM, Johnson T, Winterborn MH: Chloramphenicol and phenobarbitone. A drug interaction. Arch Dis Child 54:76–77, 1979

97. Krasinski K, Kusmiesz H, Nelson JD: Pharmacologic interactions among chloramphenicol, phenytoin, and phenobarbital. Pediatr Infect Dis 1:232–235, 1982

98. Windorfer A, Pringsheim W: Studies on the concentrations of chloramphenicol in the serum and cerebrospinal fluid of neonates, infants, and small children. Eur J Pediatr 124:129–138, 1977

99. Wilder BJ, Willmore LJ, Bruni J, Villarreal HJ: Valproic acid: Interaction with other anticonvulsant drugs. Neurology 28:892–896, 1978

100. Kapetanovic IM, Kupferberg HJ, Porter RJ, et al: Mechanism of valproate–phenobarbital interaction in epileptic patients. Clin Pharmacol Ther 29:480–486, 1981

101. Patel IH, Levy RH, Cutler RE: Phenobarbital–valproic acid interaction. Clin Pharmacol Ther 27:515–521, 1980

102. Fernandez de Gatta MR, Gonzalez ACA, Sanchez MJG, et al: Effect of sodium valproate on phenobarbital serum levels in children and adults. Ther Drug Monitor 8:416–420, 1986

103. Suganuma T, Ishizaki T, Chiba K, Hori M: The effect of concurrent administration of valproate sodium on phenobarbital plasma concentration/dosage ratio in pediatric patients. J Pediatr 99:314–317, 1981

104. Ballek RE, Reidenberg MM, Orr L: Inhibition of diphenylhydantoin metabolism by chloramphenicol. Lancet 1:150, 1973

105. Christensen LK, Skovsted L: Inhibition of drug metabolism by chloramphenicol. Lancet 2:1397–1399, 1969

106. Neuvonen PJ, Tokola RA, Kaste M: Cimetidine–phenytoin interaction: Effect on serum phenytoin concentration and antipyrine test. Eur J Clin Pharmacol 21:215–220, 1981

107. Bartle WR, Walker SE, Shapero T: Dose-dependent effect of cimetidine on phenytoin kinetics. Clin Pharmacol Ther 33:649–655, 1983

108. Levine M, Jones MW, Sheppard I: Differential effect of cimetidine on serum concentrations of carbamazepine and phenytoin. Neurology 35:562–565, 1985

109. Watts RW, Hetzel DJ, Bochner F, Hallpike JF, et al: Lack of interaction between ranitidine and phenytoin. Br J Clin Pharmacol 15:499–500, 1983

110. Hetzel DJ, Bochner F, Hallpike JF, et al: Cimetidine interaction with phenytoin. Br Med J 282:1512, 1981

111. Phillips P, Hansky J: Phenytoin toxicity secondary to cimetidine administration. Med J Aust 141:602, 1984

112. Booker HE, Tormey A, Toussaint J: Concurrent administration of phenobarbital and diphenylhydantoin: Lack of an interference effect. Neurology 21:383–385, 1971

113. Lambie DG, Nanda RN, Johnson RH, Shakir RA: Therapeutic and pharmacokinetic effects of increasing phenytoin in chronic epileptics on multiple drug therapy. Lancet 2:386–389, 1976

114. Bardy A, Hari R, Lehtovaara R, Majuri H: Valproate may lower serum-phenytoin. Lancet 2:1297–1298, 1976

115. Patsalos PN, Lascelles PT: Valproate may lower serum-phenytoin. Lancet 1:50–51, 1977

116. Windorfer A, Sauer W, Gadeke R: Elevation of diphenylhydantoin and primidone serum concentration by addition of dipropylacetate, a new anticonvulsant drug. Acta Paediatr Scand 64:771–772, 1975

117. Schmidt D: Adverse effects of antiepileptic drugs in children. Cleveland Clin 56:132–139, 1900

118. de Wolff FA, Peters ACD, van Kempen GMJ: Serum concentration and enzyme induction in epileptic children treated with phenytoin and valproate. Neuropediatrics 13:10–13, 1982

119. Menta R, David S, Cambi V: Cyclosporin A and drug interaction. Adv Exp Med Biol 252:285–296, 1989

120. Pochet JM, Pirson Y: Cyclosporin–diltiazem interaction. Lancet 2:979, 1986

121. Lindholm A, Henriesson S: Verapamil inhibits cyclosporin metabolism. Lancet 1:1262–1263, 1987

122. Ogborn MR, Crocker JFS, Grimm PC: Nifedipine, verapamil, and cyclosporine A pharmacokinetics in children. Pediatr Nephrol 3:314–316, 1989

123. Ptachcinski RJ, Venkataramanan R, Burckart GJ: Clinical pharmacokinetics of cyclosporine. Clin Pharmacokinet 11:107–132, 1986

124. Wadhwa NK, Schroeder TJ, Pesce AJ, et al: Cyclosporine drug interactions: A review. Ther Drug Monitor 9:399–406, 1987

125. Bourbigot B, Guiserix J, Aixiau J, et al: Nicardipine increases cyclosporine blood levels. Lancet 1:1447, 1986

126. Ptachcinski RJ, Carpenter BJ, Burckart GJ, et al: Effect of erythromycin on cyclosporine levels. N Engl J Med 313:1116–1117, 1985

127. Martell R, Heinrichs D, Stiller CR, et al: The effects of erythromycin in patients treated with cyclosporine. Ann Intern Med 104:660–661, 1986

128. Morgenstern GR, Powles R, Robinson B, McElwain TJ: Cyclosporin interaction with ketoconazole and melphan. Lancet 2:1342, 1982

129. Ferguson RM, Sutherland DER, Simmons RL, Najarian JS: Ketoconazole, cyclosporine metabolism, and renal transplantation. Lancet 2:882–883, 1982

130. Wadhwa NK, Schroeder TJ, O'Flaherty E, et al: The effect of oral metoclopramide on the absorption of cyclosporine. Transplantation 43:211–213, 1987

131. Freeman DJ, Laupacis A, Keowan PA, et al: Evaluation of cyclosporin–phenytoin interaction with observations on cyclosporine metabolites. Br J Clin Pharmacol 18:887–893, 1984

132. Keown PA, Laupacis A, Carruthers G: Interaction between phenytoin and cyclosporine following organ transplantation. Transplantation 38:304–306, 1984

133. Hoyer PF, Offner G, Wonigeit K, et al: Dosage of cyclosporine A in children with renal transplants. Clin Nephrol 22:68–71, 1984

134. Friedman HS: Erythromycin-induced digoxin toxicity. Chest 82:202, 1982

135. Doherty JE: A digoxin-antibiotic drug interaction. N Engl J Med 305:827, 1981

136. Morton MR, Cooper JW: Erythromycin-induced digoxin toxicity. DICP, Ann Pharmacother 23:668–669, 1989

137. Dobkins JF, Saha JR, Butler VP, et al: Digoxin-inactivating bacteria: Identification in human gut flora. Science 220:325–327, 1983

138. Maxwell DL, Gilmour-White SK, Hall MR: Digoxin toxicity due to interaction of digoxin with erythromycin. Br Med J 298:572, 1989

139. Rund DG, Lindenbaum J, Dobkins JF, et al: Decreased digoxin cardioinactive-reduced metabolites after administration as an encapsulated liquid concentrate. Clin Pharmacol Ther 34:738–743, 1983

140. Albert KS, Ayres JW, DiSanto AR, et al: Influence of kaolin–pectin suspension on digoxin bioavailability. J Pharm Sci 67:1582–1586, 1978

141. Allen MD, Greenblatt DJ, Harmatz JS, Smith TW: Effect of magnesium–hydroxide and kaolin–pectin on absorption of digoxin from tablets and capsules. J Clin Pharmacol 21:26–30, 1981

142. Moysey JO, Jaggarao NS, Grundy EN, et al: Amiodarone increases plasma digoxin concentrations. Br Med J 282:272, 1981

143. Koren G, Hesslein PS, MacLeod SL: Digoxin toxicity associated with amiodarone therapy in children. J Pediatr 104:467–470, 1984

144. Oetgens WF, Sobol SM, Tri TB, et al: Amiodarone–digoxin interaction: Clinical and experimental observations (Abstr.). Circulation 66:382, 1982

145. Nademanne K, Kannan R, Hendrickson J, et al: Amiodarone–digoxin interaction: Clinical significance, time course of devel-

opment, potential pharmacokinetic mechanisms and therapeutic implications. J Am Coll Cardiol 4:111–116, 1984

146. Belz GG, Doering W, Munkes R, et al: Interaction between digoxin and calcium antagonists and antiarrhythmic drugs. Clin Pharmacol Ther 33:410–417, 1983

147. Klein HO, Lang R, Weiss L, et al: The influence of verapamil on serum digoxin concentration. Circulation 65:998–1003, 1982

148. Pendersen KE, Dorph-Pendersen A, Hvidt S, et al: Digoxin-verapamil interaction. Clin Pharmacol Ther 30:311–316, 1981

149. Rodin SM, Johnson BF, Wilson J, et al: Comparative effects of verapamil and isradipine on steady-state digoxin kinetics. Clin Pharmacol Ther 43:668–672, 1988

150. Rameis H, Magometschnigg D, Ganzinger U: The diltiazem-digoxin interaction. Clin Pharmacol Ther 36:183–189, 1984

151. Elkayam U, Parikh K, Torkan B, et al: Effect of diltiazem on renal clearance and serum concentration of digoxin in patients with cardiac disease. Am J Cardiol 55:1293–1295, 1985

152. Kuhlmann J: Effect of nifedipine and diltiazem on plasma levels and renal excretion of beta-acetyldigoxin. Clin Pharmacol Ther 37:150–156, 1985

153. Schwartz JB, Migliore PJ: Effect of nifedipine on serum digoxin concentration and renal digoxin clearance. Clin Pharmacol Ther 36:19–24, 1984

154. Finch MB, Johnston GD, Lelly JG, McDevitt DG: Pharmacokinetics of digoxin alone and in the presence of indomethacin therapy. Br J Clin Pharmacol 17:353–355, 1984

155. Koren G: Interaction between digoxin and commonly coadministered drugs in children. Pediatrics 75:1032–1037, 1985

156. Koren G, Zarfin Y, Perlman M, MacLeod SM: Effects of indomethacin on digoxin pharmacokinetics in preterm infants. Pediatr Pharmacol 4:25–30, 1984

157. Leahey EB Jr, Reiffel JA, Drusin RE, et al: Interaction between quinidine and digoxin. JAMA 240:533–534, 1978

158. Leahey EB Jr, Bigger JT Jr, Butler VP, et al: Quinidine–digoxin interaction: Time course and pharmacokinetics. Am J Cardiol 48:1141–1146, 1981

159. Dahlqvist R, Ejvinsson G, Scheneck-Gustafsson K: Digoxin–quinidine interaction. N Engl J Med 301:727–728, 1979

160. Schenck-Gustafsson K, Dahlqvist R: Pharmacokinetics of digoxin in patients subjected to the quinidine–digoxin interaction. Br J Clin Pharmacol 11:181–186, 1981

161. Mungall DR, Ribichaux RA, Perry W, et al: Effects of quinidine on serum digoxin concentrations; a prospective study. Ann Intern Med 93:689–693, 1980

162. Doering W: Quinidine–digoxin interaction: Pharmacokinetics underlying mechanism and clinical implications. N Engl J Med 301:400–404, 1979

163. Ejvinsson G: Effect of quinidine in plasma concentrations of digoxin. Br Med J 1:279–280, 1978

164. Dahlqvist R, Ejvinsson G, Schenck-Gustafsson K: Effect of quinidine on phasma concentration and renal clearance of digoxin. Br J Clin Pharmacol 9:413–418, 1980

165. Fenster PE, Powell JR, Hager WD, et al: Onset and dose dependence of the digoxin-quinidine interaction (Abstr.). Am J Cardiol 45:413, 1980

166. Pedersen KE, Hastrup J, Hvidt S: The effect of quinidine on digoxin kinetics in cardiac patients. Acta Med Scan 207:291–295, 1980

167. Pedersen KE, Christiansen BD, Klitgaard NA, Nielsen-Kudsk F: Effect of quinidine on digoxin bioavailability. Eur J Clin Pharmacol 24:41–47, 1983

168. Ochs HR, Greenblatt DJ, Divoll M, et al: Impairment of digoxin clearance by coadministration of quinidine. J Clin Pharmacol 21:396–400, 1981

169. Leahey EB Jr, Saffidi LF, O'Connell GC, et al: Effect of quinidine on the pharmacokinetics of digoxin in normal volunteers (Abstr.). Clin Res 28:475A, 1980

170. Bigger JT Jr: The quinidine–digoxin interaction: What do we know about it? N Engl J Med 301:779–781, 1979

171. Reed RC, Schwartz HJ: Phenytoin, theophylline, quinidine interaction. N Engl J Med 308:724–725, 1983

172. Rosenberry KR, Defusco CJ, Mansnann HC, McGeady SJ: Reduced theophylline half-life induced by carbamazepine therapy. J Pediatr 102:472–474, 1983

173. Pfeifer HJ, Greenblatt DJ, Friedman P: Effect of three antibiotics on theophylline kinetics. Clin Pharmacol Ther 26:36–40, 1979

174. Maddux MS, Leeds NH, Organek HW, et al: The effect of erythromycin on theophylline pharmacokinetics at steady state. Chest 81:563–565, 1982

175. Kimelbatt BJ, Slaughter RL: Lack of effect of intravenous erythromycin lactobionate on theophylline clearance. J Allergy Clin Immunol 65:313–314, 1980

176. Hildebrandt R, Gundert-Remy U, Moller H, Weber E: Lack of clinically important interaction between erythromycin and theophylline. Eur J Clin Pharmacol 26:485–489, 1984

177. Zarowitz BJM, Szefler SJ, Lasezkay GM: Effect of erythromycin base on theophylline kinetics. Clin Pharmacol Ther 29:601–605, 1981

178. Prince RA, Wing DS, Weinberger MM, et al: Effect of erythromycin on theophylline kinetics. J Allergy Clin Immunol 68:427–431, 1981

179. Reisz G, Pingleton SK, Melethil S, Ryan PB: The effect of erythromycin on theophylline pharmacokinetics in chronic bronchitis. Am Rev Resp Dis 127:581–584, 1983

180. Kozak PP, Cummins LH, Gillman SA: Administration of erythromycin to patients on theophylline. J Allergy Clin Immunol 60:149–151, 1977

181. Murray MD, Brown BK: Theophylline-erythromycin interaction in an infant. Clin Pharm 1:107–111, 1982

182. Krstenansky PM, Javaheri S, Thomas JP, Thomas RL: Effect of continuous cimetidine infusion on steady-state theophylline concentration. Clin Pharm 8:206–209, 1989

183. Gutfield MB, Welage LS, Walawender CA, et al: The influence of intravenous cimetidine dosage regimens on the disposition of theophylline. J Clin Pharmacol 29:665–669, 1989

184. Roy AK, Cuda MP, Levine RA: Induction of theophylline toxicity and inhibition of clearance rate by ranitidine. Am J Med 85:525–527, 1988

185. Breen KJ, Bury R, Desmond PV, et al: Effects of cimetidine and ranitidine on hepatic drug metabolism. Clin Pharmacol Ther 31:297–300, 1982

186. Kelly HW: Lack of evidence for reduction of theophylline clearance by ranitidine. Am J Med 86:629–630, 1989

187. Griffith JA, Kozloski GD: Isoproterenol–theophylline interaction: Possible potentiation by other drugs. Clin Pharm 9:54–57, 1990

188. Hemstreet MP, Mile MV, Rutland RP: Effect of intravenous isoproterenol on theophylline kinetics. J Allergy Clin Immunol 69:360–364, 1982

189. O'Rouke PP, Crone RK: Effect of isoproterenol on measured theophylline levels. Crit Care Med 12:373–375, 1984

190. Jusko WJ, Gardner MJ, Mangione A, et al: Factors affecting theophylline clearance: age, tobacco, marijuana, cirrhosis, congestive heart failure, obesity, oral contraceptives, benzodiazepines, barbiturates, and ethanol. J Pharm Sci 68:1358–1366, 1979

191. Yazdani M, Kissling GE, Tran TH, et al: Phenobarbital increases the theophylline requirement of premature infants being treated for apnea. Am J Dis Child 141:97–99, 1987

192. Saccar CL, Danish M, Ragni MC, et al: The effect of phenobarbital on theophylline disposition in children with asthma. J Allergy Clin Immunol 75:716–719, 1985

193. Piafsky KM, Sitar DS, Ogilvie RI: Effect of phenobarbital on the disposition of intravenous theophylline. Clin Pharmacol Ther 22:336–339, 1977

194. Marquis J, Carruthers SG, Spence JD, et al: Phenytoin–theophylline interaction. N Engl J Med 307:1189–1190, 1982

195. Sklar SJ, Wagner JC: Enhanced theophylline clearance secondary to phenytoin therapy. Drug Intel Clin Pharm 19:34–36, 1985

196. Thomson AH, Thomson GD, Hepburn M, Whiting B: A clinically significant interaction between ciprofloxacin and theophylline. Eur J Clin Pharmacol 33:435–436, 1987

197. Rybak MJ, Bowels S, Chandrasekar PH, Edwards DJ: Increased theophylline concentrations secondary to ciprofloxacin. Drug Intel Clin Pharm 21:879–881, 1987

198. Wijnands WJA, Vree TB, Van Herwaadren CLA: The influence of quinolone derivatives on theophylline clearance. Br J Clin Pharmacol 22:677–683, 1986

199. Schwartz J, Jaureguli L, Lettieri J, Bachmann K: Impact of ciprofloxacin on theophylline clearance and steady state clearance and steady-state concentrations in serum. Antimicrob Agents Chemother 32:75–77, 1988

200. Raoof S, Wollschlager C, Khan F: Ciprofloxacin increases serum levels of theophylline. Am J Med 82:115–118, 1987

201. Bachmann K, Schwartz JI, Forney R Jr, Frogameni A, Jauregui LE: The effect of erythromycin on the disposition kinetics of warfarin. Pharmacology 28:171–176, 1984

202. Weibert RT, Lorentz SM, Townsend RJ, et al: Effect of erythromycin in patients receiving long-term warfarin therapy (Abstr.). Clin Pharmacol Ther 41:224, 1987

203. Schwartz SJ, Bachmann K, Perrigo E: Interaction between warfarin and erythromycin. S Med J 76:91–93, 1983

204. Hetzel D, Birkett D, Miners J: Cimetidine interaction with warfarin. Lancet 2:639, 1979

205. Serlin MJ, Mossman S, Sibeon RG, Breckenridge AM, et al: Cimetidine: Interaction with oral anticoagulants in man. Lancet 2:317–319, 1979

206. Serlin MJ, Sibeon RG, Breckenridge AM: Lack of effect of ranitidine on warfarin action. Br J Clin Pharmacol 12:791–794, 1981

207. O'Reilly RA: The stereoselective interaction of warfarin and metronidazole in man. N Engl J Med 295:354–357, 1976

208. Kazmier FJ: A significant interaction between metronidazole and warfarin. Mayo Clinic Proc 51:782–784, 1976

209. Dean RP, Talbert RL: Bleeding associated with concurrent warfarin and metronidazole therapy. Drug Intell Clin Pharm 14:864–866, 1980

210. O'Reilly RA: Interaction of chronic daily warfarin therapy and rifampin. Ann Intern Med 83:506–508, 1975

211. Romankiewicz JA, Ehrman M: Rifampin and warfarin: A drug interaction. Ann Intern Med 82:224–225, 1975

212. Heimark LD, Gibaldi M, Trager WF, O'Reilly RA, Goulart DA: The mechanism of the warfarin–rifampin drug interaction in humans. Clin Pharmacol Ther 42:388–394, 1987

213. Barnett DB, Hancock BW: Anticoagulant resistance: An unusual case. Br Med J 1:608–609, 1975

214. O'Reilly RO: Stereoselective interaction of trimethoprim–sulfamethoxazole with the separated enantiomorphs of a racemic warfarin in man. N Engl J Med 302:33–35, 1980

51

MANAGEMENT OF POISONING

ROBERT G. PETERSON

MEDICAL TOXICOLOGY AS A DISCIPLINE

Medical toxicology overlaps the discipline of clinical pharmacology in the area of overdose or excessive administration of drugs but extends further to interface with a number of other disciplines such as environmental toxicology, industrial medicine, and botanical and forensic toxiciology. Medical toxicology is thus focused upon the direct management of the poisoned patient, where the physician makes decisions based upon information that comes from the basic science of toxicology as well as from the numerous other medical specialties upon which the poisoning impacts.

Poisoning from food sources has been a conscious concern since the beginning of recorded history. Both the ancient Chinese and the early Egyptians were well aware of the poisoning potential of certain marine creatures. The Greeks and Romans were acquainted with both plant and animal toxins. An early text, "Poisons and Their Antidotes," intended as a practical guide to management of the poisoned patient was produced by Maimonides in 1198 A.D. Paracelsus is credited with the saying, "All substances are poisons; there is none which is not a poison. The right dose differentiates a poison."[1] This observation initiated the concept of the therapeutic index. William Withering expanded this theory best in his discourse on foxglove extract (digitalis) with the warning, "It is better the world should derive some instruction however imperfect, from my experience . . . or that a medicine of so much efficiency should be condemned and rejected as dangerous and unmanageable." A series of lectures by Claude Bernard in 1856 on the effects of toxic and medicinal substances may represent the first formal course in clinical toxicology.

The emergence of medical toxicology as a discipline has been something of a tortuous evolution. Due to modern man's increasing opportunity for exposure to an exploding array of potentially toxic substances, and the clear ethical limitations of toxicity testing in humans, much of the early literature is anecdotal and speculative. Extrapolation of animal data to humans can be extremely hazardous, since LD_{50} values for rodents can be meaningless to the child or adult human.[2] Well over a million new chemical compounds were synthesized in the last decade alone. Many of these chemicals have found their way into intentional or accidental human exposure and represent a continuing challenge to both poison prevention and medical treatment. Drug toxicity has similarly risen as the variety of drugs made available to our medication-demanding society has increased substantially. The word "drugs" in this context must include prescription and nonprescription medications as well as nonethical substances with abuse potential. While there is an obvious and substantial benefit to health associated with this expansion in pharmacotherapy, there exists, *inter alia,* a small fraction of cases in which poisoning results from drug misuse, intolerance, or accidental overdose. This has inevitably led to the substantial need for the development of systems to diagnose and manage the poisoned patient.[3-7]

The importance of medical toxicology in the area of pediatric pharmacology is considerable. Data from the American Association of Poison Control Centers National Data Collection System indicate that over 60 percent of the 1.36 million reported U.S. cases of poisonings involved chidren under 6 years of age.[8] Furthermore, with the trend toward continued employment through pregnancy, there exists a rising environmental exposure of the fetus to numerous commercial chemicals and inhalants outside the home. Heavy chemical industry employment is not the single workplace exposure that causes the principal concern. Women work throughout their pregnancies in numerous occupations where volatile solvents are used. These include hospital operating room personnel, artists, electronic factory workers, clerks, and workers in dry cleaners, among others.[9,10] Exposure may be daily at low levels or may fluctuate, and the duration of exposure may vary from one to all three trimesters. Abuse of gasoline or toluene during pregnancy also leads to the potential for serious central nervous system (CNS) injury

583

for the developing brain, such as occurs in the adult chronic abuser. Studies to date have included evaluation of "fetal solvent syndrome" in infants of toluene (glue) sniffers who have dysmorphic features and delayed neurologic development similar to fetal alcohol syndrome.[11,12] In other studies, the frequency of CNS malformations was four times higher in children whose mothers were occupationally exposed to solvents during pregnancy than in controls.[13]

CHILDHOOD POISONING: GENERAL CONCEPTS

Pediatric poisonings occur following both *accidental* and *intentional* exposures. The latter category includes both suicide attempts and other nontherapeutic intentional ingestions in which a known risk of toxicity is accepted, as in overdose associated with drug abuse. Such cases have comprised some 10–15 percent of all exposures reported to major poison control centers and occur almost exclusively in the adolescent age group. Among children age 6 and under, essentially all cases are accidents related to normal exploratory behavior. Fewer cases of poisoning occur in the age range 7–12 years, where accidental poisonings are rare and adolescent behavioral problems are not as firmly established. The reports of preteen experimentation or regular use of substances of abuse including alcohol, cocaine, marijuana, or tobacco may herald a departure from these traditional observations in this age category.[14]

There are five basic modes of exposure which, in aggregate, account for over 99 percent of all poisoning incidents. These are *ingestion,* which accounts for the vast majority of occurrences, followed by *ocular exposure, cutaneous exposure, envenomation,* and *inhalation.* The classification of poisoning cases at a U.S. regional poison control center[15] by mode of exposure demonstrates a representative distribution of childhood poisonings (Table 51–1).

To understand the scope of toxic substances involved in pediatric poisonings allows an appreciation of the broad range of information that must be available in toxicology. Table 51–2 presents categories of substances frequently ingested by children under 6 years in the United States for the year 1988.[8] The profile of pediatric poisonings differs from that of adult exposures.

The trend for the past decade has continued, with the leading causes of accidental poisonings in children being substances found frequently in the home and accessible to the toddler. From Table 51–2 a number of serious concerns are evident. Acetaminophen products represent one of the top five most frequently ingested substances by children, who comprised 75 percent of the total number of cases of acetaminophen ingestion. Less frequently ingested, stimulants and street drugs nevertheless had a substantially greater number of total fatalities associated with their exposures, and children under 6 years comprised almost one-quarter of all exposures. Clearly, one can identify cyclic antidepressants, stimulant/street

drugs, sedative hypnotics, rodenticides, and fumes/gases/vapors as among the most hazardous of these substances found in the environment of the young child.

The top 10 categories of accidental poisonings in children are uniquely childhood problems. With the exception of hydrocarbons, all 10 most common categories have a clear majority of exposures in children less than 6 years of age.

If one were to examine the data summarized in Table 51–2 by total deaths in a category along with the percentage of all exposures that occurred in children under 6 years, it could be concluded that special attention should be paid to of acetaminophen, building/construction supplies, cardiovascular medications, asthma medications, aspirin, street drugs, and narcotics for more effective preventive measures.

A further scheme for poisoning classification may be constructed according to the type of toxicity produced. For example, many drugs and chemicals have a direct toxic effect; that is, they are inherently toxic at some dose without being metabolically altered. This group includes barbiturates, narcotics, salicylates, and agents that are directly destructive to human tissues, such as strong acids and alkalis.[16]

Other agents act through interference with metabolic processes. For example, carbon monoxide combines with hemoglobin to occupy oxygen-binding sites and reduces the oxygen-carrying capacity of the blood.[17] Strontium competes with calcium for many important binding sites, including protein binding, transport through cell membranes, and bone deposition.[18]

Some other agents are only hazardous after conversion to a toxic metabolite. Methanol is converted by the body to formaldehyde and formic acid.[19] Acetaminophen poisoning following overdose results in the production of a relatively minor but highly reactive metabolite which is hepatotoxic.[20–22]

Poisonings may occur as the result of *acute* or *chronic* exposures. Most pediatric poisonings are acute and are typified by the child who surreptitiously invades the medicine cabinet or the storage area for household products.[8] Chronic poisoning is described as toxicity produced over some period of time; it refers not only to agent accumulation in the body, but also to cumulative toxicity. Chronic toxicity is exemplified by environmental pollution or the ongoing ingestion of lead or other heavy metals.[23–25] Aspirin poisoning that once occurred in infants and small children as a result of cumulative salicylate

TABLE 51–1. CLASSIFICATION OF POISONINGS BY ROUTE OF EXPOSURE

MODE OF POISONING	PERCENT (ALL CASES)	CHILDREN AGE 5 AND UNDER
Ingestion	85.0	92.7
Ocular	4.6	3.3
Inhalation	3.5	0.5
Topical	3.3	2.0
Envenomation	2.9	1.2
Other or unknown	0.7	0.3
	100.0	100.0

Adapted from Temple and Veltri,[15] with permission.

TABLE 51–2. FREQUENCY BY NUMBER OF EXPOSURES IN <6 YEARS GROUP

CATEGORY	<6 YRS	TOTAL	% <6 YRS	TOTAL DEATHS
Aspirin/narcotic	403	2,146	18.78	3
Muscle relaxants	776	4,182	18.56	5
Narcotics	995	4,048	24.58	34
Fungicides	1,344	4,549	29.54	5
Fumes/gases/vapors	1,827	17,168	10.64	39
Cyclic antidepressants	1,970	13,359	14.75	111
Anticonvulsants	2,201	6,946	31.69	6
Acetaminophen/narcotic	2,325	13,233	17.57	28
Batteries	2,988	5,664	52.75	0
Miscellaneous drugs	4,190	7,340	57.08	1
Alcohols	4,412	21,146	20.86	36
Stimulants/street drugs	4,710	19,435	24.23	101
Asthma medication	5,124	10,509	48.76	27
Aspirin	5,226	16,504	31.67	31
Sedative/hypnotic/antipsychotic	7,394	46,388	15.94	77
Tobacco products	8,697	9,246	94.06	1
Adhesives/glue	8,887	15,868	56.01	0
Cardiovascular medication	9,076	17,826	50.91	65
Rodenticide	9,406	10,626	88.52	2
Deodorizers/not personal care	9,557	10,659	89.66	1
Paints/paint strippers	10,335	17,105	60.42	0
Antihistamines	10,417	21,267	48.98	9
Bites/envenomations	10,514	47,829	21.98	1
Nsaids	13,676	29,293	46.69	6
Arts/crafts/office supplies	19,163	24,325	78.78	3
Insecticides/pesticides	22,136	41,499	53.34	12
Gastrointestinal medications	22,426	27,491	81.58	1
Hydrocarbons	26,317	52,454	50.17	8
Antimicrobials	28,058	43,374	64.69	1
Vitamins +/− iron or fluoride	30,326	36,254	83.65	1
Topical medications	40,069	49,630	80.74	3
Acetaminophen	51,668	68,259	75.69	24
Cough/cold medications	58,899	76,566	76.93	3
Plants	79,350	93,975	84.44	1
Building/construction supplies	87,393	137,240	63.68	19
Cosmetic/personal care	92,560	110,546	83.73	3

Total refers to all reported exposures in all ages, including adults. Total deaths refers to all ages, including adults.

toxic effect following administration of minimally excess drug over a period of time describes the concept of cumulative toxicity.[26] Chronic toxicity is a special problem for the physician because the source is not always obvious, the early toxicity is not always recognized, and the toxic process often proceeds surreptitiously until serious toxicity becomes evident.

CURRENT CONCEPTS IN POISONING MANAGEMENT

Whether the poisoned patient is reported by telephone or brought directly to a treatment facility, an assessment of the current or potential severity of the toxic exposure should be obtained as soon as possible. The basic historical information to obtain includes the following:

1. Confirmation that a toxic exposure has occurred
2. Identification of the toxic agent(s)
3. The route and magnitude (dose) of the exposure
4. The time of the exposure
5. The present condition of the victim, including signs and symptoms and changes in the patient's status.

On the basis of an efficient history, it is generally possible to make a judgment regarding the level of treatment required. Whenever serious poisoning is a possibility, the victim must be brought to an emergency treatment facility where appropriate management may proceed rapidly in a logical and organized manner.

For all serious exposures, the following procedures should be instituted.

Institution of Basic Life-Support Measures

Basic life-support consists of recognizing respiratory and cardiac arrest and implementing cardiopulmonary resuscitation. Such early assessment and management includes the establishment of an airway, artificial ventilation to restore breathing, and external cardiac compression to restore circulation.

Assessment of the Patient's Condition

Treatment personnel should determine heart rate, blood pressure, reflexes (deep tendon, corneal), response

TABLE 51–3. CLASSIFICATION OF COMA AND HYPERACTIVITY

COMA

Physical Findings	Coma Stage				
	0	1	2	3	4
Responds to verbal stimuli	+	0	0	0	0
Responds to minimal tactile stimuli	+	0	0	0	0
Responds to maximal tactile stimuli	+	+	0	0	0
Deep tendon reflexes present	+	+	+	0	0
Pupillary light reflexes present	+	+	+	+	0
Spontaneous respirations present	+	+	+	+	0
Stable blood pressure present	+	+	+	+	0

HYPERACTIVITY

Physical Findings	Stage			
	1	2	3	4
Restlessness, tremors, hyperreflexia	+	+	+	+
Sweating, mydriasis, flushing	+	+	+	+
Confusion, hyperactivity, tachypnea	0	+	+	+
Hypertension, hyperpyrexia	0	+	+	+
Delirium, mania, self-injury	0	0	+	+
Tachycardia, arrhythmias	0	0	+	+
Convulsions, coma, circulatory collapse	0	0	0	+

0 = absent.
+ = present.

to verbal and painful stimuli, pupil size and response to light, and state of hydration. The severity of symptoms associated with coma and hyperactivity, if present, should be assessed. The classification system shown in Table 51–3 can be used for this purpose.

Obtaining Specimens for Analytical Toxicologic Analysis

Once basic life-support measures have been instituted and while other management procedures are being instituted, blood, urine, and gastric aspirate should be collected for qualitative and quantitative toxicologic analysis, where appropriate.

Termination or Minimization of Toxic Exposure

A number of methods may be utilized to terminate the patient's exposure to a toxic substance or mitigate its effects. For inhalation, topical, and ocular exposures, removal of the victim from the toxic environment and appropriate first aid is imperative. Involved eyes should be washed for at least 15 minutes with water. For dermal exposures, the skin should be immediately washed with copious amounts of water and soap. The body should be free of all contaminated clothing. For ingestions, the principal effort is focused on prevention of absorption. This effort includes:

1. *Gastric evacuation.* The speed and extent of gastrointestinal transit and the absorption of a poison are dependent on (a) the nature of the substance, (b) the dose, (c) the volume, (d) the nature of other gastrointestinal

contents, and (e) the alimentary activity of the patient. Gastric evacuation is more effective if done within 2–4 hours. Induction of emesis is employed more commonly than gastric lavage in the removal of ingested poisons in small children and may be instituted *except when the patient has ingested caustics or is comatose, is experiencing seizures, has otherwise lost the gag reflex, or may deteriorate to any of the above states rapidly.*

The drug of choice for inducing emesis is *ipecac syrup* (not fluid extract). A dosage of 15 ml for children and 10 ml for infants under 1 year of age, given with an adequate volume of water or other liquid, will produce vomiting in over 90 percent of patients.[15–17] If vomiting does not occur within 20–30 minutes, the dose may be repeated.

In the older child or adolescent, orogastric lavage may be preferable to emesis. However, in order to carry out a satisfactory lavage, a size 24–36F or larger tube is required. Gastric contents should be aspirated *before* lavage fluid is introduced. The lavage fluid usually used is either water or 0.45 N saline. A continuous pattern of lavage fluid administration with intermittent suction should be instituted; lavage should be continued until the return is clear (usually requiring a total volume of at least 2 liters of lavage fluid).

2. *Simple dilution.* Dilution is only indicated when the toxin produces local irritancy or corrosivity. Water or milk are acceptable diluents. On the other hand, diluents should not be used for drug ingestions since they may increase absorption by increasing dissolution rates of the tablets and capsules or promote gastric emptying into the lower gastrointestinal tract.

3. *Use of activated charcoal.* Activated charcoal will minimize absorption by adsorbing a variety of poisons; its use should be considered in all cases of poisoning. Activated charcoal typically should be administered during the first hours after ingestion of the toxic agent in order to be effective. Approximately 5–10 times the amount of activated charcoal should be given for each milligram of drug or chemical ingested. A minimum 20-gm dose should be given to a child in situations where the amount of the toxic substance ingested is unknown. The activated charcoal should be mixed with a sufficient amount of water or sorbitol to make a slurry and then administered orally or by gastric tube. When used in conjunction with ipecac syrup, activated charcoal should *not* be attempted until vomiting has ceased. It should be noted that the once-advocated "universal antidote" (activated charcoal, magnesium oxide, and tannic acid) is *not recommended,* since the activity of the charcoal is inhibited by the other components. Similarly, burnt toast is *not* effective. A list of the substances known to be adsorbed by activated charcoal is provided in Table 51–4.[27]

4. *Catharsis.* After emesis or lavage, catharsis may be used to hasten the elimination of remaining ingested material. The agent of choice for this purpose is sorbitol administered with activated charcoal. Caution must be exercised in repetitive doses of charcoal/sorbitol, as the osmotic action of sorbitol may produce third-space fluid accumulation in the gut. The passage of charcoal indicates a transit of the gastrointestinal tract. Mineral oil or stimulant cathartics such as castor oil are not recom-

TABLE 51–4. SUBSTANCES KNOWN TO BE ADSORBED BY ACTIVATED CHARCOAL

Arsenic	Muscarine
Atropine	Nicotine
Barbiturates	Opium
Boric acid[3]	Oxalates
Camphor	Parathion
Cantharides	Penicillin
Chloroquine[2]	Phenol[1]
Chlorpheniramine[1]	Phenolphthalein
Chlorpromazine[2]	Phosphorus
Cocaine	Potassium hydroxide[3]
Colchicine[1]	Potassium permanganate
DDT[3]	Primaquine[1]
Dextroamphetamine sulfate[1]	Quinacrine[2]
2,4-Dichlorophenoxyacetic acid[2]	Quinidine[2]
Digitalis	Quinine[2]
Diphenylhydantoin[1]	Salicylates[1]
Ferrous sulfate[3]	Silver
Iodine[1]	Sodium hydroxide[3]
Ipecac	Sodium metasilicate[3]
Malathion[3]	Stramonium
Meprobamate[2]	Strychnine
Mercuric chloride	Sulfonamides
m-Methylcarbamate[3]	Thallium
Methylene blue	Tolbutamide[3]
Morphine	

[1]Excellent adsorption.
[2]Good adsorption.
[3]Minimal adsorption.
Adapted from Easom and Lovejoy,[27] with permission.

mended, since they may increase absorption of some poisons.[28]

5. *Whole bowel irrigation.* Balanced electrolyte solutions used for bowel preparation prior to surgery have been safely employed to wash out ingested substances from the entire gastrointestinal tract.[29] Typically, 10–12 liters in an adult or 2–4 liters in a child may be administered via nasogastric tube with the patient in an upright position at a rate that will not allow distention or emesis in the patient.

Use of Specific Systemic Antidotes

The percentage of ingestions for which a specific antidote does exist is small. Where a specific antidote can be used, it is vital that it be administered as early as possible with close attention to the recommended dosage. A partial listing of poisons with known antidotes is given in Table 51–5. Antidotes can be categorized as to their mechanism of action:[30]

1. *Antidotes can interfere with the metabolism of the poison either by blocking the metabolism of the less-toxic precursor to the active poison or by accelerating the metabolism of the poison to a nontoxic form.* The administration of ethanol to a patient suffering from methanol intoxication will competitively inhibit the metabolism of methanol to formaldehyde and formic acid. It should be noted that formic acid and formaldehyde are respectively 6 and 30 times more toxic than methanol.[31] Conversely, the administration of sodium thiosulfate

will facilitate the conversion of cyanide to the less acutely toxic thiocyanate.[32] Treatment of cyanide poisoning with sodium thiosulfate should only follow the use of sodium nitrite.[33]

2. *Antidotes can block the receptor site of action of the poison.* The administration of atropine intravenously every 10–15 minutes until atropinization is evident will effectively block the receptor site of action of acetylcholine following organophosphate insecticides.[34,35]

3. *Antidotes can compete with the poison for the receptor site of action.* The administration of 100 percent oxygen at normobaric or hyperbaric conditions will compete with carbon monoxide binding to heme in hemoglobin or cytochromes.[36] Other examples of antidotal action would include the administration of naloxone for narcotic intoxication,[37] or the usage of vitamin K_1 preparations for oral anticoagulant overdose.[38]

4. *Antidotes can chelate the poison, thus forming a nontoxic complex.* Examples of this mechanism of action include the administration of BAL (Dimercaprol) for the treatment of arsenic, copper, lead, or mercury intoxication.[39] The administration of the chelator d-penicillamine has been shown to be effective in the management of arsenic, copper, lead, or mercury intoxication.[40] Ethylenediaminetetraacetic acid (EDTA) has been shown to be of

TABLE 51–5. POISONS WITH KNOWN ANTIDOTES

ADMINISTRATION NECESSARY IN MINUTES		
Toxin	**Antidote**	**Dose**
Cyanide	Amyl nitrite	Inhalation
	Sodium nitrite	10 mg/kg
Carbon monoxide	Oxygen	–
Nitrites (nitrates)	Methylene blue	1–2 mg/kg
Arsenic	BAL	3–5 mg/kg
H_2S	Oxygen	–
	Sodium nitrite	10 mg/kg
Organophosphates Carbamates	Atropine	As needed
Narcotics	Naloxone	0.01–0.1 mg/kg

ADMINISTRATION NECESSARY IN HOURS		
Toxin	**Antidote**	**Dose**
Acetaminophen	N-Acetylcysteine (Mucomyst)	140 mg/kg P.O. 70 mg/kg/4h
Tricyclic antidepressants	Sodium bicarbonate Physostigmine	1–2 mEq/kg 0.5–4 mg I.V.
Aliphatic alcohols	Ethanol	0.75 gm/kg load 0.15 gm/kg/h
Mercury	BAL	3–5 mg/kg I.M.
Salicylates	Sodium bicarbonate	1–2 mEq/kg
Digoxin	Phenytoin	5–10 mg/kg I.V.
Iron	Desferal	10–15 mg/kg/h I.V.
Snake venom	Antiserum	3–5 vials/250 ml D_5W over 30 min I.V.

value in the therapy of lead intoxication.[41] Deferoxamine (Desferal) has a specific ability to chelate iron and is useful in treating acute iron intoxication.[42] BAL is typically administered in a dose of 3–5 mg/kg intramuscularly every 4 hours for 2 days, then every 6 hours for an additional 2 days, then every 12 hours for up to 7 additional days. d-Penicillamine, on the other hand, is administered orally at a dose of 100 mg/kg/day (maximum 1 gm) in divided doses for up to 5 days. If long-term therapy is to be used, the dose of 40 mg/kg/day should not be exceeded. EDTA can be administered either by deep intramuscular injection or by slow intravenous infusion. The dose of 75 mg/kg/day should be administered in three to six divided doses for up to 5 days; this dosage regimen may be repeated for a second course after a minimum of 2 days. Deferoxamine can be administered by careful continuous intravenous infusion or intramuscularly. The severity of the intoxication will determine the route of administration. Typically deferoxamine is given at 15 mg/kg/h as a carefully monitored infusion. Intramuscular doses in children are inconvenient due to the large volumes that must be injected. Too rapid an intravenous dose will result in hypotension.[43]

5. *Antidotes can restore function by repair or by bypassing the effect of the poison.* By restoring the sulfhydryl content of the liver that was depleted by the reactive intermediates in the metabolism of acetaminophen overdose, acetylcysteine has been proven effective in the prevention of acetaminophen-induced hepatotoxicity.[44,45] Other examples of antidotes that function by this modality include the administration of folinic acid to antagonize the toxicity of methotrexate[46] or the administration of methylene blue to reduce the ferric iron of methemoglobin back to the ferrous state.[47,48]

Enhancement of Poison Elimination

Procedures available for enhancing the elimination of an absorbed poison include ionized *diuresis* and extracorporeal drug elimination techniques. The latter consist of hemodialysis or peritoneal dialysis, hemoperfusion, exchange transfusion, or plasmapheresis. Because some risk is involved, these procedures are generally restricted to use in those cases where significant benefit can be expected in reducing morbidity in addition to improving survival.

Ionized diuresis takes advantage of the principle that net excretion is favored when a drug is in its ionized state.[49] Alkaline or acid diuresis is selected on the basis of the pK_a of the toxic agent such that the ionized drug will be trapped within the tubular lumen and not reabsorbed.[50,51] For weak acids, alkalinization of the urine would be selected. Acid diuresis similarly enhances the excretion of some weak bases. The combination of alkaline and osmotic diuresis has been shown to be beneficial in barbiturate poisoning.[52] This combination is also efficacious in adult salicylate poisoning[53]; however, satisfac-

tory alkalinization of the urine is not easily achieved in children.

The following parameters should be monitored during alkaline or acid diuresis: urine output, fluid input, Na, K, Cl, CO_2, blood urea nitrogen (BUN), Ca, P, serum osmolality, urine osmolality, and, where appropriate, central venous pressure. These parameters should be obtained prior to and at appropriate intervals during diuresis. Following the initial volume load, urine output should approximate 2–5 ml/kg/h. With the use of diuretics, urine output may reach 6–9 ml/kg/h. Diuresis can be discontinued when the patient regains consciousness, serious toxic manifestations abate, or when drug blood levels are below toxic levels.

Alkalinization of the urine is usually initiated with sodium bicarbonate at a dose of 1–2 mEq/kg intravenously over a 1- to 2-hour period. Throughout this period urine pH should be monitored. The infusion should be continued at the same rate or modified to maintain a urine pH of 7.5 or greater. As an adjunct to this therapy, when bicarbonate deficit has been corrected and arterial pH can be monitored, acetazolamide at a dose of 5 mg/kg I.V. can be given. Arterial pH should be monitored during therapy. If the arterial pH falls below 7.4, additional bicarbonate must be infused.

Acidification of the urine is usually initiated with ammonium chloride at a dose of 75 mg (2.75 mEq)/kg/dose every 6 hours via a nasogastric tube until the urine pH is equal to 5.0. As an adjunct to this therapy, ascorbic acid in a dosage range of 500 mg to 2 gm in 500 cc of fluid may be administered intravenously at a normal infusion rate.

Extracorporeal drug removal (ECDR) is used selectively in cases of severe poisoning or when renal failure is present.[54] A number of criteria must be met before dialysis is considered. These criteria include those that are *patient-related* and those that are *drug-related.* Patient-related criteria include (1) anticipated prolonged coma with the high likelihood of attendant complications, (2) development of renal failure or impairment of normal excretory pathways, and (3) progressive clinical deterioration in spite of careful medical supervision. Drug-related criteria are (1) the membrane permeability of the drug, (2) a correlation between plasma concentration and toxicity of the agent, with plasma levels in the potentially fatal range, (3) the presence of a significant quantity of an agent that is normally metabolized to a toxic substance, and (4) significant drug removal during dialysis expected.

Hemodialysis has now been used for some time in the pediatric patient and is an effective means for removal of some drugs. However, because it requires highly technical skills from both a physician and a technician, it is not universally available.

Peritoneal dialysis is less efficient than hemodialysis but offers the advantages of ready availability, simplicity, and safety; the safety is particularly evident in the management of cardiovascularly unstable small children, where dangerous blood volume fluctuations may be encountered with an extracorporeal vascular circuit. Substances that are highly protein-bound are not readily dialyzable.[54]

Gastric dialysis or continuous gastric lavage has been

used to remove agents that are actively excreted into the stomach. Drugs in this category are generally weak bases, such as mepivacaine or the tricyclics. This procedure has not been shown to remove quantitative amounts of drug.

Hemoperfusion is the process of passing blood through a cartridge containing an adsorbent, after which the detoxified blood is returned to the patient. Although there are some limitations to the extent to which hemoperfusion can be utilized, it appears to be at least as effective as and possibly more effective than hemodialysis for a number of agents.[55,56] Acidosis and electrolyte disturbances are not directly correctable with hemoperfusion. Thus, despite its apparent superiority to hemodialysis for removal of certain drugs, these additional considerations may limit its use.[54]

Exchange transfusion is indicated for substances that are not dialyzable, such as those which are tightly protein-bound, or in neonates where dialysis is not readily available. The technique has been somewhat useful in lowering blood iron levels in the case of severe acute iron poisoning,[57] and in the treatment of serious methemoglobinemia.

Other Supportive Measures

Problems requiring supportive or symptomatic care are similar to those which occur elsewhere in medicine and are managed in much the same manner. The most frequently occurring problems that occur during a poisoning are (1) central nervous system depression, (2) central nervous system stimulation, and (3) cerebral edema.

1. In *central nervous system depression,* analeptic or stimulant drugs are not recommended, since these drugs are of no real value in the treatment of the poisoning.[58] Severe depression is not reversed by reasonable doses of such drugs, and higher doses may produce convulsions. With mild depression, exposing the patient to the inherent dangers of stimulant drugs is unwarranted. The management therefore consists of using assisted ventilation when required, and volume with vasopressors as needed for support of blood pressure. Body temperature is maintained by heating or cooling, as required.

2. In *central nervous system stimulation,* one needs to terminate the seizures and provide subsequent prophylaxis. For terminating acute seizures, diazepam, lorazepam, or short-acting barbiturates are effective. Seizure prophylaxis is generally best achieved using phenobarbital or phenytoin.

3. *Cerebral edema* may occur in certain types of poisonings (carbon monoxide, cyanide) or following hypoxia with fluid overload. Cerebral edema can be managed with hyperventilation, an intravenous infusion of mannitol, and corticosteroids. The effect of mannitol is relatively short-lived and must be monitored closely. Corticosteroid therapy is thought both to reverse cerebral edema and to minimize its development. Since the steroid effect is delayed for several hours, the more immediate effects of hyperventilation or mannitol are initially required.

Table 51–6 summarizes some of the drugs and dosage regimens available for the management of selected problems associated with poisonings.

TABLE 51–6. SUPPORTIVE CARE IN THE MANAGEMENT OF POISONINGS

PURPOSE	DRUG AND DOSAGE	COMMENT
To expand blood volume	Normal saline, 10–20 ml/kg in 1 h; *or* Whole blood, 20–25 ml/kg; *or* Albumin, 5%; 0.5 gm/kg in 1 h	
To correct acidosis	Na bicarbonate, 1–3 mEq/kg I.V.	Add to maintenance fluid in mild to moderate acidosis for blood pH < 7.2
To correct hypoglycemia	50% glucose, 1–2 ml/kg I.V. push	
For hypocalcemia	10% calcium gluconate, 0.15 ml/kg I.V. slow push	
For tetany with associated hypomagnesemia	50% magnesium sulfate, 0.2 ml/kg I.V. q12h	
To terminate convulsions or extreme hyperactivity	Diazepam, 0.1–0.3 mg/kg; up to 10 mg slowly I.V. Pentobarbital, 3–5 mg/kg, slowly I.V.	Administer slowly until desired end point is reached. Respiratory arrest may occur Slowly as above
To prevent convulsions	Phenobarbital loading: 20 mg/kg followed by 3–5 mg/kg/24 h I.V. *or* Phenytoin 20 mg/kg slow I.V. infusion followed by 5 mg/kg/24 h	
To correct cerebral edema	20% mannitol, 0.5–1 gm/kg I.V. and/or Dexamethasone, 0.03–0.05 mg/kg I.V.	Infuse mannitol over 30 min; Dexamethasone should be given every 4 h
To correct hypotension	Dopamine, 5–20 µg/kg/min I.V. infusion *or* Dobutamine, 2.5–10 µg/kg/min I.V. infusion	Give parenteral fluids first. Use vasopressors if response inadequate
To reverse narcotic CNS effects	Naloxone 0.1 mg/kg up to 4 mg I.V. push	

Management of Snake Bites (Envenomation)

The basic principles include (1) adequate confirmation of envenomation by positive identification of the snake with evidence of fang puncture, pain, and edema at the site; (2) avoidance of excitement or exertion, which may accelerate the spread of the venom; (3) judicious application of a flat tourniquet proximal to the bite, which must be loosened as swelling increases and removed after antivenin is administered; (4) the administration of specific antivenin; and (5) the use of tetanus toxoid and broad-spectrum antibiotics as required.[59]

POISON CONTROL SYSTEMS

An adequate program for the management of poisonings requires a complete, up-to-date, and accessible information data base, a geographically balanced network of adequately staffed and equipped treatment facilities, education programs aimed at prevention, and adequate resources for the requirement of the region. The goal of such a regional information center is to facilitate access to:

1. Comprehensive poison information, available to both health professionals and the public, with a toll-free communications system and the provision for followup.

2. Comprehensive poisoning treatment services, including telephone consultation for patients being managed at home and for health professionals treating patients in regional medical care facilities, along with hospital facilities for treatment of critically ill poisoned patients.

3. Transportation facilities for critically ill patients and coordination of interhospital patient transfers. This includes integration with local emergency medical services.

4. A thoughtfully designed program of professional and public education.

5. An efficient system for the collection and dissemination of poisoning experience data.

DIAGNOSIS AND THERAPY FOR SELECTED COMMON DRUG OVERDOSE AND POISONING

Salicylates

Diagnosis

Differentiate acute from chronic poisoning.[26] Acute ingestion of salicylate (over a period $< 4–6$ hours) of >150 mg/kg requires assessment using plasma levels. Plasma salicylate levels should be measured 6 hours or more after ingestion and the Done nomogram utilized for

predictive value in estimating risk to the patient. Acid–base status must be assessed in all cases and fluid, sodium, potassium, and bicarbonate deficits repaired. Acute salicylate intoxication is characterized by a mixed respiratory alkalosis with metabolic acidosis. An alkaline plasma pH is present and should be preserved using I.V. sodium bicarbonate.[60]

Treatment

Provided CNS status is normal and renal function is intact, aggressive fluid therapy is indicated to repair sodium and water losses. Isotonic saline infusions followed by solutions that are 50–70 mEq/liter (mmol/liter) sodium as both chloride and bicarbonate salts are used. Sodium bicarbonate should not be added to isotonic saline infusions with resultant hyperosmolar solutions. Serum potassium requires repair, and an alkaline urine cannot be easily produced until water, sodium, and potassium losses are corrected. Urine pH > 7.5 is required to allow ion trapping and to facilitate salicylate elimination.[61] Carbonic anhydrase inhibitors should never be used to produce an alkaline urine unless fluid, electrolyte, and bicarbonate losses are completely repaired.[62] This normally requires 24 h of I.V. therapy. Bicarbonate loss is promoted by acetazolamide, thereby worsening the metabolic acidosis. Morbidity and mortality increase as salicylate enters the CNS and accelerate as plasma pH falls. Production of an alkaline urine at the expense of plasma alkalinity therefore can be expected to increase morbidity. Thus, acetazolamide use should be restricted to the second 24 hours, if it is used at all.

Hemodialysis is very effective in removing salicylate and repairing fluid, electrolyte, and acid–base disorders. It is not typically required unless the patient demonstrates renal insufficiency, severe electrolyte disturbance, or altered CNS status as a result of severe salicylism.[63]

Chronic salicylate poisoning presents with both an acid pH and an acid urine. Bicarbonate, electrolyte, and fluid losses have occurred over a period of days and renal function is more likely to be abnormal. Replacement therapy is more cautious and there must be increased concern for production of pulmonary edema or cerebral edema.[64] Judicious bicarbonate therapy is indicated for severe acidemia, and hemodialysis should be considered early in the management. Glycogen depletion can result in hypoglycemia. The mortality in chronic salicylism represents a greater risk than in appropriately treated acute salicylate ingestions. Since aggressive fluid therapy is more hazardous in *severe* chronic salicylate poisoning, hemodialysis should represent the primary therapeutic approach.[65]

Acetaminophen

Diagnosis

Diagnosis should be based on a plasma level of acetaminophen drawn at least 4 hours following ingestion.[66] In lieu of a plasma level, oral therapy may be initiated upon history of >140 mg/kg in a child or 7.5 gm in an adult.[45,67] Emesis more than 2 hours following the ingestion is not indicated. Activated charcoal is indicated at any time < 4 hours from the ingestion and does not automatically exclude oral therapy with N-acetylcysteine.

Treatment

Therapy with N-acetylcysteine is initiated for all potentially hepatotoxic acetaminophen overdoses within the first 24 hours following ingeston. Oral N-acetylcysteine is given by diluting a 20 percent solution with carbonated beverage or juice to 5 percent (1:4). The dose is 140 mg/kg as a load followed by 70 mg/kg every 4 hours. Therapy may continue to 72 hours if indicated by the continued presence of acetaminophen in plasma. Therapy should not be discontinued within the first 24 hours if any plasma level has been measured above the lower line of the Rumack-Matthew treatment nomogram.[66]

I.V. N-acetylcysteine is indicated for patients who cannot tolerate the oral route. It carries a small but real risk of anaphylactic reaction and therefore should not be utilized in the absence of a documanted toxic acetaminophen plasma level. I.V. N-acetylcysteine is most effective when given in the first 8–12 hours following ingestion but should not be withheld during the first 16–24 hours. I.V. dosages have been shown to be efficacious in the United Kingdom using a protocol of 150 mg/kg I.V. in 200 ml 5 percent dextrose water (D_5W) over 15 minutes, followed by 50 mg/kg I.V. in 500 ml D_5W over 4 hours followed by 100 mg/kg I.V. in 1000 ml D_5W over 16 hours.[68] Acetaminophen plasma levels should be remeasured at 24 hours, and therapy may require extension if plasma acetaminophen remains elevated.

Liver function should be monitored using enzymes, bilirubin, and prothrombin time. The centrilobular hepatic necrosis becomes evident over the first 72 hours. Provided the patient survives the acute injury, there is not a continuing process of hepatic dysfunction or cirrhosis.

Renal function is less commonly affected,[69] but creatinine and BUN should be followed until evidence of hepatic injury is resolved. Hemodialysis has a role in acetaminophen overdoses only for the supportive treatment of renal failure.

Overdoses that present after the first 24 hours, particularly when there is evidence of hepatic dysfunction, should be observed for evidence of progressive hepatic failure and monitored for signs of encephalopathy. Nitrogen-restricted diets, oral neomycin, and lactulose may be indicated in such patients. If encephalopathy occurs, intracranial pressure should be assessed.

Carbon Monoxide

Diagnosis

There is a history of exposure to incomplete combustion fumes, usually involving more than one person in group exposures. Headache, CNS depression, or acute gastroenteritis are frequent findings with mild to moderate exposures. More severe exposures result in seizures, coma, and evidence of lactic acidosis from tissue hypoxia.[70] Blood measurements of carboxyhemoglobin are useful in so far as carboxyhemoglobin is rarely measured in excess of 10 percent, even in heavy smokers, unless carbon monoxide poisoning has occurred. The presence of elevated carboxyhemoglobin confirms the diagnosis but will not necessarily correlate with the severity of the exposure. In this regard, time following exposure, oxygen therapy, and tissue levels are all important variables.[71,72]

Treatment

Oxygen therapy in the highest concentration available at the site should be initiated at once. Hyperbaric oxygen has been increasingly advocated for carbon monoxide poisoning, although specific indications remain controversial. Any patient with loss of consciousness, disorientation, seizures, severe metabolic acidosis, or evidence of cerebral edema or serious underlying myocardial disease is a candidate for hyperbaric oxygen. The purpose of hyperbaric oxygen is not only more rapid resolution of carboxyhemoglobin but also to facilitate tissue "washout," where carbon monoxide binding to heme in cytochromes may be responsible for substantial late toxicity and sequelae.[73]

In addition to oxygen therapy, restricted fluid intake and aggressive use of osmotic agents such as mannitol with early evidence of CNS deterioration may prove beneficial. Seizures are treated with I.V. diazepam 0.1 mg/kg over 3 minutes repeated at 10- to 15-minute intervals as required. Intubation with positive end expiratory pressure may be required to maintain both ventilation and oxygenation in patients with pulmonary edema secondary to smoke inhalation and thermal burns to the respiratory tract. Patients with severe carbon monoxide poisoning require monitoring for several days, especially if hyperbaric oxygen therapy was not available. Oxidative metabolism returns to normal baseline status only after mitochondrial cytochrome function and residual tissue hypoxic injury is normalized.[72]

Benzodiazepines

Diagnosis

Assays for detection of parent drug and/or metabolites in plasma and urine are available. Clinical presentation is that of intoxication without an odor of alcohol and includes ataxia, slurred speech, and sedation. Acute oral ingestions involving only benzodiazepines usually result in levels of intoxication that are responsive to verbal commands and without hypotension. Mixed ingestions of benzodiazepines with alcohol or other sedative hypnotic agents can be life-threatening, since benzodiazepines will potentiate the effects of the second substance.[74] I.V. benzodiazepine overdose has been associated with acute respiratory arrests. Oral benzodiazepines in children less than 2 years old may be associated with a higher incidence of severe CNS depression.

Treatment

Most cases require only careful observation and monitoring of vital signs until stable. Use of activated charcoal to prevent absorption is indicated, but more aggressive procedures such as gastric lavage are probably not indicated. An experimental benzodiazepine antagonist has had clinical evaluation and appears to facilitate reversal of benzodiazepine CNS depression, although such therapy is not often required.[75] I.V. aminophylline in low dose, 1–2 mg/kg, has been used to reverse CNS depression in documented diazepam-induced CNS depression. Hemodialysis has no role in isolated benzodiazepine overdoses.

β-BLOCKERS

Diagnosis

Plasma levels are not readily available. A history of beta blocker prescription in the presence of hypotension with bradycardia is consistent with β-blocker acute toxicity. Hypoglycemia can be an associated finding.[76,77]

Treatment

Bradycardia with accompanying hypotension should be treated with atropine, 0.01 mg/kg I.V. with repetition if unsuccessful. Use fluids cautiously. Bradycardia refractory to atropine should be treated with glucagon,[76–78] 50–100 μg/kg as a 1-minute bolus followed by an infusion of 1–5 mg/h. Isoproterenol can be used, but hypotension may be exacerbated unless a pressor agent such as dopamine is given concomitantly.[78] Isoproterenol is administered by continuous infusion of 0.05–0.5 μg/kg/minute, although larger doses may be required in extreme overdoses. Dopamine is given simultaneously as 5–20 μg/kg/minute to titrate the effects of isoproterenol on blood pressure. Patients who are refractory to glucagon and isoproterenol are candidates for temporary pacemakers. Pacing should be immediately available for all severe acute β-blocker overdoses and should be instituted as soon as failure of drug therapy to counter the overdose is evident. Pacing rate should be established to suppress ventricular ectopy and restore cardiac output.

Associated toxicity includes hypoglycemia, which should be assessed early and frequently during therapy. Treatment consists of intravenous glucose solutions; glucagon therapy as described above should also produce a favorable response. CNS depression and grand mal seizures have been seen. Nonhypoglycemic seizures are treated with I.V. diazepam, 0.1 mg/kg over 3 minutes repeated every 10–15 minutes as required. Not all β-

blockers are removed by hemodialysis (e.g., propranolol), but for cases not responding rapidly to the above treatment, hemoperfusion may rapidly remove drug from the vascular compartment,[79] including the heart, allowing stabilization.

Tricyclic Antidepressants

Diagnosis

Anticholinergic signs in the presence of widened (>0.10 seconds) QRS are pathognomonic. Anticholinergic signs include tachycardia, coma, hallucinations, seizures, xerostomia, bowel hypomotility, mydriasis, and dry, warm skin.[80]

The presence of widened QRS complexes is a sign not of the anticholinergic effects of the tricyclics but rather of their potent quinidine-like activity on heart muscle and conducting tissue.[81,82]

Treatment

A history of tricyclic antidepressant overdose in excess of 5–10 mg/kg requires observation and ECG monitoring. Coma and/or severe cardiovascular toxicity can be expected following ingestions of 10–20 mg/kg. For these reasons, prevention of absorption using gastric emptying in cases where gastric contents are likely to still contain drug and activated charcoal 25–50 gm are recommended. Activated charcoal may be repeated q4–6h provided there is evidence of G.I. motility. Osmotic cathartics such as sorbitol may be used with caution with first dose of charcoal.

Acidosis should be assessed and corrected using I.V. sodium bicarbonate. The quinidine effects of the tricyclics are more pronounced at acid pH.[82]

Therapy of the *anticholinergic* component of tricyclic poisoning includes:

Seizure Management

I.V. diazepam 0.1 mg/kg over 3 minutes, repeated q10–15min as required. Monitor respirations during therapy.
I.V. phenytoin 15–20 mg/kg (usual maximum = 1000 mg) at a rate not faster than 1 mg/kg/min. Monitor heart rate and blood pressure during infusion.
I.V. phenobarbital 15–20 mg/kg (usual maximum = 1000 mg) at a rate not faster than 0.5–1 mg/kg/min. Monitor blood pressure and respirations during infusion.

Seizures refractory to the above may require general anesthesia and use of neuromuscular blockade. Physostigmine has been used to treat refractory anticholinergic seizures but should not be used in the cardiovascular unstable patient where ventricular fibrillation or asystole may follow. The childhood dose for I.V. physostigmine is 0.5–2 mg at a rate not faster than 0.01 mg/kg/min.

Therapy of the quinidine component of tricyclic poisoning includes:

Antiarrhythmics

Caution! Do *not* use a Class 1A antiarrhythmic such as quinidine, procainamide, or disopyramide, since these drugs potentiate the conduction abnormalities of the tricyclics.

I.V. sodium bicarbonate 1–2 mEq/kg by rapid infusion has been successful in reducing QRS duration and associated ectopy.

Phenytoin in doses given for seizure control is indicated unless previously loaded.

Lidocaine, 0.5–1 mg/kg I.V. at a rate not exceeding 1 mg/kg/min as a loading dose. Continuous infusion of 20–40 μg/kg/min with careful monitoring of heart rate throughout loading and infusion.

β-Blockers may be indicated for refractory ventricular arrhythmias.

Cardiac pacemakers may be required for severe, refractory cases.

Supraventricular arrhythmias do not usually require drug therapy and will resolve with other symptoms over 12–24 hours. In those patients who cannot tolerate rapid rates, judicious use of a β-blocker may be indicated. Propranolol dose is 0.01–0.03 mg/kg I.V. over 1 minute repeated at 5- to 10-minute intervals until conversion or 0.1 mg/kg has been given.

Hypotension

Treat with I.V. fluids, correction of metabolic or respiratory acidosis, and with pure α-sympathomimetics when refractory to fluid. Norepinephrine infusions of 20–40 μg/kg/min are titrated to maintain blood pressure. Sympathomimetics with β-activity may contribute to ventricular ectopy.

Hemodialysis has no role in tricyclic poisoning due to extensive protein binding and large distribution volume. Hemoperfusion is not expected to remove substantial quantities of tricyclic following distribution but may be indicated when standard treatment outlined above is not successful.[83]

Aliphatic Alcohols: Ethylene Glycol, Isopropanol, Methanol, Ethanol

Diagnosis

Differentiate mixed ethanol ingestions with any of the above from pure ingestions of the aliphatic alcohols. Ethanol delays metabolism of the other aliphatic alcohols, since it is a better substrate for alcohol dehydrogenase, the hepatic pathway that is quantitatively the most important mechanism for alcohol elimination. Alcohols are excreted by the kidneys but are not concentrated in the urine. Delay in the metabolism of ethylene glycol and methanol will mask findings of anion gap acidosis and other more specific evidence (e.g., urinary oxalate crystals for ethylene glycol).

Isopropanol is metabolized to acetone, which is not normally considered to be more toxic than isopropanol

itself. Methanol is metabolized to formaldehyde and to formic acid. Ethylene glycol is metabolized to a family of glycoaldehydes and acids, ultimately to oxalic acid, a nephrotoxic substance. All alcohols will contribute to a gap in osmolality between calculated and measured.[84] Osmolality is calculated according to the equation:

$$Osm \text{ (mOsm/liter)} = 2 \text{ (Na}^+) + \text{(Glu)}/18 \\ + \text{(BUN)}/2.8 + \text{(EtOH)}/4.6 + \text{(MeOH)}/3.2 \\ + \text{(EtGly)}/6.2 + \text{(Iso)}/6.0$$

where

Na^+ = serum Na in mEq/liter or mmol/liter
Glu = blood glucose in mg/dl
BUN = blood urea nitrogen in mg/dl
EtOH = Blood ethanol in mg/dl
MeOH = blood methanol in mg/dl
EtGly = blood ethylene glycol in mg/dl
Iso = blood isopropyl alcohol in mg/dl

Note: When measurements are in S.I. units, no division of any value is required.

The relationship between alcohols and serum osmolality is most valid early in the course of the poisoning. As methanol and ethylene glycol are metabolized, their products will substitute for the parent alcohol's contribution to the osmolar gap, but the laboratory quantitation of parent alcohol will no longer satisfy the requirements of the equation. The numbers used to divide the alcohol concentration in mg/dl provide an estimate of the quantity of alcohol in blood for a given osmolar gap. Hence, if only methanol is present, for every 1 mOsm/liter abnormality in osmolar gap, blood methanol will be elevated by 3.2 mg/dl. Such estimates are crude and should be verified with actual laboratory measurements of alcohols.

Anion gap metabolic acidosis is present following ingestion of methanol and ethylene glycol[84] but may also be present following ethanol in some cases where lactic acidosis is produced. Anion gap is calculated from:

$$A.G. = (Na^+ + K^+) - (Cl^- + HCO_3^-)$$

An anion gap in excess of 10–14 mEq/liter (mmol/liter) is considered abnormal. Differential diagnosis of anion gap acidosis includes the following toxicologic causes: salicylates, ibuprofen, iron, isoniazid, paraldehyde, formaldehyde, methanol, ethylene glycol, carbon monoxide, cyanide, and cocaine.

In cases of industrial poisoning, the list may be extended to include numerous other chemicals not usually encounterd in routine practice, e.g., aniline dyes, nitrites, hydrogen sulfide, etc.

Treatment

Therapy consists of correcting metabolic acidosis and blocking metabolism of those alcohols which produce toxic metabolites.[85] This includes methanol and ethylene glycol. Ethanol and isopropyl alcohol are allowed to be metabolized without blockade. Sodium bicarbonate is administered intravenously to correct acidosis, although such therapy without blockade of hepatic metabolism will be transient. Methanol and ethylene glycol metabolism are blocked by administering ethanol by I.V. or oral route. A loading dose should be utilized consisting of 1 ml/kg of 95 percent ethanol diluted to a 10 percent solution in D_5W for I.V. use or in 6–8 ounces of juice for oral use. The loading dose should be administered over 15 minutes for I.V. therapy. Maintenance ethanol should be initiated immediately following the loading dose. I.V. ethanol therapy should be with a 10 percent solution in D_5W at rates varying from 0.8 ml/kg/h for young children or nondrinkers to as high as 2 ml/kg/h for some habitual alcoholics. Laboratory measurement of blood alcohol during therapy is necessary to adjust infusion to maintain blood ethanol concentration between 125 and 150 mg/dl (27–32 mmol/liter). Oral maintenance is possible for chronic drinkers but is not considered to be as reliable as I.V. therapy, since an oral dose is required hourly. Using 80 proof alcoholic beverages (40 percent ethanol by volume), the hourly adult dose is one ounce per hour.

Hemodialysis is probably indicated for every methanol or ethylene glycol ingestion where ethanol therapy is utilized. Once blockade of hepatic alcohol dehydrogenase has occurred by use of ethanol, renal elimination of methanol or ethylene glycol will require several days of therapy. This can be reduced to 8–10 hours by use of hemodialysis. Infusions of ethanol require increase during hemodialysis, usually by 1.5- to 2-fold, in order to maintain hepatic blockade.

Permanent vision loss can occur in late or inadequately treated methanol poisonings, and chronic renal failure is a consequence of late or inadequate therapy for ethylene glycol poisoning.

Hemodialysis is indicated for serious ethanol or isopropyl alcohol ingestion where respirations require support and hypotension is present.

Cocaine

Diagnosis

CNS and cardiovascular toxicity is similar to amphetamine, with excitation, aggression-combativeness, tachycardia, and hypertension. Grand mal seizures and ventricular ectopy are seen with life-threatening overdoses. Free base cocaine (crack) is pyrolized and inhaled yielding rapid plasma elevations of drug with catastrophic cardiovascular and CNS toxicity. Myocardial infarction has been observed.[86] I.V. injection of cocaine sulfate or hydrochloride salts results in similar toxicities. Cocaine smuggling involving gram quantitites in multiple ingested packets also results in comparable toxicity when rupture of the packets occurs in the GI tract.

Treatment

CNS excitation has been treated with diazepam, but effective sedation may be difficult. Chlorpromazine therapy carries a theoretical risk of seizures but may be considered for mild to moderate cocaine toxicity. I.V. diazepam and, if required, phenytoin in doses outlined for tricyclic antidepressants are indicated for treatment of sei-

zures. Intractable seizures can occur, and general anesthesia with use of neuromuscular blocking agents may be required to prevent permanent CNS damage and renal injury.[87,88] The latter may result from myoglobinuria from sustained myotonic activity. Hypertension is usually transient, and hypotension is a frequent rapid sequela to attempts to lower blood pressure. Use of β-blockers selective for β-receptors (metoprolol, atenolol) or possessing both α- and β-receptor blocking activity (e.g., labetalol)[89] may be helpful for treatment of systolic pressures in excess of 180 mmHg. Hypotension is treated with fluid and pressor agents such as dopamine, dobutamine, or norepinephrine. Ventricular ectopy is treated with phenytoin or β-blockers. Use of lidocaine or its congeners as antiarrhythmics is contraindicated, since cocaine is itself a local anesthetic. Hemodialysis or hemoperfusion is not indicated for cocaine toxicity, since hepatic and plasma metabolism is rapid.

Iron

Diagnosis

Iron supplements are ubiquitous in the household, and the diagnosis should be considered for patients presenting with abdominal pain and hematemesis. Within 4–6 hours of the ingestion, iron tablets *may* be seen on abdominal X-ray.[90,91] Serum iron in excess of the serum iron-binding capacity is evidence for potential iron toxicity. Hyperglycemia may accompany iron overdose, as may leukocytosis.

Treatment

Prevention of absorption is essential. A specific chelator, deferoxamine, is widely available but may not be capable of chelation of sufficient iron in large overdoses. Assessment of iron in the GI tract by X-ray following gastric emptying may be indicated for ingestions in excess of 60 mg/kg of elemental iron. Administration of binders of iron such as bicarbonate (2–5 percent solutions, 5–10 cc/kg) should follow gastric emptying. Aggressive volume replacement and assessment of blood loss secondary to GI hemorrhage is essential to prevent shock. Lactic acidosis may require bicarbonate replacement therapy. Serious iron ingestions require intensive care monitoring of vital signs and ECG. A history of greater than 60 mg/kg of elemental iron in the symptomatic patient and/or serum iron in excess of 350 $\mu g/dl$ (60 $\mu mol/liter$) may warrant deferoxamine treatment.[91] Due to the large volume of solution, I.M. therapy is unpleasant. I.V. therapy should be used when possible. The standard dose is 15 mg/kg/h by continuous infusion in D_5W or maintenance fluids. Too rapid administration has been associated with hypotension. *Caution* patient and family that the urine may turn red-orange during chelation of free iron. Therapy is usually continued until the color complex disappears (caution misinterpretation of very dilute urine for loss of color). Hepatic function should be monitored.[92]

Serum iron measurement may be more reliable than

urinary color complex.[93] Serious morbidity and mortality are found with serum iron in excess of 500 μg/dl (90 μmol/liter); and serum iron in excess of 1000 μg/dl (180 μmol/liter) may indicate exchange transfusion as adjunct to deferoxamine therapy.

Digoxin

Diagnosis

Acute overdose manifests as cardiac toxicity, largely disorders of A-V conduction with 1st to 3rd degree heart block. These blocks, particularly 3rd degree, in the presence of relative hypokalemia, hypercalcemia, or hypernatremia, can lead to ventricular ectopy including ventricular tachycardia and ventricular fibrillation.[94-96] Elevated serum potassium is a common occurrence in acute digoxin poisoning as Na^+,K^+-ATPase function is disrupted.

Treatment

Treatment includes the use of atropine 0.01 mg/kg I.V., repeated $\times 2$ as required for bradycardia and heart block. Phenytoin, 15–20 mg/kg I.V. no faster than 1 mg/kg/min, an antiarrhythmic whose mechanism of action is stabilization of the Na^+,K^+-ATPase, should be administered to serious digoxin overdoses. Prophylactic phenytoin administration may frequently be indicated prior to evidence of serious ventricular ectopy, due to high mortality in digoxin overdose. Transvenous pacing should be available and appropriate venous access should be ready, since rapid deterioration of rhythm is common.

When available, specific ovine Fab antibody to digoxin is indicated.[97-99] Dosage of Digibind (Burroughs Wellcome) is based on total body digoxin or estimated digoxin ingestion. Total body digoxin is estimated from plasma digoxin concentration by the equation:

$$\text{mg Body digoxin} = \text{plasma digoxin (ng/ml)} \\ \times 0.0056 \times \text{body weight (kg)}$$

The calculation using S.I. units of digoxin (nmol/liter) substitutes the constant 0.0044 for 0.0056. Plasma levels drawn prior to 6 hours from ingestion may overestimate plasma level, since distribution is usually not complete. The estimation of total body digoxin from the history of amount ingested should be:

$$\text{mg Body digoxin} = \text{mg ingested} \times 0.8$$

This will account for expected incomplete digoxin absorption. The quantity of Fab antibody in milligrams to be administered should be 60 times the total body digoxin estimate. Digibind is supplied in 40-mg vials, and therefore 1.5 vials are used for each milligram of digoxin in the body. The vial is initially diluted with 4 ml of sterile water, then further diluted with normal saline for convenient administration over 20 minutes. In the event of a life-threatening arrhythmia, the Fab product can be pushed more rapidly, but a 0.22-μm filter should always

be used. The complex requires renal elimination, although Digibind has been used in patients with renal dysfunction with satisfactory results.

Serum potassium should be monitored pre- and post-infusion, since reactivation of the digoxin-poisoned Na^+,K^+-ATPase is rapid, with response expected within 30 minutes.[98] Antibody methods for measurement of digoxin will not yield reliable estimates once Digibind has been administered.

Theophylline

Diagnosis

Toxicity is a triad of CNS, cardiac, and GI effects. GI toxicity includes nausea, vomiting, and upper GI hemorrhage. CNS toxicity is excitation and grand mal seizures.[100] Cardiac toxicity is tachycardia with myocardial ischemia possible in susceptible individuals secondary to rate. Ectopic ventricular events are also prevalent. Plasma levels of theophylline are readily available and should be used in diagnosis. The upper limit of the therapeutic range is 20 μg/ml (110 μmol/liter).

Treatment

Volume replacement is indicated for individuals with severe GI effects. Hemorrhage does not usually require blood replacement, as bleeding is diffuse leading to coffee ground emesis. Evidence of frank blood in vomitus or severe volume loss should be treated with packed cell or whole blood replacement and isotonic saline.

Seizures are managed with diazepam, phentytoin, or phenobarbital in dosages as indicated for tricyclic antidepressant poisoning. Theophylline-induced seizures may be refractory to drug therapy, and paralysis may be required if ventilation is compromised.

Ventricular ectopy is managed using phenytoin, lidocaine, or β-blockers. Dosages are indicated in the section on tricyclic antidepressant therapy.

Hemodialysis and hemoperfusion are very effective in removing theophylline, and both methods are generally available on a regional basis. The decision to use one of these methods is based upon the severity of symptomatology not responding to supportive care.[101,102]

REFERENCES

1. Doull J, Bruce MC: Origin and scope of toxicology, in Klaassen CD, Amdur MO, Doull J (eds): Casarett and Doull's Toxicology. New York, Macmillan, 1986
2. Hayes WJ: Pesticides Studied in Man. Baltimore, Williams and Wilkins, 1982
3. Temple AR: Poison control centers: Prospects and capabilities. Ann Rev Pharmacol Toxicol 17:215–222, 1977
4. Temple AR, Veltri JC: Program Guide for Regional Poison Control Programs. Prepared under Contract No. 223-75-3013 for the Public Health Service. FDA:DHEW, 1975
5. Thompson DF, Trammel HL, Robertson NJ, et al: Evaluation of regional and non-regional poison centers. N Engl J Med 308:191–194, 1983

6. American Association of Poison Control Centers: Criteria for regional poison control programs. Vet Human Toxicol 20:117–118, 1978

7. Chaffee-Bahamon C, Lovejoy FH Jr: The effectiveness of a regional poison center in reducing excess emergency room visits for children's poisonings. Pediatrics 73:164–169, 1983

8. Litovitz TL, Schmitz BF, Holm KC: 1988 Annual Report of the American Association of Poison Control Centers National Data Collection System. Am J Emerg Med 7:495–545, 1989

9. Eskenazi B, Gaylord L, Bracken MD, Brown D: In utero exposure to organic solvents and human neurodevelopment. Dev Med Child Neurol 30:492–501, 1988

10. Messite J, Bond MB: Reproductive toxicology and occupational exposure, in Zenz C (ed): Developments in Occupational Medicine. Chicago, Year Book Medical Pub., 1980

11. Kandall SR, Doberczak TM, Mauer KR, et al: Opiate vs. CNS depressant therapy in neonatal drug abstinence syndrome. Am J Dis Child 137:378–382, 1983

12. Hersh JH, Podruch PE, Rogers G, et al: Toluene embryopathy. J Pediatr 106:922–927, 1985

13. Holmberg PC, Nurminen M: Congenital defects of the central nervous system and occupational factors during pregnancy. A case reference study. Am J Indus Med 1:167–176, 1980

14. Famularo R, Stone K, Popper C: Preadolescent alcohol abuse and dependence. Am J Psychiatry 142:1187–1189, 1985

15. Temple AR, Veltri JC: One year's experience in a regional poison control center: The Intermountain Regional Poison Control Center. Clin Toxicol 12:277–289, 1978

16. Rothstein FC: Caustic injuries to the esophagus in children. Pediatr Clin No Am 33:665–674, 1986

17. Bartlett D: Pathophysiology of exposure to low concentrations of carbon monoxide. Arch Environ Health 16:719–727, 1968

18. Kulp JR, Schulert AR: Strontium-90 in man. Science 136:619–632, 1962

19. Tephly TR, Parks FE, Mannering GJ: Methanol metabolism in the rat. J Pharmacol Exp Ther 143:292–300, 1964

20. Mitchell JR, Jollow DJ, Potter WZ, et al: Acetaminophen induced hepatic necrosis: I. Role of drug metabolism. J Pharmacol Exp Ther 187:185–194, 1973

21. Jollow DJ, Mitchell JR, Potter WZ, et al: Acetaminophen induced hepatic necrosis: II. Role of covalent binding in vivo. J Pharmacol Exp Ther 187:195–202, 1973

22. Potter WZ, Davis DC, Mitchell JR, et al: Acetaminophen induced hepatic necrosis: III. Cytochrome P-450-mediated covalent binding in vitro. J Pharmacol Exp Ther 187:203–210, 1973

23. Goyer RA: Lead toxicity: A problem of environmental pathology. Am J Pathol 64:167–168, 1971

24. Wigg NR, Vimpani GV, McMichael AJ, et al: Port Pirie Cohort Study: Childhood blood lead and neuropsychological development at age two years. J Epidemiol Commun Health 42:213–219, 1988

25. McMichael AJ, Baghurst PA, Wigg NR, et al: Port Pirie Cohort Study: Environmental exposure to lead and children's abilities at the age of four years. N Engl J Med 319:468–475, 1988

26. Gaudreault P, Temple AR, Lovejoy FH Jr: The relative severity of acute versus chronic salicylate poisoning in children. Pediatrics 70:566–569, 1982

27. Easom JM, Lovejoy FH Jr: Efficacy and safety of gastrointestinal decontamination in the treatment of oral poisoning. Pediatr Clin No Am 26:827–836, 1979

28. Beckeer GL: The case against mineral oil. Am J Digest Disorder 19:344–348, 1952

29. Bock GW, Tenenbein M: Whole bowel irrigation for iron overdose. Ann Emerg Med 16:137, 1987

30. Done AK: Clinical pharmacology of systemic antidotes. Clin Pharmacol Ther 2:750–793, 1961

31. Bennett IL, Carey FH, Mitchell GL, et al: Acute methyl alcohol poisoning: A review based on experiences in an outbreak of 323 cases. Medicine 32:431–463, 1953

32. Stewart R: Cyanide poisoning. Clin Toxicol 7:561, 1974

33. Chen KK, Rose CL: Nitrite and thiosulfate therapy in cyanide poisoning. JAMA 149:113–114, 1952

34. Zavon M: Poisoning from pesticides: Diagnosis and treatment. Pediatrics 54:332–336, 1974

35. Hayes WJ: Epidemiology and general management of poisonings by pesticides. Pediatr Clin No Am 17:629–641, 1970

36. Winter PM, Miller JN: Carbon monoxide poisoning. JAMA 236:1502–1503, 1976

37. Moore RA, Rumack BH, Conner CS, et al: Naloxone: Underdosage after narcotic poisoning. Am J Dis Child 134:156–158, 1980

38. Lawson DH, Lowe GDO: Drug therapy reviews: Clincal use of anticoagulant drugs. Am J Hosp Pharm 34:1225–1234, 1977

39. Oehme FW: British Anti-Lewisite (BAL), the classic heavy metal antidote. Clin Toxicol 5:215–218, 1972

40. Aposhian HV: Penicillamine and analogous chelating agents. Ann NY Acad Sci 179:481–494, 1971

41. Piomelli S, Rosen JF, Chisolm JJ, et al: Management of childhood lead poisoning. J Pediatr 105:523–532, 1984

42. Henretig FM, Karl SR, Weintraub WH: Severe iron poisoning treated with enteral and intravenous deferoxamine. Ann Emerg Med 12:306–309, 1983

43. Westlin WF: Deferoxamine as a chelating agent. Clin Toxicol 4:597–602, 1971

44. Peterson RG, Rumack BH: Treating acute acetaminophen poisoning with acetylcysteine. JAMA 237:2406–2407, 1977

45. Peterson RG, Rumack BH: Toxicity of acetaminophen overdose. JACEP 7:202–205, 1978

46. Abelson HT, Fosburg MT, Beardsley P, et al: Methotrexate-induced renal impairment: Clinical studies and rescue from systemic toxicity with high-dose leucovorin and thymidine. J Clin Oncol 1:208–216, 1983

47. Hall AH, Kulig KW, Rumack BH: Drug and chemical induced methemoglobinemia: Clinical features and management. Med Toxicol 1:253–260, 1986

48. Harris JC, Rumack BH, Peterson RG, et al: Methemoglobinemia resulting from absorption of nitrates. JAMA 242:2869–2871, 1979

49. Milne MD, Scribner BH, Crawford MA: Non-ionic diffusion and the excretion of weak acids and bases. Am J Med 24:709–729, 1958

50. Weiner IM: Mechanics of drug absorption and excretion. Annu Rev Pharmacol 7:39–56, 1967

51. Schanker LS: Passage of drugs across body membranes. Pharmacol Rev 14:501–530, 1962

52. Linton AL, Luke RG, Speirs I, et al: Forced diuresis and haemodialysis in severe barbiturate intoxication. Lancet 1:1008–1009, 1964

53. Hill JB: Salicylate intoxication. N Engl J Med 288:1110–1113, 1973

54. Peterson RG, Peterson LM: Cleansing the blood: Hemodialysis, peritoneal dialysis, exchange transfusion, charcoal hemoperfusion, forced diuresis. Pediatr Toxicol, Pediatr Clin No Am 33:675–689, 1986

55. Rosenbaum JL, Dramer MS, Raja R: Resin hemoperfusion for acute drug intoxication. Arch Intern Med 136:263–266, 1976

56. Winchester JF, Gelfond MC, Knepshield JH, et al: Dialysis and hemoperfusion of poisons and drugs—Update. Trans Am Soc Artif Intern Organs 23:762–842, 1977

57. Robertson WO: Treatment of acute iron poisoning. Mod Treatment 8:552–560, 1971

58. Rumack BH (ed): Poisindex. Denver, Micromedex Inc., 1990

59. Russell FE: Snake Venom Poisoning. Great Neck, New York, Scholium International, 1983

60. Hill JB: Experimental salicylate poisoning: Observations on the effects of altering blood pH on tissue and plasma salicylate concentrations. Pediatrics 47:658–665, 1971

61. Summit RL, Etteldorf JN: Salicylate intoxication in children— experience with peritoneal dialysis and alkalinization of the urine. J Pediatr 64:803–814, 1964

62. Sweeney KR, Chapron DJ, Brandt JL, et al: Toxic interaction between acetazolammide and salicylate: Case reports and a pharmacokinetic explanation. Clin Pharmacol Ther 40:518–524, 1986

63. Temple AR: Acute and chronic effects of aspirin toxicity and their treatment. Arch Intern Med 141:364–369, 1981

64. Snodgrass W, Rumack BH, Peterson RG, et al: Salicylate toxicity following therapeutic doses in young children. Clin Toxicol 18:247–259, 1981

65. Jacobsen D, Wiik-Larsen E, Bredesen JE: Haemodialysis or haemoperfusion in severe salicylate poisoning. Human Toxicol 7:161–163, 1988

66. Rumack BH, Matthew H: Acetaminophen poisoning and toxicity. Pediatrics 55:871–876, 1975

67. Rumack BH, Peterson RG, Koch GG, et al: Acetaminophen overdose: 662 cases with evaluation of oral acetylcysteine treatment. Arch Intern Med 141:380–385, 1981

68. Prescott LF, Illingworth RN, Critchley JA, et al: Intravenous N-acetylcysteine: The treatment of choice for paracetamol poisoning. Br Med J 2:1097–1098, 1979

69. Prescott LF, Proudfoot AT, Cregeen RJ: Paracetamol induced acute renal failure in the absence of fulminant liver damage. Br J Med 28:21, 1982

70. Burney RE, Wu S, Nemiroff MJ, et al: Mass carbon monoxide poisoning: Clinical effects and results of treatment in 184 victims. Ann Emerg Med 11:394–399, 1982

71. Olsen KR: Carbon monoxide poisoning mechanisms, presentation, and controversies in management. J Emerg Med 1:233–243, 1984

72. Sanchez R, Fosarelli P, Felt B, et al: Carbon monoxide poisoning due to automobile exposure: Disparity between carboxyhemoglobin levels and symptoms of victims. Pediatrics 82:663–665, 1988

73. Norkool DM, Kirkpatrick JN: Treatment of acute carbon monoxide poisoning with hyperbaric oxygen: A review of 115 cases. Ann Emerg Med 14:1168–1171, 1985

74. Greenblatt DJ: Rapid recovery from massive diazepam overdose. JAMA 240:1872–1874, 1978

75. O'Sullivan GF, Wade DN: Flumazenil in the management of acute drug overdosage with benzodiazepines and other agents. Clin Pharmacol Ther 42:254–259, 1987

76. Artman M, Grayson M, Boerth R: Propranolol in children: Safety-toxicity. Pediatrics 20:30–31, 1982

77. Ward DE, Jones B: Glucagon and beta-blocker toxicity. Br Med J 2:151–152, 1976

78. Agura ED, Wexler LF, Witzburg RA: Massive propranolol overdose: Successful treatment with high-dose isoproterenol and glucagon. Am J Med 80:755–757, 1986

79. Anthony T, Jastremski M, Elliot W, et al: Charcoal hemoperfusion for the treatment of a combined diltiazem and metoprolol overdose. Ann Emerg Med 15:1344–1348, 1986

80. Biggs JT, Spiker DG, Petit JM, et al: Tricyclic antidepressant overdose. Incidence of symptoms. JAMA 238:135–141, 1977

81. Cassidy S, Henry J: Fatal toxicity of antidepressant drugs in overdose. Br Med J 295:1021–1024, 1987

82. Sasyniuk BI, Jhamandas V, Valois M, et al: Experimental amitriptyline intoxication: Treatment of cardiac toxicity with sodium bicarbonate. Ann Emerg Med 15:1052–1059, 1986

83. Heath A, Wickstrom I, Martenson E, et al: Treatment of antidepressant poisoning with resin hemoperfusion. Hum Toxicol 1:361–371, 1982

84. Jacobsen D, Bredesen JE, Eide I, et al: Anion and osmolal gaps in the diagnosis of methanol and ethylene glycol poisoning. Acta Med Scand 212:17–20, 1982

85. Ekins BR, Rollins DE, Duffy DP, et al: Standardized treatment of severe methanol poisoning with ethanol and hemodialysis. West J Med 142:337–340, 1985

86. Isner JM, Estes NAM, Thompson PD, et al: Cardiac consequences of cocaine: Premature myocardial infarction, ventricular tachyarrhythmias, myocarditis, and sudden death. Circulation 72(suppl 3):415–419, 1985

87. Jonsson S, O'Meara M, Young JB: Acute cocaine poisoning: Importance of treating seizures and acidosis. Am J Med 75:1061–1064, 1983

88. Myers JA, Earnest MP: Generalized seizures and cocaine abuse. Neurology 34:675–676, 1984

89. Bessen HA: Treatment of cocaine toxicity. Ann Emerg Med 16:922–926, 1987

90. McGuigan MA, Lovejoy FH, Marino SK, et al: Qualitative deferoxamine color test for iron ingestion. J Pediatr 94:940–942, 1979

91. Ng RCW, Perry K, Martin DJ: Iron poisoning. Assessment of radiography in diagnosis and management. Clin Pediatr 18:614–616, 1979

92. Fischer D: Acute iron poisoning in children. JAMA 218:1179–1184, 1971

93. Freeman DA, Manoguerra AS: Absence of urinary color change in a severely iron-poisoned child treated with deferoxamine. AACT/AAPCC/ABMTF Annual Scientific Meeting, August, 1981

94. Antman EM, Smith TW: Digitalis toxicity. Annu Rev Med 36:357–367, 1985

95. Bismuth L, Gaultier M, Conso F, et al: Hyperkalemia in acute digitalis poisoning: Prognostic significance and therapeutic implications. Clin Toxicol 6:153–162, 1973

96. Duke M: Atrioventricular block due to accidental digoxin ingestion treated with atropine. Am J Dis Child 124:754–756, 1972

97. Ochs HR, Smith TW: Reversal of advanced digitoxin toxicity and modification of pharmacokinetics by specific antibodies and Fab fragments. J Clin Invest 60:1303–1313, 1977

98. Wenger TL, Butler VP, Haber E, et al: Treatment of 63 severely digitalis-toxic patients with digoxin-specific antibody fragments. J Am Coll Cardiol 5:118–123, 1985

99. Zucker AR, Lacina SJ, DasGupta DS, et al: Fab fragments of digoxin-specific antibodies used to reverse ventricular fibrillation induced by digoxin ingestion in a child. Pediatrics 70:468–471, 1982

100. Baker MD: Theophylline toxicity in children. J Pediatr 109:538–542, 1986

101. Biberstein MP, Ziegler MG, Ward DM: Use of beta blockade and hemoperfusion for acute theophylline poisoning. West J Med 141:485–490, 1984

102. Ehlers SM, Zaske DE, Sawchuk RJ: Massive theophylline overdose. Rapid elimination by charcoal hemoperfusion. JAMA 240:474–475, 1978

52

THE ADVERSE EFFECTS OF COCAINE ON THE DEVELOPING HUMAN

Cocaine is currently the number one illicit drug used by women of childbearing age. The substance-abusing mother passively addicts her fetus *in utero*. For the pregnant woman abusing cocaine, one of the most profound misconceptions is that the placenta protects the unborn baby from the drug taken during pregnancy.

Recent data suggest that cocaine can disrupt the process of organogenesis in the developing fetus and subsequently give rise to congenital malformations. Furthermore, developmental and learning disabilities during the course of future ontogeny are becoming recognized in those children who were exposed to the drug *in utero*.

In September 1989, a National Drug Control Strategy issued by the federal government identified illegal drugs as the gravest present threat to the well-being of the country.[1] Cocaine is the leading illicit drug in the United States. The Senate Judiciary Committee study reported in May 1990 found that 2.2 million Americans are cocaine addicts, defined as someone using it at least once weekly. The report's state-by-state estimate of cocaine addicts placed New York in first place, followed by California, Illinois, and Texas.

A recent National Household Survey on Drug Abuse conducted by the National Institute of Drug Abuse (NIDA) found a 37 percent decrease in the number of Americans using any illegal drug on a current basis; that is, 23 million in 1985 versus 14.5 million in 1988 using a drug at least once in the 30 days preceding the survey. However, there was a 33 percent increase in the number of respondents reporting frequent use of cocaine, i.e., one or more times per week.[2]

An estimated 5 million women of childbearing age use illegal substances and 1 million use cocaine.[3] The National Association for Perinatal Addiction Research and Education, in a survey of 36 hospitals throughout the country, found the overall incidence of substance abuse in pregnancy to be 11 percent, ranging in individual hospitals from 0.4 to 27 percent.[4] This finding has been supported by the most recent NIDA Household Survey, in which approximately 9 percent of women of childbearing age admitted to having used an illegal drug during the 1 month prior to the completion of the questionnaire.[5]

Chasnoff and coworkers[6] undertook a population-based study of the prevalence of the use of illicit drugs and alcohol by 715 pregnant women who received prenatal care over a period of 6 months in Pinellas County, Florida, either at public health clinics or in private obstetrical offices. This study demonstrated that the problem of alcohol and other drug use in pregnancy crosses all racial and socioeconomic lines. The overall prevalence of a positive result on toxicologic tests of urine was 15 percent. Women enrolled in the public health clinics had an overall prevalence rate of 16 percent, whereas 13 percent of women in private obstetric care had a positive urine toxicology. The rates of positive toxicology screens did not differ between white and black women: 15 and 14 percent, respectively. The most common drugs in the urine of all women were marijuana and cocaine.

Cocaine abuse by young people has doubled in the past decade, with 17 percent of high school seniors reporting the use of the drug at least once in 1986, compared with 9 percent in 1975.[7] This finding, in association with the fact that there are approximately 500,000 births to teenagers each year in the United States,[8,9] weighs heavily on the magnitude of the problem that is well entrenched within the ranks of adolescence.

THE DRUG AND ITS PHARMACOKINETICS

Cocaine is benzoylmethylecgonine. Ecgonine is an amino alcohol base closely related to tropine, the amino alcohol in atropine. Cocaine is thus an ester of benzoic acid and a nitrogen-containing base.[10] The structural formula of cocaine is as follows:

$$H_2C-CH-CH\cdot COOCH_3$$
$$N\cdot CH_3CH\cdot OOC \text{---} \bigcirc \text{---} O$$
$$H_2C-CH-CH_2$$

Erythroxylon coca, a shrub that grows abundantly in the Andean highlands and the northwestern parts of the Amazon basin in South America, is the primary source of cocaine; the leaves of this plant contain about 0.5 percent cocaine,[11] one of the 14 alkaloids found in the leaves of the coca shrub.[12] The coca leaf has probably been used for well over a millennium, since ancient Indian legends describe its origin and supernatural powers. However, cocaine itself has only been used for approximately 100 years.[13]

Coca paste is the first product of extraction and contains approximately 80 percent cocaine.[14] Commercially, the coca alkaloids are hydrolyzed to obtain ecgonine, which is then benzoylated and methylated to the base, cocaine.[15] Conversion to the hydrochloride salt produces a powdery, white crystalline, water-soluble substance which decomposes on heating.

The drug is imported as a hydrochloride salt and sold illegally at $75 to $100 per gram, for sniffing or injection in white powder form under various street names—coke, snow, lady, or gold dust. The white powder can be adulterated with various agents to increase its volume or give the false impression of higher-grade purity. Such agents utilized are lactose, mannitol, lidocaine, procaine, arsenic, phencyclidine, heroin, and amphetamines. Cocaine purity, as a result, varies greatly, and usually diluted mixtures are only 40 percent pure with a range of 20–80 percent.

Cocaine hydrochloride will decompose if smoked, while cocaine alkaloid, or free base, will not. The drug is a tertiary amine with a pK_a of 8.6. At higher pH values the un-ionized or free base form predominates, while at more acidic pH values cocaine exists as a salt, e.g., hydrochloride.[16,17] Substance abusers can readily prepare free base from cocaine hydrochloride they purchase on the street by mixing it with an alkaline solution, usually bicarbonate of soda in water, and precipitating the alkaloidal cocaine through the process of drying in a microwave oven to form a hard substance called a "rock." The rock, as it burns during smoking, makes a cracking sound and hence the name *crack.* This alkaloidal form of cocaine is more stable on heating, vaporizes readily, and has high bioavailability when smoked.[18] Much higher blood levels of cocaine are achieved more quickly because (1) crack is a purer form of cocaine, and (2) the absorptive area of the lung is far more extensive than that of the nasal mucosa.

Cocaine, when abused by the pregnant woman, is able to cross the placental barrier by simple diffusion and can also be found in breast milk.[19,20] This facility of easy movement across the placenta as well as excretion into breast milk is due to the drug's (1) high lipid solubility, (2) low molecular weight, and (3) low ionization at physiologic pH. Cocaine and its metabolites persist in breast milk for 48 hours after last use.[20] Several reports have been published of infants with signs of cocaine intoxication such as dilated pupils, hypertension, tachycardia, and convulsions subsequent to breast feeding.[21,22]

The drug has three principal pharmacologic actions: (1) local anesthetic, (2) peripheral sympathomimetic, and (3) central nervous system (CNS) stimulant. Peripherally, cocaine inhibits the presynaptic uptake of norepinephrine and results in a transient rise of plasma catecholamine levels. This in turn promotes vasoconstriction, tachycardia, and acute blood pressure elevation. In the pregnant woman the cardiovascular effects of cocaine abuse can compromise uteroplacental function and lead to the development of abruptio placentae or fetal hypoxia.

Centrally, cocaine, like most psychoactive drugs, affects and alters brain neurochemistry. More is known about cocaine's effects on dopamine, serotonin, and norepinephrine neurotransmitter systems than other systems.[23] Dopamine levels in the brain are increased following cocaine administration because, like norepinephrine peripherally, presynaptic uptake is prevented. The elevated dopamine levels clinically promote anorexia, hyperactivity, sexual excitement, and the stereotypic "high." With continued use of the drug, dopamine reserves are eventually depleted, resulting clinically in depression, psychosis, and sexual impotence. Serotonin, which is an important neurotransmitter for the sleep–wake cycle, is also affected by cocaine. Abuse of the drug results in reduced levels and therefore decreases the requirement for sleep.

Absorption

Cocaine is well absorbed after coca chewing and nasal applications. Peak serum concentrations after oral administration generally occur 45–90 minutes after ingestion.[24,25] The reduction in the rate and extent of oral absorption is probably related to the acidic environment of the stomach.[25,26] With nasal insufflation, plasma concentrations peak in 15–60 minutes.[26] Vasoconstriction of the nasal mucosa limits the rate of absorption of cocaine when administered through this route. The bioavailability of cocaine has been estimated to range between 20 and 60 percent.[14,26,29,45]

Following intravenous or pulmonary administration, high peak plasma levels are achieved almost instantaneously. When taken intravenously, an initial intense "rush" is reported within 1–2 minutes. Following a single 32-mg intravenous dose of cocaine, plasma levels of approximately 300 ng/ml have been recorded.[13] The majority of the dose absorbed in the pulmonary circulation following smoking of free base is absorbed with the first four breaths.[14,27] Chronic free base smokers have shown plasma levels of 800–900 ng/ml 3 hours after smoking.[28] When cocaine plasma levels are compared across different routes of administration, the intravenous and smoked routes of administration yield virtually indistinguishable curves in terms of peak effect and dissipation of plasma levels.[13] Once in the systemic circulation, cocaine is in the same form, regardless of the route of administration or type of dosage preparation.[17]

Distribution

Cocaine's total volume of distribution is approximately 2 liters/kg. This degree of distribution indicates moderate tissue binding.[29]

Metabolism

Cocaine is a bicyclic alkaloid. The structures of the drug and its metabolites are illustrated in Figure 52–1. Cocaine is metabolized through two biotransformation avenues. The first and major pathway is through the hydrolysis of the two ester groups, carboxyl methyl ester and benzoate ester. The second and minor pathway is through oxidative N-demethylation. Plasma and liver esterases are responsible for the largest proportion of cocaine metabolism. Plasma cholinesterase or pseudocholinesterase and hepatic esterases mediate the enzymatic hydrolysis of cocaine to ecgonine methyl ester, while benzoyl ecgonine is a nonenzymatic hydrolysis product which is thought to result from the spontaneous hydrolysis of cocaine.[29–31] Under steady-state conditions both plasma and liver enzymes contribute equally to cocaine hydrolysis.[30] Oxidative N-demethylation of cocaine, mediated by the hepatic microsomal cytochrome P-450, produces norcocaine. Norcocaine is the only known pharmacologically active metabolite of cocaine.[16,29,32] This pathway is not considered significant in human physiology.[17]

Pseudocholinesterase activity in pregnancy is decreased.[16,33–39] This reduced enzymatic activity in pregnancy has been attributed to hemodilution, altered hepatic function, and the anticholinesterase activity of estrogen. Venkataramen and coinvestigators[38] estimated the erythrocyte and plasma cholinesterase activity in 50 normal pregnant women and 22 age-matched normal nonpregnant women. They found a significant decrease in plasma cholinesterase activity in pregnancy, with a steady decline occurring from the second to the third trimester.

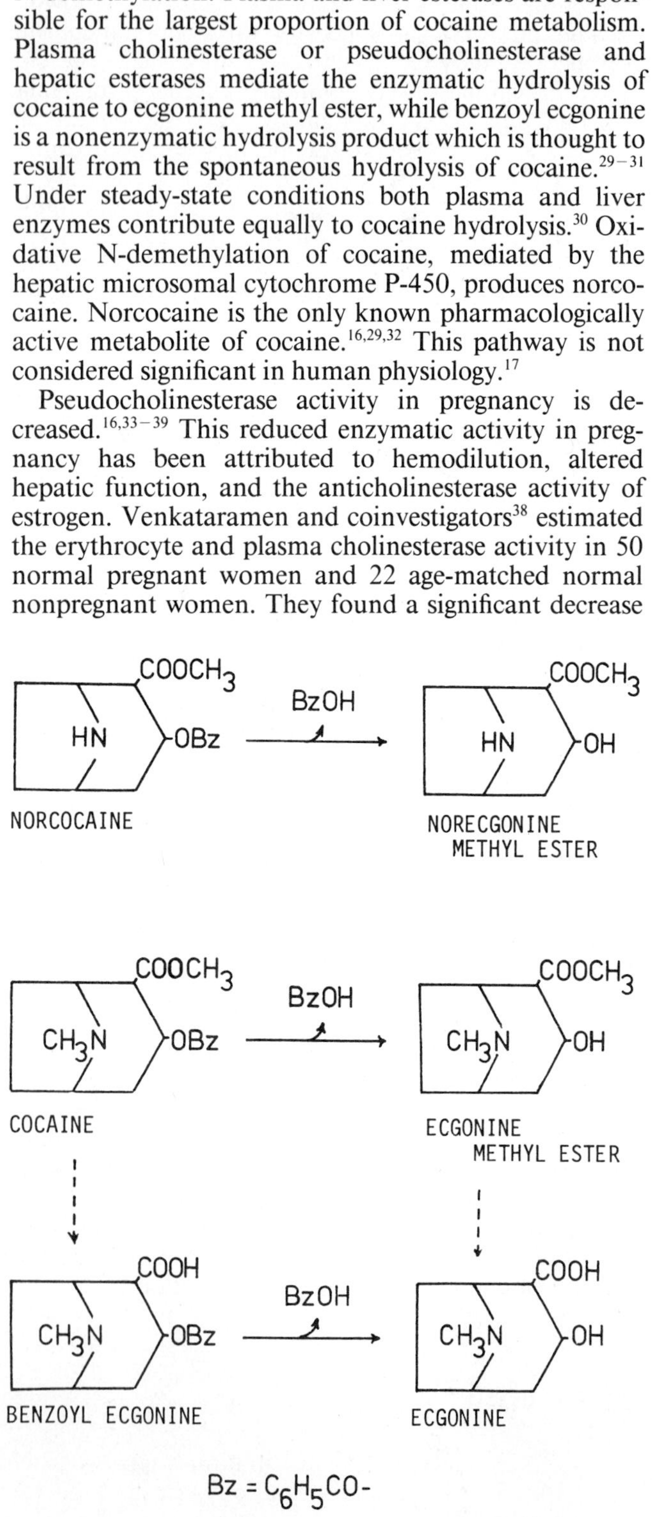

Roe and coinvestigators[40] examined the ability of the human placenta to transform cocaine into its metabolites. A dozen placentas from routine pregnancies were collected from term mothers who had uncomplicated vaginal or cesarean deliveries. The placentas were placed on ice and transported to the laboratory within 30 minutes of delivery. Placental homogenates were prepared to obtain (1) a placental supernatant and (2) a pellet of concentrated microsomal proteins. Cocaine was added to each supernatant and pellet. Two control groups were established: (1) anticholinesterase was added to a group of assay solutions to selectively inhibit placental cholinesterases, and (2) cocaine was added to phosphate buffer in the absence of placental supernatant to establish baseline spontaneous conversion of the drug.

The results of this study demonstrated a 20 percent decrease in cocaine concentration by the term placenta over a 135-minute period, with the majority of the decline occurring in the first 45-minute interval. The decrease in cocaine concentration was attributed to the action of placental cholinesterases. Cocaine levels did not decline when enzyme inhibition was achieved with anticholinesterase, and the decrease in the cocaine concentration could not be ascribed to nonenzymatic reactions because the placentas exposed to cocaine without microsomes exhibited no change.

Ecobichon and Stephens[41] investigated the perinatal development of human blood esterases. Erythrocyte acetylcholinesterase, plasma proteins, pseudocholinesterase, and arylesterase development were investigated in groups of premature infants of varying gestational ages, comparing the detected levels with those observed in groups of healthy older children and adults. A rapid increase in plasma pseudocholinesterase and arylesterase activity occurred from 28 weeks gestation to 1 year of age, with no significant changes in activities from those of adults occurring after 1 year. A rapid increase in plasma protein concentration was also evident between 28 and 40 weeks gestation, followed by a slower rate of increase until 1 year of age. Premature infant plasma degraded procaine hydrocholoride and insecticide paraoxon more slowly than plasma of full-term infants, while the rates of hydrolysis for these two groups were significantly lower than those detected for children older than 1 year or for adults. These observations would suggest that premature and full-term infants might be expected to differ significantly from older children and adults in the extent to which drugs might be protein-bound and in the rates of hydrolysis of ester-type drugs.

Genetic polymorphism for cholinesterase exists, thus creating a broad spectrum of enzymatic potential for cocaine metabolism. The frequency of depressed cholinesterase activity or inactivity in North America is 1–13 percent, according to ethnic background.[42] Cholinesterase deficiency has been associated with enhanced cocaine toxicity in the adult.[43] Roe has shown the protective effect that the term placenta can provide for the fetus by helping to metabolize cocaine, but it is possible that certain placentas, because of plasma cholinesterase genetic poly-

Bz = C_6H_5CO-

FIGURE 52–1. Structures of cocaine and its metabolites.

morphism, may not be able to offer such protection and therefore place the fetus at greater risk of suffering from cocaine's sinister effects. In fact, the ability of each fetus to metabolize cocaine will vary according to its genetic constitution as well as its degree of enzymatic maturity. Different rates of organogenesis in different fetuses may also give rise to differences in cocaine's effects.[44] The exact risk of cocaine's untoward effects to each individual pregnancy is unknown.

Elimination

Cocaine is rapidly eliminated from the body, with a biologic half-life of about 1 hour and total body clearance of about 2 liters/min.[26,45] Elimination is predominantly controlled by its biotransformation, as is suggested by its low renal clearance of 27 ml/min.[46] Approximately 85–90 percent of an administered dose of cocaine is recovered in the urine. Only 1–5 percent of cocaine is cleared unmetabolized in the urine, where it may be detected for only 3–6 hours after use. However, the two major metabolites, ecgonine methyl ester (EME) and benzoylecgonine, constitute 80–90 percent of metabolites and are detected in adult urine for 14–60 hours after cocaine administration.[16,17,47,48] In the neonate, cocaine metabolites may appear in the urine for as long as 5 days following birth to a mother who used cocaine shortly before parturition.[49] This prolonged period of metabolite excretion in the newborn is a reflection of the relative enzymatic immaturity of the pseudocholinesterases in the neonatal period.[29] Both EME and benzoylecgonine are inactive as regards their ability to block the reuptake of monoamines into presynaptic neurons and the production of pharmacologic effects in animals.[17]

THE PHARMACODYNAMIC IMPACT

The effects of cocaine use during pregnancy can lead to increased rates of (1) pregnancy loss, including spontaneous abortion and stillbirth; (2) prematurity; (3) abruptio placenta; (4) precipitous labor; and (5) intrauterine growth retardation.[50–56] The effects of in utero cocaine exposure on the fetus and newborn infant are delineated in Table 52–1.

The pathogenesis of the congenital defects associated with prenatal cocaine exposure is thought to be secondary to intermittent vascular disruption.[65,66] The uterine, placental, embryonic, and fetal vasoconstriction occurring secondary to the increased concentration of catecholamines would result in hypoperfusion and hypoxia in developing fetal tissues and therefore potentiate a disruption sequence. The congenital malformations associated with infants who were prenatally exposed to cocaine are listed in Table 52–2.

It needs to be underscored that drug abuse during pregnancy is also a marker for other multiple untoward effects that may have bearing on fetal development. A clear-cut cause-and-effect relationship between cocaine and the

TABLE 52–1. ASSOCIATED EFFECTS OF COCAINE USE ON THE FETUS AND NEONATE

Common Complications

Intrauterine growth retardation
Microcephaly
Prematurity
Infections, especially sexually transmitted disease
Neurobehavioral abnormalities*
Neurophysiologic abnormalities†
Poor feeding

Uncommon Complications

CNS bleeds and alterations in cerebral blood flow velocity
Antenatal cerebral infarction
Birth defects secondary to intermittent vascular disruptions
Myocardial infarction, ischemic changes
Necrotizing enterocolitis/ileal atresia
Neonatal abstinence syndrome
Epilepsy

*Poor organizational responses, Increased tremulousness, Irritability, State lability, Poor consolability, Poor visual attention.
†Abnormal EEGs, Abnormal visual evoked potentials, Abnormal auditory evoked potentials, Data from references 57–68, 70.

development of congenital malformations has not yet been unequivocally ascertained. Further research in this area is required.

The nature of the defect associated with vascular disruption following embryonic or fetal cocaine exposure reflects timing and location of the vasoconstriction or hemorrhage during development. Unlike the case with many teratogens, because vascular disruption may occur at any point in gestation, potential fetal damage associated with cocaine may occur in the second and third trimesters as well as in early pregnancy during the period of organogenesis.

Neonatal withdrawal from cocaine following delivery is another complication that can occur from passive in utero

TABLE 52–2. CONGENITAL MALFORMATIONS ASSOCIATED WITH PRENATAL COCAINE EXPOSURE

Skull Defects
Exencephaly
Encephalocele
Bone defects

Genitourinary
Urethral obstruction
Prune-belly syndrome
Hydronephrosis
Hypospadias
Renal agenesis

Limb Reduction Defects
Ectrodactyly (congenital absence of one or more fingers or toes)

Cardiac Defects
Pulmonary atresia
Pulmonary stenosis
ASD (atrial septal defect)
VSD (ventricular septal defect)

CNS
Basal ganglia
Frontal lobe
Posterior fossa

Data from references 57, 58, 61, 63–66, 69.

TABLE 52–3. SYMPTOMS OF NEONATAL DRUG WITHDRAWAL

W	Wakefulness
I	Irritability
T	Tremulousness, Temperature variation, Tachypnea
H	Hyperactivity, High-pitched persistent cry, Hypertonus, Hyperreflexia, Hyperacusia
D	Diarrhea, Diaphoresis, Disorganized suck
R	Rub marks, Respiratory distress, Rhinorrhea
A	Apnea, Autonomic dysfunction
W	Weight loss or failure to thrive
A	Alkalosis (respiratory)
L	Lacrimation

From AAP Committee on Drugs,[70] with permission.

drug exposure. The neonatal abstinence syndrome consists of a symptom complex in infants born to drug-addicted mothers. There is a triad of organ systems involved, namely (1) neurologic, (2) gastrointestinal, and (3) respiratory.[70] The syndrome usually commences within the first 24–48 hours of life as the child passively abstains from the drug it was chronically exposed to *in utero*. A multitude of drugs can give rise to this symptom complex, including (1) heroin, methadone, and propoxyphene; (2) meperidine and morphine; (3) alcohol; (4) diazepam, chlordiazepoxide, and meprobamate; (5) phenobarbital; (6) pentazocine and pyribenzamine ("T's and blues"); (7) phencyclidine ("PCP" or "angel dust"); (8) codeine; and (9) cocaine.

The symptoms of neonatal drug withdrawal are listed in Table 52–3. Additional symptoms include (1) abnormal sleep cycle with absence of quiet sleep and disturbance or active (REM) sleep, (2) hiccups, (3) vomiting, (4) stuffy nose, (5) sneezing, (6) yawning, (7) photophobia, and (8) twitching, myoclonic jerks, opisthotonus, and seizures.[70]

Withdrawal from cocaine does not appear to result in as severe a syndrome of abstinence as withdrawal from the narcotics. Classically, the cocaine-exposed baby is (1) lethargic and poorly responsive, (2) irritable and hypertonic when alert, (3) tremulous, and (4) disorganized in sleeping and feeding. The cocaine baby is a fragile infant who is easily overloaded by environmental stimuli and who has few self-protective mechanisms for avoiding stimulation. They require assistance to maintain control of their hyperexcitable nervous system. It is not yet fully understood whether the irritability and tremulousness found in cocaine-exposed infants is a syndrome due to withdrawal from the drug or a direct effect of cocaine on the CNS of the infant.

Chasnoff[54,55] studied two subgroups of women who abused cocaine during pregnancy. The first group consisted of 23 women who conceived during a period when cocaine was used but reached abstinence by the end of the first trimester. There was no further cocaine use during pregnancy as documented by ongoing chemical dependence evaluation and urine toxicology screens. The second group consisted of 52 women who used cocaine during the period of conception and throughout their pregnancy. These two subgroups of cocaine-abusing pregnant women were compared to a matched group of

obstetric patients with no history or evidence of substance abuse. Both groups were similar for (1) maternal age, (2) gravidity, (3) parity, (4) prenatal weight gain, (5) racial distribution, and (6) quantitative drug use patterns in those groups who abused cocaine. All neonates born to these women were examined at birth by a physician blinded to the infant's prenatal history. At 12–72 hours old, the neonatal behavioral assessment score (NBAS) was administered by trained examiners who were blinded to the infant's prenatal history.

The results of these investigations demonstrated that cessation of cocaine use in the first trimester improved obstetric outcome; that is, there was an increased proportion of pregnancies that progressed to term and fewer infants had intrauterine growth retardation develop. However, fetal exposure to cocaine during the prenatal period led to significant impairment in neonatal neurobehavioral capabilities. The neurobehavioral response deficiencies occurred in cocaine-exposed infants whether maternal cocaine use was limited to the first trimester or continued throughout pregnancy.

Hume and coinvestigators,[71] using ultrasonography, observed altered behavior in fetuses exposed to cocaine *in utero*. Disruption of normal fetal behavioral state organization and regulation was characterized by (1) hyperrigidity in extreme flexion, (2) hyperactivity with violent total body movements in response to stimulation, (3) scanning eye movements without the normal predominant rapid eye motion, and (4) alteration in fetal breathing patterns and fetal heart rate variability. All fetuses who had abnormal fetal state behavior were abnormal in state organization as newborns. Infants often were seen as "all or nothing," that is, difficult to arouse, inconsolable when aroused, and having brief or no periods of quiet alertness.

Kramer[67] in 1990 reported a disturbing group of 16 infants born to cocaine-using mothers. All 16 patients experienced clinically diagnosed seizures within 36 hours of delivery. All 16 infants had positive urine toxicology screens for cocaine metabolites. All patients had cranial computed tomography (CT) scans that were normal or demonstrated minimal cerebral atrophy. Eight patients (50 percent) had repetitive seizures during the neonatal period but did not have recurrences during the followup period of 4–12 months. The remaining eight infants (50 percent) also experienced seizures in the neonatal period but went on to develop epilepsy.

Oro and Dixon[72] reviewed the clinical course of 110 neonates born with positive results of maternal or infant toxicology screens. They found a high rate of altered behavioral patterns in neonates exposed to cocaine and/or methamphetamines, such as (1) abnormal sleep patterns, (2) poor and prolonged feeding (i.e., random sucking even when satiated, and disorganized rooting), (3) poor visual processing of faces and objects, and (4) tremors and hypertonia.

Howard[73] compared 18 prenatally drug-exposed 18-month-old toddlers with a sample of high-risk preterm toddlers who were of younger age and lighter weight. Both groups were similar in regard to (1) single-parent household, (2) ethnicity, and (3) socioeconomic status. Assessed parameters were (1) intellectual functioning, (2) quality of play, and (3) security of attachment to the parent or parent figure.

Drug-exposed toddlers had significantly lower developmental scores but were still within the low-average range. It was realized by the investigators that the standardized developmental assessment imposed an external structure in which the examiner directs the task for the child. As a result, unstructured free-play requiring (1) self-organization, (2) self-initiation, and (3) follow-through without examiner assistance was incorporated into the experimental design.

Drug-exposed children then demonstrated striking deficits in (1) less frequent and less varied representational play, and (2) increased disorganized play characterized by scattering, batting, and picking up and putting down toys. The rearing environment, by fostering attachment, mitigated the impact of prenatal drug exposure on development to some degree but did not eliminate it entirely.

SUMMARY

The problems involved in evaluating the effects of exposure to substances of maternal abuse on the developing fetus and infant are multiple. It is very difficult to determine, on a *pro rata* basis, what proportion of observed deficit in the child exposed to drugs *in utero* was due to the *in utero* impact alone and what proportion was due to the unfavorable socioeconomic milieu that coexists in any drug-using population.

The weight of evidence to date strongly suggests that cocaine has a direct impact upon fetal organogenesis, specifically CNS development. The extent to which each fetus and newborn is affected is variable and may be dependent upon (1) rates of organogenesis, (2) timing of exposure, (3) genetic polymorphism of plasma pseudocholinesterases, (4) degree of fetal pseudocholinesterase enzymatic maturity, and (5) extent of the maternal drug habit.

The presence of congenital neurobehavioral deficits compounded by the suboptimal sociologic environment of the addicted parents will devastate the ontology of a child. These children, in increasing numbers, will be at high risk for continuing developmental, educational, and societal problems.

REFERENCES

1. Office of National Drug Control Policy: National Drug Control Strategy. Executive Office of the President. Washington, DC, September 1989
2. NIDA Household Survey, 1989. National Institute of Drug Abuse. Rockville, Maryland
3. Office of the Inspector General: Crack Babies. United States Department of Health and Human Services, February 1990
4. Chasnoff IJ: Drug use and women: Establishing a standard of care. Ann NY Acad Sci 562:208–210, 1989
5. NIDA Household Survey on Drug Abuse 1988, Population Estimates. National Institute on Drug Abuse, Rockville, Maryland, 1990
6. Chasnoff IJ, Landress HJ, Barrett ME: The prevalence of illicit drug or alcohol use during pregnancy and discrepancies in mandatory reporting in Pinellas County, Florida. N Engl J Med 332:1202–1206, 1990
7. Johnson LD, et al: Drug Use by High School Seniors—The Class of 1986. United States Department of Health and Human Services. Publication No. (ADM) 87-1535. Rockville, Maryland, 1987
8. Schonberg SK (ed): Substance Abuse: A Guide for Health Professionals. American Academy of Pediatrics/Pacific Institute for Research and Education, Elk Grove Village, Illinois, 1988
9. Children's Defense Fund: The Health of America's Children. Washington, DC, 1989
10. Goodman LS, Gilman A: The Pharmacological Basis of Therapeutics. 5th ed. New York, Macmillan, 1975, p 386
11. Van Dyke C, Byck R: Cocaine. Sci Am 246:128–141, 1982
12. Mofenson HC, Caraccio TR: Cocaine. Pediatr Ann 16:864–874, 1987
13. Johanson CE, Fischman MW: The pharmacology of cocaine related to its abuse. Pharmacol Rev 41:3–52, 1989
14. Farrar HC, Kearns GL: Cocaine: Clinical pharmacology and toxicology. J Pediatr 115:665–675, 1989
15. Caldwell J, Sever PS: The biochemical pharmacology of abused drugs: I. Amphetamines, cocaine and LSD. Clin Pharmacol Ther 16:625–638, 1974
16. Fleming JA, Byck R, Barash PG: Pharmacology and therapeutic applications of cocaine. Anesthesiology 73:518–531, 1990
17. Jatlow P: Cocaine: Analysis, pharmacokinetics, and metabolic disposition. Yale J Biol Med 61:105–113, 1988
18. Grabowski J, Dworkin SI: Cocaine: An overview of current issues. Int J Addict 20:1065–1088, 1985
19. American Society for Pharmacology and Experimental Therapeutics and Committee on Problems of Drug Dependence: Scientific perspectives on cocaine abuse. Pharmacologist 29:20–27, 1987
20. Chasnoff IJ, Burns KA, Burns WJ: Cocaine use in pregnancy: Perinatal morbidity and mortality. Neurotoxicol Teratol 9:291–293, 1987
21. Chaney NE, Franke J, Waddlington WB: Cocaine convulsions in a breast-fed baby. J Pediatr 112:134–135, 1988
22. Chasnoff IJ, Lewis DE, Squires L: Cocaine intoxication in a breast-fed infant. Pediatrics 80:836–838, 1987
23. Daigle RD, Clark HW, Landry MJ: A primer on neurotransmitters and cocaine. J Psychoact Drugs 20:283–295, 1988
24. Holmstedt B, Lindgren JE, River L: Cocaine in blood of coca chewers. J Ethnopharmacol 1:69–78, 1979
25. Van Dyke C, Jatlow P, Ungerer J, Barash PG, Byck R: Oral cocaine: Plasma concentrations and central effects. Science 200:211–213, 1978
26. Wilkinson P, Van Dyke C, Jatlow P, Barash P, Byck R: Intranasal and oral cocaine kinetics. Clin Pharmacol Ther 27:386–394, 1980
27. Ellenhorn M, Barceloux D: Medical toxicology: Diagnosis and treatment of human poisoning. New York, Elsevier Science, pp 644–661, 1988
28. Perez-Reyes M, DiGuiseppi S, Ondrusek G, Jeffcoat AR, Cook CE: Free-base cocaine smoking. Clin Pharmacol Ther 32:459–465, 1982
29. Inaba T: Cocaine: Pharmacokinetics and biotransformation in man. Can J Physiol Pharmacol 67:1154–1157, 1989
30. Stewart DJ, Inaba T, Lucassen M, Kalow W: Cocaine metabolism: Cocaine and norcocaine hydrolysis by liver and serum esterases. Clin Pharmacol Ther 25:464–468, 1979
31. Leighty EG, Fentman AF Jr: Metabolism of cocaine to norcocaine and benzoylecgonine by an in-vitro microsomal enzyme system. Res Commun Chem Pathol Pharmacol 8:65–74, 1974
32. Hawks RL, Kopur IJ, Coburn RW, Thoa NB: Norcocaine: A Pharmacologically active metabolite of cocaine found in the brain. Life Sci 15:2189–2195, 1974
33. Hazel B, Monier D: Human serum cholinesterase: Variations during pregnancy and post-partum. Can Anesth Soc J 18:272–277, 1971
34. Howard JK, East NJ, Chaney JL: Plasma cholinesterase activity in early pregnancy. Arch Environ Health 33:277–279, 1978

35. Pritchard JA: Plasma cholinesterase activity in normal pregnancy and in eclamptogenic toxemias. Am J Obstet Gynecol 70:1083–1086, 1955

36. Robertson G: Serum cholinesterase deficiency. II. Pregnancy. Br J Anesth 38:361–369, 1966

37. Shnider SM: Serum cholinesterase activity during pregnancy, labour and the puerperium. Anesthesiology 26:335–391, 1965

38. Venkataramen BW, Nujer GY, Narayanan R, Thangam J: Erythrocyte and plasma cholinesterase activity in normal pregnancy. Ind J Pharmac 34:26–28, 1990

39. Kambam JR, Perry SM, Entman S, Smith BE: Effect of magnesium on plasma cholinesterase activity. Am J Obstet 159:309–311, 1988

40. Roe DA, Little BB, Bawdon RE, Gilstrap LC: Metabolism of cocaine by human placentas: Implications for fetal exposure. Am J Obstet Gynecol 163:715–718, 1990

41. Ecobichon DJ, Stephens DS: Perinatal development of human blood esterases. Clin Pharmacol Ther 14:41–47, 1972

42. Whittaker M: Cholinesterase, in Beckman L (ed): Monographs in Human Genetics. New York, Karger, pp 45–63, 1986

43. Devenyi P: Cocaine complications and pseudocholinesterase (Letter). Ann Intern Med 110:167–168, 1989

44. Lenz W: Malformations caused by drugs in pregnancy. Am J Dis Child 112:99–105, 1966

45. Barnett G, Hawks R, Resnick R: Cocaine pharmacokinetics in humans. J Ethnopharmacol 3:353–366, 1981

46. Chow MJ, Ambre JJ, Ruo TI, Atkinson AJ, Bowsher DJ, Fischman MW: Kinetics of cocaine elimination and chronotropic effects. Clin Pharmacol Ther 38:318–324, 1985

47. Jatlow PI: Drug abuse profile: Cocaine. Clin Chem 33:66B–71B, 1987

48. Kloss MW, Rosen GM, Rauckman EJ: Commentary. Cocaine-mediated hepatotoxicity. A critical review. Biochem Pharmcol 33:169–173, 1984

49. Chasnoff IJ, Lewis DE, Griffith DR, Willey S: Cocaine and pregnancy: Clinical and toxicological implications for the neonate. Clin Chem 35:1276–1278, 1989

50. Hadeed AJ, Sharon RS: Maternal cocaine use during pregnancy. Pediatrics 84:205–210, 1989

51. Zuckerman B, Frank DA, Hingson R, Amaro H, Levenson SM, Kayne H, Parker S, Vinci R, Aboagye K, Fried LE, Cabral H, Timperi R, Bauchner HB: Effects of maternal marijuana and cocaine use on fetal growth. N Engl J Med 320:762–768, 1989

52. Ryan L, Ehrlich S, Finnegan L: Cocaine abuse in pregnancy: Effects on the fetus and newborn. Neurotoxicol Teratol 9:295–299, 1987

53. Acker D, Sachs BP, Tracey KJ, Wise WE: Abruptio placenta associated with cocaine use. Am J Obstet Gynecol 146:220–221, 1983

54. Chasnoff IJ, Griffith DR: Cocaine: Clinical studies of pregnancy and the newborn. Ann NY Acad Sci 562:260–266, 1989

55. Chasnoff IJ, Griffith DR, MacGregor S, Dirkes K, Burns KA: Temporal patterns of cocaine use in pregnancy. JAMA 261:1741–1744, 1989

56. MacGregor SN, Keith LG, Chasnoff IJ, Rosner MA, Chisum GM, Shaw P, Minogue JP: Cocaine use during pregnancy: Adverse perinatal outcome. Am J Obstet Gynecol 157:686–690, 1987

57. Sproat KV (ed): Special Currents: Cocaine Babies. Ross Laboratories, 1989

58. Dixon SD, Bejar R: Echoencephalographic findings in neonates associated with maternal cocaine and methamphetamine use: Incidence and clinical correlates. J Pediatr 115:770–778, 1989

59. Chasnoff IJ, Bussey ME, Savich R, Stack CM: Perinatal cerebral infarction and maternal cocaine use. J Pediatr 108:456–459, 1986

60. Doberczak TM, Shanzer S, Senie RT, Kandall SR: Neonatal neurologic and electroencephalographic effects of intrauterine cocaine exposure. J Pediatr 113:354–358, 1988

61. Bingol N, Fuchs M, Diaz V, Stone RK, Gromisch DS: Teratogenicity of cocaine in humans. J Pediatr 110:93–96, 1987

62. Van de Bor M, Walther FJ, Sims ME: Increased cerebral blood flow velocity in infants of mothers who abuse cocaine. Pediatrics 85:733–736, 1990

63. Bingol N, Fuchs M, Holipas N, et al: Prune belly syndrome associated with maternal cocaine abuse (Abstr.). Am J Hum Genet 37:147A, 1986

64. Chasnoff IJ, Chisum GM, Kaplan WE: Maternal cocaine use and genitourinary tract malformations. Teratology 37:201–204, 1988

65. Hoyme HE, Jones KL, Dixon SD, Jewett T, Hanson JW, Robinson LK, Msall ME, Allanson JE: Prenatal cocaine exposure and fetal vascular disruption. Pediatrics 85:743–747, 1990

66. Jones KL: Developmental pathogenesis of defects associated with prenatal cocaine exposure: Fetal vascular disruption. Clin Perinatol 18:139–146, 1991

67. Kramer LD, Locke GE, Ogunyemi A, Nelson L: Neonatal cocaine-related seizures. J Child Neurol 5:60–64, 1990

68. Shih L, Cone-Wesson B, Reddix B: Effects of maternal cocaine abuse on the neonatal auditory system. Int J Pediatr Otolaryngol 15:245–251, 1988

69. Little BB, Snell LM, Klein VR, Gilstrap LC: Cocaine abuse during pregnancy: Maternal and fetal implications. Obstet Gynecol 73:157–160, 1989

70. AAP Committee on Drugs: Neonatal drug withdrawal. Pediatrics 72:895–902, 1983

71. Hume RF, O'Donnell KJ, Stranger CL, Killam AP, Gingras JL: In-utero cocaine exposure: Observations of fetal behavioral state may predict neonatal outcome. Am J Obstet Gynecol 161:685–690, 1989

72. Oro AS, Dixon SD: Prenatal cocaine and methamphetamine exposure: Maternal and neonatal correlates. J Pediatr 111:571–578, 1987

73. Howard J: Long term development of infants exposed prenatally to drugs, in Sproat KV (ed): Special Currents: Cocaine Babies. Ross Laboratories, 1989

Section VI

APPENDICES

NEONATAL AND PEDIATRIC DRUG FORMULARY

Keith W. Johnson,
Sumner J. Yaffe,
and Jacob V. Aranda

ACETAMINOPHEN (SYSTEMIC)

Pediatric dosing:
   Analgesic or
   Antipyretic -
      Oral or rectal, 1.5 grams per square meter of body surface
      a day in divided doses.

Product Availability:
   Acetaminophen Oral Solution USP [100 mg per mL; 80, 120,
      and 160 mg per 5 mL] - Children's Panadol; Children's
      Tylenol Elixir; Tempra; Generic.
   Acetaminophen Suppositories [120, 125, 300, and 325 mg] -
      Acephen; Acetaminophen Uniserts; Ty-Pap; Generic.
   Acetaminophen Oral Suspension USP [48 mg per mL] -
      Liquiprin Infants' Drops.
   Acetaminophen Tablets USP [120, 160, 300, and 325] - Ana-
      cin-3; Phenaphen; Tylenol; Generic.
   Acetaminophen Tablets USP (Chewable) [80 and 160 mg] -
      Children's Anacin-3; Children's Genapap; Children's
      Tylenol; St. Joseph Aspirin-Free Fever Reducer for Chil-
      dren; Tempra; Generic.

ACETAZOLAMIDE (SYSTEMIC)

Pediatric dosing:
   Glaucoma - Oral, 8 to 30 mg per kg of body weight, usually 10
      to 15 mg per kg, or 300 to 900 mg per square meter of body
      surface area a day in divided doses.
   Anticonvulsant - Oral, 4 to 30 mg (usually 10 mg initially) per
      kg of body weight a day in up to 4 divided doses; usually 375
      mg to 1 gram a day.

Product Availability:
   Acetazolamide Tablets USP [125 and 250 mg] - Diamox;
      Generic.

ALBUTEROL (SYSTEMIC)

Pediatric dosing:
   Bronchodilator - Bronchospasm in obstructive pulmonary
      disease (treatment):
      Children 2 to 6 years of age - Oral, 100 mcg (0.1 mg)
         (base) per kg of body weight three times a day initially,
         the dosage being increased as needed and tolerated up
         to 200 mcg (0.2 mg) per kg of body weight, not to
         exceed 4 mg, three times a day.
      Children 6 to 14 years of age - Oral, 2 mg (base) three or
         four times a day initially, the dosage being increased as
         needed and tolerated up to a maximum of 24 mg per
         day in divided doses.

Product Availability:
   Albuterol Sulfate Syrup [2 mg (base) per 5 mL] - Proventil;
      Ventolin.
   Albuterol Sulfate Tablets [2 and 4 mg (base)] - Proventil; Ven-
      tolin; Generic.

ALLOPURINOL (SYSTEMIC)

Pediatric dosing:
   Antihyperuricemic, in neoplastic disease therapy-
      Children up to 6 years of age: Oral, 50 mg three times a
         day.
      Children 6 to 10 years of age: Oral, 100 mg three times a
         day; or 300 mg as a single dose once a day.

Product Availability:
   Allopurinol Tablets USP [100 and 300 mg] - Lopurin; Zylo-
      prim; Generic.

ALPROSTADIL (SYSTEMIC)

Pediatric dosing:
   Initial -
      Intravenous, intra-arterial, or intra-aortic, 0.05 to 0.1
         mcg per kg of body weight per minute. After a satisfac-
         tory response is obtained, the rate of infusion may be
         reduced (or, rarely, increased) to the minimum level
         that will maintain the response; a possible dosage
         reduction schedule is 0.1 to 0.5 to 0.025 to 0.01 mcg
         per kg of body weight per minute.

ALPROSTADIL (SYSTEMIC)—*continued*

Maintenance -
Intravenous, intra-arterial, or intra-aortic, usually one-hundredth to one-tenth the initial dose.

Product Availability:
Alprostadil Injection USP [500 mcg (0.5 mg) per mL] - Prostin VR Pediatric.

AMANTADINE (SYSTEMIC)

Pediatric dosing:
Antiviral (systemic)-
Children 1 to 9 years of age: Oral, 1.5 to 3 mg per kg of body weight every eight hours; or 2.2 to 4.4 mg per kg of body weight every twelve hours. Maximum daily dose should not exceed 150 mg.
Children 9 to 12 years of age: Oral, 100 mg every twelve hours.

Product Availability:
Amantadine Hydrochloride Capsules USP [100 mg] - Symmetrel; Generic.
Amantadine Hydrochloride Syrup USP [50 mg per 5 mL] - Symmetrel.

AMIKACIN (SYSTEMIC)

Pediatric dosing:
Antibacterial (systemic)- Intramuscular or intravenous infusion:
Premature neonates-
Initially, 10 mg per kg of body weight, then 7.5 mg per kg of body weight every eighteen to twenty-four hours.
Neonates-
Initially, 10 mg per kg of body weight, then 7.5 mg per kg of body weight every twelve hours.
Older infants-
5 mg per kg of body weight every eight hours; or 7.5 mg per kg of body weight every twelve hours for seven to ten days.

Product Availability:
Amikacin Sulfate Injection USP [50 and 250 mg per mL] - Amikin.

AMIODARONE (SYSTEMIC)

Pediatric dosing:
Ventricular arrhythmias; or [Supraventricular arrhythmias]-
Loading:
Oral, 10 mg per kg of body weight per day or 800 mg per 1.72 square meters of body surface per day for ten days or until an initial therapeutic response or side effects occur. When adequate control or excessive side effects occur, the dose is reduced to 5 mg per kg of body weight or 400 mg per 1.72 square meters of body surface per day for several weeks and then decreased gradually to the lowest effective maintenance dose.

Maintenance: Oral, 2.5 mg per kg of body weight per day or 200 mg per 1.72 square meters of body surface per day.

Product Availability:
Amiodarone Hydrochloride Tablets [200 mg] - Cordarone.

AMITRIPTYLINE (SYSTEMIC)

Pediatric dosing:
Antidepressant-
Children 6 to 12 years of age: Oral, 10 to 30 mg, or 1 to 5 mg per kg of body weight, a day in two divided doses.
Adolescents: Oral, initially 10 mg three times a day and 20 mg at bedtime, the dosage being adjusted as needed and tolerated, up to a maximum of 100 mg a day.
[Enuresis]-
Children up to 6 years of age: Oral, 10 mg a day as a single dose at bedtime.
Children over 6 years of age: Oral, initially 10 mg a day as a single dose at bedtime, the dose being increased as needed and tolerated up to a maximum of 25 mg.

Product Availability:
Amitriptyline Hydrochloride Tablets UPS [10 and 25 mg] - Elavil; Endep; Generic.

AMOXICILLIN (SYSTEMIC)

Pediatric dosing:
Antibacterial-
Infants up to 6 kg of body weight - Oral, 25 to 50 mg every eight hours.
Infants 6 to 8 kg of body weight - Oral, 50 to 100 mg every eight hours.
Infants and children 8 to 20 kg of body weight - Oral, 6.7 to 13.3 mg per kg of body weight every eight hours.
Children 20 kg of body weight and over - Oral, 250 to 500 mg every eight hours.

Product Availability:
Amoxicillin Capsules USP [250 and 500 mg] - Amoxil; Polymox; Trimox; Wymox; Generic.
Amoxicillin for Oral Suspension USP [50 mg per mL, 125 and 250 mg per 5 mL] - Amoxil; Polymox; Trimox; Wymox; Generic.
Amoxicillin Tablets USP (Chewable) [125 and 250 mg] - Amoxil.

AMOXICILLIN AND CLAVULANATE (SYSTEMIC)

Pediatric dosing:
Antibacterial -
Infants and children up to 40 kg of body weight-
Otitis media, acute; sinusitis; pneumonia; and other severe infections: Oral, 13.3 mg (anhydrous amoxicillin) per kg of body weight every eight hours.
Other infections: Oral, 6.7 mg (anhydrous amoxicillin) per kg of body weight every eight hours.

Product Availability:
Amoxicillin and Clavulanate Potassium for Oral Suspension USP [125 mg (anhydrous amoxicillin) and 31.25 mg (cla-

vulanic acid) per 5 mL and 250 mg (anhydrous amoxicillin) and 62.5 mg (clavulanic acid) per 5 mL] - Augmentin.

Amoxicillin and Clavulanate Potassium Tablets USP [250 mg (anhydrous amoxicillin) and 125 mg (clavulanic acid) and 500 mg (anhydrous amoxicillin) and 125 mg (clavulanic acid)] - Augmentin.

Amoxicillin and Clavulanate Potassium Tablets USP (Chewable) [125 mg (anhydrous amoxicillin) and 31.25 mg (clavulanic acid) and 250 mg (anhydrous amoxicillin) and 62.5 mg (clavulanic acid)] - Augmentin.

AMPHETAMINE (SYSTEMIC)

Pediatric dosing:

Attention deficit disorder-

Children 3 to 6 years of age: Oral, 2.5 mg once a day, the dosage being increased by 2.5 mg per day at one-week intervals until the desired response is obtained.

Children 6 years of age and over: Oral, 5 mg one or two times a day, the dosage being increased by 5 mg per day at one-week intervals until the desired response is obtained.

Narcolepsy-

Children 6 to 12 years of age: Oral, 2.5 mg two times a day, the dosage being increased by 5 mg per day at one-week intervals until the desired response is obtained or until the adult dose is reached.

Children 12 years of age and over: Oral, 5 mg two times a day, the dosage being increased by 10 mg per day at one-week intervals until the desired response is obtained or until the adult dose is reached.

Product Availability:

Amphetamine Sulfate Tablets USP [5 and 10 mg] - Generic.

AMPHOTERICIN B (SYSTEMIC)

Pediatric dosing:

Antifungal (systemic)-

Intravenous infusion, initially 250 mcg (0.25 mg) per kg of body weight per day, administered in 5% dextrose injection over a period of six hours, the dosage being increased gradually (usually by 250-mcg [0.25 mg]-per-kg increments every other day) as tolerated, up to a maximum of 1 mg per kg of body weight or 30 mg per square meter of body surface per day.

Product Availability:

Amphotericin B for Injection USP [50 mg] - Fungizone Intravenous; Generic.

AMPICILLIN (SYSTEMIC)

Pediatric dosing:

Antibacterial -

Infants and children up to 20 kg of body weight - Oral, 12.5 to 25 mg per kg of body weight every six hours; or 16.7 to 33.3 mg per kg of body weight every eight hours.

Children 20 kg of body weight and over - 250 to 500 mg every six hours.

Product Availability:

Ampicillin Capsules USP [250 and 500 mg] - Polycillin; Principen; Generic.

Ampicillin for Oral Suspension USP [100 mg per mL, 125, 250, and 500 mg per 5 mL] - Polycillin; Omnipen; Generic.

ASPIRIN (SYSTEMIC)

Pediatric dosing:

Analgesic/antipyretic - Oral or rectal, 1.5 grams per square meter of body surface a day in four to six divided doses.

Antirheumatic (nonsteroidal anti-inflammatory) - Oral, 80 to 100 mg per kg of body weight a day in divided doses.

[Kawasaki disease] -

During the early febrile stage: Oral, 80 to 120 mg (average 100 mg) per kg of body weight a day in four divided doses for fourteen days or until inflammation has subsided. However, absorption may be impaired or erratic during this stage of the illness, and considerably higher doses may be required. It is recommended that dosage be adjusted to achieve and maintain a plasma salicylate concentration of 20 to 30 mg per 100 mL.

During the convalescent stage: Oral, 3 to 5 mg per kg of body weight a day as a single dose. If no coronary artery abnormalities occur, treatment is usually continued for a minimum of eight weeks. If coronary artery abnormalities occur, it is recommended that treatment be continued for at lease one year, even if the abnormalities regress, and longer if abnormalities persist.

Product Availability:

Aspirin Suppositories USP [60, 120, 200, and 325 mg] - Generic.

Aspirin Tablets USP [325 mg] - Bayer Aspirin; Generic.

Aspirin Tablets USP (Chewable) [81 mg] - Bayer Aspirin; St. Joseph Adult Chewable Aspirin; Generic.

ASTEMIZOLE (SYSTEMIC)

Pediatric dosing:

Antihistaminic (H1-receptor)-

Children 6 to 12 years of age: Oral, 5 mg once a day.

Children 12 years of age and over: Oral, 10 mg once a day.

Product Availability:

Astemizole Tablets [10 mg] - Hismanal.

AZATHIOPRINE (SYSTEMIC)

Pediatric dosing:

Immunosuppressant-

Transplant rejections, organ (prophylaxis):

Initial - Oral or intravenous, 3 to 5 mg per kg of body weight or 120 mg per square meter of body surface a day, one to three days before or at the time of surgery, the dosage being adjusted to maintain the homograft without causing toxicity.

Antirheumatic (disease-modifying)- Rheumatoid arthritis; or [Lupus erythematosus suppressant-Lupus erythematosus, systemic]-

Initial -

Oral, 1 mg per kg of body weight per day, the dosage being increased in increments of 500 mcg (0.5 mg)

AZATHIOPRINE (SYSTEMIC)—*continued*

per kg of body weight per day after six to eight weeks, then every four weeks as necessary up to a maximum dose of 2.5 mg per kg of body weight per day.

Maintenance -
Oral, the dosage being reduced to the minimum effective dose in decrements of 500 mcg (0.5 mg) per kg of body weight per day every four to eight weeks.

Product Availability:
Azathioprine Tablets USP [50 mg] - Imuran.
Azathioprine Sodium for Injection USP [100 mg] - Imuran; Generic.

AZLOCILLIN (SYSTEMIC)

Pediatric dosing:
Antibacterial -
Children with acute pulmonary exacerbation of cystic fibrosis -
Intravenous, 75 mg per kg of body weight every four hours.

Product availability:
Sterile Azlocillin Sodium USP [2, 3, and 4 grams] - Azlin.

BACAMPICILLIN (SYSTEMIC)

Pediatric dosing:
Pneumonia-
Infants and children up to 25 kg of body weight: Oral, 25 mg per kg of body weight every twelve hours.
Children 25 kg of body weight and over: Oral, 800 mg every twelve hours.
Skin and soft-tissue infections, acute otitis media, pharyngitis, sinusitis, and urinary tract infections-
Infants and children up to 25 kg of body weight: Oral, 12.5 to 25 mg per kg of body weight every twelve hours.
Children 25 kg of body weight and over: 400 to 800 mg every twelve hours.

Product Availability:
Bacampicillin Hydrochloride for Oral Suspension USP [125 mg per 5 mL] - Spectrobid.
Bacampicillin Hydrochloride Tablets USP [400 mg] - Spectrobid.

BECLOMETHASONE (INHALATION)

Pediatric dosing:
Asthma -
Children 6 to 12 years of age - 42 or 84 mcg (0.042 or 0.084 mg - 1 or 2 metered sprays) or 50 or 100 mcg (0.05 or 0.1 mg - 1 or 2 metered sprays) three or four times a day.
Alternate regimen: Oral inhalation, 168 to 200 mcg (0.168 to 0.2 mg - 4 metered sprays) two times a day.

Product Availability:
Beclomethasone Dipropionate Inhalation Aerosol [42 mcg (0.042 mg) per metered spray] - Belovent; Vanceril.

BECLOMETHASONE (NASAL)

Pediatric dosing:
Rhinitis or allergic disorders or inflammatory conditions -
Children 6 to 12 years of age - Nasal, 42 or 50 mcg (0.042 or 0.05 mg - 1 metered spray) in each nostril three or four times a day (total daily dose, 252 mcg [0.252 mg] to 400 mcg [0.4 mg]).
Children 12 years of age and over - Nasal, 42 or 50 mcg (0.042 or 0.05 mg - 1 metered spray) in each nostril two to four times a day (total daily dose, 168 to 400 mcg [0.168 to 0.4 mg]).

Product Availability:
Beclomethasone Dipropionate Nasal Aerosol [42 mcg (0.042 mg) per metered spray] - Beconase; Vancenase.

BETHAMETHASONE (SYSTEMIC)

Pediatric dosing:
Adrenocortical insufficiency -
Oral, 17.5 mcg (0.0175 mg) per kg of body weight or 500 mcg (0.5 mg) per square meter of body surface a day in three divided doses.
Intramuscular, 17.5 mcg (0.0175 mg) (base) per kg of body weight or 500 mcg (0.5 mg) (base) per square meter of body surface a day (in three divided doses) every third day; or 5.8 to 8.75 mcg (0.0058 to 0.00875 mg) (base) per kg of body weight or 166 to 250 mcg (0.166 to 0.25 mg) (base) per square meter of body surface once a day.
Other indications -
Oral, 62.5 to 250 mcg (0.0625 to 0.25 mg) per kg of body weight or 1.875 to 7.5 mg per square meter of body surface a day in three or four divided doses.
Intramuscular, 20.8 to 125 mcg (0.028 to 0.125 mg) (base) per kg of body weight or 625 mcg (0.625 mg) to 3.75 mg (base) per square meter of body surface every twelve to twenty-four hours.

Product Availability:
Bethamethasone Syrup USP [600 mcg (0.6 mg) per 5 mL] - Celestone.
Bethamethasone Tablets USP [600 mcg (0.6 mg)] - Celestone.
Bethamethasone Sodium Phosphate Injection USP [3 mg (base) per mL] - Celestone; Generic.

BETHANECHOL (SYSTEMIC)

Pediatric dosing:
Cholinergic - Oral, 200 mcg (0.2 mg) per kg of body weight or 6.7 mg per square meter of body surface three times a day.
[Treatment of gastroesophageal reflux] - Oral, 200 mcg (0.2 mg) per kg of body weight or 6.7 mg per square meter of body surface four or five times a day.

Product Availability:
Bethanechol Chloride Tablets USP [5, 10, 25, and 50 mg] - Urecholine; Generic.

BROMPHENIRAMINE (SYSTEMIC)

Pediatric dosing:
Antihistamine (H1-receptor) -
Oral, 500 mcg (0.5 mg) per kg of body weight or 15 mg

per square meter of body surface per day, in three or four divided doses, as needed.

Children up to 12 years of age: Intramuscular, intravenous, or subcutaneous, 125 mcg (0.125 mg) per kg of body weight or 3.75 mg per square meter of body surface three or four times a day as needed.

Product Availability:

Brompheniramine Maleate Elixir USP [2 mg per 5 mL] - Bromphen; Generic.

Brompheniramine Maleate Tablets USP [4 and 8 mg] - Dimetane; Generic.

Brompheniramine Maleate Injection USP [10 and 100 mg per mL] - Chlorphed; Nasahist B.

CAFFEINE, CITRATED (SYSTEMIC)

Pediatric dosing:

Neonatal apnea-
Initial:
Oral, 20 mg (10 mg of anhydrous caffeine and 10 mg of anhydrous citric acid) per kg of body weight.
Maintenance:
Oral, 5 mg (2.5 mg of anhydrous caffeine and 2.5 mg of anhydrous citric acid) per kg of body weight a day, starting forty-eight to seventy-two hours after the initial dose, the dosage being increased as needed and tolerated up to 12 mg per kg of body weight two times a day, for a serum concentration of 8 to 20 mg per liter.

Product Availability:
Citrated Caffeine Solution - Dosage form not commercially available. Compounding required.

CAPTOPRIL (SYSTEMIC)

Pediatric dosing:

Antihypertensive -
Newborns -
Initial:
Oral, 10 mcg (0.01 mg) per kg of body weight two or three times a day, the dosage being adjusted as needed and tolerated.
Children -
Initial:
Oral, 300 mcg (0.3 mg) per kg of body weight three times a day, the dosage being increased if necessary in increments of 300 mcg (0.3 mg) per kg of body weight at intervals of eight to twenty-four hours to the minimum effective dose.

Product Availability:
Captopril Tablets USP [12.5, 25, 50, and 100 mg] - Capoten.

CARBAMAZEPINE (SYSTEMIC)

Pediatric dosing:

Anticonvulsant -
Children up to 6 years of age:
Initial -
Oral, 10 to 20 mg per kg of body weight a day in two or three divided doses, the dosage being

increased by up to 100 mg a day at weekly intervals as needed and tolerated.
Maintenance -
Oral, adjusted to the minimum effective dosage, usually 250 to 350 mg a day, and generally not exceeding 400 mg a day.
Children 6 to 12 years of age:
Initial -
Oral, 100 mg two times a day on the first day, the dosage being increased by 100 mg a day at weekly intervals until the best response is obtained.
Maintenance -
Oral, adjusted to the minimum effective dosage, usually 400 to 800 mg a day.

Product Availability:
Carbamazepine Tablets USP [200 mg] - Tegretol; Generic.
Carbamazepine Tablets USP (Chewable) [100 mg] - Tegretol; Generic.
Carbamazepine Oral Suspension [100 mg per 5 mL] - Tegretol.

CARBENICILLIN (SYSTEMIC)

Pediatric dosing:

Neonates up to 2 kg of body weight - Septicemia, meningitis, pneumonia, or skin and soft-tissue infections:
Intramuscular or intravenous, 100 mg per kg of body weight initially, then 75 mg per kg of body weight every eight hours during the first week of life; followed by 100 mg per kg of body weight every six hours thereafter.

Neonates 2 kg of body weight and over - Septicemia, meningitis, pneumonia, or skin and soft-tissue infections:
Intramuscular or intravenous, 100 mg per kg of body weight initially, then 75 mg per kg of body weight every six hours during the first three days of life; followed by 100 mg per kg of body weight every six hours thereafter.
Older infants and children - Septicemia, meningitis, pneumonia, or skin and soft-tissue infections:
Intramuscular or intravenous, 50 to 83.3 mg per kg of body weight every four hours.
Urinary tract infections: Intramuscular or intravenous, 12.5 to 50 mg per kg of body weight every six hours; or 8.3 to 33.3 mg per kg of body weight every four hours.

Product Availability:
Sterile Carbenicillin Disodium USP [1, 2, 5, 10, and 30 grams] - Geopen.

CARBINOXAMINE (SYSTEMIC)

Pediatric dosing:

Antihistamine (H1-receptor) -
Children 1 to 3 years of age: Oral, 2 mg every six to eight hours as needed.
Children 3 to 6 years of age: Oral, 2 to 4 mg every six to eight hours as needed.
Children 6 years of age and over: Oral, 4 to 6 mg every six to eight hours as needed.

Product Availability:
Carbinoxamine Maleate Tablets USP [4 mg] - Clistin.

CEFACLOR (SYSTEMIC)

Pediatric dosing:
  Antibacterial -
    Infants 1 month of age and over - Oral, 6.7 to 13.4 mg per kg of body weight every eight hours.

Product Availability:
  Cefaclor Capsules USP [250 and 500 mg] - Ceclor.
  Cefaclor for Oral Suspension USP [125, 187, 250, and 375 mg per 5 mL] - Ceclor.

CEFADROXIL (SYSTEMIC)

Pediatric dosing:
  Oral -
    Group A beta-hemolytic streptococcal pharyngitis (including tonsillitis):
      15 mg per kg of body weight every twelve hours; or 30 mg per kg of body weight once a day for ten days.
    Skin and soft-tissue infections or urinary tract infections:
      15 mg per kg of body weight every twelve hours.

Product Availability:
  Cefadroxil Capsules USP [500 mg] - Duricef; Ultracef.
  Cefadroxil for Oral Suspension USP [125, 250, and 500 mg per 5 mL] - Duricef; Ultracef.
  Cefadroxil Tablets USP [1 gram] - Duricef; Ultracef.

CEFAMANDOLE (SYSTEMIC)

Pediatric dosing:
  Antibacterial -
    Infants 1 month of age and over - Intramuscular or intravenous, 8.3 to 16.7 mg per kg of body weight every four hours; 12.5 to 25 mg per kg of body weight every six hours; or 16.7 to 33.3 mg per kg of body weight every eight hours.
    Note: Perioperative prophylaxis - Children 3 months of age and over: Intramuscular or intravenous, 12.5 to 25 mg per kg of body weight one-half to one hour prior to the start of surgery; and 12.5 to 25 mg per kg of body weight every six hours following surgery.

Product Availability:
  Cefamandole Nafate for Injection USP [500 mg, 1, 2, and 10 grams] - Mandol.

CEFAZOLIN (SYSTEMIC)

Pediatric dosing:
  Antibacterial -
    Premature infants and infants up to 1 month of age:
      Less than 2000 grams of body weight, or more than 2000 grams of body weight and 7 days of age or less: Intravenous infusion, 20 mg per kg of body weight every twelve hours.
    More than 2000 grams of body weight and over 7 days of age:
      Intravenous infusion, 20 mg per kg of body weight every eight hours.
    Infants and children 1 month of age and over:
      Intramuscular or intravenous, 6.25 to 25 mg per kg of body weight every six hours, or 8.3 to 33.3 mg per kg of body weight every eight hours.

Product Availability:
  Cefazolin Sodium Injection USP [500 mg in 50 mL and 1 gram in 50 mL] - Ancef.
  Sterile Cefazolin Sodium USP [250 and 500 mg; 1, 5, 10, and 20 grams] - Ancef; Kefzol; Generic.

CEFIXIME (SYSTEMIC)

Pediatric dosing:
  Antibacterial -
    Infants up to 6 months of age - Dosage has not been established.
    Children 6 months of age and over - Oral, 4 mg per kg of body weight every twelve hours; or 8 mg per kg of body weight once a day.
    Children over 12 years of age or 50 kg of body weight - Oral, 200 mg every twelve hours; or 400 mg once a day.

Product Availability:
  Cefixime for Oral Suspension [100 mg per 5 mL] - Suprax.
  Cefixime Tablets [200 and 400 mg] - Suprax.

CEFORANIDE (SYSTEMIC)

Pediatric dosing:
  Antibacterial -
    Children 1 year of age and older - Intramuscular or intravenous, 10 to 20 mg per kg of body weight every twelve hours.

Product Availability:
  Ceforanide for Injection USP [500 mg and 1 gram] - Precef.

CEFOTAXIME (SYSTEMIC)

Pediatric dosing:
  Antibacterial -
    Neonates up to 1 week of age - Intravenous infusion, 50 mg per kg of body weight every twelve hours.
    Neonates 1 to 4 weeks of age - Intravenous infusion, 50 mg per kg of body weight every eight hours.
    Infants and children up to 50 kg of body weight - Intravenous infusion, 8.3 to 30 mg per kg of body weight every four hours; or 12.5 to 45 mg per kg of body weight every six hours.
    Children over 50 kg of body weight - Intravenous infusion, 1 to 2 grams every four to twelve hours.

Product Availability:
  Cefotaxime Sodium Injection USP [1 and 2 grams in 50 mL] - Claforan.
  Sterile Cefotaxime Sodium USP [1, 2, and 10 grams] - Claforan.

CEFOXITIN (SYSTEMIC)

Pediatric dosing:
  Antibacterial -
    Premature infants weighing 1500 grams or more to neo-

nates up to 1 week of age - Intravenous, 20 to 40 mg per kg of body weight every eight hours.

Neonates 1 to 4 weeks of age - Intravenous, 20 to 40 mg per kg of body weight every eight hours.

Infants 1 to 3 months of age - Intramuscular or intravenous, 20 to 40 mg per kg of body weight every six to eight hours.

Infants and children 3 months of age and over - Intramuscular or intravenous, 13.3 to 26.7 mg per kg of body weight every four hours; or 20 to 40 mg per kg of body weight every six hours.

Note: Perioperative prophylaxis - Infants and children 3 months of age and over: Intramuscular or intravenous, 30 to 40 mg per kg of body weight one-half to one hour prior to start of surgery; and 30 to 40 mg per kg of body weight every six hours following surgery for up to twenty-four hours.

Product Availability:

Cefoxitin Sodium Injection USP [1 and 2 grams in 50 mL] - Mefoxin.

Sterile Cefoxitin Sodium USP [1, 2, and 10 grams] - Mefoxin.

CEFTAZIDIME (SYSTEMIC)

Pediatric dosing:

Antibacterial -

Neonates up to 4 weeks of age - Intravenous infusion, 30 mg per kg of body weight every twelve hours.

Infants and children 1 month to 12 years of age - Intravenous infusion, 30 to 50 mg per kg of body weight every eight hours.

Product Availability:

Ceftazidime Injection [1 and 2 grams in 50 mL] - Fortaz.

Ceftazidime for Injection USP [500 mg; 1, 2, and 6 grams] - Fortaz; Tazicef; Tazidime.

CEFTIZOXIME (SYSTEMIC)

Pediatric dosing:

Antibacterial -

Children 6 months of age and older - Intravenous, 50 mg per kg of body weight every six to eight hours.

Product Availability:

Ceftizoxime Sodium Injection USP [1 and 2 grams in 50 mL] - Ceftizox.

Sterile Ceftizoxime Sodium USP [1, 2, and 10 grams] - Ceftizox.

CEFTRIAXONE (SYSTEMIC)

Pediatric dosing:

Antibacterial -

Intramuscular or intravenous, 25 to 37.5 mg per kg of body weight every twelve hours.

Meningitis - Intravenous, 50 mg per kg of body weight every twelve hours, with or without a loading dose of 75 mg per kg of body weight; or 80 mg per kg of body weight every twelve hours for three doses, then every twenty-four hours.

Product Availability:

Ceftriaxone Sodium Injection [1 and 2 grams in 50 mL] - Rocephin.

Sterile Ceftriaxone Sodium USP [250 and 500 mg; 1, 2, and 10 grams] - Rocephin.

CEFUROXIME (SYSTEMIC)

Pediatric dosing:

Antibacterial -

Children up to 12 years of age - Oral, 125 mg every twelve hours.

Children 12 years of age and over - Oral, 250 to 500 mg every twelve hours.

Neonates - Intramuscular or intravenous, 10 to 33.3 mg per kg of body weight every eight hours; or 15 to 50 mg per kg of body weight every twelve hours.

Infants and children 3 months of age and over - Intramuscular or intravenous, 16.7 to 33.3 mg per kg.

Bone infections - Intravenous, 50 mg per kg of body weight every eight hours.

Meningitis, bacterial (neonates) - Intravenous, 33.3 mg per kg of body weight every eight hours, or 50 mg per kg of body weight every twelve hours.

Meningitis, bacterial (infants and children 3 months of age and older) - Intravenous, 50 to 60 mg per kg of body weight every six hours; or 66.7 to 80 mg per kg of body weight every eight hours.

Product Availability:

Cefuroxime Axetil Tablets USP [125, 250, and 500 mg] - Ceftin.

Sterile Cefuroxime Sodium USP [750 mg; 1.5 and 7.5 grams] - Kefurox; Zinacef.

Cefuroxime Sodium Injection [750 mg in 50 mL and 1.5 grams in 50 mL] - Zinacef.

CEPHALEXIN (SYSTEMIC)

Pediatric dosing:

Antibacterial -

Oral, 6.25 to 25 mg per kg of body weight every six hours.

Skin and soft-tissue infections and streptococcal pharyngitis - Oral, 12.5 to 50 mg per kg of body weight every twelve hours.

Product Availability:

Cephalexin Capsules USP [250 and 500 mg] - Cefanex; Keflex; Generic.

Cephalexin for Oral Suspension USP [100 mg per mL; 125, 250, and 500 mg per 5 mL] - Keflex; Generic.

Cephalexin Tablets USP [250 and 500 mg; 1 gram] - Keflet; Generic.

Cephalexin Hydrochloride Tablets [250 and 500 mg] - Keftab.

CEPHALOTHIN (SYSTEMIC)

Pediatric dosing:

Antibacterial -

Intravenous infusion, 13.3 to 26.6 mg per kg of body weight every four hours; or 20 to 40 mg per kg of body weight every six hours.

Perioperative prophylaxis -

Intravenous infusion, 20 to 30 mg per kg of body weight one-half to one hour prior to the start of surgery; 20 to

CEPHALOTHIN (SYSTEMIC)—*continued*

30 mg per kg of body weight during surgery; and 20 to 30 mg per kg of body weight every six hours following surgery for up to twenty-four hours.

Product Availability:
Cephalothin Sodium Injection USP [1 and 2 grams in 50 mL] - Keflin.
Cephalothin Sodium for Injection USP [1, ,2, and 20 grams] - Keflin.

CEPHAPIRIN (SYSTEMIC)

Pediatric dosing:
Antibacterial -
Infants and children 3 months of age and over - Intramuscular or intravenous, 10 to 20 mg per kg of body weight every six hours.

Product Availability:
Sterile Cephapirin Sodium USP [1, 2, 4, and 20 grams] - Cefadyl; Generic.

CEPHRADINE (SYSTEMIC)

Pediatric dosing:
Antibacterial -
Oral, intramuscular, or intravenous, 6.25 to 25 mg per kg of body weight every six hours.

Product Availability:
Cephradine Capsules USP [250 and 500 mg] - Anspor; Velosef; Generic.
Cephradine for Oral Suspension USP [125 and 250 mg per 5 mL] - Anspor; Velosef; Generic.
Cephradine for Injection USP [250 and 500 mg; 1 and 2 grams] - Velosef.

CHLORAL HYDRATE (SYSTEMIC)

Pediatric dosing:
Hypnotic: Oral or rectal, 50 mg per kg of body weight or 1.5 grams per square meter of body surface at bedtime, up to a maximum of 1 gram per single dose.
Sedative:
Daytime - Oral or rectal, 8.3 mg per kg of body weight or 250 mg per square meter of body surface up to a maximum dose of 500 mg, three times a day.
Premedication prior to electroencephalographic evaluation - Oral, 20 to 25 mg per kg of body weight.

Product Availability:
Chloral Hydrate Capsules USP [250 and 500 mg] - Noctec; Generic.
Chloral Hydrate Syrup USP [250 and 500 mg per 5 mL] - Noctec; Generic.
Chloral Hydrate Suppositories [325, 500, and 650 mg] - Aquachloral Supprettes.

CHLOROQUINE (SYSTEMIC)

Pediatric dosing:
Antiprotozoal -
Malaria:
Suppressive - Oral, 8.3 mg (5 mg base) per kg of body

weight, not to exceed the adult dose, once every seven days.
Therapeutic - Oral, 41.7 mg (25 mg base) per kg of body weight administered over a period of three days as follows: 16.7 mg (10 mg base) per kg of body weight, not to exceed a single dose of 1 gram (600 mg base); then 8.3 mg (5 mg base) per kg of body weight, not to exceed a single dose of 500 mg (300 mg base) six, twenty-four, and forty-eight hours after the first dose.
Intramuscular or subcutaneous, 3.5 mg (base) per kg of body weight, repeated in six hours if necessary, not to exceed a total dose of 12.5 mg (10 mg base) per kg of body weight per twenty-four hours.
Intravenous infusion, initially 16.6 mg (13.3 mg base) per kg of body weight over eight hours, followed by 8.3 mg (6.6 mg base) per kg of body weight every six to eight hours over at least four hours.
Amebiasis, extraintestinal:
Oral, 10 mg (6 mg base) per kg of body weight (up to a maximum of 500 mg [300 mg base]) per day for three weeks.
Intramuscular, 7.5 mg (6 mg base) per kg of body weight per day for ten to twelve days.

Product Availability:
Chloroquine Phosphate Tablets USP [250 and 500 mg] - Aralen; Generic.
Chloroquine Hydrochloride Injection USP [50 mg] - Aralen HCl.

CHLORPHENIRAMINE (SYSTEMIC)

Pediatric dosing:
Antihistaminic (H1-receptor) - Oral or subcutaneous, 87.5 mcg (0.0875 mg) per kg of body weight or 2.5 mg per square meter of body surface every six hours as needed.

Product Availability:
Chlorpheniramine Maleate Syrup USP [2 mg per 5 mL] - Chlor-Trimeton; Generic.
Chlorpheniramine Maleate Tablets USP [4 mg] - Phenetron; Chlor-Trimeton; Generic.
Chlorpheniramine Maleate Tablets USP (Chewable) [2 mg] - Chlo-Amine.
Chlorpheniramine Maleate Injection USP [10 and 100 mg per mL] - Chlor-Trimeton; Generic.

CHLORPROMAZINE (SYSTEMIC)

Pediatric dosing:
Psychotic disorders -
Children 6 months of age and older:
Oral, 550 mcg (0.55 mg) (base) per kg of body weight or 15 mg per square meter of body surface every four to six hours, the dosage being adjusted as needed and tolerated.
Intramuscular, 550 mcg (0.55 mg) (base) per kg of body weight or 15 mg per square meter of body surface very six to eight hours as needed.
Rectal, 1 mg per kg of body weight every six to eight hours as needed.
Nausea and vomiting during surgery -
Intramuscular: 275 mcg (0.275 mg) (base) per kg of body weight, the dosage being repeated in thirty minutes as needed and tolerated.

Intravenous infusion: 275 mcg (0.275 mg) (base) per kg of body weight, diluted to a concentration of at least 1 mg per mL with 0.9% sodium chloride injection, administered at a rate of no more than 1 mg every 2 minutes.

Anxiety, presurgical -
Oral, 550 mcg (0.55 mg) (base) per kg of body weight or 15 mg per square meter of body surface two or three hours before surgery.
Intramuscular, 550 mcg (0.55 mg) (base) per kg of body weight one to two hours before surgery.

Tetanus -
Intramuscular: 550 mcg (0.55 mg) (base) per kg of body weight every six to eight hours.
Intravenous infusion: 550 mcg (0.55 mg) (base) per kg of body weight, diluted to a concentration of at least 1 mg per mL with 0.9% sodium chloride injection, administered at a rate of 1 mg per 2 minutes.

Product Availability:
Chlorpromazine Hydrochloride Oral Concentrate USP [30 and 100 mg (base) per mL] - Thorazine Concentrate; Generic.
Chlorpromazine Hydrochloride Syrup USP [10 mg (base) per 5 mL] - Thorazine; Generic.
Chlorpromazine Hydrochloride Tablets USP [10, 25, 50, 100, 200 mg] - Thorazine; Generic.
Chlorpromazine Hydrochloride Injection USP [25 mg (base) per mL] - Thorazine; Generic.
Chlorpromazine Suppositories USP [25 and 100 mg] - Thorazine.

CHLORTHALIDONE (SYSTEMIC)

Pediatric dosing:
Diuretic or Antihypertensive -
Oral, 2 mg per kg of body weight or 60 mg per square meter of body surface once a day for three days a week, the dosage being adjusted according to response.

Product Availability:
Chlorthalidone Tablets USP [25, 50, and 100 mg] - Hygroton; Generic.

CHORIONIC GONADOTROPIN (SYSTEMIC)

Pediatric dosing:
Prepubertal cryptorchidism - Intramuscular, 1000 to 5000 Units two to three times a week for up to several weeks, discontinuing when the desired response is achieved.
Diagnostic aid (hypogonadism) in males - Intramuscular, 2000 Units once a day for three days.

Product Availability:
Chorionic Gonadotropin for Injection USP [5000, 10,000, and 50,000 Units] - A.P.L.; Generic.

CIMETIDINE (SYSTEMIC)

Pediatric dosing:
Oral, 20 to 40 mg (base) per kg of body weight a day in divided doses four times a day, with meals and at bedtime.
Intramuscular, 5 to 10 mg (base) per kg of body weight every six to eight hours.

Intravenous, 5 to 10 mg (base) per kg of body weight every six to eight hours, diluted to a suitable volume with a compatible intravenous solution and administered over a period of not less than two minutes.
Intravenous infusion, 5 to 10 mg (base) per kg of body weight every six to eight hours, diluted to a suitable volume with a compatible intravenous solution and administered over a fifteen- to twenty-minute period.

Product Availability:
Cimetidine Tablets USP [200, 300, 400, and 800 mg] - Tagamet.
Cimetidine Hydrochloride Oral Solution [300 mg (base) per 5 mL] - Tagamet.
Cimetidine Hydrochloride Injection [300 mg (base) per 2 mL and 300 mg (base) per 50 mL] - Tagamet.

CLEMASTINE (SYSTEMIC)

Pediatric dosing:
Antihistamine (H1-receptor) -
Children up to 6 years of age: Dosage has not been established.
Children 6 to 12 years of age: Oral, 670 mcg (0.67 mg) to 1.34 mg two times a day, not to exceed 4.02 mg per day.

Product Availability:
Clemastine Fumarate Syrup [0.67 mg per 5 mL] - Tavist.
Clemastine Fumarate Tablets USP [1.34 and 2.68 mg] - Tavist.

CLINDAMYCIN (SYSTEMIC)

Pediatric dosing:
Antibacterial -
Infants up to 1 month of age: Dosage must be individualized by physician. Use with caution.
Infants 1 month of age and over: Oral, 2 to 6.3 mg per kg of body weight every six hours; or 2.7 to 8.3 mg per kg of body weight every eight hours.
[Antiprotozoal - Malaria]: Oral, 6.7 to 13.3 mg per kg of body weight three times a day for three days.
Antibacterial -
Infants up to 1 month of age - Intramuscular or intravenous, 3.75 to 5 mg per kg of body weight every six hours; or 5 to 6.7 mg per kg of body weight every eight hours.
Infants 1 month of age and over - Intramuscular or intravenous, 3.75 to 10 mg per kg of body weight or 87.5 to 112.5 mg per square meter of body surface every six hours; or 5 to 13.3 mg per kg of body weight or 116.7 to 150 mg per square meter of body surface every eight hours.
Bone infections - Intramuscular or intravenous, 7.5 mg per kg of body weight every six hours.

Product Availability:
Clindamycin Hydrochloride Capsules USP [75, 150, and 300 mg] - Cleocin; Generic.
Clindamycin Palmitate Hydrochloride for Oral Solution USP [75 mg per 5 mL] - Cleocin Pediatric.
Clindamycin Phosphate Injection USP [300 mg in 2 mL; 600 mg in 4 mL; and 900 mg in 6 mL] - Cleocin; Generic.

CLOMIPRAMINE (SYSTEMIC)

Pediatric dosing:
    Antidepressant -
        Children up to 12 years of age: Dosage has not been established.
        Adolescents: Oral, 20 to 30 mg a day, the dosage being increased by 10 mg a day as needed and tolerated.
    Antiobsessional agent -
        Children up to 10 years of age: Dosage has not been established.
        Children 10 years of age and over, and adolescents: Oral, initially 25 mg once a day, the dose being increased as needed and tolerated up to 100 mg a day or 3 mg per kg of body weight, whichever is less. The dosage may be further increased up to a maximum of 200 mg a day or 3 mg per kg of body weight, whichever is less.

Product Availability:
    Clomipramine Hydrochloride Capsules [25, 50, and 75 mg] - Anafranil.

CLOXACILLIN (SYSTEMIC)

Pediatric dosing:
    Infants and children up to 20 kg of body weight - Oral, 6.25 to 12.5 mg per kg of body weight every six hours.
    Children 20 kg of body weight and over - Oral, 250 to 500 mg every six hours.

Product Availability:
    Cloxacillin Sodium Capsules USP [250 and 500 mg] - Cloxapen; Tegopen; Generic.
    Cloxacillin Sodium for Oral Solution USP [125 mg per 5 mL] - Tegopen; Generic.

CODEINE (SYSTEMIC)

Pediatric dosing:
    Analgesic -
        Infants and children - Oral, intramuscular or subcutaneous, 500 mcg (0.5 mg) per kg of body weight or 15 mg per square meter of body surface every four to six hours as needed.
    Antidiarrheal - Oral, 500 mcg (0.5 mg) per kg of body weight up to four times a day.
    Antitussive -
        Children 2 to 5 years of age: Oral, 1 mg per kg of body weight per day, administered in four equal divided doses.
        Children 6 to 12 years of age: Oral, 5 to 10 mg every four to six hours, not to exceed 60 mg per day.

Product Availability:
    Codeine Phosphate Oral Solution [15 mg per 5 mL] - Generic.
    Codeine Phosphate Tablets USP [30 and 60 mg] - Generic.
    Codeine Sulfate Tablets USP [15, 30, and 60 mg] - Generic.
    Codeine Phosphate Injection USP [30 and 60 mg per mL] - Generic.

CORTISONE (SYSTEMIC)

Pediatric dosing:
    Adrenocortical insufficiency -
        Oral, 700 mcg (0.7 mg) per kg of body weight or 20 to 25

mg per square meter of body surface a day in divided doses.
        Intramuscular, 700 mcg (0.7 mg) per kg of body weight or 37.5 mg per square meter of body surface a day every third day; or 233.33 to 350 mcg (0.23333 to 0.350 mg) per kg of body weight or 12.5 mg per square meter of body surface once a day.
    Other indications - Oral, 2.5 to 10 mg per kg of body weight or 75 to 300 mg per square meter of body surface a day as a single dose or in divided doses.
        Intramuscular, 833 mcg (0.833 mg) to 5 mg per kg of body weight or 25 to 150 mg per square meter of body surface every twelve to twenty-four hours.

Product Availability:
    Sterile Cortisone Acetate Suspension USP [25 and 50 mg per mL] - Cortone Acetate; Generic.
    Cortisone Acetate Tablets USP [5, 10, and 25 mg] - Cortone Acetate; Generic.

CROMOLYN (INHALATION-LOCAL)

Pediatric dosing:
    Children 5 years of age and over -
    Asthma, bronchial (prophylaxis) - Oral inhalation, 1.6 or 2 mg (2 inhalations) four times a day at regular intervals, the dosage being adjusted as needed and tolerated.
    Bronchospasm (prophylaxis) - Oral inhalation, 1.6 or 2 mg (2 inhalations) as a single dose ten to fifteen (but not more than sixty) minutes before exposure to the precipitating factor; or, if used chronically, 1.6 or 2 mg (2 inhalations) four times a day at regular intervals, the dosage being adjusted as needed and tolerated.

Product Availability:
    Cromolyn Sodium Inhalation Aerosol [800 mcg (0.8 mg) per metered spray] - Intal.

CROMOLYN (NASAL)

Pediatric dosing:
    Children 6 years of age and over -
    Allergic rhinitis, perennial or seasonal (prophylaxis and treatment) - Intranasal, 5.2 mg in each nostril three or four times a day at regular intervals.

Product Availability:
    Cromolyn Sodium Nasal Solution USP [40 mg per mL (5.2 mg per metered spray)] - Nasalcrom.

CROMOLYN (SYSTEMIC)

Pediatric dosing:
    Mastocytosis -
        Term infants and children up to 2 years of age: Oral, 20 mg per kg of body weight per day in four divided doses. If control of symptoms is not achieved within two to three weeks in children six months to two years of age, dosage may be increased, if necessary, up to 30 mg per kg of body weight per day.
            Note: Use of oral cromolyn in children less than 2 years of age should be reserved for those patients with severe, incapacitating diseases.
        Children 2 to 12 years of age: Oral, 100 mg four times a day thirty minutes before meals and at bedtime. If con-

trol of symptoms is not achieved within two to three weeks, dosage may be increased, if necessary, up to 40 mg per kg of body weight per day.

Product Availability:
Cromolyn Sodium Capsules [100 mg] - Gastrocrom.

CYCLOPHOSPHAMIDE (SYSTEMIC)

Pediatric dosing:
Antineoplastic -
Initial:
Oral, 2 to 8 mg per kg of body weight or 60 to 250 mg per square meter of body surface a day in divided doses for six or more days.
Intravenous, 2 to 8 mg per kg of body weight or 60 to 250 mg per square meter of body surface a day in divided doses for six or more days (or total dose for seven days once a week).
Maintenance:
Oral, 2 to 5 mg per kg of body weight or 50 to 150 mg per square meter of body surface twice a week.
Intravenous, 10 to 15 mg per kg of body weight every seven to ten days, or 30 mg per kg of body weight at three- to four-week intervals or when bone marrow recovery occurs.
Immunosuppresent - Oral, 2.5 to 3 mg per kg of body weight per day.

Product Availability:
Cyclophosphamide Tablets USP [25, 50 mg] - Cytoxan.
Cyclophosphamide for Injection USP [100, 200, and 500 mg; 1 and 2 grams] - Cytoxan; Neosar; Generic.

CYCLOSPORINE (SYSTEMIC)

Pediatric dosing:
Initial -
Oral, 12 to 15 mg per kg of body weight per day beginning four to twelve hours before surgery and continued for one to two weeks postoperatively, then reduced, usually by 5% per week, to the maintenance dose.
Intravenous infusion, 2 to 6 mg per kg of body weight per day beginning four to twelve hours prior to surgery and continued postoperatively until the patient can tolerate the oral solution.
Maintenance -
Oral, 5 to 10 mg per kg of body weight per day.

Product Availability:
Cyclosporine Capsules [25 and 100 mg] - Sandimmune.
Cyclosporine Oral Solution USP [100 mg per mL] - Sandimmune.
Cyclosporine Concentrate for Injection USP [50 mg per mL] - Sandimmune.

CYPROHEPTADINE (SYSTEMIC)

Pediatric dosing:
Antihistaminic (H1-receptor) - Oral, 125 mcg (0.125 mg) per kg of body weight or 4 mg per square meter of body surface, every eight to twelve hours as needed; or for
Children 2 to 6 years of age: Oral, 2 mg every eight to twelve hours as needed, not to exceed 12 mg per day.

Children 6 to 14 years of age: Oral, 4 mg every eight to twelve hours as needed, not to exceed 16 mg per day.
Appetite stimulant -
Children 2 to 6 years of age: Oral, initially 2 mg two or three times a day with meals; the dosage may be increased, if necessary, but not to exceed 8 mg a day.
Children 6 to 14 years of age: Oral, initially 2 mg three or four times a day with meals. The usual maintenance dose is 4 mg two or three times a day. The dosage may be increased, if necessary, but not to exceed 16 mg a day.

Product Availability:
Cyproheptadine Hydrochloride Syrup USP [2 mg per 5mL] - Periactin; Generic.
Cyproheptadine Hydrochloride Tablets USP [4 mg] - Periactin; Generic.

DAPSONE (SYSTEMIC)

Pediatric dosing:
Leprosy (Hansen's disease) - Oral, in combination with one or more other antileprosy agents, 1.4 mg of dapsone per kg of body weight once a day.
Dermatitis herpetiformis suppressant - Oral, initially 50 mg daily. Doses may be increased up to 300 mg daily or higher if symptoms are not completely controlled. The dose should then be reduced to the lowest effective maintenance dose as soon as possible.

Product Availability:
Dapsone Tablets USP [25 and 100 mg] - Generic.

DEXAMETHASONE (INHALATION)

Pediatric dosing:
Asthma -
Oral inhalation -
Initial: 200 mcg (0.2 mg - 2 metered sprays) of dexamethasone phosphate three or four times a day.
Maintenance: Dosage to be decreased according to patient response.

Product Availability:
Dexamethasone Sodium Phosphate Inhalation Aerosol USP [100 mcg (0.1 mg) dexamethasone phosphate per metered spray] - Decadron Respihaler.

DEXAMETHASONE (NASAL)

Pediatric dosing:
Rhinitis or allergic disorders or inflammatory conditions -
Children 6 to 12 years of age - Nasal, 100 or 200 mcg (0.1 or 0.2 mg - 1 or 2 metered sprays) of dexamethasone phosphate in each nostril two times a day; (total daily dose, 400 mcg [0.4 mg] or 800 mcg [0.8 mg] of dexamethasone phosphate, respectively.

Product Availability:
Dexamethasone Sodium Phosphate Nasal Aerosol [100 mcg (0.1 mg) phosphate per metered spray] - Decadron Turbinaire.

DEXAMETHASONE (SYSTEMIC)

Pediatric dosing:
Adrenocortical insufficiency -
Oral, 23.3 mcg (0.0233 mg) per kg of body weight or 670 mcg (0.67 mg) per square meter of body surface a day in three divided doses.
Intramuscular, 23.3 mcg (0.0233 mg) (phosphate) per kg of body weight or 670 mcg (0.67 mg) (phosphate) per square meter of body surface a day (in three divided doses) every third day; or 7.76 to 11.65 mcg (0.00776 to 0.01165 mg) (phosphate) per kg of body weight or 233 to 335 mcg (0.233 to 0.335 mg) (phosphate) per square meter of body surface once a day.
Other indications -
Oral, 83.3 to 333.3 mcg (0.0833 to 0.3333 mg) per kg of body weight or 2.5 to 10 mg per square meter of body surface a day in three or four divided doses.
Intramuscular, 27.76 to 166.65 mcg (0.02776 to 0.16665 mg) (phosphate) per kg of body weight or 0.833 to 5 mg (phosphate) per square meter of body surface every twelve to twenty-four hours.

Product Availability:
Dexamethasone Elixir USP [500 mcg (0.5 mg) per 5 mL] - Decadron.
Dexamethasone Tablets USP [200, 500, and 750 mcg; 1, 1.5, 2, 4, and 6 mg] - Decadron; Dexone; Hexadrol; Generic.
Dexamethasone Sodium Phosphate Injection USP [4, 10, 20, and 24 mg (phosphate) per mL] - Hexadrol Phosphate; Decadron Phosphate; Generic.

DEXCHLORPHENIRAMINE (SYSTEMIC)

Pediatric dosing:
Antihistaminic (H1-receptor) -
Children up to 12 years of age: Oral, 150 mcg (0.15 mg) per kg of body weight or 4.5 mg per square meter of body surface per day, in four divided doses; or for:
Children 2 to 5 years of age - Oral, 500 mcg (0.5 mg) every four to six hours as needed.
Children 5 to 12 years of age - Oral, 1 mg every four to six hours as needed.

Product Availability:
Dexchlorpheniramine Maleate Syrup USP [2 mg per 5 mL] - Polaramine.
Dexchlorpheniramine Maleate Tablets USP [2 mg] - Polaramine.

DEXTROMETHORPHAN (SYSTEMIC)

Pediatric dosing:
Children up to 2 years of age - Use is not recommended.
Children 2 to 6 years of age - Oral, 2.5 to 5 mg every four hours or 7.5 mg every six to eight hours, as needed, not to exceed 30 mg per day.
Children 6 to 12 years of age - Oral, 5 to 10 mg every four hours or 15 mg every six to eight hours, as needed, not to exceed 60 mg per day.

Product Availability:
Dextromethorphan Hydrobromide Lozenges [5 mg] - Sucrets Cough Control Formula.

Dextromethorphan Hydrobromide Syrup USP [5, 7.5, 10, and 15 mg per 5 mL] - Congespirin for Children; Pertussin 8 Hour Cough Formula.
Dextromethorphan Hydrobromide Chewable Tablets [15 mg] - Mediquell.

DIAZEPAM (SYSTEMIC)

Pediatric dosing:
Antianxiety agent; anticonvulsant; skeletal muscle relaxant adjunct -
Children 6 months of age and over: Oral, 1 to 2.5 mg, 40 to 200 mcg (0.04 to 0.2 mg) per kg of body weight, or 1.17 to 6 mg per square meter of body surface, three or four times a day, the dosage being increased gradually as needed and tolerated.
Anticonvulsant - Status epilepticus and severe recurrent convulsive seizures:
Infants over 30 days of age and children up to 5 years of age - Intravenous (slow), 200 to 500 mcg (0.2 to 0.5 mg) every two to five minutes up to a maximum of 5 mg. If necessary, therapy may be repeated in two to four hours.
Children 5 years of age and over - Intravenous (slow), 1 mg every two to five minutes up to a maximum of 10 mg. If necessary, therapy may be repeated in two to four hours.
Skeletal muscle relaxant adjunct - Tetanus:
Infants over 30 days of age and children up to 5 years of age - Intramuscular or intravenous, 1 to 2 mg, the dosage being repeated every three or four hours as needed.
Children 5 years of age and over - Intramuscular or intravenous, 5 to 10 mg, the dosage being repeated every three or four hours as needed.

Product Availability:
Diazepam Oral Solution [5 mg per mL and 5 mg per 5 mL] - Diazepam Intensol; Generic.
Diazepam Tablets USP [2, 5, and 10 mg] - Valium; Generic.
Diazepam Injection USP [5 mg per mL].

DICLOXACILLIN (SYSTEMIC)

Pediatric dosing:
Infants and children up to 40 kg of body weight - Oral, 3.125 to 6.25 mg per kg of body weight every six hours.
Children 40 kg of body weight and over - Oral, 125 to 250 mg every six hours.

Product Availability:
Dicloxacillin Sodium Capsules USP [125, 250, and 500 mg] - Dycill; Dynapen; Pathocil; Generic.
Dicloxacillin Sodium for Oral Suspension USP [62.5 mg per 5 mL] - Dynapen; Pathocil.

DIGOXIN (SYSTEMIC)

Pediatric dosing:
For Elixir or Tablets -
Digitalization - The following total amounts divided into two or more doses, administered at six- to eight-hour intervals:
Premature and newborn infants up to 1 month of age - Oral, 20 to 35 mcg (0.02 to 0.035 mg) per kg of body weight.

Infants 1 month to 2 years of age - Oral, 35 to 60 mcg
(0.035 to 0.06 mg) per kg of body weight.
Children 2 to 5 years of age - Oral, 30 to 40 mcg (0.03
to 0.04 mg) per kg of body weight.
Children 5 to 10 years of age - Oral, 20 to 35 mcg
(0.02 to 0.035 mg) per kg of body weight.
Children 10 years of age and over -
Rapid: Oral, a total of 0.75 to 1.25 mg divided
into two or more doses, each ten being
administered every six to eight hours.
Slow: Oral, 125 to 500 mcg (0.125 to 0.5 mg)
once a day for seven days.
Maintenance - Oral, one-fifth to one-third of the total digitalizing dose administered once a day.
For Capsules or Injection -
Digitalization - The following total amounts divided
into three or more doses, with the initial portion
representing approximately one-half the total,
doses then being administered every four to eight
hours:
Premature neonates - Oral or intravenous, 15 to
25 mcg (0.015 to 0.025 mg) per kg of body
weight.
Full-term neonates - Oral or intravenous, 20 to
30 mcg (0.02 to 0.03 mg) per kg of body
weight.
Infants 1 month to 2 years of age - Oral or intravenous, 30 to 50 mcg (0.03 to 0.05 mg) per kg
of body weight.
Children 2 to 5 years of age - Oral or intravenous, 25 to 35 mcg (0.025 to 0.035 mg) per kg
of body weight.
Children 5 to 10 years of age - Oral or intravenous, 15 to 30 mcg (0.015 to 0.03 mg) per kg
of body weight.
Children 10 years of age and over - Oral or intravenous, 8 to 12 mcg (0.008 to 0.012 mg) per
kg of body weight.
Maintenance - Begun within 24 hours after digitalization:
Premature neonates - Oral or intravenous, 20% to
30% of the total digitalizing dose, divided and
administered in two or three equal portions per
day.
Full-term neonates, infants, and children up to 10
years of age - Oral or intravenous, 25% to 35% of
the total digitalizing dose, divided and administered in two or three equal portions per day.
Children 10 years of age and over - Oral or intravenous, 25% to 35% of the total digitalizing dose
administered once a day.

Product Availability:
Digoxin Capsules [50, 100, and 200 mcg] - Lanoxicaps.
Digoxin Elixir USP [50 mcg (0.05 mg) per mL] - Lanoxin;
Generic.
Digoxin Tablets USP [125, 250, and 500 mcg] - Lanoxin;
Generic.
Digoxin Injection USP [100 mcg (0.1 mg) per mL; 250 mcg
(0.25 mg) per mL; Lanoxin; Generic.

DIMENHYDRINATE (SYSTEMIC)

Pediatric dosing:
Antiemetic; or
Antivertigo agent -
Oral, 5 mg per kg of body weight or 150 mg per
square meter of body surface per day, in four

divided doses, as needed, not to exceed 300 mg per
day.
Intramuscular, 1.25 mg per kg of body weight or
37.5 mg per square meter of body surface every six
hours as needed, not to exceed 300 mg per day.
Intravenous, 1.25 mg per kg of body weight or 37.5
mg per square meter of body surface, in 10 mL of
0.9% sodium chloride injection, administered
slowly over a period of at least two minutes, every
six hours as needed, not to exceed 300 mg per day.
Product Availability:
Dimenhydrinate Syrup USP [12.5 mg per 4 mL] - Dramamine Liquid.
Dimenhydrinate Tablets USP [50 mg] - Dramamine;
Generic.
Dimenhydrinate Tablets USP (Chewable) [50 mg] - Dramamine Chewable.
Dimenhydrinate Injection USP [50 mg per mL] - Dramamine; Generic.

DIPHENHYDRAMINE (SYSTEMIC)

Pediatric dosing:
Antihistaminic (H1-receptor) - Oral or intramuscular, 1.25
mg per kg of body weight or 37.5 mg per square meter of
body surface, every four to six hours, not to exceed 300 mg
a day.
Antiemetic; or
Antivertigo agent - Oral or intramuscular, 1 to 1.5 mg per kg
of body weight every four to six hours as needed, not to
exceed 300 mg per day.
Antitussive -
Children 2 to 6 years of age: Oral, 6.25 mg every four to
six hours, as needed, not to exceed 25 mg per day.
Children 6 to 12 years of age: Oral, 12.5 mg every four to
six hours, as needed, not to exceed 50 mg per day.

Product Availability:
Diphenhydramine Hydrochloride Capsules USP [25 and 50
mg] - Benadryl; Generic.
Diphenhydramine Hydrochloride Elixir USP [12.5 mg per 5
mL] - Benadryl; Generic.
Diphenhydramine Hydrochloride Syrup [12.5 mg per 5 mL]
- Benylin; Hydramine; Generic.
Diphenhydramine Hydrochloride Tablets [25 and 50 mg] -
Generic.
Diphenhydramine Hydrochloride Injection USP [10 and 50
mg per mL] - Benadryl; Generic.

DIVALPROEX (SYSTEMIC)

Pediatric dosing:
Anticonvulsant -
Children 1 to 12 years of age -
Monotherapy: Oral, the equivalent of valproic acid -
Initially, 15 to 45 mg per kg of body weight a day,
the dosage being increased at one-week intervals
by 5 to 10 mg per kg of body weight a day as
needed and tolerated.
Polytherapy: Oral, the equivalent of valproic acid -
30 to 100 mg per kg of body weight a day.

Product Availability:
Divalproex Sodium Delayed-Release Capsules [125 mg] -
Depakote Sprinkle.
Divalproex Sodium Delayed-Release Tablets [125, 250, and
500 mg] - Depakote.

DOXYCYCLINE (SYSTEMIC)

Pediatric dosing:
  Antibacterial (systemic);
  Antiprotozoal -
      Children 45 kg of body weight and under:
          Oral, 2.2 mg per kg of body weight every twelve hours the first day, then 2.2 to 4.4 mg per kg of body weight once a day; or 1.1 to 2.2 mg per kg of body weight every twelve hours.
          Intravenous infusion, 4.4 mg per kg of body weight once a day or 2.2 mg per kg of body weight every twelve hours the first day; then 2.2 to 4.4 mg per kg of body weight once a day or 1.1 to 2.2 mg per kg of body weight every twelve hours.
      Children over 45 kg of body weight:
          Oral, 100 mg every twelve hours the first day, then 100 to 200 mg once a day; or 50 to 100 mg every twelve hours.
          Intravenous infusion, 200 mg once a day or 100 mg every twelve hours the first day, then 100 to 200 mg once a day; or 50 to 100 mg every twelve hours.

Product Availability:
  Doxycycline for Oral Suspension USP [25 mg per 5 mL] - Vibramycin.
  Doxycycline Calcium Oral Suspension USP [50 mg per 5 mL] - Vibramycin.
  Doxycycline Hyclate Capsules USP [50 and 100 mg] - Doxy-Caps; Vibramycin; Generic.
  Doxycycline Hyclate Delayed-Release Capsules USP [100 mg] - Doryx.
  Doxycycline Hyclate Tablets USP [100 mg] - Vibra-Tabs; Generic.
  Doxycycline Hyclate for Injection USP [100 and 200 mg] - Vibramycin.

ENALAPRIL (SYSTEMIC)

Pediatric dosing:
  Antihypertensive -
      Oral, initially 100 mcg (0.1 mg) per kg of body weight per day, the dosage being adjusted as needed and tolerated up to a maximum of 500 mcg (0.5 mg) per kg of body weight per day.

Product Availability:
  Enalapril Maleate Tablets USP [2.5, 5, 10, and 20 mg] - Vasotec.

EPINEPHRINE (SYSTEMIC)

Pediatric dosing:
  Bronchodilator; or
  Anaphylactic reactions -
      Subcutaneous, 10 mcg (0.01 mg) (base) per kg of body weight or 300 mcg (0.3 mg) per square meter of body surface up to a maximum of 500 mcg (0.5 mg) per dose, repeated every fifteen minutes for two doses, then every four hours as needed.
  Vasopressor (anaphylactic shock) -
      Intramuscular or subcutaneous, 10 mcg (0.01 mg) (base) per kg of body weight, up to a maximum of 300 mcg (0.3 mg), repeated every five minutes if necessary.
      Intravenous, 10 mcg (0.01 mg) (base) per kg of body weight every five to fifteen minutes as needed, if an inadequate response to intramuscular or subcutaneous administration.
  Cardiac stimulant -
      Intracardiac or intravenous, 5 to 10 mcg (0.005 to 0.01 mg) (base) per kg of body weight or 150 to 300 mcg (0.15 to 0.3 mg) per square meter of body surface, repeated every five minutes if necessary or followed by an intravenous infusion at an initial rate of 0.1 mcg (0.0001 mg) per kg of body weight per minute, the rate being increased in increments of 0.1 mcg (0.0001 mg) per kg of body weight per minute, if necessary, up to a maximum of 1.5 mcg (0.0015 mg) per kg of body weight per minute.

Product Availability:
  Epinephrine Injection USP [10 mcg (0.01 mg) (base) per mL; 100 mcg (0.1 mg) (base) per mL; 500 mcg (0.5 mg) (base) per mL; and 1 mg (base) per mL] - Adrenalin; EpiPen; Generic.

ERYTHROMYCIN (SYSTEMIC)

Pediatric dosing:
  Antibacterial -
      Oral, 7.5 to 12.5 mg per kg of body weight every six hours; or 15 to 25 mg per kg of body weight every twelve hours.
      Intravenous infusion, 3.75 to 5 mg per kg of body weight every six hours.
  Severe infections - 15 to 25 mg per kg of body weight every six hours.

Product Availability:
  Erythromycin Delayed-Release Capsules USP [125 and 250 mg] - Eryc; Generic.
  Erythromycin Tablets USP [250, 333, 400, and 500 mg] - Generic.
  Erythromycin Delayed-Release Tablets USP [250, 333, and 500 mg] - E-Base; Ery-Tab.
  Erythromycin Estolate Capsules USP [250 mg] - Ilosone; Generic.
  Erythromycin Estolate Oral Suspension USP [100 mg per mL; 125 and 250 mg per 5 mL] - Ilosone; Generic.
  Erythromycin Estolate Tablets USP [250 and 500 mg] - Ilosone.
  Erythromycin Estolate Tablets USP (Chewable) [125 and 250 mg] - Ilosone; Generic.
  Erythromycin Ethylsuccinate Oral Suspension USP [200 and 400 mg per 5 mL] - E.E.S.; Pediamycin; Generic.
  Erythromycin Ethylsuccinate for Oral Suspension USP [200 and 400 mg per 5 mL] - E.E.S.; EryPed; Generic.
  Erythromycin Ethylsuccinate Tablets USP [400 mg] - E.E.S.; Generic.
  Erythromycin Ethylsuccinate Tablets USP (Chewable) [200 mg] - E.E.S.
  Sterile Erythromycin Glucceptate USP [500 mg and 1 gram] - Ilotycin.
  Erythromycin Lactobionate for Injection [500 mg and 1 gram] - Erythrocin; Generic.
  Erythromycin Stearate Tablets USP [250 and 500 mg] - Erythrocin; Generic.

ERYTHROMYCIN AND SULFISOXAZOLE (SYSTEMIC)

Pediatric dosing:
 Antibacterial -
  Infants and children 2 months of age and over - The dose can be calculated, based on either the equivalent of erythromycin or sulfisoxazole base, as follows:
   Oral, 12.5 mg (erythromycin) per kg of body weight every six hours for ten days; or
   Oral, 37.5 mg (sulfisoxazole) per kg of body weight every six hours for ten days.

Product Availability:
 Erythromycin Ethylsuccinate and Sulfisoxazole Acetyl for Oral Suspension USP [200 mg of erythromycin and 600 mg of sulfisoxazole per 5 mL] - Pediazole; Generic.

ETHOSUXIMIDE (SYSTEMIC)

Pediatric dosing:
 Anticonvulsant -
  Children up to 6 years of age -
   Oral, 15 to 40 mg per kg of body weight a day; or initially 250 mg once a day, the dosage being increased by an additional 250 mg a day at four- to seven-day intervals until seizure control is obtained or until the total daily dose reaches 1 gram.
  Children 6 years of age and over -
   Oral, 15 to 30 mg per kg of body weight a day; or initially 250 mg two times a day, the dosage being increased by an additional 250 mg a day at four- to seven-day intervals until seizure control is obtained or until the total daily dose reaches 1.5 grams.

Product Availability:
 Ethosuximide Capsules USP [250 mg] - Zarontin.

FENTANYL (SYSTEMIC)

Pediatric dosing:
 Anesthesia, as primary agent in surgery -
  Children up to 2 years of age: Dosage has not been established.
  Children 2 to 12 years of age: Intravenous, 2 to 3 mcg (0.002 to 0.003 mg) (base) per kg of body weight.

Product Availability:
 Fentanyl Citrate Injection USP [50 mcg (0.05 mg) (base) per mL] - Sublimaze; Generic.

FLUDROCORTISONE (SYSTEMIC)

Pediatric dosing:
 Adrenocorticoid (mineralocorticoid) -
  Oral, 50 to 100 mcg (0.05 to 0.1 mg) per day.

Product Availability:
 Fludrocortisone Acetate Tablets USP [100 mcg (0.1 mg)] - Florinef.

FLUNISOLIDE (INHALATION)

Pediatric dosing:
 Asthma -
  Children 4 years of age and older -
   Oral inhalation, 500 mcg (0.5 - 2 metered sprays) two times a day, morning and evening.

Product Availability:
 Flunisolide Inhalation Aerosol [250 mcg (0.25 mg) per metered spray] - AeroBid.

FLUNISOLIDE (NASAL)

Pediatric dosing:
 Rhinitis or Allergic disorders or inflammatory conditions -
  Children 6 to 14 years of age -
   Initial: Nasal, 25 mcg (0.025 mg - 1 metered spray) in each nostril three times a day; or 50 mcg (0.05 mg - 2 metered sprays) in each nostril two times a day (total daily dose, 150 to 200 mcg [0.15 to 0.2 mg]).
   Maintenance: Nasal, 25 mcg (0.025 mg - 1 metered spray) in each nostril once a day (total daily dose, 50 mcg [0.05 mg]).

Product Availability:
 Flunisolide Nasal Solution USP [25 mcg (0.025 mg) per metered spray] - Nasalide.

FLUOXYMESTERONE (SYSTEMIC)

Pediatric dosing:
 Delayed puberty in males -
  Oral, 2.5 to 10 mg per day for a limited duration, usually four to six months.

Product Availability:
 Fluoxymesterone Tablets USP [2, 5, and 10 mg] - Halotestin; Generic.

FLUPHENAZINE (SYSTEMIC)

Pediatric dosing:
 Psychotic disorders -
  Oral, 250 to 750 mcg (0.25 to 0.75 mg) one to four times a day.
  Children 5 to 12 years of age:
   Intramuscular or subcutaneous, 3.125 to 12.5 mg, the dosage being repeated every one to three weeks as needed and tolerated.
  Children 12 years of age and over:
   Intramuscular or subcutaneous, initially 6.25 to 18.75 mg a week, the dosage being increased to 12.5 to 25 mg and administered every one to three weeks as needed and tolerated.

Product Availability:
 Fluphenazine Hydrochloride Elixir USP [2.5 mg per 5 mL] - Prolixin.
 Fluphenazine Hydrochloride Oral Solution USP [5 mg per mL] - Permitil Concentrate; Prolixin Concentrate.
 Fluphenazine Hydrochloride Tablets USP [1, 2.5, 5, and 10 mg] - Permitil; Prolixin; Generic.

FLUPHENAZINE (SYSTEMIC)—*continued*

Fluphenazine Decanoate Injection [25 mg per mL] - Prolixin Decanoate; Generic.

FUROSEMIDE (SYSTEMIC)

Pediatric dosing:
Diuretic -
Oral, initially 2 mg per kg of body weight as a single dose, the dosage then being increased by an additional 1 to 2 mg per kg of body weight at six- to eight-hour intervals, until the desired response is obtained.
Intramuscular or intravenous, initially 1 mg per kg of body weight as a single dose, the dosage then being increased by an additional 1 mg per kg of body weight at two-hour intervals until the desired response is obtained.
Antihypercalcemic -
Intramuscular or intravenous, 25 to 50 mg, the dosage being repeated if necessary every four hours until the desired response is obtained.

Product Availability:
Furosemide Oral Solution [8 and 10 mg per mL] - Lasix; Generic.
Furosemide Tablets USP [20, 40, and 80 mg] - Lasix; Generic.
Furosemide Injection USP [10 mg per mL] - Lasix; Generic.

GENTAMICIN (SYSTEMIC)

Pediatric dosing:
Antibacterial -
Intramuscular or intravenous infusion:
Premature or full-term neonates up to 1 week of age - 2.5 mg per kg of body weight every twelve to twenty-four hours for seven to ten days or more.
Older neonates and infants - 2.5 mg per kg of body weight every eight to sixteen hours for seven to ten days or more.
Children - 2 to 2.5 mg per kg of body weight every eight hours for seven to ten days or more.
Intralumbar or intraventricular:
Infants and children 3 months of age and over - 1 to 2 mg once a day.

Product Availability:
Gentamicin Sulfate Injection USP [2, 10, and 40 mg per mL] - Garamycin; Generic.

GRISEOFULVIN (SYSTEMIC)

Pediatric dosing:
Antifungal -
Oral, 5 mg per kg of body weight or 150 mg per square meter of body surface every twelve hours; or 10 mg per kg of body weight or 300 mg per square meter of body surface once a day.

Product Availability:
Griseofulvin Capsules USP (Microsize) [125 and 250 mg] - Grisactin.
Griseofulvin Oral Suspension USP (Microsize) [125 mg per 5 mL] - Grifulvin V.
Griseofulvin Tablets USP (Microsize) [250 and 500 mg] - Fulvicin-U/F; Grifulvin V; Grisactin.

HALOPERIDOL (SYSTEMIC)

Pediatric dosing:
Children 3 to 12 years of age and 15 to 40 kg of body weight - Psychotic disorders:
Oral, initially 50 mcg (0.05 mg) per kg of body weight a day (in two or three divided doses), the daily dose being increased as needed and tolerated by 500-mcg (0.5 mg) increments at five- to seven-day intervals up to a total of 150 mcg (0.150 mg) per kg of body weight a day.
Nonpsychotic behavior disorders and Tourette's syndrome:
Oral, initially 50 mcg (0.05 mg) per kg of body weight a day (in two or three divided doses), the daily dose being increased as needed and tolerated by 500-mcg (0.5 mg) increments at five- to seven-day intervals up to a total of 75 mcg (0.075 mg) per kg of body weight a day.
Infantile autism:
Oral, 25 mcg (0.025 mg) per kg of body weight a day, up to 50 mcg (0.05 mg) per kg of body weight a day.

Product Availability:
Haloperidol Oral Solution USP [2 mg per mL] - Haldol; Generic.
Haloperidol Tablets USP [500 mcg, 1, 2, 5, 10, and 20 mg] - Haldol; Generic.

HEPARIN (SYSTEMIC)

Pediatric dosing:
Intravenous, 50 USP Units per kg of body weight initially, then 50 to 100 USP Units per kg of body weight every four hours, or as determined by coagulation test results.
Intravenous infusion, 50 USP Units per kg of body weight as a loading dose initially, then 100 USP Units per kg of body weight added and absorbed every four hours or 20,000 USP Units per square meter of body surface every twenty-four hours, or as determined by coagulation test results.

Product Availability:
Heparin Calcium Injection USP [Derived from porcine intestinal mucosa: 25,000 USP Units per mL] -Calciparine.
Heparin Sodium Injection USP [Derived from beef lung: 1000, 5000, 10,000, and 20,000 USP Units per mL; Derived from porcine intestinal mucosa: 1000, 2500, 5000, 7500, 10,000, 15,000, 20,000, 25,000, and 40,000 USP Units per mL] - Liquaemin; Generic.

HYDRALAZINE (SYSTEMIC)

Pediatric dosing:
Antihypertensive; or
Vasodilator, congestive heart failure -
Oral, 750 mcg (0.75 mg) per kg of body weight or 25 mg per square meter of body surface a day divided into two to four doses, the dosage being increased gradually over one to four weeks as needed, up to a maximum of 7.5 mg per kg of body weight or 300 mg a day.
Intramuscular or intravenous, 1.7 to 3.5 mg per kg of body weight or 50 to 100 mg per square meter of body surface a day, divided into four to six daily doses.

Product Availability:
Hydralazine Hydrochloride Tablets USP [10, 25, 50, and 100 mg] - Apresoline; Generic.
Hydralazine Hydrochloride Injection USP [20 mg per mL] - Apresoline; Generic.

HYDROCHLOROTHIAZIDE (SYSTEMIC)

Pediatric dosing:
Antihypertensive -
Oral, 1 to 2 mg per kg of body weight or 30 to 60 mg per square meter of body surface per day, as a single dose or in two divided daily doses, the dosage being adjusted according to response.

Product Availability:
Hydrochlorothiazide Oral Solution [10 and 100 mg per mL] - Generic.
Hydrochlorothiazide Tablets USP [25, 50, and 100 mg] - Esidrix; HydroDIURIL; Generic.

HYDROCORTISONE (SYSTEMIC)

Pediatric dosing:
Adrenocortical insufficiency -
Oral, 560 mcg (0.56 mg) per kg of body weight or 15 to 20 mg per square meter of body surface a day as a single dose or in divided doses.
Intramuscular or intravenous, 186 to 280 mcg (0.186 to 0.28 mg) (base) per kg of body weight or 10 to 12 mg (base) per square meter of body surface a day in three divided doses.
Other indications -
Oral, 2 to 8 mg per kg of body weight or 60 to 240 mg per square meter of body surface a day as a single dose or in divided doses.
Intramuscular, 666 mcg (0.666 mg) to 4 mg (base) per kg of body weight or 20 to 120 mg (base) per square meter of body surface every twelve to twenty-four hours.

Product Availability:
Hydrocortisone Tablets USP [5, 10, and 20 mg] - Cortef; Hydrocortone; Generic.
Hydrocortisone Cypionate Oral Suspension USP [10 mg (base) per 5 mL] - Cortef.
Hydrocortisone Sodium Phosphate Injection USP [50 mg (base) per mL] - Hydrocortone Phosphate; Generic.
Hydrocortisone Sodium Succinate for Injection USP [100, 250, and 500 mg; 1 gram] - A-hydroCort; Solu-Cortef; Generic.

HYDROXYCHLOROQUINE (SYSTEMIC)

Pediatric dosing:
Antiprotozoal - Malaria:
Suppressive - Oral, 6.4 mg (5 mg base) per kg of body weight, not to exceed the adult dose, once every seven days.
Therapeutic - Oral, 32 mg (25 mg base) per kg of body weight administered over a period of three days as follows: 12.9 mg (10 mg base) per kg of body weight, not to exceed a single dose of 800 mg (620 mg base); then 6.4 mg (5 mg base) per kg of body weight, not to exceed

a single dose of 400 mg (310 mg base), six, twenty-four, and forty-eight hours after the first dose.

Product Availability:
Hydroxychloroquine Sulfate Tablets USP [200 mg] - Plaquenil.

HYDROXYZINE (SYSTEMIC)

Pediatric dosing:
Antianxiety agent; or
Sedative-hypnotic -
Oral, 600 mcg (0.6 mg) per kg of body weight as a single dose.
Antihistaminic (H1-receptor); or
Antiemetic -
Oral, 500 mcg (0.5 mg) per kg of body weight or 15 mg per square meter of body surface every six hours as needed.
Adjunct to narcotic medication; or
Antiemetic -
Intramuscular, 1 mg per kg of body weight, or 30 mg per square meter of body surface, as a single dose.

Product Availability:
Hydroxyzine Hydrochloride Syrup USP [10 mg per 5 mL] - Atarax; Generic.
Hydroxyzine Hydrochloride Tablets USP [10, 25, 50, and 100 mg] - Atarax; Generic.
Hydroxyzine Pamoate Capsules USP [25, 50, and 100 mg] - Vistaril; Generic.
Hydroxyzine Pamoate Oral Suspension USP [25 mg per 5 mL] - Vistaril.
Hydroxyzine Hydrochloride Injection USP [25 and 50 mg per mL] - Vistaril; Generic.

IBUPROFEN (SYSTEMIC)

Pediatric dosing:
Antirheumatic (nonsteroidal anti-inflammatory) -
Children 1 to 12 years of age: Oral, initially 30 to 40 mg per kg of body weight a day in three or four divided doses, then reduced to the lowest dose needed to control disease activity.
Antipyretic -
Children 6 months to 12 years of age: Oral, 5 mg per kg of body weight for fevers less than 39.17°C (102.5°F) and 10 mg per kg of body weight for higher fevers. Dosage may be repeated, if necessary, at intervals of 4 to 6 hours or more.

Product Availability:
Ibuprofen Oral Suspension [100 mg per 5 mL] - Children's Advil; PediaProfen.
Ibuprofen Tablets USP [200, 300, 400, 600, and 800 mg] - Motrin; Rufen; Generic.

IMIPRAMINE (SYSTEMIC)

Pediatric dosing:
Antidepressant -
Children up to 6 years of age: Use is not recommended.
Children 6 to 12 years of age: Oral, 10 to 30 mg per day in two divided doses.

IMIPRAMINE (SYSTEMIC)—*continued*

Adolescents: Oral, 25 to 50 mg a day in divided doses, the dosage being adjusted as needed and tolerated, up to 100 mg a day.

Antienuretic -

Oral, 25 mg once a day, one hour before bedtime. If a satisfactory response is not obtained within one week, the dosage may be increased to 50 mg nightly in children under 12 years of age and to 75 mg nightly in children 12 or over.

Product Availability:

Imipramine Hydrochloride Tablets USP [10, 25, and 50 mg] - Tofranil; Generic.

INDOMETHACIN (SYSTEMIC)

Pediatric dosing:

Antirheumatic (nonsteroidal anti-inflammatory) -

Oral or rectal, 1.5 to 2.5 mg per kg of body weight per day, administered in 3 or 4 divided doses, up to a maximum of 4 mg per kg of body weight per day or 150 to 200 mg per day, whichever is less.

Patent ductus arteriosus closure adjunct -

Infants up to 48 hours of age at time of first dose: Intravenous, 200 mcg (0.2 mg) of anhydrous indomethacin per kg of body weight initially. If necessary, one or two additional doses of 100 mcg (0.1 mg) of anhydrous indomethacin per kg of body weight may be given at twelve- to twenty-four-hour intervals.

Infants 2 to 7 days of age at time of first dose: Intravenous, 200 mcg (0.2 mg) of anhydrous indomethacin per kg of body weight initially. If necessary, one or two additional doses of 200 mcg (0.2 mg) of anhydrous indomethacin per kg of body weight may be given at twelve- to twenty-four-hour intervals.

Infants 7 days of age and over at time of first dose: Intravenous, 200 mcg (0.2 mg) of anhydrous indomethacin per kg of body weight initially. If necessary, one or two additional doses of 250 mcg (0.25 mg) of anhydrous indomethacin per kg of body weight may be given at twelve- to twenty-four-hour intervals.

Product Availability:

Indomethacin Capsules USP [25 and 50 mg] - Indocin; Generic.

Indomethacin Oral Suspension USP [25 mg per 5 mL] - Indocin; Generic.

Indomethacin Suppositories USP [50 mg] - Indocin.

Sterile Indomethacin Sodium [1 mg] - Indocin I.V.

ISONIAZID (SYSTEMIC)

Pediatric dosing:

Tuberculosis -

Prophylaxis: Oral or intramuscular, 10 mg per kg of body weight, up to 300 mg, once a day.

Treatment: In combination with other antituberculars - Oral or intramuscular, 10 to 20 mg of isoniazid per kg of body weight, up to 300 mg, once a day.

Product Availability:

Isoniazid Syrup USP [50 mg per 5 mL] - Laniazid; Generic.

Isoniazid Tablets USP [50, 100, and 300 mg] - Nydrazid; Generic.

Isoniazid Injection USP [100 mg per mL] - Nydrazid; Generic.

KETAMINE (SYSTEMIC)

Pediatric dosing:

Anesthetic (general) -

Induction:

Intravenous, 1 to 2 mg (base) per kg of body weight, administered as a single dose or by intravenous infusion at a rate of 500 mcg (0.5 mg) (base) per kg of body weight per minute; or

Intramuscular, 5 to 10 mg (base) per kg of body weight.

Maintenance: Intravenous, 10 to 50 mcg (0.01 to 0.05 mg) (base) per kg of body weight by continuous infusion at a rate of 1 to 2 mg per minute.

Anesthesia, local, adjunct -

Intravenous, 5 to 30 mg (base), prior to administration of the local anesthetic. May be repeated if necessary.

Sedation and analgesia -

Intravenous: 200 to 750 mcg (0.2 to 0.75 mg) (base) per kg of body weight administered over 2 to 3 minutes initially, followed by 5 to 20 mcg (0.005 to 0.02 mg) (base) per kg of body weight per minute as a continuous intravenous infusion.

Intramuscular: 2 to 4 mg (base) per kg of body weight initially, followed by 5 to 20 mcg (0.005 to 0.02 mg) (base) per kg of body weight per minute as a continuous intravenous infusion.

Product Availability:

Ketamine Hydrochloride Injection USP [10, 50, and 100 mg (base) per mL] - Ketalar; Generic.

KETOCONAZOLE (SYSTEMIC)

Pediatric dosing:

Antifungal (systemic) -

[Candidiasis, vulvovaginal]:

Children over 2 years of age - Oral, 5 to 10 mg per kg of body weight once a day for five days.

[Paronychia]; or

[Pneumonia, fungal]; or

[Septicemia, fungal]; or

[Urinary bladder infections, fungal]; or

[Urinary tract infections, fungal]:

Children over 2 years of age - Oral, 5 to 10 mg per kg of body weight once a day.

Other infections:

Children over 2 years of age - Oral, 3.3 to 6.6 mg per kg of body weight once a day.

Product Availability:

Ketoconazole Tablets USP [200 mg] - Nizoral.

Therapy should be continued for at least 1 to 2 weeks in candidiasis and for 6 months or longer in other systemic mycoses.

LEVOTHYROXINE (SYSTEMIC)

Pediatric dosing:

Children less than 6 months of age - Oral, 5 to 6 mcg (0.005 to 0.006 mg) per kg of body weight per day or 25 to 50 mcg (0.025 to 0.05 mg) per day as a single daily dose.

Children 6 to 12 months of age - Oral, 5 to 6 mcg (0.005 to 0.006 mg) per kg of body weight per day or 50 to 75 mcg (0.05 to 0.075 mg) per day as a single daily dose.

Children 1 to 5 years of age - Oral, 3 to 5 mcg (0.003 to 0.005 mg) per kg of body weight per day or 75 to 100 mcg (0.075 to 0.1 mg) per day as a single daily dose.

Children 6 to 10 years of age - Oral, 4 to 5 mcg (0.004 to 0.005 mg) per kg of body weight per day or 100 to 150 mcg (0.1 to 0.15 mg) per day as a single daily dose.

Children over 10 years of age - Oral, 2 to 3 mcg (0.002 to 0.003 mg) per kg of body weight per day as a single daily dose until the adult dose is reached (usually 150 mcg [0.15 mg] per day) up to 200 mcg (0.2 mg) per day.

Hypothyroidism - Intravenous or intramuscular, daily dose equal to 75% of the usual oral pediatric dose.

Product Availability:

Levothyroxine Sodium Tablets USP [12.5, 25, 50, 75, 100, 112, 125, 150, 175, 200, and 300 mcg] - Levothroid; Synthroid; Generic.

Levothyroxine Sodium for Injection [50, 200, and 500 mcg] - Levothroid; Synthroid; Generic.

Levothyroxine Sodium for Injection [100 and 500 mcg] - Levothroid; Generic.

LIDOCAINE (SYSTEMIC)

Pediatric dosing:

Antiarrhythmic -

Continuous intravenous infusion (usually following a loading dose), 30 mcg (range, 20 to 50 mcg) (0.03 mg; range, 0.02 to 0.05 mg) per kg of body weight per minute.

Direct intravenous injection, 1 mg per kg of body weight as a loading dose at a rate of about 25 to 50 mg per minute, the dose being repeated after five minutes if necessary but not exceeding a total dose of 3 mg per kg of body weight; usually followed by continuous intravenous infusion of lidocaine to maintain antiarrhythmic effects.

Product Availability:

Lidocaine Hydrochloride Injection USP (For Continuous Intravenous Infusion) [4% w/v (40 mg per mL); 10% w/v (100 mg per mL); 20% w/v (200 mg per mL)] - Xylocaine; Generic.

Lidocaine Hydrochloride Injection USP (For Direct Intravenous Injection) [1% w/v (10 mg per mL); 2% w/v (20 mg per mL)] - Xylocaine; Generic.

LITHIUM (SYSTEMIC)

Pediatric dosing:

Antimanic -

Children up to 12 years of age: Oral, initially 15 to 20 mg (0.4 to 0.5 mEq) per kg of body weight a day in two or three divided doses, the dosage being adjusted at weekly intervals, based on plasma lithium concentrations.

Children 12 to 18 years -

Acute mania: Oral, initially 300 to 600 mg (8 to 16 mEq) three times a day, the dosage being adjusted as needed and tolerated at weekly intervals.

Maintenance: Oral, 300 mg three or four times a day, the dosage being adjusted as needed and tolerated.

Product Availability:

Lithium Carbonate Capsules USP [150, 300, and 600 mg] - Eskalith; Lithonate; Generic.

Lithium Carbonate Tablets USP [300 mg] - Eskalith; Lithane; Lithotabs; Generic.

Lithium Citrate Syrup USP [8 mEq of lithium ion (equivalent to approximately 300 mg of lithium carbonate) per 5 mL] - Cibalith-S; Generic.

MEPERIDINE (SYSTEMIC)

Pediatric dosing:

Analgesic -

Oral, 1.1 to 1.76 mg per kg of body weight, not to exceed 100 mg, every three to four hours as needed.

Intramuscular (preferred) or subcutaneous, 1.1 to 1.76 mg per kg of body weight, not to exceed 100 mg, every three to four hours as needed.

Preoperative -

Intramuscular (preferred) or subcutaneous, 1 to 2.2 mg per kg of body weight, not to exceed 100 mg, thirty to ninety minutes prior to anesthesia.

Product Availability:

Meperidine Hydrochloride Syrup USP [50 mg per mL] - Demerol; Generic.

Meperidine Hydrochloride Tablets USP [50 and 100 mg] - Demerol; Generic.

Meperidine Hydrochloride Injection USP [25, 50, 75, and 100 mg per mL] - Demeric; Generic.

MEPHENYTOIN (SYSTEMIC)

Pediatric dosing:

Anticonvulsant -

Oral, 25 to 50 mg a day, the dosage being increased by an additional 25 to 50 mg a day at one week intervals until seizure control is obtained.

Product Availability:

Mephenytoin Tablets USP [100 mg] - Mesantoin.

METHACYCLINE (SYSTEMIC)

Pediatric dosing:

Antibacterial; antiprotozoal -

Children 8 years of age and over -

Oral, 1.65 to 3.3 mg per kg of body weight every six hours; or 3.3 to 6.6 mg per kg of body weight every twelve hours.

Product Availability:

Methacycline Hydrochloride Capsules USP [150 and 300 mg] - Rondomycin.

METHOTREXATE (SYSTEMIC)

Pediatric dosing:

Antineoplastic -

Oral or intramuscular, 20 to 40 mg per square meter of body surface, once a week.

METHOTREXATE (SYSTEMIC)—*continued*

Meningeal leukemia -

For children up to 1 year of age: Intrathecal, 6 mg (base) per square meter of body surface every two to five days until the cell count of the CSF returns to normal.

For children 1 year of age: Intrathecal, 8 mg (base) per square meter of body surface every two to five days until the cell count of the CSF returns to normal.

For children 2 years of age: Intrathecal, 10 mg (base) per square meter of body surface every two to five days until the cell count of the CSF returns to normal.

For children 3 years of age and over: Intrathecal, 12 mg (base) per square meter of body surface to a maximum of 12 mg every two to five days until the cell count of the CSF returns to normal.

Product Availability:

Methotrexate Tablets USP [2.5 mg] - Generic.

Methotrexate Sodium Injection USP [2.5 and 25 mg (base) per mL] - Folex PFS; Generic.

Methotrexate Sodium for Injection USP [20, 25, 50, 100, 250 mg; 1 gram] - Folex; Mexate; Generic.

METHYLDOPA (SYSTEMIC)

Pediatric dosing:

Antihypertensive -

Oral, initially 10 mg per kg of body weight or 300 mg per square meter of body surface, divided into two to four doses, the dosage then being adjusted, preferably at intervals of not less than two days, until the desired response is obtained, but not exceeding 65 mg per kg of body weight or 3 grams daily, whichever is less.

Intravenous infusion, 5 to 10 mg per kg of body weight in 5% dextrose injection, administered slowly over a thirty- to sixty-minute period, every six hours if necessary, but not exceeding 65 mg per kg of body weight or 3 grams daily, whichever is less.

Product Availability:

Methyldopa Oral Suspension USP [50 mg per mL] - Aldomet.

Methyldopa Tablets USP [125, 250, and 500 mg] - Aldomet; Generic.

Methyldopate Hydrochloride Injection USP [50 mg per mL] - Aldomet.

METHYLPHENIDATE (SYSTEMIC)

Pediatric dosing:

Attention-deficit hyperactivity disorder -

Children 6 years of age and over: Oral, 5 mg two times a day, before breakfast and lunch, the dosage being increased by 5 to 10 mg at one-week intervals up to a maximum of 60 mg a day.

Product Availability:

Methylphenidate Hydrochloride Tablets USP [5, 10, and 20 mg] - Ritalin; Generic.

METHYLPREDNISOLONE (SYSTEMIC)

Pediatric dosing:

Adrenocortical insufficiency -

Oral, 117 mcg (0.117 mg) per kg of body weight or

3.33 mg per square meter of body surface a day in three divided doses.

Intramuscular, 117 mcg (0.117 mg) (base) per kg of body weight or 3.33 mg (base) per square meter of body surface a day (in three divided doses) every third day; or 39 to 58.5 mcg (0.039 to 0.0585 mg) (base) per kg of body weight or 1.11 to 1.66 mg (base) per square meter of body surface once a day.

[For treatment of acute spinal cord injury] -

Intravenous, 30 mg (base) per kg of body weight administered over fifteen minutes, followed in forty-five minutes by a continuous infusion of 5.4 mg per kg of body weight per hour, for twenty-three hours.

Other indications -

Oral, 417 mcg (0.417 mg) to 1.67 mg per kg of body weight or 12.5 to 50 mg per square meter of body surface per day in three or four divided doses.

Intramuscular, 139 to 835 mcg (0.139 to 0.835 mg) (base) per kg of body weight or 4.16 to 25 mg (base) per square meter of body surface every twelve to twenty-four hours.

Product Availability:

Methylprednisolone Tablets USP [2, 4, 8, 16, 24, and 32 mg] - Medrol; Generic.

Methylprednisolone Sodium Succinate for Injection USP [40, 125, and 500 mg (base); 1 and 2 grams (base)] - A-methaPred; Solu-Medrol; Generic.

METHYLTESTOSTERONE (SYSTEMIC)

Pediatric dosing:

Delayed puberty in males - Buccal, 2.5 to 12.5 mg per day for a limited duration, usually four to six months.

Product Availability:

Methyltestosterone Tablets USP (Buccal) [5 and 10 mg] - Metandren; Oreton; Generic.

METOCLOPRAMIDE (SYSTEMIC)

Pediatric dosing:

Gastrointestinal emptying (delayed) adjunct; or

Peristaltic stimulant -

Children 5 to 14 years of age: Oral, 2.5 to 5 mg three times a day thirty minutes before meals.

Children up to 6 years of age: Intravenous, 100 mcg (0.1 mg) per kg of body weight as a single dose.

Children 6 to 14 years of age: Intravenous, 2.5 to 5 mg as a single dose.

Product Availability:

Metoclopramide Tablets USP [5 and 10 mg] - Reglan; Generic.

Metoclopramide Hydrochloride Syrup [5 mg (base) per 5 mL] - Reglan; Generic.

Metoclopramide Injection USP [5 mg per mL] - Reglan; Generic.

METRONIDAZOLE (SYSTEMIC)

Pediatric dosing:

Antiprotozoal -

Amebiasis: Oral, 11.6 to 16.7 mg per kg of body weight three times a day for ten days.

[Balantidiasis]: Oral, 11.6 to 16.7 mg per kg of body weight three times a day for five days.

[Giardiasis]: Oral, 5 mg per kg of body weight three times a day for five to seven days.

Trichomoniasis: Oral, 5 mg per kg of body weight three times a day for seven days.

[Anthelmintic (systemic)-Dracunculiasis] - Oral, 8.3 mg per kg of body weight, up to a maximum of 250 mg, three times a day for ten days.

Product Availability:
Metronidazole Tablets USP [250 and 500 mg] - Flagyl; Generic.

MEZLOCILLIN (SYSTEMIC)

Pediatric dosing:
Intramuscular or intravenous -
Infants 7 days of age and under: 75 mg per kg of body weight every twelve hours.
Infants 8 to 30 days of age: 75 mg per kg of body weight every six to eight hours.
Infants over 1 month of age and children up to 12 years of age: 50 mg per kg of body weight every four hours.

Product Availability:
Sterile Mezlocillin Sodium USP [1, 2, 3, 4, and 20 grams] - Mezlin.

MIDAZOLAM (SYSTEMIC)

Pediatric dosing:
Sedation, preoperative, and amnesia - Dosage must be individualized; however, as a general guideline:
Intramuscular, 80 to 200 mcg (0.08 to 0.2 mg) per kg of body weight.
Sedation, conscious (endoscopic or cardiovascular procedures) - dosage must be individualized by physician.
Anesthesia, general, adjunct (prior to administration of other general anesthetics) - Dosage must be individualized; however, as a general guideline: Intravenous, 50 to 200 mcg (0.05 to 0.2 mg) per kg of body weight.

Product Availability:
Midazolam Hydrochloride Injection [1 and 5 mg (base) per mL] - Versed.

MINOCYCLINE (SYSTEMIC)

Pediatric dosing:
Antibacterial; antiprotozoal -
Children 8 years of age and over -
Oral or intravenous infusion, 4 mg per kg of body weight initially, then 2 mg per kg of body weight every twelve hours.

Product Availability:
Minocycline Hydrochloride Capsules USP [50 and 100 mg] - Minocin.
Minocycline Hydrochloride Pellet-Filled Capsules [50 and 100 mg] - Minocin.
Minocycline Hydrochloride Oral Suspension USP [50 mg per 5 mL] - Minocin.

Minocycline Hydrochloride Tablets USP [50 and 100 mg] - Minocin.
Sterile Minocycline Hydrochloride USP [100 mg] - Minocin.

MINOXIDIL (SYSTEMIC)

Pediatric dosing:
Children up to 12 years of age -
Initial: Oral, 200 mcg (0.2 mg) per kg of body weight a day as a single dose or as two divided doses, the dosage being adjusted as required (i.e., in increments of 100, 150, 200 mcg per kg of body weight, etc.), up to 50 mg a day.
Maintenance: Oral, 250 mcg (0.25 mg) to 1 mg per kg of body weight a day, as a single dose or in divided daily doses, up to 50 mg a day.

Product Availability:
Minoxidil Tablets USP [2.5 and 10 mg] - Loniten; Generic.

MOXALACTAM (SYSTEMIC)

Pediatric dosing:
Antibacterial -
Intramuscular or intravenous -
Neonates up to 1 week of age: 50 mg per kg of body weight every twelve hours.
Neonates 1 to 4 weeks of age: 50 mg per kg of body weight every eight hours.
Infants: 50 mg per kg of body weight every six hours.
Children: 50 mg per kg of body weight every six to eight hours.

Product Availability:
Moxalactam Disodium for Injection USP [1, 2, and 10 grams] - Moxam.

MUROMONAB-CD3 (SYSTEMIC)

Pediatric dosing:
Immunosuppressant -
Children less than 12 years of age - Intravenous (rapid), 100 mcg (0.1 mg) per kg of body weight per day for ten to fourteen days.

Product Availability:
Muromonab-CD3 Injection [1 mg per mL] - Orthoclone OKT3.

NAFCILLIN (SYSTEMIC)

Pediatric dosing:
Antibacterial -
Neonates -
Oral, 10 mg per kg of body weight every six to eight hours.
Intramuscular, 10 to 20 mg per kg of body weight every twelve hours.
Intravenous, 10 to 20 mg per kg of body weight every four hours; or 20 to 40 mg per kg of body weight every eight hours.
Older infants and children -
Oral, 6.25 to 12.5 mg per kg of body weight every six hours.

NAFCILLIN (SYSTEMIC)—*continued*

Intramuscular, 25 mg per kg of body weight every twelve hours.

Intravenous, 10 to 20 mg per kg of body weight every four hours; or 20 to 40 mg per kg of body weight every eight hours.

Product Availability:
Nafcillin Sodium Capsules USP [250 mg] - Unipen.
Nafcillin Sodium for Oral Solution USP [250 mg per 5 mL] - Unipen.
Nafcillin Sodium Tablets USP [500 mg] - Unipen.
Nafcillin Sodium for Injection USP [500 mg; 1, 2, and 10 grams] - Nafcil; Unipen; Generic.

NALOXONE (SYSTEMIC)

Pediatric dosing:
Neonates -
Opioid-induced depression: Intravenous via the umbilical vein (preferred), intramuscular, or subcutaneous, 10 mcg (0.01 mg) per kg of body weight. The intravenous dose may be repeated at two- to three-minute intervals until the desired response is obtained.
Children -
Opioid toxicity: Intravenous (preferred in emergencies), intramuscular, or subcutaneous, 10 mcg (0.01 mg) per kg of body weight. The intravenous dose may be repeated at two- to three-minute intervals for one or two additional doses.
Postoperative opioid depression: Intravenous, 5 to 10 mcg (0.005 to 0.01 mg) every two to three minutes until adequate ventilation and alertness without significant pain are obtained. If necessary, dosage may be repeated at one- or two-hour intervals.

Product Availability:
Naloxone Hydrochloride Injection USP [20 mcg (0.02 mg) per mL, 400 mcg (0.4 mg) per mL, and 1 mg per mL] - Narcan; Generic.

NAPROXEN (SYSTEMIC)

Pediatric dosing:
Antirheumatic (nonsteroidal anti-inflammatory) - Oral, 10 mg per kg of body weight per day, given in two divided doses.

Product Availability:
Naproxen Oral Suspension [125 mg per 5 mL] - Naprosyn.
Naproxen Tablets USP [250, 373, and 500 mg] - Naprosyn.

NETILMICIN (SYSTEMIC)

Pediatric dosing:
Antibacterial (systemic) - Intramuscular or intravenous:
Neonates up to 6 weeks of age - 2 to 3.25 mg per kg of body weight every twelve hours for seven to fourteen days.
Infants and children 6 weeks to 12 years of age - 1.83 to 2.67 mg per kg of body weight every eight hours;

or 2.75 to 4 mg per kg of body weight every twelve hours for seven to fourteen days.

Product Availability:
Netilmicin Sulfate Injection USP [10 and 100 mg per mL] - Netromycin.

NICLOSAMIDE (SYSTEMIC)

Pediatric dosing:
Diphyllobothrium latum, [Dipylidium caninum], Taenia saginata, and [T. solium] infections -
Children 11 to 34 kg of body weight: Oral, 1 gram as a single dose. May be repeated in seven days if required.
Children over 34 kg of body weight: Oral, 1.5 grams as a single dose. May be repeated in seven days if required.
Hymenolepis nana and [H. diminuta] infections -
Children 11 to 34 kg of body weight: Oral, 1 gram as a single dose the first day, then 500 mg once a day for the next six days. May be repeated in seven to fourteen days in H. nana infections if required.
Children over 34 kg of body weight: Oral, 1.5 grams as a single dose the first day, then 1 gram once a day for the next six days. May be repeated in seven to fourteen days in H. Nana infections if required.

Product Availability:
Niclosamide Chewable Tablets [500 mg] - Niclocide.

NITROFURANTOIN (SYSTEMIC)

Pediatric dosing:
Antibacterial -
Infants and children 1 month of age and over - Oral, 0.75 to 1.75 mg per kg of body weight every six hours.

Product Availability:
Nitrofurantoin Capsules USP [25, 50, and 100 mg] - Macrodantin; Generic.
Nitrofurantoin Oral Suspension USP [25 mg per 5 mL] - Furadantin.
Nitrofurantoin Tablets USP [50 and 100 mg] - Furadantin; Generic.

NORTRIPTYLINE (SYSTEMIC)

Pediatric dosing:
Antidepressant -
Children 6 to 12 years of age: Oral, 10 to 20 mg (base), or 1 to 3 mg per kg of body weight, a day in divided doses.
Adolescents: Oral, 25 to 50 mg, or 1 to 3 mg per kg of body weight, a day in divided doses, the dosage being adjusted as needed and tolerated.

Product Availability:
Nortriptyline Hydrochloride Capsules USP [10, 25, 50, and 75 mg] - Aventyl; Pamelor.
Nortriptyline Hydrochloride Oral Solution USP [10 mg (base) per 5 mL] - Aventyl; Pamelor.

OCTREOTIDE (SYSTEMIC)

Pediatric dosing:
Antidiarrheal (gastrointestinal tumor) -
Subcutaneous, 1 to 10 mcg (0.001 to 0.01 mg) per kg of body weight per day.

Product Availability:
Octreotide Acetate Injection [0.05, 0.1, and 0.5 mg per mL] - Sandostatin.

OXACILLIN (SYSTEMIC)

Pediatric dosing:
Children up to 40 kg of body weight - Oral, intramuscular, or intravenous, 12.5 to 25 mg per kg of body weight every six hours.
Children 40 kg of body weight and over - Oral, intramuscular, or intravenous, 500 mg to 1 gram every four to six hours.

Product Availability:
Oxacillin Sodium Capsules USP [250 and 500 mg] - Bactocill; Prostaphlin; Generic.
Oxacillin Sodium for Oral Solution USP [250 mg per 5 mL] - Prostaphlin; Generic.
Oxacillin Sodium for Injection USP [250, 500 mg; 1, 2, 4, and 10 grams] - Bactocill; Prostaphlin; Generic.

OXANDROLONE (SYSTEMIC)

Pediatric dosing:
Anabolic steroid -
Oral, 250 mcg (0.25 mg) per kg of body weight per day.
[Turner's syndrome] -
Oral, 50 mcg to 125 mcg (0.05 to 0.125 mg) per kg of body weight per day. Generally, the patient should be started and maintained on the lowest effective dose to minimize the potential for adverse effects.

Product Availability:
Oxandrolone Tablets USP [2.5 mg] - Anavar.

PANCRELIPASE (SYSTEMIC)

Pediatric dosing:
Enzyme (pancreatic) replenisher; and
Digestant -
Oral, contents of 1 to 3 capsules with meals, the dosage being adjusted as needed and tolerated.

Product Availability:
Pancrelipase Capsules USP [8000 USP Units of lipase, 30,000 USP Units of protease, and 30,000 USP Units of amylase per capsule] - Cotazym.
Pancrelipase Tablets USP [8000 USP Units of lipase, 30,000 USP Units of protease, and 30,000 USP Units of amylase per tablet; 11,000 USP Units of lipase, 30,000 USP Units of protease, and 30,000 USP Units of amylase per tablet] - Viokase, Ilozyme.

PARAMETHADIONE (SYSTEMIC)

Pediatric dosing:
Anticonvulsant -
Children up to 2 years of age: Oral, 100 mg three times a day.
Children 2 to 6 years of age: Oral, 200 mg three times a day.
Children 6 years of age and over: Oral, 300 mg three times a day.

Product Availability:
Paramethadione capsules USP
150 mg (Paradione)
300 mg (Paradione tartrazine)
Paramethadione oral solution USP
300 mg per mL (Paradione-alcohol 65%)

PEMOLINE (SYSTEMIC)

Pediatric dosing:
Children 6 years of age and over: Oral, 37.5 mg as a single dose each morning, the dosage being increased by 18.75 mg a day at one-week intervals until the desired response is obtained, up to a maximum of 112.5 mg a day.

Product Availability:
Pemoline Tablets [18.75, 37.5, and 75 mg] - Cylert.
Pemoline Chewable Tablets [37.5 mg] - Cylert Chewable.

PENICILLAMINE (SYSTEMIC)

Pediatric dosing:
Chelating agent -
Infants over 6 months of age and young children: Oral, 250 mg as a single dose administered in fruit juice.
Older children - Oral, 250 mg four times a day.
Antiurolithic -
Oral, 7.5 mg per kg of body weight four times a day.
Antidote (to heavy metals) -
Oral, 30 to 40 mg per kg of body weight or 600 to 750 mg per square meter of body surface per day for one to six months.

Product Availability:
Penicillamine Capsules USP [125 and 250 mg] - Cuprimine.
Penicillamine Tablets USP [250 mg] - Depen.

PENICILLIN G (SYSTEMIC)

Pediatric dosing:
Antibacterial -
Infants and children up to 12 years of age - Oral, 4167 to 15,000 Units (2.5 to 9.3 mg) per kg of body weight every four hours; 6250 to 22,500 Units (3.75 to 14 mg) per kg of body weight every six hours; or 8333 to 30,000 Units (5 to 18.7 mg) per kg of body weight every eight hours.
Children 12 years of age and over - Oral, 200,000 to 500,000 Units (125 to 312 mg) every six to eight hours.

PENICILLIN G (SYSTEMIC)—*continued*

Premature and full-term neonates - Intramuscular or intravenous, 30,000 Units per kg of body weight every twelve hours.

Older infants and children - Intramuscular or intravenous, 4167 to 16,667 Units per kg of body weight every four hours; or 6250 to 25,000 Units per kg of body weight every six hours.

[Lyme disease] -

Intravenous, 41,667 to 100,000 Units every four hours for ten to fourteen days.

Product Availability:

Penicillin G Potassium for Oral Solution USP [200,000 Units (125 mg) per 5 mL and 400,000 Units (250 mg) per 5 mL] - Pentids; Generic.

Penicillin G Potassium Tablets USP [200,000 Units (125 mg); 250,000 Units (156 mg); 400,000 Units (250 mg); 500,000 Units (312 mg); 800,000 Units (500 mg)] - Pentids; Generic.

Penicillin G Potassium for Injection USP [1,000,000; 5,000,000; 10,000,000; 20,000,000 Units] - Pfizerpen; Generic.

PENICILLIN V (SYSTEMIC)

Pediatric dosing:

Antibacterial -

Infants and children up to 12 years of age - Oral, 2.5 to 9.3 mg (4167 to 15,000 Units) per kg of body weight every four hours; 3.75 to 14 mg (6250 to 22,500 Units) per kg of body weight every six hours; or 5 to 18.7 mg (8333 to 30,000 Units) per kg of body weight every eight hours.

Children 12 years of age and over - Oral, 125 to 500 mg (200,000 to 800,000 Units) every six to eight hours.

Product Availability:

Penicillin V Potassium for Oral Solution USP [125 mg (200,000 Units) per 5 mL; 250 mg (400,000 Units) per 5 mL] - Pen Vee K; V-Cillin K; Generic.

Penicillin V Potassium Tablets USP [125 mg (200,000 Units); 250 mg (400,000 Units); 500 mg (800,000 Units)] - Pen Vee K; V-Cillin K; Generic.

PENTAMIDINE (SYSTEMIC)

Pediatric dosing:

Pneumonia, Pneumocystis carinii -

Intramuscular or intravenous infusion, over one to two hours, 4 mg per kg of body weight once a day for fourteen days or longer in patients with AIDS.

[Leishmaniasis, visceral] -

Intramuscular or intravenous infusion, over one to two hours, 2 to 4 mg per kg of body weight once a day for up to fifteen days. May be repeated in one to two weeks if required.

[Leishmaniasis, cutaneous] -

Intramuscular or intravenous infusion, over one to two hours, 2 to 4 mg per kg of body weight once or twice a week until the lesions heal.

[Trypanosomiasis, African (without CNS involvement)] -

Treatment: Intramuscular or intravenous overinfusion, over one to two hours, 4 mg per kg of body weight once a day for ten days.

Product Availability:

Sterile Pentamidine Isethionate [300 mg] - Pentam 300.

PHENOBARBITAL (SYSTEMIC)

Pediatric dosing:

Anticonvulsant -

Oral, 1 to 6 mg (base) per kg of body weight per day, as a single dose or in divided doses.

Neonates:

Intravenous:

Loading dose: 10 to 20 mg per kg slow pace for 10 minutes.

Maintenance: 2 to 5 mg per kg every 12 hours usually 12 to 24 hours after the loading dose. Give orally when patient is stable.

Sedative-hypnotic -

Hypnotic: Dosage must be individualized by physician.

Sedative:

Daytime - Oral, 2 mg (base) per kg of body weight or 60 mg per square meter of body surface three times a day.

Preoperative - Oral, 1 to 3 mg (base) per kg of body weight.

[Antihyperbilirubinemia] -

Neonates: Oral, 5 to 10 mg (base) per kg of body weight per day for the first few days after birth.

Children up to 12 years of age: Oral, 1 to 4 mg (base) per kg of body weight three times a day.

Product Availability:

Phenobarbital Capsules [16 mg] - Solfoton.

Phenobarbital Elixir USP [20 mg per 5 mL] - Generic.

Phenobarbital Tablets USP [8, 15, 16, 30, 32, 60, 65, 100 mg] - Solfoton; Generic.

PHENYTOIN (SYSTEMIC)

Pediatric dosing:

Anticonvulsant -

Initial: Oral, 5 mg per kg of body weight a day, divided into two or three doses, the dosage being adjusted as needed and tolerated but not to exceed 300 mg a day.

Maintenance: Oral, 4 to 8 mg per kg of body weight or 250 mg per square meter of body surface a day, divided into two or three doses.

Anticonvulsant in status epilepticus -

Intravenous, direct, 15 to 20 mg per kg of body weight, or 250 mg per square meter of body surface area, administered at a rate of 1 to 3 mg per kg of body weight per minute, not exceeding 50 mg a minute.

Product Availability:

Phenytoin Oral Suspension USP [30 and 125 mg per 5 mL] - Dilantin.

Phenytoin Tablets USP (Chewable) [50 mg] - Dilantin Infatabs.

Extended Phenytoin Sodium Capsules USP [30 and 100 mg] - Dilantin Kapseals; Generic.

Prompt Phenytoin Sodium Capsules USP [30 and 100 mg] - Diphenylan; Generic.

Phenytoin Sodium Injection USP [50 mg per mL] - Dilantin; Generic.

PIMOZIDE (SYSTEMIC)

Pediatric dosing:

Children 12 years of age and over -

Tourette's disorder -

Oral, initially 1 to 2 mg a day in divided doses, the dosage being increased gradually every other day as needed and tolerated.

[Psychotic disorders] -

Oral, 2 to 4 mg once a day, the dosage being increased at weekly intervals by 2 to 4 mg a day.

Product Availability:

Pimozide Tablets USP [2 mg] - Orap.

POTASSIUM CITRATE AND CITRIC ACID (SYSTEMIC)

Pediatric dosing:

Alkalizer, urinary -

Oral, initially 5 to 15 mL (1.1 to 3.3 grams of potassium citrate [10 to 30 mEq of potassium ion]) four times a day, after meals and at bedtime, the dosage being adjusted as needed and tolerated.

Product Availability:

Potassium Citrate and Citric Acid Oral Solution USP [1.1 grams of potassium citrate (10 mEq of potassium ion) and 334 mg of citric acid per 5 mL] - Polycitra-K.

POTASSIUM PHOSPHATES (SYSTEMIC)

Pediatric dosing:

Electrolyte replenisher -

Children up to 4 years of age: Oral, the equivalent of 200 mg (6.4 mmol) of phosporus in 60 mL of water four times a day, after meals and at bedtime.

Children 4 years of age and over: Oral, 1 gram (228 mg or 7.4 mmol of phosphorus) in 180 to 240 mL of water four times a day, with meals and at bedtime.

Product Availability:

Monobasic Potassium Phosphate Tablets for Oral Solution [500 mg (114 mg [3.7 mmol] of phosphorus)] - K-Phos Original.

Potassium Phosphates Capsules for Oral Solution [1.45 grams (250 mg [8 mmol] of phosphorus)] - Neutra-Phos-K.

Potassium Phosphates for Oral Solution [71 grams (250 mg [8 mmol] of phosphorus)] - Neutra-Phos-K.

PRAZOSIN (SYSTEMIC)

Pediatric dosing:

Antihypertensive -

Children under 7 years of age -

Oral, initially 250 mcg (0.25 mg) (base) two or

three times a day, adjusted according to response.

Children 7 to 12 years of age -

Oral, initially 500 mcg (0.5 mg) (base) two or three times a day, adjusted according to response.

Product Availability:

Prazosin Hydrochloride Capsules USP [1, 2, and 5 mg] - Minipress; Generic.

Prazosin Hydrochloride Tablets [1, 2, and 5 mg] - Minipress.

PREDNISOLONE (SYSTEMIC)

Pediatric dosing:

Adrenocortical insufficiency -

Oral, 140 mcg (0.14 mg) per kg of body weight or 4 mg per square meter of body surface a day in three divided doses.

Intramuscular, 140 mcg (0.14 mg) per kg of body weight or 4 mg per square meter of body surface a day (in three divided doses) every third day; or 46 to 70 mcg (0.046 to 0.07 mg) per kg of body weight or 1.33 to 2 mg per square meter of body surface once a day.

Other indications -

Oral, 500 mcg (0.5 mg) to 2 mg per kg of body weight or 15 to 60 mg per square meter of body surface a day in three or four divided doses.

Intramuscular, 166 mcg (0.166 mg) to 1 mg per kg of body weight or 5 to 30 mg per square meter of body surface every twelve to twenty-four hours.

Product Availability:

Prednisolone Syrup USP [15 mg per 5 mL] - Prelone.

Prednisolone Tablets USP [5 mg] - Delta-Cortef; Generic.

Prednisolone Sodium Phosphate Oral Solution [5 mg (base) per mL] - Pediapred.

Sterile Prednisolone Acetate Suspension USP [25 and 50 mg per mL] - Predicort-50; Generic.

Prednisolone Sodium Phosphate Injection USP [20 mg (phosphate) per mL] - Hydeltrasol; Generic.

PREDNISONE (SYSTEMIC)

Pediatric dosing:

For nephrosis -

Children 18 months to 4 years of age: Oral, initially 7.5 to 10 mg four times a day.

Children 4 to 10 years of age: Oral, initially 15 mg four times a day.

Children 10 years of age and older: Oral, initially 20 mg four times a day.

For rheumatic carditis, leukemia, tumors -

Oral, 500 mcg (0.5 mg) per kg of body weight or 15 mg per square meter of body surface four times a day for two to three weeks; then 375 mcg (0.375 mg) per kg of body weight or 11.25 mg per square meter of body surface four times a day for four to six weeks.

For tuberculosis (with concurrent antitubercular therapy) -

Oral, 500 mcg (0.5 mg) per kg of body weight or 15 mg per square meter of body surface four times a day for two months.

PREDNISONE (SYSTEMIC)—*continued*

Product Availability:
Prednisone Oral Solution USP [5 mg per 5 mL and 5 mg per mL] - Predisone; Generic.
Prednisone Syrup USP [5 mg per 5 mL] - Liquid Pred.
Prednisone Tablets USP [1, 2.5, 5, 10, 20, 25, and 50 mg] - Meticorten; Orasone; Generic.

PRIMAQUINE (SYSTEMIC)

Pediatric dosing:
Malaria -
Oral, 680 mcg (390 mcg base) (0.68 mg [0.39 mg base]) per kg of body weight once a day for fourteen days.

Product Availability:
Primaquine Phosphate Tablets USP [26.3 mg (15 mg base)] - Generic.

PRIMIDONE (SYSTEMIC)

Pediatric dosing:
Anticonvulsant -
Children up to 8 years of age:
Initial - Oral, 50 mg at bedtime for the first three days, the daily dose being increased to 50 mg two times a day for the fourth, fifth, and sixth days and then increased to 100 mg two times a day for the seventh, eighth, and ninth days.
Maintenance - Oral, on the tenth day, 125 to 250 mg three times a day (or 10 to 25 mg per kg of body weight a day given in divided doses), the dosage being adjusted according to patient needs and tolerance.
Children 8 years of age and over -
Initial - Oral, 100 or 125 mg once a day at bedtime for the first three days, the daily dose being increased to 100 to 125 mg two times a day for the fourth, fifth, and sixth days, and then increased to 100 or 125 mg three times a day for the seventh, eighth, and ninth days. On the tenth day, a maintenance dosage of 250 mg three times a day may be established and then adjusted according to patient needs and tolerance but not to exceed 2 grams a day.
Maintenance - Oral, 250 mg three or four times a day.

Product Availability:
Primidone Oral Suspension USP [250 mg per 5 mL] - Mysoline.
Primidone Tablets USP [50 and 250 mg] - Mysoline; Generic.

PROBENECID (SYSTEMIC)

Pediatric dosing:
Antibiotic therapy adjunct -
Penicillin or cephalosporin therapy (general):
Children up to 2 years of age - Use is not recommended.
Children 2 to 14 years of age or

Children weighing up to 50 kg - Oral, initially 25 mg per kg of body weight or 700 mg per square meter of body surface area, then 10 mg per kg of body weight or 300 mg per square meter of body surface area, four times a day.
Children weighing over 50 kg - Oral, 500 mg four times a day.
Treatment of gonorrhea: Postpubertal children and/or those weighing over 45 kg - Oral, 25 mg per kg of body weight, up to a maximum of 1 gram, as a single dose administered simultaneously or concurrently with appropriate antibiotic therapy.

Product Availability:
Probenecid Tablets USP [500 mg] - Benemid; Generic.

PROCAINAMIDE (SYSTEMIC)

Pediatric dosing:
Antiarrhythmic -
Oral, 12.5 mg per kg of body weight or 375 mg per square meter of body surface four times a day.

Product Availability:
Procainamide Hydrochloride Capsules USP [250, 375, and 500 mg] - Pronestyl; Generic.
Procainamide Hydrochloride Tablets USP [250, 375, and 500 mg] - Pronestyl; Generic.

PROCHLORPERAZINE (SYSTEMIC)

Pediatric dosing:
Psychotic disorders -
Children 2 to 12 years of age:
Oral, 2.5 mg (base) two or three times a day.
Intramuscular, 132 mcg (0.132 mg) (base) per kg of body weight.
Children 12 years of age and over: Oral, 5 to 10 mg (base) three or four times a day, the dosage being gradually increased every two to three days as needed and tolerated.
Nausea and vomiting -
Children 9 to 13 kg of body weight: Oral or rectal, 2.5 mg (base) one or two times a day, not to exceed 7.5 mg per day.
Children 14 to 17 kg of body weight: Oral or rectal, 2.5 mg (base) two or three times a day, not to exceed 10 mg per day.
Children 18 to 39 kg of body weight: Oral or rectal, 2.5 mg (base) three times a day or 5 mg two times a day, not to exceed 15 mg per day.
Children 2 to 12 years of age: Intramuscular, 132 mcg (0.132 mg) (base) per kg of body weight.

Product Availability:
Prochlorperazine Edisylate Syrup USP [5 mg (base) per 5 mL] - Compazine.
Prochlorperazine Maleate Tablets USP [5, 10, and 25 mg] - Compazine; Generic.
Prochlorperazine Edisylate Injection USP [5 mg (base) per mL] - Compazine; Generic.
Prochlorperazine Suppositories USP [2.5, 5, and 25 mg] - Compazine.

PROMETHAZINE (SYSTEMIC)

Pediatric dosing:
  Children 2 years of age and older -
    Antihistaminic (H1-receptor): Oral, intramuscular, or rectal, 125 mcg (0.125 mg) per kg of body weight or 3.75 mg per square meter of body surface every four to six hours, or 500 mcg (0.5 mg) per kg of body weight or 15 mg per square meter of body surface at bedtime as needed; or 5 to 12.5 mg three times a day or 25 mg at bedtime as needed.
    Antiemetic: Oral, intramuscular, or rectal, 250. to 500 mcg (0.25 to 0.5 mg) per kg of body weight or 7.5 to 15 mg per square meter of body surface every four to six hours as needed; or 10 to 25 mg every four to six hours as needed.
    Antivertigo agent: Oral or rectal, 500 mcg (0.5 mg) per kg of body weight or 15 mg per square meter of body surface every twelve hours as needed; or 10 to 25 mg two times a day as needed.
    Sedative-hypnotic: Oral, intramuscular, or rectal, 500 mcg (0.5 mg) to 1 mg per kg of body weight or 15 to 30 mg per square meter of body surface as needed; or 10 to 25 mg as needed.

Product Availability:
  Promethazine Hydrochloride Syrup USP [6.25 and 25 mg per 5 mL] - Phenergan; Generic.
  Promethazine Hydrochloride Tablets USP [12.5, 25, and 50 mg] - Phenergan; Generic.
  Promethazine Hydrochloride Injection USP [25 and 50 mg per mL] - Phenergan; Generic.
  Promethazine Hydrochloride Suppositories USP [12.5, 25, and 50 mg] - Phenergan; Generic.

PROPRANOLOL (SYSTEMIC)

Pediatric dosing:
  Antiarrhythmic; or
  Antihypertensive -
    Initial: Oral, 500 mcg (0.5 mg) to 1 mg per kg of body weight per day in two to four divided doses has been used as an initial dose, the dosage being adjusted as necessary to treat hypertension and prevent supraventricular tachycardia.
    Maintenance: Oral, 2 to 4 mg per kg per day in two divided doses.
  Antiarrhythmic -
    Slow intravenous, 10 to 100 mcg (0.01 to 0.1 mg) per kg of body weight (up to a maximum of 1 mg per dose), repeated every six to eight hours if necessary.

Product Availability:
  Propranolol Hydrochloride Oral Solution [4, 8, and 80 mg per mL] - Generic.
  Propranolol Hydrochloride Tablets USP [10, 20, 40, 60, 80, and 90 mg] - Inderal; Generic.
  Propranolol Hydrochloride Injection USP [1 mg per mL] - Inderal; Generic.

PROPYLTHIOURACIL (SYSTEMIC)

Pediatric dosing:
  Hyperthyroidism -
    Initial:
        Children 6 to 10 years of age - Oral, 50 to 150 mg a day as one to four divided daily doses.
        Children 10 years of age and over - Oral, 50 to 300 mg a day as one to four divided daily doses.
    Maintenance: Oral, determined by response.
  Neonatal thyrotoxicosis: Oral, 10 mg per kg of body weight a day in divided daily doses.

Product Availability:
  Propylthiouracil Tablets USP [50 mg] - Generic.

PROTRIPTYLINE (SYSTEMIC)

Pediatric dosing:
  Antidepressant -
        Adolescents: Oral, initially 5 mg three times a day, the dosage being adjusted as needed and tolerated.

Product Availability:
  Protriptyline Hydrochloride Tablets USP [5 and 10 mg] - Vivactil.

PYRANTEL (ORAL-LOCAL)

Pediatric dosing:
  Children 2 years of age and over-
  Ascariasis -
        Oral, 11 mg (base) per kg of body weight as a single dose. May be repeated in two to three weeks if required.
  Enterobiasis -
        Oral, 11 mg (base) per kg of body weight as a single dose. Repeat in two to three weeks.
  [Hookworm infection] -
        Oral, 11 mg (base) per kg of body weight once a day for three days.
  [Trichostrongyliasis] -
        Oral, 11 mg (base) per kg of body weight as a single dose.

Product Availability:
  Pyrantel Pamoate Oral Suspension USP [250 mg (base) per 5 mL] - Antiminth.

PYRAZINAMIDE (SYSTEMIC)

Pediatric dosing:
  Tuberculosis -
    In combination with other antitubercular drugs -
        Oral, 7.5 to 15 mg per kg of body weight twice a day; or 15 to 30 mg per kg of body weight once a day.

Product Availability:
  Pyrazinamide Tablets USP [500 mg] - Generic.

PYRIMETHAMINE (SYSTEMIC)

Pediatric dosing:
Malaria -
Treatment:
Chloroquine-resistant P. falciparum malaria - Oral, 1.25 mg per kg of body weight of pyrimethamine in combination with 25 mg per kg of body weight of sulfadoxine as a single dose on day three of quinine therapy.
Chloroquine-resistant P. falciparum malaria acquired in Southeast Asia, Bangladesh, East Africa, or the Amazon basin - Oral, 1 mg per kg of body weight of pyrimethamine in combination with 10 mg per kg of body weight of mefloquine and 20 mg per kg of body weight of sulfadoxine as a single dose.
Presumptive treatment, for self-treatment of febrile illness when medical care is not immediately available:
Children 5 to 10 kg of body weight - Oral, 12.5 mg of pyrimethamine and 250 mg of sulfadoxine combination (1/2 tablet) as a single dose.
Children 11 to 20 kg of body weight - Oral, 25 mg of pyrimethamine and 500 mg of sulfadoxine combination (1 tablet) as a single dose.
Children 21 to 30 kg of body weight - Oral, 37.5 mg of pyrimethamine and 750 mg of sulfadoxine combination (1 1/2 tablets) as a single dose.
Children 31 to 45 kg of body weight - Oral, 50 mg of pyrimethamine and 1 gram of sulfadoxine combination (2 tablets) as a single dose.
Children greater than 45 kg of body weight - Oral, 75 mg of pyrimethamine and 1.5 grams of sulfadoxine combination (3 tablets) as a single dose.
Toxoplasmosis - In combination with the usual pediatric dose of a sulfapyrimidine-type sulfonamide: Oral, 1 mg of pyrimethamine per kg of body weight once a day for one to three days; then 0.5 mg of pyrimethamine per kg of body weight once a day for four to six weeks.

Product Availability:
Pyrimethamine Tablets USP [25 mg] - Daraprim.

QUINACRINE (SYSTEMIC)

Pediatric dosing:
Giardiasis -
Oral, 2 mg per kg of body weight three times a day for five to seven days.

Product Availability:
Quinacrine Hydrochloride Tablets USP [100 mg] - Atabrine.

QUINIDINE (SYSTEMIC)

Pediatric dosing:
Antiarrhythmic -
Oral, 6 mg per kg of body weight or 180 mg per square meter of body surface five times a day.

Product Availability:
Quinidine Sulfate Capsules USP [200 and 300 mg] - Cin-Quin; Generic.
Quinidine Sulfate Tablets USP [100, 200, and 300 mg] - Cin-Quin; Quinora; Generic.

RANITIDINE (SYSTEMIC)

Pediatric dosing:
Oral, 2 to 4 mg per kg of body weight, two times a day up to a maximum dose fo 300 mg per day.

Product Availability:
Ranitidine Tablets USP [150 and 300 mg] - Zantac.
Ranitidine Hydrochloride Syrup [150 mg (base) per 10 mL] - Zantac.

RESERPINE (SYSTEMIC)

Pediatric dosing:
Antihypertensive -
Oral, 5 to 20 mcg (0.005 to 0.02 mg) per kg of body weight or 150 to 600 mcg (0.15 to 0.6 mg) per square meter of body surface a day in one or two divided daily doses.

Product Availability:
Reserpine Tablets USP [100 mcg (0.1 mg); 250 mcg (0.25 mg); and 1 mg] - Serpalan; Serpasil; Generic.

RIBAVIRIN (SYSTEMIC)

Pediatric dosing:
Respiratory syncytial virus (RSV) infection, lower respiratory tract -
Oral inhalation, via a Viratek Small Particle Aerosol Generator (SPAG) Model SPAG-2 utilizing a 20-mg-per-mL ribavirin concentration in the reservoir, over a twelve- to eighteen-hour period per day for a least three to a maximum of seven days.

Product Availability:
Ribavirin for Inhalation Aerosol [6 grams] - Virazole.

RIFAMPIN (SYSTEMIC)

Pediatric dosing:
Infants up to 1 month of age -
Tuberculosis: In combination with other antituberculars -
Oral or intravenous, 10 to 20 mg per kg of body weight once a day.
Meningococcal carriers (asymptomatic):
Oral or intravenous, 5 mg per kg of body weight every twelve hours for four doses.
Children 1 month of age and over -
Tuberculosis: In combination with other antituberculars -
Oral or intravenous, 10 to 20 mg per kg of body weight once a day.
Meningococcal carriers (asymptomatic):
Oral or intravenous, 10 mg per kg of body weight every twelve hours for four doses.

Product Availability:
Rifampin Capsules USP [150 and 300 mg] - Rifadin; Rimactane.
Rifampin for Injection USP [600 mg] - Rifadin IV.

SOMATREM (SYSTEMIC)

Pediatric dosing:
Hormone, growth, human -
Intramuscular or subcutaneous, initially 0.025 to 0.05 mg (0.065 to 0.13 International Units [IU]) per kg of body weight every other day or three times a week.

Product Availability:
Somatrem for Injection [5 mg (approximately 13 IU) per vial] - Protropin.

SOMATROPIN, RECOMBINANT (SYSTEMIC)

Pediatric dosing:
Hormone, growth, human -
Intramuscular or subcutaneous, initially 0.025 to 0.05 mg (0.065 to 0.13 International Unit [IU]) per kg of body weight every other day or three times a week.

Product Availability:
Somatropin, Recombinant, for Injection [5 mg (approximately 13 IU)] - Humatrope.

SPECTINOMYCIN (SYSTEMIC)

Pediatric dosing:
Antibacterial -
Children up to 45 kg of body weight - Intramuscular, 40 mg per kg of body weight as a single dose.
Children 45 kg of body weight and over - Intramuscular, 2 grams as a single dose.

Product Availability:
Sterile Spectinomycin Hydrochloride for Suspension USP [2 and 4 grams] - Trobicin.

SPIRONOLACTONE (SYSTEMIC)

Pediatric dosing:
Diuretic or antihypertensive - Edema, ascites, or hypertension:
Initial -
Oral, 1 to 3 mg per kg of body weight or 30 to 90 mg per square meter of body surface a day as a single daily dose or in two to four divided doses, the dosage being readjusted after five days. Dosage may be increased up to three times the initial dose.
Maintenance: oral 1.65 to 3.3 mg of spironolactone and of hydrochlorthiazide per kg of body weight a day in divided doses

Product Availability:
Spironolactone Tablets USP [25, 50, and 100 mg] - Aldactone; Generic.

STANOZOLOL (SYSTEMIC)

Pediatric dosing:
Angioedema prophylactic -
Children up to 6 years of age - Oral, 1 mg a day, to be administered only during an attack.
Children 6 to 12 years of age - Oral, up to 2 mg a day, to be administered only during an attack.

Product Availability:
Stanozolol Tablets USP [2 mg] - Winstrol.

STREPTOMYCIN (SYSTEMIC)

Pediatric dosing:
Antibacterial (antimycobacterial) - Tuberculosis:
Intramuscular - In combination with other antimycobacterials, 20 mg per kg of body weight once a day. Maximum dose per day should not exceed 1 gram.
Antibacterial (systemic) - Other infections:
Intramuscular - In combination with other antibacterials, 5 to 10 mg per kg of body weight every six hours; or 10 to 20 mg per kg of body weight every twelve hours.

Product Availability:
Streptomycin Sulfate Injection USP [400 mg per mL] - Generic.
Sterile Streptomycin Sulfate USP [1 and 5 grams] - Generic.

SULFADOXINE AND PYRIMETHAMINE (SYSTEMIC)

Pediatric dosing:
Malaria -
Acute attack: The following amounts as a single dose, administered alone or sequentially with quinine:
Infants up to 1 month of age: Use is contraindicated since sulfonamides may cause kernicterus in neonates.
Infants and children 1 month to 4 years of age: Oral, 1/2 tablet.
Children 4 to 8 years of age: Oral, 1 tablet.
Children 9 to 14 years of age: Oral, 2 tablets.
Chemoprophylaxis:
Infants up to 2 months of age - Use is contraindicated since sulfonamides may cause kernicterus in neonates.
Infants and children 2 months to 4 years of age - Oral, 1/4 tablet once every seven days; or 1/2 tablet once every fourteen days.
Children 4 to 8 years of age - Oral, 1/2 tablet once every seven days; or 1 tablet once every fourteen days.
Children 9 to 14 years of age - Oral, 3/4 tablet once every seven days; or 1 1/2 tablets once every fourteen days.

Product Availability:
Sulfadoxine and Pyrimethamine Tablets USP [500 mg of sulfadoxine and 25 mg of pyrimethamine] - Fansidar.

SULFAMETHOXAZOLE (SYSTEMIC)

Pediatric dosing:
Antibacterial -
Infants and children 2 months of age and over - Oral, 50 to 60 mg per kg of body weight (maximum - 2 grams) initially, then 25 to 30 mg per kg of body weight every twelve hours.

Product Availability:
Sulfamethoxazole Oral Suspension USP [500 mg per 5 mL] - Gantanol.
Sulfamethoxazole Tablets USP [500 mg] - Gantanol; Generic.

SULFAMETHOXAZOLE AND TRIMETHOPRIM (SYSTEMIC)

Pediatric dosing:
Antibacterial (systemic) -
Infants and children up to 40 kg of body weight: Oral, 4 mg of trimethoprim and 20 mg of sulfamethoxazole per kg of body weight every twelve hours.
Children 40 kg of body weight and over: Oral, 160 mg of trimethoprim and 800 mg of sulfamethoxazole every twelve hours.
Intravenous infusion, 2 to 2.5 mg of trimethoprim and 10 to 12.5 mg of sulfamethoxazole per kg of body weight every six hours; 2.7 to 3.3 mg of trimethoprim and 13.3 to 16.7 mg of sulfamethoxazole per kg of body weight every eight hours; or 4 to 5 mg of trimethoprim and 20 to 25 mg of sulfamethoxazole per kg of body weight every twelve hours.
Antiprotozoal - Pneumocystis carinii pneumonia:
Oral, 3.75 to 5 mg of trimethoprim and 18.75 to 25 mg of sulfamethoxazole per kg of body weight every six hours.
Intravenous infusion, 3.75 to 5 mg of trimethoprim and 18.75 to 25 mg of sulfamethoxazole per kg of body weight every six hours; or 5.0 to 6.7 mg of trimethoprim and 25 to 33.3 mg of sulfamethoxazole per kg of body weight every eight hours.

Product Availability:
Sulfamethoxazole and Trimethoprim Oral Suspension USP [40 mg of trimethoprim and 200 mg of sulfamethoxazole per 5 mL] - Bactrim; Septra; Generic.
Sulfamethoxazole and Trimethoprim Tablets USP [80 mg of trimethoprim and 400 mg of sulfamethoxazole; 160 mg of trimethoprim and 800 mg of sulfamethoxazole] - Bactrim; Septra; Generic.
Sulfamethoxazole and Trimethoprim Concentrate for Injection USP [80 mg of trimethoprim and 400 mg of sulfamethoxazole per 5 mL] - Bactrim; Septra; Generic.

SULFASALAZINE (SYSTEMIC)

Pediatric dosing:
Bowel disease (inflammatory) suppressant -
Infants 2 years of age and over:
Initial - Oral, 6.7 to 10 mg per kg of body weight every four hours; 10 to 15 mg per kg of body weight every six hours; or 13.3 to 20 mg per kg of body weight every eight hours.
Maintenance - Oral, 7.5 to 10 mg per kg of body weight every six hours.

Product Availability:
Sulfasalazine Oral Suspension [250 mg per 5 mL] - Azulfidine.
Sulfasalazine Tablets USP [500 mg] - Azulfidine; Generic.

SULFISOXAZOLE (SYSTEMIC)

Pediatric dosing:
Antibacterial:
Infants and children 2 months of age and over - Oral, 75 mg per kg of body weight or 2 grams per square meter of body surface initially, then 25 mg per kg of body weight or 667 mg per square meter of body surface every four hours; or 37.5 mg per kg of body weight or 1 gram per square meter of body surface every six hours.

Product Availability:
Sulfisoxazole Tablets USP [500 mg] - Gantrisin; Generic.
Sulfisoxazole Acetyl Oral Suspension USP [500 mg per 5 mL] - Gantrisin.
Sulfisoxazole Acetyl Oral Syrup [500 mg per 5 mL] - Gantrisin.

TETRACYCLINE (SYSTEMIC)

Pediatric dosing:
Antibacterial (systemic); or
Antiprotozoal -
Children 8 years of age and over:
Oral, 6.25 to 12.5 mg per kg of body weight every six hours; or 12.5 to 25 mg per kg of body weight every twelve hours.
Intramuscular, 5 to 8.3 mg per kg of body weight every eight hours; or 7.5 to 12.5 mg per kg of body weight every twelve hours. Maximum daily dose should not exceed 250 mg.
Intravenous, 5 to 10 mg per kg of body weight every twelve hours.

Product Availability:
Tetracycline Oral Suspension USP [125 mg per 5 mL] - Achromycin V; Sumycin; Generic.
Tetracycline Hydrochloride Capsules USP [250 and 500 mg] - Achromycin; Sumycin; Generic.
Tetracycline Hydrochloride Tablets USP [250 and 500 mg] - Sumycin.
Tetracycline Hydrochloride for Injection USP (Intramuscular) [100 and 250 mg] - Achromycin.
Tetracycline Hydrochloride for Injection USP (Intravenous) [500 mg] - Achromycin.

THEOPHYLLINE (SYSTEMIC)

Pediatric dosing:
Bronchodilator -
Acute Attack:
Loading dose -
For patients not currently receiving theophylline preparations: Children up to 16 years of age - Oral, the equivalent of 5 to 6 mg of anhydrous theophylline per kg of body weight.
For patients currently receiving theophylline preparations: A serum theophylline measure-

ment should be obtained immediately, if possible. The loading dose for theophylline is based on the principle that each 0.5 mg of theophylline per kg of lean (ideal) body weight will result in a 1 (range, 0.5 to 1.6) mcg per mL increase in serum theophylline concentration. If a serum theophylline measurement cannot be obtained rapidly and the patient's condition requires immediate therapy, a single dose of the equivalent of 2.5 mg of anhydrous theophylline per kg of body weight may be administered if there are no symptoms of theophylline toxicity.

Maintenance (in acute attack) -
Children up to 6 months of age: Oral, the equivalent of anhydrous theophylline - Dose in mg per kg of body weight every eight hours = (0.07) (age in weeks) + 1.7.
Children 6 months to 1 year of age: Oral, the equivalent of anhydrous theophylline - Dose in mg per kg of body weight every six hours = (0.05) (age in weeks) + 1.25.
Children 1 to 9 years of age: Oral, the equivalent of anhydrous theophylline - 5 mg per kg of body weight every six hours.
Children 9 to 12 years of age: Oral, the equivalent of anhydrous theophylline - 4 mg per kg of body weight every six hours.
Children 12 to 16 years of age: Oral, the equivalent of anhydrous theophylline - 3 mg per kg of body weight every six hours.
Chronic therapy: Oral, the equivalent of anhydrous theophylline - Initially, 16 mg per kg of body weight, up to a maximum of 400 mg, per day in three or four divided doses at six- to eight-hour intervals. The dosage may be increased, if tolerated, in approximately 25% increments at two- to three-day intervals, up to the following maximum doses without measurement of serum concentration:
Children up to 1 year of age - Dose in mg per kg of body weight per day = (0.3) (age in weeks) + 8.0.
Children 1 to 9 years of age - 22 mg per kg of body weight per day.
Children 9 to 12 years of age - 20 mg per kg of body weight per day.
Adolescents 12 to 16 years of age - 18 mg per kg of body weight per day.
Adolescents 16 years of age and over - 13 mg per kg of body weight or 900 mg per day, whichever is less.

Product Availability:
Theophylline Capsules USP [100, 200, 250, and 260 mg] - Somophyllin-T; Generic.
Theophylline Elixir [27 and 50 mg (equivalent of anhydrous theophylline) per 5 mL] - Accurbron; Generic.
Theophylline Oral Solution [27 and 53.3 mg (equivalent of anhydrous theophylline) per 5 mL] - Aerolate.
Theophylline Oral Suspension [100 mg (equivalent of anhydrous theophylline) per 5 mL] - Elixicon.
Theophylline Syrup [27 and 50 mg (equivalent of anhydrous theophylline) per 5 mL] - Accurbron; Solu-Phyllin.
Theophylline Tablets USP [100, 125, 200, 250, and 300 mg] - Slo-Phyllin; Theolair; Generic.
Theophylline Sodium Glycinate Elixir USP [110 mg (equivalent to 55 mg of anhydrous theophylline) per 5 mL] - Synophylate.

THIORIDAZINE (SYSTEMIC)

Pediatric dosing:
Psychotic disorders -
Children 2 to 12 years of age: Oral, 250 mcg (0.25 mg) to 3 mg (hydrochloride) per kg of body weight or 7.5 mg per square meter of body surface four times a day; or 10 to 25 mg two or three times a day.
Children 12 years of age and over -
Initial: Oral, 25 to 100 mg (hydrochloride) three times a day, the dosage being adjusted gradually as needed and tolerated.
Maintenance: Oral, 10 to 200 mg (hydrochloride) two to four times a day.

Product Availability:
Thioridazine Oral Suspension [25 and 100 mg (hydrochloride) per 5 mL] - Mellaril-S.
Thioridazine Hydrochloride Oral Solution USP [30 and 100 mg per mL] - Mellaril Concentrate; Generic.
Thioridazine Hydrochloride Tablets USP [10, 15, 25, 50, 100, 150, and 200 mg] - Mellaril; Generic.

TICARCILLIN (SYSTEMIC)

Pediatric dosing:
Neonates up to 2 kg of body weight - Septicemia, pneumonia, skin and soft-tissue, intra-abdominal, and genitourinary tract infections: Intramuscular or intravenous, 100 mg per kg of body weight initially, then 75 mg per kg of body weight every eight hours during the first week of life; followed by 100 mg per kg of body weight every four hours thereafter.
Neonates 2 kg of body weight and over - Septicemia, pneumonia, skin and soft-tissue, intra-abdominal, and genitourinary tract infections: Intramuscular or intravenous, 100 mg per kg of body weight initially, then 75 mg per kg of body weight every four to six hours during the first two weeks of life; followed by 100 mg per kg of body weight every four hours thereafter.
Children up to 40 kg of body weight -
Septicemia, pneumonia, skin and soft-tissue, intra-abdominal, and genitourinary tract infections: Intravenous infusion, 33.3 to 50 mg per kg of body weight every four hours; or 50 to 75 mg per kg of body weight every six hours.
Urinary tract infections, bacterial (complicated): Intravenous infusion, 25 to 33.3 mg per kg of body weight every four hours; or 37.5 to 50 mg per kg of body weight every six hours.
Urinary tract infections, bacterial (uncomplicated): Intramuscular or intravenous, 12.5 to 25 mg per kg of body weight every six hours; or 16.7 to 33.3 mg per kg of body weight every eight hours.

Product Availability:
Sterile Ticarcillin Disodium USP [1, 3, 6, 20, and 30 grams] - Ticar.

TOBRAMYCIN (SYSTEMIC)

Pediatric dosing:
Antibacterial (systemic)-
Intramuscular or intravenous infusion:
Premature or full-term neonates up to 1 week of age - Up to 2 mg per kg of body weight every twelve to twenty-four hours.

TOBRAMYCIN (SYSTEMIC)—*continued*

Older infants and children - 1.5 to 1.9 mg per kg of body weight every six hours; or 2 to 2.5 mg per kg of body weight every eight to sixteen hours.

Product Availability:
Tobramycin Sulfate Injection USP [10 and 40 mg per mL] - Nebcin; Generic.
Sterile Tobramycin Sulfate USP [1.2 grams] - Nebcin.

TOLMETIN (SYSTEMIC)

Pediatric dosing:
Antirheumatic (nonsteroidal anti-inflammatory) -
Children 2 years of age and over -
Initial - Oral, 20 mg (free acid) per kg of body weight a day in divided doses.
Maintenance - Oral, 15 to 30 mg (free acid) per kg of body weight a day in divided doses.

Product Availability:
Tolmetin Sodium Capsules USP [400 mg] - Tolectin DS.
Tolmetin Sodium Tablets USP [200 and 600 mg] - Tolectin.

TRAZODONE (SYSTEMIC)

Pediatric dosing:
Antidepressant -
Children 6 to 18 years of age: Oral, initially 1.5 to 2 mg per kg of body weight a day in divided doses, the dosage being increased gradually at three- or four-day intervals, as needed and tolerated up to a maximum of 6 mg per kg of body weight a day.

Product Availability:
Trazodone Hydrochloride Tablets [50, 100, 150, and 300 mg] - Desyrel; Generic.

TRIAMCINOLONE (INHALATION)

Pediatric dosing:
Asthma -
Children 6 to 12 years of age - Oral inhalation, 100 to 200 mcg (0.1 to 0.2 mg - one or two metered sprays) three or four times a day. Dosage must be adjusted according to patient response.

Product Availability:
Triamcinolone Acetonide Inhalation Aerosol [100 mcg (0.1 mg) per metered spray] - Azmacort.

TRIAMCINOLONE (SYSTEMIC)

Pediatric dosing:
Adrenocortical insufficiency -
Oral, 117 mcg (0.117 mg) per kg of body weight or 3.3 mg per square meter of body surface a day as a single dose or in divided doses.
Other indications -
Oral, 416 mcg (0.416 mg) to 1.7 mg per kg of body weight or 12.5 to 50 mg per square meter of body surface a day as a single dose or in divided doses.

Children 6 to 12 years of age -
Intra-articular, intrabursal, or tendon-sheath injection, 2.5 to 15 mg, repeated as needed.
Intramuscular, 40 mg, repeated at four-week intervals if necessary; or 30 to 200 mcg (0.03 to 0.2 mg) per kg of body weight or 1 to 6.25 mg per square meter of body surface, repeated at one- to seven-day intervals.

Product Availability:
Triamcinolone Tablets USP [1, 2, 4, 8, and 16 mg] - Aristocort; Kenacort; Generic.
Triamcinolone Diacetate Syrup USP [2 mg (diacetate) per 5 mL; 4.85 mg anhydrous diacetate (4 mg base) per 5 mL] - Aristocort; Kenacort Diacetate.
Sterile Triamcinolone Acetonide Suspension USP [3, 10, and 40 mg per mL] - Kenalog; Tiramonide; Generic.

TRIAMTERENE (SYSTEMIC)

Pediatric dosing:
Diuretic -
Initial: Oral, 2 to 4 mg per kg of body weight or 120 mg per square meter of body surface a day or on alternate days in divided doses.
Maintenance: Oral, increased to 6 mg per kg of body weight a day according to individual requirements up to a maximum of 300 mg a day in divided doses.

Product Availability:
Triamterene Capsules USP [50 and 100 mg] - Dyrenium.

TRIKATES (SYSTEMIC)

Pediatric dosing:
Potassium replacement -
Oral, 15 to 30 mEq of potassium per square meter of body surface or 2 to 3 mEq per kg of body weight a day, administered in divided doses and well diluted in water or juice.

Product Availability:
Trikates Oral Solution USP [15 mEq of potassium per 5 mL] - Tri-K; Generic.

TRIMEPRAZINE (SYSTEMIC)

Pediatric dosing:
Antihistaminic (H1-receptor) -
Children 2 to 3 years of age: Oral, 1.2 mg (base) at bedtime or three times a day as needed.
Children 3 years of age and over: Oral, 2.5 mg (base) at bedtime or three times a day as needed.

Product Availability:
Trimeprazine Tartrate Syrup USP [2.5 mg (base) per 5 mL] - Temaril; Generic.
Trimeprazine Tartrate Tablets USP [2.5 mg (base)] - Temaril.

TRIMETHADIONE (SYSTEMIC)

Pediatric dosing:
Anticonvulsant -
Oral, 13 mg per kg of body weight or 335 mg per square meter of body surface three times a day; or for
Children up to 2 years of age: Oral, 100 mg three times a day.
Children 2 to 6 years of age: Oral, 200 mg three times a day.
Children 6 years of age and over: Oral, 300 mg three or four times a day.

Product Availability:
Trimethadione Capsules USP [300 mg] - Tridione.
Trimethadione Oral Solution USP [200 mg per 5 mL] - Tridione.
Trimethadione Tablets USP [150 mg] - Tridione Dulcets.

TRIMETHOBENZAMIDE (SYSTEMIC)

Pediatric dosing:
Antiemetic -
Oral or rectal, 15 mg per kg of body weight a day as needed, divided into three or four doses.

Product Availability:
Trimethobenzamide Hydrochloride Capsules USP [100 and 250 mg] - Tigan; Generic.
Trimethobenzamide Hydrochloride Suppositories [100 and 200 mg] - Tigan; Generic.

TRIMIPRAMINE (SYSTEMIC)

Pediatric dosing:
Antidepressant -
Adolescents: Oral, initially 50 mg (base) a day in divided doses, the dosage being adjusted as needed and tolerated, up to a maximum of 100 mg a day.

Product Availability:
Trimipramine Maleate Capsules [25, 50, and 100 mg] - Surmontil; Generic.

TRIPELENNAMINE (SYSTEMIC)

Pediatric dosing:
Antihistaminic (H1-receptor) -
Oral, 1.25 mg per kg of body weight or 37.5 mg per square meter of body surface every six hours as needed, not to exceed 300 mg per day.

Product Availability:
Tripelennamine Hydrochloride Tablets USP [25 and 50 mg] - PBZ; Generic.

TRIPROLIDINE (SYSTEMIC)

Pediatric dosing:
Antihistaminic (H1-receptor) -
Children 4 months to 2 years of age: Oral, 312 mcg (0.312 mg) every six to eight hours as needed.

Children 2 to 4 years of age: Oral, 625 mcg (0.625 mg) every six to eight hours as needed.
Children 4 to 6 years of age: Oral, 937 mcg (0.937 mg) every six to eight hours as needed.
Children 6 to 12 years of age: Oral, 1.25 mg every six to eight hours as needed.

Product Availability:
Triprolidine Hydrochloride Syrup USP [1.25 mg per 5 mL] - Actidil; Generic.
Triprolidine Hydrochloride Tablets USP [2.5 mg] - Actidil; Alleract.

VALPROIC ACID (SYSTEMIC)

Pediatric dosing:
Anticonvulsant -
Children 1 to 12 years of age -
Monotherapy: Oral, initially, 15 to 45 mg per kg of body weight a day, the dosage being increased at one-week intervals by 5 to 10 mg per kg of body weight a day as needed and tolerated.
Polytherapy: Oral, 30 to 100 mg per kg of body weight a day.

Product Availability:
Valproic Acid Capsules USP [250 mg] - Depakene; Generic.
Valproic Acid Syrup USP [250 mg per 5 mL] - Depakene; Generic.

VANCOMYCIN (ORAL-LOCAL)

Pediatric dosing:
Antibiotic-associated pseudomembranous colitis caused by Clostridium difficile; or
Staphylococcal enterocolitis -
Oral, 11 mg per kg of body weight every six hours for five to ten days. May be repeated if necessary.

Product Availability:
Vancomycin Hydrochloride Capsules USP [125 and 250 mg] - Vancocin.
Vancomycin Hydrochloride for Oral Solution USP [250 mg per 5 mL; 500 mg per 6 mL] - Vancocin.

VANCOMYCIN (SYSTEMIC)

Pediatric dosing:
Prophylaxis - Prophylaxis of endocarditis in penicillin-allergic patients with prosthetic heart valves or congenital, rheumatic, or other acquired valvular heart disease who are undergoing:
Dental procedures or surgical procedures of the upper respiratory tract - Intravenous infusion, 20 mg per kg of body weight, beginning one hour prior to the procedure and repeated in eight hours.
[Gastrointestinal and genitourinary tract procedures] - Intravenous infusion, 20 mg per kg of body weight, beginning one hour prior to the procedure, and given concurrently with either gentamicin, 2 mg per kg of body weight intramuscularly or intravenously, or streptomycin, 20 mg per kg of body weight intra-

VANCOMYCIN (SYSTEMIC)—*continued*

muscularly, beginning one-half to one hour prior to the procedure; both are repeated in eight hours.

Treatment -

Neonates up to 1 week of age - Intravenous infusion, 15 mg per kg of body weight initially, followed by 10 mg per kg of body weight every twelve hours.

Neonates and infants 1 week to 1 month of age - Intravenous infusion, 15 mg per kg of body weight initially, followed by 10 mg per kg of body weight every eight hours.

Children - Intravenous infusion, 10 mg per kg of body weight every six hours; or 20 mg per kg of body weight every twelve hours.

Product Availability:
Sterile Vancomycin Hydrochloride USP [500 mg; 1 and 5 grams] - Vancoled; Generic.

VERAPAMIL (SYSTEMIC)

Pediatric dosing:
Antiarrhythmic; or
Antihypertensive -

For infants less than 1 year and children 1 to 15 years of age - Oral, 4 to 8 mg per kg of body weight per day in divided doses.

The following doses should be intravenously administered slowly over a two-minute period, with continuous ECG monitoring. If response is not adequate, a repeat dose may be administered thirty minutes after completion of initial dose.

Infants up to 1 year of age - Initially, 100 to 200 mcg (0.1 to 0.2 mg) per kg of body weight (usual single dose range, 0.75 to 2 mg).

Children 1 to 15 years of age - Initially, 100 to 300 mcg (0.1 to 0.3 mg) per kg of body weight (usual single dose range, 2 to 5 mg) not to exceed a total of 5 mg. For repeat dose, thirty minutes after initial dose, do not exceed 10 mg as a single dose.

Product Availability:
Verapamil Tablets USP [40, 80, and 120 mg] - Calan; Isoptin; Generic.
Verapamil Injection USP [2.5 mg (HCl) per mL] - Calan; Isoptin; Generic.

ZIDOVUDINE (SYSTEMIC)

Pediatric dosing:
Children 3 months to 12 years of age - Oral, 180 mg/m^2 every six hours.
Children 13 years of age and older -
Symptomatic HIV infection - Oral, 100 mg every four hours (600 mg per day).
Asymptomatic HIV infection - Oral, 100 mg every four hours while awake (500 mg per day).
120 mg/m^2, infused over one hour, every six hours.

Product Availability:
Zidovudine Capsules [100 mg] - Retrovir.
Zidovudine Syrup [50 mg per 5 mL] - Retrovir.
Zidovudine Injection [200 mg per 20 mL] - Retrovir.

ACKNOWLEDGEMENT: We thank Ms. Rita Barrafato for her invaluable assistance in the preparation of this formulary.

Revised Pharmacokinetic Constants for use Under Système International

ROBERT G. PETERSON

INTRODUCTION

Clinical pharmacologic estimations of alterations in dosage based upon laboratory-measured plasma levels are commonly used in medical practice. There exist both empirical and measured relationships between desired therapeutic effect and plasma levels as well as with undesired or toxic side effects at plasma levels above the "therapeutic range" for many drugs. The mathematical relationships are usually expressed in straightforward equations. For example, to estimate a loading dose to be administered to achieve a desired plasma concentration (usually selected to be within the therapeutic range) the following relationship may be used:

$$\text{loading dose (mg/kg)} = V_D \text{ (l/kg)} \times C_p \text{ (mg/l)}.$$

The appropriate loading dose to administer is estimated by multiplying a constant referred to as the "apparent volume of distribution" (V_D) for the drug times the desired plasma level (C_p) to be achieved. Clinical judgment dictates the selection of the desired plasma level and usually the intention would be to place the patient into the low, mid, or upper limits of the therapeutic range for the drug based upon severity of illness, past medical history, and other clinical data. V_D is available in many reference sources[1-4] and is simply inserted into the equation. Table 1 gives an alphabetical listing of drugs with the kinetic constants discussed in this article and is based upon data from those reference sources.

V_D is a pharmacologic term. It may be looked upon as the volume in the body into which any amount of a given drug that is administered will be diluted. Thus, if V_D of phenytoin is 0.64 l/kg and a desired plasma level is 15 mg/l the estimated loading dose would be:

$$\text{loading dose (mg/kg)} = 0.64 \text{ l/kg} \times 15 \text{ mg/l}$$
$$= 9.6 \text{ mg/kg}$$

This would be an appropriate dose to administer to a patient not currently receiving phenytoin. For patients who already have a pre-existing plasma level of phenytoin, but where the clinical decision has been to raise this to a higher, perhaps more aggressive level (as an example,

to raise a level of 15 mg/l to 19 mg/l), the calculation is:

$$\text{incremental loading dose (mg/kg)} = V_D \text{ (l/kg)} \times \Delta C_p \text{ (mg/l)},$$

where ΔC_p is the change in the desired plasma level; in this example $19 - 15 = 4$ mg/l.

$$\text{Incremental loading dose} = 0.64 \text{ l/kg} \times 4 \text{ mg/l}$$
$$= 2.56 \text{ mg/kg}$$

The calculations are simple, but the concept of V_D is more complex. Rarely can one discover the actual "volume" referred to in the body. It may appear that the drug is diluted or "distributed" into this volume, hence the terminology "apparent volume of distribution," but in reality the drug is diluted not only by plasma, extracellular fluid and other *real* fluid compartments, but it is bound to proteins or lipids and concentrated in cells, at times manyfold higher than in plasma. The result is that the volume referred to as V_D is purely a pharmacologic quantity and not intended to be an actual physiologic volume. This results in some drugs having apparently very large V_D values. Take digoxin, for example. Its V_D is 7 l/kg in humans. A 70-kg man would have an apparent volume into which any digoxin was administered of more than 500 liters! Since 1 liter of water weighs 1 kg this is a physical impossibility; however, if one calculates the appropriate loading dose for digoxin (in practice given as divided doses over a "digitalization" period), the use of this large distribution volume is pharmacologically accurate.

USE OF SYSTEME INTERNATIONAL IN CLINICAL PHARMACOLOGY

A unique system of reporting for laboratory values was introduced into clinical use in the 1970s largely in European countries. This was an extension of the metric system already used in medicine. Under système international (SI) the standard quantity for substrate or drug is the mole. In practice, this becomes the millimole, micromole, and nanomole as well because a volume must always be in liters. Therefore, a small concentration of a drug in plasma, as in the case of digoxin, would be reported as 1.5×10^{-9} mol/l or 1.5 nmol/l. The mole, of course, is related to a drug's molecular weight insofar as a quantity of a drug in grams that is equal to its molecular

Text continued on page 646

From Developmental Pharmacology and Therapeutics 11:338–346, 1988. Copyright © S. Karger AG, Basel, Switzerland. Reprinted with permission.

TABLE I.   KINETIC CONSTANTS

Molecular Weight	Generic Drug Name	V_D l/kg	Cl_p l/kg/h	V_{DSI}	Cl_{SI}
336.43	Acebutolol	1.2	0.408	0.4037	0.1373
151.16	Acetaminophen	0.95	0.3	0.1436	0.0453
180.15	Acetylsalicylic acid	0.15	0.558	0.027	0.1005
225.21	Acyclovir	0.69	0.2022	0.1554	0.0455
308.77	Alprazolam	1.03	0.084	0.318	0.0259
249.34	Alprenolol	3.3	0.9	0.8228	0.2244
585.62	Amikacin	0.27	0.078	0.1581	0.0457
277.39	Amitriptyline	14	0.75	3.8835	0.208
365.41	Amoxicillin	0.41	0.318	0.1498	0.1162
924.11	Amphotericin B	4	0.0258	3.6964	0.0238
349.42	Ampicillin	0.28	0.102	0.0978	0.0356
187.2	Amrinone	1.2	0.258	0.2246	0.0483
266.34	Atenolol	0.55	0.0462	0.1465	0.0123
277.29	Azathioprine	0.81	3.42	0.2246	0.9483
392.45	Betamethasone	1.4	0.174	0.5494	0.0683
414.37	Bretylium tosylate	5.9	0.612	2.4448	0.2536
246.31	Busulfan	0.99	0.27	0.2438	0.0665
194.19	Caffeine	0.61	0.084	0.1185	0.0163
217.28	Captopril	0.7	0.762	0.1521	0.1656
236.26	Carbamazepine	1.4	0.078	0.3308	0.0184
378.42	Carbenicillin	0.18	0.0408	0.0681	0.0154
214.04	Carmustine (BCNU)	3.3	3.36	0.7063	0.7192
462.5	Cefamandole	0.16	0.168	0.074	0.0777
454.5	Cefazolin	0.12	0.057	0.0545	0.0259
542.56	Cefonicid	0.11	0.0192	0.0597	0.0104
645.68	Cefoperazone	0.09	0.072	0.0581	0.0465
519.56	Ceforanide	0.14	0.0156	0.0727	0.0081
455.48	Cefotaxime	0.24	0.0804	0.1093	0.0366
427.46	Cefoxitin	0.31	0.198	0.1325	0.0846
546.58	Ceftazidime	0.23	0.063	0.1257	0.0344
383.4	Ceftizoxime	0.36	0.066	0.138	0.0253
424.4	Cefuroxime	0.19	0.0564	0.0806	0.0239
347.4	Cephalexin	0.26	0.258	0.0903	0.0896
396.44	Cephalothin	0.26	0.402	0.1031	0.1594
445.45	Cephapirin	0.13	0.258	0.0579	0.1149
349.41	Cephradine	0.25	0.306	0.0874	0.1069
304.23	Chlorambucil	0.86	0.033	0.2616	0.01
323.14	Chloramphenicol	0.94	0.144	0.3038	0.0465

TABLE I. KINETIC CONSTANTS (*Continued*)

Molecular Weight	Generic Drug Name	V_D l/kg	Cl_p l/kg/h	V_{DSI}	Cl_{SI}
299.75	Chlordiazepoxide	0.3	0.0324	0.0899	0.0097
295.72	Chlorothiazide	0.2	0.27	0.0591	0.0798
318.88	Chlorpromazine	21	0.516	6.6965	0.1645
276.75	Chlorpropamide	0.097	0.0018	0.0268	0.0005
338.78	Chlorthalidone	3.9	0.096	1.3212	0.0325
252.34	Cimetidine	1	0.462	0.2523	0.1166
300.05	Cisplatin	0.51	1.02	0.153	0.3061
424.98	Clindamycin	0.66	0.21	0.2805	0.0892
242.71	Clofibrate	0.11	0.0072	0.0267	0.0017
315.72	Clonazepam	3.2	0.093	1.0103	0.0294
230.1	Clonidine	2.1	0.186	0.4832	0.0428
332.74	Clorazepate	0.33	0.108	0.1098	0.0359
435.88	Cloxacillin	0.094	0.132	0.041	0.0575
303.35	Cocaine	2.1	2.1	0.637	0.637
261.1	Cyclophosphamide	0.78	0.078	0.2037	0.0204
243.22	Cytarabine	3	0.78	0.7297	0.1897
248.3	Dapsone	1.5	0.0384	0.3725	0.0095
266.37	Desipramine	34	1.8	9.0566	0.4795
392.45	Dexamethasone	0.82	0.222	0.3218	0.0871
284.76	Diazepam	1.1	0.0228	0.3132	0.0065
230.7	Diazoxide	0.21	0.0036	0.0484	0.0008
470.33	Dicloxacillin	0.086	0.096	0.0404	0.0452
764.92	Digitoxin	0.54	0.0033	0.4131	0.0025
750.92	Digoxin	7	0.0528	5.2564	0.0396
414.52	Diltiazem	5.3	0.69	2.197	0.286
255.35	Diphenhydramine	6.5	0.588	1.6598	0.1501
339.47	Disopyramide	0.59	0.072	0.2003	0.0244
301.39	Dobutamine	0.2	3.54	0.0603	1.0669
279.37	Doxepin	20	0.84	5.5874	0.2347
462.46	Doxycycline	0.75	0.0318	0.3468	0.0147
246.15	Edrophonium	1.1	0.576	0.2708	0.1418
733.92	Erythromycin	0.78	0.546	0.5725	0.4007
204.31	Ethambutol	1.6	0.516	0.3269	0.1054
46.07	Ethanol	0.54	7.44	0.0249	0.3428
141.17	Ethosuximide	0.72	0.0114	0.1016	0.0016
336.46	Fentanyl	4	0.78	1.3458	0.2624
313.3	Flunitrazepam	3.3	0.21	1.0339	0.0658
130.08	Fluorouracil	0.25	0.96	0.0325	0.1249

Table continued on following page

TABLE I. KINETIC CONSTANTS (*Continued*)

Molecular Weight	Generic Drug Name	V_D l/kg	Cl_p l/kg/h	V_{DSI}	Cl_{SI}
387.89	Flurazepam	22	0.27	8.5336	0.1047
330.77	Furosemide	0.11	0.12	0.0364	0.0397
375.88	Haloperidol	17.8	0.708	6.6907	0.2661
236.26	Hexobarbital	1.2	0.234	0.2835	0.0553
160.18	Hydralazine	1.5	3.36	0.2403	0.5382
297.72	Hydrochlorothiazide	0.83	0.294	0.2471	0.0875
206.27	Ibuprofen	0.15	0.045	0.0309	0.0093
280.4	Imipramine	23	0.9	6.4492	0.2524
357.81	Indomethacin	0.26	0.12	0.093	0.0429
137.15	Isoniazid	0.67	0.222	0.0919	0.0304
236.14	Isosorbide dinitrate	1.5	2.7	0.3542	0.6376
237.74	Ketamine	2.9	1.146	0.6894	0.2725
254.29	Ketoprofen	0.11	0.072	0.028	0.0183
328.41	Labetalol	10	1.32	3.2841	0.4335
234.33	Lidocaine	1.1	0.552	0.2578	0.1294
321.16	Lorazepam	1.3	0.066	0.4175	0.0212
370.92	Lorcainide	6.4	1.05	2.3739	0.3895
305.2	Melphalan	0.62	0.312	0.1892	0.0952
247.35	Meperidine	4.4	1.02	1.0883	0.2523
152.19	Mercaptopurine	0.56	0.66	0.0852	0.1004
345.9	Methadone	3.8	0.084	1.3144	0.0291
284.3	Methohexital	2.2	0.654	0.6255	0.1859
454.46	Methotrexate	0.96	0.096	0.4363	0.0436
211.22	Methyldopa	0.37	0.186	0.0782	0.0393
374.46	Methylprednisolone	0.84	0.228	0.3145	0.0854
267.38	Metoprolol	4.2	0.9	1.123	0.2406
171.16	Metronidazole	1.1	0.078	0.1883	0.0134
179.27	Mexiletine	9.5	0.618	1.7031	0.1108
457.49	Minocycline	0.4	0.018	0.183	0.0082
209.25	Minoxidil	12	0.009	2.511	0.0019
295.33	Morphine	3.3	0.9	0.9746	0.2658
520.48	Moxalactam	0.25	0.06	0.1301	0.0312
309.42	Nadolol	2.1	0.174	0.6498	0.0538
436.46	Nafcillin	0.35	0.45	0.1528	0.1964
327.37	Naloxone	2	1.5	0.6547	0.4911
230.26	Naproxen	0.16	0.0078	0.0368	0.0018
209.29	Neostigmine	0.7	0.504	0.1465	0.1055
475.6	Netilmicin	0.2	0.078	0.0951	0.0371

TABLE I. KINETIC CONSTANTS (*Continued*)

Molecular Weight	Generic Drug Name	V_D l/kg	Cl_p l/kg/h	V_{DSI}	Cl_{SI}
162.23	Nicotine	2.6	1.11	0.4218	0.1801
346.34	Nifedipine	1.2	0.618	0.4156	0.214
281.26	Nitrazepam	1.9	0.0516	0.5344	0.0145
227.09	Nitroglycerin	3.3	13.8	0.7494	3.1338
263.37	Nortriptyline	18	0.432	4.7407	0.1138
401.44	Oxacillin	0.33	0.366	0.1325	0.1469
286.74	Oxazepam	1	0.072	0.2867	0.0206
732.7	Pancuronium	0.26	0.108	0.1905	0.0791
232.23	Phenobarbital	0.54	0.0037	0.1254	0.0009
308.37	Phenylbutazone	0.097	0.0014	0.0299	0.0004
252.26	Phenytoin	0.64	0.45	0.1614	0.1135
248.32	Pindolol	2.3	0.498	0.5711	0.1237
517.57	Piperacillin	0.18	0.156	0.0932	0.0807
324.83	Prazepam	14.4	8.4	4.6776	2.7286
382.42	Prazosin	0.6	0.18	0.2295	0.0688
360.44	Prednisolone	1.5	0.522	0.5407	0.1881
358.44	Prednisone	0.97	0.216	0.3477	0.0774
218.25	Primidone	0.59	0.0564	0.1288	0.0123
271.79	Procainamide	1.9	0.162	0.5164	0.044
259.34	Propranolol	3.9	0.72	1.0114	0.1867
263.37	Protriptyline	22	0.216	5.7941	0.0569
261.14	Pyridostigmine	1.1	0.51	0.2873	0.1332
248.71	Pyrimethamine	2.9	0.0246	0.7213	0.0061
324.41	Quinidine	2.7	0.282	0.8759	0.0915
324.41	Quinine	1.8	0.114	0.5839	0.037
314.41	Ranitidine	1.8	0.624	0.5659	0.1962
822.96	Rifampin	0.97	0.21	0.7983	0.1728
138.12	Salicylic acid	0.17	0.0528	0.0235	0.0073
581.58	Streptomycin	0.18	0.0234	0.1047	0.0136
250.28	Sulfadiazine	0.29	0.033	0.0726	0.0083
253.31	Sulfamethoxazole	0.21	0.0192	0.0532	0.0049
267.3	Sulfisoxazole	0.15	0.0198	0.0401	0.0053
300.74	Temazepam	1.06	0.0522	0.3188	0.0157
225.29	Terbutaline	1.4	0.18	0.3154	0.0406
444.43	Tetracycline	1.5	0.1002	0.6666	0.0445
180.17	Theophylline	0.5	0.039	0.0901	0.007
264.33	Thiopental	2.3	0.234	0.608	0.0619
384.43	Ticarcillin	0.21	0.12	0.0807	0.0461

Table continued on following page

TABLE I. KINETIC CONSTANTS (*Continued*)

Molecular Weight	Generic Drug Name	V_D l/kg	Cl_p l/kg/h	V_{DSI}	Cl_{SI}
316.42	Timolol	2.1	0.438	0.6645	0.1386
467.54	Tobramycin	0.26	0.0396	0.1216	0.0185
192.26	Tocainide	3	0.156	0.5768	0.03
270.34	Tolbutamide	0.15	0.018	0.0406	0.0049
257.3	Tolmetin	0.09	0.078	0.0232	0.0201
343.22	Triazolam	1.1	0.498	0.3775	0.1709
290.32	Trimethoprim	1.8	0.132	0.5226	0.0383
681.66	Tubocurarine	0.3	0.138	0.2045	0.0941
144.21	Valproic acid	0.13	0.0066	0.0187	0.001
1,449.22	Vancomycin	0.39	0.0654	0.5652	0.0948
454.59	Verapamil	4	0.708	1.8184	0.3218
308.32	Warfarin	0.11	0.0027	0.0339	0.0008

Source: From Peterson RG: Revised pharmacokinetic constants for use under SI, Developmental Pharmacology and Therapeutics, Basel, Switzerland, S. Karger AG, 1988. Reprinted with permission.

V_D apparent volume of distribution in mass units: liters/kilogram
C_p plasma concentration in mass units: milligrams/liter
SI système international: extended metric system of units where volumes are in liters and quantities are in moles, millimoles, micromoles, and nanomoles
V_{DSI} volume of distribution 'SI': a composite kinetic constant incorporating the apparent volume of distribution and the drug's molecular weight, units become liter·microdaltons/kilogram
C_{pSI} plasma concentration in SI units: e.g. micromoles/liter
Cl_p plasma clearance in mass units of volume per weight per time, typically liters/kilogram/hour
k_{el} elimination rate constant, the fraction of the amount of drug in plasma that is eliminated in a given time; units are simply reciprocal time, e.g. 0.154/h for theophylline = 15.4% elimination per hour
Cl_{SI} plasma clearance in SI units, the units become liter·microdaltons/kilogram/hour

weight is 1 mole. In 1983, 7 of the 10 Canadian provinces had changed to SI units for reporting clinical laboratory values. A motivating factor was to have a common system for interchange of information between countries and followed Canada's more universal change to metric as a standard system for all measurements. This created immediate difficulties in the use of standard clinical pharmacokinetic estimations. Consider the previous example of phenytoin loading dose:

$$\text{loading dose} = V_D \times C_{pSI}$$
$$= 0.64 \text{ l/kg} \times 60 \text{ } \mu\text{mol/l}$$
$$= 38.4 \text{ } \mu\text{mol/kg}$$

Unfortunately, the clinician cannot find a phenytoin preparation that is provided in SI units. Medications continue to be marketed as mass units of milligrams, grams, etc. Thus, if after looking up V_D for phenytoin, the clinician also looked up the molecular weight of the drug (not all drugs *have* a discrete molecular weight; e.g., gentamicin is a mixture of several individual components), one could multiply the loading dose in SI units by the molecular weight:

$$38.4 \text{ } \mu\text{mol/kg} \times 252.26 \text{ } \mu\text{g/}\mu\text{mol} = 9,686.8 \text{ } \mu\text{g/kg}$$
$$= 9.69 \text{ mg/kg}$$

and certainly arrive at an appropriate loading dose. To calculate any required increment in plasma level, the lab-

oratory values reported in SI units must be converted as above. Of note is that a large number of the drug standards that are used for instrument calibration are obtained from the United States where they are supplied as milligram/liter (mass units). Thus, the clinical pharmacologist working in this system knows that the laboratory probably measures the plasma drug level in mass units and then does a calculation to convert it to SI units. The clinical pharmacologist must effectively convert the reported value back to mass units in order to use the traditional pharmacokinetic constants.

There are two principal kinetic constants that are affected by SI unit reporting, the first is the volume of distribution. Since this constant no longer affords a direct relationship between reported plasma level in SI units and dosage in milligram/kilogram, it seemed reasonable to incorporate the necessary conversion factor into V_D and define a kinetic constant referred to as V_{DSI}. The relationship between V_D and V_{DSI} is as follows:

$$V_{DSI} = \frac{V_D \times \text{molecular weight}}{1,000}$$

The molecular weight is necessary to accommodate the molar units of SI plasma levels and the factor of 1,000 is necessary in addition to the molecular weight to convert micromolar units to milligram units.

The intuitive understanding of the meaning of V_D

becomes more difficult when this transformation occurs. The units are now:

$$\frac{\text{liter} \cdot \text{microdaltons}}{\text{kilogram}}$$

The loading dose will calculate to milligram/liter provided the plasma level is in micromoles/liter. Despite a great amount of argument as to the "simplification" of units under SI, in clinical pharmacologic terms there is still the necessity to accommodate millimoles/liter, micromoles/liter, and nanomoles/liter. Thus, if the plasma level is nanomoles/liter, the plasma level will calculate to be micrograms/kilogram, e.g., the incremental loading dose of digoxin to raise a plasma level by 2 nmol/l is estimated as:

$$\begin{aligned} \text{loading dose} &= V_{DSI} \times C_{pSI} \\ &= 5.25 \times 2 \\ &= 10.5 \ \mu g/kg \end{aligned}$$

Conversely, if the plasma level is millimoles/liter, the loading dose will be grams/kilogram, e.g., the loading dose to achieve a plasma level of 30 mmol/l of ethanol is

$$\text{loading dose} = 0.025 \times 30 \ mmol/l = 0.75 \ g/kg.$$

The second kinetic constant which requires revision is plasma clearance. This is a pharmacokinetic quantity which describes the volume of plasma from which all of the drug can be removed in a given time. The plasma clearance for theophylline in adults is approximately 0.075 l/kg/h. The estimation of a continuous infusion of aminophylline to produce a desired plasma level is made with the following equation:

$$\text{infusion rate (mg/kg/h)} = Cl_p \ l/kg/h \times C_p \ (mg/l)$$

If one wished to achieve a plasma level of 10 mg/l of theophylline, the estimation would be:

$$\begin{aligned} \text{infusion rate} &= 0.075 \ l/kg/h \times 10 \ mg/l \\ &= 0.75 \ mg/kg/h \end{aligned}$$

Keep in mind that this would be a theophylline infusion. Since it is the ethylenediamine salt of theophylline:aminophylline, which we infuse, the salt effect on the molecular weight (1.2:1) requires that 0.9 mg/kg/h of aminophylline be infused.

In order to use an appropriate plasma level in SI units for the same infusion, the equation requires the use of a modified plasma clearance term, Cl_{SI}. Cl_p is related to V_D by the following equation:

$$Cl_p = V_D \times k_{el}$$

where the term k_{el} represents the elimination rate constant for the drug. Rate constants are not affected by SI and therefore Cl_{SI} can be defined simply as:

$$Cl_{SI} = V_{DSI} \times k_{el}$$

To repeat the aminophylline infusion example with SI units, the following estimation would apply:

$$\begin{aligned} \text{infusion rate (mg/kg/h)} \\ = Cl_{SI} \ (1 \cdot \text{microdaltons/kg/h}) \times C_{pSI} \ (\mu mol/l) \\ = 1.39 \times 10^{-2} \times 55 \\ = 0.76 \ mg/kg/h \ \text{theophylline} \\ = 0.91 \ mg/kg/h \ \text{aminophylline} \end{aligned}$$

DISCUSSION

There are many convincing arguments for the introduction and use of the SI units.[5,6] For many physiologic substances there can be increased appreciation of the relationship of one endogenous substance to another; for example, lactate and pyruvate.

Arguments for the use of SI units in clinical pharmacology suffer from several factors. First, the pharmaceutical industry has not converted units of dosage to molarity. In part this could lead to reformulation of pharmaceutical products that might not withstand close scrutiny of the relicensing procedure. As well, if this were voluntary on the part of industry there would not be a uniform conversion and one company's drug converted to SI units would not necessarily be equivalent to another competitor's identical product that is marketed in mass units.

The proposal that drug-receptor interactions or drug-albumin binding association constants will be more completely understood under SI units is a non sequitur. Molarities of drug receptor proteins would be required for complete appreciation of such interactions and until the molecular weights of these membrane proteins are known, molarity cannot be calculated. Even in the case of albumin where a molecular weight is known, SI has not uniformly used molarity; albumin is often reported as grams/liter. In addition, partial conversion within a country can produce major problems, particularly for regionalized Poison and Drug Information Centers.

A possible solution to better accommodate SI units in clinical pharmacology is to use the kinetic constants defined in this appendix. Conversions are incorporated into the SI kinetic constants, and therefore mass unit dosages can be related to SI plasma levels. The intuitive understanding of the pharmacologic concepts becomes more difficult and the units for the constants do become further removed from reality. Perhaps this may be acceptable in the overall benefits to be derived from SI units.

This discussion should not belittle the very serious confusion that exists in the United States with respect to units used for reporting plasma levels. Physicians are continuously confused by laboratories in one hospital where a drug like phenobarbital is reported in micrograms/milliliter and another affiliated hospital where phenobarbital is reported as milligram/deciliter or milligram percent. A phenobarbital value of 9 $\mu g/ml$ is subtherapeutic. A value of 9 mg/dl is highly toxic.

A great improvement in reporting of drug levels in mass units could be made by universally adopting the SI convention of liters as the only volume unit to be reported. Thus, micrograms/milliliter would be reported as milligrams/liter (the numeric value is unchanged). Nanograms/milliliter would become micrograms/liter and again the numeric value would not change. Mass units using percents or deciliters should be abandoned. In this manner uniformity could be achieved, traditional pharmacologic terms maintained and, if in the future a total change of SI is legislated and this included *drug dosage* conversion to molar quantities, the complete adoption of SI units could more easily replace the current metric mass units.

For those countries already converted to SI units for drug plasma level reporting, the kinetic constants described in this article may paradoxically make interpretation of their laboratory values more rational.

REFERENCES

1. Benet LZ, Sheiner LB: Design and optimization of dosage regimens; pharmacokinetic data. Appendix II; in Gilman AG, Goodman LS, Rall TW, Murad F, Goodman and Gilman's pharmacologic basis of therapeutics; 7th edition (Macmillan, New York 1985).
2. Rumack BH: Poisindex, A computer generated poison information system (Micromedix, Denver 1987).
3. Riegelman S, Loo J, Rowland M: Concept of a volume of distribution and possible errors in evaluation of this parameter. J Pharm Sci 57:128 (1968).
4. Wagner JG, Northram JI: Estimation of volume of distribution and half-life of a compound after rapid intravenous injection. J Pharm Sci 56:529 (1967).
5. McQueen MJ: SI (Systeme International) unit myths and monsters. Can Med Assoc J 124:537–539 (1981).
6. McQueen MJ: Conversion to SI units, the Canadian experience. J Am Med Assoc 256:3001–3002 (1986).

INDEX

Note: Page numbers in *italics* refer to illustrations; page numbers followed by t refer to tables.

649